Nursing Theorists AND THEIR WORK

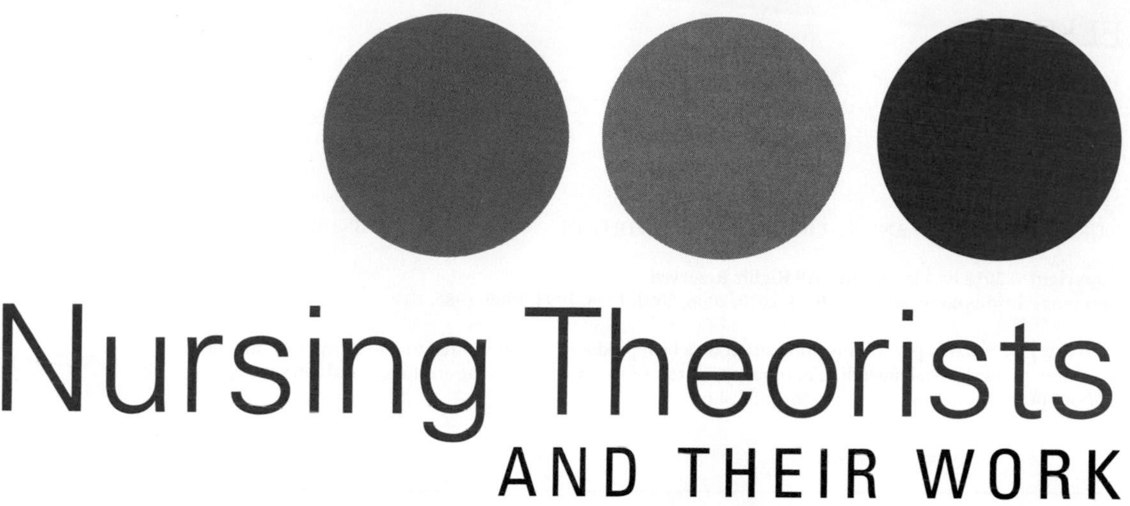

Nursing Theorists
AND THEIR WORK

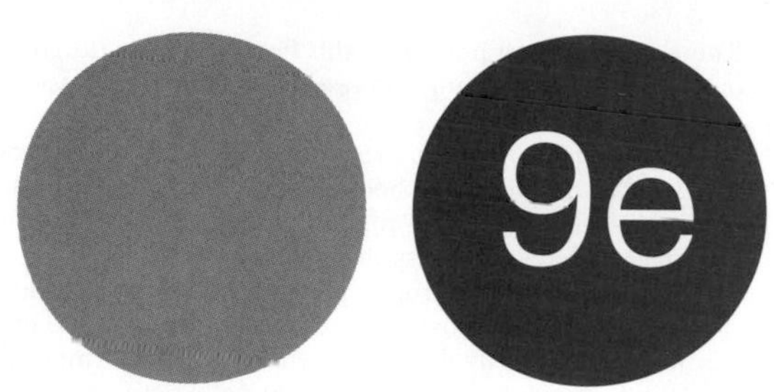

Martha Raile Alligood, PhD, RN, ANEF
Professor Emeritus
College of Nursing
East Carolina University
Greenville, North Carolina

ELSEVIER

ELSEVIER

3251 Riverport Lane
St. Louis, Missouri 63043

NURSING THEORISTS AND THEIR WORK, NINTH EDITION ISBN: 978-0-323-40224-8

Notices

Knowledge and best practice in this field are constantly changing. As new research and experience broaden our understanding, changes in research methods, professional practices, or medical treatment may become necessary.

Practitioners and researchers must always rely on their own experience and knowledge in evaluating and using any information, methods, compounds, or experiments described herein. In using such information or methods they should be mindful of their own safety and the safety of others, including parties for whom they have a professional responsibility.

With respect to any drug or pharmaceutical products identified, readers are advised to check the most current information provided (i) on procedures featured or (ii) by the manufacturer of each product to be administered, to verify the recommended dose or formula, the method and duration of administration, and contraindications. It is the responsibility of practitioners, relying on their own experience and knowledge of their patients, to make diagnoses, to determine dosages and the best treatment for each individual patient, and to take all appropriate safety precautions.

To the fullest extent of the law, neither the Publisher nor the authors, contributors, or editors, assume any liability for any injury and/or damage to persons or property as a matter of products liability, negligence or otherwise, or from any use or operation of any methods, products, instructions, or ideas contained in the material herein.

International Standard Book Number: 978-0-323-40224-8

Director, Traditional Education, Nursing Books: Kristin Geen
Content Development Manager: Billie Sharp, Lisa Newton
Associate Content Development Specialist: Samantha Dalton
Publishing Services Manager: Julie Eddy
Project Manager: Mike Sheets
Design Direction: Brian Salisbury

Printed in the United States of America

Last digit is the print number: 9 8 7 6 5 4 3 2 1

Dedicated to the memory of my parents:
George Fredrick Raile and Winifred Havener Raile, RN
They met one snowy night (he was her patient)
At Good Samaritan Hospital
Zanesville, Ohio

CONTRIBUTORS

Herdis Alvsvåg, RN, Cand Polit
Professor
VID Specialized University
Oslo, Norway

Mary T. Antonelli, PhD(c), RN
PhD Candidate
Boston College
Chestnut Hill, Massachusetts

Donald E. Bailey, Jr., PhD, RN, FAAN
Associate Professor
School of Nursing
Duke University
Durham, North Carolina

Barbara E. Banfield, PhD, RN
Associate Professor
Madonna University
Livonia, Michigan

Violeta A. Berbiglia, EdD, MSN
Associate Professor, Retired
School of Nursing
The University of Texas Health Science Center at San Antonio
San Antonio, Texas

Debra A. Bournes, RN, PhD
Chief Nursing Executive and Vice President Clinical Programs
The Ottawa Hospital
Ottawa, Canada

Nancy Brookes, PhD, RN, MSc(A)
Nurse Scholar
Adjunct Professor
University of Ottawa Faculty of Health Sciences—Nursing
Ottawa, Canada

Karen A. Brykczynski, PhD, RN, FNP, FAAN
Professor, Retired
School of Nursing at Galveston
The University of Texas Medical Branch
Galveston, Texas

Sandra Schmidt Bunkers, PhD, RN, FAAN
Adjunct Professor of Nursing
South Dakota State University
Brookings, South Dakota

Sherrilyn Coffman, PhD, RN, COI
Professor
School of Nursing
Nevada State College
Henderson, Nevada

Thérèse Dowd, PhD, RN
Associate Professor Emeritus
College of Nursing
University of Akron
Akron, Ohio

Margaret E. Erickson, PhD, RN, CNS, APHN-BC
CEO
American Holistic Nurses Credentialing Corporation
Cedar Park, Texas

Mary Gunther, PhD, RN
Associate Dean
Academic Affairs
University of Tennessee
Knoxville, Tennessee

Dana M. Hansen, PhD, APRN, ACHPN
Assistant Professor
College of Nursing
Kent State University
Kent, Ohio

Sonya R. Hardin, PhD, RN, CCRN, NP-C
Professor
College of Nursing
East Carolina University
Greenville, North Carolina

Robin Harris, PhD, ANP-BC, ACNS-BC
Clinical Assistant Professor
College of Nursing
University of Tennessee
Knoxville, Tennessee

Bonnie Holaday, PhD, RN, FAAN
Professor Emerita
School of Nursing
Clemson University
Clemson, South Carolina

Eun-Ok Im, PhD, MPH, RN, CNS, FAAN
Professor & Mary T. Champagne Professor
School of Nursing
Duke University
Durham, North Carolina

Dorothy Jones, EdD, MSN, BSN
Senior Nurse Scientist
Massachusetts General Hospital
Boston, Massachusetts
Professor
Boston College
Chestnut Hill, Massachusetts

Lisa Kitko, PhD, RN, FAHA
Assistant Professor
College of Nursing
The Pennsylvania State University
University Park, Pennsylvania

Theresa Gunter Lawson, PhD, APRN, FNP-BC, CNE
Visiting Professor
Chamberlain College of Nursing
Family Nurse Practitioner
Neuman Systems Model Trustees Group
Anderson Free Clinic
Anderson, South Carolina

Danielle Leone-Sheehan, MSN, RN
PhD Candidate
Connell School of Nursing
Boston College
Chestnut Hill, Massachusetts

Unni Å. Lindström, PhD, RN
Professor Emerita
Department of Caring Science
Åbo Academy University
Vasa, Finland

M. Katherine Maeve, PhD, RN
Adjunct Faculty
Augusta University
Augusta, Georgia
Mental Health Outpatient Case Manager
Charlie Norwood Veterans Medical Center
Augusta, Georgia

Marilyn R. McFarland, PhD, RN, FNP-BC, CTN-A
Professor of Nursing and Family Nurse Practitioner, Advanced Certified Transcultural Nurse, Author
Department of Nursing
University of Michigan—Flint
Flint, Michigan

Gwen McGhan, PhD, RN
Assistant Professor
School of Nursing
University of Alabama at Birmingham
Birmingham, Alabama

Linda C. Mefford, PhD, APRN, NNP-BC, RNC-NIC
Associate Professor
Bellarmine University
Louisville, Kentucky

Molly Meighan, PhD, RNC-e
Professor Emerita
Division of Nursing
Carson-Newman University
Jefferson City, Tennessee

Patricia R. Messmer, PhD, MA, MSN, FAAN
Consultant for Nursing Research & Education
Benjamín León School of Nursing
Miami Dade College
Miami, Florida

Gail J. Mitchell, RN, PhD
Professor
School of Nursing
York University
Toronto, Canada

Julie L. Murphy, MSN, RN
Doctoral Candidate
College of Nursing
The Pennsylvania State University
University Park, Pennsylvania

Lisbet Lindholm Nyström, PhD, RN
Associate Professor, Retired
Department of Caring Science
Åbo Academy University
Vasa, Finland

Janice Penrod, PhD, RN, FGSA, FAAN
Professor
College of Nursing
The Pennsylvania State University
University Park, Pennsylvania

Susan A. Pfettscher, PhD, RN
Clinical Nurse
PD Program
DaVita
Templeton, California

Kenneth D. Phillips, PhD, RN
Professor and Associate Dean for Research
College of Nursing
East Tennessee State University
Johnson City, Tennessee

Marie E. Pokorny, PhD, RN
Professor Emerita of Nursing
College of Nursing
East Carolina University
Greenville, North Carolina

Marguerite J. Purnell, PhD, RN, AHN-BC
Professor Emeritus
Christine E. Lynn College of Nursing
Florida Atlantic University
Boca Raton, Florida

Pamela G. Reed, PhD, MSN, MA, FAAN
Professor
College of Nursing
The University of Arizona
Tucson, Arizona

Teresa J. Sakraida, PhD, RN
Associate Professor
Christine E. Lynn College of Nursing
Florida Atlantic University
Boca Raton, Florida

Ann M. Schreier, PhD, RN
Associate Professor
College of Nursing
East Carolina University
Greenville, North Carolina

Carrie Scotto, PhD, RN
Associate Professor
College of Nursing
University of Akron
Akron, Ohio

Christina Leibold Sieloff, PhD, RN
Associate Professor
College of Nursing
Montana State University
Bozeman, Montana

Cynthia K. Snyder, MSN, RN
Doctoral Student
The Pennsylvania State University
University Park, Pennsylvania

Janet L. Stewart, PhD, RN
Dean
Faculty of the Health Sciences
Kibogora Polytechnic Institute
Kirambo, Rwanda, Africa

Danny G. Willis, DNS, RN, PMHCNS-BC
Associate Professor & Department Chair
Connell School of Nursing
Boston College
Chestnut Hill, Massachusetts

Jane C. Wilson, MSN, RN
Assistant Professor of Nursing
Palm Beach Atlantic University
West Palm Beach, Florida

Danuta M. Wojnar, PhD, RN, FAAN
Professor & Associate Dean
Undergraduate Education
College of Nursing
Seattle University
Seattle, Washington

Joan E. Zetterlund, PhD, RN
Professor Emerita
School of Nursing
North Park University
Chicago, Illinois

REVIEWERS

Karen E. Alexander, PhD, RN, CNOR
Program Director and Assistant Professor RN-BSN
University of Houston - Clear Lake
Houston, Texas

ChengChing Hiya Liu, RN, PhD, MBA
Assistant Professor
College of Nursing
Michigan State University
East Lansing, Michigan

Ronda Mintz-Binder, DNP, RN, CNE
Clinical Associate Professor
College of Nursing Health Innovation
University of Texas at Arlington
Arlington, Texas

Karen Pennington, PhD, RN
Director RN-BSN and MS Leadership Programs
Loretto Heights School of Nursing
Regis University
Denver, Colorado

Lynda F. Turner, EdD, MSN, RN, ACNS-BC, CNE
Associate Professor and Director of BSN Program
Marshall University
Huntington, West Virginia

Wendy Wheeler, RN, BScN, MN
Instructor
Red Deer College
Alberta, Canada

Sarah J. Williams, BSN, MA, MSN, PhD
Professor and Director RN-BSN-MSN Nursing Program
Ila Faye Miller School of Nursing and Health Professions
University of the Incarnate Word
San Antonio, Texas

ABOUT THE EDITOR

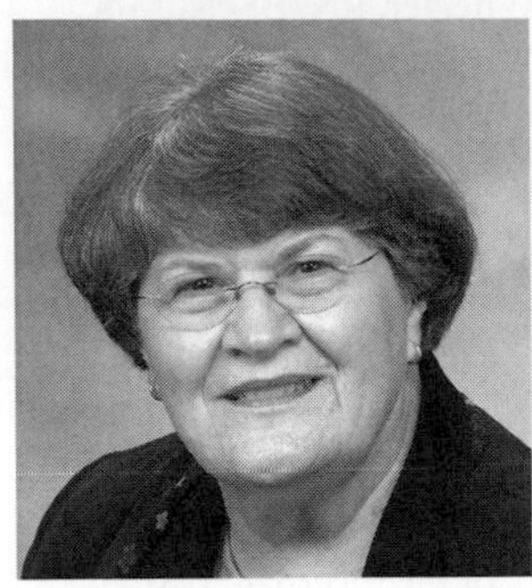

Martha Raile Alligood is professor emeritus at East Carolina University College of Nursing in Greenville, North Carolina, where she was Director of the Nursing PhD program. A graduate of Good Samaritan School of Nursing, she also holds a bachelor of sacred literature (BSL) from Johnson University, a bachelor of science in nursing (BSN) from University of Virginia, a master of science (MS) with a major in nursing from The Ohio State University, and a doctorate of philosophy (PhD) in nursing science from New York University.

Her career in nursing education began in Rhodesia, (now Zimbabwe) Africa and has included graduate faculty appointments at the University of Florida, University of South Carolina, University of Tennessee and East Carolina University. Among professional memberships are Epsilon and Beta Nu Chapters of Sigma Theta Tau International (STTI) and Society of Rogerian Scholars (SRS).

A recipient of numerous awards and honors, she is a National League for Nursing (NLN) Academy of Nursing Education Fellow (ANEF). She received the SNRS Leadership in Research Award, and the East Carolina University Chancellors's Women of Distinction Award. As a member of the Board of Trustees at Johnson University, Dr. Alligood chairs the Academic Affairs Committee.

She is known nationally and internationally for expertise in nursing theory, was contributing editor for the Theoretical Concerns column, *Nursing Science Quarterly,* vol. 24, 2011, and Consultant and Interviewer for *The Nurse Theorists: Portraits of Excellence,* vol. II, 2008 and vol. III, 2016, video series for Fitne, Inc. Athens, OH. She is author and editor of *Nursing Theory: Utilization & Application,* fifth edition, as well as this ninth edition of *Nursing Theorists and Their Work.*

Photo credit: Center for Health Sciences Communication, Brody School of Medicine, East Carolina University, Greenville, NC

PREFACE

This book is a tribute to nursing theorists and a classic in theoretical nursing literature. It presents many major thinkers in nursing, reviews their important knowledge-building ideas, lists their publications, and points the reader to those using the works and writing about them in their own theoretical publications.

The Unit I opener introduces the reader to a graphic that is a new feature in this ninth edition. This graphic illustrates the type of theoretical work presented in that Unit in relation to the types of works in the other Units. Unit I highlights the core: person, environment, health & nursing, the metaparadigm concepts forming nursing's disciplinary boundaries.

Unit I has been reorganized to better introduce the reader to the organization of the text. A brief history of nursing knowledge development and its significance to the discipline and practice of the profession is presented in Chapter 1. Chapter 2 continues the historical introduction with 10 works from earlier editions of *Nursing Theorists and Their Work* presented briefly as nursing theorists of historical significance. They are Peplau; Henderson; Abdellah; Wiedenbach; Hall; Travelbee; Barnard; Adam; Orlando; and the work of Roper, Logan, Tierney. An introduction to the history and philosophy of science, logical reasoning, and theory development processes are presented in Chapters 3 and 4. Finally Chapter 5 presents an introduction to nursing knowledge, types of knowledge, the framework used for analysis of each theoretical work, and the content outline for Chapters 6–36.

In Unit II, the philosophies of Nightingale, Watson, Ray, Benner, Martinsen, and Eriksson are presented. Unit III includes nursing models by Levine, Rogers, Orem, King, Neuman, Roy, and Johnson. The work of Boykin and Schoenhofer begins Unit IV on nursing theory, followed by the works of Meleis; Pender; Leininger; Newman; Parse; Erickson, Tomlin, and Swain; and the Husteds. Unit V presents middle-range theoretical works of Mercer; Mishel; Reed; Wiener and Dodd; Eakes, Burke, and Hainsworth; Barker; Kolcaba; Beck; Swanson; Ruland; and Moore. Unit VI offers three perspectives on the status of the art and science of nursing theory: expansion of the philosophy of nursing science, the advance of theory development in this theory utilization era, and the global evidence of nursing theoretical works in the nursing literature worldwide.

The works of nurse theorists from around the world are featured in this text, including works by international theorists that have been translated into English. *Nursing Theorists and Their Work* has also been translated into numerous languages for nursing faculty and students in other parts of the world as well as nurses in practice.

Nurses and students at all stages of their education and nursing career are interested in learning about nursing theory and the use of theoretical works from around the world. Those just beginning their nursing education, such as associate degree and baccalaureate students, will find the life of the theorists, their conceptual focus, definitions, and theoretical assertions interesting. Graduate students, at the master and doctoral levels, will be more attracted to the logical form, acceptance by the nursing community, the theoretical sources for theory development, the use of empirical data, and the analyses of each work. The references and bibliographies are particularly useful to graduate students for locating primary and secondary sources that augment the websites specific to the theorist. The following comprehensive websites are excellent resources for information about theory research and links to the individual theorists featured in this book:

- Nursing Theory Link Page, Clayton College and State University, Department of Nursing: http://www.clayton.edu/nursing/Nursing-Theory
- Nursing Theory and Research page, Hahn School of Nursing and Health Science, University of San Diego: https://www.sandiego.edu/nursing/research/nursing-theory-research.php
- A comprehensive collection of nursing theory media, *The Nurse Theorists: Portraits of Excellence, Vol. I, Vol. II, Vol. III* and *Nurse Theorists: Excellence in Action:* https://www.fitne.net/nurse_theorists.jsp

The works of the theorists presented in this text have stimulated phenomenal growth in nursing literature and enriched the professional lives of nurses around the world by guiding nursing research, education, administration, and practice. The professional growth continues to increase as we analyze and synthesize these works, generate new ideas, and develop new theory and applications for education in the discipline and high quality care in practice by nurses.

ACKNOWLEDGMENTS

I am thankful to the theorists who critiqued the original and subsequent chapters about themselves to keep the content current and accurate. The work of Paterson and Zderad was omitted at their request.

I am very grateful to those who have contributed or worked behind the scenes with previous editions to develop this text over the years. In the third edition, I joined Ann Marriner Tomey, serving as a contributing author, to reorder the chapters and edit for consistency with the new organization of the text. Subsequently I was invited by Mosby personnel to design and coedit a practice-focused nursing theory text, *Nursing Theory: Utilization and Application*. Beginning with the fifth edition of this text, Ann Marriner Tomey invited me to coedit and contribute to two more editions (fifth and sixth) of *Nursing Theorists and Their Work*. After Ann retired, I completed the seventh, eighth, and ninth editions. I recognize Ann Marriner Tomey for her vision to develop this book. Her mentorship, wisdom, and collegial friendship contributed to the development of my professional career. She is to be commended for initiating this text that continues to make valuable global contributions to the discipline and the profession of nursing.

I want to thank Dr. Marie E. Pokorny, whom I consulted on the reorganization of Unit I. She provided support and wise counsel to better reflect the flow of history for the beginning student in Unit I of this ninth edition.

As in most new editions, I welcome new chapter authors and doctoral student contributors to this ninth edition: Dr. Danny Willis and Danielle M. Leone-Sheehan to Chapter 7 on Jean Watson, Dr. Linda Mefford to Chapter 12 on Myra Estrin Levine, Jane Wilson to Chapter 21 on Nola J. Pender, Dr. Dorothy Jones and Mary Antonelli to Chapter 23 on Margaret Newman, Dr. Sandra Bunkers to Chapter 24 on Rosemary Parse, Dr. Pam Reed to Chapter 29 on Pam Reed, and Julie L. Murphy and Cynthia K. Snyder to Chapter 30 on Carolyn L. Wiener and Marilyn J. Dodd.

Finally, I would like to thank the publishers at Elsevier for their guidance and assistance through the years to bring this text to this ninth edition. The external reviews requested by Elsevier editors have contributed to the successful development of each new edition. The chapter authors, who over the years have contributed their expert knowledge of the theorists and their work, continue to make a most valuable contribution.

Martha Raile Alligood

CONTENTS

UNIT I

Evolution of Nursing Theories

- Nurse scholars led the search for specialized theoretical nursing knowledge to guide education, professional practice, research, and administration.
- Nursing history and significant developments demonstrate the incredible influence theory has had on nursing as a specialized field of practice (the profession) and a division of education (the discipline).
- Nursing followed a developmental path from concepts to conceptual frameworks to models to theories to practice-level middle-range theories in the theory utilization era.
- Knowledge of the role of concepts in the theory development process contributes to an understanding of the theoretical works of the discipline of nursing.
- Theory plays a major role in knowledge development by specifying the question and the approach and guiding the research process.
- Analysis facilitates learning through systematic review and critical reflection of the theoretical works of the discipline.
- Theory analysis begins the process of identifying a decision-making framework for nursing practice or research.

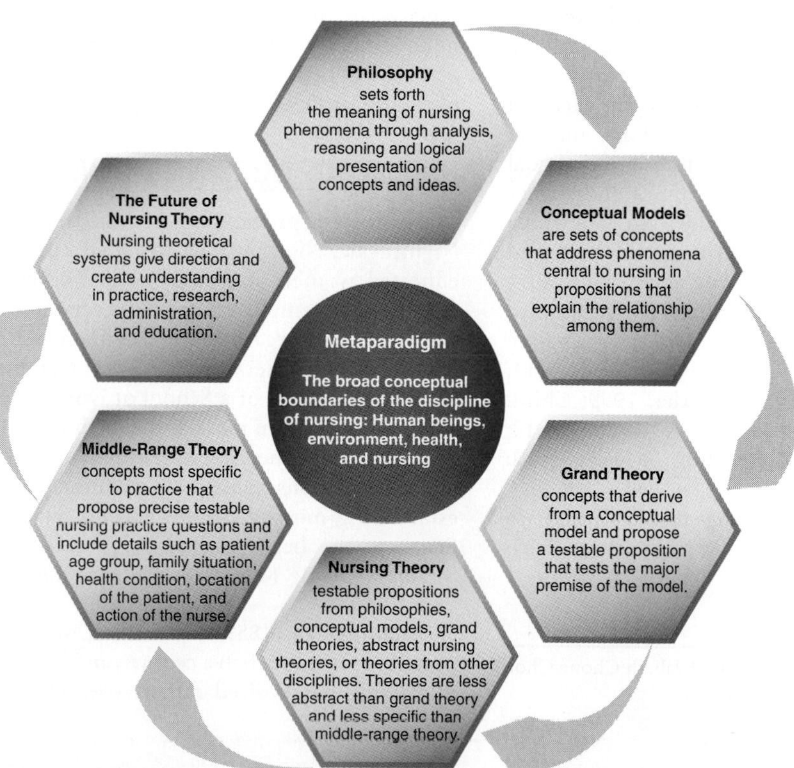

Philosophy
sets forth the meaning of nursing phenomena through analysis, reasoning and logical presentation of concepts and ideas.
Conceptual Models
are sets of concepts that address phenomena central to nursing in propositions that explain the relationship among them.
Grand Theory
concepts that derive from a conceptual model and propose a testable proposition that tests the major premise of the model.
Nursing Theory
testable propositions from philosophies, conceptual models, grand theories, abstract nursing theories, or theories from other disciplines. Theories are less abstract than grand theory and less specific than middle-range theory.
Middle-Range Theory
concepts most specific to practice that propose precise testable nursing practice questions and include details such as patient age group, family situation, health condition, location of the patient, and action of the nurse.
The Future of Nursing Theory
Nursing theoretical systems give direction and create understanding in practice, research, administration, and education.
Metaparadigm
The broad conceptual boundaries of the discipline of nursing: Human beings, environment, health, and nursing

1

Introduction to Nursing Theory: Its History and Significance

*Martha Raile Alligood**

"The systematic accumulation of knowledge is essential to progress in any profession . . . however theory and practice must be constantly interactive. Theory without practice is empty and practice without theory is blind."

(Cross, 1981, p. 110)

This text is designed to introduce nursing theorists and their work. Nursing theory became a major theme in the last half of the 20th century, and it continues to stimulate phenomenal professional growth globally and expansion of nursing literature and education around the world. The nursing theorists presented in this text are selected to introduce students at all levels of nursing to a broad range of nurse theorists and various theoretical works. Although nurses of early eras often delivered excellent care to patients, much of what was known about nursing was not tested or used uniformly in practice or education. Rather ideas that were passed on through education focused on skills and functional tasks about nursing practices that seemed effective. Therefore a major goal was put forth by nursing leaders in the 20th century for the development of nursing knowledge on which to base nursing practice, improve quality of care, and gain recognition of nursing as a profession. The history of nursing clearly documents sustained efforts toward that goal of developing a specialized body of nursing knowledge to guide nursing practice (Alligood, 2014; Alligood & Tomey, 1997; Bixler & Bixler, 1959; Chinn & Kramer, 2015; George, 2011; Im & Chang, 2012; Judd & Sitzman, 2013; McCrae, 2012; Meleis, 2012; Shaw, 1993).

This chapter introduces nursing theory from two important perspectives: history and significance. Each contributes meaning to an understanding of the contributions of the nurse theorists and their work. A brief **history** of nursing development from vocational to professional presents a description of the search for substantive nursing knowledge on which to base nursing practice. The progressive search ultimately led to this exciting time of theory utilization in nursing history. The history of this development provides context and perspective to understand the continuing **significance** of nursing theory. As nursing advanced, the significance of nursing theory became more clear for both the discipline and profession of nursing.

HISTORY OF NURSING THEORY

The history of professional nursing began with Florence Nightingale. Nightingale envisioned nurses as a body of educated women at a time when women were neither educated nor employed in public service. After her wartime service of organizing and caring for the wounded in Scutari during the Crimean War, Nightingale's vision and establishment of a School of Nursing at St. Thomas' Hospital in London marked the birth of modern nursing. Nightingale's pioneering activities in nursing practice and education and her subsequent writings became a guide for establishing nursing schools and hospitals in the United States at the beginning of the 20th century (Judd & Sitzman, 2013; Kalisch & Kalisch, 2003; Nightingale, 1859/1969).

Nightingale's (1859/1969) vision of nursing has been practiced for more than a century, and theory development in nursing has evolved rapidly over the past 6 decades,

*Previous authors: Martha Raile Alligood, Elizabeth Chong Choi, Juanita Fogel Keck, and Ann Marriner Tomey.

leading to the recognition of nursing as an academic discipline with a specialized body of knowledge (Alligood, 2014; Bixler & Bixler, 1959; Chinn & Kramer, 2015; Fawcett & DeSanto-Medeya, 2013; Im & Chang, 2012; Walker & Avant, 2011). It was during the mid-1800s that Nightingale recognized the unique focus of nursing and declared nursing knowledge as distinct from medical knowledge. She described a nurse's proper function as putting the patient in the best condition for nature (God) to act upon him or her. She set forth the following: that care of the sick is based on knowledge of persons and their surroundings—a different knowledge base than that used by physicians in their practice (Nightingale, 1859/1969). Despite this early edict from Nightingale in the 1850s, it was 100 years later, during the 1950s, when nursing profession leaders began serious discussion of the need to develop nursing knowledge apart from medical knowledge to guide nursing practice. This awareness of the need to develop nursing knowledge continued to grow (Alligood, 2014; Chinn & Kramer, 2015; Meleis, 2012; Walker & Avant, 2011). Until the proposal of nursing as a science in the 1950s, nursing practice was based on principles and traditions that were handed down through an apprenticeship model of education and individual hospital procedure manuals (Alligood, 2014; Kalisch & Kalisch, 2003). Although some nursing leaders aspired for nursing to be recognized as a profession and become an academic discipline, nursing practice reflected its vocational heritage more than its professional vision. The transition from vocation to profession is described here in successive eras of history as nurses began developing a body of specialized knowledge on which to base nursing practice. Nurses began with a strong emphasis on practice, and worked throughout the century toward the development of nursing as a profession. Progress in each of these eras toward the goal of a specialized basis for nursing practice demonstrates the seriousness of this drive toward professional development (Alligood, 2014).

The **curriculum era** addressed the question of what content nurses should study to learn how to be a nurse. During this era, the emphasis was on what courses nursing students should take, with the goal of arriving at a standardized curriculum (Alligood, 2014). By the mid-1930s, a standardized curriculum had been published and adopted by many diploma nursing programs, where nursing was taught at the time. The idea of moving nursing education from hospital-based diploma programs into colleges and universities began to emerge during this era (Ervin, 2015; Judd & Sitzman, 2013). However, despite this early concept of nursing education, it was the middle of the century before most states acted upon this goal, and the second half of the 20th-century diploma programs began closing and significant numbers of nursing education programs opened in colleges and universities (Ervin, 2015; Judd & Sitzman, 2013; Kalisch & Kalisch, 2003). The curriculum era emphasized course selection and content for nursing programs and gave way to the research era, which focused on the research process and the long-range goal of acquiring substantive knowledge to guide nursing practice.

As nurses increasingly sought degrees in higher education, the **research emphasis era** began to emerge. During the midcentury more nurse leaders embraced higher education and arrived at an understanding of the scientific age and that research was the path to new nursing knowledge. Nurses began to participate in research, and research courses were included in nursing curricula in early graduate nursing programs (Alligood, 2014). In the mid-1970s, an evaluation of the first 25 years of the journal *Nursing Research* revealed that nursing studies lacked conceptual connections and theoretical frameworks, accentuating their necessity for the development of specialized nursing knowledge (Batey, 1977). Awareness of the need for concept and theory development coincided with two other milestones in the evolution of nursing theory: the standardization of curricula for a nursing master's education by the National League for Nursing accreditation criteria for baccalaureate and higher-degree programs, and the decision that doctoral education for nurses should be in nursing (Alligood, 2014).

The research era and the **graduate education era** developed in tandem. Master's degree programs in nursing emerged across the country to meet the public need for nurses for specialized clinical nursing practice. Many of these graduate programs included a course that introduced the student to the research process. Also during this era, nursing master's programs began to include courses in concept development and nursing models, introducing students to early nursing theorists and knowledge development processes (Alligood, 2014). The development of nursing knowledge was a major force at this time. The baccalaureate degree began to gain wider acceptance as the educational level for professional nursing, and nursing attained nationwide recognition and acceptance as an academic discipline in higher education. Nurse researchers worked to develop and clarify a specialized body of nursing knowledge, with the goals of improving the quality of patient care, providing a professional style of practice, and achieving recognition as a profession. There were debates and discussions in the 1960s regarding the proper direction and appropriate discipline for nursing knowledge development. In the 1970s, nursing continued to make the transition from vocation to profession as nurse leaders debated whether nursing should be other-discipline based or nursing based. History records the outcome: that nursing practice is to be based on nursing science (Alligood, 2014; Fawcett, 1978; Nicoll, 1986). It is as Meleis (2007) noted, "theory is not a luxury in the discipline of nursing . . . but an integral part of the nursing lexicon in education, administration, and practice" (p. 4). An important precursor to the theory era was the general acceptance of nursing as a profession and an academic discipline in its own right.

The **theory era** was a natural outgrowth of the research and graduate education eras (Alligood, 2014; Im & Chang, 2012). The explosive proliferation of nursing doctoral programs from the 1970s and nursing theory literature substantiated that nursing doctorates should be in nursing rather than in other disciplines (Nicoll, 1986, 1992, 1997; Reed & Shearer, 2009, 2012; Reed, Shearer, & Nicoll, 2003). As understanding of research and knowledge development increased, it became obvious that research without conceptual and theoretical frameworks produced isolated information rather than a body of nursing knowledge. Understanding that both research and theory were required to produce nursing science moved nurses forward toward their goal (Batey, 1977; Fawcett, 1978; Hardy, 1978). Doctoral education in nursing began to develop with a strong emphasis on theory development and testing. The theory era accelerated as early works developed as frameworks for curricula and advanced practice guides began to be recognized as theory. In fact, the Nurse Educator Nursing Theory Conference in New York City in 1978 presented a group of nursing theorists in a program together for the first time (Alligood, 2014; Fawcett, 1984).

The 1980s was a period of major developments in nursing theory that has been characterized as a transition from the preparadigm to the paradigm period in nursing (Fawcett, 1984; Hardy, 1978; Kuhn, 1970). The prevailing nursing paradigms (models) provided perspectives for education, nursing practice, research, administration, and further theory development. In the 1980s, Fawcett's seminal proposal of four global nursing concepts as a nursing metaparadigm served as an organizing structure for existing nursing frameworks and introduced a way of organizing individual theoretical works in a meaningful structure (Fawcett, 1978, 1984, 1993). Classifying the nursing models as paradigms within metaparadigm concepts of **person, environment, health,** and **nursing** systematically united nursing theoretical works for the discipline. This system clarified and improved comprehension of knowledge development by positioning the theorists' works in a larger context, thus greatly facilitating the growth of nursing science (Fawcett, 2005). The body of nursing science in research, education, administration, and practice continues to expand through nursing scholarship. In the last decades of the 20th century, emphasis shifted from learning about the theorists to use of the theoretical works to generate research questions, guide practice, and organize curricula. Evidence of this growth of theoretical works has proliferated in podium presentations at national and international conferences, and in newsletters, journals, and books written by nurse scientists who are members of societies or communities of scholars for nursing models and theories. Members contribute to the general nursing literature and communicate their research and practice with a certain paradigm model or framework at conferences of the societies where they present their scholarship and move the science of the selected paradigm forward (Alligood, 2014; Fawcett & Garity, 2009; Im & Chang, 2012; Smith & Parker, 2014).

These observations of nursing theory development progress bring Kuhn's (1970) description of normal science to life. His philosophy of science clarifies an understanding of the evolution of nursing theory through paradigm science. It is important historically to understand that what we view collectively today as nursing models and theories is the work of individuals who originally published their ideas and conceptualizations of nursing in various areas of the country and around the world. These works later were viewed collectively within a systematic structure of knowledge according to analysis and evaluation (Fawcett, 1984, 1993, 2005). Theory development emerged as a process and product of professional scholarship and growth among nurse leaders, administrators, educators, and practitioners who sought higher education. These leaders recognized limitations of theory from other disciplines to describe, explain, or predict nursing outcomes, and they labored to establish a scientific basis for nursing curricula, practice, research, and management. The development and use of theory led to what is recognized today as the nursing theory era (Alligood, 2014; Nicoll, 1986, 1992, 1997; Reed & Shearer, 2012; Reed, Shearer, & Nicoll, 2003; Wood, 2014). It was as Fitzpatrick and Whall (1983) had said, "nursing is on the brink of an exciting new era" (p. 2). This awareness ushered in the **theory utilization era.**

The accomplishments of normal science accompanied the theory utilization era as emphasis shifted to theory application in nursing practice, education, research, and administration (Alligood, 2014; Wood, 2014). In this era, middle-range theory and the value of a nursing framework for thought and action in nursing practice was realized. The shift in emphasis to the application of nursing theory was extremely important for theory-based nursing, evidence-based practice, and future theory development (Alligood, 2010, 2014; Alligood & Tomey, 1997, 2002, 2006; Chinn & Kramer, 2015; Fawcett, 2005; Fawcett & Garity, 2009). The fifth edition of *Nursing Theory: Utilization*

TABLE 1.1 Historical Eras of Nursing's Search for Specialized Knowledge

Historical Era	Major Question	Emphasis	Outcomes	Emerging Goal
Curriculum era: 1900–1940s	What curriculum content should student nurses study to be nurses?	Courses included in nursing programs.	Standardized curricula for diploma programs.	Develop specialized knowledge and higher education.
Research era: 1950–1970s	What is the focus for nursing research?	Role of nurses and what to research.	Problem studies and studies of nurses.	Isolated studies do not yield unified knowledge.
Graduate education era: 1950–1970s	What knowledge is needed for the practice of nursing?	Carving out an advanced role and basis for nursing practice.	Nurses have an important role in health care.	Focus graduate education on knowledge development.
Theory era: 1980–1990s	How do these frameworks guide research and practice?	There are many ways to think about nursing.	Nursing theoretical works shift the focus to the patient.	Theories guide nursing research and practice.
Theory utilization era: 21st century	What new theories are needed to produce evidence for quality care?	Nursing theory guides research, practice, education, and administration.	Middle-range theory may be from quantitative or qualitative approaches.	Nursing frameworks produce knowledge (evidence) for quality care.

Alligood, M. R. (2014). *Nursing theory: Utilization & application.* St Louis: Mosby-Elsevier.

& Application (Alligood, 2014) offers numerous case applications of nursing theoretical works in practice. Table 1.1 presents a summary of the eras of nursing's search for specialized nursing knowledge. Within each era, the pervading question "What is the nature of the knowledge that is needed for the practice of nursing?" was addressed at the prevailing level of understanding at the time (Alligood, 2014).

This brief history provides some background and context for the study of nursing theorists and their work. The theory utilization era continues to emphasize the development and use of nursing theory and to produce evidence for quality professional practice. New theory and new methodologies from qualitative research approaches continue to expand Carper's (1978) ways of knowing among nurse scientists. The use of nursing philosophies, models, theories, and middle-range theories for the thought and action of nursing practice contributes important evidence for quality care in all areas of current practice (Alligood, 2014; Fawcett, 2005; Fawcett & Garity, 2009; Peterson & Bredow, 2014; Smith & Leihr, 2013; Wood, 2014). Practice in nursing today requires knowledge of and use of the theoretical works of the discipline (Alligood, 2014). Not only is theory relevant in the history of nursing's progress toward specialized nursing knowledge, but that knowledge also contributed to recognition of nursing as a profession and a discipline.

The achievements of the profession over the past century were highly relevant to nursing science development, but they did not come easily. History shows that many nurses pioneered the cause of human health and challenged the status quo with creative ideas for both the health of people and the development of nursing. Their achievements ushered in this exciting time (Kalisch & Kalisch, 2003; Meleis, 2012; Shaw, 1993). Since the publication of the first edition of *Nursing Theorists and Their Work* (1986), the volume of theoretical works has expanded considerably. There are nurses who made significant contributions during the preparadigm period of nursing knowledge development (Hardy, 1973, 1978). However, references to those early works in the literature became increasingly limited despite their important contributions. Therefore in the sixth edition of this text (2006), a chapter of ten selected exemplars from that early development were recognized for their significant nursing knowledge contributions. Chapter 2 of this text presents those selected exemplars (Box 1.1) of early works and their updates to further explore the history and significance of nursing theory in the discipline of nursing. Those interested in learning more about these early nursing pioneers or any theorist whose work is included in this

BOX 1.1 Early Theorists of Historical Significance

Hildegard E. Peplau	1909–1999
Virginia Henderson	1897–1996
Faye Glenn Abdellah	1919 to present
Earnestine Wiedenbach	1900–1996
Lydia Hall	1906–1969
Joyce Travelbee	1926–1973
Kathryn E. Barnard	1938 to present
Evelyn Adam	1929 to present
Nancy Roper*	1918–2004
Winifred Logan*	
Alison J. Tierney*	
Ida Jean Orlando Pelletier	1926–2007

*Roper, Logan, and Tierney collaborated on The Roper-Logan-Tierney Model of Nursing.

text are referred to their original publications. Nursing theoretical works represent the most comprehensive presentation of systematic nursing knowledge and are therefore vital to the future of both the discipline and the profession of nursing.

SIGNIFICANCE OF NURSING THEORY

At the beginning of the 20th century, nursing was not recognized as an academic discipline or a profession, but the accomplishments of the past century led to recognition of nursing in both areas. The terms *discipline* and *profession* are interrelated, and some may use them interchangeably; however, they are not the same. It is important to note their differences and specific meaning, as presented in Box 1.2.

BOX 1.2 The Meaning of a Discipline Versus a Profession

- A *discipline* is specific to academia and refers to a branch of education, a department of learning, or a domain of knowledge.
- A *profession* refers to a specialized field of practice, founded on the theoretical structure of the science or knowledge of that discipline and accompanying practice abilities.

Data from Donaldson, S. K., & Crowley, D. M. (1978). The discipline of nursing. *Nursing Outlook,* 26(2), 1113–1120; Orem, D. (2001). *Nursing: Concepts of practice* (6th ed.). St Louis: Mosby; Styles, M. M. (1982). *On nursing: Toward a new endowment.* St Louis: Mosby.

Significance for the Discipline

When nurses entered baccalaureate and higher-degree programs in universities during the last half of the 20th century, the goal of developing knowledge as a basis for nursing practice began to be realized. University baccalaureate programs proliferated, master's programs in nursing were developed, and a standardized curriculum was realized through accreditation. Nursing had passed through eras of gradual development, and nursing leaders offered their perspectives on the development of nursing science. They addressed significant disciplinary questions about whether nursing was an applied science or a basic science (Donaldson & Crowley, 1978; Johnson, 1959; Rogers, 1970). History provides evidence of the consensus that was reached, and nursing doctoral programs began to open to generate nursing knowledge.

The 1970s was a significant period of development. In 1977 after the journal *Nursing Research* had been published for 25 years, studies were reviewed comprehensively and their strengths and weaknesses reported. Batey (1977) called attention to the importance of nursing conceptualization in the research process and the role of a conceptual framework in research design for the production of science. This emphasis led to the theory development era and moved nursing forward to new nursing knowledge for nursing practice. Soon nursing theoretical works began to be recognized to address Batey's call (Johnson, 1968, 1974; King, 1971; Levine, 1969; Neuman, 1974; Orem, 1971; Rogers, 1970; Roy, 1970). In 1978 Fawcett presented her double helix metaphor, now a classic publication, clarifying the interdependent relationship of theory and research. Also at this time, nurse scholars such as Henderson, Nightingale, Orlando, Peplau, and Wiedenbach were recognized for the theoretical nature of their earlier writings. These early works were developed by educators as frameworks for nursing practice or to structure curriculum content in nursing programs. Orlando's (1961, 1972) theory was derived from the report of an early nationally funded research project that was designed to study nursing practice.

At the Nurse Educator Nursing Theory Conference in New York City in 1978, the theorists were brought together on the same stage for the first time, although most of them denied they were theorists, and understanding of the significance of the works for nursing was limited at the time. Also noteworthy at this time, Donaldson and Crowley (1978) presented the keynote address at the Western Commission of Higher Education in Nursing Conference in 1977, just as the nursing doctoral program at the University of Washington was about to open. They discussed the nature of nursing science and the nature of knowledge needed for the discipline and the profession. The published version of their keynote address remains a classic for students to learn the difference between the discipline and the profession of nursing. They called for both basic and applied research, asserting that each type of knowledge was vital to nursing as a discipline and as a profession. They argued that the discipline and the profession are inextricably linked, but failure to separate them from each other anchors nursing in a vocational rather than a professional view. The current development of Doctor of Nursing Practice (DNP) programs, not to be confused with nursing research Philosophy Doctorates (PhD), is apropos to their point.

Soon nursing conceptual frameworks began to be used to organize curricula in nursing programs and were recognized as models that address the values and concepts of nursing. The creative conceptualization of a nursing metaparadigm (person, environment, health, and nursing) and a structure of knowledge clarified the related nature of the collective works of major nursing theorists as conceptual frameworks and paradigms of nursing (Fawcett, 1984). This approach organized nursing works into a system of theoretical knowledge, developed by theorists at different times and in different parts of the country. Each nursing conceptual model was classified on the basis of a set of analysis and evaluation criteria (Fawcett, 1984, 1993). Recognition of the separate nursing works collectively with a metaparadigm umbrella enhanced the recognition and understanding of nursing theoretical works as a body of nursing knowledge. In short, the significance of theory for the discipline of nursing is that the discipline is dependent on theory for its continued existence—that is, nursing can be a vocation, or nursing can be a discipline with a professional style of theory-based practice. The theoretical works have taken nursing to higher levels of education and practice as nurses moved from the functional focus, with an emphasis on what nurses do, to a patient focus, emphasizing what nurses know for thought, decision making, and action.

Frameworks and theories are structures about human beings and their health; these structures provide nurses with a perspective of the patient for professional practice. Professionals provide public service in a practice focused on those whom they serve. The nursing process is useful in practice, but the primary focus is the patient, or human being. Knowledge of persons, health, and environment forms the basis for recognition of nursing as a discipline, and this knowledge is taught to those who enter the profession. Every discipline or field of knowledge includes theoretical knowledge. Therefore nursing as an academic discipline depends on the existence of nursing knowledge (Alligood, 2011a; Grace et al., 2016; McCrae, 2012). For those entering the profession, this knowledge is basic for their practice. Kuhn (1970), noted philosopher of science, stated, "The study of paradigms . . . is what mainly prepares the student for membership in the particular scientific community with which he [or she] will later practice" (p. 11). This is significant for all nurses, but it is particularly important to those who are entering the profession because "in the absence of a paradigm . . . all of the facts that could possibly pertain to the development of a given science are likely to seem equally relevant" (Kuhn, 1970, p. 15). Finally, with regard to the priority of paradigms, Kuhn (1970) states, "By studying them and by practicing with them, the members of their corresponding community learn their trade" (p. 43). Master's and Doctor of Nursing Practice (DNP) students apply and test theoretical knowledge in nursing practice. Doctoral (PhD) students studying to become nurse scientists develop nursing theory, test theory, and contribute nursing science in theory-based and theory-generating research studies (Grace et al., 2016).

Significance for the Profession

Not only is theory essential for the existence of nursing as an academic discipline, it is also vital to the practice of professional nursing (McCrae, 2012). Recognition as a profession seemed to be a less urgent issue as the 20th century ended because of consistent progress in the nursing theory era to solidify professional status. Nursing is recognized as a profession today because its development was guided by the criteria for a profession. Bixler and Bixler (1959) published a set of criteria for a profession tailored to nursing in the *American Journal of Nursing* (Box 1.3). These criteria have historical value for enhancing our understanding of the developmental path that nurse leaders followed. For example, a knowledge base that is well defined, organized, and specific to the discipline was formalized during the last half of the 20th century. And this knowledge is not static; rather, it continues to grow in relation to the nursing profession's goals for the human and social welfare of the society. Theories and research are vital to the discipline and the profession, so that new theory-based knowledge continues to be generated (Grace et al., 2016; McCrae, 2012). The application of nursing knowledge in practice is the criterion for a profession that is currently at the forefront, with emphasis on quality, accountability, theory-based or informed evidence, and recognition of middle-range theory for professional nursing practice (Alligood, 2014).

In the last decades of the 20th century, in anticipation of the new millennium, ideas were targeted toward moving nursing forward. Styles (1982) called for a distinction between the collective nursing profession and the individual professional nurse and for internal developments

BOX 1.3 Criteria for Development of the Professional Status of Nursing

1. Utilizes in its practice a well-defined and well-organized body of specialized knowledge [that] is on the intellectual level of the higher learning
2. Constantly enlarges the body of knowledge it uses and improves its techniques of education and service through use of the scientific method
3. Entrusts the education of its practitioners to institutions of higher education
4. Applies its body of knowledge in practical services vital to human and social welfare
5. Functions autonomously in the formulation of professional policy and thereby in the control of professional activity
6. Attracts individuals with intellectual and personal qualities of exalting service above personal gain who recognize their chosen occupation as a life work
7. Strives to compensate its practitioners by providing freedom of action, opportunity for continuous professional growth, and economic security

Data from Bixler, G. K., & Bixler, R. W. (1959). The professional status of nursing. *American Journal of Nursing, 59*(8), 1142–1146.

based on nursing ideals and beliefs for continued professional development. Similarly, Fitzpatrick (1983) presented a historical chronicle of 20th-century achievements that has led to the professional status of nursing. Both Styles (1982) and Fitzpatrick (1983) referenced a detailed history specific to the development of nursing as a profession. With recognition of nursing as a profession, emphasis in this text is on the relationship between nursing theoretical works and the status of nursing as a profession. Similarities and differences may exist in sets of criteria to evaluate professions, but they all call for a body of knowledge that is foundational to the practice of the given profession (Styles, 1982).

As individual nurses grow in their professional status, the use of substantive knowledge for theory-based evidence for nursing is a quality that is characteristic of their practice (Butts & Rich, 2011). This commitment to theory-based evidence for practice is beneficial to patients in that it guides systematic, knowledgeable care. It serves the profession as nurses are recognized for the contributions they make to the health care of society. As noted previously in relation to the discipline of nursing, the development of knowledge is a vital activity for nurse scholars to pursue. It is important that nurses have continued recognition and respect for their scholarly discipline and their contributions to the health of society.

Finally, the continued recognition of nursing theory as a tool for reasoning, critical thinking, and decision making is required for quality nursing practice. Professional nursing practice requires a systematic approach that is focused on the patient, and the theoretical works provide perspectives of the patient. The theoretical works presented in this text illustrate those various perspectives. Philosophies of nursing, conceptual models of nursing, nursing theories, and middle-range theories provide the nurse with a view of the patient and a guide for data processing, evaluation of evidence, and decisions regarding actions to take in practice (Alligood, 2014; Butts & Rich, 2011; Chinn & Kramer, 2015; Fawcett & Garity, 2009; Masters, 2015). Globally, nurses have recognized the rich heritage of the works of nursing theorists; that is, the philosophies, conceptual models, theories, and middle-range theories of nursing have become more and more numerous in the nursing literature worldwide. The publication of this text in multiple (at least 10) languages also reflects the global use of theory. The contributions of global theorists present nursing as a discipline and provide a knowledge structure for further development. Theory-based research contributes to evidence-based practice. That is, when nursing theory-based research is supported, it informs evidence. There is worldwide recognition of the rich diversity of nursing values represented in nursing models and theories. Today we see added clarification of the theoretical works in the nursing literature as more and more nurses learn and use theory-based practice. The philosophies, models, theories, and middle-range theories are used broadly in all areas—nursing education, practice, research, and administration. McCrae (2012) argues that nursing theoretical knowledge takes on greater importance, because evidence-based practice and multidisciplinary health care require nurses to articulate a sound basis for their contributions to other professionals.

The theoretical works exhibit the criteria for normal science (Kuhn, 1970; Wood, 2014). The scholarship of the past 5 decades has greatly expanded the volume of nursing literature around the philosophies, models, theories, and middle-range theories. In addition, the philosophy of science for nursing knowledge development has expanded with new research approaches. More and more nurses are acquiring higher education and understanding the value of nursing theory. The use of theory amplifies knowledge development and enhances the quality of nursing practice (Alligood, 2011a, 2011b, 2014; Chinn & Kramer, 2015; Fawcett & Garity, 2009; George, 2011; Grace et al., 2016; Im & Chang, 2012; McCrae, 2012; Reed & Shearer, 2012; Wood, 2014).

SUMMARY

This chapter has introduced the vital nature of nursing theoretical knowledge from the perspective of its history and significance. History traces the progression toward professional status with a focus on development of knowledge on which to base nursing practice and verifies that nurses increase their professional power when using systematic theoretical evidence for critical thinking and decision making (McCrae, 2012). The significance of nursing theory is verified as nurses use theory and theory-based evidence to structure their practice and quality of care improves. They are able to not only sort patient data quickly, decide on appropriate nursing action, deliver care, and evaluate outcomes but also discuss the nature of their practice clearly with other health professionals, which is vital for nurse participation in interdisciplinary care. Finally, considering nursing practice in a theory context for education helps students develop analytical skills and critical thinking ability as they clarify their values and assumptions. Theory guides education, practice, research, and administration (Alligood, 2014; Chinn & Kramer, 2015; Fawcett & DeSanto-Madeya, 2012; Meleis, 2012).

POINTS FOR FURTHER STUDY

- Donaldson, S. K., & Crowley, D. M. (1978). The discipline of nursing. *Nursing Outlook, 26*(2), 1113–1120.
- Fawcett, J. (1984). The metaparadigm of nursing: Current status and future refinements. *Image: The Journal of Nursing Scholarship, 16,* 84–87.
- *The Nursing Theory Page at Hahn School of Nursing, University of San Diego.* Retrieved from http://www.sandiego.edu/nursing/research/nursing-theory-research.php

REFERENCES

Alligood, M. R. (2011a). The power of theoretical knowledge. *Nursing Science Quarterly, 24*(4), 304–305.

Alligood, M. R. (2011b). Theory-based practice in a major medical centre. *The Journal of Nursing Management, 19,* 981–988.

Alligood, M. R. (2010). *Nursing theory: Utilization & application* (4th ed.). St Louis: Mosby-Elsevier.

Alligood, M. R. (2014). *Nursing theory: Utilization & application* (5th ed.). St Louis: Mosby-Elsevier.

Alligood, M. R., & Tomey, A. M. (Eds.). (1997). *Nursing theory: Utilization & application.* St Louis: Mosby.

Alligood, M. R., & Tomey, A. M. (Eds.). (2002). *Nursing theory: Utilization & application* (2nd ed.). St Louis: Mosby.

Alligood, M. R., & Tomey, A. M. (Eds.). (2006). *Nursing theory: Utilization & application* (3rd ed.). St Louis: Mosby.

Batey, M. V. (1977). Conceptualization: Knowledge and logic guiding empirical research. *Nursing Research, 26*(5), 324–329.

Bixler, G. K., & Bixler, R. W. (1959). The professional status of nursing. *American Journal of Nursing, 59*(8), 1142–1146.

Butts, J. B., & Rich, K. L. (2011). *Philosophies and theories for advanced nursing practice.* Sudbury, MA: Jones & Bartlett.

Carper, B. A. (1978). Fundamental patterns of knowing in nursing. *Advances in Nursing Science, 1*(1), 13–23.

Chinn, P. L., & Kramer, M. K. (2015). *Knowledge development in nursing theory and process* (9th ed.). St Louis: Elsevier-Mosby.

Cross, K. P. (1981). *Adults as learners.* Washington, DC: Jossey-Bass.

Donaldson, S. K., & Crowley, D. M. (1978). The discipline of nursing. *Nursing Outlook, 26*(2), 1113–1120.

Ervin, S. (2015). History of nursing education in the United States. In S. B. Keating (Ed.), *Curriculum development & evaluation* (3rd ed., pp. 5–32). New York: Springer.

Fawcett, J. (1978). The relationship between theory and research: A double helix. *Advances in Nursing Science, 1*(1), 49–62.

Fawcett, J. (1984). The metaparadigm of nursing: Current status and future refinements. *Image: The Journal of Nursing Scholarship, 16,* 84–87.

Fawcett, J. (1993). *Analysis and evaluation of nursing theories.* Philadelphia: F. A. Davis.

Fawcett, J. (2005). *Contemporary nursing knowledge: Conceptual models of nursing and nursing theories.* Philadelphia: F. A. Davis.

Fawcett, J., & DeSanto-Madeya, S. (2013). *Contemporary nursing knowledge: Conceptual models of nursing and nursing theories* (3rd ed.). Philadelphia: F. A. Davis.

Fawcett, J., & Garity, J. (2009). *Evaluating research for evidence-based nursing practice.* Philadelphia: F. A. Davis.

Fitzpatrick, M. L. (1983). *Prologue to professionalism.* Bowie, MD: Robert J. Brady.

Fitzpatrick, J., & Whall, A. (1983). *Conceptual models of nursing.* Bowie, MD: Robert J. Brady.

George, J. (2011). *Nursing theories* (6th ed.). Upper Saddle River, NJ: Pearson.

Grace, P., Willis, D., Roy, C. & Jones, D. (2016). Profession at the crossroads: A dialog concerning the preparation of nursing scholars and leaders. *Nursing Outlook, 64*(1), 61–70.

Hardy, M. E. (1973). Theories: components, development, evaluation. *Nursing Research, 23*(2), 100–107.

Hardy, M. E. (1978). Perspectives on nursing theory. *Advances in Nursing Science, 1,* 37–48.

Im, E. O., & Chang, S. J. (2012). Current trends in nursing theories. *Journal of Nursing Scholarship*, *44*(2), 156–164.

Johnson, D. (1959). The nature of a science of nursing. *Nursing Outlook*, *7*, 291–294.

Johnson, D. (1968). *One conceptual model for nursing*. Nashville, TN: Unpublished paper presented at Vanderbilt University.

Johnson, D. (1974). Development of the theory: A requisite for nursing as a primary health profession. *Nursing Research*, *23*, 372–377.

Judd, D., & Sitzman, K. (2013). *A history of American nursing* (2nd ed.). Boston: Jones & Bartlett.

Kalisch, P. A., & Kalisch, B. J. (2003). *American nursing: A history* (4th ed.). Philadelphia: Lippincott.

King, I. (1971). *Toward a theory of nursing*. New York: Wiley.

Kuhn, T. S. (1970). *The structure of scientific revolutions*. Chicago: University of Chicago Press.

Levine, M. (1969). *Introduction to clinical nursing*. Philadelphia: F. A. Davis.

Marriner, A. (1986). *Nursing theorists and their work*. St Louis: Mosby.

Masters, K. (2015). *Role development in professional nursing practice* (4th ed.). Burllington, MA: Jones & Bartlett.

McCrae, N. (2012). Whither nursing models? The value of nursing theory in the context of evidence-based practice and multidisciplinary health care. *Journal of Advanced Nursing*, *68*(1), 222–229.

Meleis, A. (2007). *Theoretical nursing: Development and progress* (4th ed.). Philadelphia: Lippincott.

Meleis, A. (2012). *Theoretical nursing: Development and progress* (5th ed.). Philadelphia: Lippincott.

Neuman, B. (1974). The Betty Neuman health systems model: A total person approach to patient problems. In J. P. Riehl & C. Roy (Eds.), *Conceptual models for nursing practice* (pp. 94–114). New York: Appleton-Century-Crofts.

Nicoll, L. (1986). *Perspectives on nursing theory*. Boston: Little, Brown.

Nicoll, L. (1992). *Perspectives on nursing theory* (2nd ed.). Philadelphia: Lippincott Williams & Wilkins.

Nicoll, L. (1997). *Perspectives on nursing theory* (3rd ed.). Philadelphia: Lippincott Williams & Wilkins.

Nightingale, F. (1859/1969). *Notes on nursing: What it is and what it is not*. New York: Dover. (Originally published 1859.)

Orem, D. (1971). *Nursing: Concepts of practice*. St Louis: Mosby.

Orem, D. (2001). *Nursing: Concepts of practice* (6th ed.). St Louis: Mosby.

Orlando, I. (1961). *The dynamic nurse-patient relationship*. New York: Putnam.

Orlando, I. (1972). *The discipline and teaching of nursing process*. New York: Putnam.

Peterson, S., & Bredow, T. (2014). *Middle-range theories: Applications to nursing research* (3rd ed.). Philadelphia: Lippincott Williams & Wilkins.

Reed, P., & Shearer, N. (2009). *Perspectives on nursing theory* (5th ed.). New York: Lippincott Williams & Wilkins.

Reed, P., & Shearer, N. (2012). *Perspectives on nursing theory* (6th ed.). New York: Lippincott Williams & Wilkins.

Reed, P., Shearer, N., & Nicoll, L. (2003). *Perspectives on nursing theory* (4th ed.). Philadelphia: Lippincott Williams & Wilkins.

Rogers, M. E. (1970). *An introduction to the theoretical basis of nursing*. Philadelphia: F. A. Davis.

Roy, C. (1970). Adaptation: A conceptual framework for nursing. *Nursing Outlook*, *18*, 42–45.

Shaw, M.C. (1993). The discipline of nursing: Historical roots, current perspectives, future directions. *Journal of Advanced Nursing*, *18*, 1651–1656.

Smith, M., & Leihr, P. (2013). *Middle range theory for nursing* (3rd ed.). New York: Springer.

Smith, M., & Parker, M. (2014). *Nursing theory and nursing practice* (4th ed.). Philadelphia: F. A. Davis.

Styles, M. M. (1982). *On nursing: Toward a new endowment*. St Louis: Mosby.

Walker, L. O., & Avant, K. C. (2011). *Strategies for theory construction in nursing* (5th ed.). Boston: Prentice Hall.

Wood, A. F. (2014). Nursing models: Normal science for nursing practice. In M. R. Alligood (Ed.), *Nursing theory: Utilization & application* (5th ed., pp. 13–39). St Louis: Mosby-Elsevier.

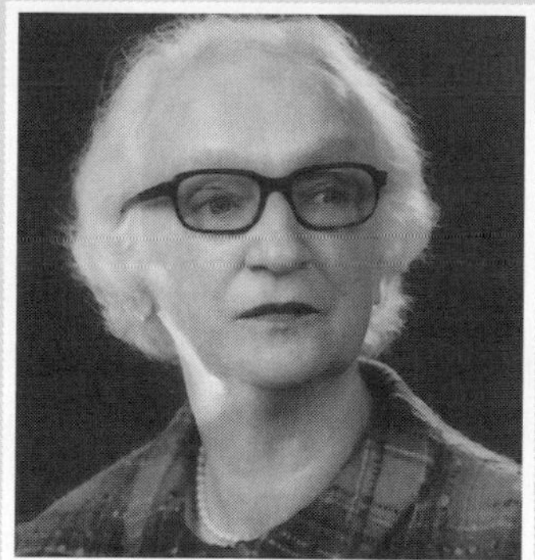

Hildegard E. Peplau
1909–1999

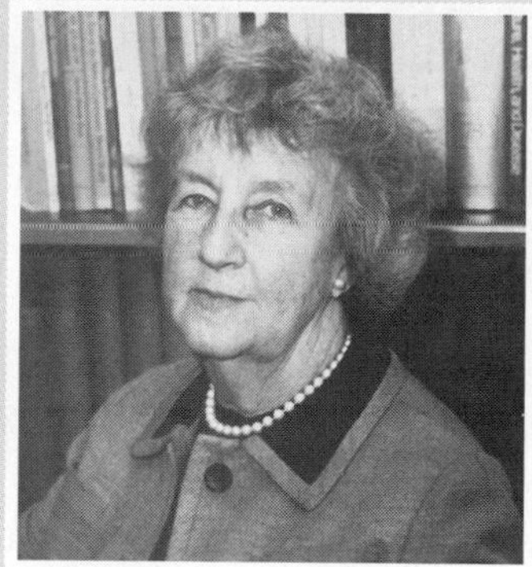

Virginia Henderson
1897–1996

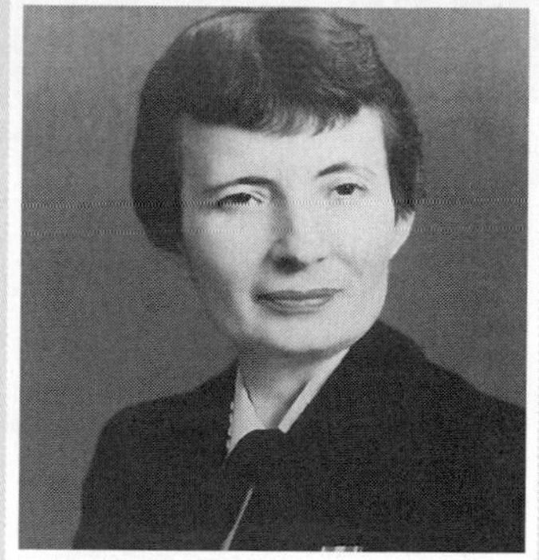

Faye Glenn Abdellah
1919–Present

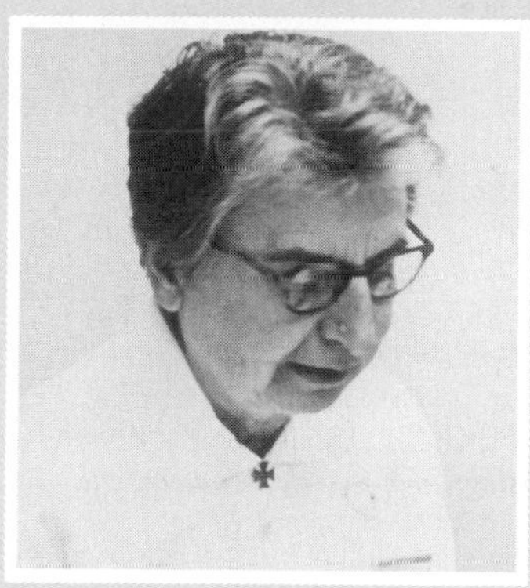

Ernestine Wiedenbach
1900–1996

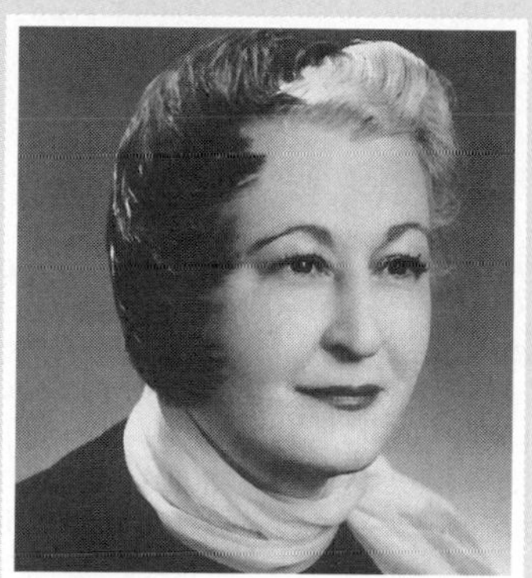

Lydia Hall
1906–1969

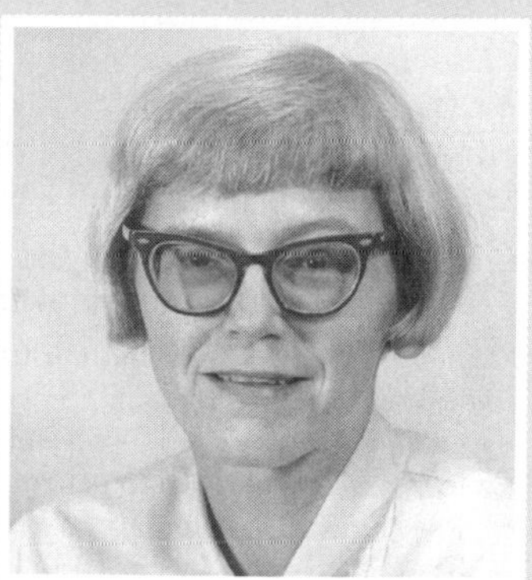

Joyce Travelbee
1926–1973

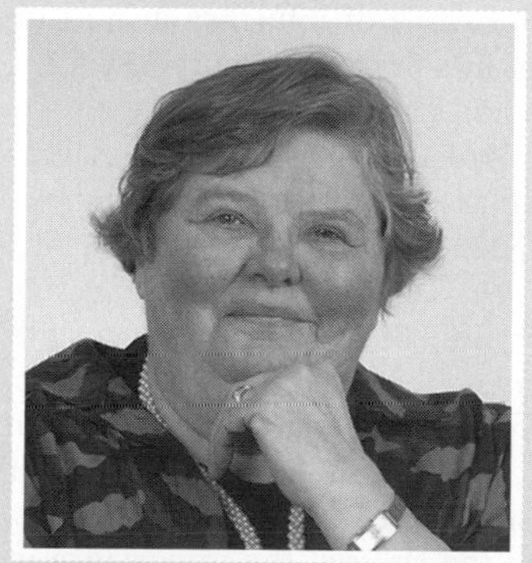

Kathryn E. Barnard
1938–2015

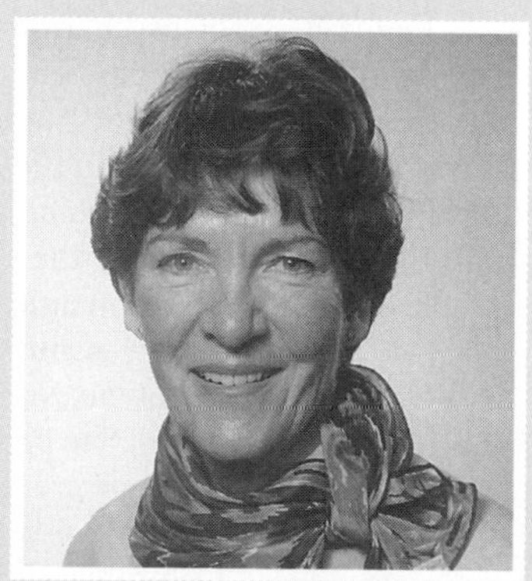

Evelyn Adam
1929–Present

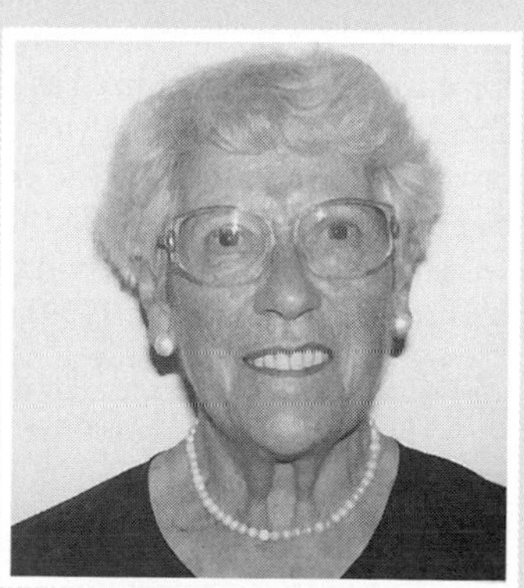

Nancy Roper
1918–2004

2

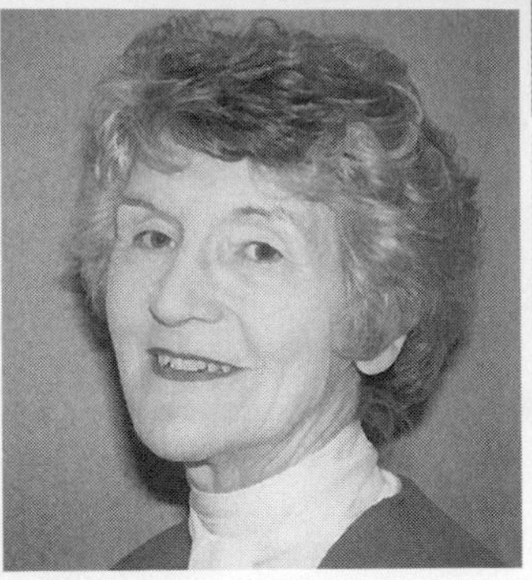
Winifred W. Logan
1931–2010

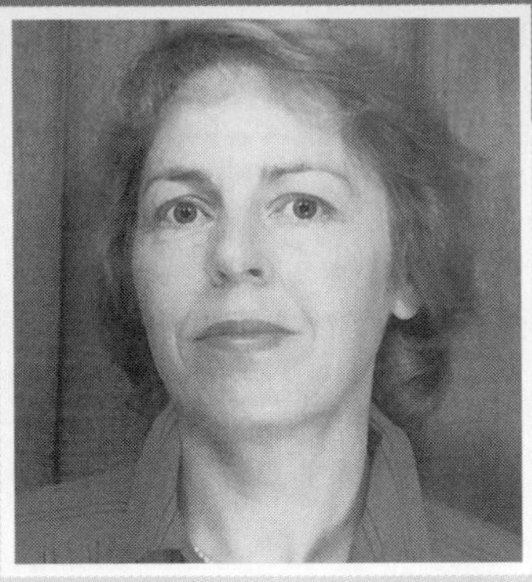
Alison J. Tierney

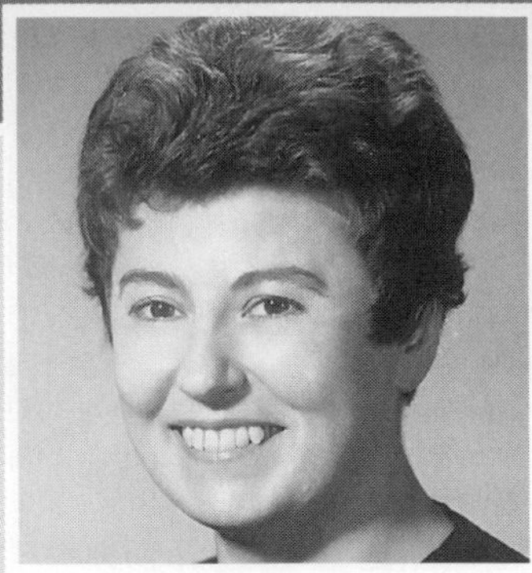
Ida Jean (Orlando) Pelletier
1926–2007

Nursing Theorists of Historical Significance

*Marie E. Pokorny**

"The idea of nursing, historically rooted in the care of the sick and in the provision of nurturance for those vulnerable to ill health, is foundational to the profession."

(Wolf, 2006, p. 301)

This chapter presents selected theorists noted for developing nursing theoretical works during the preparadigm period and for making important early contributions to the development of specialized nursing knowledge. National health sociological studies recommended that nursing be developed as a profession (Ervin, 2015), and, as presented in Chapter 1, a body of specialized knowledge was required for nursing to be recognized as such. Ultimately criteria for a profession were tailored to nursing, and guidance was provided in the process. One criterion that called for specialized nursing knowledge and knowledge structure served as an important driving force throughout the 20th century (Bixler & Bixler, 1959). The criterion reads:

> Utilizes in its practice a well-defined and well-organized body of specialized knowledge [that] is on the intellectual level of the higher learning (p. 1143).

Photo Credit (Joyce Travelbee): Louisiana State University Health Sciences Center, School of Nursing, New Orleans, LA.
*Previous author: Ann Marriner Tomey

HILDEGARD E. PEPLAU

Theory of Interpersonal Relations

Hildegard E. Peplau has been described as the mother of psychiatric nursing because her theoretical and clinical work led to the development of the distinct specialty field of psychiatric nursing. Her scope of influence in nursing includes her contributions as a psychiatric nursing expert, educator, author, and nursing leader and theorist.

Peplau provided major leadership in the professionalization of nursing. She served as executive director and president of the American Nurses Association (ANA). She was instrumental in the 1980 ANA definition of nursing that was nursing's declaration of a social contract with society in *Nursing: A Social Policy Statement* (Butts & Rich, 2015). She promoted professional standards and regulation through credentialing. Peplau taught the first classes for graduate psychiatric nursing students at Teachers College, Columbia University, and she stressed the importance of nurses' ability to understand their own behavior to help others identify perceived difficulties. Her seminal book,

Interpersonal Relations in Nursing (1952), describes the importance of the nurse-patient relationship as a "significant, therapeutic interpersonal process" (p. 16) and is recognized as the first nursing theory textbook since Nightingale's work in the 1850s. She discussed four psychobiological experiences that compel destructive or constructive patient responses, as follows: needs, frustrations, conflicts, and anxieties. Peplau identified four phases of the nurse-patient relationship—**orientation, identification, exploitation,** and **resolution** (Fig. 2.1); diagrammed changing aspects of nurse-patient relationships (Fig. 2.2), and proposed and described six nursing roles: **stranger, resource person, teacher, leader, surrogate,** and **counselor** (Fig. 2.3).

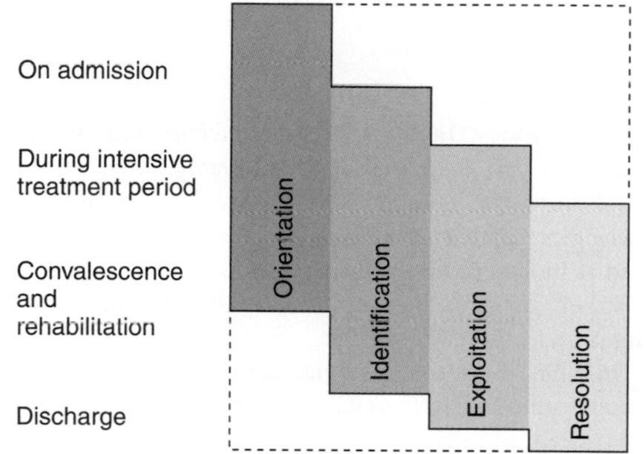

FIG 2.1 Overlapping phases in nurse-patient relationships. (From Peplau, H. E. [1952]. *Interpersonal relations in nursing*. New York: Putnam.)

Peplau had professional relationships with others in psychiatry, medicine, education, and sociology that influenced her view of what a profession is and does and what it should be (Sills, 1998). Her work was influenced by Freud's, Maslow's, and Sullivan's interpersonal relationship theories and by the contemporaneous psychoanalytical model. She borrowed the psychological model to synthesize her Theory of Interpersonal Relations (Haber, 2000). Her work on nurse-patient relationships is known well internationally and continues to influence nursing practice and research. Recent publications using her model include research on the effect of communication on nurse-patient relationships (Arungwa, 2014), observing and analyzing empathy in Brazilian nursing professionals (Trevizan et al., 2015), assisting nursing students to understand holistic communication skills during their encounters with older adults (Deane & Fain, 2016), applying her theory to simulation learning in undergraduate nursing students (Searl et al., 2014), illustrating the roles played by nurses caring for children with complex needs in the home setting in Ireland (Doyle & Buckley, 2012), generating best-practice knowledge for working with children of incarcerated parents (Falk, 2014), describing identity concerns in those who experienced adolescent dating violence (Draucker et al., 2012), developing a framework to support the evaluation of Nurse Practitioner-Aged Care Models of Practice in Australia (Hungerford, Prosser, & Davey, 2015), describing home health care nurse therapeutic interactions with homebound geriatric patients with depression and disability (Liebel, Powers, & Hauenstein, 2015), highlighting aspects of her theory in emergency and rural nursing (Senn,

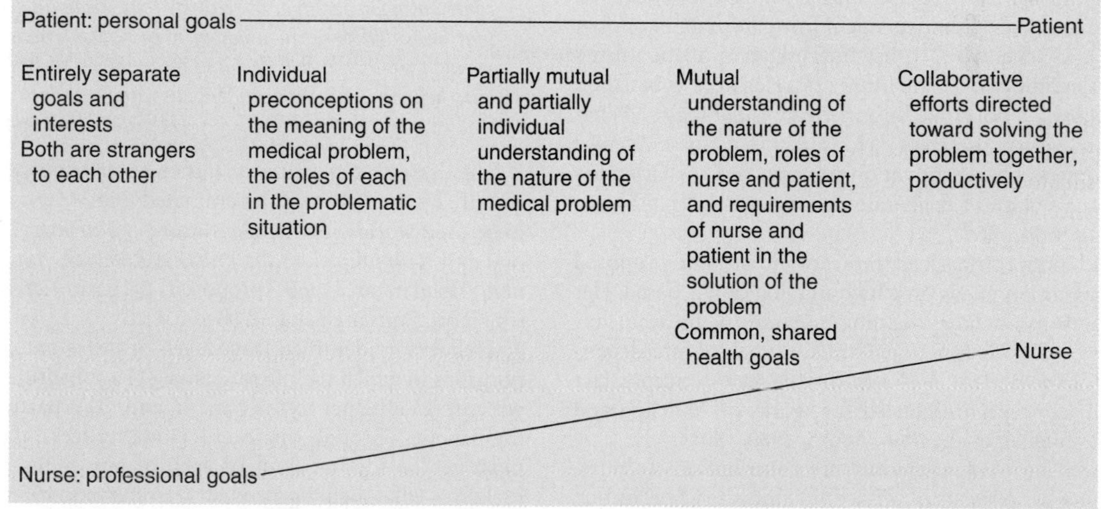

FIG 2.2 Changing aspects of nurse-patient relationships. (From Peplau, H. E. [1952]. *Interpersonal relations in nursing*. New York: Putnam.)

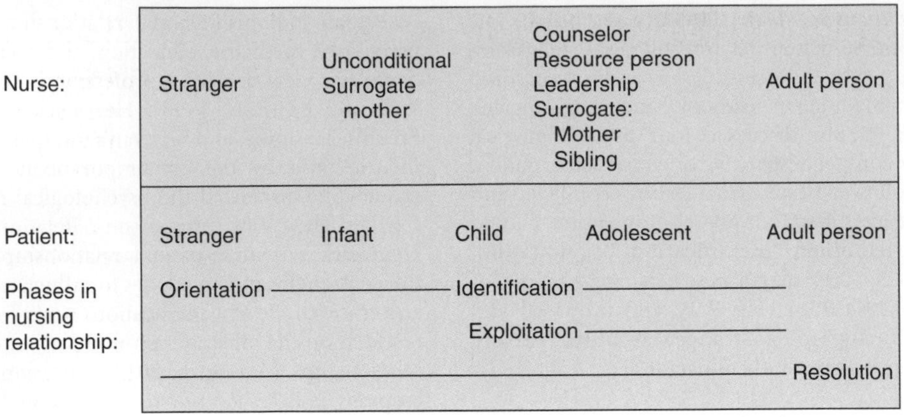

Nurse:	Stranger	Unconditional Surrogate mother		Counselor Resource person Leadership Surrogate: Mother Sibling	Adult person
Patient:	Stranger	Infant	Child	Adolescent	Adult person
Phases in nursing relationship:	Orientation ———		Identification ———		
			Exploitation ———		
	———				Resolution

FIG 2.3 Phases and changing roles in nurse-patient relationships. (From Peplau, H. E. [1952]. *Interpersonal relations in nursing.* New York: Putnam.)

2013), developing an auditory hallucinations interview guide for psychiatric–mental health nurses (Trygstad et al., 2015), and applying her theory to the preceptor–new graduate relationship and measuring the strength and presence of that relationship (Washington, 2013). Peplau's work is specific to the nurse-patient relationship and is a theory for the practice of nursing.

VIRGINIA HENDERSON

Definition of Nursing

Virginia Henderson viewed the patient as an individual who requires help toward achieving independence and completeness or wholeness of mind and body. She clarified the practice of nursing as independent from the practice of physicians and acknowledged her interpretation of the nurse's role as a synthesis of many influences. Her work is based on (1) Edward L. Thorndike, an American psychologist; (2) her experiences with the Henry House Visiting Nurse Agency; (3) experience in rehabilitation nursing; and (4) Orlando's conceptualization of deliberate nursing action (Henderson, 1964; Orlando, 1961).

Henderson emphasized the art of nursing and proposed 14 basic human needs on which nursing care is based. Her contributions include defining nursing, delineating autonomous nursing functions, stressing goals of interdependence for the patient, and creating self-help concepts. Her self-help concepts influenced the works of Abdellah and Adam (Abdellah et al., 1960; Adam, 1980, 1991).

Henderson made extraordinary contributions to nursing during her 60 years of service as a nurse, teacher, author, and researcher, and she published extensively throughout those years. Henderson wrote three books that have become nursing classics: *Textbook of the Principles and Practice of Nursing* (1955), *Basic Principles of Nursing Care* (1960), and *The Nature of Nursing* (1966). Her major contribution to nursing research was an 11-year Yale-sponsored Nursing Studies Index Project published as a four-volume annotated index of nursing's biographical, analytical, and historical literature from 1900 to 1959.

In 1958, the nursing service committee of the International Council of Nurses (ICN) asked Henderson to describe her concept of nursing. This now historical definition, published by the ICN in 1961, represented her final crystallization on the subject:

> *"The unique function of the nurse is to assist the individual, sick or well, in the performance of those activities contributing to health or its recovery (or to peaceful death) that he would perform unaided if he had the necessary strength, will, or knowledge; and to do this in such a way as to help him gain independence as rapidly as possible."*
>
> ***(Henderson, 1964, p. 63)***

Henderson's definition of nursing was adopted subsequently by the ICN and disseminated widely; it continues to be used worldwide. In *The Nature of Nursing: A Definition and Its Implications for Practice, Research, and Education,* Henderson (1966) proposed 14 basic needs upon which nursing care is based (Box 2.1).

Henderson identified three levels of nurse-patient relationships in which the nurse acts as: (1) a substitute for the patient, (2) a helper to the patient, and (3) a partner with the patient. Through the interpersonal process, the nurse must get "inside the skin" of each of her or his patients to know what help is needed (Henderson, 1955, p. 5). Although she believed that the functions of nurses and physicians overlap, Henderson asserted that the nurse

BOX 2.1 Henderson's Fourteen Needs

1. Breathe normally.
2. Eat and drink adequately.
3. Eliminate body wastes.
4. Move and maintain desirable postures.
5. Sleep and rest.
6. Select suitable clothes; dress and undress.
7. Maintain body temperature within a normal range by adjusting clothing and modifying the environment.
8. Keep the body clean and well groomed and protect the integument.
9. Avoid dangers in the environment and avoid injuring others.
10. Communicate with others in expressing emotions, needs, fears, or opinions.
11. Worship according to one's faith.
12. Work in such a way that there is a sense of accomplishment.
13. Play or participate in various forms of recreation.
14. Learn, discover, or satisfy the curiosity that leads to normal development and health, and use the available health facilities.

From Henderson, V. A. (1991). *The nature of nursing: Reflections after 25 years* (pp. 22–23). New York: National League for Nursing Press.

works in interdependence with other health care professionals and with the patient.

In *The Nature of Nursing: Reflections after 25 Years,* Henderson (1991) added addenda to each chapter of the 1966 edition with changes in her views and opinions. Henderson said of her theory that "the complexity and quality of the service is limited only by the imagination and the competence of the nurse who interprets it" (Henderson, 2006, p. 26). Her theory has been applied to research in the specialized area of organ donation (Nicely & DeLario, 2011) and framed a discussion of remembering the art of nursing in a technological age (Henderson, 1980; Timmins 2011). More recently her theory framed the research investigating the association between physical mobility demands and social and clinical variables of the elderly living in community (Clares, de Frietas, & Borges, 2014) and research investigating hematology and oncology nurses' experiences and perceptions of "do not resuscitate" orders (Pettersson, Hedström, & Höglund, 2014). Her components of nursing care were used to specify the variable aspects of the concept of care and to develop the Care Dependency Scale for measuring basic human needs (Dijkstra et al., 2012) and to evaluate home care nursing for elderly people in Cyprus (Kouta et al., 2015). Henderson's work is viewed as a nursing philosophy of purpose and function.

FAYE GLENN ABDELLAH

Twenty-One Nursing Problems

Faye Glenn Abdellah is recognized as a leader in the development of nursing research and nursing as a profession within the U.S. Public Health Service (PHS) and as an international expert on health problems. She was named a "living legend" by the American Academy of Nursing in 1994 and was inducted into the National Women's Hall of Fame in 2000 for a lifetime spent establishing and leading essential health care programs for the United States. In 2012 Abdellah was inducted into the ANA Hall of Fame for a lifetime of contributions to nursing and to honor her legacy of more than 60 years of accomplishments that live on nationally and globally (ANA, 2012).

Abdellah has been active in professional nursing associations and is a prolific author, with more than 150 publications. During her 40-year career as a Commissioned Officer in the U.S. PHS (1949–1989), she served as Chief Nurse Officer (1970–1987) and was the first nurse to achieve the rank of a two-star Flag Officer (Abdellah, 2004) and the first woman and nurse Deputy Surgeon General (1982–1989). After retirement, Abdellah founded and served as the first dean in the Graduate School of Nursing (GSN) at the Uniformed Services University of the Health Sciences (USUHS).

Abdellah (2004) considers her greatest accomplishment being able to "play a role in establishing a foundation for nursing research as a science" (p. iii). Her book, *Patient-Centered Approaches to Nursing,* emphasizes the science of nursing and has elicited changes throughout nursing curricula. Her work, which is based on the problem-solving method, serves as a vehicle for delineating nursing (patient) problems as the patient moves toward a healthy outcome.

Abdellah views nursing as an art and a science that mold the attitude, intellectual competencies, and technical skills of the individual nurse into the desire and ability to help individuals cope with their health needs, whether they are ill or well. She formulated 21 nursing problems based on a review of nursing research studies (Box 2.2). She used Henderson's 14 basic human needs (see Box 2.1) and nursing research to establish the classification of nursing problems.

Abdellah's work is a set of problems formulated in terms of nursing-centered services, which are used to determine the patient's needs. Her contribution to nursing theory development is the systematic analysis of research reports and creation of 21 nursing problems that guide comprehensive nursing care. The typology of her 21 nursing problems first appeared in *Patient-Centered Approaches to Nursing* (Abdellah et al., 1960). It evolved into *Preparing for Nursing Research in the 21st Century: Evolution,*

BOX 2.2 Abdellah's Typology of Twenty-One Nursing Problems

1. To maintain good hygiene and physical comfort
2. To promote optimal activity: exercise, rest, sleep
3. To promote safety through prevention of accident, injury, or other trauma and through prevention of the spread of infection
4. To maintain good body mechanics and prevent and correct deformity
5. To facilitate the maintenance of a supply of oxygen to all body cells
6. To facilitate the maintenance of nutrition for all body cells
7. To facilitate the maintenance of elimination
8. To facilitate the maintenance of fluid and electrolyte balance
9. To recognize the physiological responses of the body to disease conditions—pathological, physiological, and compensatory
10. To facilitate the maintenance of regulatory mechanisms and functions
11. To facilitate the maintenance of sensory function
12. To identify and accept positive and negative expressions, feelings, and reactions
13. To identify and accept interrelatedness of emotions and organic illness
14. To facilitate the maintenance of effective verbal and nonverbal communication
15. To promote the development of productive interpersonal relationships
16. To facilitate progress toward achievement and personal spiritual goals
17. To create or maintain a therapeutic environment
18. To facilitate awareness of self as an individual with varying physical, emotional, and developmental needs
19. To accept the optimum possible goals in the light of limitations, physical and emotional
20. To use community resources as an aid in resolving problems that arise from illness
21. To understand the role of social problems as influencing factors in the cause of illness

From Abdellah, F. G., Beland, I. L., Martin, A., & Matheney, R. V. (1960). *Patient-centered approaches to nursing.* New York: Macmillan. Reprinted with the permission of Scribner, a division of Simon & Schuster.

Methodologies, and Challenges (Abdellah & Levine, 1994). The 21 nursing problems progressed to a second-generation development referred to as patient problems and patient outcomes. Abdellah educated the public on Acquired Immuno Deficiency Syndrome (AIDS), drug addiction, violence, smoking, and alcoholism. Her classification framework for identifying nursing problems was used to determine how to reduce peripheral intravenous catheter infiltration to increase the longevity of peripheral intravenous catheters (Banks, 2015). Her work is a problem-centered approach or philosophy of nursing. Abdellah's papers are available at http://www.nlm.nih.gov/hmd/manuscripts/msc.html (National Library of Medicine, 1988).

ERNESTINE WIEDENBACH

The Helping Art of Clinical Nursing

Ernestine Wiedenbach is known for her work in theory development and maternal infant nursing developed while teaching maternity nursing at the School of Nursing, Yale University. Wiedenbach taught with Ida Orlando at Yale University and wrote, with philosophers Dickoff and James, a classic work on theory in a practice discipline that is used by those studying the evolution of nursing theory (Dickoff, James, & Wiedenbach, 1968a, 1968b). She directed the major curriculum in maternal and newborn health nursing when the Yale School of Nursing established a master's degree program (Kaplan & King, 2000) and authored books used widely in nursing education. Her definition of nursing reflects her nurse-midwife background as follows: "People may differ in their concept of nursing, but few would disagree that nursing is nurturing or caring for someone in a motherly fashion" (Wiedenbach, 1964, p. 1).

Wiedenbach's orientation is a philosophy of nursing that guides the nurse's action in the art of nursing. She specified four elements of clinical nursing: **philosophy, purpose, practice,** and **art.** She postulated that clinical nursing is directed toward meeting the patient's perceived need for help in a vision of nursing that reflects considerable emphasis on the art of nursing. She followed Orlando's theory of deliberate rather than automatic nursing and incorporated the steps of the nursing process. In her book (1964), *Clinical Nursing: A Helping Art,* Wiedenbach outlines nursing steps in sequence.

Wiedenbach proposes that nurses identify patients' need for help in the following ways:

1. Observing behaviors consistent or inconsistent with their comfort
2. Exploring the meaning of their behavior
3. Determining the cause of their discomfort or incapability
4. Determining whether they can resolve their problems or have a need for help

The nurse then administers the help needed (Fig. 2.4) and validates that the need for help was met (Fig. 2.5)

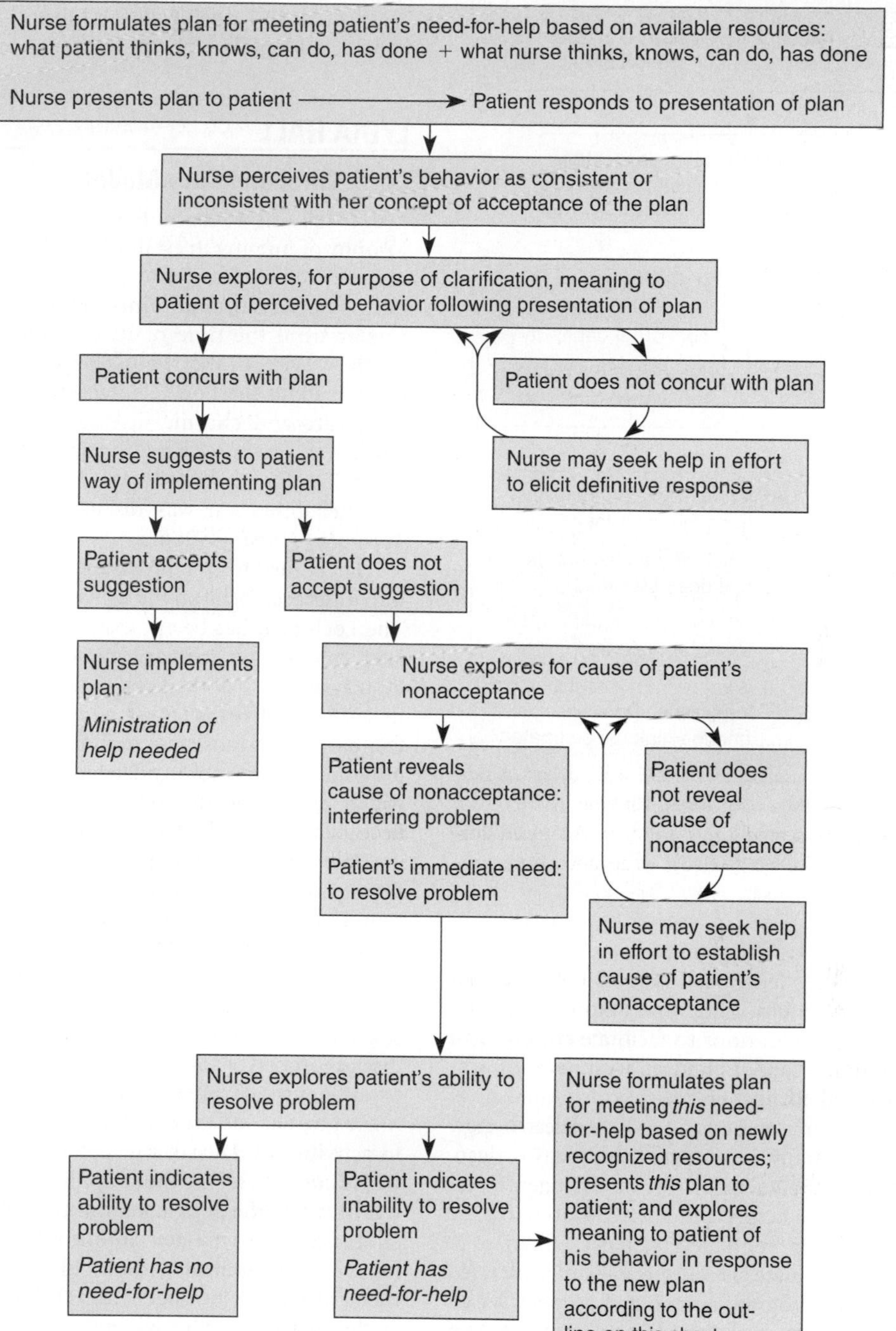

FIG 2.4 Ministration of help. (From Wiedenbach, E. [1964]. *Clinical nursing: A helping art* [p. 61]. New York: Springer.)

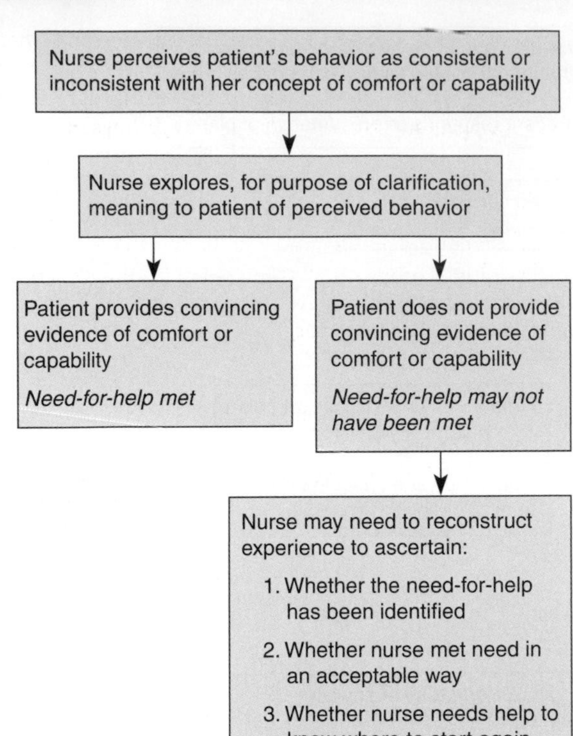
Nurse perceives patient's behavior as consistent or inconsistent with her concept of comfort or capability
Nurse explores, for purpose of clarification, meaning to patient of perceived behavior
Patient provides convincing evidence of comfort or capability
Need-for-help met
Patient does not provide convincing evidence of comfort or capability
Need-for-help may not have been met
Nurse may need to reconstruct experience to ascertain:
1. Whether the need-for-help has been identified
2. Whether nurse met need in an acceptable way
3. Whether nurse needs help to know where to start again and then take appropriate action

FIG 2.5 Validation that the need-for-help was met. (From Wiedenbach, E. [1964]. *Clinical nursing: A helping art* [p. 62]. New York: Springer.)

(Wiedenbach, 1964). Wiedenbach (1970) proposed that prescriptive theory would guide and improve nursing practice. Program interventions to facilitate coping with the demands of home care of children with heart disease were conceptualized using her framework (Amakali & Small, 2014). Her framework was used to research how mothers of newborns transition into motherhood (Corrigan, Kwasky, & Groh, 2015), to access the knowledge of oral care practices of nurses before and after education on the oral care practices for ventilated patients (Cherian & Karkada, 2015), to evaluate the effectiveness of a planned cardiac rehabilitation program among staff nurses (Degavi & Bjupali, 2015), to evaluate the effectiveness of foot massage on level of pain among patients with cancer (Doss, 2014), to access the effectiveness of massage on respiratory status among toddlers with lower respiratory tract infections (Martina, Beulah, & David, 2015), and to develop a model of facilitation of emotional intelligence to promote wholeness in neophyte critical care nurses in South Africa (Towell, Nel, & Muller, 2015). Her work is considered a philosophy of the art of nursing.

LYDIA HALL

Core, Care, and Cure Model

Lydia Hall was a rehabilitation nurse who used her philosophy of nursing to establish the Loeb Center for Nursing and Rehabilitation at Montefiore Hospital in New York. She served as administrative director of the Loeb Center from the time of its opening in 1963 until her death in 1969. In the 1960s, she published more than 20 articles about the Loeb Center and her theories of long-term care and chronic disease control. In 1964 Hall's work was presented in "Nursing: What Is It?" in *The Canadian Nurse*. In 1969 the Loeb Center for Nursing and Rehabilitation was discussed in the *International Journal of Nursing Studies*.

Hall argued for the provision of hospital beds grouped into units that focus on the delivery of therapeutic nursing. The Loeb plan has been considered to be similar to what later emerged as "primary nursing" (Wiggins, 1980). An evaluation study of the Loeb Center for Nursing published in 1975 revealed that those admitted to the nursing unit compared with those in a traditional unit were readmitted less often, were more independent, had higher postdischarge quality of life, and were more satisfied with their hospital experience (Hall et al., 1975).

Hall used three interlocking circles to represent aspects of the patient and nursing functions. The care circle represents the patient's body, the cure circle represents the disease that affects the patient's physical system, and the core circle represents the inner feelings and management of the person (Fig. 2.6). The three circles change in size and overlap in relation to the patient's phase in the disease process. A nurse functions in all three circles but to different degrees. For example, in the care phase, the nurse gives hands-on bodily care to the patient in relation to activities of daily living such as toileting and bathing. In the cure phase, the nurse applies medical knowledge to treatment of the person, and in the core phase, the nurse addresses the social and emotional needs of the patient for effective communication and a comfortable environment (Touhy & Birnbach, 2001). Nurses also share the circles with other providers. Lydia Hall's theory was used to show improvement in patient-nurse communication, self-growth, and self-awareness in patients whose heart failure was managed in the home setting (McCoy, Davidhizar, & Gillum, 2007) and for the nursing process and critical thinking linked to disaster preparedness (Bulson & Bulson, 2011).

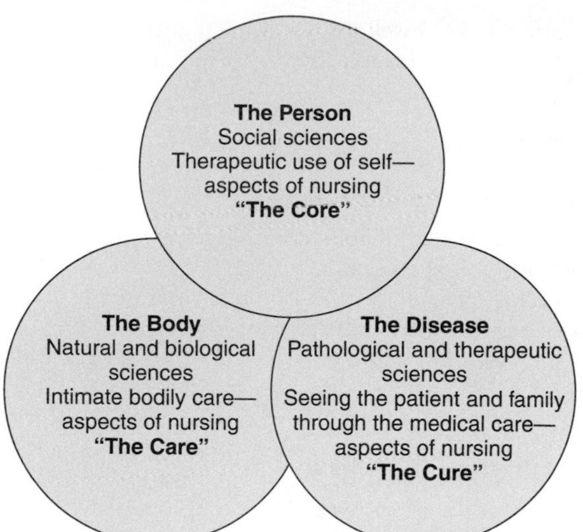

FIG 2.6 Core, care, and cure model. (From Hall, L. [1964]. Nursing: What is it? *The Canadian Nurse, 60*[2], 151.)

Hall believed that professional nursing care hastened recovery, and as less medical care was needed, more professional nursing care and teaching were necessary. She stressed the autonomous function of nurses. Her contribution to nursing theory was the development and use of her philosophy of nursing care at the Loeb Center for Nursing and Rehabilitation in New York. She recognized professional nurses and encouraged them to contribute to patient outcomes. Hall's work is viewed as a philosophy of nursing.

JOYCE TRAVELBEE

Human-to-Human Relationship Model

Joyce Travelbee presented her Human-to-Human Relationship Theory in her book *Interpersonal Aspects of Nursing* (1966, 1971). She published predominantly in the mid-1960s and died at a young age in 1973. Travelbee proposed that the goal of nursing was to assist an individual, family, or community to prevent or cope with the experiences of illness and suffering and, if necessary, to find meaning in these experiences, with the ultimate goal being the presence of hope (Travelbee, 1966, 1971). She discussed her theory with Victor Frankel (1963), whom she credits along with Rollo May (1953) for influencing her thinking (Meleis, 2012). Travelbee's work was conceptual, and she wrote about illness, suffering, pain, hope, communication, interaction, empathy, sympathy, rapport, and therapeutic use of self. She proposed that nursing was accomplished through human-to-human relationships that began with (1) the original encounter and progressed through stages of (2) emerging identities, (3) developing feelings of empathy and, later, (4) sympathy, until (5) the nurse and the patient attained rapport in the final stage (Fig. 2.7). Travelbee believed that it was as important to sympathize as it was to empathize if the nurse and the patient were to develop a **human-to-human** relationship (Travelbee, 1964). She was explicit about the patient's and the nurse's spirituality, observing the following:

> *"It is believed the spiritual values a person holds will determine, to a great extent, his perception of illness. The spiritual values of the nurse or her philosophical beliefs about illness and suffering will determine the degree to which he or she will be able to help ill persons find meaning, or no meaning, in these situations."*
>
> ***(Travelbee, 1971, p. 16)***

Travelbee's theory extended the interpersonal relationship theories of Peplau and Orlando, and her unique synthesis of their ideas differentiated her work in terms of the therapeutic human relationship between nurse and patient. Travelbee's emphasis on caring stressed empathy, sympathy, rapport, and the emotional aspects of nursing (Travelbee, 1963, 1964). Rich (2003) revisited Travelbee's argument on the value of sympathy in nursing and updated it with a reminder that compassion is central to holistic nursing care. Bunkers (2012) examined her human relationship model to explore the meaning of presence. Travelbee's work is categorized a nursing theory.

KATHRYN E. BARNARD

Child Health Assessment

Kathryn E. Barnard was an internationally recognized pioneer in the field of infant mental health, which studies the social and emotional development of children during their first 5 years of life. She was a renowned researcher, teacher, and innovator (*The Washington Nurse,* 2015). She published extensively since the mid-1960s about improving the health of infants and their families. She remained at the University of Washington for her career where she founded The Barnard Center on Infant Mental Health and Development. Her pioneering work to improve the physical and mental health outcomes of infants and young children earned her numerous honors, including the Gustav O. Leinhard Award from the Institute of Medicine, and the Episteme Award and the Living Legend Award in 2006

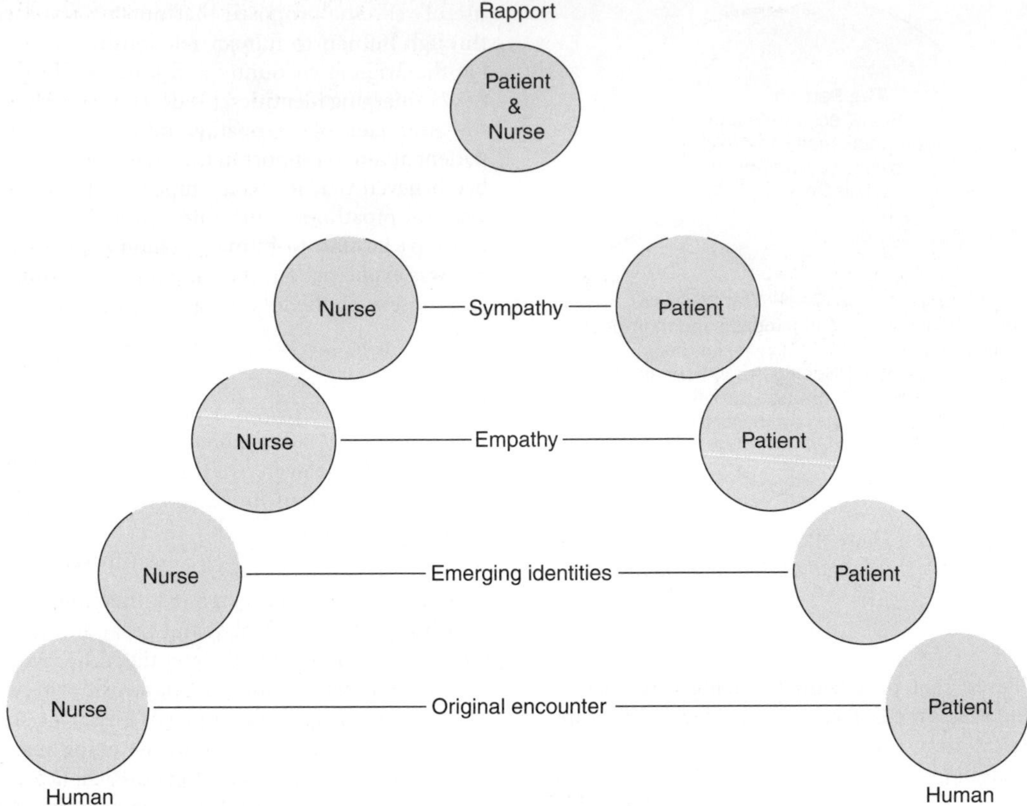

FIG 2.7 Human-to-human relationship. (Conceptualized by William Hobble and Theresa Lansinger, based on Joyce Travelbee's writings.)

from the American Academy of Nursing and the ZERO TO THREE Lifetime Achievement Award. Barnard began by studying mentally and physically handicapped children and adults, moved into the activities of the well child, and expanded to methods of evaluating the growth and development of children and mother-infant relationships, and finally how environment influences development for children and families (Barnard, 2004). She was the founder of the Nursing Child Assessment Satellite Training Project (NCAST), providing health care workers around the globe with guidelines for assessing infant development and parent-child interactions.

Although Barnard never intended to develop theory, her longitudinal nursing child assessment study provided the basis for a Child Health Assessment Interaction Theory (Fig. 2.8). Barnard (1978) proposed that individual characteristics of members influence the parent-infant system, and adaptive behavior modifies those characteristics to meet the needs of the system. Her theory borrows from psychology and human development and focuses on mother-infant interaction with the environment. Barnard's theory is based on scales designed to measure the effects of feeding, teaching, and environment (Kelly & Barnard, 2000). Her theory remains population specific; it was originally designed to be applicable to interactions between the caregiver and the child in the first year and has been expanded to 3 years of life (Masters, 2015). With continual research, Barnard refined the theory and has provided a close link to practice that has transformed the way health care providers evaluate children in light of the parent-child relationship. She modeled the role of researcher in clinical practice and engaged in theory development in practice for the advancement of nursing science. Her sleep-activity record of the infant's sleep-wake cycle was used in research on infant and mother circadian rhythm (Tsai et al., 2011, 2012). She explored the mechanisms of emotion coregulation in parent-child dyads (Guo et al., 2015). Barnard's work is a theory of nursing.

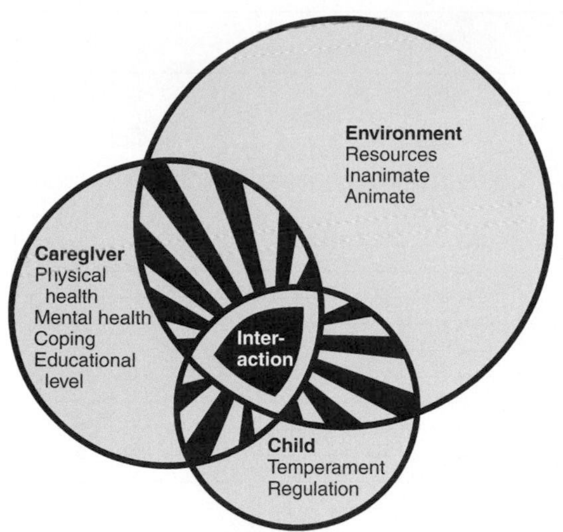

FIG 2.8 Child health assessment model. (From Sumner, G., & Spietz, A. [Eds.]. [1994]. *NCAST caregiver/parent-child interaction teaching manual* [p. 3]. Seattle: NCAST Publications, University of Washington School of Nursing.)

EVELYN ADAM

Conceptual Model for Nursing

Evelyn Adam is a Canadian nurse who started publishing in the mid-1970s. Her work focuses on the development of models and theories on the concept of nursing (1983, 1987, 1999). She uses a model that she learned from Dorothy Johnson. In her book, *To Be a Nurse* (1980), she applies Virginia Henderson's definition of nursing to Johnson's model and identifies the assumptions, beliefs, and values, as well as major units. In the latter category, Adam includes the goal of the profession, the beneficiary of the professional service, the role of the professional, the source of the beneficiary's difficulty, the intervention of the professional, and the consequences. She expanded her work in a 1991 second edition. Her classic paper titled simply "Modèles conceptuels" argues their importance in shaping a way of thinking and providing a framework for practice (Adam, 1999). Adam's work is a good example of using a unique basis of nursing for further expansion. Adam's argument for an ideological framework in nursing was described in a health telematics education conference (Tallberg, 1997). She contributed to theory development with clear explanation and use of earlier works. Adam's work is a theory of nursing.

NANCY ROPER, WINIFRED W. LOGAN, AND ALISON J. TIERNEY

A Model for Nursing Based on a Model of Living

Nancy Roper is described as a practical theorist who produced a simple nursing theory, "which actually helped bedside nurses" (Dopson, 2004; Scott, 2004, p. 28). After 15 years as a principal tutor in a school of nursing in England, Roper began her career as a full-time book writer during the 1960s and published several popular textbooks, including *Principles of Nursing* (1967). She investigated the concept of an identifiable "core" of nursing for her MPhil research study, published in a monograph titled *Clinical Experience in Nurse Education* (1976). This work served as the basis for her work with theorists Winifred Logan and Alison Tierney. Roper worked with the European and Nursing and Midwifery Unit, where she was influential in developing European Standards for Nursing (Hallett & Wagner, 2011; Roper, 1977). She authored *The Elements of Nursing* in 1980, 1985, and 1990. The trio collaborated in the fourth and most recent edition of *The Elements of Nursing: A Model for Nursing Based on a Model of Living* (1996). During the 1970s, they conducted research to discover the core of nursing, based on a Model of Living (Fig. 2.9). Three decades of study of the elements of nursing by Roper evolved into a model for nursing with five main factors that influenced activities of living (ALs) (Fig. 2.10 and Table 2.1).

Rather than revising the fourth edition of their textbook, these theorists prepared a monograph (Roper, Logan, & Tierney, 2000) about the model titled *The Roper-Logan-Tierney Model of Nursing: Based on Activities of Living,* without application of the model. Holland, Jenkins, Solomon, and Whittam (2008) explored the use of the Roper-Logan-Tierney Model of Nursing. They used case studies and exercises about adult patients with a variety of health problems in acute care and community-based settings to help students develop problem-solving skills.

In the Model of Nursing, the ALs include maintaining a safe environment, communicating, breathing, eating and drinking, eliminating, personal cleansing and dressing, controlling body temperature, mobilizing, working and playing, expressing sexuality, sleeping, and dying. Life span ranges from birth to death, and the dependence-independence continuum ranges from total dependence to total independence. The five groups of factors that influence the ALs are biological, psychological, sociocultural, environmental, and politicoeconomic. Individuality of living is the way in which the individual attends to the ALs in regard to the individual's place in the life span; on the dependence-independence continuum; and as influenced by biological, psychological, sociocultural, environmental,

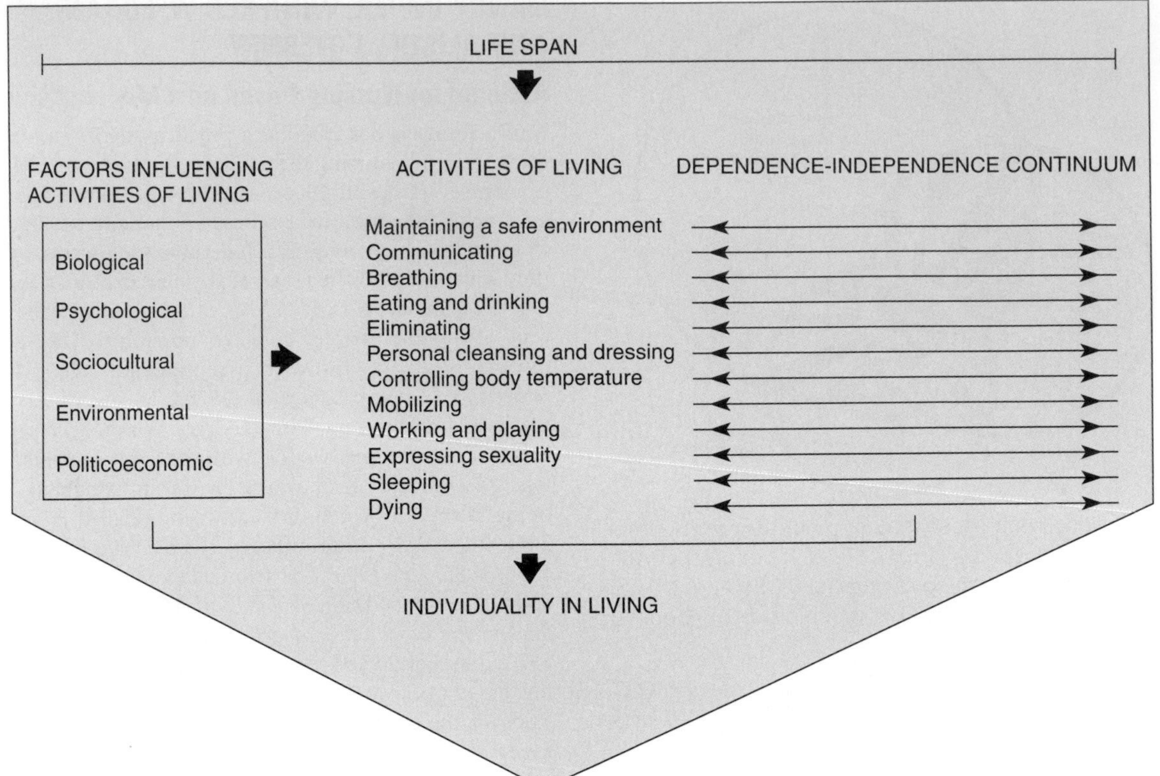

FIG 2.9 Diagram of the model of living. (From Roper, N., Logan W. W., & Tierney, A. J. [1996]. *The elements of nursing: A model for nursing based on a model of living* [4th ed., p. 20]. Edinburgh: Churchill Livingstone.)

and politicoeconomic factors. The five components can be used to describe the individual in relation to maintaining health, preventing disease, coping during periods of sickness and rehabilitation, coping positively during periods of chronic ill health, and coping when dying. Individualizing nursing is accomplished by using the process of nursing, which involves four phases: (1) assessing, (2) planning, (3) implementing, and (4) evaluating. Nursing process is a method of logical thinking that should be used with an explicit nursing model, and the patient's individuality in living must be borne in mind during all four phases of the process. The Roper, Logan, and Tierney Model was applied on the management of thalamic hemorrhage in the critical care setting (Chan, 2015) and to plan nursing care for patients receiving mechanical ventilation in complex neurological settings (Venkatesaperumal et al., 2013) and to set out terms to be used in diagnosis/outcomes statements and in nursing interventions for senior patients (de Medeiros & da Nóbrega, 2013). This model has been used as a guide for nursing practice, research, and education.

IDA JEAN (ORLANDO) PELLETIER

Nursing Process Theory

Ida Jean Orlando developed her theory from a study conducted at the Yale University School of Nursing, integrating mental health concepts into a basic nursing curriculum. The study was carried out by observing and participating in experiences with patients, students, nurses, and instructors and was derived inductively from field notes for this study. Orlando analyzed the content of 2000 nurse-patient contacts and created her theory based on analysis of these data (Schmieding, 1993). Meleis (2012) has noted, "Orlando was one of the early thinkers in nursing who proposed that patients have their own meanings and interpretations of situations and therefore nurses must validate their inferences and analyses with patients before drawing conclusions" (p. 243). The theory was published in *The Dynamic Nurse-Patient Relationship* (Orlando, 1961), which was an outcome of the project. Her book purposed a contribution to concerns about the nurse-patient relationship,

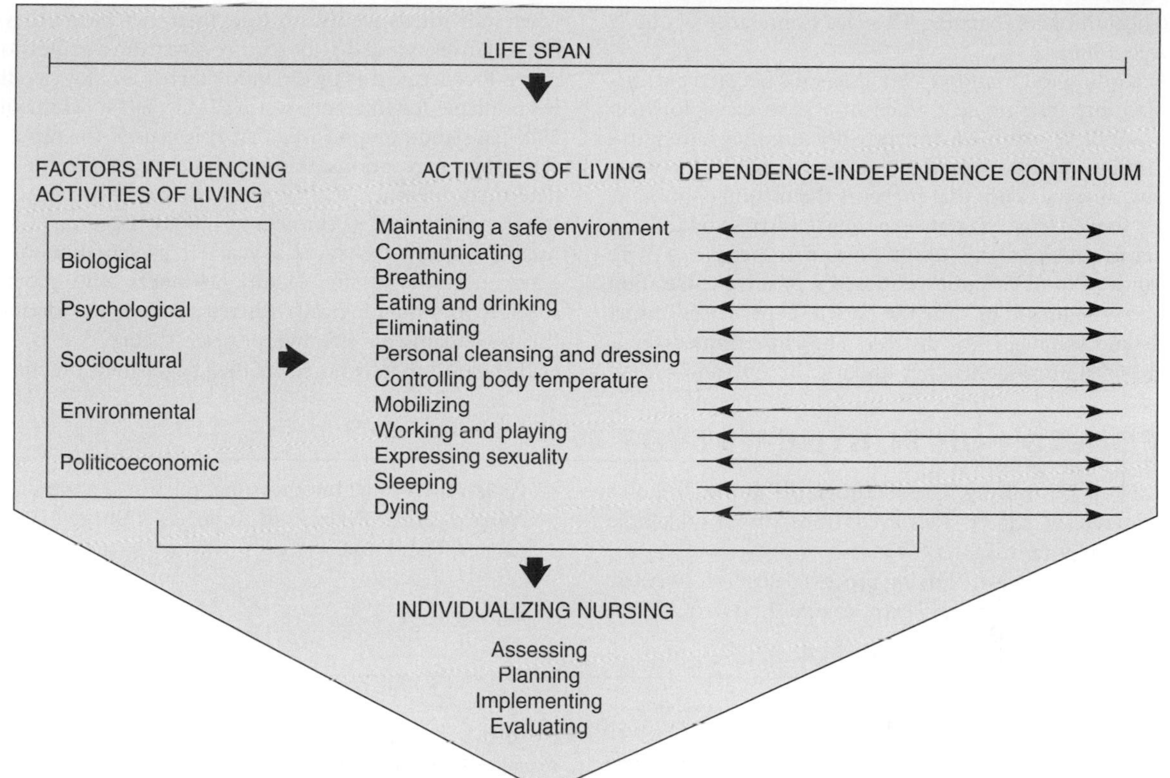

FIG 2.10 Diagram of the model for nursing. (From Roper, N., Logan, W. W., & Tierney, A. J. [1996]. *The elements of nursing: A model for nursing based on a model of living* [4th ed., p. 34]. Edinburgh: Churchill Livingstone.)

TABLE 2.1 Comparison of Main Concepts in the Model of Living and Model for Nursing

Model of Living	Model for Nursing
12 ALs	12 ALs
Life span	Life span
Dependence-independence continuum	Dependence-independence continuum
Factors influencing the ALs	Factors influencing the ALs
Individuality in living	Individualizing nursing

From Roper, N., Logan, W. W., & Tierney, A. J. (1996). *The elements of nursing: A model for nursing based on a model of living* (4th ed., p. 33). Edinburgh: Churchill Livingstone.
AL, Activities of living.

the nurse's professional role and identity, and the knowledge development distinct to nursing (Schmieding, 1993). In 1990 the National League for Nursing (NLN) reprinted Orlando's 1961 publication. In the preface to the NLN edition, Orlando states: "If I had been more courageous in 1961, when this book was first written, I would have proposed it as 'nursing process theory' instead of as a 'theory of effective nursing practice'" (Orlando, 1990, p. vii). Orlando (1972) continued to develop and refine her work, and in her second book, *The Discipline and Teaching of Nursing Process: An Evaluative Study*, she redefined and renamed deliberative nursing process as nursing process discipline.

Orlando's nursing theory stresses the reciprocal relationship between patient and nurse. What the nurse and the patient say and do affects them both. Orlando (1961) views the professional function of nursing as finding out and meeting the patient's immediate need for help. She was one of the first nursing leaders to identify and emphasize the elements of nursing process and the critical importance of the patient's participation in the nursing process. Orlando's theory focuses on how to produce improvement in the patient's behavior. Evidence of relieving the patient's distress is seen as positive changes in the patient's observable behavior. Orlando may have facilitated the development of nurses as logical thinkers (Nursing Theories Conference Group & George, 1980).

According to Orlando (1961), persons become patients who require nursing care when they have needs for help that cannot be met independently because they have physical limitations, have negative reactions to an environment, or have an experience that prevents them from communicating their needs. Patients experience distress or feelings of helplessness as the result of unmet needs for help (Orlando, 1961). Orlando proposed a positive correlation between the length of time the patient experiences unmet needs and the degree of distress. Therefore immediacy is emphasized throughout her theory. In Orlando's view, when individuals are able to meet their own needs, they do not feel distress and do not require care from a professional nurse. Practice guided by Orlando's theory employs a reflexive principle for inference testing (May, 2014; Schmieding, 2006). Orlando emphasizes that it is crucial for nurses to share their perceptions, thoughts, and feelings so they can determine whether their inferences are congruent with the patient's need (Schmieding, 2006). Boschini (2015) used Orlando's theory as a visual representation of the experiences of nursing faculty members who provided support to psychologically distressed students. Orlando's theory remains an effective practice theory that is especially helpful to new nurses as they begin their practice.

POINTS FOR FURTHER STUDY

- Kaplan, D., & King, C. (2000). *Guide to the Ernestine Wiedenbach papers.* Retrieved from http://hdl.handle.net/10079/fa/mssa.ms.1647.
- Orlando interview: Nursing process discipline. In *Nurse theorists: Portraits of excellence,* Volume 1 (video). Athens, OH: Fitne.
- Peplau Interview: Interpersonal relations in nursing. In *Nurse theorists: Portraits of excellence,* Volume 1 (video). Athens, OH: Fitne.

REFERENCES

Abdellah, F. G. (2004). Interview with Rear Admiral Faye Glenn Abdellah. Interview by Captain Melvin Lessing. *Military Medicine, 169*(11), iii–xi.

Abdellah, F. G., Beland, I. L., Martin, A., & Matheney, R. V. (1960). *Patient-centered approaches to nursing.* New York: Macmillan.

Abdellah, F. G., & Levine, E. (1994). *Preparing for nursing research in the 21st century: Evolution, methodologies, challenges.* New York: Springer.

Adam, E. (1980). *To be a nurse.* Philadelphia: Saunders.

Adam, E. (1983). Frontiers of nursing in the 21st century: Development of models and theories on the concept of nursing. *Journal of Advanced Nursing, 8,* 41–45.

Adam, E. (1987). Nursing theory: What it is and what it is not. Nursing papers. *Perspectives in Nursing, 19,* 5–14.

Adam, E. (1991). *To be a nurse* (2nd ed.). Montreal: Saunders.

Adam, E. (1999). Conceptual models. *Canadian Journal of Nursing Research, 30,* 103–114.

Amakali, K., & Small, L. F. (2014). Beyond routine care for children with heart diseases from the vulnerable context: A clinical practice perspective. *Journal of Nursing Education and Practice, 4,* 43–49.

American Nurses Association. (June 14, 2012). *Six registered nurses to be inducted into ANA hall of fame for lifetime of contributions to nursing.* Retrieved April 16, 2016 from http://nursingworld.org/FunctionalMenuCategories/MediaResources/PressReleases/ANAHallofFamePR-June2012.pdf.

Arungwa, O. T. (2014). The relevance of continuing education among nurses in national orthopaedic hospital, Igbobi, Lagos. *West African Journal of Nursing, 25*(2), 63–74.

Banks, J. (2015). Identifying risk factors for high incidence of peripheral intravenous catheters complications: Reducing infiltration rate within the hospital. *Walden University Scholar Works.* Walden University: Walden Dissertations and Doctoral Studies.

Barnard, K. E. (1978). *Nursing child assessment and training: Learning resource manual.* Seattle: University of Washington.

Barnard, K. E. (2004). *Welcome and Opening Plenary. Proceedings from AMCHP '04: Mental health—Promoting a new paradigm for MCH public health practice.* Retrieved from http://128.248.232.90/archives/mchb/amchp2004/p1/transcripts/session09f.htm.

Bixler, G. K., & Bixler, R. W. (1959). The professional status of nursing. *American Journal of Nursing, 59*(8), 1142–1146.

Boschini, D. J. (2015). *Nursing faculty experiences with providing support to psychologically distressed students: A phenomenological approach* (Doctoral dissertation, California State University, Fresno).

Bulson, J. A., & Bulson, T. (2011). Nursing process and critical thinking linked to disaster preparedness. *Journal of Emergency Nursing, 37,* 477–483.

Bunkers, S. S. (2012). Presence: The eye of the needle. *Nursing Science Quarterly, 25,* 10–14.

Butts, J. B., & Rich, K. L. (2015). *Philosophies and theories for advanced nursing practice* (2nd ed.). Burlington, MA: Jones & Bartlett Learning.

Chan, C. (2015). Applying the Roper, Logan and Tierney Model on the management of thalamic haemorrhage in the critical care setting: A case study. *Singapore Nursing Journal, 42*, 22–28.

Cherian, S., & Karkada, S. (2015). Effect of education related to oral care practices on nurses' knowledge, practice and clinical outcomes of mechanically ventilated patients in Dubai. *International Journal of Nursing Research and Practice, 2*, 9–14.

Clares, J. W. B., de Freitas, M. C., & Borges, C. L. (2014). Social and clinical factors causing mobility limitations in the elderly. *Acta Paulista de Enfermagem, 27*, 237–242.

Corrigan, C., Kwasky, A., & Groh, C. (2015). Social support, postpartum depression and professional assistance: A survey of mothers in the midwestern United States. *The Journal of Perinatal Education, 24*, 48–60.

de Medeiros, A. T., & da Nóbrega, M. L. (2013). Terminological subsets of the International Classification for Nursing Practice—ICNPA® for senior patients: A methodological study. *Online Brazilian Journal of Nursing, 12*, 590–592.

Deane, W. H., & Fain, J. A. (2016). Incorporating Peplau's Theory of Interpersonal Relations to promote holistic communication between older adults and nursing students. *Journal of Holistic Nursing, 34*, 35–41.

Degavi, G., & Bjupali, P. (2015). Knowledge regarding cardiac rehabilitation among staff nurses. *Asian Journal of Nursing Education and Research, 5*, 87–93.

Dickoff, J., James, P., & Wiedenbach, E. (1968a). Theory in a practice discipline, part I: Practice oriented research. *Nursing Research, 17*, 415–444.

Dickoff, J., James, P., & Wiedenbach, E. (1968b). Theory in a practice discipline, part II: Practice oriented research. *Nursing Research, 17*, 545–554.

Dijkstra, A., Yönt, G. H., Korhan, E. A., Muszalik, M., Kedziora-Kornatowska, K., & Suzuki, M. (2012). The care dependency scale for measuring basic human needs: An international comparison. *Journal of Advanced Nursing, 68*, 2341–2348.

Dopson, L. (October 15, 2004). Obituary: Nancy Roper. *The Independent.* Retrieved from http://www.independent.co.uk.

Doss, J. (2014). Effectiveness of foot massage on level of pain among patients with cancer. *Asian Journal of Nursing Education & Research, 4*, 228–231.

Doyle, C., & Buckley, S. (2012). An account of nursing a child with complex needs in the home. *Nursing Children and Young People, 24*, 19–22.

Draucker, C. B., Cook, C. B., Martsolf, D. S., & Stephenson, P. S. (2012). Adolescent dating violence and Peplau's dimensions of the self. *Journal of the American Psychiatric Nurses Association, 18*, 175–188.

Ervin, S. (2015). History of nursing education in the United States. In Sarah B. Keating (Ed.), *Curriculum development & evaluation* (3rd ed., pp. 5–32). New York: Springer Publishing Company.

Falk, K. J. (2014). Appreciative inquiry with nurses who work with children of incarcerated parents. *Nursing Science Quarterly, 27*(4), 315–323.

Frankel, V. (1963). *Man's search for meaning: An introduction to logotherapy*. New York: Washington Square Press.

Guo, Y., Leu, S.-Y., Barnard, K. E., Thompson, E. A., & Spieker, S. J. (2015). An examination of changes in emotion co-regulation among mother and child dyads during the strange situation. *Infant and Child Development, 24*, 256–273.

Haber, J. (2000). Hildegard E. Peplau: The psychiatric nursing legacy of a legend. *Journal of the American Psychiatric Nurses Association, 6*, 56–62.

Hall, L. E. (1964). Nursing: What is it? *The Canadian Nurse, 60*, 150–154.

Hall, L. E. (1969). The Loeb Center for Nursing and Rehabilitation. *International Journal of Nursing Studies, 6*, 81–95.

Hall, L. E., Alfano, G. J., Rifkin E., & Levine, H. S. (1975). *Longitudinal effects of an experimental nursing process (final report).* New York: Loeb Center for Nursing and Rehabilitation.

Hallett, D. C., & Wagner, L. (2011). Promoting the health of Europeans in a rapidly changing world: A historical study of the implementation of World Health Organization policies by the nursing and midwifery unit, European regional office, 1970–2003. *Nursing Inquiry, 18*, 359–368.

Henderson, V. (1955). *Textbook of the principles and practice of nursing* (5th ed.). New York: Macmillan.

Henderson, V. (1960). *Basic principles of nursing care*. London: International Council of Nurses.

Henderson, V. (1964). The nature of nursing. *American Journal of Nursing, 64*, 62–68.

Henderson, V. (1966). *The nature of nursing: A definition and its implications for practice, research, and education*. New York: Macmillan.

Henderson V. (1980). Preserving the essence of nursing in a technological age. *Journal of Advanced Nursing, 5*, 245–260.

Henderson, V. A. (1991). *The nature of nursing: Reflections after 25 years*. New York: National League for Nursing Press.

Henderson, V. (2006). The concept of nursing. *Journal of Advanced Nursing, 53*, 21–31.

Holland, K., Jenkins, J., Solomon, J., & Whittam, S. (2008). *Applying the Roper-Logan-Tierney Model in practice* (2nd ed.). Edinburgh: Churchill Livingstone Elsevier Health Sciences.

Hungerford, C., Prosser, B., & Davey, R. (2015). The key role of nurse researchers in the evaluation of nurse practitioner models of practice. *Research and Theory for Nursing Practice, 29*, 214–225.

Kaplan, D., & King, C. (2000). *Guide to the Ernestine Wiedenbach papers*. Retrieved from http://hdl.handle.net/10079/fa/mssa.ms.1647.

Kelly, J. F., & Barnard, K. E. (2000). Assessment of parent-child interaction: implications for early intervention. In S. Shonkoff & S. J. Meisels (Eds.), *Handbook of early childhood intervention* (pp. 258–289). Cambridge: Cambridge University Press.

Kouta, C., Kaite, C. P., Papadopoulos, I., & Phellas, C. N. (2015). Evaluation of home care nursing for elderly people in Cyprus. *International Journal of Caring Sciences, 8*(2), 376–384.

Liebel, D. V., Powers, B. A., & Hauenstein, E. J. (2015). Home health care nurse interactions with homebound geriatric patients with depression and disability. *Research in Gerontological Nursing, 8*(3), 130–139.

Martina, H., Beulah, H., & David, A. (2015). Effectiveness of massage therapy on respiratory status among toddlers with lower respiratory tract infections. *Nitte University Journal of Health Science, 5*, 49–54.

Masters, K. (2015). *Nursing theories: A framework for professional practice*. Burlington, MA: Jones & Bartlett Learning.

May, B. A. (2014). Orlando's nursing process theory and nursing practice. In M. R. Alligood (Ed.), *Nursing theory: Utilization & application* (5th ed., pp. 285–302). St Louis: Mosby-Elsevier.

May, R. (1953). *Man's search for himself*. New York: W. W. Norton.

McCoy, M. L., Davidhizar, R., & Gillum, D. R. (2007). A correlational pilot study of home health nurse management of heart failure patients and hospital readmissions. *Home Health Care Management and Practice, 19*, 392–396.

Meleis, A. (2012). *Theoretical nursing: Development and progress* (5th ed.). Philadelphia: Wolters Kluwer Health, Lippincott Williams & Wilkins.

National Library of Medicine. (1988). *Finding aid to the Faye Glenn Abdellah papers, 1952–1989*. (NIH Collection No. MS C 424). Bethesda, MD: National Library of Medicine. Retrieved from http://www.nlm.nih.gov/hmd/manuscripts/ead/abdellah.html.

Nicely, B., & DeLario, G. T. (2011). Virginia Henderson's principles and practice of nursing applied to organ donation after brain death. *Progress in Transplantation, 21*, 72–77.

Nursing Theories Conference Group & George, J. B. (Chairperson). (1980). *Nursing theories: The base for professional practice*. Englewood Cliffs, NJ: Prentice-Hall.

Orlando, I. J. (1961). *The dynamic nurse-patient relationship: Function, process and principles of professional nursing practice*. New York: Putnam.

Orlando, I. J. (1972). *The discipline and teaching of nursing process: An evaluative study*. New York: Putnam.

Orlando, I. J. (1990). *The dynamic nurse-patient relationship: Function, process, and principles* (Pub. No. 15-2341). New York: National League for Nursing.

Peplau, H. E. (1952). *Interpersonal relations in nursing*. New York: Putnam.

Pettersson, M., Hedström, M., & Höglund, A. T. (2014). Striving for good nursing care: Nurses' experiences of do not resuscitate orders within oncology and hematology care. *Nursing Ethics, 21*(8), 902–915.

Rich, K. (2003). Revisiting Joyce Travelbee's question: What's wrong with sympathy? *Journal of the American Psychiatric Association, 9*(6), 202–205.

Roper, N. (1967). *Principles of nursing*. Edinburgh: Churchill Livingstone.

Roper, N. (1976). *Clinical experience in nurse education* (Research monograph). Edinburgh: Churchill Livingstone.

Roper, N. (1977). *Paper (and working documents) on the assessment of patient/client needs for nursing care*. NMU Archive Box 2, Kolding, Denmark.

Roper, N. (1985). *The elements of nursing: A model for nursing* (2nd ed.). Edinburgh: Churchill Livingstone.

Roper, N. (1990). *The elements of nursing: A model for nursing based on a model of living* (3rd ed.). Edinburgh: Churchill Livingstone.

Roper, N., Logan, W. W., & Tierney, A. J. (1996). *The elements of nursing: A model for nursing based on a model of living* (4th ed.). Edinburgh: Churchill Livingstone.

Roper, N., Logan, W. W., & Tierney, A. J. (2000). *The Roper-Logan-Tierney model of nursing: Based on activities of living*. Edinburgh: Churchill Livingstone.

Schmieding, N. J. (1993). *Ida Jean Orlando: A nursing process theory*. Newbury Park, CA: Sage Publications.

Schmieding, N. J. (2006). Ida Jean Orlando (Pelletier): Nursing process theory. In A. M. Tomey & M. R. Alligood (Eds.), *Nursing theorists and their work* (6th ed., pp. 431–451). St Louis: Mosby.

Scott, H. (2004). Nancy Roper (1918–2004): A great Nursing pioneer. *British Journal of Nursing, 19*, 1121.

Searl, K. R., McAllister, M., Dwyer, T., Krebs, K. L., Anderson, C., Quinney, L., & McLellan, S. (2014). Little people, big lessons: An innovative strategy to develop interpersonal skills in undergraduate nursing students. *Nurse Education Today, 34*, 1201–1206.

Senn, J. F. (2013). Peplau's theory of interpersonal relations: Application in emergency and rural nursing. *Nursing Science Quarterly, 26*, 31–35.

Sills, G. M. (1998). Peplau and professionalism: The emergence of the paradigm of professionalization. *Journal of Psychiatric and Mental Health Nursing, 5*, 167–171.

Tallberg, M. (1997). Supporting the nursing process—an aim for education in nursing informatics. In J. Mantas (Ed.), *Health telematics education: Studies in health technology and informatics*, vol 41 (pp. 291–296). Amsterdam: IOS Press.

Timmins, F. (2011). Remembering the art of nursing in a technological age. *Nursing in Critical Care, 16*, 161–163.

Touhy, T. A., & Birnbach, N. (2001). Lydia Hall: The care, core, cure model. In M. E. Parker (Ed.), *Nursing theories and nursing practice* (pp. 135–137). Philadelphia: F. A. Davis.

Towell, A., Nel, W., & Muller, A. (2015). Model of facilitation of emotional intelligence to promote wholeness in neophyte critical care nurses in South Africa. *Health SA Gesondheid, 20*, 1–10.

Travelbee, J. (1963). What do we mean by rapport? *American Journal of Nursing, 63*, 70–72.

Travelbee, J. (1964). What's wrong with sympathy? *American Journal of Nursing, 64*, 68–71.

Travelbee, J. (1966). *Interpersonal aspects of nursing*. Philadelphia: F. A. Davis.

Travelbee, J. (1971). *Interpersonal aspects of nursing* (2nd ed.). Philadelphia: F. A. Davis.

Trevizan, M. A., Almeida, R. G. D. S., Souza, M. C., Mazzo, A., Mendes, I. A. C., & Martins, J. C. A. (2015). Empathy in Brazilian nursing professionals: A descriptive study. *Nursing Ethics, 22*, 367–376.

Trygstad, L. N., Buccheri, R. K., Buffum, M. D., Ju, D., & Dowling, G. A. (2015). Auditory hallucinations interview guide: Promoting recovery with an interactive assessment tool. *Journal of Psychosocial Nursing & Mental Health Services, 53*, 20–28.

Tsai, S. Y., Barnard, K. E., Lentz, M. J., & Thomas, K. A. (2011). Mother-infant activity synchrony as a correlate of the emergence of circadian rhythm. *Biological Research for Nursing, 1*, 80–88.

Tsai, S., Thomas, K. A., Lentz, M. J., & Barnard, K. E. (2012). Light is beneficial for infant circadian entrainment: An actigraphic study. *Journal of Advanced Nursing, 68*, 1738–1747.

Venkatesaperumal, R., D'Souza, M. S., Balachandran, S., & Radhakrishnan, J. (2013). Role of a nurse in noninvasive positive pressure ventilation: A conceptual model for clinical practice. *International Journal of Nursing Education, 5*, 119–123.

Washington, G. T. (2013). The theory of interpersonal relations applied to the preceptor-new graduate relationship. *Journal for Nurses in Professional Development, 29*, 24–29.

The Washington Nurse. (July 2, 2015). UW nursing prof Kathryn Barnard, pioneer for babies, dies at 77. *The Seattle Times.*

Wiedenbach, E. (1964). *Clinical nursing: A helping art.* New York: Springer.

Wiedenbach, E. (1970). Nurses' wisdom in nursing theory. *American Journal of Nursing, 70*, 1057–1062.

Wiggins, R. L. (1980). Lydia Hall's place in the development of theory of nursing. *Image: Journal of Nursing Scholarship, 12*, 10–12.

Wolf, K. A. (2006). Advancing the profession. In L. C. Andrist, P. K. Nicholas, & K. A. Wolf (Eds.), *A history of nursing ideas* (pp. 301–304). Sudbury, MA: Jones & Bartlett.

3

History of Nursing Science

Sonya R. Hardin

"Philosophy in its broadest sense is wondering and being curious about the 'big' or fundamental questions that humans have grappled with throughout history. Questions about 'what is real?' (ontology), 'what is knowable?' (epistemology), 'is this just?' (ethics), and 'is there an art to caring?' (aesthetics) are considered indispensable reflections in nursing practice."

(Bruce, Rietze, & Lim, 2014, p. 65)

Why is science important? Science is a method for describing, explaining, and predicting causes or outcomes of interventions. Scientific activity has helped to establish the evidence we use to guide practice in the delivery of nursing care. We desire to understand the unknown and identify the cause, the effect, and the significant difference that an intervention can make to increase the longevity of life (Bronowski, 1979; Gale, 1979; Piaget, 1970). Since the 1960s, nursing leaders have strategized to be considered a scientific discipline. Being a scientific discipline means identifying nursing's unique knowledge for the care of patients, families, and communities. It means that nurses can conduct clinical and basic nursing research to establish the scientific base for the care of individuals, families, communities, and populations. Recent research, for example, revealed that extubation success in preterm infants who were younger than 28 weeks' gestational age was associated with greater gestational age and lower preextubation partial pressure carbon dioxide (Pco_2). Furthermore, extubation failure was associated with death; bronchopulmonary dysplasia; severe retinopathy of prematurity; patent ductus arteriosus ligation; and longer durations of respiratory support, oxygen supplementation, and hospitalization. Other items studied that did not influence the success of extubation were preextubation fraction of inspired oxygen (Fio_2), age at extubation, and birth weight. Infants with extubation failure were more likely to die (Manley et al., 2016). This study is just one example of nursing science; nurses should be familiar with the long history of the science of nursing.

HISTORICAL VIEWS OF THE NATURE OF SCIENCE

To formalize the science of nursing, basic questions must be considered, such as: What is science, knowledge, and truth? What methods produce scientific knowledge? The answers to these questions are influenced by one's philosophy. The particular philosophical perspective selected to answer these questions will influence how researchers perform scientific activities, how they interpret outcomes, and even what they regard as science and knowledge (Brown, 1977; Foucault, 1973).

Two competing philosophical perspectives used in science are rationalism and empiricism. Each is a type of **epistemology** that is a theory of knowledge for understanding how to uncover the answer to a question. Gale (1979) labeled these alternative epistemologies as centrally concerned with the power of reason and the power of sensory experience. Gale noted similarity in the divergent views of science in the time of the classical Greeks. For example, Aristotle believed that advances in biological science would develop through systematic observation of objects and events in the natural world, whereas Pythagoras believed that knowledge of the natural world would develop from mathematical reasoning (Brown, 1977; Gale, 1979).

Nursing science has been characterized by two branching philosophies of knowledge as the discipline developed. Various terms are used to describe these two stances: (1) **empiricist, mechanistic, quantitative,** and **deductive** or (2) **interpretive, holistic, qualitative,** and **inductive** forms of science. Understanding the nature of these different philosophical stances facilitates appreciation for what each form contributes to nursing knowledge.

Rationalism

Rationalist epistemology (scope of knowledge) emphasizes the importance of *a priori* reasoning as the appropriate method for advancing knowledge. A priori reasoning uses deductive logic by reasoning from the cause to an effect or from a generalization to a particular instance. An example in nursing is to reason that a lack of social support (cause) results in hospital readmission (effect). This causal reasoning is a theoretical assertion until tested and disproven. The traditional approach proceeds by explaining hospitalization with a systematic explanation (theory) of a given phenomenon (Gale, 1979). Theoretical assertions derived by deductive reasoning are then subjected to experimental testing to corroborate the theory. Reynolds (1971) labeled this approach the **theory-then-research strategy.** If the research findings fail to correspond with the theoretical assertions, additional research is conducted or modifications are made in the theory and further tests are devised; otherwise, the theory is discarded in favor of an alternative explanation (Gale, 1979; Zetterberg, 1966). Popper (1962) argued that science would evolve more rapidly through devising research in an attempt to refute new ideas. For example, his point is simple; you can never prove that all individuals without social support have frequent rehospitalizations, because there might be one individual who presents with no rehospitalization. A single person with no social support that does not have a readmission disproves the theory that *all* individuals with a lack of social support have hospital readmissions. From Popper's perspective, "research consists of generating general hypotheses and then attempting to refute them" (Lipton, 2005, p. 1263). Thus the hypothesis that a lack of social support results in hospital readmission would be the topic of interest to be refuted.

The rationalist view is most clearly evident in the work of Einstein, the theoretical physicist, who made extensive use of mathematical equations in developing his theories. The theories Einstein constructed offered an imaginative framework, which has directed research in numerous areas (Calder, 1979). As Reynolds (1971) noted, if someone believes that science is a process of inventing descriptions of phenomena, the appropriate strategy for theory construction is the theory-then-research strategy. In Reynolds' view, "as the continuous interplay between theory construction (invention) and testing with empirical research progresses, the theory becomes more precise and complete as a description of nature and, therefore, more useful for the goals of science" (Reynolds, 1971, p. 145).

Empiricism

The empiricist view is based on the central idea that scientific knowledge can be derived only from sensory experience (i.e., seeing, feeling, hearing facts). Francis Bacon (Gale, 1979) received credit for popularizing the basis for the empiricist approach to inquiry. Bacon believed that scientific truth was discovered through generalizing observed facts in the natural world. This approach, called the **inductive method,** is based on the idea that the collection of facts precedes attempts to formulate generalizations, or as Reynolds (1971) called it, the **research-then-theory strategy.** One of the best examples to demonstrate this form of logic in nursing has to do with formulating differential diagnoses. Formulating a differential diagnosis requires collecting the facts and then devising a list of possible theories to explain the facts.

The strict empiricist view is reflected in the work of the behaviorist Skinner. In a 1950 paper, Skinner asserted that advances in the science of psychology could be expected if scientists would focus on the collection of empirical data. He cautioned against drawing premature inferences and proposed a moratorium on theory building until further facts were collected. Skinner's (1950) approach to theory construction was clearly inductive. His view of science and the popularity of behaviorism have been credited with influencing psychology's shift in emphasis from the building of theories to the gathering of facts between the 1950s and 1970s (Snelbecker, 1974). The difficulty with the inductive mode of inquiry is that the world presents an infinite number of possible observations, and, therefore, scientists bring their own ideas to their experiences to decide what to observe and what to exclude (Steiner, 1977). With induction it is important not to end the observations too soon and arrive at a premature conclusion that is faulty.

In summary, deductive inquiry uses the theory-then-research approach, and inductive inquiry uses the research-then-theory approach. Both approaches are used in the field of nursing.

EARLY 20TH CENTURY VIEWS OF SCIENCE AND THEORY

During the first half of the 20th century, **philosophers** focused on the analysis of theory structure, whereas **scientists** focused on empirical research (Brown, 1977). There was minimal interest in the history of science, the nature of scientific discovery, or the similarities between the philosophical view of science and the scientific methods (Brown, 1977). **Positivism,** a term first used by Comte, emerged as the dominant view of modern science (Gale, 1979). Modern logical positivists believed that empirical research and logical analysis (deductive and inductive) were two approaches that would produce scientific knowledge (Brown, 1977).

The logical empiricists offered a more lenient view of logical positivism and argued that theoretical propositions (propositions that affirm or deny something) must be tested through observation and experimentation (Brown, 1977). This perspective is rooted in the idea that empirical facts exist independently of theories and offer the only basis for objectivity in science (Brown, 1977). In this view, objective truth exists independently of the researcher, and the task of science is to discover it, which is an inductive method (Gale, 1979). This view of science is often presented in research method courses as: "The scientist first sets up an experiment; observes what occurs . . . reaches a preliminary hypothesis to describe the occurrence; runs further experiments to test the hypothesis [and] finally corrects or modifies the hypothesis in light of the results" (Gale, 1979, p. 13).

The increasing use of computers, which permit the analysis of large data sets, may have contributed to the acceptance of the positivist approach to modern science (Snelbecker, 1974). However, in the 1950s, the literature began to reflect an increasing challenge to the positivist view, thereby ushering in a new view of science in the late 20th century (Brown, 1977).

EMERGENT VIEWS OF SCIENCE AND THEORY IN THE LATE 20TH CENTURY

In the latter years of the 20th century, several authors presented analyses challenging the positivist position, thus offering the basis for a new perspective of science (Brown, 1977; Foucault, 1973; Hanson, 1958; Kuhn, 1962; Toulmin, 1961). Foucault (1973) published his analysis of the **epistemology** (knowledge) of human sciences from the 17th to the 19th centuries. His major thesis stated that empirical knowledge was arranged in different patterns at a given time and in a given culture and that humans were emerging as objects of study.

In 1977, Brown argued for an intellectual revolution in philosophy that emphasized the history of science was replacing formal logic as the major analytical tool in the philosophy of science. One of the major perspectives in the new philosophy emphasized that science was a process of continuously building research rather than a product of findings. In this emergent epistemology, emphasis shifted to understanding scientific discovery and process as theories change over time.

Empiricists view phenomena objectively, collect data, and analyze it to inductively propose theory (Brown, 1977). This position is based upon objective truth existing in the world, waiting to be discovered. Brown (1977) set forth a new epistemology challenging the empiricist view, proposing that theories play a significant role in determining what the scientist observes and how it is interpreted. The following story (created by the author) illustrates Brown's premise that observations are concept laden; that is, an observation is influenced by the values and ideas in the mind of the observer:

> *"An elderly patient has been in a trauma and appears to be crying. The nurse on admission observes that the patient has marks on her body and believes that she has been abused; the orthopedist has viewed an x-ray and believes that the crying patient is in pain due to a fractured femur that will not require surgery only a closed reduction; the chaplain observes the patient crying and believes the patient needs spiritual support. Each observation is concept laden."*

Brown (1977) presented the example of a chemist and a child walking together past a steel mill. The chemist perceived the odor of sulfur dioxide and the child smelled rotten eggs. Both observers in the examples responded to the same observation but with distinctly different interpretations. Concepts and theories set up boundaries and specify pertinent phenomena for reasoning about specific observed patterns. These examples represent different ideas that emerge for each person.

If scientists perceive patterns in the empirical world based on their presupposed theories, how can new patterns ever be perceived or new discoveries become formulated? Gale (1979) answered by proposing that the scientist is able to perceive forceful intrusions from the environment that challenge his or her *a priori* mental set, thereby raising questions regarding the current theoretical perspective. Brown (1977) maintained that a presupposed theoretical framework influences perception; however, theories are not the single determining factor of the scientist's perception. He identified the following three different views of the relationship between theories and observation:

1. Scientists are merely passive observers of occurrences in the empirical world. Observable data are objective truth waiting to be discovered.
2. Theories structure what the scientist perceives in the empirical world.
3. Presupposed theories and observable data interact in the process of scientific investigation. (Brown, 1977, p. 298)

Brown's argument for an interactionist's perspective coincides with the scientific consensus in the study of pattern recognition in how humans process information. The following distinct minitheories have directed research efforts in this area: (1) the data-driven, or bottom-up, theory and (2) the conceptually driven, or top-down, theory (Norman, 1976). In the former, cognitive expectations (what is known or ways of organizing meaning) are used to select input and process incoming information from the environment. The second, top-down theory, asserts that incoming data are perceived as unlabeled input and analyzed as raw data with increasing levels of complexity until all the data are classified. Current research evidence suggests that human pattern recognition progresses through the interaction of both data-driven and conceptually driven processes, and uses sources of information in currently organized, cognitive categories as well as stimuli from the sensory environment. The interactionist's perspective also is clearly reflected in Piaget's theory of human cognitive functioning:

> *"Piagetian man actively selects and interprets environmental information in the construction of his own knowledge, rather than passively copying the information just as it is presented to his senses. While paying attention to and taking account of the structure of the environment during knowledge seeking, Piagetian man reconstrues and reinterprets that environment [according to] his own mental framework. . . . The mind neither copies the world . . . nor does it ignore the world [by] creating a private mental conception of it out of whole cloth. The mind meets the environment in an extremely active, self-directed way."*
>
> ***(Flavell, 1977, p. 6)***

In the new epistemology, science is viewed as an ongoing process. Much importance is given to the idea of consensus among scientists. As Brown (1977) concluded, it is a myth that science can establish final truths. Tentative consensus based on reasoned judgments about the available evidence is what can be expected. In this view, scientific knowledge is what the consensus of scientists in any given historical era regard as scientific knowledge (Brown, 1977). This consensus is possible through the collaboration of many scientists as they make their work available for public review and debate and as they build upon previous scientific discoveries (Randall, 1964). It is through this evidence that we begin to understand evidence-based science. Nursing uses evidence-based science to support the interventions performed in the care of patients.

In any given era and in any given discipline, science is structured by an accepted set of presuppositions that define the topic for study and define the best methods for data collection and interpretation (Brown, 1977; Foucault, 1973; Kuhn, 1962). These presuppositions set the boundaries for the scientific enterprise in a particular field. In Brown's view of the transactions between theory and empirical observation:

> *"Theory determines what observations are worth making and how they are to be understood, and observation provides challenges to accepted theoretical structures. The continuing attempt to produce a coherently organized body of theory and observation is the driving force of research, and the prolonged failure of specific research projects leads to scientific revolutions."*
>
> ***(Brown, 1977, p. 167)***

What we understand today as the best approach to patient care based upon current science may change with time. When new problems or a new way to interpret observations emerges, a change in the way we think and do things occurs (Kuhn, 1962). According to Kuhn, science progresses from a prescience, to a normal science, to a crisis, to a revolution, and then to a new normal science. Once normal science develops, the process begins again when a crisis erupts and leads to revolution, and a new normal science emerges once again (Kuhn, 1970; Nyatanga, 2005). This is what Kuhn refers to as *paradigm shift* in the scientific development within a discipline. For example, recent research supports that early mobilization of critically ill patients shows better patient outcomes (Schweickert & Kress, 2011).

INTERDEPENDENCE OF THEORY AND RESEARCH

Traditionally, theory building and research have been presented to students in separate courses. Often, this separation has caused problems for students in understanding the nature of theories and in comprehending the relevance of research efforts (Winston, 1974). Although theory and research can be viewed as distinct operations, they are regarded more appropriately as interdependent components of the scientific process (Dubin, 1978). In constructing a theory, the theorist must be knowledgeable about available empirical findings and be able to take these into account because theory is, in part, concerned with organizing and formalizing available knowledge of a given phenomenon. The theory is subject to revision if hypotheses fail to correspond with empirical findings, or the theory may be abandoned in favor of an alternative explanation that accounts for the new information (Brown, 1977; Dubin, 1978; Kuhn, 1962).

In any scientific discipline, it is not appropriate to judge a theory on the basis of authority, faith, or intuition; it should be judged on the basis of scientific consensus

(Randall, 1964). For example, if a specific nursing theory is deemed acceptable, this judgment should not be made because a respected nursing leader advocates the theory. Instead, the theory should be judged acceptable on the basis of logical and conceptual or empirical grounds. The scientific community (nursing) makes these judgments (Gale, 1979).

The advancement of science is thus a collaborative endeavor in which many researchers evaluate and build on the work of others. Theories, procedures, and findings from empirical studies must be made available for critical review by scientists for evidence to be cumulative. The same procedures can be used to support or refute a given analysis or finding. A theory is accepted when scientists agree that it provides a description of reality that captures the phenomenon based on current research findings (Brown, 1977). The acceptance of a scientific hypothesis depends on the coherence of theory, which involves efforts to relate the theory to observable phenomena in practice through research (Steiner, 1978).

The consensus regarding the correspondence of the theory is, therefore, not based on a single study. Repeated testing is crucial. The study must be replicated under the same conditions, and the theoretical assertions must be explored under different conditions or with different measures. Consensus is, therefore, based on accumulated evidence (Giere, 1979). When the theory does not appear to be supported by research, the scientific community may not necessarily reject it. Rather than agreeing that a problem exists with the theory itself, the community may make judgments about the validity or the reliability of the measures used in testing the theory or about the appropriateness of the research design. These possibilities are considered in critically evaluating all attempts to test a given theory.

Scientific consensus is necessary in three key areas for any given theory: (1) agreement on the boundaries of the theory; that is, the phenomenon it addresses and the phenomena it excludes (criterion of coherence), (2) agreement on the logic used in constructing the theory to further understanding from a similar perspective (criterion of coherence), and (3) agreement that the theory fits the data collected and analyzed through research (criterion of correspondence) (Brown, 1977; Dubin, 1978; Steiner, 1977, 1978). Essentially, consensus in these three areas constitutes an agreement among scientists to "look at the same 'things,' to do so in the same way, and to have a level of confidence certified by an empirical test" (Dubin, 1978, p. 13). Therefore the theory must meet these criteria to be operationalized.

Scientific questioning involves testing a given theory, developing new applications of a theory, or extending a given theory. Occasionally, a new theory with different assumptions is developed that could replace previous theories. Hence, one previously accepted theory is abandoned for another theory if it fails to correspond with empirical findings or if it does not present clear directions for further research. The scientific community judges the selected alternative theory to account for available data and to suggest further lines of questioning (Brown, 1977; Kuhn, 1962). Hence, a new worldview is formed.

In the social and behavioral sciences such as nursing, there is some challenge to the assumptions underlying the accepted methods of experimental design, measurement, and statistical analysis that emphasizes the search for universal laws and the use of procedures for the random assignment of subjects across contexts. Mishler (1979) argued that, in studying human behavior, researchers should develop methods and procedures that are dependent on context for meaning rather than eliminate context by searching for laws that hold across contexts. This critique of the methods and assumptions of research is emerging from phenomenological theorists who view the scientific process differently (Bowers, 1992; Hudson, 1972; Mishler, 1979; Pallikkathayil & Morgan, 1991). One such worldview is called **phenomenology,** which describes how we experience the objects of the external world and provides an explanation of how we construct objects of experience. In phenomenology, the researcher posits that all objects exist because people perceive and construct them as such. An example of phenomenology is to attempt to understand a patient through listening to his or her lived experience and appreciate each individual holistically.

Consensus has emerged in nursing that the knowledge base for nursing practice is based upon the **postpositivist** and **interpretive** philosophies (Ford-Gilboe, Campbell, & Berman, 1995). Postpositivism focuses on discovering patterns that may describe, explain, and predict phenomena. It rejects the older, traditional positivist views of an ultimate objective knowledge that is observable only through the senses (Ford-Gilboe et al., 1995; Weiss, 1995). The interpretive paradigm tends to promote understanding by addressing the meanings of the participants' social interaction that emphasize the situation, context, and multiple cognitive constructions individuals create from everyday experiences (Ford-Gilboe et al., 1995). A critical paradigm for knowledge development in nursing also has been described as an emergent, postmodern paradigm. This paradigm is focused on the interaction between social, political, economic, gender, and cultural factors and the experiences of health and illness (Ford-Gilboe et al., 1995). A broad conception of postmodernism includes the particular philosophies that challenge the "objectification of knowledge," such as phenomenology, hermeneutics, feminism, critical theory, and poststructuralism (Omery, Kasper, & Page, 1995).

The philosophy of nursing has been developing over a 150-year period. The philosophy of caring, naturalism, and holism has themes that can be found in the literature. Numerous authors have written about caring. Caring involves the wholeness of the patient's situation, which implies that nursing care requires interpretation, understanding, and hermeneutic experience. The philosophy of caring involves knowledge, skills, patient trust, and the ability to manage all elements simultaneously in the context of care (Adams, 2016).

Wholism is another philosophy in understanding the patient (Hennessey, 2011). Wholistic nursing views the biophysical, psychological, and sociological subsystems as related but separate; thus the whole is equal to the sum of the parts. Holistic nursing recognizes that multiple subsystems are in continuous interaction and that mind-body relationships do exist (Aghebati et al., 2015).

Naturalism has a metaphysical component that implies that the natural world exists; there is no nonnatural or supranatural realm. The natural world is open, because it depends on what method the inquiry requires. Naturalism insists that knowledge and beliefs are gained by one's senses guided by reason, and by the various methods of science (Hussey, 2011). Although these philosophies are proposed in the literature, nursing science is still in the early stages of scientific development.

As the discipline of nursing moves forward, there is abundant evidence that a greater number of nurse scholars are actively engaged in the advancement of knowledge for the discipline of nursing through research and scholarly dialogue. This can be seen with the emergence of middle-range theories that use inductive, deductive, and synthesis theories from nursing and other disciplines (Peterson & Bredow, 2017; Sieloff & Frey, 2007; Smith & Liehr, 2013). This new century of nursing scholarship by nurse scientists and scholars explores nursing phenomena of interest and provides research evidence for quality nursing practice.

SCIENCE AS A SOCIAL ENTERPRISE

The process of scientific inquiry may also be viewed as a social enterprise (Mishler, 1979). In Gale's words, "Human beings do science" (Gale, 1979, p. 290). Therefore it might be anticipated that social, economic, or political factors may influence the scientific enterprise (Brown, 1977). For example, the popularity of certain ideologies influences how phenomena are viewed and which problems that are selected for study (Hudson, 1972). Science progresses by the diversity of dialogue within the discipline of nursing. The use of a single paradigm, multiple paradigms, or the creation of a merged paradigm from many paradigms is considered in relation to the advancement in the epistemology of nursing.

POINTS FOR FURTHER STUDY

- 100 Basic Philosophical Terms: http://www.str.org/articles/100-basic-philosophical-terms#.V1N0fyGIxS0
- Edmund Husserl: http://plato.stanford.edu/entries/husserl/
- Kant's Philosophy of Science: http://plato.stanford.edu/entries/kant-science/
- Rationalism vs Empiricism: http://plato.stanford.edu/entries/rationalism-empiricism/
- Phenomenology: http://plato.stanford.edu/entries/phenomenology/
- Naturalism: http://plato.stanford.edu/entries/naturalism/

REFERENCES

Adams, L. Y. (2016). The conundrum of caring in nursing. *International Journal of Caring Sciences, 9*(1), 1–8.

Aghebati, N., Mohammadi, E., Ahmadi, F., & Noaparast, K. B. (2015). Principle-based concept analysis: Intentionality in holistic nursing theories. *Journal of Holistic Nursing, 33*, 68–83.

Bowers, L. (1992). Ethnomethodology I: An approach to nursing research. *International Journal of Nursing Studies, 29*(1), 59–67.

Bronowski, J. (1979). *The visionary eye: Essays in the arts, literature and science.* Cambridge, MA: MIT Press.

Brown, H. (1977). *Perception, theory and commitment: The new philosophy of science.* Chicago: University of Chicago Press.

Bruce, A., Rietze, L., & Lim, A. (2014). Understanding philosophy in a nurse's world: What, where and why? *Nursing and Health, 2*(3), 65–71.

Calder, N. (1979). *Einstein's universe.* New York: Viking.

Dubin, R. (1978). *Theory building.* New York: Free Press.

Flavell, J. H. (1977). *Cognitive development.* Englewood Cliffs, NJ: Prentice-Hall.

Ford-Gilboe, M., Campbell, J., & Berman, H. (1995). Stories and numbers: Coexistence without compromise. *Advances in Nursing Science, 18*(1), 14–26.

Foucault, M. (1973). *The order of things: An archaeology of the human sciences.* New York: Vintage Books.

Gale, G. (1979). *Theory of science: An introduction to the history, logic and philosophy of science.* New York: McGraw-Hill.

Giere, R. N. (1979). *Understanding scientific reasoning.* New York: Holt, Rhinehart, & Winston.
Hanson, N. R. (1958). *Patterns of discovery.* Cambridge, MA: Cambridge University Press.
Hennessey, S. (2011). Wholism: Another perspective. *California Journal of Oriental Medicine, 22*(2), 7–11.
Hudson, L. (1972). *The cult of the fact.* New York: Harper & Row.
Hussey, T. (2011). Naturalistic nursing. *Nursing Philosophy, 12*, 45–52.
Kuhn, T. S. (1962). *The structure of scientific revolutions.* Chicago: University of Chicago Press.
Kuhn, T. S. (1970). *The structure of scientific revolutions* (2nd ed.). Chicago: University of Chicago Press.
Lipton, P. (2005). The Medawar lecture 2004: The truth about science. *Philosophical Transactions of the Royal Society, 360*, 1259–1269.
Manley, B. J., Doyle, L. W., Owen, L. S., & Davis, P. G. (2016) Extubating extremely preterm infants: Predictors of success and outcomes following failure. *Journal of Pediatrics, 173*, 45–49.
Mishler, E. G. (1979). Meaning in context: Is there any other kind? *Harvard Educational Review, 49*, 1–19.
Norman, D. A. (1976). *Memory and attention: An introduction to human information processing.* New York: Wiley.
Nyatanga, L. (2005). Nursing and the philosophy of science. *Nurse Education Today, 25*(8), 670–674.
Omery, A., Kasper, C. E., & Page, G. G. (1995). *In search of nursing science.* Thousand Oaks, CA: Sage.
Pallikkathayil, L., & Morgan, S. (1991). Phenomenology as a method for conducting clinical research. *Applied Nursing Research, 4*(4), 195–200.
Peterson, S. J., & Bredow, T. S. (2017). *Middle range theories: Application to nursing research* (3rd ed.). Philadelphia: Lippincott Williams & Wilkins.
Piaget, J. (1970). *The place of the sciences of man in the system of sciences.* New York: Harper & Row.
Popper, K. (1962). *Conjectures and refutations.* New York: Basic Books.
Randall, J. H. (1964). *Philosophy: An introduction.* New York: Barnes & Noble.
Reynolds, P. (1971). *A primer in theory construction.* Indianapolis, IN: Bobbs-Merrill.
Schweickert, W. D., & Kress J. P. (2011). Implementing early mobilization interventions in mechanically ventilated patients in the ICU. *Chest, 140*, 1612–1617.
Sieloff, C. L., & Frey, M. A. (Eds.). (2007). *Middle range theory development using King's conceptual system.* New York: Springer.
Skinner, B. F. (1950). Are theories of learning necessary? *Psychological Review, 57*, 193–216.
Smith, M. J., & Liehr, P. R. (2013). *Middle range theory for nursing* (3rd ed.). New York: Springer.
Snelbecker, G. (1974). *Learning theory, instructional theory, and psychoeducational design.* New York: McGraw-Hill.
Steiner, E. (1977). *Criteria for theory of art education.* Unpublished monograph presented at Seminar for Research in Art Education. Bloomington: Indiana University School of Education.
Steiner, E. (1978). *Logical and conceptual analytic techniques for educational researchers.* Washington, DC: University Press.
Toulmin, S. (1961). *Foresight and understanding.* New York: Harper & Row.
Weiss, S. J. (1995). Contemporary empiricism. In A. Omery, C. E. Kasper, & G. G. Page (Eds.), *In search of nursing science.* (pp. 13–26) Thousand Oaks, CA: Sage.
Winston, C. (1974). *Theory and measurement in sociology.* New York: Wiley.
Zetterberg, H. L. (1966). *On theory and verification in sociology.* Totowa, NJ: Bedminster Press.

4

Theory Development Process

Sonya R. Hardin

"To advance nursing science, it is critical for nurses to have a comprehensive understanding of the philosophical and theoretical foundations of the discipline."
(Yancey, 2015, p. 278)

Nursing theories that clearly set forth understanding of nursing phenomena (i.e., self-care, therapeutic communication, chronic sorrow) guide nursing practice and research. Once a nursing theory is proposed to address a phenomenon of interest, several considerations follow, such as its completeness and logic, internal consistency, correspondence with empirical findings, and whether it has been operationally defined for testing. Analyses of these lead logically to the further development of the theory. Scientific evidence accumulates through repeated rigorous research that supports or refutes theoretical assertions and guides modifications or extensions of the theory. Nursing theory development is not a mysterious activity, but a scholarly endeavor pursued systematically. Rigorous development of nursing theories, then, is a high priority for the future of the discipline and the practice of the profession of nursing (McCrae, 2012).

Nurses in practice see patterns that often lead to protocols or decision-making trees. The focus of these protocols and decision-making trees is the phenomenon that is of interest in patient care. A conceptual model or framework to understand and define phenomena of interest is the first step in theory development. Building relationships with linkages between related concepts is the second step. Last, the relationship statements or propositions are developed to build a theory.

THEORY COMPONENTS

Development of theory requires understanding of selected scholarly terms, definitions, and assumptions so that scholarly review and analysis may occur. Attention is given to terms and defined meanings to understand the theory development process that was used. Therefore the clarity of terms, their scientific utility, and their value to the discipline are important considerations in the process.

Hage (1972) identified six theory components and specified the contributions they make to theory (Table 4.1). Three categories of theory components are presented as a basis for understanding the function of each element in the theory-building process: concepts and definitions, relational statements, and the linkages and ordering.

Concepts and Definitions

Concepts, the building blocks of theories, classify the phenomena of interest (Kaplan, 1964). It is crucial that concepts are considered within the theoretical system in which they are embedded and from which they derive their meaning, because concepts may have different meanings in various conceptual frameworks or theoretical systems. Scientific progress is based on critical review and testing of a researcher's work by the scientific community.

Concepts may be abstract or concrete. Abstract concepts are mentally constructed independent of a specific time or place, whereas concrete concepts are directly experienced and relate to a particular time or place (Chinn & Kramer, 2015; Hage, 1972; Reynolds, 1971) (Table 4.2).

The stretcher, stroke, wheelchair, and hospital ambulance are examples of concrete concepts of the abstract concept *transport*. In a given theoretical system, the definition, characteristics, and functioning of a nurse competency clarify more specific instances, such as medication administration nurse competency.

TABLE 4.1 Theory Components and Their Contributions to the Theory

Theory Components	Contributions to the Theory	Examples	
Concepts and Definitions			
Concepts	Describe phenomena	Age	Exercise
Theoretical definitions of concept	Establish meaning	How long someone has been alive	A person being active
Operational definitions of concept	Provide measurement	Years of life	Number of hours of being active
Relational Statements			
Theoretical statements	Relate concepts to one another; permit analysis	Exercise decreases with age.	
Operational statements	Relate concepts to measurements	The hours of activity decrease with more years of life.	
Linkages and Ordering			
Linkages of theoretical statements	Provide rationale of why theoretical statements are linked; add plausibility	A 2013 CDC study reported that more than 30% of adults aged 65 or older report no leisure-time physical activity (CDC, 2013).	
Linkages of operational statements	Provide rationale for how measurement variables are linked; permit testability	Self-reports of amount (hours) are practical, easy to administer to large groups, and cost-efficient. They are also generally well accepted and place relatively low burden on and interfere little with the usual habits of the individual. However, they are prone to either overestimation or underestimation because of inaccurate recall, social desirability, and misinterpretation (Falck et al., 2016).	
Organization of concepts and definitions into primitive and derived terms	Eliminates overlap (tautology)	Older adults would be healthier if they exercised.	
Organization of statements and linkages into premises and derived hypotheses and equations	Eliminates inconsistency	Older adults participate in fewer hours of exercise in a week. Older adults have increased risk of health problems. Therefore a decrease in exercise increases the risk of health problems.	

CDC, Centers for Disease Control and Prevention.

TABLE 4.2 Concepts: Abstract Versus Concrete

Abstract Concepts	Concrete Concepts
Transport	Stretcher, wheelchair, hospital bed, ambulance
Vascular disease	Stroke, myocardial infarction, peripheral vascular disease
Telemetry	Electrocardiogram, Holter monitor
Loss of relationship	Divorce, widowhood, suicide
Nurse competency	Cultural, IV insertion, drug calculation

Theories may be used as a series of nonvariable discrete concepts (and subconcepts) to build typologies. Typologies are systematic arrangements of concepts within a given category. For example, a typology on marital status could be partitioned into marital statuses in which a population is classified as married, divorced, widowed, or single. These discrete categories could be partitioned further to permit the classification of an additional variable in this typology. A typology of marital status and sex is shown in Table 4.3. The participants are either one sex or the other, because there are no degrees of how much they are in this discrete category. Taking the illustration further, the typology could be partitioned by

TABLE 4.3 Typology of Marital Status and Gender

	MARITAL STATUS			
Participants	**Single**	**Married**	**Divorced**	**Widowed**
Male	15	75	23	6
Female	25	72	41	13
Total	40	147	64	19

TABLE 4.4 Published Concept Analyses Using Walker and Avant (2011) Approach

Selected Examples of Concept Analyses	Author(s)
Spiritual care in nursing	Ramezani et al. (2014)
Quality of life in old age	Boggatz (2016)
Music therapy	Murrock & Bekhet (2016)
Body image	Rhoten (2016)
Concealed pregnancy	Murphy, Tighe, & Lalor (2016)

adding the discrete concept of children. Participants would be classified for gender, marital status, and as having or not having children.

A **continuous concept,** on the other hand, permits classification of dimensions or gradations of a phenomenon, indicating degree of marital conflict. Marital couples may be classified with a range representing degrees of marital conflict in their relationships from low to high.

Degree of Marital Conflict

0 ⟷ 120

Low High

Other continuous concepts that may be used to classify couples might include amount of communication, number of shared activities, or number of children. Examples of continuous concepts used to classify patients are degree of temperature, level of anxiety, or age. Another example is how nurses conceptualize pain as a continuous concept when they ask patients to rate their pain on a scale from 0 to 10 to better understand their pain threshold or pain experience.

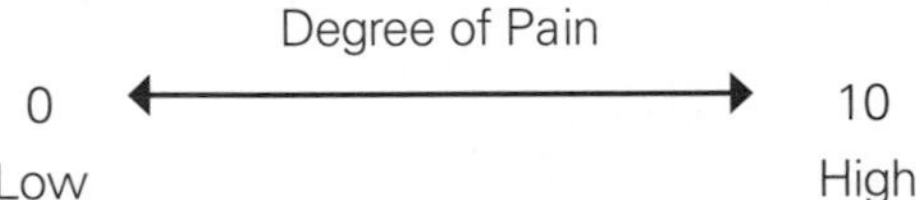

The development of concepts, then, permits description and classification of phenomena (Hage, 1972). The labeled concept specifies boundaries for selecting phenomena to observe and for reasoning about the phenomena of interest. New concepts may focus attention on new phenomena or facilitate thinking about phenomena in a different way (Hage, 1972). The concept analysis continues to flourish, with many examples in the nursing literature. See Table 4.4 for references to analyses carried out using different approaches.

Concept analysis is an important beginning step in the process of theory development to create a conceptual definition. It is crucial that concepts are clearly defined within the conceptual model or framework to reduce ambiguity in the given concept or set of concepts. To eliminate perceived differences in meaning, explicit definitions are necessary. As the theory develops, theoretical and operational definitions provide the theorist's meaning of the concept and the basis for the empirical indicators. Theories are tested in reality; therefore the concepts must be linked to operational definitions that relate the concepts to observable phenomena specifying empirical indicators. Table 4.5 provides examples of concepts with their theoretical and operational definitions. These linkages are vital to the logic of the theory, its observation, and its measurement.

Relational Statements

Statements in a theory may state definitions or relations among concepts. Whereas definitions provide descriptions of the concept, relational statements propose relationships between and among two or more concepts. Concepts must be connected with one another in a series of theoretical statements to devise a nursing theory.

In the connections between variables, one variable may be proposed to influence a second. In this case the first variable may be viewed as the antecedent or determinate (independent) variable and the second as the consequent or resultant (dependent) variable (Giere, 1997). An example of an antecedent and a consequent variable is explained with the concept of *well* in older adults, where the antecedents were identified as connecting with others, imagining opportunities, recognizing strengths, and seeking meaning. The consequences identified were living values and being well. These antecedents (prior condition) and consequences (outcome) were developed from the literature (McMahon & Fleury, 2012).

Theoretical assertions are either a necessary or sufficient condition, or both. These labels of necessary or sufficient condition characterize conditions that help explain the nature of the relationship between two variables in theoretical statements. For example, a relational statement expressed as a sufficient condition could be: If nurses

TABLE 4.5 Examples of Theoretical and Operational Definitions

Concept	Theoretical Definition	Operational Definition
Body temperature	Homeothermic range of one's internal environment maintained by the thermoregulatory system of the human body	Degree of temperature measured by oral thermometer taken for 1 minute under the tongue
Quality of life	A subjective state characterized by the attributes of life satisfaction and emotional balance	Diener's Life Satisfaction Scale (Diener & Lucas, 1999). This scale measures the judgmental component of subjective well-being.
Workplace spirituality	Spiritual expressions at work	The Daily Spiritual Experiences Scale (Underwood & Teresi, 2002). This scale is intended to measure a person's perception of the transcendent (God, the divine) in daily life and his or her perception of his or her interaction with or involvement of the transcendent in life.

react with approval (NA) of patients' self-care behaviors, patient self-care activity efforts (PSC) increase. This is a type of compound statement linking antecedent and consequent variables. The statement does not assert the truth of the antecedent. Rather, the assertion is made that if the antecedent is true, then the consequent is true (Giere, 1979).

A sufficient condition means that one variable results in another variable occurring. It does not claim it is the only variable that can result in the occurrence of the other variable. This statement asserts that nurse approval of a patient's self-care behaviors is sufficient for the occurrence of the patient's self-care activities. However, patient assumption of self-care activities resulting from other factors, such as the patient's health status and personality variables, is not ruled out. There may be other antecedent conditions sufficient for the patient's assumption of self-care activities.

A statement in the form of a necessary condition asserts that one variable is required for the occurrence of another variable. For example: If patients are motivated to get well (wellness motivation), then they adhere to their prescribed treatment regimen.

This means that adherence to a treatment regimen never occurs unless wellness motivation occurs. It is not asserted that the patients' adherence to the treatment regimen stems from their wellness motivation. However, it is asserted that if the wellness motivation is absent, patients will not assume strict adherence to their treatment regimens. The wellness motivation is a necessary, but not a sufficient, condition for the occurrence of this consequent.

The term *if* is generally used to introduce a sufficient condition, whereas *only if* and *if . . . then* are used to introduce necessary conditions (Giere, 1979). Usually conditional statements are not both necessary and sufficient. However, it is possible for a statement to express both conditions. In such instances, the term *if and only if* is used to imply that conditions are both necessary and sufficient for one another. In this case (1) the consequent never occurs in the absence of the antecedent and (2) the consequent always occurs when the antecedent occurs (Giere, 1979). It should be noted that not all conditional statements are causal. For example, "If this month is November, then the next month is December," does not assert that November causes December to occur; rather, the sequence of months suggests that December follows November (Dubin, 1978; Giere, 1979).

An example is a study that was conducted on the effect of participation in an incentive-based wellness program on exercise. The theoretical assertion was that wellness motivation would promote healthy behaviors. When individuals were motivated with an incentive such as $20 monthly, participants had roughly one half more exercise days per week than nonparticipants. Offering a motivation for exercise at a fitness center increased physical activity (Crespin, Abraham, & Rothman, 2016).

Linkages and Ordering

Specification of linkages is a vital part of the development of theory. Although the theoretical statements assert connections between concepts, the rationale for the stated connections must be developed and clearly presented. Development of theoretical linkages provides an explanation of why the variables are connected in a certain manner; that is, the theoretical reason for particular relationships. Operational linkages contribute testability to the theory by specifying how measurement variables are connected. Operational definitions specify the measurability of the concepts, and operational linkages provide the testability of the assertions. It is the operational linkages that contribute a perspective for understanding the nature of the relationship between concepts, to know whether the relationship between the concepts is negative or positive, linear, or curvilinear. A theory may be considered fairly complete if it identifies its conceptual framework and presents the concepts, definitions, relational statements, and linkages. Complete development of a theory, however, requires organizing the concepts, definitions, relational statements, and linkages into premises and hypotheses (Hage, 1972).

In the study noted previously by Crespin, Abraham, and Rothman (2016), the rationale for the stated connection of motivation promoting healthy behaviors was based upon previous research. The RAND CORPORATION found that 35% of businesses with 50 or more employees encouraged participation in exercise with financial incentives for the purpose of promoting healthy behaviors (Mattke et al., 2013). The operational linkages in the study were that two self-reported measures of exercise were used to compare participants and nonparticipants. They measured vigorous exercise by asking how many days per week the participant did 20 minutes or more of vigorous exercise such as running, aerobics, or stair/ski/rowing machine. The operational definition of exercise was the number of self-reported exercise days. In this study a positive relationship existed between the concepts of motivation and exercise. Their hypothesis was that if individuals were given a financial motivation, then more exercise would occur.

Reynolds (1971) concluded that the set-of-laws approach provides for classification of phenomena or prediction of relationships between selected variables, but it does not lead to further understanding or advance science, because it is based on what is already known. Finally, Reynolds (1971) notes that each statement or law is considered to be independent, because the various statements have not been interrelated into a system of description and explanation or evolved from an organized conceptual model or framework. Therefore each statement must be tested—because the statements are not interrelated, one statement does not provide support for another statement. This set of laws may be useful to begin theory development; however, research efforts must be more extensive. Table 4.6 describes the principles of theory development: laws, hypotheses, and theory.

The **organization** of a theory is an interrelated, logical system. Specifically, a theory consists of explicit definitions, a set of, a set of existence statements, and a set of relationship statements arranged in hierarchical order (Reynolds, 1971). The concepts may include abstract, intermediate, and concrete concepts. The set-of-existence statements describe situations in which the theory is applicable. Statements that delineate the boundaries describe the scope of the theory (Dubin, 1978; Hage, 1972; Reynolds, 1971). Relational statements consist of axioms and propositions. Abstract theoretical statements, or axioms, are at the top of the hierarchy of relational statements. The other propositions are developed through logical deduction from the axioms or from research findings in the literature (Table 4.7). This results in a highly interrelated, explanatory system.

The distinguishing feature of the **causal process** form of theory development is the theoretical statements that specify causal mechanisms between independent and dependent variables. Hence the statements are, to some degree, attempting to predict. This form of theory organization consists of a set of concepts, a set of definitions, a set of existence statements, and a set of theoretical statements specifying a causal process (Reynolds, 1971). Causal statements specify the hypothesized effects of one variable upon one or more other variables for testing. In complex causal processes, feedback loops and paths of influence through several variables are hypothesized in a set of interrelated causal statements (Mullins, 1971; Nowak, 1975). Reynolds (1971) concludes that the causal process form of theory provides for testing an explanation of the process of how events happen. This is a highly advanced form of theory development that builds successively on previous research findings in the researchers' area of research with extensive theory building and testing over time. An example is a middle-range theory developed by Dobratz (2016) using Roy's Adaptation Model for the theory of adaptive

TABLE 4.6 Theory Development Principles

Principle	Definition	Proof
Scientific laws	A statement of fact meant to describe an action or a set of actions	Simple, true, universal, and absolute
Hypothesis	An educated guess based upon observation	Has not been proved
Theory	One or more hypotheses that explains a set of related observations or events and has been verified multiple times	Accepted as true and proved

TABLE 4.7 Theory Development in the Scientific Method

Steps	Example
Observation: Start with an observation that evokes a question.	Early mobilization of ICU patients seems to improve patient outcomes.
Logical hypothesis: Using abductive, inductive, or deductive logic, state a possible answer (hypothesis).	Patients receiving early mobilization in the ICU will have less days in the ICU.
Testing: Perform an experiment or test.	Measure the average length of stay of ICU patients receiving early mobilization and compare length of stay to those who did not receive early mobilization.
Dissemination: Publish your findings for the discipline.	Perme, C., & Chandrashekar, R. (2009). Early mobility and walking program for patients in intensive care units: Creating a standard of care. *American Journal of Critical Care, 18*(3):212–221.
Replication: Other scientists will read your published work and try to duplicate it (verification).	Hodgson, C. L., Bailey, M., Bellomo, R. et al. (2016). The trial of early activity and mobilization study Investigators: A binational multicenter pilot feasibility randomized controlled trial of early goal-directed mobilization in ICU. *Critical Care Medicine,44*(6),1145–1152.
Theory: If experiments from other researchers support your hypothesis, it will become a theory.	Early mobilization, comprising early active exercises during mechanical ventilation, decreases length of stay.

ICU, Intensive care unit.

TABLE 4.8 Middle Range Theory of Adaptive Spirituality

Theoretical statements	1. Spirituality influenced supportive coping for individuals in caregiver roles related to terminal illness and dementia. 2. Spirituality enhanced psychological adjustment and well-being and improved quality of life for persons who experienced cancer, chronic illness, and life closure. 3. Spirituality improved self-image and reduced depression in younger individuals who were adapting to trauma and overcoming substance abuse. 4. Spirituality provided support for working nurses and helped during times of moral conflict. 5. Spirituality assisted African American and Mexican American populations to cope with illness challenges and life transitions. 6. Spirituality can be difficult to express in older adults who are challenged with chronic illness.
Conceptual definition	1. Adaptive spiritually is integrating one's beliefs and values, religious practices, and cultural values in adapting to physical illness, loss, and life transitions.
Hypotheses	1. Spirituality has a positive effect on psychological adjustment, well-being, supportive coping, and quality of life. 2. Spirituality has a positive effect on caregiver coping. 3. Spirituality is inversely related to depression and PTSD.

Modified from Dobratz, M. C. (2016). Building a middle-range theory of adaptive spirituality. *Nursing Science Quarterly, 29*(2), 146–153.
PTSD, Posttraumatic stress disorder.

spirituality. Dobratz's work is based upon 21 empirical studies that investigated religion/spirituality. The work includes six theoretical statements, a conceptual definition of adaptive spirituality, and three hypotheses for future testing. Table 4.8 summarizes a middle-range theory of adaptive spirituality.

Middle-range theory was described very early in the nursing literature by a sociologist (Merton, 1967). He proposed that it focused on specific phenomena (rather than attempting to address a broader range of phenomena) and comprised hypotheses with two or more concepts that are linked together in a conceptual system. Today in the nursing literature, many middle-range theories are developed qualitatively from practice observations and interviews and quantitatively from nursing conceptual models or theories. Middle-range theory is pragmatic at the practice level and contains specific aspects about the practice situation as follows:

- The situation or health condition involved
- Client population or age group
- Location or area of practice (such as community)
- Action of the nurse or the intervention

It is these specifics that make middle-range theory so applicable to nursing practice (Alligood, 2014). Therefore the development of middle-range theory facilitates conceptions of relationships among theory, nursing practice, and patient outcomes in focused areas.

In 1996, Lenz (in Liehr & Smith, 1999) identified the following six approaches for devising middle-range theories:

1. Inductive approach through research
2. Deductive approach from grand nursing theories
3. Integration of nursing and nonnursing theories
4. Derivative (retroductive) approach from nonnursing theories
5. Theories devised from guidelines for clinical practice
6. Synthesis approach from research findings

The nursing literature abounds with a range of different approaches to middle-range theory building and development. The recent nursing literature emphasizes the importance of relating middle-range theories to broader nursing theories and conceptual models and continuing to pursue empirical testing and the replication of studies to advance nursing knowledge (McCrae, 2012).

CONTEMPORARY ISSUES IN NURSING THEORY DEVELOPMENT

Theoretical Boundaries and Levels to Advance Nursing Science

Since Fawcett's (1984) seminal proposal of the four metaparadigm concepts—person, environment, health, and nursing—general agreement has emerged among nursing scholars such that the proposed framework is now used without reference to the author for the development of nursing science. In general, a metaparadigm should specify the broad boundaries of the phenomenon of concern in a discipline, for example, to set nursing apart from other disciplines, such as medicine, clinical exercise physiology, or sociology. Fawcett (2005) proposed that a metaparadigm defines the totality of phenomena inherent in the discipline in a parsimonious way, as well as being perspective-neutral and international in scope. Her definition of *perspective-neutral* is that the metaparadigm concepts reflect nursing but not any particular nursing conceptual model or paradigm. This criterion is clearly illustrated in the way the nursing models and paradigms include the metaparadigm concepts but define each in distinctly different ways. This supports their generic nature as broad metaparadigm concepts but with specificity within each conceptual theory or paradigm. It is important to grasp the significance of Fawcett's point. Because the metaparadigm is the highly philosophical level in the structure of knowledge, models and theories define the terms specifically within each of their works, and differences among them are anticipated. In the discipline of nursing, the earlier focus on theory development has evolved to an emphasis on theory use, with development and use of middle-range theories focused at the practice level.

Nursing Theory, Practice, and Research

Theory-testing research may lead one nursing theory to fall aside as new theory is developed that explains nursing phenomena more adequately. Therefore it is critical that theory-testing research continues to advance the discipline. Nursing scholars have presented criteria for evaluating theory-testing research in nursing (Acton, Irvin, & Hopkins, 1991; Silva, 1986). These criteria emphasize the importance of using a nursing framework to design the purpose and focus of the study, to derive hypotheses, and to relate the significance of the findings back to nursing. In addition to the call for more rigorous theory-testing research in nursing, nursing scholars and practitioners call for increased attention to the relationships among theory, research, and practice. Their recommendations include the following:

- Continued development of nursing theories that are relevant to nurses' specialty practice
- Increased collaboration between scientists and practitioners (Lorentzon, 1998)
- Encouraging nurse researchers to communicate research findings to practitioners
- Increased efforts to relate middle-range theories to nursing paradigms
- Increased emphasis on clinical research
- Increased use of nursing theories for theory-based practice and clinical decision making

(See Chinn & Kramer, 2015; Cody, 1999; Hoffman & Bertus, 1991; Liehr & Smith, 1999; Lutz, Jones, & Kendall, 1997; Reed, 2000; Sparacino, 1991.)

Within nursing education, some programs use one specific nursing theory to guide their nursing curricula, whereas others use a framework of the four metaparadigm concepts (person, health, nursing, and environment). Yancey (2015) and others have urged increased attention to nursing theory–based research and strengthening of nursing theory–based curricula in undergraduate, master's, and doctoral programs.

SUMMARY

In summary, contemporary nursing scholars are emphasizing the following in theory-building processes:

- Continued development of theoretical inquiry in nursing
- Continued scholarship with middle-range theories and situation-specific theories, including efforts to relate to nursing theories and paradigms
- Greater attention to synthesizing nursing knowledge
- Development of stronger nursing theory-research-practice linkages

The discipline of nursing has evolved to an understanding of the relationships among theory, practice, and research that no longer separates them into distinct categories. Rather, their complementary interrelationships foster the development of new understanding about practice as theory is used to guide practice and practice innovations drive new middle-range theory. Similarly, nurse scientists have reached a new understanding of the relationship of theory to research as quantitative study reports include explicit descriptions of their frameworks and qualitative researchers interpret their findings in the context of nursing frameworks. The complementary nature of these relationships is fostering nursing science growth in this theory utilization era. Thus emphasis on theory is important because theory development in nursing is an essential component in nursing scholarship to advance the knowledge of the discipline (McCrae, 2012).

CRITICAL THINKING ACTIVITIES

1. Examine a photograph from the Zwerdling Postcard Collection: Pictures of Nursing, located at the U.S. National Library of Medicine, https://www.nlm.nih.gov/exhibition/picturesofnursing/. Look at the photograph for a minute, and ask yourself, What do I see? Make a list. Come back to the photo a second time, and ask yourself if this list is accurate. Then ask yourself what question comes to mind when looking at the photo. What is missing from the photo? What is missing from the situation? How did the situation in the photo occur and why? Each type of question will lead to different types of thinking.
2. Move thinking from dualist to contextual with this exercise. Use the analogy of a building. Take a piece of paper and draw a building. At the foundation of the building, write *paradigm.* Label the walls *conceptual models.* Conceptual models are the structure supported by the foundational paradigm. Then color the interior walls inside the building and label this *theory.* Theories are similar to interior wall configuration. Some configurations have a clear purpose, and others do not. All interior walls are bound by outside walls (conceptual models) and supported by the foundation (paradigm). Draw the inside of a room with all of its décor. The unique concepts of theories are similar to the unique aspects of the décor. The décor is observable, as are the concepts of a conceptual model.
3. Identify a concept that you have read about and observed in nursing practice. Write a theoretical definition and an operational definition (hint: for the operational definition you will need to find a way to measure the chosen concept).

(From Hanna, D. R. [2011]. Teaching theoretical thinking for a sense of salience. *Journal of Nursing Education, 50*[8], 479–482.)

POINTS FOR FURTHER STUDY

- Webber, P. B. (2008). Yes, Virginia, nursing does have laws. *Nurse Science Quarterly, 21*(1), 68–73.
- Classic References:
  - Dubin, R. (1978). *Theory building.* New York: Free Press.
  - Hage, J. (1972). *Techniques and problems of theory construction in sociology.* New York, Wiley.
  - Kaplan, A. (1964). *The conduct of inquiry: Methodology for behavioral science.* New York: Chandler.
  - Mullins, N. (1971). *The art of theory: Construction and use.* New York: Harper & Row.
  - Wilson, J. (1969). *Thinking with concepts.* Cambridge: Cambridge University Press.

REFERENCES

Acton, G., Irvin, B., & Hopkins, B. (1991). Theory-testing research: Building the science. *Advances in Nursing Science, 14*(1), 52–61.

Alligood, M. R. (2014). Areas for further development of theory-based nursing practice. In M. R. Alligood (Ed.), *Nursing theory: Utilization & application* (5th ed., pp. 413–424). St Louis: Elsevier.

Boggatz, T. (2016). Quality of life in old age—a concept analysis. *International Journal of Older People Nursing, 11*(1), 1748–3743.

Centers for Disease Control and Prevention (CDC). (2013). *The state of aging and health in America 2013.* Atlanta, GA: Centers for Disease Control and Prevention, U.S. Department of Health and Human Services.

Chinn, P., & Kramer, M. (2015). *Integrated theory and knowledge development in nursing* (9th ed.). St Louis: Mosby.

Cody, W. (1999). Middle range theories: Do they foster the development of nursing science? *Nursing Science Quarterly, 12*(1), 9–14.

Crespin, D. J., Abraham, J. M., & Rothman, A. J. (2016). The effect of participation in an incentive-based wellness program on self-reported exercise. *Preventive Medicine, 82*, 92–98.

Diener, E., & Lucas, R. E. (1999). Personality and subjective well-being. In D. Kahneman, E. Diener, & N. Schwarz (Eds.), *Well-being: The foundations of a hedonic psychology* (pp. 213–229). New York, NY: Russell Sage Foundation.

Dobratz, M. C. (2016). Building a middle-range theory of adaptive spirituality. *Nursing Science Quarterly, 29*(2), 146–153.

Dubin, R. (1978). *Theory building*. New York: Free Press.

Falck R. S., Mcdonald S. M., Beets M. W., Brazendale K., & Liu-Ambrose T. (2015). Measurement of physical activity in older adult interventions: A systematic review. *British Journal of Sports Medicine, 50*(8), 464–470.

Fawcett, J. (1984). The metaparadigm of nursing: Present status and future refinements. *Image: The Journal of Nursing Scholarship, 16*(3), 84–87.

Fawcett, J. (2005). *Analysis and evaluation of contemporary nursing knowledge: Nursing models and theories* (2nd ed.). Philadelphia: F. A. Davis.

Giere, R. N. (1979). *Understanding scientific reasoning*. New York: Holt, Rhinehart, & Winston.

Giere, R. N. (1997). *Understanding scientific reasoning* (4th ed.). Fort Worth, TX: Harcourt.

Hage, J. (1972). *Techniques and problems of theory construction in sociology*. New York: John Wiley & Sons.

Hanna, D. R. (2011). Teaching theoretical thinking for a sense of salience. *Journal of Nursing Education, 50*(8), 479–482.

Hoffman, A., & Bertus, P. (1991). Theory and practice: Bridging scientists' and practitioners' roles. *Archives of Psychiatric Nursing, 7*(1), 2–9.

Hodgson, C. L., Bailey, M., Bellomo, R., et al.; The Trial of Early Activity and Mobilization Study Investigators. (2016). A binational multicenter pilot feasibility randomized controlled trial of early goal-directed mobilization in ICU. *Critical Care Medicine, 44*(6), 1145–1152.

Kaplan, A. (1964). *The conduct of inquiry: Methodology for behavioral science*. New York: Chandler.

Lenz, E. (1996). *Middle range theory—Role in research and practice.* In *Proceedings of the Sixth Rosemary Ellis Scholar's Retreat, Nursing Science Implications for the 21*st Century. Cleveland, OH: Frances Payne Bolton School of Nursing, Case Western Reserve University.

Liehr, P., & Smith, M. J. (1999). Middle range theory: Spinning research and practice to create knowledge for the new millennium. *Advances in Nursing Science, 21*(4), 8–91.

Lorentzon, M. (1998). The way forward: Nursing research or collaborative health care research? *Journal of Advanced Nursing, 27*, 675–676.

Lutz, K., Jones, K., & Kendall, J. (1997). Expanding the praxis debate: Contributions to clinical inquiry. *Advances in Nursing Science, 20*(2), 13–22.

Mattke, S., Liu, H., & Caloyeras, J.P., et al. (2013). Workplace Wellness Programs Study Final Report, Rand Health, Santa Monica, CA. Retrieved from http://www.rand.org/content/dam/rand/pubs/research_reports/RR200/RR254/RAND_RR254.pdf.

McCrae, N. (2012). Whither nursing models? The value of nursing theory in the context of evidence-based practice and multidisciplinary health care. *Journal of Advanced Nursing, 68*(1), 222–229.

McMahon, S., & Fleury, J. (2012). Wellness in older adults: A concept analysis. *Nursing Forum, 47*(1), 39–51.

Merton, R. K. (1967). *On theoretical sociology*. New York: Free Press.

Mullins, N. (1971). *The art of theory: Construction and use*. New York: Harper & Row.

Murphy Tighe, S., & Lalor, J. G. (2016). Concealed pregnancy: A concept analysis. *Journal of Advanced Nursing, 72*(1), 1365–2648.

Murrock, C. J., & Bekhet, A. K. (2016). Concept analysis: Music therapy. *Research and Theory for Nursing Practice, 30*(1), 44–59.

Nowak, S. (1975). Causal interpretations of statistical relationships in social research. In H. Blalock (Ed.), *Quantitative sociology: International perspectives on mathematical and statistical modeling* (pp. 79–132). New York: Academic Press.

Perme, C., & Chandrashekar, R. (2009). Early mobility and walking program for patients in intensive care units: Creating a standard of care. *American Journal of Critical Care, 18*(3), 212–221.

Ramezani, M., Ahmadi, F., Mohammadi, E., & Kazemnejad, A. (2014). Spiritual care in nursing: A concept analysis. *International Nursing Review, 61*(2), 211–219.

Reed, P. (2000). Nursing reformation: Historical reflections and philosophic foundations. *Nursing Science Quarterly, 13*(2), 129–136.

Reynolds, P. (1971). *A primer in theory construction*. Indianapolis, IN: Bobbs-Merrill.

Rhoten, B. A. (2016). Body image disturbance in adults treated for cancer—a concept analysis. *Journal of Advanced Nursing, 72*(5), 1001–1011.

Silva, M. (1986). Research testing nursing theory: State of the art. *Advances in Nursing Science, 9*(10), 1–11.

Sparacino, P. (1991). The reciprocal relationship between practice and theory. *Clinical Nurse Specialist, 5*(3), 138.

Underwood, L. G., & Teresi, J. A. (2002). The daily spiritual experience scale: Development, theoretical description, reliability, exploratory factor analysis, and preliminary construct validity using health-related data. *Annals of Behavioral Medicine, 24*(1), 22–33.

Walker, L., & Avant, K. (2011). *Strategies for theory construction in nursing* (5th ed.). Upper Saddle River, NJ: Prentice Hall.

Wilson, J. (1969). *Thinking with concepts*. Cambridge, MA: Cambridge University Press.

Yancey, N. R. (2015). Why teach nursing theory? *Nursing Science Quarterly, 28*(4), 274–278.

5

The Structure and Analysis of Specialized Nursing Knowledge

Martha Raile Alligood

"The art of nursing is the creative use of the science of nursing for human betterment."
(Rogers, 1990, p. 5)

As presented in Chapter 1, development of the body of specialized knowledge required for nursing to be recognized as a profession was a driving force in the 20th century. Because of the importance of nurses to the nation's health, studies of nursing were legislated early in the century and conducted by sociologists who recommended that nursing be developed as a profession. The criteria for a profession provided guidance in this process (Bixler & Bixler, 1959; Kalisch & Kalisch, 2003). The criterion that called for specialized nursing knowledge and knowledge structure was a particularly important driving force in the recognition of nursing as a profession (Bixler & Bixler, 1959). The criterion reads: "Utilizes in its practice a well-defined and well-organized body of specialized knowledge [that] is on the intellectual level of the higher learning" (p. 1143).

This chapter presents the structure and analysis of specialized nursing knowledge to explain the organization of the text. Specifically, the structure of knowledge that was used to organize the units of the text and the definitions of the analysis criteria used for the review process of the theoretical works in each chapter.

A STRUCTURE OF NURSING KNOWLEDGE

The theoretical works presented in Chapters 6–36 are nursing frameworks that have been organized into types. Box 5.1 lists the theorists who have been selected for each type. The identification of selected works within each of the types is arbitrary at best. Effort has been made to reflect the level of abstraction for each type or preference of the theorist. Types of knowledge, levels, and examples of each within the structure are illustrated in Table 5.1 and discussed in the following text.

The first type is the metaparadigm level that includes the broad conceptual boundaries of nursing knowledge, human beings, health, nursing, and environment (Fawcett, 1984, 2000; Fawcett & DeSanto-Madeya, 2013).

The next type is nursing philosophy. Philosophy is an abstract type that sets forth the meaning of nursing phenomena through analysis, reasoning, and logical presentation. Early works that predate the nursing theory era, such as Nightingale (1969/1859), contributed to knowledge development by providing direction or a basis for subsequent developments. Later works reflect contemporary science methods and approaches (Alligood, 2014b; Chinn & Kramer, 2015; Meleis, 2012). Selected works for the classification of nursing philosophies are presented in Unit II, Chapters 6–11.

The next type, nursing conceptual models, comprises nursing works by theorists referred to by some as pioneers in nursing (Chinn & Kramer, 2015; Meleis, 2012). Conceptual models are a set of concepts that address phenomena central to nursing in propositions that explain relationships among them (Fawcett & DeSanto-Madeya, 2013). The nursing models are comprehensive, and each addresses the metaparadigm concepts of person, environment, health, and nursing (Fawcett, 1984, 2000; Fawcett & DeSanto-Madeya, 2013). The nursing conceptual models have explicit theories derived from them by theorists or other nurse scholars and implicit theories within them yet to be developed (Alligood, 2014a; Wood, 2014). Works classified as nursing models are discussed in Unit III, Chapters 12–18. Theorists who developed nursing conceptual models often proposed a grand theory from their model.

The grand theory level derives from the conceptual model and proposes an abstract testable theory. These theories have the capacity to threaten the solvency of the conceptual model from which they are derived,

BOX 5.1 Types of Nursing Theoretical Works

Nursing Philosophies	
Nightingale	Pender
Watson	Leininger
Ray	Newman
Benner	Parse
Martinsen	Erickson, Tomlin, and Swain
Eriksson	Husted and Husted

Nursing Conceptual Models	Middle-Range Nursing Theories
Levine	Mercer
Rogers	Mishel
Orem	Reed
King	Wiener and Dodd
Neuman	Eakes, Burke, and Hainsworth
Roy	Barker
Johnson	Kolcaba
Nursing Theories and Grand Theories	Beck
Boykin and Schoenhofer	Swanson
Meleis	Ruland and Moore

TABLE 5.1 Knowledge Structure Levels With Selected Examples for Illustration

Structure Level	Examples
Metaparadigm	Human beings, environment, health, and nursing
Philosophy	Nightingale's philosophy
Conceptual models	Neuman's systems model
Grand theory	Neuman's optimal client stability
Theory	Flexible line of defense moderate optimal client stability
Middle-range theory	Maintaining optimal client stability with structured activity (body recall) in a community setting for healthy aging

Modified from Alligood, M. R. (2014). *Nursing theory: Utilization & application* (5th ed.). St Louis: Mosby; Fawcett, J., & DeSanto Madeya, S. (2013). *Contemporary nursing knowledge: Conceptual models of nursing and nursing theories* (3rd ed.). Philadelphia: F. A. Davis.

because they test the major premise of the conceptual model. Examples of this level of grand theory are Roy's theory of the person as an adaptive system, King's theory of goal attainment, and Neuman's theory of optimal client stability (Alligood, 2014b). Interestingly, each of these grand theories has been and continues to be supported.

The nursing theory type comprises works derived from nursing philosophies, conceptual models, grand theories, abstract nursing theories, or works in other disciplines (Alligood, 2014b; Wood, 2014). A work classified as a nursing theory is developed from some conceptual framework or grand theory and is generally not as specific as a middle-range theory. Although some use the terms *model* and *theory* interchangeably, theories propose a testable action (Alligood 2014a, 2014b; Wood, 2014). An example of a grand theory derived from a nursing model is in Roy's work (see Chapter 17) in which she derives the person as an adaptive system from her adaptation model. The abstract level of the grand theory in this example facilitates derivation of theories and middle-range theories specific to nursing practice from it (Alligood 2014a, 2014b). Theories may be specific to a particular aspect or setting of nursing practice. Another example is Meleis's transition theory (see Chapter 20), which is specific to changes in a person's life process in health and illness. Nursing theories are presented in Unit IV, Chapters 19–26.

The last type, middle-range theory, has the most specific focus and is concrete in its level of abstraction (Alligood 2014a, 2014b; Chinn & Kramer, 2015; Fawcett & DeSanto-Madeya, 2013). Middle-range theories propose precise testable nursing practice questions. They address the specifics of nursing situations within the perspective of the model, grand theory, or theory from which they originate (Alligood, 2014a, 2014b; Fawcett & DeSanto-Madeya, 2013; Wood, 2014). The specifics in middle-range theories are such things as the age group of the patient; the family situation; the patient's health condition; the location of the patient; and, most important, the action of the nurse (Alligood, 2014b; Wood, 2014). There are many examples of middle-range theories in the nursing literature that have been developed inductively as well as deductively. Selected middle-range theories are presented in Unit V, Chapters 27–36.

The second aspect of this introduction to Chapters 6–36 and Units II–V is analysis of theory, an essential systematic process of critical reflection that is a vital aspect of review of theoretical works (Chinn & Kramer, 2015). Criteria for analysis of the works of theorists are presented, along with a brief discussion of how each criterion contributes to a deeper understanding of the work (Chinn & Kramer, 2015).

ANALYSIS OF THEORY

Analysis, critique, and evaluation are methods used to study nursing theoretical works critically. Analysis of theory is carried out to acquire knowledge of theoretical adequacy. It is an important process and the first step in applying nursing theoretical works to education, research, administration, or practice. The analysis criteria used for each theoretical work in this text are included in Box 5.2 with the questions that guide the critical reflection of analysis.

The analysis process is useful for learning about the works and is essential for nurse scientists who intend to test, expand, or extend the works. When nurse scientists consider their research interests in the context of one of the theoretical works, areas for further development are discovered through the processes of critique, analysis, and critical reflection. Therefore analysis is an important process for learning, for developing research projects, and for expanding the science associated with the theoretical works of nursing in the future. Understanding a theoretical framework is vital to applying it in practice.

Clarity

Clarity and structure are reviewed in terms of semantic clarity and consistency and structural clarity and consistency. Clarity speaks to the meaning of terms used, and definitional consistency and structure speak to the consistent structural form of terms in the theory. Analysis begins as the major concepts and subconcepts and their definitions are identified. Words have multiple meanings within and across disciplines; therefore a word should be defined specifically according to the framework (philosophy, conceptual model, theory, or middle-range theory) within which it is used. Clarity and consistency are facilitated with diagrams and examples. The logical development and type of structure used should be clear, and assumptions should be stated clearly and be consistent with the goal of the theory (Chinn & Kramer, 2015).

Simplicity

Simplicity is highly valued in nursing theory development. Chinn and Kramer (2015) discuss degrees of simplicity and call for simple forms of theory, such as middle range, to guide practice. Complex practice situations may call for more complex theory. A theory should be sufficiently comprehensive, presented at a level of abstraction to provide guidance, and have as few concepts as possible with as simplistic relations as possible to aid clarity.

BOX 5.2 Questions for Analysis and Critical Reflection of Theoretical Works

- Clarity: How clear is this theory?
- Simplicity: How simple is this theory?
- Generality: How general is this theory?
- Accessibility: How accessible is this theory?
- Importance: How important is this theory?

From Chinn, P. L., & Kramer, M. K. (2015). *Knowledge development in nursing: Theory and process* (9th ed., p. 199). St Louis: Elsevier-Mosby.

Generality

The generality of a theory speaks to the scope of application and the purpose within the theory (Chinn & Kramer, 2015). The generality of a theoretical work varies by how abstract or concrete it is (Fawcett & DeSanto-Madeya, 2013). Understanding the levels of abstraction by doctoral students and nurse scientists has facilitated the use of abstract frameworks and the development of middle-range theories. Rogers' (1986) theory of accelerating change is an example of an abstract theory from which numerous middle-range theories have been generated.

Accessibility

"*Accessible* addresses the extent to which empiric indicators for the concepts can be identified and to what extent the purposes of the theory can be attained" (Chinn & Kramer, 2015, p. 205).

Accessibility is vital to developing nursing research to test a theory. Accessibility facilitates testing, because the empirical indicators provide linkage to practice for testability and ultimate use of a theory to describe and test aspects of practice (Chinn & Kramer, 2015).

Importance

A parallel can be drawn between outcome and importance. Chinn and Kramer (2015) say the central question is, "Does this theory create understanding that is important to nursing?" (p. 207). Because research, theory, and practice are closely related, nursing theory lends itself to research testing, and research testing leads itself to knowledge for practice. Nursing theory guides research and practice, generates new ideas, and differentiates the focus of nursing from other service professions (Chinn & Kramer, 2015).

The five criteria for the analysis of theory—clarity, simplicity, generality, accessibility, and importance—guide the critical reflection of each theoretical work discussed in Chapters 6–36. These broad criteria facilitate the analysis of theoretical works, whether they are applied to works at the level of philosophies, conceptual models, grand theories, theories, or middle-range theories. Box 5.3 describes the content provided in each chapter of Units II–V.

Finally, the content headings in the theorist chapters (6–36) are the same in each chapter to facilitate uniformity for review and comparison of the theorists and their works. A list of the chapter content headings is presented in Box 5.4.

BOX 5.3 Descriptive Content of Divider Pages for Units II-V at a Glance

Unit II: Nursing Philosophies

- Nursing philosophy sets forth the meaning of nursing phenomena through analysis, reasoning, and logical argument.
- Philosophies contribute to nursing knowledge with direction for the discipline, forming a basis for professional scholarship that leads to new theoretical understandings.
- Nursing philosophies represent early works predating the theory era and contemporary works of a philosophical nature.
- Philosophies are works that provide broad understandings that advance the discipline of nursing and its professional applications.

Unit III: Nursing Conceptual Models

- Nursing conceptual models are concepts and their relationships that specify a perspective and produce evidence among phenomenon specific to the discipline.
- Conceptual models address broad metaparadigm concepts (human beings, health, nursing, and environment) that are central to their meaning in the context of a particular framework and the discipline of nursing.
- Nursing conceptual models provide perspectives with different foci for critical thinking about persons, families, and communities and for making knowledgeable nursing decisions.
- Nursing conceptual models provide a nursing perspective for theory development at various levels of abstraction.

Unit IV: Theories and Grand Theories

- Nursing theories describe, explain, or predict outcomes based on relationships among the concepts of nursing phenomena.
- Theories propose relationships by framing a nursing issue and defining relevant terms.
- Nursing theories may be developed at various levels of abstraction.
- Grand nursing theories are considered theory because although they are nearly as abstract as a conceptual model, they propose a testable outcome that tests the major premise of the grand theory.
- Examples of grand theories from nursing models are Roy's theory of the person as an adaptive system, Neuman's theory of optimal client stability, and King's theory of goal attainment. Other grand theory examples might be Erickson's modeling and role modeling, or Meleis's theory of transitions.

Unit V: Middle-Range Theories

- Middle-range theories are the least abstract theory level for concrete practice applications.
- Middle-range theories include the characteristics of nursing practice or situations.
- Middle-range theories are theoretical evidence of applicability and outcome.
- Middle-range theories develop evidence for nursing practice outcomes.
- Middle-range theories are recognizable as such because they contain characteristics of nursing practice.
- Characteristics of middle-range theories include:
  - The situation or health condition of the client/patient
  - Client/patient population or age group
  - Location or area of practice (e.g., community)
  - Action of the nurse or intervention
  - The client/patient outcome anticipated

Presented with thanks from Dr. Alligood to the reviewer who suggested Box 5.3

BOX 5.4 Major Content Headings in Chapters 6–36

- Credentials and Background
- Theoretical Sources for Theory Development
- Use of Empirical Evidence
- Major Concepts and Definitions
- Major Assumptions
- Theoretical Assertions
- Logical Form
- Acceptance by the Nursing Community
- Further Development
- Critique of the Work
- Summary
- Case Study Based on the Work
- Critical Thinking Activities
- Points for Further Study
- References and Bibliography

REFERENCES

Alligood, M. R. (2014a). Areas for further development of theory-based nursing practice. In M. R. Alligood (Ed.), *Nursing theory: Utilization & application* (5th ed., pp. 414–424). St Louis: Mosby-Elsevier.

Alligood, M. R. (2014b). Models and theories: Critical thinking structures. In M. R. Alligood (Ed.), *Nursing theory: Utilization & application* (5th ed., pp. 40–62). St Louis: Mosby-Elsevier.

Bixler, G. K., & Bixler, R. W. (1959). The professional status of nursing. *American Journal of Nursing, 59*(8), 1142–1146.

Chinn, P. L., & Kramer, M. K. (2015). *Integrated knowledge development in nursing* (9th ed.). St Louis: Elsevier-Mosby.

Fawcett, J. (1984). The metaparadigm of nursing: Current status and future refinements. *Image: The Journal of Nursing Scholarship, 16*, 84–87.

Fawcett, J. (2000). *Contemporary nursing knowledge: Conceptual models of nursing and nursing theories*. Philadelphia: F. A. Davis.

Fawcett, J., & DeSanto-Madeya, S. (2013). *Contemporary nursing knowledge: Conceptual models of nursing and nursing theories* (3rd ed.). Philadelphia: F. A. Davis.

Kalisch, P. A., & Kalisch, B. J. (2003). *American nursing: A history* (4th ed.). Philadelphia: Lippincott.

Meleis, A. (2012). *Theoretical nursing: Development and progress* (5th ed.). Philadelphia: Lippincott.

Nightingale, F. (1969). *Notes on nursing: What it is and what it is not*. New York: Dover. (Originally published in 1859.)

Rogers, M. E. (1986). Science of unitary human beings. In V. Malinski (Ed.), *Explorations on Martha Rogers' science of unitary human beings* (pp. 3–14). Norwalk, CT: Appleton, Century, Crofts.

Rogers, M. E. (1990). Nursing: Science of unitary, irreducible human beings. Update 1990. In E. Barrett (Ed.), *Visions of Rogers' science based nursing* (pp. 5–11). New York: National League for Nursing.

Wood, A. F. (2014). Nursing models: Normal science for nursing practice. In M. R. Alligood (Ed.), *Nursing theory: Utilization & application* (5th ed., pp. 13–39). St Louis: Mosby-Elsevier.

UNIT II

Nursing Philosophies

- Nursing philosophy sets forth the meaning of nursing phenomena through analysis, reasoning, and logical argument.
- Philosophies contribute to nursing knowledge with direction for the discipline, forming a basis for professional scholarship leading to new theoretical understandings.
- Nursing philosophies represent early works predating the theory era as well as contemporary works of a philosophical nature.
- Philosophies are works that provide broad understandings that advance the discipline of nursing and its professional applications.

Philosophy
sets forth the meaning of nursing phenomena through analysis, reasoning and logical presentation of concepts and ideas.
Conceptual Models
are sets of concepts that address phenomena central to nursing in propositions that explain the relationship among them.
Grand Theory
concepts that derive from a conceptual model and propose a testable proposition that tests the major premise of the model.
Nursing Theory
testable propositions from philosophies, conceptual models, grand theories, abstract nursing theories, or theories from other disciplines. Theories are less abstract than grand theory and less specific than middle-range theory.
Middle-Range Theory
concepts most specific to practice that propose precise testable nursing practice questions and include details such as patient age group, family situation, health condition, location of the patient, and action of the nurse.
The Future of Nursing Theory
Nursing theoretical systems give direction and create understanding in practice, research, administration, and education.
Metaparadigm
The broad conceptual boundaries of the discipline of nursing: Human beings, environment, health, and nursing

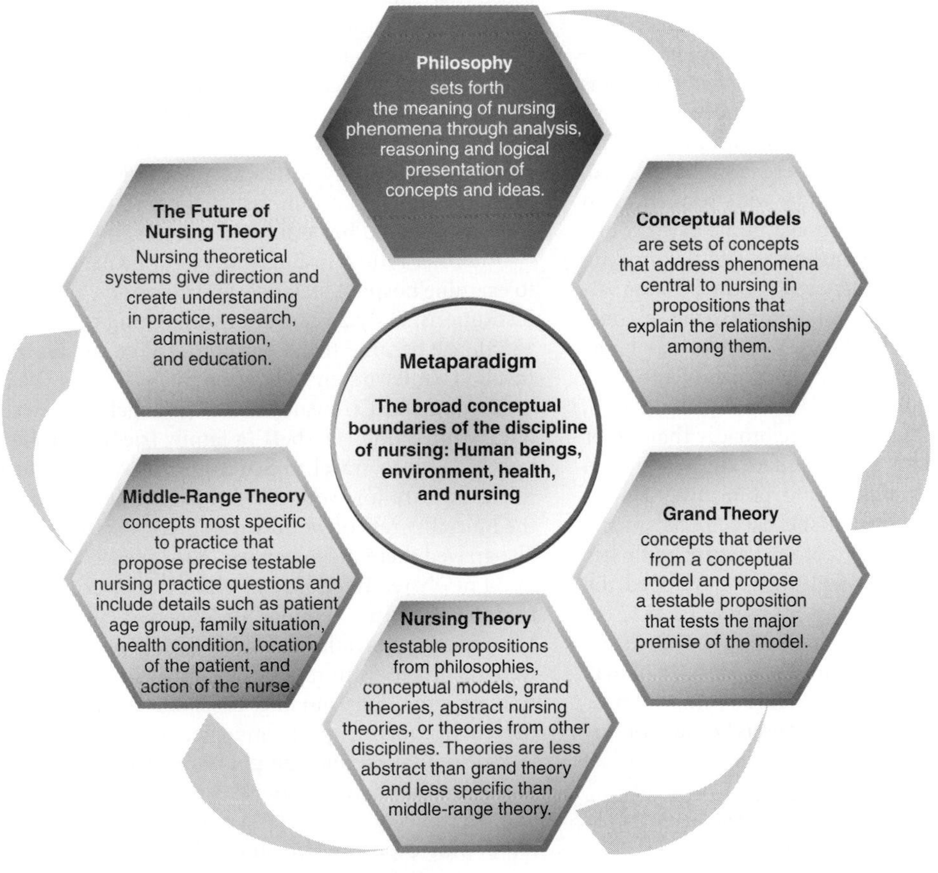

6

Modern Nursing

*Susan A. Pfettscher**

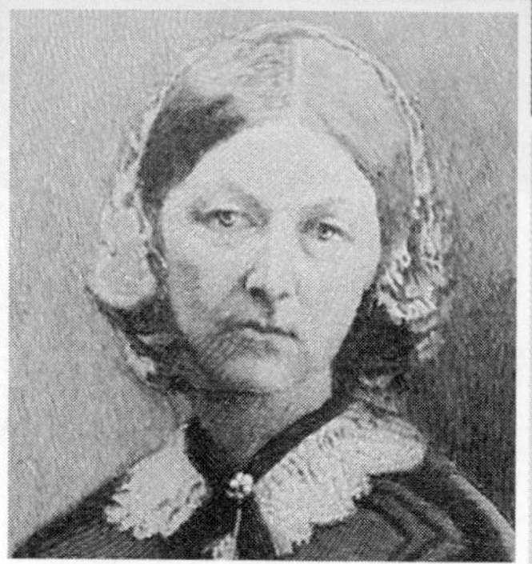

Florence Nightingale
1820–1910

"Recognition of nursing as a professional endeavor distinct from medicine began with Nightingale."

(Chinn & Kramer, 2015, p. 26)

CREDENTIALS AND BACKGROUND OF THE THEORIST

Florence Nightingale, the founder of modern nursing, was born on May 12, 1820, in Florence, Italy, while her parents were on an extended European tour; she was named after her birthplace. The Nightingales were a well-educated, affluent, aristocratic Victorian family with residences in Derbyshire (Lea Hurst was their primary home in the country near the family's tanning business) and Hampshire (Embley Park). This latter residence was near London, allowing the family to participate in London's social seasons.

Although the extended Nightingale family was large, the immediate family included only Florence Nightingale and her older sister, Parthenope. During her childhood, Nightingale's father educated her more broadly than other girls of the time. Her father and others tutored her in mathematics, languages, religion, and philosophy (influences on her lifework). Although she participated in the usual Victorian social activities commensurate with her status during her adolescence, Nightingale developed the sense that her life should become more useful. In 1837 (at age 17), Nightingale wrote about her "calling" in her diary: "God spoke to me and called me to his service" (Holliday & Parker, 1997, p. 491). Although she had suitors who proposed marriage, she rejected their proposals because of this sense that she should do something else in her life. The nature of her calling was unclear to her for some time; her family attempted to dissuade her from such an idea and plan. After she understood that she was called to become a nurse, she was finally able to complete her nursing training in 1851 (at age 31) at Kaiserwerth, Germany, a Protestant religious community with a hospital facility. She was there for approximately 3 months; at the end of that time, her teachers declared her trained as a nurse.

After her return to England, Nightingale was employed to examine hospital facilities, reformatories, and charitable institutions. Only 2 years after completing her training (in 1853), she became the superintendent of the Hospital for Invalid Gentlewomen in London.

During the Crimean War, Nightingale received a request from Sidney Herbert (a family friend and the Secretary of War) to travel to Scutari, Turkey, with a group of nurses to care for wounded British soldiers; at that time, the mortality rate of wounded soldiers was incredibly high. She arrived there in November 1854 (age 34) accompanied by 34 newly recruited nurses who met her criteria for professional nursing—young, middle-class women with a basic general education (not the usual type of women who were identified as nurses in England). To achieve her mission of providing nursing care, she needed to address the environmental problems that existed, including the lack of sanitation and the presence of filth (few chamber pots, contaminated water, contaminated bed linens, and overflowing cesspools). In addition, the soldiers were faced with exposure, frostbite, louse infestations, wound

---

*Previous authors: Karen R. de Graff, Ann Marriner Tomey, Cynthia L. Mossman, and Maribeth Slebodnik.

infections, and opportunistic diseases as they recovered from their battle wounds.

Nightingale's work in improving these deplorable environmental conditions made her a popular and revered person to the soldiers, but the support of physicians and military officers was less enthusiastic. She was called The Lady of the Lamp, as immortalized in the poem "Santa Filomena" (Longfellow, 1857), because she made ward rounds during the night, providing emotional comfort to the soldiers. In Scutari, Nightingale became critically ill with Crimean fever, which might have been typhus or brucellosis and which may have affected her physical condition for years afterward.

After the war, Nightingale returned to England to great accolades, particularly from the royal family (Queen Victoria), the soldiers who had survived the Crimean War, their families, and the families of those who died at Scutari. She rejected much of the attention and arrived at the family home in Lea Hurst without any announcement or fanfare. She was awarded funds in recognition of her work, which she used to establish schools for nursing training at St. Thomas's Hospital and King's College Hospital in London. Within a few years, the Nightingale School began to receive requests to establish new schools at hospitals worldwide, and Florence Nightingale's reputation as the founder of modern nursing was established.

Nightingale devoted her energies not only to the development of nursing as a vocation (profession), but even more to local, national, and international societal issues in an attempt to improve the living environment of the poor and to create social change. She continued to concentrate on army sanitation reform, the functions of army hospitals, sanitation in India, and sanitation and health care for the poor in England. Her writings, *Notes on Matters Affecting the Health, Efficiency, and Hospital Administration of the British Army Founded Chiefly on the Experience of the Late War* (Nightingale, 1858b), *Notes on Hospitals* (Nightingale, 1858a), and *Report on Measures Adopted for Sanitary Improvements in India, from June 1869 to June 1870* (Nightingale, 1871), reflect her continuing concern about these issues.

Shortly after her return to England, Nightingale confined herself to her residence in London, citing her continued ill health. However, she remained most productive in that state of health and isolation. Until 80 years of age, she wrote between 15,000 and 20,000 letters to friends, acquaintances, allies, and opponents. Her strong, clear written words conveyed her beliefs, observations, and plans for change in health care and in society. Through these writings, she was able to influence issues in the world that concerned her. When necessary and when her health allowed, Nightingale received powerful visitors in her home to maintain dialogue, plot strategies to support causes, and carry out her work.

During her lifetime, Nightingale's work was recognized through the many awards she received from her own country and from many others. She was able to work into her 80s until she lost her vision; she died in her sleep on August 13, 1910, at 90 years of age.

Modern biographers and essayists have attempted to analyze Nightingale's lifework through her family relationships, notably with her parents and sister. Film dramatizations commonly and inaccurately focus on her personal relationships with family and friends. Although her personal and public life holds great intrigue for many, these retrospective analyses are often very negative and harshly critical or overly positive in their descriptions of this Victorian leader and founder of modern nursing. Many biographies have been written to describe Nightingale's life and work. Cook (1913) wrote the first original and comprehensive biography of Nightingale, which was based on her written papers, but it may have been biased by her family's involvement in and oversight of the project. It remains the most positive biography written. Shortly thereafter, Strachey (1918) described her negatively as arrogant and manipulative in his book, *Eminent Victorians.* O'Malley (1931) wrote a more positive biography that focused on her life from 1820 to 1856; however, the second volume, which would have described the rest of her life and activities, was never published. Woodham-Smith's (1951) book chronicled her entire life and was drawn primarily from original documents made available by her family. This is the biography with which most Americans are familiar; it has endured as the definitive biography of Nightingale's life, and although it is more balanced, it maintains a positive tone. F. B. Smith (1982) wrote *Florence Nightingale: Reputation and Power,* which is critical of Nightingale's character and her work. Small (1998) published yet another Nightingale biography titled *Florence Nightingale: Avenging Angel.* Although he is critical of specific aspects of her character and work, Small is more balanced in his presentation. He notes that Nightingale's life "is better documented than perhaps any previous life in history" because of the vast quantity of family and personal papers that remain available today (Small, 2000). His concerns and disagreements with other biographers have been noted in reviews (Small, 2008). Small continues to study Nightingale and updates his website with additional information about the Crimean War and Nightingale. The controversy and intrigue about Nightingale's role, her status, and her confined lifestyle continue; a London newspaper recently reported on newly found letters related to the conflicts Nightingale had with Sir John Hall (chief British army medical officer in the Crimea) (Kennedy, 2007). An

Internet search reveals thousands of sites that provide various articles, resources, and commentaries about Nightingale. Clearly, the world still is fascinated by this unique woman.

The nursing community in the United States remains similarly fascinated by the life and work of Nightingale. During their professional careers, Kalisch and Kalisch (1983a, 1983b, 1987) published several critiques of media portrayals that provide a better understanding of the many histories of Florence Nightingale; their techniques may provide methods of analyzing more recent publications and events for persons interested in studying Nightingale's life and work. Dossey's (2000) comprehensive book, *Florence Nightingale: Mystic, Visionary, Healer,* provides another in-depth history and interpretation of Nightingale's personal life and work. Using quotes from Nightingale's own writings (diaries and letters) and from people with whom she interacted and corresponded during her lifetime, Dossey focused on interpreting the spiritual nature of her being and her lifework, creating yet another way of looking at Nightingale. In an introduction/prelude to her descriptions of spirituality for nurses' lives based on Nightingale's writings, Macrae (2001) explores Nightingale's personal spirituality as she interprets it after review of writings and documents. Lorentzon (2003) more recently has provided a review and analysis of letters written between Nightingale and one of her former students that clearly demonstrate her role as mentor.

Finally, all of Nightingale's surviving writings are in the process of being published as *The Collected Works of Florence Nightingale.* All 16 volumes have been published under the leadership of sociologist and Nightingale scholar Lynn McDonald (2001–2012). This large project and other newly discovered and released documents continue to spawn articles and books that explore, interpret, and speculate on Nightingale's life and work. In addition, she has published a new biography of Nightingale (McDonald, 2010a).

THEORETICAL SOURCES FOR THEORY DEVELOPMENT

Many factors influenced the development of Nightingale's philosophy of nursing. Her personal, societal, and professional values and concerns all were integral to the development of her beliefs. She combined her individual resources with societal and professional resources available to her to produce immediate and long-term change throughout the world.

As noted, Nightingale's education was an unusual one for a Victorian girl. Her tutelage by her well-educated, intellectual father in subjects such as mathematics and philosophy provided her with knowledge and conceptual thinking abilities that were unique for women of her time. Although her parents initially opposed her desire to study mathematics, they relented and allowed her to receive additional tutoring from well-respected mathematicians. Her aunt Mai, a devoted relative and companion, described her as having a great mind; this is not a description that was used at the time for Victorian women, but it is one that was accepted for Nightingale. It remains unknown whether or not Nightingale was a genius who would have been a great leader and thinker under any circumstance, or whether her unique, formal education and social status were necessary for this to occur at the time. Would Nightingale become such a leader if born today? What would nursing be today if she had not been born at that time and in that place?

The Nightingale family's aristocratic social status provided her with easy access to people of power and influence. Many were family friends, such as Stanley Herbert, who remained an ally and staunch supporter until his death. Nightingale learned to understand the political processes of Victorian England through the experiences of her father during his short-lived political career and through his continuing role as an aristocrat involved in the political and social activities of his community. She most likely relied on this foundation and on her own experiences as she waged political battles for her causes.

Nightingale also recognized the societal changes of her time and their impact on the health status of individuals. The industrial age had descended upon England, creating new social classes, new diseases, and new social problems. Dickens' social commentaries and novels provided English society with scathing commentaries on health care and the need for health and social reform in England. In his serialized novel (1843–44), *Martin Chuzzlewit* (Dickens, 1987), Dickens' portrayal of Sairey Gamp as a drunken, untrained nurse provided society with an image of the horrors of Victorian nursing practice. Nightingale's alliance with Dickens undoubtedly influenced her definitions of nursing and health care and her theory for nursing; that relationship also provided her with a forum for expressing her views about social and health care issues (Dossey, 2000; Kalisch & Kalisch, 1983a; Woodham-Smith, 1951).

Similar dialogues with political leaders, intellectuals, and social reformers of the day (John Stuart Mill, Benjamin Jowett, Edwin Chadwick, and Harriet Marineau) advanced Nightingale's philosophical and logical thinking, which is evident in her philosophy and theory of nursing (Dossey, 2000; Kalisch & Kalisch, 1983a; Woodham-Smith, 1951). These dialogues likely inspired her to strive to change the things she viewed as unacceptable in the society in which she lived.

Finally, Nightingale's religious affiliation and beliefs were especially strong sources for her nursing theory. Reared as a Unitarian, her belief that action for the benefit of others is a primary way of serving God served as the foundation for defining her nursing work as a religious calling. In addition, the Unitarian community strongly supported education as a means of developing divine potential and helping people move toward perfection in their lives and in their service to God. Nightingale's faith provided her with personal strength throughout her life and with the belief that education was a critical factor in establishing the profession of nursing. Also, religious conflicts of the time, particularly between the Anglican and Catholic Churches in the British Empire, may have led to her strongly held belief that nursing could and should be a secular profession (Dossey, 2000; Helmstadter, 1997; Nelson, 1997; Woodham-Smith, 1951). Despite her strong religious beliefs and her acknowledgment of her calling, this was not a requirement for her nurses. Indeed, her opposition to the work of the nuns in Crimea (she reported that they were proselytizing) escalated the conflict to the level of involvement of the Vatican (Dossey, 2000; Woodham-Smith, 1951). Nelson's review of pastoral care in the 19th century provides an interesting historical view of the role of religious service in nursing (Nelson, 1997).

MAJOR CONCEPTS & DEFINITIONS

Nightingale's theory focused on environment; however, Nightingale used the term *surroundings* in her writing. She defined and described the concepts of *ventilation, warmth, light, diet, cleanliness,* and *noise*—components of surroundings usually referred to as *environment* in discussions of her work. When reading *Notes on Nursing* (Nightingale, 1969), one can easily identify an emphasis on the physical environment. In the context of issues Nightingale identified and struggled to improve (war-torn environments and workhouses), this emphasis appears to be most appropriate (Gropper, 1990). Her concern about healthy surroundings involved hospital settings in Crimea and England, and also extended to the public in their private homes and to the physical living conditions of the poor. She believed that healthy surroundings were necessary for proper nursing care and the restoration and maintenance of health. Her theoretical work on five essential components of environmental health (*pure air, light, cleanliness, efficient drainage,* and *pure water*) is as relevant today as it was 150 years ago.

1. Pure air. Proper ventilation for the patient seemed to be of greatest concern to Nightingale; her charge to nurses was to "keep the air he breathes as pure as the external air, without chilling him" (Nightingale, 1969, p. 12). Nightingale's emphasis on proper ventilation indicates that she recognized the surroundings as a source of disease and recovery. In addition to discussing ventilation in the room or home, Nightingale provided a description for measuring the patient's body temperature through palpation of extremities to check for heat loss (Nightingale, 1969). The nurse was instructed to manipulate the surroundings to maintain ventilation and patient warmth by using a good fire, opening windows, and properly positioning the patient in the room.
2. Light. The concept of light was also of importance in Nightingale's theory. In particular, she identified direct sunlight as a particular need of patients. She noted that "light has quite as real and tangible effects upon the human body. . . . Who has not observed the purifying effect of light, and especially of direct sunlight, upon the air of a room?" (Nightingale, 1969, pp. 84–85). To achieve the beneficial effects of sunlight, nurses were instructed to move and position patients to expose them to sunlight.
3. Cleanliness is another critical component of Nightingale's environmental theory (Nightingale, 1969). In this regard, she specifically addressed the patient, the nurse, and the physical environment. She noted that a dirty environment (floors, carpets, walls, and bed linens) was a source of infection through the organic matter it contained.
4. Efficient drainage. Even if the environment was well ventilated, the presence of organic material created a dirty area; therefore appropriate handling and disposal of bodily excretions and sewage were required to prevent contamination of the environment.
5. Pure water. Finally, Nightingale advocated bathing patients on a frequent, even daily, basis at a time when this practice was not the norm. She required that nurses also bathe daily, that their clothing be clean, and that they wash their hands frequently (Nightingale, 1969). This concept held special significance for individual patient care, and it was critically important in improving the health status of the poor who were living in crowded, environmentally inferior conditions with inadequate sewage and limited access to pure water (Nightingale, 1969).

Nightingale included the concepts of *quiet* and *diet* in her theory. The nurse was required to assess the need for quiet and to intervene as needed to maintain it (Nightingale,

Continued

MAJOR CONCEPTS & DEFINITIONS—cont'd

1969). Noise created by physical activities in the areas around a patient's room was to be prevented, because it could harm the patient. Nightingale was also concerned about the patient's diet (Nightingale, 1969). She instructed nurses to assess not only dietary intake, but also the meal schedule and its effect on the patient. She believed that patients with chronic illness could be starved to death unintentionally and that intelligent nurses successfully met patients' nutritional needs.

Another component of Nightingale's writing was a description of petty management (nursing administration) (Nightingale, 1969). She pointed out that the nurse was in control of the environment both physically and administratively. The nurse was to protect the patient from receipt of upsetting news, seeing visitors who could negatively affect recovery, and experiencing sudden disruptions of sleep. In addition, Nightingale recognized that pet visits (small animals) might be of comfort to the patient. Nightingale believed that the nurse remained in charge of the environment, even when she was not physically present, because she should oversee others who worked in her absence.

USE OF EMPIRICAL EVIDENCE

Nightingale's reports describing health and sanitary conditions in Crimea and in England identify her as an outstanding scientist and empirical researcher. Her expertise as a statistician is evident in the reports that she generated throughout her lifetime on the varied subjects of health care, nursing, and social reform.

Nightingale's carefully collected information that illustrated the efficacy of her hospital nursing system and organization during the Crimean War is perhaps her best-known work. Her report of her experiences and collected data was submitted to the British Royal Sanitary Commission in *Notes on Matters Affecting the Health, Efficiency, and Hospital Administration of the British Army Founded Chiefly on the Experience of the Late War* (Nightingale, 1858b). This Commission had been organized in response to Nightingale's charges of poor sanitary conditions. The data in this report provided a strong argument in favor of her proposed reforms in the Crimean hospital barracks. According to Cohen (1984), she created the polar area diagram to represent dramatically the extent of needless death in British military hospitals in Crimea. In this article, Cohen summarized the work of Nightingale as both a researcher and a statistician by noting that "she helped to pioneer the revolutionary notion that social phenomena could be objectively measured and subjected to mathematical analysis" (1984, p. 128). Palmer (1977) described Nightingale's research skills as including recording, communicating, ordering, coding, conceptualizing, inferring, analyzing, and synthesizing. The observation of social phenomena at both individual and systems levels was especially important to Nightingale and served as the basis of her writings. Nightingale emphasized the concurrent use of observation and performance of tasks in the education of nurses and expected them to continue to use both of these activities in their work.

MAJOR ASSUMPTIONS

Nursing

Nightingale believed that every woman, at one time in her life, would be a nurse in the sense that nursing is being responsible for someone else's health. Nightingale wrote *Notes on Nursing,* published originally in 1859, to provide women with guidelines for caring for their loved ones at home and to give advice on how to "think like a nurse" (Nightingale, 1969, p. 4). Trained nurses, however, were to learn additional scientific principles to be applied in their work and were to be more skilled in observing and reporting patients' health status while providing care as the patient recovered.

Person

In most of her writings, Nightingale referred to the person as a *patient.* Nurses performed tasks to and for the patient and controlled the patient's environment to enhance recovery. For the most part, Nightingale described a passive patient in this relationship. However, specific references are made to the patient performing self-care when possible and, in particular, being involved in the timing and substance of meals. The nurse was to ask the patient about his or her preferences, which reveals the belief that Nightingale saw each patient as an individual. However, Nightingale (1969) emphasized that the nurse was in control of and responsible for the patient's environmental surroundings. Nightingale had respect for persons of various backgrounds and was not judgmental about social worth.

Health

Nightingale defined health as being well and using every power (resource) to the fullest extent in living life. In addition, she saw disease and illness as a reparative process that nature instituted when a person did not attend to health concerns. Nightingale envisioned the maintenance of health through prevention of disease by environmental control and social responsibility. What she described led to public health nursing and the more modern concept of health promotion. She distinguished the concept of health nursing as different from nursing a sick patient to enhance recovery, and from living better until peaceful death. Her concept of health nursing exists today in the role of district nurses and health workers in England and in other countries where lay health care workers are used to maintain health and teach people how to prevent disease and illness. Her concept of health nursing is a model used by many public health agencies and departments in the United States.

Environment

Nightingale's concept of environment emphasized that nursing was to assist nature in healing the patient. Little, if anything, in the patient's world is excluded from her definition of environment. Her admonition to nurses, both those providing care in the home and trained nurses in hospitals, was to create and maintain a therapeutic environment that would enhance the comfort and recovery of the patient. Her treatise on rural hygiene includes an incredibly specific description of environmental problems and their results, as well as practical solutions to these problems for households and communities (Halsall, 1997).

Nightingale's assumptions and understanding about the environmental conditions of the day were most relevant to her philosophy. She believed that sick poor people would benefit from environmental improvements that would affect both their bodies and their minds. She believed that nurses could be instrumental in changing the social status of the poor by improving their physical living conditions.

Many aristocrats of the time were unaware of the living conditions of the poor. Nightingale's mother, however, had visited and provided care to poor families in the communities surrounding their estates; Nightingale accompanied her on these visits as a child and continued them when she was older. Thus Nightingale's understandings of physical surroundings and their effect on health were acquired through first-hand observation and experience beyond her own comfortable living situation.

THEORETICAL ASSERTIONS

Nightingale believed that disease was a reparative process; disease was nature's effort to remedy a process of poisoning or decay, or it was a reaction against the conditions in which a person was placed. Although these concepts seem ridiculous today, they were more scientific than the prevailing ones of the time (e.g., disease as punishment). She often capitalized the word *Nature* in her writings, thereby suggesting that it was synonymous with God. Her Unitarian religious beliefs would support this view of God as nature. However, when she used the word *nature* without capitalization, it is unclear whether or not the intended meaning is different and perhaps synonymous with an organic pathological process. Nightingale believed that the role of nursing was to prevent an interruption of the reparative process and to provide optimal conditions for its enhancement, thus ensuring the patient's recovery.

Nightingale was totally committed to nursing education (training). She wrote *Notes on Nursing* (1969) for women caregivers, making a distinction between the role of household servants and those trained specifically as nurses to provide care for the sick person. Nightingale (1969) believed that nurses needed to be excellent observers of patients and the environment; observation was an ongoing activity for trained nurses. In addition, she believed that nurses should use common sense in practice, coupled with observation, perseverance, and ingenuity. Finally, Nightingale believed that people desired good health, that they would cooperate with the nurse and nature to allow the reparative process to occur, and that they would alter their environment to prevent disease.

Although Nightingale has been ridiculed for saying she didn't embrace the germ theory, she very clearly understood the concept of contagion and contamination through organic materials from the patient and the environment. Many of her observations are consistent with the concepts of infection and the germ theory; for example, she embraced the concept of vaccination against various diseases. Small (2008) argues that Nightingale did indeed believe in a germ theory but not in the one that suggests that disease germs cause inevitable infection. Such a theory was antithetical to her belief that sanitation and good hygiene could prevent infection. Her belief that appropriate manipulation of the environment could prevent disease underlies modern sanitation activities.

Nightingale did not explicitly discuss the caring behaviors of nurses. She wrote very little about interpersonal relationships, except as they influence the patient's reparative processes. She did describe the phenomenon of being called to nursing and the need for commitment to nursing work. Her own example of nursing practice in Crimea provides evidence of caring behaviors. These include her commitment to observing patients at night, a new concept and practice; sitting with them during the dying process; standing beside them during surgical procedures; writing letters for them; and providing a reading room and materials during their recuperation. Finally, she wrote letters to soldiers' families after their deaths. Watson (2010) defines Nightingale's descriptions and behaviors as a "blueprint for transpersonal meanings and models of caring" (p. 107). Neils (2010) describes a nursing role of caring as a liaison nurse based on Nightingale's description of rounding. She interprets this activity as a way of expressing caring and spiritual support while also achieving other nursing observations. Straughair (2012) reports that a loss of compassion in nursing (as a component of caring) was identified by patients in the National Health Service in England and pleads for nursing attention to this aspect of Nightingale's Christian ideal of professional nursing.

Similarly, both Burkhart and Hogan (2008) and Wu and Lin (2011) have conducted research to identify the spiritual care in nursing practice as first described by Nightingale. The settings of these studies (United States and Taiwan) reflect the universality of Nightingale's work. Straughair (2012) makes the case that there needs to be a rediscovery of the compassion that appears to be diminishing in modern nursing. Finally, Wagner and White (2010) explore and analyze "caring relationships" in Nightingale's own writings. This historical study contributes to our understanding of how Nightingale described the modern concept of caring.

Nightingale believed that nurses should be moral agents. She addressed their professional relationship with their patients; she instructed them on the principle of confidentiality and advocated for care of the poor to improve their health and social situations. In addition, she commented on patient decision making, a component of a relevant modern ethical concept. Nightingale (1969) called for concise and clear decision making by the nurse and physician regarding the patient, noting that indecision (irresolution) or changing the mind is more harmful to the patient than the patient having to make a decision. Hoyt (2010) analyzed how Nightingale defined nursing as an ethical profession and the ethical practices embedded in nursing.

LOGICAL FORM

Nightingale used inductive reasoning to extract laws of health, disease, and nursing from her observations and experiences. Her childhood education, particularly in philosophy and mathematics, may have contributed to her logical thinking and inductive reasoning abilities. For example, her observations of the conditions in the Scutari hospital led her to conclude that the contaminated, dirty, dark environment led to disease. Not only did she prevent disease from flourishing in such an environment, but she also validated the outcome by careful record keeping. From her own training, her brief experience as a superintendent in London, and her experiences in Crimea, she made observations and established principles for nurse training and patient care (Nightingale, 1969).

ACCEPTANCE BY THE NURSING COMMUNITY

Practice

Nightingale's nursing principles remain the foundation of nursing practice today. The environmental aspects of her theory (i.e., ventilation, warmth, quiet, diet, and cleanliness) remain integral components of nursing care. As nurses practice in the 21st century, the relevance of her concepts continues; in fact, they have increased relevance as a global society faces new issues of disease control. Although modern sanitation and water treatment have controlled traditional sources of disease fairly successfully in the United States, contaminated water resulting from environmental changes or from the introduction of uncommon contaminants remains a health issue in many communities. Global travel has altered dramatically the actual and potential spread of disease. Modern sanitation, adequate water treatment, and recognition and control of other methods of disease transmission remain challenges for nurses worldwide.

New environmental concerns have been created by modern architecture (e.g., sick-building syndrome); nurses need to ask whether modern, environmentally controlled buildings meet Nightingale's principle of good ventilation. On the other hand, controlled environments increasingly protect the public from second-hand cigarette smoke, toxic gases, automobile emissions, and other environmental hazards. Disposal of these wastes, including toxic waste, and the use of chemicals in modern society challenge professional nurses and other health care professionals to reassess the concept of a healthy environment (Butterfield, 1999; Gropper, 1990; Sessler, 1999). Shaner-McRae, McRae, and Jas (2007) described environmental conditions of our hospitals that affect not only the individual patient environment but also the larger environment, incorporating multiple environmental concepts identified by Nightingale. Although they focus on Western hospitals, it is evident that this is a global challenge for nurses.

In health care facilities, the ability to control room temperature for an individual patient is increasingly difficult. This environment may also create significant noise through activities and the technology (equipment) used to assist the patient's reparative process. Nurses have taken a scholarly look at these problems as they continue to affect patients and the health care system (McCarthy, Ouimet, & Daun, 1991; McLaughlin et al., 1996; Pope, 1995).

Monteiro (1985) provided the American public health community with a comprehensive review of Nightingale's work as a sanitarian and a social reformer, reminding them of the extent of her impact on health care in various settings and her concern about poverty and sanitation issues. Although other disciplines in the United States have increasingly addressed such issues, it is clear that nurses and nursing have an active role in providing direct patient care and in becoming involved in the social and political arenas to ensure healthy environments for all citizens.

McPhaul and Lipscomb (2005) have applied Nightingale's environmental principles to practice in occupational health nursing. These nurse specialists have increasingly recognized current environmental health problems at local, regional, and global levels. Modern changes in travel, migration, and the physical environment are causing health problems for many.

Infectious diseases (e.g., HIV, tuberculosis [TB], West Nile virus, Ebola, and Zika) are examples of these changes. In addition, nurses are confronted by an epidemic of toxic substances and nosocomial infections and the development of resistant organisms (e.g., methicillin-resistant *Staphylococcus aureus* [MRSA]) in their patient care environments; first-line prevention measures of handwashing and environmental cleanliness harken back to Nightingale's original environmental theory and principles. Other problems created by environmental changes and pollution might astound Nightingale, but she would probably approach them in a typically aggressive fashion for control. As health care systems and providers struggle to promote patient safety through prevention of infection in health care facilities, this work can be framed in these words of Florence Nightingale: "It seems a strange principle to enunciate, as the very first requirement, in a hospital that it should Do the Sick No Harm" (Vincent, 2010, p. 5).

Although some of Nightingale's rationales have been modified or disproved by medical advances and scientific discovery, many of her concepts have endured the tests of time and technological advances. It is clear that much of her theory remains relevant for nursing today. Concepts from Nightingale's writings, from political commentary to scholarly research, continue to be cited in the nursing literature (Medeiros et al., 2015).

Several authors have analyzed Nightingale's petty management concepts and actions, identifying the timelessness and universality of some of her management style (Decker & Farley, 1991; Henry, Woods, & Nagelkerk, 1990; Monteiro, 1985). Lorentzon (2003) focused specifically on Nightingale's role as a mentor to a former student in her review and analysis of letters written between her and her former student Rachel Williams. This analysis provides a review of mentoring approaches based on Nightingale's theories; her comments on management as offered to Rachel Williams would stimulate good discussion about the needs of nurses today for mentoring and professional development. Lannon (2007) and Narayanasamy and Narayanasamy (2007) based their examinations of nursing staff and leadership development on Nightingale's statements about the essential need for continued learning in nursing practice.

Finally, several writers have analyzed Nightingale's role in the suffrage movement, especially in the context of feminist theory development. Although she has been criticized for not actively participating in this movement, Nightingale indicated in a letter to John Stuart Mill that she could do work for women in other ways (Woodham-Smith, 1951). Her essay *Cassandra* (Nightingale, 1852) reflects support for the concept that is now known as feminism. Scholars continue to assess and analyze her role in the feminist movement of this modern era (Dossey, 2000; Hektor, 1994; Holliday & Parker, 1997; Selanders, 2010a; Welch, 1990). Selanders (2010a) argues powerfully that Nightingale was a feminist and that her beliefs as a feminist were integral to the development of modern professional nursing.

Education

Nightingale's principles of nurse training (instruction in scientific principles and practical experience for the mastery of skills) provided a universal template for early nurse training schools, beginning with St. Thomas's Hospital and King's College Hospital in London. Using the Nightingale model of nurse training, three experimental schools were established in the United States in 1873 (Ashley, 1976):

1. Bellevue Hospital in New York
2. New Haven Hospital in Connecticut
3. Massachusetts Hospital in Boston

The influence of this training system and of many of its principles is still evident in today's nursing programs. Although Nightingale advocated independence of the nursing school from a hospital to ensure that students would not become involved in the hospital's labor pool as part of their training, American nursing schools were unable to achieve such independence for many years (Ashley, 1976). Nightingale (Decker & Farley, 1991) believed that the art of nursing could not be measured by licensing examinations, but she used testing methods, including case studies (notes), for nursing probationers at St. Thomas's Hospital.

Clearly, Nightingale understood that good practice could result only from good education. This message resounds throughout her writings on nursing. Nightingale historian Joanne Farley responded to a modern nursing student by noting that "Training is to teach a nurse to know her business. . . . Training is to enable the nurse to act for the best . . . like an intelligent and responsible being" (Decker & Farley, 1991, pp. 12–13). It is difficult to imagine what the care of sick human beings would be like if Nightingale had not defined the educational needs of nurses and established these first schools.

Research

Nightingale's interest in scientific inquiry and statistics continues to define the scientific inquiry used in nursing research. She was exceptionally efficient and resourceful in her ability to gather and analyze data; her ability to represent data graphically was first identified in the polar diagrams, the graphical illustration style that she invented (Agnew, 1958; Cohen, 1984; McDonald, 2010b). Her empirical approach to solving problems of health care delivery is obvious in the data that she included in her numerous reports and letters.

When Nightingale's writings are defined and analyzed as theory, they are seen to present a philosophical approach that is applicable in modern nursing today. Concepts that Nightingale identified serve as the basis for research, adding to modern nursing science and practice throughout the world. Most notable is her focus on surroundings (environment) and their importance to nursing.

Current nurse writers and researchers have described this aspect of Nightingale's work as her "Environmental Theory." Medeiros et al. (2015) organized her writings about surroundings and environment and conducted an analysis of theory based on Johnson and Webber's model; they determined that Nightingale's environmental theory serves today's parameters with landmark relevance. Similarly, Zborowsky (2014) refers to Nightingale's environmental theory and its resonance on today's health care environments. Finally, Selanders (2010b) describes nursing practice as one "environmental adaptation."

FURTHER DEVELOPMENT

Nightingale's philosophy and theory of nursing are stated clearly and concisely in *Notes on Nursing* (1969), Nightingale's most widely known and read work. In this writing, she provides guidance for care of the sick and in so doing clarifies what nursing is and what it is not. The content of the text seems most amenable to theory analysis. Hardy (1978) proposed that Nightingale formulated a grand theory that explains the totality of behavior. As knowledge of nursing theory has developed, Nightingale's work has come to be recognized as a philosophy of nursing. Although some formulations have been tested, most often principles are derived from anecdotal situations to illustrate their meaning and support their claims. Her work is often discussed as a theory, and it is clear that Nightingale's premises provide a foundation for the development of both nursing practice and current nursing theories. Tourville and Ingalls (2003) described Nightingale as the trunk of the living tree of nursing theories.

CRITIQUE

Clarity

Nightingale's work is clear and easily understood. It addresses three major relationships:

1. Environment to patient
2. Nurse to environment
3. Nurse to patient

Nightingale believed that the environment was the main factor that created illness in a patient and regarded disease as "the reactions of kindly nature against the conditions in which we have placed ourselves" (Nightingale, 1969, p. 56). She recognized the potential harmfulness of an environment and emphasized the benefit of a good environment in preventing disease.

The nurse's practice includes manipulation of the environment in a number of ways to enhance patient recovery. Elimination of contamination and contagion and exposure to fresh air, light, warmth, and quiet were identified as elements to be controlled or manipulated in the environment. Nightingale began to develop relationships between some of these elements in her discussions of contamination and ventilation, light and patient position in the room, cleanliness and darkness, and noise and patient stimulation. She also described the relationship between the sickroom and the rest of the house and the relationship between the house and the surrounding neighborhood.

The nurse-patient relationship may be the least well defined in Nightingale's writings. Yet cooperation and collaboration between the nurse and patient are suggested in her discussions of a patient's eating patterns and preferences, the comfort of a beloved pet to the patient, protection of the patient from emotional distress, and conservation of energy while allowing the patient to participate in self-care. Finally, it is interesting to note that Nightingale discussed the concept of observation extensively, including its use to guide the care of patients and to measure improvement or lack of response to nursing interventions.

Simplicity

Nightingale provides a descriptive, explanatory theory. Its environmental focus, along with its epidemiological components, has predictive potential. Nightingale could be said to have tested her theory in an informal manner by collecting data and verifying improvements. She used brief case studies, possible exemplars, to illustrate a number of the concepts that she identified in *Notes on Nursing* (1969). Her intent was to provide general rules and explanations that would result in good nursing care for patients. Thus her objective of setting forth general rules for the practice and development of nursing was met through this simple theory.

Generality

Nightingale's theories have been used to provide general guidelines for all nurses since she introduced them more than 150 years ago. Although some activities that she described are no longer relevant, the universality and timelessness of her concepts remain pertinent. Nurses are increasingly recognizing the role of observation and measurement of outcomes as an essential component of nursing practice. Burnes-Bolton and Goodenough (2003), Erlen (2007), Robb et al. (2007), and Weir-Hughes (2007) all have written about the measurement of patient outcomes and methods of quality improvement based on Nightingale's notions of observation. The relation concepts (nurse, patient, and environment) remain applicable in all nursing settings today. Therefore they meet the criterion of generality.

Empirical Precision

Concepts and relationships within Nightingale's theory typically are stated implicitly and are presented as truths rather than as tentative, testable statements. In contrast to her quantitative research on mortality performed in Crimea, Nightingale advised the nurses of her day that their practice should be based on their observations and experiences. Her concepts are amenable to studies with the qualitative approaches of today as well as quantitative methods.

Derivable Consequences

To an extraordinary degree, Nightingale's writings direct the nurse to take action on behalf of the patient and the nurse. These directives encompass the areas of practice, research, and education. Her principles to shape nursing practice are the most specific. She urges nurses to provide physicians with "not your opinion, however respectfully given, but your facts" (Nightingale, 1969, p. 122). Similarly, she advises that "if you cannot get the habit of observation one way or other, you had better give up being a nurse, for it is not your calling, however kind and anxious you may be" (Nightingale, 1969, p. 113).

Nightingale's view of humanity was consistent with her theory of nursing. She believed in a creative, universal humanity with the potential and ability for growth and change (Dossey, 2000; Hektor, 1994; Palmer, 1977). Deeply religious, she viewed nursing as a means of doing the will of her God. The zeal and self-righteousness that come from being a reformer might explain some of her beliefs and the practices that she advocated. Finally, the period and place in which she lived, Victorian England, must be considered if one is to understand and interpret her views.

Nightingale's basic principles of environmental manipulation and care of the patient can be applied in contemporary nursing settings. Although subjected to some criticisms, her theory and her principles are relevant to the professional identity and practice of nursing.

The statements and observations made by Nightingale in *Notes on Nursing* can have great significance for the world of nursing today. Vidrine et al. (2002) have identified one of these observations as the guiding theory for their work with equine-facilitated group psychotherapy: "a small pet animal is often an excellent companion for the sick, for long chronic cases especially" (Nightingale, 1969, p. 102). Although a horse may not qualify as a "small animal in the sickroom," these authors have found that their therapy is successful with their patients. Indeed, Nightingale is a testament to her own theory; it is reported that she had 60 cats over her lifetime (she was chronically ill for much of her adult life and lived to 90 years of age).

SUMMARY

Florence Nightingale is a unique figure in the history of the world. Her picture appeared on the English 10-pound note for 100 years. No other woman has been and still is revered as an icon by so many people in so many diverse geographical locations. Few other figures continue to stimulate such interest in, controversy about, and interpretation of their lives and work. The nursing profession embraces her as the founder of modern nursing.

Nightingale defined the skills, behaviors, and knowledge required for professional nursing. Remnants of these descriptions serve the nursing profession well today, although their origins probably are not known by today's nurses.

Because of scientific and social changes that have occurred in the world, some of Nightingale's observations have been rejected, only to find after closer analysis that her underlying beliefs, philosophy, and observations continue to be valid. Nightingale did not consciously attempt to develop what is considered a theory of nursing; she provided the first definitions from which nurses could develop theory and the conceptual models and frameworks that inform professional nursing today. Professionals increasingly identify her as their matriarch. Mathematicians revere her for her work as an outstanding statistician. Epidemiologists, public health professionals, and lay health care workers trace the origins of their disciplines to Nightingale's descriptions of people who perform health promotion and disease prevention. Sociologists acknowledge her leadership role in defining communities and their social ills, and in working to correct problems of society as a way of improving the health of its members.

On the centennial of her death, nursing communities throughout the world gave special attention to her life and work. In particular, the *Journal of Holistic Nursing* published multiple articles (cited in this chapter). Of special note is Beck's (2010) article identifying seven recommendations for 21st-century nursing practice based on Nightingale's philosophy, offering a clarion call for nurses throughout the world to emulate the work of Nightingale.

Nurses, both students and practitioners, would be wise to become familiar with Nightingale's original writings and to review the many books and documents that are available (McDonald, 2001–2012). Rereading *Notes on Nursing* will reveal new and inspirational ideas and provide a brief look at her wry sense of humor. The logic and common sense that are embodied in Nightingale's writings serve to stimulate productive thinking for the individual nurse and the nursing profession. To emulate the life of Nightingale is to become a good citizen and leader in the community, the country, and the world. It is only right that Nightingale should continue to be recognized as the brilliant and creative founder of modern nursing and its first nursing theorist. What would Nightingale say about nursing today? Whatever she would say, she undoubtedly would provide an objective, logical, and revealing analysis and critique.

CASE STUDY

You are caring for an 82-year-old woman who has been hospitalized for several weeks for burns that she sustained on her lower legs during a cooking accident. Before the time of her admission, she lived alone in a small apartment. The patient reported on admission that she has no surviving family. Her support system appears to be other elders who live in her neighborhood. Because of transportation difficulties, most of them are unable to visit frequently. One of her neighbors has reported that she is caring for the patient's dog, a Yorkshire terrier. As you care for this woman, she begs you to let her friend bring her dog to the hospital. She says that none of the other nurses have listened to her about such a visit. As she asks you about this, she begins to cry and tells you that they have never been separated. You recall that the staff discussed their concern about this woman's well-being during report that morning. They said that she has been eating very little and seems to be depressed.

1. Based on Nightingale's work, identify specific interventions that you would provide in caring for this patient.
2. Describe what action, if any, you would take regarding the patient's request to see her dog. Discuss the theoretical basis of your decision and action based on your understanding of Nightingale's work.
3. Describe and discuss what nursing diagnoses you would make and what interventions you would initiate to address the patient's nutritional status and emotional well-being.
4. As the patient's primary nurse, identify and discuss the planning you would undertake regarding her discharge from the hospital. Identify members of the discharge team and their roles in this process. Describe how you would advocate for the patient based on Nightingale's observations and descriptions of the role of the nurse.

CRITICAL THINKING ACTIVITIES

1. Your community is at risk for a specific type of natural disaster (e.g., tornado, flood, hurricane, earthquake). Use Nightingale's principles and observations to develop an emergency plan for one of these events. Outline the items you would include in the plan.
2. Using Nightingale's concepts of *ventilation, light, noise,* and *cleanliness,* analyze the setting in which you are practicing nursing as an employee or student.
3. You are participating in a quality improvement project in your work setting. Share how you would develop ideas to present to the group based on a Nightingale approach.

POINTS FOR FURTHER STUDY

- Florence Nightingale: *The nurse theorists: Portraits of excellence,* The Helene Fuld Health Trust (1990), Studio Three Productions, a division of Samuel Merritt College, Oakland, CA. (Video/DVD available from Fitne, Inc., Athens, OH.)
- McDonald, L. (Ed.). (2001–2012). *The collected works of Florence Nightingale.* Ontario, Canada: Wilfred Laurier University (WLU) Press. Retrieved from http://www.uoguelph.ca/~cwfn/ightingale, F. (1969). *Notes on nursing: What it is and what it is not.* New York: Dover (first published in 1859).
- *The Florence Nightingale Museum.* Retrieved from http://www.florence-nightingale.co.uk.

REFERENCES

Agnew, L. R. (1958). Florence Nightingale, statistician. *American Journal of Nursing, 58,* 644.

Ashley, J. A. (1976). *Hospitals, paternalism, and the role of the nurse.* New York: Teachers College Press.

Beck, D. M. (2010). Expanding our Nightingale horizon: Seven recommendations for 21st century nursing practice. *Journal of Holistic Nursing, 28*(4), 317–326.

Burkhart, L., & Hogan, N. (2008). An experiential theory of spiritual care in nursing practice. *Qualitative Health Research, 18*(7), 928–938.

Burnes-Bolton, L., & Goodenough, A. (2003). A Magnet nursing service approach to nursing's role in quality improvement. *Nursing Administration Quarterly, 27*(4), 344–354.

Butterfield, P. (1999). Integrating environmental health into clinical nursing. *Journal of the New York State Nurses Association, 30*(1), 24–27.

Chinn, P., & Kramer, M. (2015). *Theory and nursing: A systematic approach* (8th ed.). St Louis: Mosby-Elsevier.

Cohen, I. B. (1984). Florence Nightingale. *Scientific American, 250*(3), 128–137.

Cook, E. T. (1913). *The life of Florence Nightingale.* London: Macmillan.

Decker, B., & Farley, J. K. (1991, May/June). What would Nightingale say? *Nurse Educator, 16*(3), 12–13.

Dickens, C. (1987). *Life and adventures of Martin Chuzzlewit.* London: New Oxford Press.

Dossey, B. M. (2000). *Florence Nightingale: Mystic, visionary, healer.* Springhouse, PA: Springhouse.

Erlen, J. A. (2007). Patient safety, error reduction, and ethical practice. *Orthopaedic Nursing, 26*(2), 130–133.

Gropper, E. I. (1990). Florence Nightingale: Nursing's first environmental theorist. *Nursing Forum, 25*(3), 30–33.

Halsall, P. (1997). *Modern history sourcebook: Florence Nightingale: rural hygiene.* Retrieved from http://www.fordham.edu/halsall/mod/nightingale-rural.html.

Hardy, M. (1978). Perspectives on nursing theory. *Advances in Nursing Science, 1,* 37–48.

Hektor, M. (1994). Florence Nightingale and the women's movement: Friend or foe? *Nursing Inquiry, 1*(1), 38–45.

Helmstadter, C. (1997). Doctors and nurses in the London teaching hospitals: Class, gender, religion, and professional expertise, 1850–1890. *Nursing History Review, 5,* 161–167.

Henry, B., Woods, S., & Nagelkerk, J. (1990). Nightingale's perspective of nursing administration. *Nursing and Health Care, 11*(4), 200–206.

Holliday, M. E., & Parker, D. L. (1997). Florence Nightingale, feminism and nursing. *Journal of Advanced Nursing, 28,* 483–488.

Hoyt, S. (2010). Florence Nightingale's contribution to contemporary nursing ethics. *Journal of Advanced Nursing, 28*(4), 331–332.

Kalisch, B. J., & Kalisch, P. A. (1983a). Heroine out of focus: Media images of Florence Nightingale. Part I: Popular biographies and stage productions. *Nursing and Health Care, 4*(4), 181–187.

Kalisch, B. J., & Kalisch, P. A. (1983b). Heroine out of focus: Media images of Florence Nightingale. Part II: Film, radio, and television dramatizations. *Nursing and Health Care, 4*(5), 270–278.

Kalisch, P. A., & Kalisch B. J. (1987). *The changing image of the nurse.* Menlo Park, CA: Addison-Wesley.

Kennedy, M. (2007). *Angel of mercy or power-crazed meddler? Unseen letters challenge view of pioneer nurse.* Retrieved from http://www.guardian.co.uk/uk/2007/sep/03/health.healthandwellbeing/print.

Lannon, S. L. (2007). Leadership skills beyond the classic: Professional development classes for the staff nurse. *Journal of Continuing Education in Nursing, 38*(1), 17–21.

Longfellow, H. W. (1857). Santa Filomena. *Atlantic Monthly, 1*(1), 22–23.

Lorentzon, M. (2003). Florence Nightingale as "mentor of matrons": Correspondence with Rachel Williams at St. Mary's Hospital. *Journal of Nursing Management, 11,* 266–274.

Macrae, J. A. (2001). *Nursing as a spiritual practice: A contemporary application of Florence Nightingale's views.* New York: Springer.

McCarthy, D. O., Ouimet, M. E., & Daun, J. M. (1991). Shades of Florence Nightingale: Potential impact of noise stress on wound healing. *Holistic Nursing Practice, 5*(4), 39–48.

McDonald, L. (Ed.). (2001–2012). *The collected works of Florence Nightingale.* Ontario, Canada: Wilfred Laurier University Press.

McDonald, L. (2010a). *Florence Nightingale at First Hand.* Waterloo, ON: Wilfrid Laurier University Press.

McDonald, L. (2010b). Florence Nightingale: Passionate statistician. *Journal of Holistic Nursing, 28*(1), 92–98.

McLaughlin, A., McLaughlin, B., Elliott, J., & Campalani, G. (1996). Noise levels in a cardiac surgical intensive care unit: A preliminary study conducted in secret. *Intensive and Critical Care Nursing, 12*(4), 226–230.

McPhaul, K. M., & Lipscomb, J. A. (2005). Incorporating environmental health into practice. *AAO-HN Journal, 53*(1), 31–36.

Medeiros, A., Enders, B., & De Carvalho Lira, A. (2015). The Florence Nightingale's environmental theory: A critical analysis. *Escola Anna Nery*, 19(3). Brazil. http://dx.doi.org/10.5935/1414-8145.20150069.

Monteiro, L. A. (1985). Response in anger. Florence Nightingale on the importance of training for nurses. *Journal of Nursing History*, 1(1), 11–18.

Narayanasamy, A., & Narayanasamy, M. (2007). Advancing nursing development and progression in nursing. *British Journal of Nursing, 16*(7), 384–388.

Neils, P. E. (2010). The influence of Nightingale rounding by the liaison nurse on surgical patient families with attention to differing cultural needs. *Journal of Holistic Nursing, 28*(4), 235–243.

Nelson, S. (1997). Pastoral care and moral government: Early nineteenth century nursing and solutions to the Irish question. *Journal of Advanced Nursing, 26*, 6–14.

Nightingale, F. (1852). *Cassandra*. Collected Works of Florence Nightingale (Vol. 11). Toronto: WLU Press.

Nightingale, F. (1858a). *Notes on hospitals: Being two papers read before the National Association for the Promotion of Social Science, at Liverpool, in October 1858. With evidence given to the Royal Commissioner on the state of the army in 1857*. London: John W. Park and Son.

Nightingale, F. (1858b). *Notes on matters affecting the health, efficiency, and hospital administration of the British army founded chiefly on the experience of the late war. Presented by request to the Secretary of State for War*. London: Harrison & Sons.

Nightingale, F. (1871). *Report on measures adopted for sanitary improvements in India, from June 1870 to June 1871*. London: George Edward Eye and William Spottiswoode.

Nightingale, F. (1969). *Notes on nursing: What it is and what it is not*. New York: Dover Publications.

O'Malley, I. B. (1931). *Life of Florence Nightingale, 1820–1956*. London: Butterworth.

Palmer, I. S. (1977). Florence Nightingale: Reformer, reactionary, researcher. *Nursing Research, 26*, 84–89.

Pope, D. S. (1995). Music, noise, and the human voice in the nurse-patient environment. *Image: The Journal of Nursing Scholarship, 27*, 291–295.

Robb, E., Mackie, S., & Elcock, K. (2007). Monitoring quality. *Nursing Management, 14*(5), 22–26.

Selanders, L. (2010a). Florence Nightingale: the evolution and social impact of feminist values in nursing. *Journal of Holistic Nursing, 28*(1), 70–78.

Selanders, L. (2010b). The power of environmental adaptation: Florence Nightingale's original theory for nursing practice. *Journal of Holistic Nursing, 28*(1), 81–88.

Sessler, A. (1999). Doing more than doing no harm: Nursing professionals turn their attention to the environment. *On-Call, 2*(4), 20–23.

Shaner-McRae, H., McRae, G., & Jas, V. (2007). Environmentally safe health care agencies: Nursing's responsibility, Nightingale's legacy. *Online Journal of Issues in Nursing, 12*(2), 1.

Small, H. (1998). *Avenging angel*. New York: St. Martin's Press.

Small, H. (2000). *Florence Nightingale's 20th century biographies*. Paper originally presented to the Friends of Florence Nightingale Museum, London. Retrieved from http://www.florence-nightingale-avenging-angel.co.uk/biograph.htm.

Small, H. (2008). *Florence Nightingale, avenging angel* (book review). Retrieved from http://www.florence-nightingale-avenging-angel.co.uk/Nightingale.html.

Smith, F. B. (1982). *Florence Nightingale: Reputation and power*. New York: St. Martin.

Strachey, L. (1918). *Eminent Victorians*. London: Chatto & Windus.

Straughair, C. (2012). Exploring compassion: Implications for contemporary nursing. Part 1. *British Journal of Nursing, 21*(3), 160–164.

Tourville, C., & Ingalls, K. (2003). The living tree of nursing theories. *Nursing Forum, 38*(3), 21–30.

Vidrine, M., Owen-Smith, P., & Faulkner, P. (2002). Equine-facilitated group psychotherapy: Applications for therapeutic vaulting. *Issues in Mental Health Nursing, 23*, 587–603.

Vincent, C. (2005). *Patient safety*. London: Churchill Livingstone Elsevier.

Wagner, D. J., & White, B. (2010). An exploration of the nature of caring relationships in the writings of Florence Nightingale. *Journal of Holistic Nursing, 28*(4), 225–234.

Watson, J. (2010). Florence Nightingale and the enduring legacy of transpersonal human caring-healing. *Journal of Holistic Nursing, 28*(1), 107–108.

Weir-Hughes, D. (2007). Reviewing nursing diagnoses. *Nursing Management, 14*(5), 32–35.

Welch, M. (1990). Florence Nightingale—the social construction of a Victorian feminist. *Western Journal of Nursing Research, 12*(3), 404–407.

Woodham-Smith, C. (1951). *Florence Nightingale*. New York: McGraw-Hill.

Wu, L-F., & Lin, L-Y. (2011). Exploration of clinical nurses' perceptions of spirituality and spiritual care. *Journal of Nursing Research, 19*(4), 250–256.

Zborowsky, T. (2014). The legacy of Florence Nightingale's environmental theory: Nursing research focusing on the impact of healthcare environments. *HERD, 7*(4), 19–34.

BIBLIOGRAPHY

Primary Sources

Books

Nightingale, F. (1911). *Letters from Miss Florence Nightingale on health visiting in rural districts*. London: King.

Nightingale, F. (1954). *Selected writings* [Compiled by Lucy R. Seymer]. New York: Macmillan.

Nightingale, F. (1957). *Notes on nursing*. Philadelphia: Lippincott. [Originally published in1859.]

Nightingale, F. (1969). *Notes on nursing: What it is and what it is not*. New York: Dover.

Nightingale, F. (1974). *Letters of Florence Nightingale in the history of nursing archive*. Boston: Boston University Press.
Nightingale, F. (1976). *Notes on hospitals*. New York: Gordon.
Nightingale, F. (1978). *Notes on nursing*. London: Duckworth.
Nightingale, F. (1992). *Notes on nursing*. Philadelphia: Lippincott. [Commemorative edition with commentaries by contemporary nursing leaders.]

Journal Articles
Nightingale, F. (1930, July). Trained nursing for the sick poor. *International Nursing Review, 5*, 426–433.
Nightingale, F. (1954, May). Maternity hospital and midwifery school. *Nursing Mirror, 99*, ix–xi, 369.
Nightingale, F. (1954). The training of nurses. *Nursing Mirror, 99*, iv–xi.

Secondary Sources
Books
Aiken, C. A. (1915). *Lessons from the life of Florence Nightingale*. New York: Lakeside.
Aldis, M. (1914). *Florence Nightingale*. New York: National Organization for Public Health Nursing.
Andrews, M. R. (1929). *A lost commander*. Garden City, NY: Doubleday.
Baly, M. E. (1986). *Florence Nightingale: The nursing legacy*. New York: Methuen.
Barth, R. J. (1945). *Fiery angel: The story of Florence Nightingale*. Coral Gables, FL: Glade House.
Bishop, W. J. (1962). *A bio-bibliography of Florence Nightingale*. London: Dawson's of Pall Mall.
Boyd, N. (1982). *Three Victorian women who changed their world*. New York: Oxford.
Bull, A. (1985). *Florence Nightingale*. North Pomfret, VT: David and Charles.
Bullough, V. L., Bullough, B., & Stanton, M. P. (Eds.). (1990). *Florence Nightingale and her era: A collection of new scholarship*. New York: Garland.
Calabria, M., & Macrae, J. (Eds.). (1994). *Suggestions for thought by Florence Nightingale: Selections and commentaries*. Philadelphia: University of Pennsylvania Press.
Collins, D. (1985). *Florence Nightingale*. Milford, MI: Mott Media.
Columbia University Faculty of Medicine and Department of Nursing. (1937). *Catalogue of the Florence Nightingale collection*. New York: Author.
Cook, E. T. (1913). *The life of Florence Nightingale*. London: Macmillan.
Cook, E. T. (1941). *A short life of Florence Nightingale*. New York: Macmillan.
Cope, Z. (1958). *Florence Nightingale and the doctors*. Philadelphia: Lippincott.
Cope, Z. (1961). *Six disciples of Florence Nightingale*. New York: Pitman.
Davies, C. (1980). *Rewriting nursing history*. London: Croom Helm.
Dossey, B. M. (2000). *Florence Nightingale: mystic, visionary, healer*. Springhouse, PA: Springhouse.
Editors of RN. (1970). *Florence Nightingale: Rebel with a cause*. Oradell, NJ: Medical Economics.
French, Y. (1953). *Six great Englishwomen*. London: H. Hamilton.
Goldie, S. (1987). *I have done my duty: Florence Nightingale in the Crimea War, 1854–1856*. London: Manchester University Press.
Goldsmith, M. L. (1937). *Florence Nightingale: The woman and the legend*. London: Hodder and Stoughton.
Gordon, R. (1979). *The private life of Florence Nightingale*. New York: Atheneum.
Hall, E. F. (1920). *Florence Nightingale*. New York: Macmillan.
Hallock, G. T., & Turner, C. E. (1928). *Florence Nightingale*. New York: Metropolitan Life Insurance Company.
Herbert, R. G. (1981). *Florence Nightingale: Saint, reformer, or rebel?* Melbourne, FL: Krieger.
Holmes, M. (n.d.). *Florence Nightingale: A cameo lifesketch*. London: Woman's Freedom League.
Huxley, E. J. (1975). *Florence Nightingale*. London: Putnam.
Hyndman, J. A. (1969). *Florence Nightingale: Nurse to the world*. Cleveland, OH: World.
Keele, J. (Ed.). (1981). *Florence Nightingale in Rome*. Philadelphia: American Philosophical Society.
Lammond, D. (1935). *Florence Nightingale*. London: Duckworth.
Macrae, J. A. (2001). *Nursing as a spiritual practice: A contemporary application of Florence Nightingale's views*. New York: Springer.
McDonald, L. (2010). *Florence Nightingale at first hand*. Waterloo, ON: Wilfrid Laurier University Press.
Miller, B. W. (1947). *Florence Nightingale: The lady with the lamp*. Grand Rapids, MI: Zondervan.
Miller, M. (1987). *Florence Nightingale*. Minneapolis: Bethany House.
Mosby, C. V. (1938). *Little journey to the home of Florence Nightingale*. New York: Mosby.
Muir, D. E. (1946). *Florence Nightingale*. Glasgow: Blackie and Son.
Nash, R. (1937). *A sketch for the life of Florence Nightingale*. London: Society for Promoting Christian Knowledge.
O'Malley, I. B. (1931). *Life of Florence Nightingale, 1820–1856*. London: Butterworth.
Pollard, E. (1902). *Florence Nightingale: The wounded soldiers' friend*. London: Partridge.
Presbyterian Hospital School of Nursing. (1937). *Catalogue of the Florence Nightingale collection*. New York: Author.
Quiller-Couch, A. T. (1927). *Victor of peace*. New York: Nelson.
Quinn, V., & Prest, J. (Eds.). (1987). *Dear Miss Nightingale: A selection of Benjamin Jowett's letters to Florence Nightingale, 1860–1893*. Oxford: Clarendon Press.
Rappe, E. C. (1977). *God bless you, my dear Miss Nightingale*. Stockholm: Almqvist och Wiksell.
Sabatini, R. (1934). *Heroic lives*. Boston: Houghton.
Saint Thomas's Hospital. (1960). *The Nightingale training school: St. Thomas's Hospital, 1860–1960*. London: Author.
Selanders, L. C. (1993). *Florence Nightingale: An environmental adaptation theory*. Newbury Park, CA: Sage.
Seymer, L. R. (1951). *Florence Nightingale*. New York: Macmillan.
Shor, D. (1987). *Florence Nightingale*. Lexington, NH: Silver.
Small, H. (1998). *Avenging angel*. New York: St. Martin's Press.
Smith, F. B. (1982). *Florence Nightingale: Reputation and power*. New York: St. Martin's Press.

Stark, M. (1979). *Introduction to Cassandra: An essay by Florence Nightingale*. Old Westbury, NY: Feminist Press.

Stephenson, G. E. (1924). *Some pioneers in the medical and nursing world*. Shanghai: Nurse Association of China.

Strachey, L. (1918). *Eminent Victorians*. London: Chatto & Windus.

Tooley, S. A. (1905). *The life of Florence Nightingale*. New York: Macmillan.

Turner, D. (1986). *Florence Nightingale*. New York: Watts.

Vicinus, M., & Nergaard, B. (1990). *Ever yours, Florence Nightingale*. Cambridge, MA: Harvard University Press.

Wilson, W. G. (1940). *Soldier's heroine*. Edinburgh: Missionary Education Movement.

Woodman-Smith, C. (1983). *Florence Nightingale*. New York: Atheneum.

Woodham-Smith, C. B. (1951). *Florence Nightingale, 1820–1910*. New York: McGraw-Hill.

Woodham-Smith, C. B. (1951). *Lonely crusader: The life of Florence Nightingale, 1820–1910*. New York: Whittlesey House.

Woodham-Smith, C. B. (1956). *Lady-in-chief*. London: Methven.

Woodham-Smith, C. B. (1977). *Florence Nightingale, 1820–1910*. London: Collins.

Unpublished Dissertations

Hektor, L. M. (1992). *Nursing, science, and gender: Florence Nightingale and Martha E. Rogers*. Unpublished doctoral dissertation, University of Miami, Miami.

Newton, M. E. (1949). *Florence Nightingale's philosophy of life and education*. Unpublished doctoral dissertation, Stanford University, Stanford, CA.

Selanders, L. C. (1992). *An analysis of the utilization of power by Florence Nightingale*. Unpublished doctoral dissertation, Western Michigan University, Kalamazoo, MI.

Tschirch, P. (1992). *The caring tradition: Nursing ethics in the United States, 1890–1915*. Unpublished doctoral dissertation, The University of Texas at Galveston, Graduate School of Biomedical Science, Galveston, TX.

Journal Articles

A criticism of Miss Florence Nightingale. (1907, Feb.). *Nursing Times, 3*, 89.

Address by the Archbishop of York. (1970, May). Florence Nightingale. *Nursing Times, 66*, 670.

Address given at fiftieth anniversary of founding by Florence Nightingale of first training school for nurses at St. Thomas's Hospital, London, England. (1911, Feb.). *American Journal of Nursing, 11*, 331–361.

A passionate statistician. (1931, May). *American Journal of Nursing, 31*, 566.

Attewell, A. (1998). Florence Nightingale's relevance to nurses. *Journal of Holistic Nursing, 16*, 281–291.

Baly, M. (1986). Shattering the Nightingale myth. *Nursing Times, 82*(24), 16–18.

Baly, M. E. (1969, Jan.). Florence Nightingale's influence on nursing today. *Nursing Times, 65*(Suppl.), 1–4.

Barber, E. M. (1935, July). A culinary campaign. *Journal of the American Dietetic Association, 11*, 89–98.

Barber, J. A. (1999). Concerning our national honour: Florence Nightingale and the welfare of Aboriginal Australians. *Collegian: Journal of the Royal College of Nursing Australia, 6*(1), 36–39.

Barker, E. R. (1989, Oct.). Caregivers as casualties: War experiences and the postwar consequences for both Nightingale- and Vietnam-era nurses. *Western Journal of Nursing Research, 11*, 628–631.

Barritt, E. R. (1973). Florence Nightingale's values and modern nursing education. *Nursing Forum, 12*, 7–47.

Berentson, L. (1982, April/May). Florence Nightingale: Change agent. *Registered Nurse, 6*(2), 3, 7.

Bishop, W. J. (1957). Florence Nightingale's letters. *American Journal of Nursing, 57*(5), 607.

Bishop, W. J. (1960, May). Florence Nightingale's message for today. *Nursing Outlook, 8*, 246.

Blanc, E. (1980). Nightingale remembered: Reflections on times past. *California Nurse, 75*(10), 7.

Blanchard, J. R. (1939, June). Florence Nightingale: A study in vocation. *New Zealand Nursing Journal, 32*, 193–197.

Boylen, J. O. (1974, April). The Florence Nightingale–Mary Stanley controversy: Some unpublished letters. *Medical History, 18*(2), 186–193.

Bridges, D. C. (1954, April). Florence Nightingale centenary. *International Nurses Review, 1*, 3.

Brow, E. J. (1954, April). Florence Nightingale and her international influence. *International Nursing Review, 1*, 17–19.

Brown, E. (2000). Nightingale's values live on. *Kai Tiaki: Nursing New Zealand, 6*(3), 31.

Carlisle, D. (1989). A nightingale sings: Florence Nightingale: Unknown details of her life story. *Nursing Times, 85*(50), 38–39.

Charatan, F. B. (1990). Florence Nightingale: The most famous nurse in the world. *Today's OR Nurse, 12*(2), 25–30.

Cherescavich, G. (1971). Florence, where are you? *Nursing Clinics of North America, 6*(2), 217–223.

Choa, G. H. (1971, May). Speech by Dr. the Hon. G. H. Choa at the Florence Nightingale Day Celebration on Wednesday, 12th May, 1971, at City Hall, Hong Kong. *Nursing Journal, 10*, 33–34.

Clayton, R. E. (1974, April). How men may live and not die in India: Florence Nightingale. *Australian Nurses Journal, 2*(33), 10–11.

Coakley, M. L. (1989). Florence Nightingale: A one-woman revolution. *Journal of Christian Nursing, 6*(1), 20–25.

Cohen, S. (1997). Miss Loane, Florence Nightingale, and district nursing in late Victorian Britain. *Nursing History Review, 5*, 83–103.

de Guzman, G. (1935, July). Florence Nightingale. *Filipino Nurse, 10*, 10–14.

Dennis, K. E., & Prescott, P. A. (1985). Florence Nightingale: Yesterday, today, and tomorrow. *Advances in Nursing Science, 7*(2), 66–81.

de Tornayay, R. (1976). Past is prologue: Florence Nightingale. *Pulse, 12*(6), 9–11.

Dwyer, B. A. (1937, Jan.). The mother of our modern nursing system. *Filipino Nurse, 12*, 8–10.

Florence Nightingale: Rebel with a cause. (1970, May). *Registered Nurse, 33*, 39–55.

Florence Nightingale: The original geriatric nurse. (1980). *Oklahoma Nurse, 25*(4), 6.

Gibbon, C. (1997). The influence of Florence Nightingale's image on Liverpool nurses 1945–1995. *International History of Nursing Journal, 2*(3), 17–26.
Gordon, J. E. (1972). Nurses and nursing in Britain. 21. The work of Florence Nightingale. I. For the health of the army. *Midwife Health Visitor and Community Nurse, 8*(10), 351–359.
Gordon, J. E. (1972, Nov.). Nurses and nursing in Britain. 22. The work of Florence Nightingale. II. The establishment of nurse training in Britain. *Midwife Health Visitor and Community Nurse, 8*(11), 391–396.
Gordon, J. E. (1973, Jan.). Nurses and nursing in Britain. 23. The work of Florence Nightingale. III. Her influence throughout the world. *Midwife Health Visitor and Community Nurse, 9*(1), 17–22.
Hoole, L. (2000). Florence Nightingale must remain as nursing's icon. *British Journal of Nursing, 4,* 189.
Ifemesia, C. C. (1976). Florence Nightingale (1820–1910). *Nigerian Nurse, 8*(3), 26–34.
Kelly, L. Y. (1976). Our nursing heritage: Have we renounced it? (Florence Nightingale). *Image: The Journal of Nursing Scholarship, 8*(3), 43–48.
Large, J. T. (1985). Florence Nightingale: A multifaceted personality. *Nursing Journal of India, 76*(5), 110, 114.
LeVasseur, J. (1998). Student scholarship: Plato, Nightingale, and contemporary nursing. *Image: The Journal of Nursing Scholarship, 30,* 281–285.
Light, K. M. (1997). Florence Nightingale and holistic philosophy. *Journal of Holistic Nursing, 15*(1), 25–40.
Macmillan, K. (1994). Brilliant mind gave Florence her edge: Florence Nightingale. *Registered Nurse, 6*(2), 29–30.
Macrae, J. (1995, Spring). Nightingale's spiritual philosophy and its significance for modern nursing. *Image: The Journal of Nursing Scholarship, 27*(1), 8–10.
McDonald, L. (1998). Florence Nightingale: Passionate statistician. *Journal of Holistic Nursing, 16,* 267–277.
Monteiro, L. A. (1985). Response in anger: Florence Nightingale on the importance of training for nurses. *Journal of Nursing History, 1*(1), 11–18.
Rabstein, C. (2000). Patron saint or has-been? Role models: Is Florence Nightingale holding us back? *Nursing, 30*(1), 8.
Selanders, L. C. (1998). Florence Nightingale: The evolution and social impact of feminist values in nursing. *Journal of Holistic Nursing, 16*(2), 227–243.
Selanders, L. C. (1998). The power of environmental adaptation: Florence Nightingale's original theory for nursing practice. *Journal of Holistic Nursing, 16,* 247–263.
Sparacino, P. S. A. (1994). Clinical practice: Florence Nightingale: a CNS role model. *Clinical Nurse Specialist, 8*(2), 64.
Stronk, K. (1997). Florence Nightingale: Mother of all nurses. *Journal of Nursing Jocularity, 7*(2), 14.
Watson, J. (1998). Reflections: Florence Nightingale and the enduring legacy of transpersonal human caring. *Journal of Holistic Nursing, 16,* 292–294.
Welch, M. (1986). Nineteenth-century philosophic influences on Nightingale's concept of the person. *Journal of Nursing History, 1*(2), 3–11.
Wheeler, W., & Walker, M. (1999). Florence: Death of an icon: Florence Nightingale. *Nursing Times, 95*(19), 24–26.
Widerquist, J. G. (1992). The spirituality of Florence Nightingale. *Nursing Research, 41*(1), 49–55.
Widerquist, J. G. (1997). Sanitary reform and nursing: Edwin Chadwick and Florence Nightingale. *Nursing History Review, 5,* 149–160.
Williams, B. (2000). Florence Nightingale: A relevant heroine for nurses today? *California Nurse, 96*(1), 9, 27.

7

Watson's Philosophy and Theory of Transpersonal Caring

*Danny G. Willis and Danielle M. Leone-Sheehan**

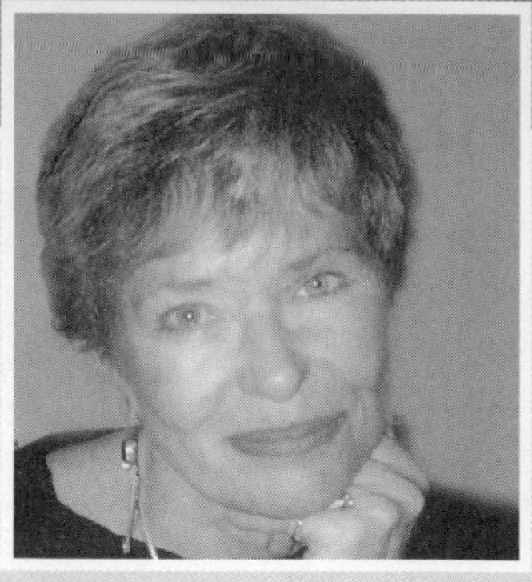

Jean Watson (1940–Present)

"We are the light in institutional darkness, and in this model we get to return to the light of our humanity."

(Jean Watson, 2012)

CREDENTIALS AND BACKGROUND OF THE THEORIST

Margaret Jean Harman Watson, PhD, RN, AHN-BC, FAAN, was born and grew up in the small town of Welch, West Virginia. The youngest of eight children, she was surrounded by an extended family–community environment.

Watson attended high school in West Virginia and the Lewis Gale School of Nursing in Roanoke, Virginia. After graduation in 1961, she married Douglas Watson and moved to his native state of Colorado. Douglas, whom Watson describes as her physical and spiritual partner, and her best friend, died in 1998. She has two grown daughters, Jennifer and Julie, and five grandchildren. Jean lives in Boulder, Colorado.

After moving to Colorado, Watson continued her nursing education at the University of Colorado. She earned a baccalaureate degree in nursing in 1964, a master's degree in 1966, and a doctorate in educational psychology and counseling in 1973. After completing her doctorate, she joined the School of Nursing faculty at the University of Colorado Health Sciences Center, serving in both faculty and administrative positions. In 1981 and 1982, she pursued international sabbatical studies in New Zealand, Australia, India, Thailand, and Taiwan; in 2005, she took a sabbatical for a walking pilgrimage in the Spanish El Camino.

In the 1980s, Watson and her colleagues established the Center for Human Caring at the University of Colorado, the nation's first interdisciplinary center using human caring knowledge for clinical practice, scholarship, administration, and leadership (Watson, 1986). At the center, Watson and others sponsored clinical, educational, and community scholarship activities with national and international scholars in residence, as well as with international colleagues around the world, in Australia, Brazil, Canada, Korea, Japan, New Zealand, the United Kingdom, Scandinavia, Thailand, and Venezuela, among others.

The Watson Caring Science evolved and the Watson Caring Science Institute (WCSI) was established from groundwork laid by the Center for Human Caring. WCSI exists as a nonprofit organization devoted to advancing caring science in Global World Caring Science programs and projects. The Watson Caring Science Center established at the University of Colorado is an interdisciplinary center for nurses and health professionals. This center is operationally and philosophically aligned with WCSI in partnership. In line with the University of Colorado initiatives in Watson Caring Science, the Watson Endowed Chair in Caring Science was recently established at the University of Colorado (Watson, personal communication, April 6, 2016).

At the University of Colorado School of Nursing, Watson served as chairperson and assistant dean of the undergraduate program, implementing the nursing PhD program, and served as director of the PhD program from 1978 to 1981. Watson was Dean of the University of Colorado School of Nursing and Associate Director of Nursing Practice at the University Hospital from 1983 to 1990. As dean, she developed a postbaccalaureate

*Previous authors: D. Elizabeth Jesse, Martha R. Alligood, Ruth M. Neil, Ann Marriner Tomey, Tracey J. F. Patton, Deborah A. Barnhart, Patricia M. Bennett, Beverly D. Porter, and Rebecca S. Sloan. These authors wish to thank Dr. Jean Watson for her assistance in updating the chapter.

nursing curriculum in human caring, health, and healing that led to a Nursing Doctorate (ND), a clinical doctorate that became the Doctor of Nursing Practice (DNP) in 2005.

Watson has been active in many community programs, such as founder and member of the Board of Boulder County Hospice, and numerous other area health care facilities. Watson has received research and education federal grants, numerous university and private grants, and extramural funding for faculty and administrative projects and scholarships in human caring.

She received numerous honors and awards from national and international universities and organizations, including honorary degrees, appointed positions of leadership, and honoraria for her ongoing work and service. She has received 13 honorary degrees, nine from international universities, including Göteborg University in Sweden, Luton University in London, and the University of Montreal in Quebec, Canada. In 2015 she received an honorary doctorate from Erciyes University in Kayseri, Turkey (Watson, personal communication, April 6, 2016). In 1993 she received the National League for Nursing (NLN) Martha E. Rogers Award. From 1993 to 1996, Watson served on the Executive Committee and Governing Board for the NLN, and she served as president from 1995 to 1996. In 1997 the NLN awarded her an honorary lifetime holistic nurse certificate.

The University of Colorado School of Nursing honored Watson as a distinguished professor in 1992; Watson was recognized in 1998 as a Distinguished Nurse Scholar by New York University and in 1999 received the Fetzer Institute's national Norman Cousins Award in recognition of her commitment to developing, maintaining, and exemplifying relationship-centered care practices (Watson, personal communication, August 14, 2000). In 1999 Watson assumed the Murchison-Scoville Endowed Chair of Caring Science at the University of Colorado. In 2015 she received the Helene Hildebrand Center of Compassionate Care in Medicine Award from Notre Dame University as well as an award from the Academy of Integrative Healing Medicine. In 2016 she was honored by the United Nations via the Nightingale Global Health Initiative 60th session on Commission of Women. Also in 2016 she was Honorary Chair Emerita of the International Society for Caring and Peace in Japan (Watson, personal communication, April 6, 2016).

Watson has served as a Distinguished and Endowed Lecturer at national universities, including Boston College, Catholic University, Adelphi University, Columbia University–Teachers College, State University of New York, and at universities in numerous foreign countries. Her international activities include an International Kellogg Fellowship in Australia (1982), a Fulbright Research and Lecture Award in Sweden and other parts of Scandinavia (1991), and a lecture tour in the United Kingdom (1993). Watson has been involved in international projects and received invitations to New Zealand, India, Thailand, Taiwan, Israel, Japan, Venezuela, and Korea. She is featured in at least 20 nationally distributed audiotapes, videotapes, and CDs on nursing theory, a few of which are listed in Points for Further Study at the end of the chapter.

Jean Watson has authored 11 books, shared authorship of 9 books, and published countless articles in nursing and interdisciplinary journals. The following publications reflect the evolution of her theory of caring.

Her first book, *Nursing: The Philosophy and Science of Caring* (1979), was reprinted in 1985 and translated into Korean and French. Yalom's 11 curative factors stimulated Watson to use 10 carative factors as the organizing framework for her book (Watson, 1979), "central to nursing" (p. 9), and a moral ideal. Watson's early work embraced 10 carative factors but evolved to include "caritas," making explicit connections between caring and love in the 2008 revised edition of this seminal text.

Her second book, *Nursing: Human Science and Human Care—A Theory of Nursing* (1985) reprinted in 1988 and 1999, addressed her conceptual and philosophical problems in nursing. Her second book has been translated into Chinese, German, Japanese, Korean, Swedish, Norwegian, and Danish.

Her third book, *Postmodern Nursing and Beyond* (1999), presented a model to bring nursing practice into the 21st century. Watson describes two personal life-altering events that contributed to her writing. In 1997 she experienced an accidental injury that resulted in the loss of her left eye, and soon after, in 1998, her husband died. Watson states that she has "attempted to integrate these wounds into my life and work. One of the gifts through the suffering was the privilege of experiencing and receiving my own theory through the care from my husband and loving nurse friends and colleagues" (Watson, personal communication, August 31, 2000). This third book has been translated into Portuguese and Japanese. *Instruments for Assessing and Measuring Caring in Nursing and Health Sciences* (2002), her fourth book, comprises a collection of 21 instruments to assess and measure caring and received the *American Journal of Nursing* Book of the Year Award.

Her fifth book, *Caring Science as Sacred Science* (2005), describes her personal journey to enhance understanding about caring science, spiritual practice, the concept and practice of care, and caring-healing work. In this book, she leads the reader through thought-provoking experiences and the sacredness of nursing by emphasizing deep inner reflection and personal growth, communication skills, use of self-transpersonal growth, and attention to both caring science and healing through forgiveness, gratitude, and surrender. It received the *American Journal of Nursing* 2005 Book of the Year Award.

Recent books include *Measuring Caring: International Research on Caritas as Healing* (Nelson & Watson, 2011); *Creating a Caring Science Curriculum* (Hills & Watson, 2011); *Human Caring Science: A Theory of Nursing* (Watson, 2012); and *Caring Science, Mindful Practice: Implementing Watson's Human Caring Theory* (Sitzman & Watson, 2013).

THEORETICAL SOURCES

Watson's work has been called a philosophy, blueprint, ethic, paradigm, worldview, treatise, conceptual model, framework, and theory (Watson, 1996). Watson (1988) defines *theory* as "an imaginative grouping of knowledge, ideas, and experience that are represented symbolically and seek to illuminate a given phenomenon" (p. 1). She draws on the Latin meaning of *theory* "to see" and concludes, "It (Human Science) is a theory because it helps me 'to see' more broadly (clearly)" (p. 1). Watson acknowledges a phenomenological, existential, and spiritual orientation from the sciences and humanities as well as philosophical and intellectual guidance from feminist theory, metaphysics, phenomenology, quantum physics, wisdom traditions, perennial philosophy, and Buddhism (Watson, 1995, 1997, 1999, 2005, 2008, 2012). She cites as background for her theory nursing philosophies and theorists, including Nightingale, Henderson, Leininger, Peplau, Rogers, and Newman and the work of Gadow, a nursing philosopher and health care ethicist (Watson, 1985, 1997, 2005, 2012).

Watson attributes her emphasis on the interpersonal and transpersonal qualities of congruence, empathy, and warmth to Carl Rogers and more recent writers of transpersonal psychology. Watson points out that Carl Rogers's phenomenological approach, with his view that nurses are not here to manipulate and control others but rather to understand, was profoundly influential at a time when "clinicalization" (therapeutic control and manipulation of the patient) was considered the norm (Watson, personal communication, August 31, 2000). In her book, *Caring Science as Sacred Science*, Watson (2005) describes the wisdom of French philosopher Emmanuael Levinas (1969) and Danish philosopher Knud Løgstrup (1995) as foundational to her work.

Watson's main concepts include the 10 carative factors (see Major Concepts & Definitions box and Table 7.1) and the transpersonal healing and transpersonal caring relationship, caring moment, caring occasion, caring healing modalities,

TABLE 7.1 Carative Factors and Caritas Processes

Carative Factors	Caritas Processes
"The formation of a humanistic-altruistic system of values"	"Practice of loving-kindness and equanimity within the context of caring consciousness"
"The instillation of faith-hope"	"Being authentically present and enabling and sustaining the deep belief system and subjective life-world of self and one being cared for"
"The cultivation of sensitivity to one's self and to others"	"Cultivation of one's own spiritual practices and transpersonal self, going beyond the ego self"
"Development of a helping-trust relationship"; became "development of a helping-trusting, human caring relation" (in the 2004 Watson website)	"Developing and sustaining a helping trusting authentic caring relationship"
"The promotion and acceptance of the expression of positive and negative feelings"	"Being present to, and supportive of, the expression of positive and negative feelings as a connection with deeper spirit and self and the one-being-cared for"
"The systematic use of the scientific problem solving method for decision making"; became "systematic use of a creative problem solving caring process" (in the 2004 Watson website)	"Creative use of self and all ways of knowing as part of the caring process; to engage in the artistry of caring-healing practices"
"The promotion of transpersonal teaching-learning"	"Engaging in genuine teaching-learning experience that attends to unity of being and meaning, attempting to stay within others' frame of reference"
"The provision of supportive, protective, and (or) corrective mental, physical, societal, and spiritual environment"	"Creating healing environment at all levels (physical as well as non-physical, subtle environment of energy and consciousness, whereby wholeness, beauty, comfort, dignity, and peace are potentiated)"
"The assistance with gratification of human needs"	"Assisting with basic needs, with an intentional caring consciousness, administering 'human care essentials,' which potentiate alignment of mind body spirit, wholeness, and unity of being in all aspects of care"
"The allowance for existential-phenomenological forces"; became "allowance for existential-phenomenological-spiritual forces" (in the 2004 Watson website)	"Opening and attending to spiritual-mysterious and existential dimensions of one's own life-death; soul care for self and the one-being-cared for"

Modified from Watson, J. (1979). *Nursing: The philosophy and science of caring* (pp. 9–10). Boston: Little, Brown (carative factors), and Watson, J. (2008) *Nursing: The philosophy and science of caring. Revised & Updated Edition.* Boulder, CO: University Press of Colorado (caritas processes).

caring consciousness, caring consciousness energy, and phenomenal file/unitary consciousness. Watson expanded the carative factors to *caritas,* and offered a translation of the original carative factors into clinical caritas processes that suggested open ways they could be considered (see Table 7.1).

Watson (1999) describes a "transpersonal caring relationship" as foundational to her theory; it is a "special kind of human care relationship—a union with another person—high regard for the whole person and their being-in-the-world" (p. 63). Development and maintenance of the transpersonal relationship is actualized through the application of the 10 caritas processes that guide the relationship and set the foundation for the caring-loving relationship essential to nursing practice (Watson, 2008).

MAJOR CONCEPTS & DEFINITIONS

Ten Caritas Processes

Watson originally based her theory for nursing practice on 10 carative factors. Since the initial publication of the theory, the factors have evolved into what are now described as the 10 caritas processes that include a decidedly spiritual dimension and overt evocation of love and caring (Watson, 2008). One essential shift from carative to caritas is the explication of Caritas Consciousness, defined as "an awareness and intentionality" that forms the foundation for the caritas nurse (Watson, 2008, p. 43). (See Table 7.1 for the original carative factors and for caritas process interpretation.)

1. Cultivating the Practice of Loving-Kindness and Equanimity Toward Self and Other as Foundational to Caritas Consciousness.

Humanistic and altruistic values are learned early in life but can be influenced greatly by nurse educators and clinical experience. This process can be defined as satisfaction through giving and extension of the sense of self and an increased understanding of the impact of love and caring on self and other (Watson, 2008).

2. Being Authentically Present: Enabling, Sustaining, and Honoring the Faith, Hope, and Deep Belief System and the Inner-Subjective World of Self/Other.

This process, incorporating humanistic and altruistic values, facilitates the promotion of holistic nursing care and positive health within the patient population. It also describes the nurse's role in developing effective nurse-patient interrelationships and in promoting wellness by helping the patient adopt health-seeking behaviors (Watson, 2008).

3. Cultivation of One's Own Spiritual Practices and Transpersonal Self, Going Beyond Ego-Self.

The recognition of feelings leads to self-actualization through self-acceptance for both the nurse and patient. As nurses acknowledge their sensitivity and feelings, they become more genuine, authentic, and sensitive to others. The nurse also goes beyond feelings in a lifelong exploration of personal values and belief systems with the goal of increased mindfulness in caring actions (Watson, 2008).

4. Development and Sustaining a Helping-Trust Caring Relationship.

The development of a helping-trust relationship between the nurse and patient is crucial for transpersonal caring. A trusting relationship promotes and accepts the expression of both positive and negative feelings. It involves congruence, empathy, nonpossessive warmth, and effective communication. Congruence involves being real, honest, genuine, and authentic. Empathy is the ability to experience and thereby understand the other person's perceptions and feelings and to communicate those understandings. Nonpossessive warmth is demonstrated by a moderate speaking volume, a relaxed open posture, and facial expressions that are congruent with other communications. Effective communication has cognitive, affective, and behavior response components (Watson, 2008).

5. Being Present to, and Supportive of, the Expression of Positive and Negative Feelings.

The sharing of feelings is a risk-taking experience for both nurse and patient. The nurse must be prepared for either positive or negative feelings. The nurse must recognize that intellectual and emotional understandings of a situation differ (Watson, 2008).

6. Creative Use of Self and All Ways of Knowing as Part of the Caring Process; Engage in the Artistry of Caritas Nursing.

The process of nursing requires application of various ways of knowing, including "creative, intuitive, aesthetic, ethical, personal and even spiritual" (Watson, 2008, p. 107). This process moves most significantly away from a singular perspective on scientific knowledge as essential for nursing practice and calls upon the nurse to use knowledge creatively in practicing caritas nursing (Watson, 2008).

Continued

MAJOR CONCEPTS & DEFINITIONS

Ten Caritas Processes—cont'd

7. Engage in Genuine Teaching-Learning Experience that Attends to Unity of Being and Subjective Meaning—Attempting to Stay Within the Other's Frame of Reference.

This factor is an important concept for nursing in that it separates caring from curing. It allows the patient to be informed and shifts the responsibility for wellness and health to the patient. The nurse facilitates this process with teaching-learning techniques that are designed to enable patients to provide self-care, determine personal needs, and provide opportunities for their personal growth (Watson, 2008).

8. Creating a Healing Environment at All Levels.

Nurses must recognize the influence that internal and external environments have on the health and illness of individuals. Concepts relevant to the internal environment include the mental and spiritual well-being and sociocultural beliefs of an individual. In addition to epidemiological variables, other external variables include comfort, privacy, safety, and clean, esthetic surroundings (Watson, 2008).

9. Administering Sacred Nursing Acts of Caring-Healing by Tending to Basic Human Needs.

The nurse recognizes the biophysical, psychophysical, psychosocial, and intrapersonal needs of self and patient. Patients must satisfy lower-order needs before attempting to attain higher-order needs. Food, elimination, and ventilation are examples of lower-order biophysical needs, whereas activity, inactivity, and sexuality are considered lower-order psychophysical needs. Achievement and affiliation are higher-order psychosocial needs. Self-actualization is a higher-order intrapersonal-interpersonal need (Watson, 2008).

10. Opening and Attending to Spiritual/Mysterious and Existential Unknowns of Life-Death.

Watson considers this process the most difficult to understand and can be best understood through her own words.

"Our rational minds and modern science do not have all the answers to life and death and all the human conditions we face: thus, we have to be open to unknowns we cannot control, even allowing for what we may consider a 'miracle' to enter our life and work. This process also acknowledges that the subjective world of the inner-life experiences of self and other is ultimately a phenomenon, an ineffable mystery, affected by many, many factors that can never be fully explained."

(Watson, 2008, p. 191)

USE OF EMPIRICAL EVIDENCE

Watson's research into caring incorporates empiricism but emphasizes approaches that begin with nursing phenomena rather than with the natural sciences (Leininger, 1979). For example, she has used human science, empirical phenomenology, and transcendent phenomenology. She has investigated metaphor and poetry to communicate, convey, and elucidate human caring and healing (Watson, 1987, 2005). In her inquiry and writing, she increasingly incorporated her conviction that a sacred relationship exists between humankind and the universe (Watson, 1997, 2005).

MAJOR ASSUMPTIONS

Watson calls for joining of science with humanities so that nurses have a strong liberal arts background and understand other cultures as a requisite for using caring science and a mind-body-spiritual framework. She believes that study of the humanities expands the mind and enhances thinking skills and personal growth. Watson has compared the status of nursing with the mythological Danaides, who attempted to fill a broken jar with water, only to see water flow through the cracks. She proposed that the study of sciences and humanities was required to seal similar cracks in the scientific basis of nursing knowledge (Watson, 1981, 1997).

Watson describes assumptions for a transpersonal caring relationship extending to multidisciplinary practitioners:

- Moral commitment, intentionality, and caritas consciousness by the nurse protect, enhance, and potentiate human dignity, wholeness, and healing, thereby allowing a person to create or cocreate his or her own meaning for existence.
- The conscious will of the nurse affirms the subjective and spiritual significance of the patient while seeking to sustain caring in the midst of threat and despair—biological, institutional, or otherwise. The result is honoring of an *I-thou relationship* rather than an *I-it relationship.*
- The nurse seeks to recognize, accurately detect, and connect with the inner condition of spirit of another through genuine presence and by being centered in the caring moment; actions, words, behaviors, cognition, body language, feelings, intuition, thoughts, senses, the

energy field, and so forth all contribute to the transpersonal caring connection.

- The nurse's ability to connect with another at this transpersonal spirit-to-spirit level is translated via movements, gestures, facial expressions, procedures, information, touch, sound, verbal expressions, and other scientific, technical, esthetic, and human means of communication, into nursing human art and acts or intentional caring-healing modalities.
- The caring-healing modalities within the context of transpersonal caring/caritas consciousness potentiate harmony, wholeness, and unity of being by releasing some of the disharmony—that is, the blocked energy that interferes with natural healing processes; thus the nurse helps another through this process to access the healer within, in the fullest sense of Nightingale's view of nursing.
- Ongoing personal and professional development and spiritual growth, as well as personal spiritual practice, assist the nurse in entering into this deeper level of professional healing practice, allowing for awakening to a transpersonal condition of the world and fuller actualization of the "ontological competencies" necessary at this level of advanced practice of nursing.
- The nurse's own life history, previous experiences, opportunities for focused study, having lived through or experienced various human conditions, and having imagined others' feelings in various circumstances are valuable teachers for this work; to some degree, the nurse can gain the knowledge and consciousness needed through work with other cultures and study of the humanities (e.g., art, drama, literature, personal story, or narratives of illness or journeys), along with exploration of one's own values; deep beliefs; and relationship with self, others, and one's world.
- Other facilitators are personal growth experiences such as psychotherapy, transpersonal psychology, meditation, bioenergetics work, and other models for spiritual awakening.
- Continuous growth for developing and maturing within a transpersonal caring model is ongoing. The notion of health professionals as wounded healers is acknowledged as part of the necessary growth and compassion called forth within this theory and philosophy (Watson, 2006b).

THEORETICAL ASSERTIONS

Nursing

According to Watson (1988), the word *nurse* is both a noun and a verb. To her, nursing consists of "knowledge, thought, values, philosophy, commitment, and action, with some degree of passion" (p. 53). Nurses are interested in understanding health, illness, and the human experience; promoting and restoring health; and preventing illness. Watson's theory calls nurses to go beyond procedures, tasks, and techniques in practice, the **trim** of nursing, in contrast to the **core** of nursing, those aspects of the nurse-patient relationship resulting in a therapeutic outcome included in the transpersonal caring process (Watson, 2005, 2012). Using the 10 carative factors, the nurse provides care to various patients. Each carative factor and the clinical caritas processes describe how a patient attains or maintains health or dies a peaceful death. Conversely, Watson described **curing** as a medical term that refers to the elimination of disease (Watson, 1979). As Watson's work evolved, she increased her focus on the human care process and the transpersonal aspects of caring-healing in a transpersonal caring relationship (1999, 2005).

Watson's evolving work continues to make explicit that humans cannot be treated as objects and that humans cannot be separated from self, other, nature, and the larger universe. Caring-healing is located within a cosmology that is metaphysical and transcendent with the coevolving human in the universe.

Personhood (Human Being)

Watson uses interchangeably the terms **human being, person, life, personhood,** and **self.** She views the person as "a unity of mind/body/spirit/nature" (1996, p. 147), and she says that "personhood is tied to notions that one's soul possesses a body that is not confined by objective time and space" (Watson, 1988, p. 45). Watson states, "I make the point to use mind, body, soul or unity within an evolving emergent world view-connectedness of all, sometimes referred to as Unitary Transformative Paradigm-Holographic thinking. It is often considered dualistic because I use the *three* words 'mind, body, soul,' but my intention is to make explicit spirit/metaphysical—which is silent in other models" (Watson, personal communication, April 12, 1994).

Health

Watson's (1979) definition of **health** has evolved. It was originally derived from the World Health Organization as "The positive state of physical, mental, and social well-being with the inclusion of three elements: (1) a high level of overall physical, mental, and social functioning; (2) a general adaptive-maintenance level of daily functioning; (3) the absence of illness (or the presence of efforts that lead to its absence)" (p. 220). Later, she defined *health* as "unity and harmony within the mind, body, and soul"; associated with the "degree of congruence between the self as perceived and the self as experienced" (Watson, 1988, p. 48).

Watson (1988) stated further, "illness is not necessarily disease; [instead it is a] subjective turmoil or disharmony within a person's inner self or soul at some level of disharmony within the spheres of the person, for example, in the mind, body, and soul, either consciously or unconsciously" (p. 47). "While illness can lead to disease, illness and health are [a] phenomenon that is not necessarily viewed on a continuum. Disease processes can also result from genetic, constitutional vulnerabilities and manifest themselves when disharmony is present. Disease in turn creates more disharmony" (Watson, 1988, p. 48).

Environment

Watson speaks to the nurse's role in the environment as "attending to supportive, protective, and/or corrective mental, physical, societal, and spiritual environments" (Watson, 1979, p. 10) in the original carative factors. In later work, a much broader view of environment states: "the caring science is not only for sustaining humanity, but also for sustaining the planet. . . . Belonging is to an infinite universal spirit world of nature and all living things; it is the primordial link of humanity and life itself, across time and space, boundaries and nationalities" (Watson, 2003, p. 305). She says that "healing spaces can be used to help others transcend illness, pain, and suffering," emphasizing the environment and person connection: "when the nurse enters the patient's room, a magnetic field of expectation is created" (Watson, 2003, p. 305).

LOGICAL FORM

The theory is presented in a logical form. It contains broad ideas that address health-illness phenomena. Watson's definition of **caring** as opposed to **curing** is to delineate nursing from medicine and classify the body of nursing knowledge as a separate science.

Since 1979, the development of the theory has been toward clarifying the person of the nurse and the person of the patient. Another emphasis has been on existential-phenomenological and spiritual factors. Her works (2005) remind us of the "spirit-filled dimensions of caring work and caring knowledge" (p. x).

Watson's theory has foundational support from theorists in other disciplines, such as Carl Rogers, Erikson, and Maslow. She has been adamant that nursing education incorporate holistic knowledge from many disciplines integrating the humanities, arts, and sciences and that the increasingly complex health care systems and patient needs require nurses to have a broad, liberal education (Sakalys & Watson, 1986).

Watson incorporated dimensions of a postmodern paradigm shift throughout her theory of transpersonal caring. Her theoretical underpinnings associated with concepts such as steady-state maintenance, adaptation, linear interaction, and problem-based nursing practice were replaced with a postmodern approach, leading to a more holistic, humanistic, open system, wherein harmony, interpretation, and self-transcendence emerge, reflecting a epistemological shift.

APPLICATION BY THE NURSING COMMUNITY

Practice

Watson's theory has been validated in outpatient, inpatient, and community health clinical settings and with various populations, including recent applications with attention to patient care essentials (Pipe et al., 2012), living on a ventilator (Lindahl, 2011), simulating care (Diener & Hobbs, 2012), mothers struggling with mental illness (Blegen, Eriksson, & Bondas, 2014), and women with infertility (Arslan-Ozkan, Okumus, & Buldukoglu, 2014; Ozan, Okumus, & Lash, 2015). Jesse and Alligood (2014) provide examples of the application of Watson's theory in nursing practice.

The Attending Nursing Caring Model (ANCM) exemplifies the application of Watson Caring Science to practice, initially described in Watson and Foster (2003) as an application of theory to practice. The ANCM was a unique pilot project in a Denver children's hospital that is modeled after the "attending" physician model. However, unlike a medical cure model, the ANCM is concerned with the nursing care model. "It is constructed as a Nursing-Caring Science, theory-guided, evidence based, collaborative practice model for applying it to the conduct and oversight of pain management on a 37-bed, postsurgical unit" (Watson & Foster, 2003, p. 363). Nurses who participate in the project learn about Watson's caring theory, carative factors, caring consciousness, intentionality, and caring-healing practices. The mission of the ANCM is to have a continuous caring relationship with children in pain and their families. The ANCM is made visible in a caring-healing presence throughout the hospital. The influence and presence of Watson's theory continues to be applicable and transformative in hospital systems applying for initial and ongoing Magnet status. The list of Caring Science hospitals is growing and continually evolving; examples of those who have achieved this status include Stanford Health (Palo Alto, CA), Brigham and Women's (Boston, MA), Veterans Administration (District of Columbia), Veterans Administration (Tampa, FL), Memorial Beacon Health (Indiana), Colorado Children's Hospital (Denver, CO); those in process include Denver Health and Hospitals (Denver, CO) and Craig Rehabilitation Hospital (Denver, CO) (Watson, personal communication, April 6, 2016).

(See Watson's website [http://www.watsoncaringscience.org] for examples of this theory in practice.)

Administration and Leadership

Watson's theory calls for administrative practices and business models to embrace caring (Watson, 2006a), even in a health care environment of increased acuity levels of hospitalized individuals, short hospital stays, increasing complexity of technology, and rising expectations in the "task" of nursing. These challenges call for solutions that address health care system reform at a deep and ethical level and that enable nurses to follow their own professional practice model rather than short-term solutions, such as increasing numbers of beds, sign-on bonuses, and relocation incentives for nurses. Many hospitals seeking Magnet status are meeting these challenges by using Watson's theory of human caring for administrative change. Others call for sustaining a professional environment based on the definition of *patient care essentials* (Pipe et al., 2012). This and other examples of caring administrative practices are described on her website and in her article, "Caring Theory as an Ethical Guide to Administrative and Clinical Practices" (Watson, 2006a). Recent advances in Watson's theory relevant to administration include an effort toward linking caring science and quantum leadership, which includes the work of Tim Porter O'Grady, Teri Pipe, and Kathy Malloch at Arizona State University (personal communication, April 6, 2016).

Education

Watson's writings focus on educating graduate nursing students and providing them with ontological, ethical, and epistemological bases for their practice, along with research directions (Hills & Watson, 2011). Watson's caring theory has been taught in numerous baccalaureate nursing curricula, including Bellarmine College in Louisville, Kentucky; Indiana State University in Terre Haute; Oklahoma City University; and Florida Atlantic University. In addition, the concepts are used in international nursing programs in Australia, Japan, Brazil, Finland, Saudi Arabia, Sweden, and the United Kingdom, to name a few. At the University of Colorado students can pursue a PhD in nursing with a caring science focus, and the WCSI supports postdoctoral training in caring science. More initiatives are developing in South America and the Middle East (United Arab Emirates). Additional grassroot efforts aim to integrate caring science with nursing educational developments, for example with Mary Jo Kreitzer at the University of Minnesota and Mary Kothian at the University of Arizona. There are pockets of excellent creative caring science nursing programs in the United States: Viterbo University (La Crosse, Wisconsin), Nevada State College (Henderson, Nevada), and Florida Atlantic University (Boca Raton, Florida), which has the longest caring science academic program in the United States (Watson, personal communication, April 6, 2016).

Research

Qualitative, naturalistic, and phenomenological methods have been identified as particularly relevant to the study of caring and to the development of nursing as a human science (Nelson & Watson, 2011; Watson, 2012). Watson suggests that a combination of qualitative-quantitative inquiry, what is known broadly as mixed-methods design, may be useful for furthering the exploration and testing of the theory (Watson, 2008). There is a growing body of national and international research that tests, expands, and evaluates the theory (DiNapoli et al., 2010; Nelson & Watson, 2011). Smith (2004) published a review of 40 research studies that specifically used Watson's theory. Mason et al. (2014) presented the results of a mixed-methods pilot study in which Watson's theory was influential in the development of an intervention aimed at increasing nurse retention and reducing compassion fatigue and moral distress in a surgical trauma intensive care unit. As Watson's theory advances in the literature, researchers are providing statistical validation supporting the impact of the theory with randomized controlled trials. One such trial provided evidence in support of the efficacy of nursing care guided by Watson's theory to reduce distress experienced by infertile women (Arslan-Ozkan, Okumus, & Buldukoglu, 2014).

Measurement of outcomes associated with Watson's theory and the application of theory to clinical practice and hospital organizations have been major weak areas of research, with particular focus on survey development. Nelson and Watson (2011) report on studies carried out in seven countries. Nelson and Watson (2011) present eight caring surveys and other research tools for caritas research, such as differences among international perceptions of caring, nurse and patient relationships, and guidelines for hospitals seeking Magnet status. Development of measures to quantify the outcomes of caring science has received significant ongoing attention with the development of the Watson Caritas Patient Score (Brewer & Watson, 2015). Further, Watson is currently working with Press Ganey on a pilot program under way in five health care systems whereby five caritas items are being included in the Press Ganey survey to link the relationship between patients' experiences of caring and outcomes, beyond problem-focused data (Watson, personal communication, April 6, 2016).

A number of PhD dissertations and DNP projects have been conducted since 2013; a search of the Proquest Dissertations and Theses database yielded 29 such publications. A wide range of topics were researched that were grounded in or informed by Watson Caring Science. Topics reflected primarily the domains of nursing education and clinical practice, including, but not limited to, faculty-student caring relationships, caring health care leadership, Watson's caring theory translation bridging the theory-practice gap, emancipatory nursing experiences, and clinicians' and patients' perspectives and experiences of caring, including patient satisfaction.

FURTHER DEVELOPMENT

Jean Watson is currently working with more than 20 different countries that are involved in caring science in education, doctoral programs, clinical practice, or clinical care models. There is an ongoing commitment to global programs of caring science, with current work focused on the future unveiling of a formal Watson Caring Science Global Associate network. There are membership commitments from the Middle East, Japan, Italy, South America (Peru), China, and Mexico. Programs, projects, or systems pending are South Africa, Portugal, Spain, Canada (Quebec), Korea, Singapore, Thailand, the Philippines, and Taiwan.

Watson envisions Watson Caring Science influencing interdisciplinary realms of knowledge and practice, given that Watson Caring Science and unitary views are universal and transdisciplinary, beyond all health and healing professions, so it can be held as a hopeful paradigm for all health and healing professions and educational and human service programs. The paradigm is a guide toward honoring the whole person, preserving human dignity, and sustaining and evolving human consciousness, humanity, and views and informed moral action toward authentic human caring, healing, and health for self, other, and planet (personal communication, April 6, 2016).

On the horizon, Watson is creating a Watson Caring Science World Portal, evolving as a dream network of global programs, projects, and systems networking with one another with their unique programs, able to access a common portal of others' works, and to have virtual programs/webcasts from different countries sharing their work and helping one another as a resource for the 19 million nurses and midwifes as well as health and healing professions. Other future visions include creating new standards and criteria for hospitals and clinical agencies, including academic programs to be fully and formally credentialed as authentic Watson Caring Science organizations, with new forms of evidence beyond empirics alone, perhaps guided by evidence of new concepts such as "human flourishing"; caring-healing presence, consciousness, intentionality, evidence of caritas processes lived out at multiple levels in systems, and new outcome measures (caritas items).

CRITIQUE

Clarity

Watson uses nontechnical, sophisticated, fluid, and evolutionary language to artfully describe her concepts, such as caring-love, and caritas processes and consciousness. Paradoxically, abstract and simple concepts such as caring-love are difficult to practice, yet practicing and experiencing these concepts leads to greater understanding. At times, lengthy phrases and sentences are best understood if read more than once. Watson's inclusion of metaphors, personal reflections, artwork, and poetry make her concepts more tangible and more esthetically appealing. She has continued to refine her theory and has revised the original carative factors as caritas processes. Critics of Watson's work have concentrated on her use of undefined or changing/shifting definitions and terms and her focus on the psychosocial rather than the pathophysiological aspects of nursing. Watson (1985) has addressed the critiques of her work in the preface of *Nursing: The Philosophy and Science of Caring* (1979, 2008), in the preface of *Nursing: Human Science and Human Care—A Theory of Nursing* (1985, 1988), and in *Caring Science as Sacred Science* (2005).

Simplicity

Watson draws on a number of disciplines to formulate her theory. The theory is more about *being* than about *doing*, and the nurse must internalize it thoroughly if it is to be actualized in practice. To understand the theory as it is presented, it is best for the reader to be familiar with the broad subject matter. This theory is viewed as complex when the existential-phenomenological nature of her work is considered, particularly for nurses who have a limited liberal arts background. Although some consider her theory complex, many find it easy to understand and to apply in practice.

Generality

Watson's theory is best understood as a moral and philosophical basis for nursing. The scope of the theory encompasses broad aspects of health and illness phenomena. In addition, the theory addresses aspects of health promotion, preventing illness, and experiencing peaceful death, thereby increasing its generality. The caritas processes provide guidelines for nurse-patient interactions, an important aspect of patient care.

One critique is that the theory does not furnish explicit direction about what to do to achieve authentic caring-healing relationships. Nurses who want concrete guidelines may not feel secure when trying to use this theory alone. Some have suggested that it takes too much time to incorporate the caritas into practice, and some note that Watson's personal growth emphasis is a quality "that while appealing to some may not appeal to others" (Drummond, 2005, p. 218).

Empirical Precision

Watson describes her theory as descriptive; she acknowledges the evolving nature of the theory and welcomes input from others (Watson, 2012). Although the theory does not lend itself easily to research conducted through traditional scientific methods, recent work focused on intervention development and measurement stretch to validate the theory through quantitative or mixed-method design. In addition to this work, ongoing development with qualitative nursing approaches is appropriate and needed to adequately explore concepts central to the theory. Recent work on measurement reviews a broad array of international studies and provides research guidelines, design recommendations, and instruments for caring research (Nelson & Watson, 2011).

Derivable Consequences

Watson's theory continues to provide a useful and important metaphysical orientation for the delivery of nursing care (Watson, 2007). Watson's theoretical concepts, such as use of self, patient-identified needs, the caring process, and the spiritual sense of being human, may help nurses and their patients to find meaning and harmony during a period of increasing complexity. Watson's rich and varied knowledge of philosophy, the arts, the human sciences, and traditional science and traditions, joined with her prolific ability to communicate, has enabled professionals in many disciplines to share and recognize her work.

SUMMARY

Jean Watson began developing her theory while she was assistant dean of the undergraduate program at the University of Colorado, and it evolved into planning and implementation of its nursing PhD program. Her first book started as class notes that emerged from teaching in an innovative, integrated curriculum. She became coordinator and director of the PhD program when it began in 1978 and served until 1981. While she was serving as Dean of the University of Colorado, School of Nursing, a postbaccalaureate nursing curriculum in human caring was developed that led to a professional clinical doctoral degree (ND). This curriculum was implemented in 1990 and was later transitioned into the DNP degree. Watson initiated the Center for Human Caring, the nation's first interdisciplinary center with a commitment to develop and use knowledge of human caring for practice and scholarship. She worked from Yalom's 11 curative factors to formulate her 10 carative factors. She modified the 10 factors slightly over time and developed the caritas processes, which have a spiritual dimension and use a more fluid and evolutionary language.

CASE STUDY

A 62-year-old inmate is admitted to this hospital from prison with a complaint of chest pain. The patient is being worked up for possible myocardial infarction and admitted to the cardiac unit. Because the patient is an inmate, while he is in the hospital a prison guard will be posted outside of the patient's room and the patient will be handcuffed to the bed rail. During the initial assessment, the admission nurse finds the patient to be withdrawn. The nurse discovers the patient has a past medical history significant for abuse of multiple substances. The patient describes how the addictive behaviors led to his incarceration and estrangement from his family. The patient expresses to the nurse interest in meeting with a chaplain while in the hospital.

- Describe examples of the how the nurse can provide care to this patient as guided by each of the 10 caritas processes.

CRITICAL THINKING ACTIVITIES

1. Review the values and beliefs in your own philosophy of person, environment, health, and nursing and compare your beliefs with Watson's 10 caritas processes.
2. Create a list of caring behaviors in your own nursing practice. Review *Measuring Caring: International Research on Caritas as Healing* (Nelson & Watson, 2011), and compare your list with the caring behaviors from instruments designed to measure caring included in that text.
3. Plan a time and place to meditate for 10 minutes each week, closing your eyes and listening to quiet music. Reflect on ways to feel compassionate, intentional, calm, and peaceful. Consider ways to incorporate ideas from your reflection into your nursing practice.

POINTS FOR FURTHER STUDY

- Hill, M., & Watson, J. (2011). *Creating a caring sequence curriculum.* New York: Springer.
- Jesse, D. E., & Alligood, M. R. (2014). Watson's philosophy in nursing practice. In M. R. Alligood, *Nursing theory: Utilization application* (5th ed., pp. 96–117). St Louis: Mosby-Elsevier.
- Watson, J. (1989). *The nurse theorists: Portraits of excellence* [Videotape, CD, DVD]. Available from Fitne, Inc., Athens, OH, at http://www.fitne.net/.
- Watson, J. (2005). *Caring science as sacred science.* Philadelphia: F. A. Davis.
- Watson, J. (2012). *Human caring science: A theory of nursing.* Boston: Jones & Bartlett.
- Additional resources, references, and updates on the state of Watson Caring Science can be found at http://www.watsoncaringscience.org.

REFERENCES

Arslan-Ozkan, I., Okumus, H., & Buldukoglu, K. (2014). A randomized controlled trial of the effects of nursing care based on Watson's theory of human caring on distress, self-efficacy and adjustment in infertile women. *Journal of Advanced Nursing, 70*(8), 1801–1812.

Blegen, N. E., Eriksson, K., & Bondas, T. (2014). Through the depths and heights of darkness; mothers as patients in psychiatric care. *Scandinavian Journal of Caring Sciences, 28*(4), 852.

Brewer, B. B., & Watson, J. (2015). Evaluation of authentic human caring professional practices. *JONA: The Journal of Nursing Administration, 45*(12), 622–627.

Diener, E., & Hobbs, N. (2012). Simulating care: Technology-mediated learning in twenty-first century education. *Nursing Forum, 47*(1), 34–38.

DiNapoli, P., Nelson, J., Turkel, M., & Watson, J. (2010). Measuring the caritas processes: Caring factor survey. *International Journal for Human Caring, 14*(3), 17–20.

Drummond, J. (2005). Caring science as sacred science. [Book review.] *Nursing Philosophy, 6*, 218–220.

Hills, M., & Watson, J. (2011). *Creating a caring science curriculum: An emancipatory pedagogy for nursing.* New York: Springer.

Jesse, D. E., & Alligood, M. R. (2014). Watson's philosophy in nursing practice. In M. R. Alligood (Ed.), *Nursing theory: Utilization & application* (5th ed., pp. 96–117). St Louis: Mosby-Elsevier.

Leininger, M. (1979). Preface. In J. Watson (Ed.), *Nursing: The philosophy and science of caring.* Boston: Little, Brown.

Levinas, E. (1969). *Totality and infinity.* (A. Lingis, Trans.) Pittsburgh, PA: Duquesne University.

Lindahl, B. (2011). Experiences of exclusion when living on a ventilator: Reflections based on the application of Julia Kristev's philosophy of caring. *Nursing Philosophy, 12*(1), 12–21.

Løgstrup, K. E. (1995). *Metaphysics* (Vol. 1). Milwaukee: Marquette University.

Mason, V. M., Leslie, G., Clark, K., Lyons, P., Walke, E., Bulter, C., & Griffin, M. (2014). Compassion fatigue, moral distress, and work engagement in surgical intensive care unit trauma nurses. *Dimensions of Critical Care Nursing, 33*(4), 215–225.

Nelson, J., & Watson, J. (2011). *Measuring caring: International research on caritas as healing.* New York: Springer.

Ozan, Y. D., Okumus, H., & Lash, A. A. (2015). Implementation of Watson's theory of human caring: A case study. *International Journal of Caring Sciences*, 8(1), 25–35.

Pipe, T., Connolly, T., Spahr, N., Lendzion, N., Buchda, V., Jury, R., et al. (2012). Bringing back the basics of nursing: Defining patient care. *Nursing Administration Quarterly, 36*(3), 225–233.

Sakalys, J., & Watson, J. (1986). Professional education: Post-baccalaureate education for professional nursing. *Journal of Professional Nursing, 2*(2), 91–97.

Sitzman, K., & Watson, J. (2013). *Caring science, mindful practice: Implementing Watson's human caring theory.* New York: Springer.

Smith, M. (2004). Review of research related to Watson's theory of caring. *Nursing Science Quarterly, 17*(1), 13–25.

Watson, J. (1979). *Nursing: The philosophy and science of caring.* Boston: Little, Brown.

Watson, J. (1981). Nursing's scientific quest. *Nursing Outlook, 29*, 413–416.

Watson, J. (1985). *Nursing: Human science and human care—a theory of nursing.* Norwalk, CT: Appleton-Century-Crofts.

Watson, J. (1986, Dec.). The dean speaks out: Center for human caring established. *The University of Colorado School of Nursing News*, 1–6.

Watson, J. (1987). Nursing on the caring edge: Metaphorical vignettes. *Advances in Nursing Science, 10*(1), 10–18.

Watson, J. (1988). *Nursing: Human science and human care: A theory of nursing.* New York: National League for Nursing.

Watson, J. (1995). Post modernism and knowledge development in nursing. *Nursing Science Quarterly, 8*(2), 60–64.

Watson, J. (1996). Watson's theory of transpersonal caring. In P. J. Walker & B. Neuman (Eds.), *Blueprint for use of nursing models: Education, research, practice and administration* (pp. 141–184). New York: National League for Nursing Press.

Watson, J. (1997). The theory of human caring: Retrospective and prospective. *Nursing Science Quarterly, 10*(1), 49–52.

Watson, J. (1999). *Postmodern nursing and beyond.* Edinburgh: Churchill Livingstone.

Watson, J. (2002). *Instruments for assessing and measuring caring in nursing and health sciences.* New York: Springer.

Watson, J. (2003). Caring science: Belonging before being as ethical cosmology. *Nursing Science Quarterly, 18*(4), 304–305.

Watson, J. (2005). *Caring science as sacred science.* Philadelphia: F. A. Davis.

Watson, J. (2006). Caring theory as an ethical guide to administrative and clinical practices. *Nursing Administration Quarterly, 30*(1), 48–55.

Watson, J. (2007). Theoretical questions and concerns: Response from a caring science framework. *Nursing Science Quarterly, 20*(1), 13–15.

Watson, J. (2008). *Nursing: The philosophy and science of caring. Revised & Updated Edition.* Boulder, CO: University Press of Colorado.

Watson, J. (2012). *Human caring science: A theory of nursing.* Boston: Jones & Bartlett.

Watson, J., & Foster, R. (2003). The attending nurse caring model: Integrating theory, evidence, and advanced caring-healing therapeutics for transforming professional practice. *Journal of Clinical Nursing, 12,* 360–365.

Watson Caring Science Institute, International Caritas Consortium. Retrieved from http://www.watsoncaringscience.org.

BIBLIOGRAPHY

Primary Sources

Books

Bevis, E. O., & Watson, J. (1989). *Toward a caring curriculum: A new pedagogy for nursing.* New York: National League for Nursing.

Bevis, E. O., & Watson, J. (2000, reprinted). *Toward a caring curriculum: A new pedagogy for nursing.* Sudbury, MA: Jones & Bartlett.

Chinn, P., & Watson, J. (Eds.). (1994). *Art and aesthetics of nursing.* New York: National League for Nursing.

Leininger, M., & Watson, J. (Eds.). (1990). *The caring imperative in education.* New York: National League for Nursing.

Lane, M. R., Samuels, M. & Watson, J. (2012). *The caritas path to peace: A guide for creating world peace with caring, love, and compassion,* Gainesville, FL: M.R. Lane publisher.

Taylor, R., & Watson, J. (Eds.). (1989). *They shall not hurt: Human suffering and human caring.* Boulder, CO: University Press of Colorado.

Watson, J. (Ed.). (1994). *Applying the art and science of human caring.* New York: National League for Nursing.

Watson, J. (2002). *Assessing and measuring caring in nursing and health sciences.* New York: Springer.

Watson, J. (2008). *Nursing: The philosophy and science of caring. Revised & Updated Edition.* Boulder, CO: University Press of Colorado.

Watson, J. (2011). *Postmodern nursing and beyond. New edition.* Boulder, CO: Watson Caring Science Institute.

Chapters and Monographs

Newman, M., Roy, C., & Watson, J. (2005). Dialogue with nursing theorists. In C. Picard & D. Jones (Eds.), *Giving voice to what we know.* Boston: Jones and Bartlett.

Watson, J. (2000). *Monograph of instruments for measuring and assessing caring.* New York: Springer.

Watson, J. (2000). Postmodern nursing and beyond. In N. L. Chaska (Ed.), *The nursing profession: Tomorrow's vision and beyond* (pp. 299–308). Thousand Oaks, CA: Sage.

Watson, J. (2001). Jean Watson: Theory of human caring. In M. E. Parker (Ed.), *Nursing theories and nursing practice* (pp. 344–354). Philadelphia: F. A. Davis.

Watson, J. (2002). Illuminating the spiritual journey: Jean Watson tells her story. In P. Burkhardt & M. G. Nagai-Jackson (Eds.), *Spirituality: Living our connectedness* (pp. 181–186). New York: Delmar.

Watson, J. (2003). Meditation: Contemplative practice. In K. Wren & C. Norred (Eds.), *Real-world nursing survival guide: Complementary and alternative therapies* (pp. 156–160). St Louis: Harcourt.

Watson, J. (2005). Watson's theory of human caring. In J. Fawcett & S. Desanto-Madeya (Ed.), *Contemporary nursing knowledge: Analysis and evaluation of nursing models and theories.* Philadelphia: F. A. Davis.

Watson, J. (2006). Jean Watson's theory of human caring. In M. Parker (Ed.), *Nursing theories and nursing practice* (2nd ed., pp. 295–301). Philadelphia: F. A. Davis.

Watson, J. (2007). Leadership is… visionary conversations and reflections on my journey into the heart of nursing: Human caring-healing. In T. Hansen-Turton, S. Sherman, & V. Ferguson (Eds.), *Conversations with leaders* (pp. 174–183). Indianapolis, IN: Sigma Theta Tau International.

Watson, J. (2011). Jean Watson: Personal experience and background in being a nurse theorist. In K. L. Sitzman & L. W. Eichelberger (Eds.), *Understanding the work of nurse theorists* (2nd ed., pp. 55–58). Boston: Jones & Barlett.

Watson, J. (2013). Curriculum and student advisement reflection. In D. D. Hunt (Ed.), *The new nurse educator.* New York: Springer.

Watson, J. (2014). Social/moral justice from caring science cosmology. In P. N. Kagan, M. C. Smith, & P. L. Chinn (Eds.), *Philosophies and practices of emancipatory nursing: Social justice as praxis* (101–105). Oxford, UK: Routledge.

Watson, J. (2014). Integrative nursing: Caring science—human caring and peace. In M. J. Kreitzer & M. Koithan (Eds.), *Integrative nursing.* Oxford, UK: Oxford University Press.

Journal Articles

Clarke, P. N., Watson, J., & Brewer, B. (2009). From theory to practice: Caring science according to Watson and Brewer. *Nursing Science Quarterly, 22*(3), 339–345.

Cowling, R. Smith, M., Watson, J., & Newman, M. (2008). The power of wholeness, consciousness, and caring. A dialogue on nursing science, art, and healing. *Advances in Nursing Science, 31*(1), E41–E51.

Giovannoin, J., McCoy, K. T., Mays, M., & Watson, J. (2015). Probation officers reduce their stress by cultivating the practice of loving-kindness with self and others. *International Journal of Caring Sciences, 8*(2), 325–343.

Hemsley, M. S., Glass, N., & Watson, J. (2006). Taking the eagle's view: Using Watson's conceptual model to investigate the extraordinary and transformative experiences of nurse healers. *Journal of Holistic Nursing Practice, 20*(2), 85–94.

Howie, L., Rankin, J., & Watson, J. (2013). An evaluation of the Scottish multiprofessional maternity development programme (SMMDP). *Midwifery Matters, 138*, 5–6.

Ozkan, I. A., Okumus, H., Buldukoglu, K., & Watson, J. (2013). A case study based on Watson's theory of human caring: Being an infertile woman in Turkey. *Nursing Science Quarterly, 26*(4), 352–359.

Persky, G. J., Nelson, J. W., Watson, J., & Bent, K. (2008). Creating a profile of a nurse effective in caring. *Nursing Administration Quarterly, 32*(1), 15–20.

Quinn, J., Smith, M., Swanson, K., Ritenbaugh, C., & Watson, J. (2003). The healing relationship in clinical nursing: Guidelines for research. *Journal of Alternative Therapies*, 9(3), A65–A79.

Turkel, M. C., & Watson, J. (2014). Advancing caring science through international collaboration and partnerships. *International Journal of Human Caring, 18*(4), 65.

Watson, J. (2000). Leading via caring-healing: The fourfold way toward transformative leadership. *Nursing Administration Quarterly, 25*(1), 1–6.

Watson, J. (2000). Philosophical perspectives in home care: Reconsidering caring. *Journal of Geriatric Nursing, 21*(6), 330–331.

Watson, J. (2000). Reconsidering caring in the home. *Journal of Geriatric Nursing, 21*(6), 330–333.

Watson, J. (2000). Via negative: Considering caring by way of non-caring. *Australian Journal of Holistic Nursing, 7*(1), 4–8.

Watson, J. (2001). Post-hospital nursing: Shortages, shifts, and script. *Nursing Administration Quarterly, 25*(3), 77–82.

Watson, J. (2002). Caring and healing our living and dying. *The International Nurse, 14*(2), 4–5.

Watson, J. (2002). Holistic nursing and caring: A values-based approach. *Journal of Japan Academy of Nursing Science, 22*(2), 69–74.

Watson, J. (2002). Intentionality and caring-healing consciousness: A theory of transpersonal nursing. *Holistic Nursing Journal, 16*(4), 12–19.

Watson, J. (2002). Metaphysics of virtual caring communities. *International Journal of Human Caring, 6*(1), 41–45.

Watson, J. (2002, Spring). Nursing: Seeking its source and survival. [Guest editorial.] *ICU Nursing Web Journal, 9*, 1–7. Retrieved from http://www.nursing.gr/J.W.editorial.pdf.

Watson, J. (2003). Love and caring: Ethics of face and hand. *Nursing Administration Quarterly, 27*(3), 197–202.

Watson, J. (2004). Caritas and communitas: An ethic for caring science. *Journal Japan Academy of Nursing Science, 24*(1), 66–71.

Watson, J. (2004). The relational core of nursing practice as partnership. [Invited commentary.] *Journal of Advanced Nursing, 47*(3), 241–250.

Watson, J. (2005). Caring for our future: An interview with Jean Watson. [Interview by Carla Mariano.] *Beginnings* (American Holistic Nurses' Association), *25*(3), 1, 12–14.

Watson, J. (2005). Caring science: Belonging before being as ethical cosmology. *Nursing Science Quarterly, 18*(4), 304–305.

Watson, J. (2005). Commentary on Shattell, M. (2004). Nurse-patient interaction: A review of the literature. *Journal of Clinical Nursing, 14*, 530–532.

Watson, J. (2005). What, may I ask, is happening to nursing knowledge and professional practices? What is nursing thinking at this turn in human history? *Journal of Clinical Nursing, 14*(8), 913–914.

Watson, J. (2005). Current issues and haunting concerns for survival of nursing profession. *Japanese Journal of Nursing Science, 30*(11), 50–53.

Watson, J. (2005). *An overview of Watson's theory of human caring.* Tokyo, Japan: Bulletin of Japanese Red Cross University College of Nursing.

Watson, J. (2006). Can an ethic of caring be maintained? *Journal of Advanced Nursing, 54*(3), 257–259.

Watson, J. (2006). Carative factors—Caritas processes guide to professional nursing. *Danish Clinical Nursing Journal, 20*(3), 21–27.

Watson, J. (2006). Caring theory as an ethical guide to administrative and clinical practices. *JONAS Healthcare Law, Ethics and Regulation, 8*(3), 87–93.

Watson, J. (2006). Caring theory as an ethical guide to administrative and clinical practices. *Nursing Administration Quarterly, 30*(1), 48–55.

Watson, J. (2006). Frontline and backstage caring: American nurse/world-wide nurses. *American Nurse Today, 1*(1), 24–28.

Watson, J. (2006). Walking pilgrimage as caritas action in the world. *Journal of Holistic Nursing, 24*(4), 289–296.

Watson, J. (2007). Theoretical questions and concerns: Response from a caring science framework. *Nursing Science Quarterly, 20*(1), 13–15.

Watson, J. (2007). Watson's theory of human caring and subjective living experiences: Disciplinary guide to professional nursing practice. *Brazilian Clinical Nursing Journal: Texto and Contexto, 16*(1), 129–135.

Watson, J. (2008). Social justice and caring: A model of caring science as a hopeful paradigm for moral justice for humanity. *Creative Nursing: A Journal of Values, Issues, Experience & Collaboration, 32*(1), 15–20.

Watson, J. (2009). Caring as the essence of nursing and health care. *Mundo da Saude, 3*(2), 143–149.

Watson, J. (2009). Caring science and human caring theory: Transforming personal/professional practice in nursing and healthcare. *Journal of Health and Human Services Administration. Symposium issue, 31*(4), 466–482.

Watson, J. (2010). Florence Nightingale and the enduring legacy of transpersonal human caring-healing. *Journal of Holistic Nursing, 28*(1), 107–108.

Watson, J. (2010 Spring). Caring science: The next decade of holistic healing. *Beginnings, 30*(2), 14–16.

Watson, J. (2012). Next generation of caring theory. Editorial. *International Journal of Human Caring, 16*(2), xx.

Watson, J. (2012). Touching the heart of our humanity: The caritas path of peace. *Japanese Journal of Nursing Research, 45*(6), 528–537.

Watson, J. (2014). Caring science in nursing: Coming of age in theory-practice-research. *Chinese Journal of Nursing Science, 29*(1), 1–3.

Watson, J. (2015). The fourfold way toward global leadership. *Chinese Nursing Management Journal, 15*(3), 257–258.

Watson, J. (2015). Editorial: Human caring research in nursing. *Revista Enfermia* Bogota Colomia UnivJaverina. Journal Online, *17*(2), 13–16.

Watson, J. (2015). Human caring research in nursing. *Inicio, 17*(2), 13–16.

Watson, J., Bauer, R., & Biley, F. (2002). Bavarian nursing secret: An inside view. *Reflections on Nursing Leadership: Sigma Theta Tau International Magazine, 28*(1), 26–28.

Watson, J., Biley, F. C., & Biley, A. M. (2001). Aesthetics, post-modern nursing, complementary therapies and more: An Internet dialogue. *Theoria: Journal of Nursing Theory, 10*(3), 13–16.

Watson, J., Biley, F. C., & Biley, A. M. (2002). Aesthetics, postmodern nursing, complementary therapies, and more: An Internet dialogue. *Complementary Therapies in Nursing and Midwifery, 8*, 81–83.

Watson, J., & Brewer, B. (2015). Caring science research, criteria, evidence, measurement. *Journal of Nursing Administration, 45*(5), 235–236.

Watson, J., & Foster, R. (2003). The Attending Nurse Caring Model: Integrating theory, evidence, and advanced caring-healing therapeutics for transforming professional practice. *Journal of Clinical Nursing, 12*, 360–365.

Watson, J., & Smith, M. C. (2002). Caring science and the science of unitary human beings: A trans-theoretical discourse for nursing knowledge development. *Journal of Advanced Nursing, 7*(5), 452–461.

Watson, J., Russel, M., Creanery, P., Walker, L., & Walsh, M. (2014). Peer review in supervision. *Midwives, 17*(5), 52–53.

8

Theory of Bureaucratic Caring

Sherrilyn Coffman

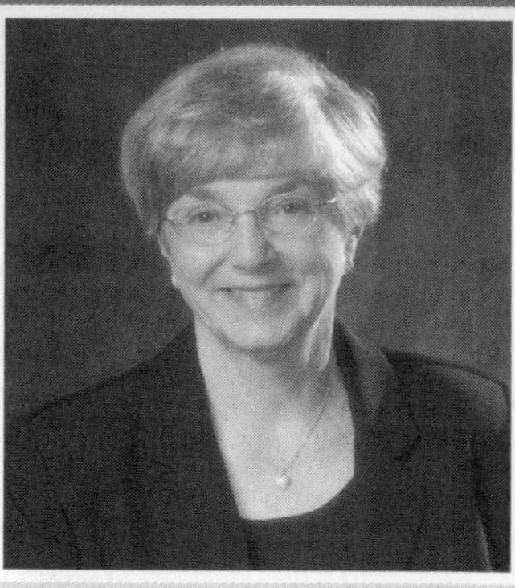

Marilyn Anne Ray (1938–Present)

"Improved patient safety, infection control, reduction in medication errors, and overall quality of care in complex bureaucratic health care systems cannot occur without knowledge and understanding of complex organizations, such as the political and economic systems, and spiritual-ethical caring, compassion and right action for all patients and professionals."

(Ray, personal communication, May 15, 2012)

CREDENTIALS AND BACKGROUND OF THE THEORIST

Marilyn Anne (Dee) Ray was born in Hamilton, Ontario, Canada, and grew up in a family of six children. When Ray was 15 years old, her father became seriously ill, was hospitalized, and almost died. A nurse saved his life. Marilyn decided that she would become a nurse so that she could help others and perhaps save lives, too.

In 1958, Marilyn Ray graduated from St. Joseph Hospital School of Nursing, Hamilton, and left for Los Angeles, California, where she worked at the University of California, Los Angeles Medical Center on several different patient units. While working with African American and Latino patients, Ray noted how important cultures were in the development of people's views about nursing and the world.

In 1965, Ray returned to school for her BSN and MSN at the University of Colorado School of Nursing, where she met Dr. Madeleine Leininger, a nurse anthropologist and Director of the Federal Nurse-Scientist program. Through mentorship, Leininger influenced Ray's life to take a special interest in nursing, anthropology, childhood, and culture. She studied organizations as small cultures, and her graduate school project involved the study of a children's hospital as a small culture. While at the University of Colorado, Ray practiced with children and adults in critical care, renal dialysis, and occupational health nursing.

In the 1960s, Ray became a citizen of the United States and afterward was commissioned as an officer in the U.S. Air Force Reserve, Nurse Corps (and Air National Guard). She graduated as a flight nurse from the School of Aerospace Medicine at Brooks Air Force Base, San Antonio, Texas, and served as an aero-medical evacuation nurse. She cared for combat casualties and other patients on board various types of aircraft during the Vietnam War. Ray served more than 30 years in different positions in the U.S. Air Force—flight nurse, clinician, administrator, educator, and researcher—and held the rank of colonel. Her interest in space nursing stimulated her to attend the program for educators at Marshall Space Flight Center in Huntsville, Alabama. She remains a charter member of the Space Nursing Society. In 1990 Ray went to the Soviet Union with the Aerospace Medical Association, when the USSR opened its space operations to American space engineers and physicians. Ray returned to active duty during the Persian Gulf War in 1991 and was assigned to Eglin Air Force Base, Valparaiso, Florida, where she orchestrated discharge planning and conducted research.

Ray is the recipient of multiple medals, including an Air Force commendation for nursing education and research

Photo credit: M. Dauley, Artistic Images, Littleton, CO.

developments received during her Air Force career. Most notably, in 2000 she received the Federal Nursing Services Essay Award from the Association of Military Surgeons of the United States for research on the impact of TRICARE/Managed Care on Total Force Readiness. This award recognized her research program on economics and the nurse-patient relationship that received nearly $1 million from the TriService Military Nursing Research Council. In 2008 she received the TriService Nursing Research Program Coin for excellence in nursing research.

Ray's first nursing faculty positions were at the University of San Francisco and the University of California San Francisco with Glaser and Strauss, authors of the grounded theory method. She was intrigued by the study of nursing as a culture and had opportunities to teach students from various American and Asian cultures. She traveled to Mexico in 1971 with colleagues to study anthropology and health.

From 1973 to 1977, Ray returned to Canada to be with family and joined the nursing faculty at McMaster University in Hamilton, Ontario. This was an exciting time, because McMaster University Health Sciences Center was initiating evidence-based teaching, education, and practice. Ray completed a Master of Arts in Cultural Anthropology at McMaster University, studying human relationships, decision making and conflict, and the hospital as an organizational culture. Dr. Leininger invited her to apply for the first transcultural nursing doctoral program at the University of Utah. Ray's doctoral dissertation (1981b) was a study on caring in the complex hospital organizational culture. From this research, the theory of bureaucratic caring, the focus of this chapter, was developed.

During doctoral studies, Ray married James L. Droesbeke, her inspiration and friend, and the love of her life. He was a constant source of support and helped her over the course of her career until his untimely death from cancer in 2001. After completing her doctorate in 1981, Ray rejoined the University of Colorado School of Nursing, where she worked with Jean Watson, who developed the theory and practice of human caring in nursing. With Watson and other scholars, Ray helped found the International Association for Human Caring, which recognized her with its Lifetime Achievement Award in 2008.

In the 1980s, at the University of Colorado, Ray continued her study of phenomenology and qualitative research approaches and directed dissertation work. In 1989 Ray was appointment the Christine E. Lynn Eminent Scholar at Florida Atlantic University, College of Nursing, a position she held until 1994. Florida Atlantic University developed the Center for Caring, which has been housing caring archives since the inception of the International Association for Human Caring in 1978. Ray held the position of Yingling Visiting Scholar Chair at Virginia Commonwealth University School of Nursing from 1994 to 1995, and she was a visiting professor at the University of Colorado from 1989 to 1999. Ray has been visiting professor at universities in Australia, New Zealand, and Thailand, advancing the teaching and research of human caring (Ray, 1994b, 2000, 2010b, 2016; Ray & Turkel, 2000, 2015). She authored several theoretical and research publications in transcultural caring, transcultural ethics, and caring inquiry.

Ray continues as Professor Emeritus at the Florida Atlantic University Christine E. Lynn College of Nursing as a part-time faculty member in the PhD program and faculty mentor. Ray's interest in transcultural nursing remains a theme in her research, teaching, and practice. With Dr. Sherrilyn Coffman, she completed a grounded theory research study of high-risk pregnant African American women (Coffman & Ray, 1999, 2002). Learning about vulnerable populations gave Ray a deeper understanding of their needs, particularly the importance of access to health care and caring communities. Ray was vice president of Floridians for Health Care (universal health care) from 1998 to 2000. She is a Certified Transcultural Nurse and a member of the International Transcultural Nursing Society. She has made international presentations in China, Saudi Arabia, Sweden, Finland, England, Switzerland, Thailand, and Vietnam. In 1984 Ray received the Leininger Transcultural Nursing Award for excellence in transcultural nursing. In 2005 she was named a Transcultural Nursing Scholar by the International Transcultural Nursing Society. Ray is listed in *Who's Who in America* and *Who's Who in the World* and gave a paper in 2010 on caring organizations at the World Universities Forum in Davos, Switzerland (Ray, 2010a). She attended a program of study at the United Nations related to implementation of the 2015 millennium goals. Ray serves on review boards of the *Journal of Transcultural Nursing* and *Qualitative Health Research.* She also published *Transcultural Caring Dynamics in Nursing and Health Care* (Ray, 2010c) which was revised in 2016. Her coedited book, *Nursing, Caring, and Complexity Science: For Human-Environment Well-Being,* received a 2011 American Journal of Nursing Book of the Year award.

Ray's research interests continue to focus on nurses, nurse administrators, and patients in critical care and intermediate care, and in nursing administration in complex hospital organizational cultures. She developed research with Dr. Marian Turkel to study the nurse-patient relationship as an economic resource, funded by the TriService Nursing Research Program (Turkel & Ray, 2000, 2001, 2003). With Turkel, Ray has published about complex caring relational theory, organizational transformation through caring and ethical choice making, instrument development on organizational caring, economic and political caring, and caring organization creation. They recently proposed renaming the nursing process to the language of caring in *Nursing Science Quarterly* (Turkel, Ray, & Kornblatt, 2012). Continued involvement at Florida Atlantic University has given Ray opportunities to influence complex organizations and caring organizations and environments in local, national, and global contexts. Her contributions to nursing education were recognized in 2005 with an honorary degree from Nevada State College and in 2007 with the Distinguished Alumna Award from University of Utah College of Nursing. Ray is a Sustaining Fellow in the Society for Applied Anthropology. In 2013 she was inducted as a Fellow of the American Academy of Nursing (FAAN).

THEORETICAL SOURCES FOR THEORY DEVELOPMENT

Ray's interest in caring as a topic of nursing scholarship was stimulated by her work with Leininger in 1968, focused on transcultural nursing and ethnographic-ethnonursing research methods. She used ethnographic methods in combination with phenomenology and grounded theory to generate substantive and formal grounded theories, resulting in the overarching theory of bureaucratic caring (Ray, 1981b, 1984, 1989, 1994b, 2010b, 2011; Ray & Turkel, 2015), which focuses on nursing in complex organizations such as hospitals. She distinguishes organizations as cultures based on anthropological study of how people behave in communities and the significance or meaning of work life (Louis, 1985). Organizational cultures, viewed as social constructions, are formed symbolically through meaning in interaction (Smircich, 1985).

Ray's work (1981a, 1989, 2010b; Moccia, 1986) was influenced by Hegel, who posited the interrelationship among thesis, antithesis, and synthesis. In Ray's theory, the thesis of caring (humanistic, spiritual, and ethical) and the antithesis of bureaucracy (technological, economic, political, and legal) are reconciled and synthesized into the unitive force, bureaucratic caring. The synthesis, as a process of becoming, is a transformation that continues to repeat itself, always changing, emerging, and transforming.

As she continued to develop her formal theory, Ray (2001, 2006; Ray & Turkel, 2015) discovered that her study findings fit well with explanations from chaos theory. Chaos theory describes simultaneous order and disorder, and order within disorder. An underlying order or interconnectedness exists in apparently random events (Peat, 2002). Mathematical studies have shown that what may seem random is actually part of a larger pattern. Application of this theory to organizations demonstrates that within a state of chaos, the system is held within boundaries that are well ordered (Wheatley, 2006). Furthermore, chaos is necessary for new creative ordering. The creative process as described by Briggs and Peat is as follows:

> *"[W]hen we enter the vital turbulence of life, we realize that, at bottom, everything is always new. Often we have simply failed to notice this fact. When we're being creative, we take notice."*
>
> **(Briggs & Peat, 1999, p. 30)**

Ray compares change in complex organizations with this creative process and challenges nurses to step back and renew their perceptions of everyday events, to discover embedded meanings. This is particularly important during organizational change. Complexity is a broader concept than chaos and focuses on wholeness or holonomy. Complex systems, such as organizations, have many agents interacting in multiple ways. As a result, these systems are dynamic and always changing. Systems behave in nonlinear fashion because they do not react proportionately to inputs. For example, a simple intervention such as asking a colleague for help may be accommodated easily or may be seen as unreasonable on a busy day, making human behavior in complex systems impossible to predict (Davidson, Ray, & Turkel, 2011; Vicenzi, White, & Begun, 1997). Briggs and Peat (1999) describe "chaotic wholeness" as "full of particulars, active and interactive, animated by nonlinear feedback and capable of producing everything from self-organized systems to fractal self-similarity to unpredictable chaotic disorder" (pp. 156–157). Their ideas influenced Ray's ongoing development of bureaucratic caring theory, which suggests that multiple system inputs are interconnected with caring in the organizational culture (Davidson, Ray, & Turkel, 2011; Ray, Turkel, & Cohn, 2011).

Ray's idea of the theory of bureaucratic caring as holographic was influenced by the revolution taking place in science based on the holographic worldview (Davidson, Ray, & Turkel, 2011; Ray, 2001, 2006, 2016; Ray & Turkel, 2015). The discovery of interconnectedness among apparently unrelated subatomic events has intrigued scientists. Scientists concluded that systems possess the capacity to self-organize; therefore attention is shifting away from parts to a focus on the totality as an actual process (Wheatley, 2006). The conceptualization of the hologram portrays how every structure interpenetrates and is interpenetrated by other structures—so the part is the whole, and the whole reflects every part (Talbot, 1991). The hologram provided scientists with a new way of understanding order. Bohm conceptualized the universe as a kind of giant, flowing hologram (Davidson, Ray, & Turkel, 2011; Talbot, 1991). He asserted that our day-to-day reality is an illusion, like a holographic image. Bohm termed our conscious level of existence **explicate,** or **unfolded order,** and the deeper layer of reality of which humans are usually unaware **implicate,** or **enfolded order.**

In the theory of bureaucratic caring, Ray compares the health care structures of political, legal, economic, educational, physiological, social-cultural, and technological systems with the explicate order and spiritual-ethical caring with the implicate order. A case manager's decisions about obtaining resources for a client's care in the home is an example. At first, explicate structures such as the legal managed care contract or the physical needs of the client appear to provide enough information. However, through the case manager's caring relationship with the client, implicate issues emerge, such as the client's values and desires. In truth, nursing situations involve an endless enfolding and unfolding of information that may be viewed as explicate and implicate order and are important to consider in the decision-making process.

Making things work in a health care organizational system requires knowledge and understanding of bureaucracy and the complexity of change. Bureaucracy and complexity may seem like the antithesis, but in reality the structure of bureaucracy (illuminating the political, economic, legal, and technological systems in organizations) works in conjunction with the complex relational process of networks to cocreate patterns of human behavior and patterns of caring. Bureaucracy and complexity influence the ways in which diverse participants describe and intuitively live out their life world experience in the system. No one thing or person in a system is independent; rather, they are interdependent. The system is holographic as whole and part are intertwined. Thus bureaucracy and complexity cocreate and transform each other. The theory of bureaucratic caring is a representation of the relatedness of system and caring factors.

MAJOR CONCEPTS & DEFINITIONS

Theoretical processes of awareness of viewing truth, or seeing the good of things (caring), and of communication are central to the theory. The dialectic of spiritual-ethical caring (the implicate order) in relation to the surrounding structures of political, legal, economic, educational, physiological, social-cultural, and technological (the explicate order) illustrates the interconnection with caring and the system as a macrocosm of the culture. In the model (see Fig. 8.2) everything is infused with spiritual-ethical caring (the center) by integrative and relational connection to the structures of organizational life. Spiritual-ethical caring involves different political, economic, and technological processes.

Holography means that everything is a *whole* in one context and a *part* in another—with each part being in the whole and the whole being in the part (Talbot, 1991). Spiritual-ethical caring is both a part and a whole. Every part secures its meaning from each part, also seen as wholes.

Caring

Caring is defined as a complex transcultural, relational process grounded in an ethical, spiritual context. Caring is the relationship between charity and right action, between love as compassion in response to suffering and need and justice or fairness in terms of what ought to be done. Caring occurs within a culture or society, including personal culture, hospital organizational culture, and societal and global culture (Ray, 2010b, 2016).

Spiritual-Ethical Caring

Spirituality involves creativity and choice and is revealed in attachment, love, and community. The **ethical** imperatives of caring join with the spiritual and are related to moral obligations toward others. This means never treating people as a means to an end but as beings with the capacity to make choices. Spiritual-ethical caring for nursing focuses on the facilitation of choices for the good of others (Ray, 1989, 1997a, 2016).

Educational

Formal and informal **educational** programs, use of audiovisual media to convey information, and other forms of teaching and sharing information are examples of educational factors related to the meaning of caring (Ray, 1981b, 1989, 2010a).

Physical

Physical factors are related to the physical state of being, including biological and mental patterns. Because the mind and body are interrelated, each pattern influences the other (Ray, 2001, 2006).

Social-Cultural

Examples of **social** and **cultural** factors are ethnicity and family structures; intimacy with friends and family; communication; social interaction and support; understanding interrelationships, involvement, and intimacy; and structures of cultural groups, community, and society (Ray, 1981b, 1989, 2001, 2006, 2016).

Legal

Legal factors related to the meaning of caring include responsibility and accountability; rules and principles to

Continued

MAJOR CONCEPTS & DEFINITIONS—cont'd

guide behaviors, such as policies and procedures; informed consent; rights to privacy; malpractice and liability issues; client, family, and professional rights; and the practice of defensive medicine and nursing (Gibson, 2008; Ray, 1981b, 1989, 2010b, 2016).

Technological

Technological factors include nonhuman resources, such as the use of machinery to maintain the physiological well-being of the patient, diagnostic tests, pharmaceutical agents, and the knowledge and skill needed to use these resources (Davidson, Ray, & Turkel, 2011; Ray, 1987, 1989). Also included with technology are computer-assisted practice and documentation as well as social media and virtual reality (Campling, Ray, & Lopez-Devine, 2011; Ray, 2016; Swinderman, 2011; Wu & Ray, 2016).

Economic

Factors related to the meaning of caring include money, budget, insurance systems, limitations, and guidelines imposed by managed care organizations and the 2010 Patient Protection and Affordable Care Act, and, in general, allocation of scarce human and material resources to maintain the economic viability of the organization (Ray, 1981b, 1989, 2016). Caring as an interpersonal resource should be considered, as well as goods, money, and services (Ray, Turkel, & Cohn, 2011; Turkel & Ray, 2000, 2001, 2003).

Political

Political factors and the power structure within health care administration influence how nursing is viewed in health care and include patterns of communication and decision making in the organization; role and gender stratification among nurses, physicians, and administrators; union activities, including negotiation and confrontation; government and insurance company influences; uses of power, prestige, and privilege; and, in general, competition for scarce human and material resources (Ray, 1989, 2010b, 2016).

USE OF EMPIRICAL EVIDENCE

The theory of bureaucratic caring was generated from qualitative research involving health professionals and clients in the hospital setting. This research focuses on caring in the organizational culture and first appeared in the doctoral dissertation in 1981, and in other literature in 1984 and 1989. The dissertation research generated a theory of the dynamic structure of caring in a complex organization. Methods used were grounded theory, phenomenology, and ethnography to elicit the study participants' meaning of caring. The grounded theory process results in the evolution of substantive theory (caring data generated from experience) and formal theory (integrated synthesis of caring and bureaucratic structures). Ray studied caring in all areas of a hospital, from nursing practice to materials management to administration, including nursing administration. More than 200 respondents participated in the purposive and convenience sample. The principal question asked was "What is the meaning of caring to you?" Through dialogue, caring evolved from in-depth interviews, participant observation, caregiving observation, and documentation (Ray, 1989).

Ray's discovery of bureaucratic caring began as a substantive theory and evolved to a formal theory. The substantive theory emerged as differential caring—that is, the meaning of caring differentiates itself by its context. Dominant caring dimensions vary in terms of areas of practice or hospital units. For example, an intensive care unit has a dominant value of technological caring (e.g., monitors, ventilators, treatments, and pharmacotherapeutics), and an oncology unit has a value of a more intimate, spiritual caring (e.g., family focused, comforting, compassionate). Staff nurses valued caring in relation to patients, and administrators valued caring in relation to the system, such as the economic well-being of the hospital.

The formal theory of bureaucratic caring symbolized a dynamic structure of caring. This structure emerged from the dialectic between the thesis of caring as humanistic (i.e., social, education, ethical, and religious-spiritual structures) and the antithesis of caring as bureaucratic (i.e., economic, political, legal, and technological structures). The dialectic of caring illustrates that everything is interconnected and that the organization is a macrocosm of the culture.

The evolution of Ray's theory is illustrated in Fig. 8.1, with diagrams of the bureaucratic caring structure published in 1981 and 1989. In the original grounded theory (see Fig. 8.1*A*), political and economic structures occupied a larger dimension to illustrate their increasing influence on the nature of institutional caring (Ray, 1981b). Subsequent research conducted in intensive care and intermediate care units (Ray, 1989) emphasized the differential nature of caring, as seen through its competing structures of political, legal, economic, technological-physiological, spiritual-religious, ethical, and educational-social elements (see Fig. 8.1*B*). In her 1987 article on technological caring, Ray noted that "critical care nursing is intensely human,

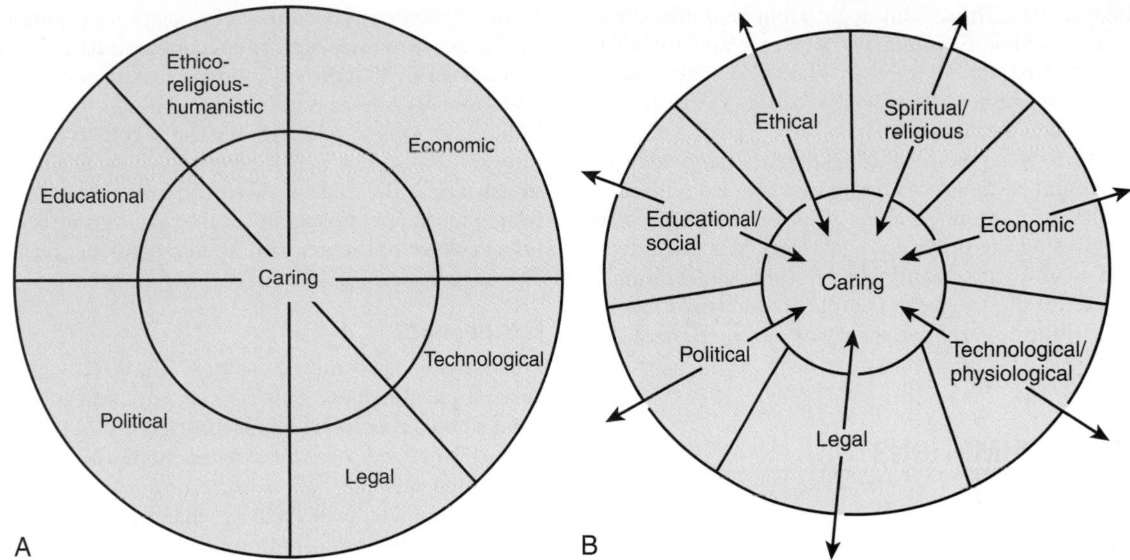

FIG. 8.1 (A) The original grounded theory of bureaucratic caring. **(B)** Subsequent grounded theory revealing differential caring. (A, From Ray, M. A. [1981a]. A study of caring within an institutional culture. Dissertation Abstracts International, 42[06]. [University Microfilm No. 8127787.]. B, From Parker, M. E. [2006]. Nursing theories and nursing practice [3rd ed.]. Philadelphia: F. A. Davis. Graphics redrawn from originals by J. Castle and B. Jensen, Nevada State College, Henderson, NV.)

moral, and technocratic" (p. 172). Ray encouraged other researchers to study this area to enhance nursing's understanding of the advantages and limitations of technology in critical care. The *Dimensions of Critical Care Nursing* journal recognized Ray as Researcher of the Year in 1987 for her groundbreaking work.

With continued reflection and analysis, combined with research on the economics of the nurse-patient relationship, Ray began to illuminate the ethical-spiritual realm of nursing (Fig. 8.2) (Ray, 2001). Spiritual-ethical caring became a dominant modality because of discoveries that focused on the nurse-patient relationship. Qualitatively different systems, such as political, economic, social-cultural, and physiological, when viewed as open and interactive wholes, operate through the choice making of nurses (Davidson & Ray, 1991; Ray, 1994a). Spiritual-ethical caring proposes how choice making for the good of others can be accomplished in nursing practice.

Ray's research reveals that in complex organizations, nursing as caring is practiced and lived out at the margin between the humanistic-spiritual dimension and the systemic dimension. These findings are consistent with worldviews from the science of complexity, which proposes antithetical phenomena coexistence (Briggs & Peat,

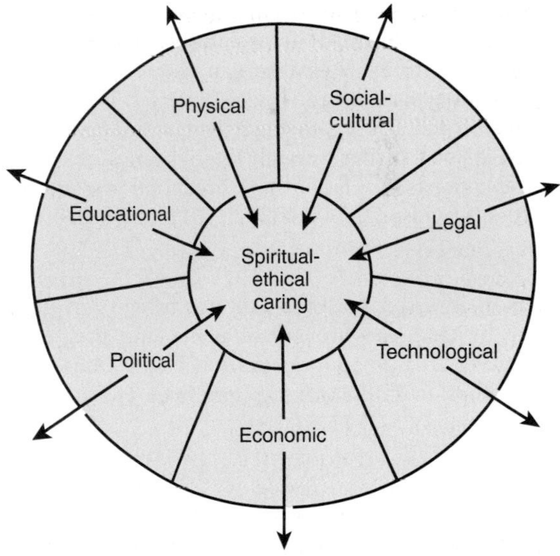

FIG. 8.2 The holographic theory of bureaucratic caring. (From Parker, M. E. [2006]. Nursing theories and nursing practice [3rd ed.]. Philadelphia: F. A. Davis. Graphics redrawn from originals by J. Castle and B. Jensen, Nevada State College, Henderson, NV.)

1999; Ray, 1998). Thus technological and humanistic systems exist together. Complexity theory explains the resolution of the paradox between differing systems (thesis and antithesis) represented in the synthesis or the theory of bureaucratic caring.

In summary, the theory of bureaucratic caring emerged using a grounded theory methodology, blended with phenomenology and ethnography. The initial theory was examined using the philosophy of Hegel. The theory was revisited in 2001 after continuing research and examination in light of the science of complexity and chaos theory, resulting in the holographic theory of bureaucratic caring (see Fig. 8.2).

MAJOR ASSUMPTIONS

Nursing

Nursing is holistic, relational, spiritual, and ethical caring that seeks the good of self and others in complex community, organizational, and bureaucratic cultures. Dwelling with the nature of caring reveals that love is the foundation of spiritual caring. Through knowledge of the inner mystery of the inspirational life, love calls forth a responsible ethical life enabling the expression of concrete actions of caring in the lives of nurses. As such, caring is cultural and social. Transcultural caring encompasses beliefs and values of compassion or love and justice or fairness, which has significance in the social realm, where relationships are formed and transformed. Transcultural caring serves as a unique lens through which human choices are seen and understanding in health and healing emerges. Thus through compassion and justice, nursing strives toward excellence in the activities of caring through the dynamics of complex cultural contexts of relationships, organizations, and communities (Davidson, Ray, & Turkel, 2011; Ray, 2016).

Person

A person is a spiritual and cultural being. Persons are created by God, the Mystery of Being, and they engage cocreatively in human organizational and transcultural relationships to find meaning and value (Ray, personal communication, May 25, 2004).

Health

Health provides a pattern of meaning for individuals, families, and communities. In all human societies, beliefs and caring practices about illness and health are central features of culture. Health is not simply the consequence of a physical state of being. People construct their reality of health in terms of biology; mental patterns; characteristics of their image of the body, mind, and soul; ethnicity and family structures; structures of society and community (political, economic, legal, and technological); and experiences of caring that give meaning to lives in complex ways. The social organization of health and illness in society (the health care system) determines the way that people are recognized as sick or well. It determines how health professionals and individuals view health and illness. Health is related to the way people in a cultural group or organizational culture or bureaucratic system construct reality and give or find meaning (Ray, 2016).

Environment

Environment is a complex spiritual, ethical, ecological, and cultural phenomenon. This conceptualization of environment embodies knowledge and conscience about the beauty of life forms and symbolic (representational) systems or patterns of meaning. These patterns are transmitted historically and are preserved or changed through caring values, attitudes, and communication. Functional forms identified in the social structure or bureaucracy (e.g., political, legal, technological, and economic) play a role in facilitating understanding of the meaning of caring, cooperation, and conflict in human cultural groups and complex organizational environments. Nursing practice in environments embodies the elements of the social structure and spiritual and ethical caring patterns of meaning (Davidson, Ray, & Turkel, 2011; Ray, 2016).

THEORETICAL ASSERTIONS

Person, nursing, environment, and health are integrated into the structure of the theory of bureaucratic caring. The theory implies a dialectical relationship (thesis, antithesis, synthesis) among humans (person and nurse), the dimension of spiritual-ethical caring, and the structural (nursing, environment) dimensions of the bureaucracy or organizational culture (technological, economic, political, legal, and social). For Ray, the dialectic of caring and bureaucracy is synthesized into a theory of bureaucratic caring. Bureaucratic caring, the synthetic margin between the human and structural dimensions, is where nurses, patients, and administrators integrate person, nursing, health, and environment.

Theoretical assertions within the theory of bureaucratic caring are as follows:

1. The meaning of caring is highly differential, depending on its structures (social-cultural, educational, political, economic, physical, technological, legal). The substantive theory of differential caring states that caring in nursing is contextual and is influenced by organizational structure or culture. Thus the meaning of caring is varied in the emergency department, intensive care

unit, oncology unit, and other areas of the hospital as influenced by the role and position that a person holds. The meaning of caring emerged as differential because no one definition or meaning of caring was identified (Ray, 1984, 1989, 2010b). The theoretical statement that describes the substantive theory of differential caring is formulated as:

> *"In a hospital, differential caring is a dynamic social process that emerges as a result of the various values, beliefs, and behaviors expressed about the meaning of caring. Differential Caring relates to competing [cooperating] educational, social, humanistic, religious/spiritual, and ethical forces as well as political, economic, legal, and technological forces within the organizational culture that are influenced by the social forces within the dominant American [world] culture."*
>
> ***(Ray, 1989, p. 37)***

2. Caring is bureaucratic as well as spiritual/ethical, given the extent to which its meaning can be understood in relation to the organizational structure (Davidson, Ray, & Turkel, 2011; Ray, 1989, 2006; Ray & Turkel, 2015). In the theoretical model (see Fig. 8.2), everything is infused with spiritual-ethical caring by its integrative and relational connection to the structures of organizational life (e.g., political, educational). Spiritual-ethical caring is both a part and a whole, just as each of the organizational structures is both a part and a whole. Every part secures its purpose and meaning from the other parts. Understanding of spiritual-ethical caring in the bureaucratic organizational system, as a holographic formation, facilitates improvement in patient outcomes and transformation of human environmental well-being (Ray, personal communication, April 13, 2008; Ray, 2016).
3. Caring is the primordial construct and consciousness of nursing. Spiritual-ethical caring and the organizational structures in Fig. 8.2, when integrated, open, and interactive, are whole and operate by conscious choice. Nurses' choice making occurs with the interest of humanity at heart, using ethical principles as the compass in deliberations. Ray (2001) states, "Spiritual-ethical caring for nursing does not question whether or not to care in complex systems, but intimates how sincere deliberations and ultimately the facilitation of choices for the good of others can or should be accomplished" (p. 429).

LOGICAL FORM

The formal theory of bureaucratic caring was induced primarily by comparative analysis and insight into the whole of the experience. Review of the literature on nursing, philosophy, social processes, and organizations was combined with the substantive theory, differential caring, that Ray discovered with ethnography, phenomenology, and grounded-theory research. These ideas were analyzed and integrated through a process that was inductive and logical—inductively building on the substantive theory and logically drawing upon the philosophical argument of Hegel's dialectic (Moccia, 1986; Ray, 1989, 2006, 2010b) and complexity science to synthesize caring and bureaucracy to a new theoretical formulation (Davidson, Ray, & Turkel, 2011; Ray, 2001; Ray & Turkel, 2015).

ACCEPTANCE BY THE NURSING COMMUNITY

Practice

The theory of bureaucratic caring has direct application for nursing. In the clinical setting, staff nurses are challenged to integrate knowledge, skills, and caring (Turkel, 2001). This synthesis of behaviors and knowledge reflects the holistic nature of the theory of bureaucratic caring. At the edge of chaos, contemporary issues such as inflation of health care costs serve as the catalyst for change within corporate health care organizations. The ethical component embedded in spiritual-ethical caring (see Fig. 8.2) addresses nurses' moral obligations to others. Ray (2001) emphasizes that "transformation can occur even in the businesslike atmosphere of today if nurses reintroduce the spiritual and ethical dimensions of caring. The deep values that underlie choice to do good will be felt both inside and outside organizations" (p. 429).

Deborah McCray-Stewart, a correction health service administrator at Telfair State Prison in Helena, Georgia, described how nurses in correctional health care settings integrate the theory of bureaucratic caring into the framework of their practice (McCray-Stewart, personal communication, April 5, 2008). Nurses in correctional facilities must understand the culture, see prisoners as human beings, and have the ability to communicate, educate, and rehabilitate in this area of health care. In the correctional system, economic strategies included conducting health services at the facility level as opposed to transporting patients to a hospital. Radiology, laboratory, and telemedicine are introduced into the system requiring nurses to work in all areas. Dr. Dana Lusk, DNP Graduate of Regis University, Denver, Colorado, used Ray's theory of bureaucratic caring as a guide to educate new employees of the Veterans' Administration (VA) Hospital in Denver (Lusk, personal communication, June 15, 2015). She found the theory useful to inform new nurses about the complex organization of the hospital and the VA system. Colonel Marcia Potter, DNP Graduate of Chamberlain University, used Ray's theory of bureaucratic caring as a guide to study nurse-directed primary care, focusing on quality improvement of outcomes such as health-healing, time, and economic resources. She was able to accomplish significant economic resource savings for the U.S. Air Force Joint-Base Andrews in Washington, DC (Potter, personal communication, June 10, 2015). Dr. Carol Conroy, Chief Nursing Officer, Southwestern Vermont Medical Center, Bennington, Vermont, applied the theory of bureaucratic caring to the Vermont Health Care System in the study of how staff ascribe value to practice innovation. She studied the effect of organizational culture on the implementation and uptake of evidence-based practice (Conroy, personal communication, May 2, 2016).

Ray (2016) has addressed the interface of diverse cultures within the health care system. The Transcultural Communicative Caring Tool provides guidelines to help nurses understand the needs, adversity, problems, and questions that arise in culturally dynamic health care situations (Ray, 2016; Ray & Turkel, 2000). The dimensions of this tool are as follows:

1. Compassion
2. Advocacy
3. Respect
4. Interaction
5. Negotiation
6. Guidance

Administration

Ray's research has shown that nurses, patients, and administrators value the caring intentionality that is cocreated in the nurse-patient or administrator-nurse relationship. By creating ethical caring relationships, administrators and staff can transform the work environment (Ray, Turkel, & Cohn, 2011; Ray, Turkel, & Marino, 2002). The theory of bureaucratic caring proposes that organizations fostering ethical choices, respect, and trust will become the successful organizations of the future.

Nyberg studied with Ray and acknowledged the impact of Ray's ideas in her book, *A Caring Approach in Nursing Administration* (Nyberg, 1998). Nyberg urged nurse administrators to create a caring and compassionate system, while being accountable for organizational management, costs, and economic forces. Turkel and Ray (2003) conducted a study with U.S. Air Force personnel that led to increased awareness of issues between civilian and military policy makers.

At the National University of Colombia in Bogota, Colombia, Professor Olga J. Gomez and her nursing students studied Ray's theory of bureaucratic caring, focusing on the hospital nursing administration role (Gomez, personal communication, April 5, 2008). As they studied the paradox between the concepts of human caring and economics, the students developed a framework for phenomenological research and explored the perceptions of executive nurses about the relationships among human care, economics, and control of health costs. An outcome of the study was recognition of the importance of working together in university and practice settings for empowerment and satisfaction of clients in the hospital environment. Finally, the theory of bureaucratic caring was adopted in 2012 by Iowa Health, Des Moines (three hospitals) for implementation as a theory guide for professional nursing practice at their hospitals in preparation for application for Magnet Recognition Status as centers for excellence (Turkel, 2004).

Education

The theory of bureaucratic caring is useful in nursing education for its broad focus on caring in nursing and the health care system. The holographic theory combines differentiation of structures within a holistic framework. Discussion of the structures or forces within complex organizations (e.g., legal, economic, social-cultural) provides an overview of factors involved in nursing situations. Infusion of these structures with spiritual-ethical caring emphasizes the moral imperatives of practice and the choice making of nurses.

When developing a new baccalaureate nursing program at Nevada State College, the faculty was particularly drawn to the theory because of its description of the dimensions relevant to nursing within a philosophy of caring. The conceptual framework of the new nursing program combined Ray's theory of bureaucratic caring with theoretical ideas from Watson (1985) and Johns (2000). Fig. 8.3 depicts the ways nurses and clients interact in the health care system and how reflection on practice influences this process. A description of the conceptual framework for the curriculum illustrated in Fig. 8.3 is as follows:

> *"[T]he holographic theory of caring recognizes the interconnectedness of all things, and that everything is a whole in one context and a part of the whole in another context. Spiritual-ethical caring, the focus for communication, infuses all nursing phenomena, including physical, social-cultural, legal, technological, economic, political, and educational forces. The arrows reflect the dynamic nature of spiritual-ethical caring by the nurse and the forces that influence the changing structure of the health care system. These forces impact both the client/patient and the nurse."*
>
> ***(Nevada State College, 2010, p. 2)***

In the health care system, the client-patient and the nurse come together in a dynamic transpersonal caring relationship (Watson, 1985). The nurse, through communication, views the person as having the capacity to make

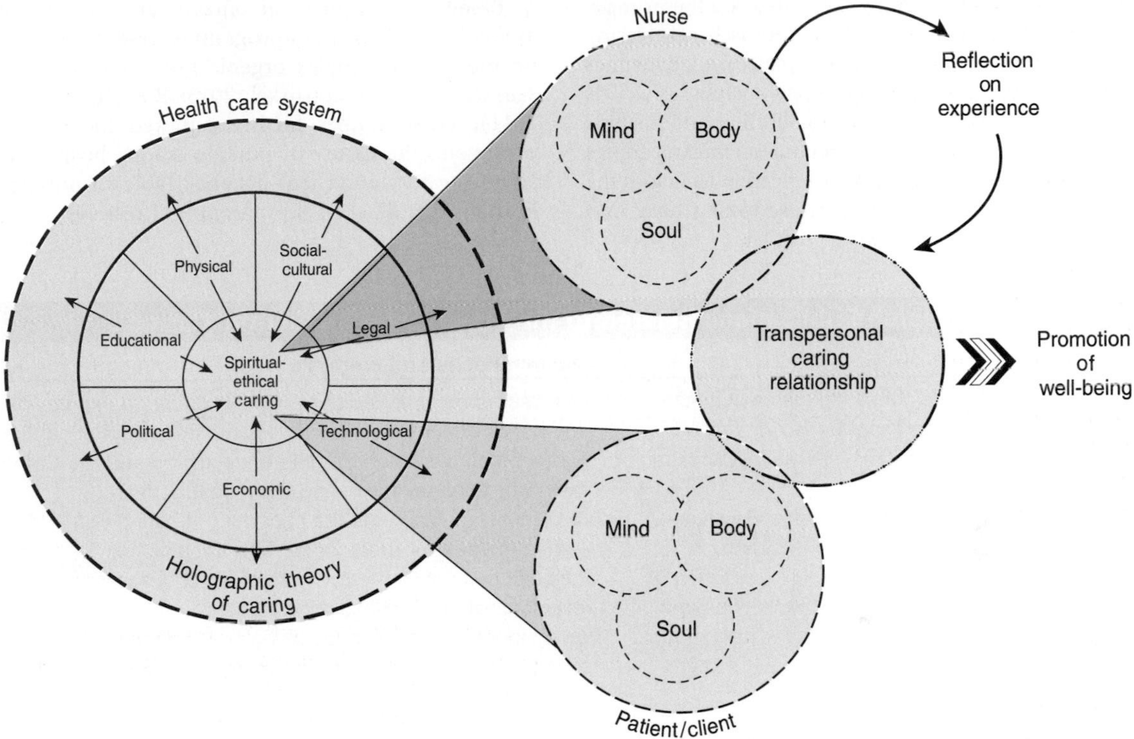

FIG. 8.3 Nevada State College nursing organizing framework. (Reprinted with permission from Nevada State College School of Nursing, Henderson, NV, 2010. Graphics redrawn from originals by J. Castle, Nevada State College, Henderson, NV.)

choices. Through reflection on experience, the nurse assesses which force has the most influence on the nursing situation (Johns, 2000). The nurse draws upon empirical, ethical, and personal knowledge to inform and influence the esthetic response to the patient. Through the nurse's caring activities within the transpersonal relationship, the goal of nursing can be achieved—the promotion of well-being through caring (Nevada State College, 2010).

The theory of bureaucratic caring is being used to guide curriculum development in the master's program in nursing administration and in the master's Doctor of Philosophy and Doctor of Nursing Practice (PhD and DNP) programs at Florida Atlantic University and Capital University. Structures from the theory, including ethical, spiritual, economic, technological, legal, political, and social, serve as a framework for exploration of current health care issues. Students are challenged to analyze the contemporary economic structure of health care from the perspective of caring. Caring within the health care delivery system is a key concept in nursing courses (Ray, personal communication, May 2012; Turkel, 2001). Ray taught bureaucratic caring theory to students at Kobe University School of Nursing, and Japanese nursing scholars such as Dr. Naohiro Hohashi introduced the theory in texts in the Japanese nursing literature.

Research

From her research that resulted in the theory of bureaucratic caring, Ray developed a phenomenological-hermeneutic approach and a caring inquiry approach that has continued to guide her studies (Ray, 1985, 1991, 1994b, 2011, 2013). This research approach is particularly significant because it is grounded in the philosophy of humanism and caring, and it encourages nurses to use phenomenological hermeneutics through the lens of caring. The evolution of Ray's research methods began with ethnography-ethnonursing, grounded theory, and phenomenology, culminating in caring inquiry and complex caring dynamics approaches (Ray, 2011). These approaches consist of the generation of data by inquiry into the meaning of participants' life-world and relational experiences. Interviews and narrative discourse are the primary methods of data generation in these approaches. In caring inquiry, an ontology of caring in complex caring dynamics includes qualitative data generation and analysis, as well as complex quantitative research data collection and analysis techniques. The researcher dwells on the essential meanings of phenomena and through further reflection facilitates the interpretation of interview data, transforming data into interpretative themes and metathemes. The ultimate goals are to capture the unity of meaning and to synthesize meanings into a theory.

Based on the theory of bureaucratic caring, Ray and Turkel have developed a program of research that focuses on nursing in complex organizations (Davidson, Ray, & Turkel, 2011; Ray & Turkel, 2015; Ray, Turkel, & Cohn, 2011). These studies further explored the meaning of caring and the nature of nursing among hospital nurses, administrators, and client-patients. Table 8.1 outlines publications that describe this program of research.

TABLE 8.1 Research Publications Related to the Theory of Bureaucratic Caring

Year	Citation	Research Focus and Findings
1981	Ray, M. A. Study of caring within an institutional culture. *Dissertation Abstracts International, 42*(06). (University Microfilm No. 8127787.)	The dissertation analyzed the meaning of caring expressions and behaviors among 192 participants in a hospital culture. The substantive theory of differential caring and the formal theory of bureaucratic caring were abstracted.
1984	Ray, M. The development of a classification system of institutional caring. In M. Leininger (Ed.), *Care: The essence of nursing and health.* Thorofare, NJ: Slack.	The discussion examines the construct of caring within the cultural context of the hospital. The classification system included cultural caring symbols of psychological, practical, interactional, and philosophical factors.
1987	Ray, M. Technological caring: A new model in critical care. *Dimensions in Critical Care Nursing, 6*(3), 166–173.	This phenomenological study examined the meaning of caring to critical care unit nurses. The study showed that ethical decisions, moral reasoning, and choice undergo a process of growth and maturation.
1989	Ray, M. A. The theory of bureaucratic caring for nursing practice in the organizational culture. *Nursing Administration Quarterly, 13*(2), 31–42.	Caring within the organizational culture was the focus of the study. It describes the substantive theory of differential caring and the formal theory of bureaucratic caring. With caring at the center of the model, the study included ethical, spiritual-religious, economic, technological-physiological, legal, political, and educational-social structures.
1989	Valentine, K. Caring is more than kindness: Modeling its complexities. *Journal of Nursing Administration,* 19(11), 28–34.	Nurses, patients, and corporate health managers provided quantitative and qualitative data to define caring. Data were organized using the categorization schema developed by Ray (1984).
1993	Ray, M. A. A study of care processes using total quality management as a framework in a USAF regional hospital emergency service and related services. *Military Medicine, 158*(6), 396–403.	This descriptive study investigated access to care processes in a military regional hospital emergency service using a total quality management framework. The study lends support to the need for a decentralized, coordinated health care system with greater authority and control given to local commands.
1997	Ray, M. The ethical theory of existential authenticity: The lived experience of the art of caring in nursing administration. *Canadian Journal of Nursing Research, 29*(1), 111–126.	Existential authenticity was uncovered as the unity of meaning of caring by nurse administrators. This was described as an ethic of living and caring for the good of nursing staff members and the good of the organization.
1998	Ray, M. A. A phenomenological study of the interface of caring and technology in intermediate care: Toward a reflexive ethics for clinical practice. *Holistic Nursing Practice, 12*(4), 69–77.	This phenomenological study examined the meaning of caring for technologically dependent patients. Results revealed that vulnerability, suffering, and the ethical situations of moral blurring and moral blindness were the dynamics of caring for these patients.

TABLE 8.1 Research Publications Related to the Theory of Bureaucratic Caring—cont'd

Year	Citation	Research Focus and Findings
2000	Turkel, M., & Ray, M. Relational complexity: A theory of the nurse-patient relationship within an economic context. *Nursing Science Quarterly, 13*(4), 307–313.	The formal theory of relational complexity illuminated that the caring relationship is complex and dynamic, is both process and outcome, and is a function of both economic and caring variables that, as a mutual process, is lived all at once as relational and system self-organization.
2001	Ray, M., & Turkel, M. Impact of TRICARE/managed care on total force readiness. *Military Medicine, 166*(4), 281–289.	A phenomenological study was conducted to illuminate the life world descriptions of experiences of USAF active duty and reserve personnel with managed care in the military and civilian health care systems. The research illuminated the need for policy change to better meet the health care needs of these personnel and their families.
2001	Turkel, M., & Ray, M. Relational complexity: From grounded theory to instrument theoretical testing. *Nursing Science Quarterly, 14*(4), 281–287.	The article describes a series of studies that examined the relationships among caring, economics, cost, quality, and the nurse-patient relationship. The results of theory testing revealed relational caring as a process and the strongest predictor of the outcome—relational self-organization that is aimed at well-being.
2002	Ray, M., Turkel, M., & Marino, F. The transformative process for nursing in workforce redevelopment. *Nursing Administration Quarterly, 26*(2), 1–14.	Relational self-organization is a shared, creative response to a continuously changing and interconnected work environment. Strategies of respecting, communicating, maintaining visibility, and engaging in participative decision making are the transformative processes leading to growth and transformation.
2003	Turkel, M. A journey into caring as experienced by nurse managers. *International Journal for Human Caring, 7*(1), 20–26.	The purpose of this phenomenological study was to capture the meaning of caring as experienced by nurse managers. Essential themes that emerged were growth, listening, support, intuition, receiving gifts, and frustration.
2003	Turkel, M., & Ray, M. A process model for policy analysis within the context of political caring. *International Journal for Human Caring, 7*(3), 17–25.	This phenomenological study illuminated the experiences of USAF personnel with managed care in the military and civilian health care systems. A model outlining the process of policy analysis was generated.

USAF, U.S. Air Force.

FURTHER DEVELOPMENT

Development of the theory of bureaucratic caring is ongoing in Ray's program of research and scholarship. Her work is a synthesis of nursing science, transcultural nursing, ethics, philosophy, complexity science, economics, and organizational management. Ray's most recent program of research was sponsored by the TriService Nursing Research program (Turkel & Ray, 2001). It included instrument development and psychometric testing of the original Nurse-Patient Relationship Resource Analysis Tool, now referred to as the Relational Caring Questionnaire (Professional Form) and the Relational Caring Questionnaire (Patient Form) (Ray & Turkel, 2012; Watson, 2009). These tools are Likert-type questionnaires for health care professionals (nurses and nonnurses and nurse-administrators) and patients that measure the nurse-patient relationship as an administrative and interpersonal resource. These tools will help researchers link the noneconomic (interpersonal) resources of caring with the administrative system resources (including economic and budgetary procedures). The tools are being translated into Swedish and Portuguese and are being tested. This interdisciplinary cutting-edge research will enhance understanding of the concepts and relationships outlined in the theory of bureaucratic caring.

CRITIQUE OF THE WORK

Clarity

The major structures—spiritual-religious, ethical, technological-physiological, social, legal, economic, political, and educational—are defined clearly in Ray's 1989 publication. These definitions are consistent with definitions commonly used by practicing nurses. They have semantic consistency in that concepts are used in ways consistent with their definitions (Chinn & Kramer, 2015). Most terms did not change from the 1989 article to the 2001 and 2006 publications; however, some concepts combined or separated as Ray's development of the theory evolved (Ray, 2010c; Ray & Turkel, 2015) and concepts were updated (Wu & Ray, 2016). Therefore for this chapter currently used terms were clarified with the theorist. Furthermore, the formal definitions of the terms **spiritual-ethical caring, social-cultural, physical,** and **technological,** as they relate to the theory, are published for the first time in this chapter.

The diagram presented in Fig. 8.2 enhances clarity. The interrelationship of spiritual-ethical caring with the other structures and the openness of the system are depicted by the organization of concepts and the dynamic arrows. Ray's description of the theory (Ray & Turkel, 2015) assists the reader in perceiving the theory relationships as holographic.

Simplicity

Ray's theory simplifies the dynamics of complex bureaucratic organizations. From numerous descriptions of the inductive grounded theory study, Ray derived the integrative concept of spiritual-ethical caring and the seven interrelated concepts of **physical, social-cultural, legal, technological, economic, political,** and **educational** structures. Given the complexity of bureaucratic organizations, the number of concepts is minimal.

Generality

The theory of bureaucratic caring is a philosophy that addresses the nature of nursing as caring. Alligood (2014) notes, "Nursing philosophy sets forth the meaning of nursing phenomena through analysis, reasoning, and logical argument" (p. 59). Ray's theory addresses questions such as "What is the nature of caring in nursing?" and "What is the nature of nursing practice as caring?" Philosophies are broad and provide direction for the discipline (Alligood, 2014). The theory of bureaucratic caring proposes that nurses are choice makers guided by spiritual-ethical caring, in relation to legal, economic, technological, and other structures.

The theory of bureaucratic caring provides a unique view of health care organizations and how nursing phenomena interrelate as wholes and parts of the system. Concepts are derived logically with inductive research. Ray's analysis incorporates ideas from complexity science. The conceptualization of the health care system as holographic emphasizes the holistic nature of concepts and relationships. As nurses in all areas of practice study these new conceptualizations, they may be led to question the cause-and-effect stance of older linear ideas. Therefore the theory of bureaucratic caring has the potential to change the paradigm or way of thinking of practicing nurses.

Accessibility

Because the theory of bureaucratic caring is generated using grounded theory and has undergone continued revisions based largely on research, empirical precision is high with concepts grounded in observable reality. The theory corresponds directly to the research data that are summarized in published reports (Ray, 1981a, 1981b, 1984, 1987, 1989, 1997b, 1998; Ray & Turkel, 2012).

Ray, Turkel, and Marino used this theory in a program of research into the nurse-patient relationship as an economic resource (Ray, 1998; Ray, Turkel, & Marino, 2002; Turkel, 2003; Turkel & Ray, 2000, 2001, 2003). These studies provide guidance for nursing practice and enhance nurses' understanding of the dynamics of health care organizations. Ray (2001) proposes that bureaucratic caring culminates "in a vision for understanding the deeper reality of nursing life" (p. 426).

Importance

The issues that confront nurses today include economic constraints in the economic, technological, and political environments and the effects of these constraints (e.g., staffing ratios, electronic health records) on the nurse-patient relationship. These are the very issues that the theory of bureaucratic caring addresses. Nurses in administrative, research, and clinical roles can use the political and economic dimensions of the theory as a framework to inform their practice. This theory is relevant to the contemporary work world of nurses.

Ray and Turkel have generated middle-range theories through their program of research based on the theory of bureaucratic caring. Ray uncovered the theory of existential authenticity (1997b) as the unity of meaning for the nurse-administrator caring art, and Sorbello (2008) adapted it more recently. Nurse administrators described an ethic of living, caring for the good of their staff nurses and for the good of the organization. Relational (caring) complexity focuses on the nurse-patient relationship within an economic context (Davidson, Ray, & Turkel, 2011; Ray & Turkel, 2014; Ray, Turkel, & Cohn, 2011; Turkel & Ray, 2000, 2001). Study data show that relational caring among administrators, nurses, and patients is the strongest predictor of relational self-organization aimed at well-being. Relational self-organization is a shared, creative response that involves growth and transformation (Ray, Turkel, & Marino, 2002). Transformative processes that can lead to relational self-organization include respecting, communicating, maintaining visibility, and engaging in participative decision making in the workplace. Finally, Ray's work emphasizes the need for reflexive ethics for clinical practice, to enhance understanding of how deep values and moral interactions shape ethical decisions (Ray, 1998, 2016).

SUMMARY

The theory of bureaucratic caring challenges participants in nursing to think beyond their usual frame of reference and envision the world holistically, while considering the universe as a hologram. Appreciation of the interrelatedness of persons, environments, and events is key to understanding this theory. The theory provides a unique view of how health care organizations and nursing phenomena interrelate as wholes and parts in the system. Unique constructs within Ray's theory include technological and economic caring. Theory development by Ray's colleagues and other scholars continues. Ray challenges nurses to envision the spiritual and ethical dimensions of caring and complex organizational health care systems so the theory of bureaucratic caring may inform nurse creativity and transform the work world.

CASE STUDY

Mrs. Smith was a 73-year-old widow who lived alone with no significant social support. She had been suffering from emphysema for several years and had had frequent hospitalizations for respiratory problems. On the last hospital admission, her pneumonia quickly progressed to organ failure. Death appeared to be imminent, and she went in and out of consciousness, alone in her hospital room. The medical-surgical nursing staff and the nurse manager focused on making Mrs. Smith's end-of-life period as comfortable as possible. Upon consultation with the vice president for nursing, the nurse manager and the unit staff nurses decided against moving Mrs. Smith to the palliative care unit, although considered more economical, because of the need to protect and nurture her because she was already experiencing signs and symptoms of the dying process. Nurses were prompted by an article they read on human caring as the "language of nursing practice" (Turkel, Ray, & Kornblatt, 2012) in their weekly caring practice meetings.

The nurse manager reorganized patient assignments. She felt that the newly assigned clinical nurse leader who was working between both the medical and surgical units could provide direct nurse caring and coordination at the point of care (Sherman, 2012). Over the next few hours, the clinical nurse leader and a staff member who had volunteered her assistance provided personal care for Mrs. Smith. The clinical nurse leader asked the nurse manager whether there was a possibility that Mrs. Smith had any close friends who could "be there" for her in her final moments. One friend was discovered and came to say goodbye to Mrs. Smith. With help from her team, the clinical nurse leader turned, bathed, and suctioned Mrs. Smith. She spoke quietly, prayed, and sang hymns softly in Mrs. Smith's room, creating a peaceful environment that expressed compassion and a deep sense of caring for her. The nurse manager and nursing unit staff were calmed and their "hearts awakened" by the personal caring that the clinical nurse leader and the volunteer nurse provided. Mrs. Smith died with caring persons at her bedside, and all members of the unit staff felt comforted that she had not died alone.

Davidson, Ray, and Turkel (2011) note that caring is complex, and caring science includes the art of practice, "an aesthetic which illuminates the beauty of the dynamic nurse-patient relationship, that makes possible authentic spiritual-ethical choices for transformation—healing, health, well-being, and a peaceful death" (p. xxiv). As the clinical nurse leader and the nursing staff in this situation engaged in caring practice that focused on the well-being of the patient, they simultaneously created a caring-healing environment that contributed to the well-being of the *whole*—the emotional atmosphere of the unit, the ability of the clinical nurse leader and staff nurses to practice caringly and competently, and the quality of care the staff were able to provide to other patients. The bureaucratic nature of the hospital included leadership and management systems that conferred power, authority, and control to the nurse manager, the clinical nurse leader, and the nursing staff in partnership with the vice president for nursing. The actions of the nursing administration, clinical nurse leader, and staff reflected values and beliefs, attitudes, and behaviors about the nursing care they would provide, how they would use technology, and how they would deal with human relationships. The ethical and spiritual choice making of the whole staff and the way they communicated their values both reflected and created a caring community in the workplace culture of the hospital unit.

CRITICAL THINKING ACTIVITIES

Based on this case study, consider the following questions.

1. What caring behaviors prompted the nurse manager to assign the clinical nurse leader to engage in direct caring for Mrs. Smith? Describe the clinical nurse leader role established by the American Association of Colleges of Nursing in 2004.
2. What issues (ethical, spiritual, legal, social-cultural, economic, and physical) from the structure of the theory of bureaucratic caring influenced this situation? Discuss end-of-life issues in relation to the theory.
3. How did the nurse manager balance these issues? What considerations went into her decision making? Discuss the role and the value of the clinical nurse leader on nursing units. What is the difference between the nurse manager and the clinical nurse leader in terms of caring practice in complex hospital care settings? How does a clinical nurse leader fit into the theory of bureaucratic caring for implementation of a caring practice?
4. What interrelationships are evident between persons in this environment—that is, how were the vice president for nursing, nurse manager, clinical nurse leader, staff, and patient connected in this situation? Compare and contrast the traditional nursing process with Turkel, Ray, and Kornblatt's (2012) language of caring practice within the theory of bureaucratic caring.

POINTS FOR FURTHER STUDY

- International Association for Human Caring at www.humancaring.org.
- Marilyn Ray website at: http://marilynray.com.
- Ray, M. (2016). *Transcultural caring dynamics in nursing and health care* (2nd ed.). Philadelphia: F.A. Davis Company. (EBOOK with Instructor Guide). Retrieved from http://www.davisplus.com.
- Transcultural Nursing Society at www.tcns.org.

REFERENCES

Alligood, M. R. (2014). *Nursing theorists and their work* (8th ed.). St Louis: Mosby-Elsevier.

Briggs, J., & Peat, F. D. (1999). *Seven life lessons of chaos: Spiritual wisdom from the science of change*. New York: HarperCollins.

Campling, A., Ray, M., & Lopez-Devine, J. (2011). Implementing change in nursing informatics practice. In A. Davidson, M. Ray, & M. Turkel (Eds.), *Nursing, caring, and complexity science: For human-environment well-being* (pp. 325–339). New York: Springer.

Chinn, P. L., & Kramer, M. K. (2015). *Integrated theory and knowledge development in nursing* (9th ed.). St Louis: Mosby.

Coffman, S., & Ray, M. A. (1999). Mutual intentionality: A theory of support processes in pregnant African American women. *Qualitative Health Research, 9*(4), 479–492.

Coffman, S., & Ray, M. A. (2002). African American women describe support processes during high-risk pregnancy and postpartum. *Journal of Obstetric, Gynecologic, and Neonatal Nursing, 31*(5), 536–544.

Davidson, A., & Ray, M. (1991). Studying the human-environment phenomenon using the science of complexity. *Advances in Nursing Science,14*(2), 73–87.

Davidson, A., Ray, M., & Turkel, M. (2011). *Nursing, caring and complexity science: For human-environment well-being*. New York: Springer.

Gibson, S. (2008). Legal caring: Preventing retraumatization of abused children through the caring nursing interview using Roach's six Cs. *International Journal for Human Caring, 12*(4), 32–37.

Johns, C. (2000). *Becoming a reflective practitioner*. Oxford, UK: Blackwell Science.

Louis, M. (1985). An investigator's guide to workplace culture. In P. Frost, L. Moore, M. Louis, L. C. Lundberg, & J. Martin (Eds.), *Organizational culture* (pp. 73–93). Beverly Hills, CA: Sage.

Moccia, P. (1986). *New approaches to theory development* (Pub. No. 15-1992). New York: National League for Nursing.

Nevada State College. (2010). *Nursing organizing framework*. Henderson, NV: Author.

Nyberg, J. J. (1998). *A caring approach in nursing administration*. Niwot, CO: University Press of Colorado.

Peat, F. (2002). *From certainty to uncertainty: The story of science and ideas in the twentieth century*. Washington, DC: Joseph Henry Press.

Ray, M. (1981a). A philosophical analysis of caring within nursing. In M. Leininger (Ed.), *Caring: An essential human need* (pp. 25–36). Thorofare, NJ: Slack.

Ray, M. (1981b). A study of caring within an institutional culture. *Dissertation Abstracts International,* 42(06). (University Microfilms No. 8127787.)

Ray, M. (1984). The development of a classification system of institutional caring. In M. Leininger (Ed.), *Care: The essence of nursing and health* (pp. 95–112). Thorofare, NJ: Slack.

Ray, M. A. (1985). A philosophical method to study nursing phenomena. In M. Leininger (Ed.), *Qualitative research methods in nursing* (pp. 81–92). New York: Grune & Stratton.

Ray, M. (1987). Technological caring: A new model in critical care. *Dimensions in Critical Care Nursing, 6*(3), 166–173.

Ray, M. (1989). The Theory of Bureaucratic Caring for nursing practice in the organizational culture. *Nursing Administration Quarterly, 13*(2), 31–42.

Ray, M. A. (1991). Caring inquiry: The esthetic process in the way of compassion. In D. Gaut & M. Leininger (Eds.), *Caring: The compassionate healer* (pp. 181–189). New York: National League for Nursing.

Ray, M. A. (1994a). Complex caring dynamics: A unifying model for nursing inquiry. *Theoretic and Applied Chaos in Nursing, 1*(1), 23–32.

Ray, M. A. (1994b). The richness of phenomenology: Philosophic, theoretic, and methodologic concerns. In J. Morse (Ed.), *Critical issues in qualitative research methods* (pp. 116–135). Newbury Park, CA: Sage.

Ray, M. A. (1997a). Consciousness and the moral ideal: A transcultural analysis of Watson's theory of transpersonal caring. *Advanced Practice Nursing Quarterly, 3*(1), 25–31.

Ray, M. A. (1997b). The ethical theory of existential authenticity: The lived experience of the art of caring in nursing administration. *Canadian Journal of Nursing Research, 29*(1), 111–126.

Ray, M. A. (1998). A phenomenologic study of the interface of caring and technology: A new reflexive ethics in intermediate care. *Holistic Nursing Practice, 12*(4), 71–79.

Ray, M. A. (2000). Transcultural assessment of older adults. In S. Garratt & S. Koch (Eds.), *Assessing older people: A practical guide for health professionals*. Sydney, Australia: MacLennan & Petty.

Ray, M. A. (2001). The Theory of Bureaucratic Caring. In M. Parker (Ed.), *Nursing theories and nursing practice* (pp. 422–431). Philadelphia: F. A. Davis.

Ray, M. A. (2006). The Theory of Bureaucratic Caring. In M. Parker (Ed.), *Nursing theories and nursing practice* (2nd ed., pp. 360–368). Philadelphia: F. A. Davis.

Ray, M. (2010a). Creating caring organizations and cultures through communitarian ethics. *Journal of the World Universities Forum, 3*(5), 41–52.

Ray, M. (2010b). *A study of caring within the institutional culture: The discovery of the Theory of Bureaucratic Caring*. Saarbrucken, Germany: Lambert Academic Press.

Ray, M. (2010c). *Transcultural caring dynamics in nursing and health care*. Philadelphia: F. A. Davis.

Ray, M. (2011). Complex caring dynamics: A unifying model for nursing inquiry. In A. Davidson, M. Ray, & M. Turkel (Eds.), *Nursing, caring, and complexity science: For human-environment well-being* (pp. 31–52). New York: Springer.

Ray, M. (2013). Caring inquiry: The esthetic process in the way of compassion. In M. Smith & M. Parker (Eds.), *Nursing theories and nursing practice* (4th ed., pp. 461–482). Philadelphia: F. A. Davis.

Ray, M. (2016). *Transcultural caring dynamics in nursing and health care* (2nd ed.). Philadelphia: F. A. Davis.

Ray, M. A., & Turkel, M. C. (2000). Culturally based caring. In L. Dunphy & J. Winland-Brown (Eds.), *Advanced practice nursing: A holistic approach* (pp. 43–55). Philadelphia: F. A. Davis.

Ray, M., & Turkel, M. (2012). A transtheoretical evolution of caring science within complex systems. *International Journal for Human Caring, 16*(2), 28–49.

Ray, M., & Turkel, M. (2014). Caring as emancipatory nursing praxis: The theory of relational caring complexity. *Advances in Nursing Science, 37*(2), 132–146.

Ray, M., & Turkel, M. (2015). Marilyn Anne Ray's Theory of Bureaucratic Caring. In M. Smith & M. Parker (Eds.), *Nursing theories and nursing practice* (4th ed., pp. 461–482). Philadelphia: F. A. Davis.

Ray, M., Turkel, M., & Cohn, J. (2011). Relational caring complexity: The study of caring and complexity in health care hospital organizations. In A. Davidson, M. Ray, & M. Turkel (Eds.), *Nursing, caring, and complexity science: For human-environment well-being* (pp. 95–117). New York: Springer.

Ray, M., Turkel, M., & Marino, F. (2002). The transformative process for nursing in workforce redevelopment. *Nursing Administration Quarterly, 26*(2), 1–14.

Sherman, R. (2012). Lessons in innovations: Role transition experiences of clinical nurse leaders. *Journal of Nursing Administration, 40*(12), 547–554.

Smircich, L. (1985). Is the concept of culture a paradigm for understanding organizations and ourselves? In P. Frost, L. Moore, M. Louis, L. C. Lundberg, & J. Martin (Eds.), *Organizational culture* (pp. 55–72). Beverly Hills, CA: Sage.

Sorbello, B. (2008). The nurse administrator as caring person: A synoptic analysis applying caring philosophy, Ray's ethical theory of existential authenticity, the ethic of justice, and the ethic of care. *International Journal for Human Caring, 12*(1), 44–49.

Swinderman, T. (2011). Technological change in health care electronic documentation as facilitated by the science of complexity. In A. Davidson, M. Ray, & M. Turkel (Eds.), *Nursing, caring, and complexity science: For human-environment well-being* (pp. 309–319). New York: Springer.

Talbot, M. (1991). *The holographic universe*. New York: Harper Collins.

Turkel, M. (2001). Applicability of bureaucratic caring theory to contemporary nursing practice: The political and economic dimensions. In M. Parker (Ed.), *Nursing theories and nursing practice* (pp. 433–444). Philadelphia: F. A. Davis.

Turkel, M. (2003). A journey into caring as experienced by nurse managers. *International Journal for Human Caring, 7*(1), 20–26.

Turkel, M. (2004). *Magnet status: Assessing, pursuing, and achieving nursing excellence*. Marblehead, MA: HCPro.

Turkel, M., & Ray, M. (2000). Relational complexity: A theory of the nurse-patient relationship within an economic context. *Nursing Science Quarterly, 13*(4), 307–313.

Turkel, M., & Ray, M. (2001). Relational complexity: From grounded theory to instrument development and theoretical testing. *Nursing Science Quarterly, 14*(4), 281–287.

Turkel, M., & Ray, M. (2003). A process model for policy analysis within the context of political caring. *International Journal for Human Caring, 7*(3), 17–25.

Turkel, M. C., Ray, M. A., & Kornblatt, L. (2012). Instead of reconceptualizing the nursing process let's re-name it. *Nursing Science Quarterly, 25*(2), 194–198.

Vicenzi, A. E., White, K. R., & Begun, J. W. (1997). Chaos in nursing: Make it work for you. *American Journal of Nursing, 97*(10), 26–31.

Watson, J. (1985). *Nursing: Human science and human care.* Norwalk, CT: Appleton-Century-Crofts.

Watson, J. (2009). *Assessing and measuring caring in nursing and health science* (2nd ed.). New York: Springer.

Wheatley, M. J. (2006). *Leadership and the new science: Discovering order in a chaotic world* (2nd ed.). San Francisco: Berrett-Koehler.

Wu, J., & Ray, M. (2016). Technological caring for healthcare complexities of patients with cardiac disease comorbid with diabetes. *International Journal for Human Caring, 20*(2), 1–5.

BIBLIOGRAPHY

Primary Sources

Books

Watson, J., & Ray, M. (Eds.). (1988). *The ethics of care and the ethics of cure: Synthesis in chronicity*. New York: National League for Nursing.

Book Chapters

France, N., & Ray, M. (2014). Studying caring science in nursing: The foundation of the discipline and profession of nursing at Florida Atlantic University, USA. In L. Pellico, M. Oermann, D. Hrabe, N. France, M. Ray et al. (Authors), *Nursing for the curious—Why study nursing* (Chapter 12)? New York: Amazon Digital Services.

Ray, M. A. (1990). Phenomenological method in nursing research. In N. Chaska (Ed.), *The nursing profession: Turning points* (pp. 173–179). New York: McGraw-Hill.

Ray, M. A. (1992). Phenomenological method for nursing research. In J. Poindexter (Ed.), *Nursing theory. Research & Practice Summer Research Conference monograph* (pp. 163–174). Detroit: Wayne State University.

Ray, M. A. (1994). Environmental encountering through interiority. In E. Schuster & C. Brown (Eds.), *Exploring our environmental connections* (pp. 113–118). New York: National League for Nursing Press.

Ray, M. A. (1994). The quality of authentic presence: Transcultural caring inquiry in primary care. In J. Wang & P. Simoni (Eds.), *Proceedings of First International and Interdisciplinary Health Research Symposium* (pp. 69–72). At Peking Union Medical College Hospital, Beijing, China, and Zhejiang Medical University, Hangzhou, China (Chinese translation). Morgantown, WV: West Virginia University.

Ray, M. A. (1995). Transcultural health care ethics: Pathways to progress. In J. Wang (Ed.), *Health care and culture* (pp. 3–9). Morgantown, WV: West Virginia University.

Ray, M. A. (1997). Illuminating the meaning of caring: Unfolding the sacred art of divine love. In M. S. Roach (Ed.), *Caring from the heart: the convergence between caring and spirituality* (pp. 163–178). New York: Paulist Press.

Ray, M. A. (1999). Caring foundations of deacony. In T. Ryokas & K. Keissling (Eds.), *Spiritus-Lux-Caritas* (pp. 225–236). Lahti, Finland: Deaconal Institution of Lahti.

Ray, M. A. (1999). Critical theory as a framework to enhance nursing science. In E. Polifroni & M. Welch (Eds.), *Perspectives on philosophy of science in nursing* (pp. 382–386). Philadelphia: Lippincott.

Ray, M. A. (2001). Complex culture and technology: Toward a global caring communitarian ethics of nursing. In R. Locsin (Ed.), *Concerning technology and caring* (pp. 41–52). Westport, CT: Greenwood.

Ray, M. (2007). Technological caring as a dynamic of complexity in nursing practice. In A. Barnard & R. Locsin (Eds.), *Perspectives on technology and nursing practice*. United Kingdom: Palgrave.

Ray, M. (2013). The theory of bureaucratic caring. In M. Smith, M. Turkel, & Z. Wolf (Eds.), *Caring in nursing classics: An essential resource* (pp. 309–320). New York: Springer.

Ray, M., Morris, E., & McFarland, M. (2013). Ethnonursing method of Dr. Madeleine Leininger. In C. Beck (Ed.), *Encyclopedia of qualitative research methods* (pp. 213–229). New York: Routledge.

Ray, M. A., & Turkel, M. C. (2000). Culturally based caring. In L. Dunphy & J. Winland-Brown (Eds.), *Advanced practice nursing: A holistic approach* (pp. 43–55). Philadelphia: F. A. Davis.

Ray, M., & Turkel, M. (2015). Marilyn Anne Ray's Theory of Bureaucratic Caring. In M. Smith & M. Parker (Eds.), *Nursing theories and nursing practice* (4th ed., pp. 461–482). Philadelphia: F. A. Davis Company.

Journal Articles

Douglas, M. K., Kemppainen, J. K., McFarland, M. R., Papadopoulos, I., Ray, M. A., Roper, J. M., et al. (2010). Chapter 10: Research methodologies for investigating cultural phenomena and evaluating interventions. *Journal of Transcultural Nursing, 21*(4), S373– S405.

Grumme, V., Barry, C., Gordon, S., & Ray, M. (2016). On virtual presence. *Advances in Nursing Science.* doi: 10.1097/ANS.000000000000103.

Ray, M. (1999). Transcultural caring in primary care. *National Academies of Practice Forum, 1*(1), 177–182.

Ray, M. A. (1987). Technological caring: A new model in critical care. *Dimensions of Critical Care Nursing, 2*(3), 166–173.

Ray, M. A. (1989). A theory of bureaucratic caring for nursing practice in the organizational culture. *Nursing Administration Quarterly, 13*(2), 31–42.

Ray, M. A. (1992). Critical theory as a framework to enhance nursing science. *Nursing Science Quarterly, 5*(3), 98–101.

Ray, M. A. (1993). A study of care processes using Total Quality Management as a framework in a USAF regional hospital emergency service and related services. *Military Medicine, 158*(6), 396–403.

Ray, M. A. (1993). A theory of bureaucratic caring for nursing practice in the organizational culture. *The Japanese Journal of Nursing Research, 1*, 14–24.

Ray, M. A. (1994). Communal moral experience as the research starting point for health care ethics. *Nursing Outlook, 42*(3), 104–109.

Ray, M. A. (1994). Complex caring dynamics: A unifying model for nursing inquiry. *Theoretic and Applied Chaos in Nursing, 1*(1), 23–32.

Ray, M. A. (1994). Interpretive analysis of Olson's book, The life of illness: One woman's journey. *Qualitative Health Research, 2*(2), 250–253.

Ray, M. A. (1994). Transcultural nursing ethics: A framework and model for transcultural ethical analysis. *Journal of Holistic Nursing, 12*(3), 251–264.

Ray, M. A. (1997). Consciousness and the moral ideal: Transcultural analysis of Watson's Transpersonal Caring Theory. *Advanced Nursing Practice Journal, 3*(1), 25–31.

Ray, M. A. (1997). The ethical theory of Existential Authenticity: The lived experience of the art of caring in nursing administration. *Canadian Journal of Nursing Research, 22*(1), 111–126.

Ray, M. A. (1998). Complexity and nursing science. *Nursing Science Quarterly, 11*(3), 91–93.

Ray, M. A. (1998). The interface of caring and technology: A new reflexive ethics in intermediate care. *Holistic Nursing Practice, 12*(4), 71–79.

Ray, M. A. (1999). The future of caring in the challenging health care environment. *International Journal for Human Caring, 3*(1), 7–11.

Ray, M. A. (2011). A celebration of a life of commitment to transcultural nursing: Opening of the Madeleine M. Leininger Collection on Human Caring and Transcultural Nursing. *Journal of Transcultural Nursing, 22*(1), 97.

Ray, M. (2015). Rootedness in holistic nursing: The ontologic mystery and structure of caring. *Beginnings, 35*(2), 12–14.

Ray, M. A., Didominic, V. A., Dittman, P. W., Hurst, P. A., Seaver, J. B., Sorbello, B. C., et al. (1995). The edge of chaos: caring and the bottom line. *Nursing Management, 9*, 48–50.

Ray, M., & Turkel, M. (2001). Impact of TRICARE/managed care on total force readiness. *Military Medicine, 166*(4), 281–289.

Ray, M., Turkel, M., & Marino, F. (2002). The transformative process for nursing in workforce redevelopment. *Nursing Administration Quarterly, 26*(2), 1–14.

Turkel, M., & Ray, M. (2000). Relational complexity: A theory of the nurse-patient relationship within an economic context. *Nursing Science Quarterly, 13*(4), 307–313.

Turkel, M., & Ray, M. (2001). Relational complexity: From grounded theory to instrument development and theoretical testing. *Nursing Science Quarterly, 14*(4), 281–287.

Turkel, M., & Ray, M. (2003). A process model for policy analysis within the context of political caring. *International Journal for Human Caring, 7*(3), 17–25.

Turkel, M., & Ray, M. (2004). Creating a caring practice environment through self-renewal. *Nursing Administration Quarterly, 28*(4), 249–254.

Turkel, M., & Ray, M. A. (2005). Models of caring practice. [Editorial.] *International Journal for Human Caring, 9*(3), 7–8.

Secondary Sources

Book Chapters

Coffman, S. (2015). Caring. In A. Berman & S. Snyder (Eds.), *Kozier & Erb's fundamentals of nursing: Concepts, process, and practice* (10th ed., pp. 448–461). Upper Saddle River, NJ: Prentice Hall.

Turkel, M. (2006). Applications of Marilyn Ray's Theory of Bureaucratic Caring. In M. Parker (Ed.), *Nursing theories and nursing practice* (2nd ed., pp. 369–379). Philadelphia: F. A. Davis.

Journal Articles

Andrews, M., Backstrand, J. R., Boyle, J. S., Campinha-Bacote, J., Davidhizar, R. E., Doutrich, D., et al. (2010). Chapter 3: Theoretical basis for transcultural care. *Journal of Transcultural Nursing, 21*(4), S53–S136.

Dyess, S. M., Prestia, A. S., & Smith, M. C. (2015). Support for caring and resiliency among successful nurse leaders. *Nursing Administrative Quarterly, 39*(2), 104–116.

Honda, J., Ray, M., & Hohashi, N. (2013). Ray's Theory of Bureaucratic Caring and nursing organization management. *Health Care, 55*(12), 819–825.

Johnson, P. (2015). Ray's Theory of Bureaucratic Caring: A conceptual framework for APRN primary care providers and the homebound population. *International Journal for Human Caring, 19*(2), 41–44.

Martin, M. (2015). Gender equality and the empowerment of women in Arab countries: A transcultural caring perspective. *International Journal for Human Caring, 19*(1), 13–18.

Prestia, A. (2015). Chief nursing officer sustainment: A phenomenological inquiry. *Journal of Nursing Administration, 45*(11), 575–581.

Prestia, A. (2016). Existential authenticity: Caring strategies for living leadership presence. *International Journal for Human Caring, 20*(11), 8–11.

Turkel, M. (2007). Dr. Marilyn Ray's Theory of Bureaucratic Caring. *International Journal for Human Caring, 11*(4), 57–70.

Theses and Dissertations

Eggenberger, T. (2011). *Holding the frontline: The experience of being a charge nurse in an acute care setting.* PhD Dissertation, Florida Atlantic University, Boca Raton, Florida.

Hilsenbeck, J. R. (2006). *Unveiling the mystery of covenantal trust: The theory of the social process between the nurse manager and the chief nursing officer.* DNS dissertation, Florida Atlantic University, United States—Florida. Retrieved from ProQuest Digital Dissertations database. (Publication No. AAT3244888).

9

Caring, Clinical Wisdom, and Ethics in Nursing Practice

*Karen A. Brykczynski**

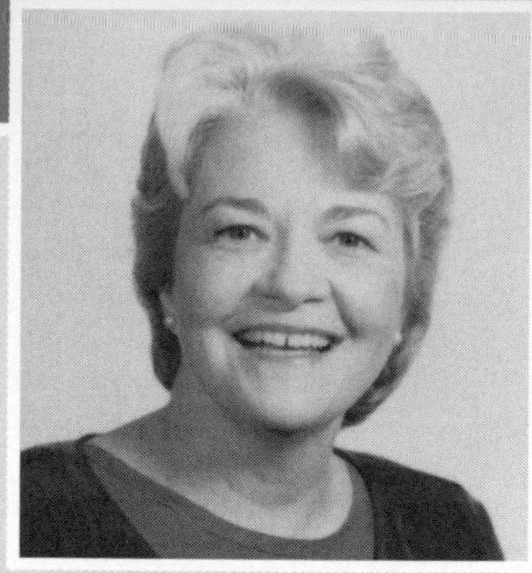

Patricia Benner

"The nurse-patient relationship is not a uniform, professionalized blueprint but rather a kaleidoscope of intimacy and distance in some of the most dramatic, poignant, and mundane moments of life."

(Benner, 1984a)

CREDENTIALS AND BACKGROUND OF THE PHILOSOPHER

Patricia Benner was born in Hampton, Virginia, and spent her childhood in California, where she received her early and professional education. She obtained a baccalaureate of arts degree in nursing from Pasadena College in 1964. In 1970 she earned a master's degree in nursing, with major emphasis in medical-surgical nursing, from the University of California, San Francisco (UCSF) School of Nursing. Her PhD in stress, coping, and health was conferred in 1982 at the University of California, Berkeley, and her dissertation was published in 1984 (Benner, 1984b). Benner has a range of clinical experience, including acute medical-surgical, critical care, and home health care.

Benner has a rich background in research and began this part of her career in 1970 as a postgraduate nurse researcher in the School of Nursing at UCSF. Upon completion of her doctorate in 1982, Benner became an associate professor in the Department of Physiological Nursing at UCSF and a tenured professor in 1989. In 2002 she moved to the Department of Social and Behavioral Sciences at UCSF, as the first occupant of the Thelma Shobe Cook Endowed Chair in Ethics and Spirituality. She taught at the doctoral and master's levels and served on three to four dissertation committees per year. Benner retired from full-time teaching in 2008 as professor emerita from UCSF but continues with presentations, consultation, and visiting professorships as well as writing and research projects. She is currently Chief Development Officer for educatingnurses.com and works with Dr. Pat Hooper-Kyriakidis on continued development of the textbook replacement learning program, NovEx.

Benner published extensively and is the recipient of numerous honors and awards, the most recent being induction into the Danish Nursing Society as an Honorary Member and the Sigma Theta Tau International Book Author award, shared with her coeditors for *Interpretive Phenomenology in Health Care Research* (Chan et al., 2010). She was honored in 1984, 1989, 1996, 1999, and 2011 with *American Journal of Nursing* Book of the Year awards for *From Novice to Expert: Excellence and Power in Clinical Nursing Practice* (1984a), *The Primacy of Caring: Stress and Coping in Health and Illness* (1989, with Wrubel), *Expertise in Nursing Practice: Caring, Clinical Judgment, and Ethics* (1996, with Tanner and Chesla), *Clinical Wisdom and Interventions in Critical Care: A Thinking-in-Action Approach* (1999, with Hooper-Kyriakidis & Stannard), and the second edition of *Clinical Wisdom* (2011), respectively. *The Crisis of Care: Affirming and Restoring Caring Practices in the Helping Professions* (1994), edited by Susan S. Phillips and Patricia Benner, was selected for the CHOICE list of Outstanding Academic Books in 1995. Benner's books and

*Previous authors: Jullette C. Mitre, Sr., Judith E. Alexander, and Susan L. Keller. The author wishes to express appreciation to Patricia Benner for reviewing this chapter.

several of her articles have been translated into 10 languages. Benner received the *American Journal of Nursing* media CD-ROM of the year award for *Clinical Wisdom and Interventions in Critical Care: A Thinking-in-Action Approach* (2001, with Hooper-Kyriakidis & Stannard).

In 1985, Benner was inducted into the American Academy of Nursing. She received the National League for Nursing's Linda Richards Award for leadership in education in 1989 and both the National League for Nursing (NLN) Excellence in Leadership Award for Nursing Education and the NLN President's Award for Creativity and Innovation in Nursing Education in 2010. In 1990 she received the Excellence in Nursing Research and Excellence in Nursing Education Award from the California Organization of Nurse Executives. She also received the Alumnus of the Year Award from Point Loma Nazarene College (formerly Pasadena College) in 1993. In 1994 Benner became an Honorary Fellow in the Royal College of Nursing, United Kingdom. In 1995 she received the Helen Nahm Research Lecture Award from the faculty at UCSF for her contribution to nursing science and research. Benner received an award for outstanding contributions to the profession from the National Council of State Boards of Nursing in 2002, for developing an instrument, Taxonomy of Error, Root Cause and Practice (TERCAP), an electronic data collection tool used to capture the sources and nature of nursing errors (Benner et al., 2002).

In 2002, The Institute for Nursing Healthcare Leadership commemorated the impact of the landmark book *From Novice to Expert* (1984a) with an award acknowledging 20 years of collecting and extending clinical wisdom, experiential learning, and caring practices and a celebration at the conference "Charting the Course: The Power of Expert Nurses to Define the Future." Benner received the American Association of Critical Care Nurses Pioneering Spirit Award in May 2004 for her work on skill acquisition and articulating nursing knowledge in critical care. In 2007 she was selected for the UCSF School of Nursing's Centennial Wall of Fame and she received the American Organization of Nurse Executives (AONE) excellence in research award. In 2008 Benner was ranked as the fourth most influential nurse in the past 60 years by the readership of the journal *Nursing Standard* in the United Kingdom. She was a visiting professor at the University of Pennsylvania School of Nursing in 2009 and Seattle University School of Nursing in 2013. Along with her husband and colleague, Richard Benner, Patricia Benner consults around the world regarding clinical practice development models (CPDMs) (Benner & Benner, 1999). Benner was appointed Nursing Education Study Director for the Carnegie Foundation's Preparation for the Professions Program (PPP) in March 2004. The book published from The Carnegie Foundation for the Advancement of Teaching National Nursing Education Study, *Educating Nurses: A Call for Radical Transformation*, was awarded the *American Journal of Nursing* Book of the Year Award for 2010 and the Prose Award for Scholarly Writing. This was a nationwide study of professional education and the shift from technical professionalism to civic professionalism. In 2011 the American Academy of Nursing honored Patricia Benner as a Living Legend.

PHILOSOPHICAL SOURCES

Benner acknowledges that her thinking in nursing was influenced greatly by Virginia Henderson. Benner studies clinical nursing practice in an attempt to discover and describe the knowledge embedded in nursing practice. She maintains that knowledge accrues over time in a practice discipline and is developed through experiential learning, situated thinking, and reflection on practice in particular practice situations. She refers to this work as **articulation research,** defined as: "describing, illustrating, and giving language to taken-for-granted areas of practical wisdom, skilled know-how, and notions of good practice" (Benner, Hooper-Kyriakidis, & Stannard, 1999, p. 5). One of the first philosophical distinctions that Benner made was to differentiate between practical and theoretical knowledge. She stated that knowledge development in a practice discipline "consists of extending practical knowledge (know-how) through theory-based scientific investigations and through the charting of the existent 'know-how' developed through clinical experience in the practice of that discipline" (1984a, p. 3). Benner believes that nurses have been delinquent in documenting their clinical learning, and "this lack of charting of our practices and clinical observations deprives nursing theory of the uniqueness and richness of the knowledge embedded in expert clinical practice" (Benner, 1983, p. 36).

Citing Kuhn (1970) and Polanyi (1958), philosophers of science, Benner (1984a) emphasizes the difference between "knowing how," a practical knowledge that may elude precise abstract formulations, and "knowing that," which lends itself to theoretical explanations. Clinical situations are always more varied and complicated than theoretical accounts; therefore clinical practice is an area of inquiry and a source of knowledge development. By studying practice, nurses uncover new knowledge. Nurses must develop the knowledge base of practice (know-how), and, through investigation and observation, begin to record and develop the know-how of clinical expertise. Ideally, practice and theory dialogue creates new possibilities. Theory is derived from practice, and practice is extended by theory.

Hubert Dreyfus introduced Benner to phenomenology. Stuart Dreyfus, in operations research, and Hubert Dreyfus, in philosophy, both professors at the University of California at Berkeley, developed the Dreyfus Model of Skill Acquisition (Dreyfus & Dreyfus, 1980, 1986), which Benner applied in her work, *From Novice to Expert* (1984a). She credits Jane Rubin's (1984) scholarship, teaching, and colleagueship as sources of inspiration and influence, especially in relation to the works of Heidegger (1962) and Kierkegaard (1962). Richard Lazarus (Lazarus, 1985; Lazarus & Folkman, 1984) mentored her in the field of stress and coping. Judith Wrubel was a participant and coauthor with Benner for years, collaborating on the ontology of caring and caring practices (Benner & Wrubel, 1989). Additional philosophical and ethical influences on Benner's work include Dunne (1993), Løgstrup (1995a, 1995b, 1997), MacIntyre (1981, 1999), Martinsen (Alvsvåg, 2014), Merleau-Ponty (1962), O'Neill (1996), and Taylor (1971, 1989, 1991, 1993, 1994).

Benner (1984a) adapted the Dreyfus model to clinical nursing practice. The Dreyfus brothers developed the skill acquisition model by studying the performance of chess masters and airline pilots (Dreyfus & Dreyfus, 1980, 1986). Benner's model is situational and describes five levels of skill acquisition and development: (1) novice, (2) advanced beginner, (3) competent, (4) proficient, and (5) expert. The model posits that changes in four aspects of performance occur in movement through the levels of skill acquisition: (1) movement from a reliance on abstract principles and rules to the use of past, concrete experience; (2) shift from reliance on analytical, rule-based thinking to intuition; (3) change in the learner's perception of the situation from viewing it as a compilation of equally relevant bits to viewing it as an increasingly complex whole, in which certain parts stand out as more or less relevant; and (4) passage from a detached observer, standing outside the situation, to one of a position of involvement, fully engaged in the situation (Benner, Tanner, & Chesla, 1992).

Because the model is situation-based and not trait-based, the level of performance is not an individual characteristic of an individual performer, but a function of a given nurse's familiarity with a particular situation in combination with her or his educational background. The performance level can be determined only by consensual validation of expert judges and by assessment of outcomes of the situation (Benner, 1984a). In applying the model to nursing, Benner noted that "experience-based skill acquisition is safer and quicker when it rests upon a sound educational base" (1984a, p. xix). Benner (1984a) defines skill and skilled practice as implementing skilled nursing interventions and clinical judgment skills in actual clinical situations. It does not refer to context-free psychomotor skills or other demonstrable enabling skills outside the context of nursing practice.

In subsequent research undertaken to further explicate the Dreyfus model, Benner identified two interrelated aspects of practice that also distinguish the levels of practice from advanced beginner to expert (Benner, Tanner, & Chesla, 1992, 1996). First, clinicians at different levels of practice live in different clinical worlds, recognizing and responding to different situated needs for action. Second, clinicians develop what Benner terms *agency*, or the sense of responsibility toward the patient, and evolve into fully participating members of the health care team. The skills acquired through nursing experience and the perceptual awareness that expert nurses develop as decision makers from the "gestalt of the situation" lead them to follow hunches as they search for evidence to confirm the subtle changes they observe in patients (1984a, p. xviii).

The concept that experience is defined as the outcome when preconceived notions are challenged, refined, or refuted in actual situations is based on the works of Heidegger (1962) and Gadamer (1970). As the nurse gains experience, clinical knowledge becomes a blend of practical and theoretical knowledge. Expertise develops as the clinician tests and modifies principle-based expectations in the actual situation. Heidegger's influence is evident in this and in Benner's subsequent writings on the primacy of caring. Benner refutes the dualistic Cartesian descriptions of mind-body person and espouses Heidegger's phenomenological description of person as a self-interpreting being who is defined by concerns, practices, and life experiences. Persons are always **situated**—that is, they are engaged meaningfully in the context of where they are. Heidegger (1962) termed **practical knowledge** as the kind of knowing that occurs when an individual is involved in the situation. By virtue of being humans, we have embodied intelligence, meaning that we come to know things by being in situations. When a familiar situation is encountered, there is embodied recognition of its meaning. For example, having previously witnessed someone developing a pulmonary embolus, a nurse notices qualitative nuances and has recognition ability for observing it before those nurses who have never seen it. Benner and Wrubel (1989) state, "Skilled activity, which is made possible by our embodied intelligence, has been long regarded as 'lower' than intellectual, reflective activity" but argue that intellectual, reflective capacities are dependent on **embodied knowing** (p. 43). Embodied knowing and the meaning of being are premises for the capacity to care; things matter and "cause us to be involved in and defined by our concerns" (p. 42).

While engaged in her doctoral studies at Berkeley, Benner was a research assistant to Richard S. Lazarus (Lazarus, 1985; Lazarus & Folkman, 1984), who is known for his stress and coping theory. As part of Lazarus' larger study, Benner studied midcareer males' meaning of work and coping that was published as *Stress and Satisfaction on the Job: Work Meanings and Coping of Mid-Career Men* (1984b). Lazarus' theory of stress and coping is described as phenomenological, because the person is understood to constitute and be constituted by meanings. Stress is the disruption of meanings, and coping is what the person does about the disruption. Both doing something and refraining from doing something are ways of coping. Coping is bound by the meanings inherent in what the person interprets as stressful. Different possibilities arise from the way the person is in the situation. In applying this concept to clinical nursing practice, Benner theorized that nurses make a difference by being in a situation in a caring way.

Benner's approach to knowledge development that began with *From Novice to Expert* (1984a) began a growing, living tradition for learning from clinical nursing practice through collection and interpretation of exemplars (Benner, 1994; Benner & Benner, 1999; Benner, Tanner & Chesla, 1996; Benner, Hooper-Kyriakidis, & Stannard, 1999). Benner and Benner (1999) stated the following:

> *"Effective delivery of patient/family care requires collective attentiveness and mutual support of good practice embedded in a moral community of practitioners seeking to create and sustain good practice . . . This vision of practice is taken from the Aristotelian tradition in ethics (Aristotle, 1985) and the more recent articulation of this tradition by Alasdair MacIntyre (1981), where practice is defined as a collective endeavor that has notions of good internal to the practice . . . However, such collective endeavors must be comprised of individual practitioners who have skilled know how, craft, science, and moral imagination, who continue to create and instantiate good practice."*
>
> **(pp. 23–24)**

MAJOR CONCEPTS & DEFINITIONS

Novice

In the **novice** stage of skill acquisition in the Dreyfus model, the person has no background experience of the situation in which he or she is involved. Context-free rules and objective attributes must be given to guide performance. There is difficulty discerning between relevant and irrelevant aspects of a situation. Generally, this level applies to students of nursing, but Benner has suggested that nurses at higher levels of skill in one area of practice could be classified at the novice level if placed in an area or situation completely foreign to them, such as moving from general medical-surgical adult care to neonatal intensive care (Benner, 1984a).

Advanced Beginner

The **advanced beginner** stage in the Dreyfus model develops when the person can demonstrate marginally acceptable performance, having coped with enough real situations to note, or to have pointed out by a mentor, the recurring meaningful components of the situation. The advanced beginner has enough experience to grasp aspects of the situation (Benner, 1984a). Unlike attributes and features, aspects cannot be objectified completely, because they require experience based on recognition in the context of the situation.

Nurses functioning at this level are guided by rules and are oriented by task completion. They have difficulty grasping the current patient situation in terms of the larger perspective. However, Dreyfus and Dreyfus (1996) state the following:

> *"Through practical experience in concrete situations with meaningful elements which neither the instructor nor student can define in terms of objective features, the advanced beginner starts intuitively to recognize these elements when they are present. We call these newly recognized elements 'situational' to distinguish them from the objective elements of the skill domain that the beginner can recognize prior to seeing concrete examples."*
>
> *(p. 38)*

Clinical situations are viewed by nurses in the advanced beginner stage as a test of their abilities and the demands of the situation placed on them rather than in terms of patient needs and responses (Benner et al., 1992). Advanced beginners feel highly responsible for managing patient care, yet still rely on the help of those who are more experienced (Benner et al., 1992). Benner places most newly graduated nurses at this level.

Competent

Through learning from actual practice situations and by following the actions of others, the advanced beginner moves to the **competent** level (Benner, Tanner, & Chesla, 1992). The competent stage of the Dreyfus model is typified by conscious and deliberate planning that determines which

Continued

MAJOR CONCEPTS & DEFINITIONS—cont'd

aspects of current and future situations are important and which can be ignored (Benner, 1984a).

Consistency, predictability, and time management are important in competent performance. A sense of mastery is acquired through planning and predictability (Benner, Tanner, & Chesla, 1992). The level of efficiency is increased, but "the focus is on time management and the nurse's organization of the task world rather than on timing in relation to the patient's needs" (Benner, Tanner, & Chesla, 1992, p. 20). The competent nurse may display hyper-responsibility for the patient, often more than is realistic, and may exhibit an ever-present and critical view of self (Benner, Tanner, & Chesla, 1992).

The competent stage is most pivotal in clinical learning, because the learner begins to recognize patterns and determine which elements of the situation warrant attention and which can be ignored. The competent nurse devises new rules and reasoning procedures for a plan, while applying learned rules for action on the basis of relevant facts of that situation. To become proficient, the competent performer allows the situation to guide responses (Dreyfus & Dreyfus, 1996). Studies point to the importance of active teaching and learning in the competent stage for nurses making the transition from competency to proficiency (Benner, 2005; Benner, Hooper-Kyriakidis, & Stannard, 1999; Benner, Malloch, & Sheets, 2010; Benner, Tanner, & Chesla, 1996). The competent stage of learning is pivotal in the formation of the everyday ethical comportment of the nurse (Benner, 2005).

Anxiety is now more tailored to the situation than it was at the novice or advanced beginner stage, when general anxiety exists over learning and performing well without making mistakes. Coaching at this point should encourage competent-level nurses to follow through on a sense that things are not as usual, or even on vague feelings of foreboding or anxiety, because they have to learn to decide what is relevant with no rules to guide them. Nurses at this stage feel exhilarated when they perform well and feel remorse when they recognize that their performance could have been more effective or more prescient because they had paid attention to the wrong things or had missed relevant subtle signs and symptoms. These emotional responses are the formative stages of esthetic appreciation of good practice. These feelings of satisfaction and uneasiness with performance act as a moral compass that guides experiential ethical and clinical learning. "There is a built-in tension between the deliberate rule- and maxim-based strategies of organizing, planning, and prediction and developing a more response-based practice, as noted in our study of critical-care nurses" (Benner, 2005, p. 195).

Proficient

At the **proficient** stage of the Dreyfus model, the performer perceives the situation as a whole (the total picture) rather than in terms of aspects, and the performance is guided by maxims. The proficient level is a qualitative leap beyond the competent. Now the performer recognizes the most salient aspects and has an intuitive grasp of the situation based on background understanding (Benner, 1984a).

Nurses at this level demonstrate a new ability to see changing relevance in a situation, including recognition and implementation of skilled responses to the situation as it evolves. They no longer rely on preset goals for organization and demonstrate increased confidence in their knowledge and abilities (Benner, Tanner, & Chesla, 1992). At the proficient stage, there is much more involvement with the patient and family. The proficient stage is a transition into expertise (Benner, Tanner, & Chesla, 1996).

Expert

The fifth stage of the Dreyfus model is achieved when "the expert performer no longer relies on analytical principle (i.e., rule, guideline, maxim) to connect an understanding of the situation to an appropriate action" (Benner, 1984a, p. 31). Benner described the **expert** nurse as having an intuitive grasp of the situation and as being able to identify the region of the problem without losing time considering a range of alternative diagnoses and solutions. There is a qualitative change as the expert performer "knows the patient," meaning knowing typical patterns of responses and knowing the patient as a person. Key aspects of expert practice include the following (Benner, Tanner, & Chesla, 1996):

- Demonstrating a clinical grasp and resource-based practice
- Possessing embodied know-how
- Seeing the big picture
- Seeing the unexpected

The expert nurse has the ability to recognize patterns on the basis of deep experiential background. For the expert nurse, meeting the patient's actual concerns and needs is of utmost importance, even if it means planning and negotiating for a change in the plan of care. There is almost a transparent view of the self (Benner, Tanner, & Chesla, 1992).

Aspects of a Situation

The **aspects** are the recurring meaningful situational components recognized and understood in context because the nurse has previous experience (Benner, 1984a).

MAJOR CONCEPTS & DEFINITIONS—cont'd

Attributes of a Situation
The **attributes** are measurable properties of a situation that can be explained without previous experience in the situation (Benner, 1984a).

Competency
Competency is "an interpretively defined area of skilled performance identified and described by its intent, functions, and meanings" (Benner, 1984a, p. 292). This term is unrelated to the competent stage of the Dreyfus model.

Domain
The **domain** is an area of practice having a number of competencies with similar intents, functions, and meanings (Benner, 1984a).

Exemplar
An **exemplar** is an example of a clinical situation that conveys one or more intents, meanings, functions, or outcomes easily translated to other clinical situations (Benner, 1984a).

Experience
Experience is not a mere passage of time, but an active process of refining and changing preconceived theories, notions, and ideas when confronted with actual situations; it implies there is a dialogue between what is found in practice and what is expected (Benner & Wrubel, 1982).

Maxim
Maxim is a cryptic description of skilled performance that requires a certain level of experience to recognize the implications of the instructions (Benner, 1984a).

Paradigm Case
A **paradigm case** is a clinical experience that stands out and alters the way the nurse will perceive and understand future clinical situations (Benner, 1984a). Paradigm cases create new clinical understanding and open new clinical perspectives and alternatives.

Salience
Salience describes a perceptual stance or embodied knowledge whereby aspects of a situation stand out as more or less important (Benner, 1984a).

Ethical Comportment
Ethical comportment is good conduct born out of an individualized relationship with the patient. It involves engagement in a particular situation and entails a sense of membership in the relevant professional group. It is socially embedded, lived, and embodied in practices, ways of being, and responses to a clinical situation that promote the well-being of the patient (Day & Benner, 2002). "Clinical and ethical judgments are inseparable and must be guided by being with and understanding the human concerns and possibilities in concrete situations" (Benner, 2000, p. 305).

Hermeneutics
Hermeneutics means "interpretive." The term derives from biblical and judicial exegesis. As used in research, hermeneutics refers to describing and studying "meaningful human phenomena in a careful and detailed manner as free as possible from prior theoretical assumptions, based instead on practical understanding" (Packer, 1985, pp. 1081–1082).

Formation
"Transformation and **formation** . . . address the development of senses, esthetics, perceptual acuities, relational skills, knowledge and dispositions that take place as student nurses form professional identity" (Day et al., 2009, p. 87). It goes beyond content knowledge and role enactment to development of moral character, self-understanding, and identity as a nurse.

Situated Coaching
Situated coaching was identified as the signature pedagogy in nursing from the *Educating Nurses* study (Benner et al., 2010). It occurs in particular clinical situations in which the teacher describes his or her understanding of the situation for students, including what is perceived as most relevant and salient (Benner, 2015). Situated coaching enables students to learn to make qualitative distinctions and recognize trends and changes in the patient's responses (Day & Benner, 2014).

USE OF EMPIRICAL EVIDENCE

From 1978 to 1981, Benner was the author and project director of a federally funded grant, Achieving Methods of Intraprofessional Consensus, Assessment and Evaluation, known as the AMICAE project. This research led to the publication of *From Novice to Expert* (1984a). Benner directed the AMICAE project to develop evaluation methods for participating schools of nursing and hospitals in the San Francisco area. It was an interpretive, descriptive study that led to the use of Dreyfus' five levels of competency to describe skill acquisition in clinical nursing practice. Benner (1984a) explains that the interpretive approach seeks a rich description of nursing practice from observation and narrative accounts of actual nursing practice to provide text for interpretation (hermeneutics).

Nurses' descriptions of patient care situations in which they made a positive difference "present the uniqueness of nursing as a discipline and an art" (Benner, 1984a, p. xxvi). More than 1200 nurse participants completed questionnaires and interviews as part of the AMICAE project. Paired interviews with preceptors and preceptees were "aimed at discovering if there were distinguishable, characteristic differences in the novice's and expert's descriptions of the same clinical incident" (Benner, 1984a, p. 14). Additional interviews and participant observations were conducted with 51 nurse-clinicians and other newly graduated nurses and senior nursing students to "describe characteristics of nurse performance at different stages of skill acquisition" (Benner, 1984a, p. 15). The purpose "of the inquiry has been to uncover meanings and knowledge embedded in skilled practice. By bringing these meanings, skills, and knowledge into public discourse, new knowledge and understandings are constituted" (Benner, 1984a, p. 218).

Thirty-one competencies emerged from the analysis of transcripts of interviews about nurses' detailed descriptions of patient care episodes that included their intentions and interpretations of events. From these competencies, which were identified from actual practice situations, the following seven domains were derived inductively on the basis of similarity of function and intent (Benner, 1984a):

1. The helping role
2. The teaching-coaching function
3. The diagnostic and patient monitoring function
4. Effective management of rapidly changing situations
5. Administering and monitoring therapeutic interventions and regimens
6. Monitoring and ensuring the quality of health care practices
7. Organizational work role competencies

Each domain was developed using the related competencies from actual practice situation descriptions. Benner presented the domains and competencies of nursing practice as an open-ended interpretive framework for enhancing the understanding of the knowledge embedded in nursing practice. As a result of the socially embedded, relational, and dialogical nature of clinical knowledge, domains and competencies should be adapted for use in each institution through the study of clinical practice at each specific locale (Benner & Benner, 1999). Such adaptations have been implemented in many institutions for nursing staff in hospitals around the world (Alberti, 1991; Balasco & Black, 1988; Brykczynski, 1998; Dolan, 1984; Gaston, 1989; Gordon, 1986; Hamric, Whitworth, & Greenfield, 1993; Lock & Gordon, 1989; Nuccio et al., 1996; Silver, 1986a, 1986b). The domains and competencies have also been useful for ongoing articulation of the knowledge embedded in advanced practice nursing (Brykczynski, 1999; Fenton, 1985; Fenton & Brykczynski, 1993; Lindeke, Canedy, & Kay, 1997; Martin, 1996).

Benner and Wrubel (1989) have further explained and developed the background to the ongoing study of the knowledge embedded in nursing practice in *The Primacy of Caring: Stress and Coping in Health and Illness.* They note that the primacy of caring is three-pronged "as the producer of both stress and coping in the lived experience of health and illness as the enabling condition of nursing practice (indeed any practice), and the ways that nursing practice based in such caring can positively affect the outcome of an illness" (1989, p. 7).

Benner extended the research reported in *From Novice to Expert* (1984a) in *Expertise in Nursing Practice: Caring, Clinical Judgment, and Ethics* (Benner, Tanner, & Chesla, 1996, 2009). This book presents a 6-year study of 130 hospital nurses, primarily critical care nurses, examining the acquisition of clinical expertise and the nature of clinical knowledge, clinical inquiry, clinical judgment, and expert ethical comportment. The key aims of the extension of this research were as follows:

- Delineate the practical knowledge embedded in expert practice.
- Describe the nature of skill acquisition in critical care nursing practice.
- Identify institutional impediments and resources for the development of expertise in nursing practice.
- Begin to identify educational strategies that encourage the development of expertise.

In the introduction to the 1996 book, Benner stated, "In the study we found that examining the nature of the nurse's agency, by which we mean the sense and possibilities for acting in particular clinical situations, gave new insights about how perception and action are both shaped by a practice community" (Benner, Tanner, & Chesla, 1996, p. xiii). This study resulted in a clearer understanding of the distinctions between engagement with a problem or situation and the requisite nursing skills of interpersonal involvement. It appears that these nursing skills are learned over time experientially. The skill of involvement seems central in gaining nursing expertise. Understanding of the interlinkage of clinical and ethical decision making (i.e., how an individual's notions of good and poor outcomes and visions of excellence shape clinical judgments and actions) was enhanced by this research. This study represents phase one of the articulation project designed to describe the nature of critical care nursing practice.

Phase two took place from 1996 to 1997 and included 76 nurses (32 of them advanced practice nurses) from six different hospitals. This work is presented in *Clinical Wisdom and Interventions in Acute and Critical Care: A Thinking-in-Action Approach,* which was published in 1999 then updated and enlarged in 2011 by Benner, Hooper-Kyriakidis, and Stannard. The following nine domains of critical care nursing practice were identified as broad themes in this work:

1. Diagnosing and managing life-sustaining physiological functions in acute and unstable patients
2. Using the skilled know-how of managing a crisis
3. Providing comfort measures for the acute critically ill
4. Caring for patients' families
5. Preventing hazards in a technological environment
6. Facing death: end-of-life care and decision making
7. Communicating and negotiating multiple perspectives
8. Monitoring quality and managing breakdown
9. Using the skilled know-how of clinical leadership and the coaching and mentoring of others

These nine domains of critical care nursing practice were used as broad themes to interpret the data and incorporate descriptions of the following nine aspects of clinical judgment and skillful comportment:

1. Developing a sense of salience
2. Situated learning and integration of knowledge acquisition and knowledge use
3. Engaged reasoning-in-transition
4. Skilled know-how
5. Response-based practice
6. Agency
7. Perceptual acuity and interpersonal engagement with patients
8. Integrating clinical and ethical reasoning
9. Developing clinical imagination

Identification of clinical grasp and clinical forethought (two pervasive habits of thought linked with action in nursing practice in phase two of this articulation project) enriched the understanding of clinical judgment (Benner, Hooper-Kyriakidis, & Stannard, 1999). Benner explained that clinical grasp is "clinical inquiry in action that includes problem identification and clinical judgment across time about the particular transitions of particular patients and families. It has four components: making qualitative distinctions, engaging in detective work, recognizing changing clinical relevance, and developing clinical knowledge in specific patient populations" (Benner, Hooper-Kyriakidis, & Stannard, 1999, p. 317).

Benner added that although clinical forethought plays a role in clinical grasp, it "also plays an essential role in structuring the practical logic of clinicians. Clinical forethought refers to at least four habits of thought and action: future think, clinical forethought about specific diagnoses and injuries, anticipation of risks for particular patients, and seeing the unexpected" (Benner, Hooper-Kyriakidis, & Stannard, 1999, p. 317).

MAJOR ASSUMPTIONS

Benner incorporates the following assumptions (as delineated in Brykczynski's 1985 dissertation) in her ongoing articulation research:

- There are no interpretation-free data. This abandons the assumption from natural science that there is an independent reality whose meaning can be represented by abstract terms or concepts (Taylor, 1982).
- There are no nonreactive data. This abandons the false belief from natural science that one can neutrally observe brute data (Taylor, 1982).
- Meanings are embedded in skills, practices, intentions, expectations, and outcomes. They are taken for granted and often are not recognized as knowledge. According to Polanyi (1958), a context possesses existential meaning, and this distinguishes it from "denotative or, more generally, representative meaning" (p. 58). He claims that transposing a significant whole in terms of its constituent parts deprives it of any purpose or meaning.
- People who share a common cultural and language history have a background of common meanings that allow for understanding and interpretation. Heidegger (1962) refers to this as *primordial understanding,* after the writings of Dilthey (1976) in the late 1800s and early 1900s, asserting that cultural organization and meanings precede and influence individual understanding.
- The meanings embedded in skills, practices, intentions, expectations, and outcomes cannot be made completely explicit; however, they can be interpreted by someone who shares a similar language and cultural background and can be validated consensually by participants and relevant practitioners. Humans are self-interpreting beings (Heidegger, 1962). Hermeneutics is the interpretation of cultural contexts and meaningful human action.
- Humans are integrated, holistic beings. The mind-body split is abandoned. Embodied intelligence enables skilled activity that is transformed through experience and mastery (Dreyfus & Dreyfus, 1980, 1986). Benner stated, "This model assumes that all practical situations are far more complex than can be described by formal models, theories and textbook descriptions" (1984a, p. 178). The hierarchical elevation of intellectual,

reflective activity above embodied skilled activity ignores the point that skilled action is a way of knowing and that the skilled body may be essential for the more highly esteemed levels of human intelligence (Dreyfus, 1979).

Benner and her collaborators explicated the themes of *nursing, person, health,* and *situation* in their publications.

Nursing

Nursing is described as a caring relationship, an "enabling condition of connection and concern" (Benner & Wrubel, 1989, p. 4). "Caring is primary because caring sets up the possibility of giving help and receiving help" (Benner & Wrubel, 1989, p. 4). "Nursing is viewed as a caring practice whose science is guided by the moral art and ethics of care and responsibility" (Benner & Wrubel, 1989, p. xi). Benner and Wrubel (1989) understand nursing practice as the care and study of the lived experience of health, illness, and disease and the relationships among these three elements.

Person

Benner and Wrubel (1989) use Heidegger's phenomenological description of person, which they describe as: "A person is a self-interpreting being, that is, the person does not come into the world predefined but gets defined in the course of living a life. A person also has an effortless and nonreflective understanding of the self in the world" (p. 41). "The person is viewed as a participant in common meanings" (Benner & Wrubel, 1989, p. 23).

Finally, the person is embodied. Benner and Wrubel (1989) conceptualized the following four major aspects of understanding that the person must deal with:

1. The role of the situation
2. The role of the body
3. The role of personal concerns
4. The role of temporality

Together, these aspects of the person make up the person in the world. This view of the person is based on the works of Heidegger (1962), Merleau-Ponty (1962), and Dreyfus (1979, 1991). Their goal is to overcome Cartesian dualism, the view that the mind and body are distinct, separate entities (Visintainer, 1988).

Benner and Wrubel (1989) define *embodiment* as the capacity of the body to respond to meaningful situations. Based on the work of Merleau-Ponty (1962), Dreyfus (1979, 1991), and Dreyfus and Dreyfus (1986), they outline the following five dimensions of the body (Benner & Wrubel, 1989):

1. The unborn complex, unacculturated body of the fetus and newborn baby
2. The habitual skilled body complete with socially learned postures, gestures, customs, and skills evident in bodily skills such as sense perception and "body language" that are "learned over time through identification, imitation, and trial and error" (Benner & Wrubel, 1989, p. 71)
3. The projective body that is set (predisposed) to act in specific situations (e.g., opening a door or walking)
4. The actual projected body indicating an individual's current bodily orientation or projection in a situation that is flexible and varied to fit the situation, such as when an individual is skillful in using a computer
5. The phenomenal body, the body aware of itself with the ability to imagine and describe kinesthetic sensations

Benner and Wrubel (1989) point out that nurses attend to all of these dimensions of the body and seek to understand the role of embodiment in particular situations of health, illness, and recovery.

Health

On the basis of the work of Heidegger (1962) and Merleau-Ponty (1962), Benner and Wrubel focus "on the lived experience of being healthy and being ill" (1989, p. 7). **Health** is defined as what can be assessed, whereas **well-being** is the human experience of health or wholeness. Well-being and being ill are understood as distinct ways of being in the world. Health is described as not just the absence of disease and illness. Also, on the basis of the work of Kleinman et al. (1978), a person may have a disease and not experience illness, because illness is the human experience of loss or dysfunction, whereas disease is what can be assessed at the physical level (Benner & Wrubel, 1989).

Situation

Benner and Wrubel (1989) use the term **situation** rather than **environment,** because situation conveys a social environment with social definition and meaningfulness. They use the phenomenological terms **being situated** and **situated meaning,** which are defined by the person's engaged interaction, interpretation, and understanding of the situation. "Personal interpretation of the situation is bounded by the way the individual is in it" (Benner & Wrubel, 1989, p. 84). This means that each person's past, present, and future, which include her or his own personal meanings, habits, and perspectives, influence the current situation.

THEORETICAL ASSERTIONS

Benner (1984a) stated that there is always more to any situation than theory predicts. The skilled practice of nursing exceeds the bounds of formal theory. Concrete experience facilitates learning about the exceptions and shades of meaning in a situation. The knowledge embedded in practice can lead to discovering and interpreting theory, precedes and extends theory, and synthesizes and adapts theory in caring nursing practice. Benner has taken a hermeneutical approach to uncover the knowledge in clinical nursing practice. Dunlop (1986) stated, "As she does this, she is also uncovering the nursing-caring with which it is deeply intertwined" (p. 668). Dunlop also noted that Benner's approach "does not provide us with any universal truths about caring in general or about nursing-caring in particular—indeed it does not make any such pretension" (p. 668).

As such, the competencies within each domain are in no way intended as an exhaustive list. Instead, the situation-based interpretive approach to describing nursing practice seeks to overcome some of the problems of reductionism and the problem of global and overly general descriptions based on nursing process categories (Benner, 1984a). In a further description of this approach, Benner (1992) examined the role of narrative accounts for understanding the notion of good or ethical caring in expert clinical nursing practice. "The narrative memory of the actual concrete event is taken up in embodied know-how and comportment, complete with emotional responses to situations. The narrative memory can evoke perceptual or sensory memories that enhance pattern recognition" (p. 16). Some of the relationship statements included in Benner's work follow:

- "Discovering assumptions, expectations, and sets can uncover an unexamined area of practical knowledge that can then be systematically studied and extended or refuted" (Benner, 1984a, p. 8).
- Clinical knowledge is embedded in perceptions rather than precepts.
- "Perceptual awareness is central to good nursing judgment and [for the expert] begins with vague hunches and global assessments that initially bypass critical analysis; conceptual clarity follows more often than it precedes" (Benner, 1984a, p. xviii).
- Formal rules are limited and discretionary judgment is needed in actual clinical situations.
- Clinical knowledge develops over time, and each clinician develops a personal repertoire of practice knowledge that can be shared in dialogue with other clinicians.
- "Expertise develops when the clinician tests and refines propositions, hypotheses, and principle based expectations in actual practice situations" (Benner, 1984a, p. 3).

LOGICAL FORM

Through qualitative descriptive research, Benner used the Dreyfus model of skill acquisition to better understand skill acquisition in clinical nursing practice. By following the model's logical sequence, Benner was able to identify the performance characteristics and teaching-learning needs inherent at each skill level. In reporting her research, Benner used exemplars taken directly from interviews and observation of clinical nurses at different skill levels to help the reader form a clear picture of practice. Guidelines for describing exemplars or clinical narratives, first termed "critical incidents," were presented in *From Novice to Expert* (1984a) and are developed further in *Clinical Wisdom and Interventions in Acute and Critical Care: A Thinking-in-Action Approach* (Benner, Hooper-Kyriakidis, & Stannard, 2011). The approach for describing clinical narratives is consistent throughout the body of Benner's work whether the narratives are used in research, practice, or education. The goal of Benner's research is to bring meanings and knowledge embedded in skilled practice into public discourse. Benner (1984a) claims that new knowledge and understanding are constituted by articulating meanings, skills, and knowledge that previously were taken for granted and embedded in clinical practice.

ACCEPTANCE BY THE NURSING COMMUNITY

Practice

Benner describes clinical nursing practice using an interpretive phenomenological approach. *From Novice to Expert* (1984a) includes several examples of the application of her work in practice settings as follows: Dolan (1984) describes its usefulness for preceptor development, orientation programs, and career development; Huntsman et al. (1984) detail their implementation of a clinical ladder to recognize and retain experienced staff nurses; Ullery (1984) presents its usefulness for conducting annual excellence symposia where nurses present their clinical narratives to recognize and further develop clinical knowledge; and Fenton (1984) reported the use of Benner's approach in an ethnographic study of the performance of clinical nurse-specialists.

Balasco and Black (1988) and Silver (1986a, 1986b) used Benner's work as a basis for differentiating clinical knowledge development and career progression in nursing. Neverveld (1990) used Benner's rationale and format in the development of basic and advanced preceptor workshops. Farrell and Bramadat (1990) used Benner's paradigm case analysis in a collaborative educational project between a university school of nursing and a tertiary care teaching hospital to better understand the development of clinical reasoning skills in actual practice situations. Crissman and Jelsma (1990) applied Benner's findings to develop a cross-training program to address staffing imbalances. They delineated specific cross-training performance objectives for novice nurses and provided support for experiential judgment needed to function in unfamiliar settings by designating a preceptor in the clinical area. The aim was for the novice to perform more like an advanced beginner with an experienced nurse available as a resource.

Benner's approach continues to be used in the development of clinical promotion ladders, new graduate orientation programs, and clinical knowledge development seminars (Benner & Benner, 1999; Benner, Tanner, & Chesla, 2009; Coyle, 2011; Hargreaves et al., 2010). Mauleon and colleagues (2005) conducted an interpretive phenomenological analysis of problematic situations experienced by nurse anesthetists in anesthesia care of elderly patients which indicated a need for ethical forums for dealing with moral distress arising from their experiences. Uhrenfeldt's (2009) study of how first-line nurse leaders care for their nursing staff was based on Benner and Wrubel's (1989) caring framework. Cathcart (2010) articulated the experientially acquired knowledge, skill, and ethics embedded in nurse manager practice after Benner's approach.

Benner has been cited extensively in nursing literature regarding nursing practice concerns and the role of caring in such practice. She continues to advance understanding of the knowledge embedded in clinical situations through her publications (Benner 1985a, 1985b, 1987; Benner, Hooper-Kyriakidis, & Stannard, 1999, 2011; Benner & Tanner, 1987; Benner, Tanner, & Chesla, 1996, 2009). Benner edited a clinical exemplar series in the *American Journal of Nursing* during the 1980s. In 2001 she began editing a series called "Current Controversies in Critical Care" in the *American Journal of Critical Care*. Benner's work with the National Council of State Boards of Nursing constitutes a major contribution to error recognition and safety of nursing practice (Benner et al., 2002). This research examines practice breakdowns from a systems perspective with the goal of transforming the culture of blame in the health care system to reduce health care errors (Benner, Malloch, & Sheets, 2010).

Education

Benner (1982) critiqued the concept of competency-based testing by contrasting it with the complexity of the proficient and expert stages described in the Dreyfus model of skill acquisition and the 31 competencies described in the AMICAE project (Benner, 1984a). In summary, she stated, "Competency-based testing seems limited to the less situational, less interactional areas of patient care where the behavior can be well defined and patient and nurse variations do not alter the performance criteria" (1982, p. 309).

Fenton (1984, 1985) applied the domains of clinical nursing practice as a basis for studying skilled performance of clinical nurse specialists (CNSs). Her analysis validated all seven of the original domains in the CNSs studied. She identified additional areas of skilled performance for CNSs, including the consulting role. Brykczynski's (1985/1999) study used the research approach presented in *From Novice to Expert* to address the question: "Where is the nurse in nurse practitioner?" That study produced an adaptation of Benner's original domains and competencies for nurse practitioners (NPs). This adaptation of the domains and competencies for NP practice formed the framework for the National Organization of Nurse Practitioner Faculties (NONPF, 1990) curriculum guidelines. Fenton and Brykczynski (1993) later compared the findings from their studies of CNSs and NPs to uncover commonalities and distinctions between these advanced practice nurses that were relevant for graduate curriculum planning.

According to Barnum (1990), it was not Benner's development of the seven domains of nursing practice that has had the greatest impact on nursing education, but the "appreciation of the utility of the Dreyfus model in describing learning and thinking in our discipline" (p. 170). As a result of Benner's application of the Dreyfus model, nursing educators have realized that learning needs at the early stages of clinical knowledge development are different from those required at later stages. These differences need to be acknowledged and valued to develop nursing education programs appropriate for the background experience of the students.

In *Expertise in Nursing Practice,* Benner et al. (1996) emphasized the importance of learning the skills of involvement and caring through practical experience, the articulation of knowledge with practice, and the use of narratives in undergraduate education. This work supports the thesis that it is better to place a new graduate with a competent nurse preceptor who can explain nursing practice in ways that the beginner comprehends, rather than with the expert, whose intuitive knowledge may elude beginners who do not have the experienced know-how to grasp the situation. This work, now in its second edition (Benner, Tanner, & Chesla, 2009), led to the development of internship and orientation programs for newly graduated nurses and to clinical development programs for more experienced nurses.

In *Clinical Wisdom in Critical Care,* Benner et al. (1999) urged greater attention to experiential learning and presented the work as a guide to teaching. They designed a highly interactive CD-ROM to accompany the book (Benner, Stannard, & Hooper-Kyriakidis, 2001). The second edition (Benner, Hooper-Kyriakidis, & Stannard,

2011) includes a chapter on the educational implications and recommended teaching strategies from this research on knowledge embedded in acute and critical care nursing from *Educating Nurses: A Call for Radical Transformation* (Benner et al., 2010). The two major types of integrative strategies presented in that 2011 edition are examples of coaching-situated-learning and a thinking-in-action approach of integrating classroom with clinical teaching.

A national study of nursing education was designed to identify and describe "signature pedagogies" that maximize the nurse's ability to cope with the challenges of nursing that have developed during the 30 years since the last national study of nursing education (Schwartz, 2005). The book *Educating Nurses* (Benner et al., 2010) reports details of this national study of nursing education, and it concludes that nursing education is in need of a major transformation. An education gap has developed from the difficulty of addressing competing demands and keeping pace with the increasing complexity of practice driven by research and new technologies. The authors recommend that nurse educators make four major shifts in their focus: (1) from covering abstract knowledge to emphasizing teaching for particular situations, (2) from separations between clinical and classroom teaching to integration of these components, (3) from critical thinking to clinical reasoning, and (4) from emphasizing socialization and role-taking to professional identity formation. These findings and recommendations have been presented at national and international conferences and to faculty at many schools of nursing.

McNiesh et al. (2011) studied how students in an accelerated master's entry program experientially learned the practice of nursing. They found that independent care of a patient was pivotal in the development of students' identity and agency as nurses. Crider and McNiesh (2011) incorporated a three-pronged apprenticeship approach (Benner et al., 2010) that integrates intellectual, practical, and ethical aspects of the professional role in teaching students in psychiatric nursing to develop practical reasoning skills.

Research

Benner maintains that there is excellence and power in clinical nursing practice made visible through **articulation research.** Intricate nuanced descriptions of situational contexts (clinical narratives) are the essence of this research approach, which dictates data be collected through situation-based dialogue and observation of actual practice. The situational context guides interpretation of meanings so there is agreement among interpreters. This is a holistic approach that emphasizes identification and description of meanings embedded in clinical practice. The holistic approach is maintained throughout the research process. The situational context is maintained as narratives are interpreted through dialogue among researchers and clinicians.

Benner's numerous studies and projects with research colleagues and graduate students have created a community of interpretive phenomenological scholars. Benner (1994) edited and contributed to *Interpretive Phenomenology: Embodiment, Caring, and Ethics in Health and Illness*, a collection of essays and studies selected from that community of researchers that she has inspired and taught during her career. The book offers a philosophical introduction to interpretive phenomenology as a qualitative research method, a guide to understanding the strategies and processes of this approach, and a selection of studies that conveys its resemblances and variations. Interpretive phenomenology cannot be explained as a set of procedures and techniques. Instead, "each interpreter enters the interpretive circle by examining preunderstandings and confronting otherness, silence, similarities, and commonalities from his or her own particular historical, cultural, and personal stance" (Benner, 1994, p. xviii).

A second volume of interpretive phenomenological readings and studies edited by Chan et al. (2010) arose from a *Festschrift* (retirement celebration for a scholar) honoring the impact and significance of the research tradition Benner established. That second volume presents the interpretive phenomenology philosophy and research approach that continues to evolve. The first section explores theoretical and philosophical discourses and issues within the interpretive phenomenological tradition, whereas the second section is a collection of studies that exemplifies the similarities and variations in the approaches across studies.

Benner and colleagues (De Jong et al., 2010) conducted a large-scale collaborative study with The TriService Military Nursing Research group to investigate knowledge development and experiential learning from nursing practice during the Iraq and Afghanistan Wars. It describes how nurses learned to improve clinical practice and care delivery during mass casualty events. That research was followed by a study describing the evolution of case management for service members wounded in Iraq and Afghanistan (Kelley et al., 2015). The new types of injuries, in-field treatment, immediate transport to multiple care centers, and new technologies required expansion of case management practice to include family support, reentry, and life coaching for extremely altered life circumstances.

FURTHER DEVELOPMENT

The separation of academic course work from clinical learning developed over time as nursing education moved from hospital schools to colleges and universities with the eventual result that nursing faculty and students have come to be regarded as "guests in the house" (Glass, 1975). The ever-increasing complexity of technology and clinical nursing practice coupled with the separation between education and practice sets the stage for new graduate nurses to face a major transition upon graduation. Implementation of the findings from Benner and colleagues' extensive body of work articulating the knowledge developed in clinical practice and describing ways to teach nursing that integrate theory and decontextualized content with practical context-dependent know-how requires extensive transformation of nursing education. The hidden curriculum described by Day and Benner (2014, p. 140) as "the implicit and unconscious devaluing of practice-based learning in context and the privileging of theory-based" abstract learning must be recognized and augmented with integrated approaches that recontextualize teaching and learning. There are many examples of how to teach nursing using integrated approaches that emphasize knowledge acquisition and knowledge use in practice, such as team-based and problem-based learning, simulation, narrative pedagogy, and unfolding case studies. Nursing faculty require ongoing continuing education and coaching to develop the skills and knowledge needed to incorporate these approaches into their teaching.

Benner initiated an educational newsletter to share *Educating Nurses* study recommendations and create an ongoing dialogue with nurse educators. Benner (2012) discussed the progress in implementing study recommendations, reporting that several states have implemented suggested changes in nursing education and many hospitals and health science campuses have instituted nurse residency programs. Two websites have been created to facilitate dissemination and implementation of the study recommendations, which are listed in the Points for Further Study at the end of this chapter.

CRITIQUE

Clarity

The clarity of Benner's novice to expert model has led to its use among nurses around the world. An identification with the idea of clinical wisdom and varying levels of clinical expertise development progressed very quickly. The research approach differentiated Benner's work from other theoretical approaches at the time. Altmann (2007) addressed the question of whether the work was a philosophy or theory. Benner's work not only contributed to appreciative understanding of clinical practice but also revealed nursing knowledge embedded in practice. Benner's perspective is phenomenological, not cognitive. She stated, "Clinical judgment and caring practices require attendance to the particular patient across time, taking into account changes and what has been learned. In this vision of clinical judgment, skilled know-how and action are linked" (Benner, 1999, p. 316). There has been ongoing debate over cognitive interpretations of Benner's concepts of expertise and intuition (Benner, 1996b; Cash, 1995; Darbyshire, 1994; English, 1993; Paley, 1996). Scholarly debate around these concepts has contributed to clarification of the nature of the research approach (Brykczynski & Benner, 2010).

Simplicity

Benner developed interpretive descriptive accounts of clinical nursing practice. The model is relatively simple with regard to the five stages of skill acquisition, and it provides a comparative guide for identifying levels of nursing practice from individual nurse descriptions and observations and interpretations validated by consensus. A degree of complexity is encountered in the subconcepts for differentiation among the levels of competency and the need to identify meanings and intentions. This interpretive approach is designed to overcome the constraints of the rational-technical approach to the study and description of nursing practice. Although a decontextualized (object) description of the novice level of performance is possible, such a description of expert performance would be difficult, if not impossible, and is of limited usefulness because of the limits of objectification. In other words, the philosophical problem of infinite regress would be encountered in attempts to specify all the aspects of expert practice. Rather, a holistic understanding of the particular situation is required for expert performance.

Generality

The novice-to-expert skill acquisition model has universal characteristics; that is, it is not restricted by age, illness, health, or location of nursing practice. However, the characteristics of theoretical universality imply properties of operationalization for prediction that are not a part of this perspective. Indeed, this phenomenological perspective critiques the limits of universality in studies of human practices. The interpretive model of nursing practice has the potential for universal application as a framework, but the descriptions are limited by dependence on the actual clinical nursing situations from which they must be derived. Its use depends on an understanding of the five levels of competency and the ability to identify the characteristic intentions and meanings inherent at each level of practice.

Generalization is approached through an understanding of common meanings, skills, practices, and embodied capacities. Preferred strategies for generalization in clinical practice are based on the skilled knowledge, intent, content, and notion of good in clinical knowledge depicted by exemplars that illustrate the role of the situation. The generalizations possible with the interpretive approach are depicted through exemplars that demonstrate relational and contextually relevant intents and aspects of clinical knowledge. Benner (1984a) believes that the scope and complexity of nursing practice are too extensive for nurses to rely on idealized, decontextualized views of practice or experiments.

To capture the contextual and relational aspects of practice, Benner uses narrative accounts of actual clinical situations and maintains that this approach enables the reader to recognize similar intents and meanings, although the objective circumstances may be quite different. An example of generalizability or transferability as used here follows: Upon reading or hearing a narrative about a nurse connecting with a family whose child is dying, other nurses can relate the knowledge and meanings conveyed to the experiences they may have had with families of patients of any age who were dying.

Accessibility

Clinical nurses around the world enthusiastically received *From Novice to Expert* (1984a). They found understanding of their practice in terms of what they did in specific patient situations validated and enhanced by this work, which taught them to listen to their voices as nurses. Subsequent research suggests that the framework is applicable and useful for continued development of knowledge embedded in nursing practice. This approach to knowledge development honors the primacy of caring and the central ethic of care and responsibility embedded in expert nursing practice (Benner, 1999). The qualitative interpretive approach describes expert nursing practice with narrative exemplars. Benner's work is considered hypothesis generating rather than hypothesis testing. Benner provides a methodology for uncovering and entering into the situated meaning of expert nursing care.

Importance

The landmark research reported in *From Novice to Expert* has influenced major changes in nursing practice, research, teaching, and administration. The thesis of the work was revolutionary in that it advocated developing knowledge from clinical nursing practice. This was a complete change from the time-honored approach of applying theory to practice. This represented what Kuhn (1970) referred to as a *paradigm shift*. It is an example of articulation research wherein knowledge develops through dialogue (Benner, 1999) that provides a way of recognizing aspects of nursing that are relational, contextual, basic, and pervasive. *From Novice to Expert* gave voice and visibility to nursing's embedded caring practices that are often taken for granted, unrecognized, and unrewarded yet are essential to maintaining dignity, humanity, and safety in the cost-driven high-tech world of hospital nursing practice.

Benner claims that nurses need to overcome the limits of subject-object descriptions. Her call is to "increase public storytelling" to validate nursing as an ethical caring practice, and "to extend, alter, and preserve ethical distinctions and concerns" (Benner, 1992, pp. 19–20). Benner (1996a) stated, "We have overlooked practitioner stories that demonstrate that compassion can be wise and, in the long run, less costly than 'defensive' adversarial commodified technocures" (pp. 35–36). Benner's work is useful in that it frames nursing practice in the context of what a nurse actually is and does. The significance of Benner's research findings lies in her conclusion that "a nurse's clinical knowledge is relevant to the extent to which its manifestation in nursing skills makes a difference in patient care and patient outcomes" (Benner & Wrubel, 1982, p. 11).

SUMMARY

Benner maintains that caring practices are imbued with knowledge and skill about everyday human needs, and that to be experienced as caring, these practices must be attuned to the particular person who is being cared for and to the particular situation as it unfolds. Benner's philosophy of nursing practice is a dynamic, emerging holistic perspective that holds philosophy, practice, research, and theory as interdependent, interrelated, and hermeneutic. Her hope, voiced in the preface of *From Novice to Expert* (1984a), that domains and competencies would not be deified by system builders seems to have been largely realized, because those who have sought to apply these concepts have honored the contextual background on which they are based. Benner's work exemplifies the interrelationship of philosophy, practice, research, theory, and education and the resources she and her colleagues have developed for teacher training, curriculum development, and online student learning integrate practical and theoretical knowledge.

CASE STUDY

This case study from the peer-identified nurse expert project illustrates Benner's approach to knowledge development in clinical nursing practice (Brykczynski, 1993–1995, 1998). The project was undertaken to identify and describe expert staff nursing practices. Exemplars were obtained and participant observations conducted to yield narrative text that was interpreted through Benner's multiphase interpretive phenomenological process (Benner, 1984a, 1994). In the final phase of data analysis, Benner's (1984a) domains and competencies of nursing practice were an interpretive framework. A critical aspect of using Benner's practice approach is that domains and competencies form a dynamic evolving interpretive framework, which is used to interpret the narrative and observational data collected. The nurse who described this situation had approximately 8 years of experience in critical care. She shared that her project participation was significant to her practice because it taught her how to integrate care of a family in crisis along with care of a critically ill patient. Thus this was a paradigm case for that nurse, who learned many things from it that affected her future practice.

"Mrs. Walsh, a woman in her 70s, was in critical condition after repeat coronary artery bypass graft (CABG) surgery. Her family lived nearby when Mrs. Walsh had her first CABG surgery. They had moved out of town but returned to our institution, where the first surgery had been performed successfully. Mrs. Walsh remained critically ill and unstable for several weeks before her death. Her family was very anxious because of Mrs. Walsh's unstable and deteriorating condition, and a family member was always with her 24 hours a day for the first few weeks.

The nurse became involved with this family while Mrs. Walsh was still in surgery, because family members were very anxious that the procedure was taking longer than it had the first time and made repeated calls to the critical care unit to ask about the patient. The nurse met with the family and offered to go into the operating room to talk with the cardiac surgeon to better inform the family of their mother's status.

One of the helpful things the nurse did to assist this family was to establish a consistent group of nurses to work with Mrs. Walsh, so that family members could establish trust and feel more confident about the care their mother was receiving. This eventually enabled family members to leave the hospital for intervals to get some rest. The nurse related that this was a family whose members were affluent, educated, and well informed, and that they came in prepared with lists of questions. A consistent group of nurses who were familiar with Mrs. Walsh's particular situation helped both family members and nurses to be more satisfied and less anxious. The family developed a close relationship with the three nurses who consistently cared for Mrs. Walsh and shared with them details about Mrs. Walsh and her life.

The nurse related that there was a tradition in this particular critical care unit not to involve family members in care. She broke that tradition when she responded to the son's and the daughter's helpless feelings by teaching them some simple things that they could do for their mother. They learned to give some basic care, such as bathing her. The nurse acknowledged that involving family members in direct patient care with a critically ill patient is complex and requires knowledge and sensitivity. She believes that a developmental process is involved when nurses learn to work with families.

She noted that after a nurse has lots of experience and feels very comfortable with highly technical skills, it becomes okay for family members to be in the room when care is provided. She pointed out that direct observation by anxious family members can be disconcerting to those who are insecure with their skills when family members ask things like, "Why are you doing this? Nurse 'So and So' does it differently." She commented that nurses learn to be flexible and to reset priorities. They should be able to let some things wait that do not need to be done right away to give the family some time with the patient. One of the things that the nurse did to coordinate care was to meet with the family to see what times worked best for them; then she posted family time on the patient's activity schedule outside her cubicle to communicate the plan to others involved in Mrs. Walsh's care.

When Mrs. Walsh died, the son and daughter wanted to participate in preparing her body. This had never been done in this unit, but after checking to see that there was no policy forbidding it, the nurse invited them to participate. They turned down the lights, closed the doors, and put music on; the nurse, the patient's daughter, and the patient's son all cried together while they prepared Mrs. Walsh to be taken to the morgue. The nurse took care of all intravenous lines and tubes while the children bathed her. The nurse provided evidence of how finely tuned her skill of involvement was with this

CASE STUDY—cont'd

family when she explained that she felt uncomfortable at first because she thought that the son and daughter should be sharing this time alone with their mother. Then she realized that they really wanted her to be there with them. This situation taught her that families of critically ill patients need care as well. The nurse explained that this was a paradigm case that motivated her to move into a CNS role, with expansion of her sphere of influence from her patients during her shift to other shifts, other patients and their families, and other disciplines" (Brykczynski, 1998, pp. 351–359).

Domain: The Helping Role of the Nurse

This narrative exemplifies the meaning and intent of several competencies in this domain, in particular creating a climate for healing and providing emotional and informational support to patients' families (Benner, 1984a). Incorporating the family as participants in the care of a critically ill patient requires a high level of skill that cannot be developed until the nurse feels competent and confident in technical critical care skills. This nurse had many years of experience in this unit, and she felt that providing care for their mother was so important to these children that she broke tradition in her unit and taught them how to do some basic comfort and hygiene measures. The nurse related that the other nurses in this critical care unit held the belief that active family involvement in care was intrusive and totally out of line. A belief such as this is based on concerns for patient safety and efficiency of care, yet it cuts the family off from being fully involved in the caring relationship. This nurse demonstrated moral courage, commitment to care, and advocacy in going against the tradition in her unit of excluding family members from direct care. She had 8 years of experience in this unit, and her peers respected her, so she was able to change practice by starting with this one patient-family situation and involving the other two nurses who were working with them.

Chesla's (1996) research points to a gap between theory and practice with respect to including families in patient care. Eckle (1996) studied family presence with children in emergency situations and concluded that in times of crisis, the needs of families must be addressed to provide effective and compassionate care. The skilled practice of including the family in care emerged as significantly meaningful in the narrative text from the peer-identified nurse expert study. This was defined as an additional competency in the domain called the *helping role of the nurse* and was named *maximizing the family's role in care* (Brykczynski, 1998). The intent of this competency is to assess each situation as it arises and develops over time, so that family involvement in care can adequately address specific patient-family needs, and so they are not excluded from involvement nor do they have participation thrust upon them.

This narrative illustrates how Benner's approach is dynamic and specific for each institution. The belief that being attuned to family involvement in care is in part a developmental process is supported by Nuccio and colleagues' (1996) description of this aspect of care at their institution. They observed that novice nurses begin by recognizing their feelings associated with family-centered care, whereas expert nurses develop creative approaches to include patients and families in care. The intricate process of finely tuning the nurse's collaboration with families in critical care is delineated further by Levy (2004) in her interpretive phenomenological study that articulates the practices of nurses with critically burned children and their families.

CRITICAL THINKING ACTIVITIES

1. Discuss the clinical narrative provided here using the unfolding case study format to promote situated learning of clinical reasoning (Benner, Hooper-Kyriakidis, & Stannard, 2011).
2. Regarding the various aspects of the case as they unfold over time, consider questions that encourage thinking, increase understanding, and promote dialogue, such as: What are your concerns in this situation? What aspects stand out as salient? What would you say to the family at given points in time? How would you respond to your nursing colleagues who may question your inclusion of the family in care?
3. Using Benner's approach, describe the five levels of competency and identify the characteristic intentions and meanings inherent at each level of practice.

POINTS FOR FURTHER STUDY

- Brykczynski, K. A. (2014). Benner's philosophy in nursing practice. In M. R. Alligood (Ed.), *Nursing theory: Utilization & application* (5th ed., pp. 118–137). St Louis: Elsevier Mosby.

Videotapes and Web Media

- Benner, P., Tanner, C., & Chesla, C. (1992). *From beginner to expert: Clinical knowledge in critical care nursing* (Video). New York: Helene Fuld Trust Fund; Athens OH: Fitne, Inc. Available at Fitne.net
- EducatingNurses.com: Provides videotaped teaching resources, curriculum development, and training resources: http://www.educatingnurses.com.
- NovicetoExpert.org: Online textbook replacement learning system. Demonstration of online clinical simulation of unfolding case studies: http://www.NovicetoExpert.org.
- Benner, P., Stannard, D., & Hooper-Kyriakidis, P. (2001). *Clinical wisdom and interventions in critical care: A thinking-in-action approach* (CD-ROM). Philadelphia: Saunders.
- Patricia Benner, Novice to Expert (2008). Video interview. *The Nurse Theorists Portraits of Excellence,* Volume 2. Athens, OH: FITNE, Inc. Available at Fitne.net.

REFERENCES

Alberti, A. M. (1991). Advancing the scope of primary nurses in the NICU. *Journal of Perinatal and Neonatal Nursing, 5*(3), 44–50.

Altmann, T. K. (2007). An evaluation of the seminal work of Patricia Benner: Theory or philosophy? *Contemporary Nurse, 25*(1–2), 114–123.

Alvsvåg, H. (2014). Kari Martinsen: Philosophy of caring. In M. R. Alligood (Ed.), *Nursing theorists and their work* (8th ed., pp. 147–170). St Louis: Mosby.

Aristotle. (1985). *Nicomachean ethics* [T. Irwin, Trans.]. Indianapolis, IN: Hackett.

Balasco, E. M., & Black, A. S. (1988). Advancing nursing practice: Description, recognition, and reward. *Nursing Administration Quarterly, 12*(2), 52–62.

Barnum, B. J. (1990). *Nursing theory: Analysis, application, evaluation*. Glenview, IL: Scott, Foresman.

Benner, P. (1982). Issues in competency-based training. *Nursing Outlook, 20*(5), 303–309.

Benner, P. (1983). Uncovering the knowledge embedded in clinical practice. *Image: The Journal of Nursing Scholarship, 15*(2), 36–41.

Benner, P. (1984a). *From novice to expert: Excellence and power in clinical nursing practice*. Menlo Park, CA: Addison-Wesley.

Benner, P. (1984b). *Stress and satisfaction on the job: Work meanings and coping of mid-career men*. New York: Praeger.

Benner, P. (1985a). The oncology clinical nurse specialist: An expert coach. *Oncology Nursing Forum, 12*(2), 40–44.

Benner, P. (1985b). Quality of life: A phenomenological perspective on explanation, prediction, and understanding in nursing science. *Advances in Nursing Science, 8*(1), 1–14.

Benner, P. (1987). A dialogue with excellence. *American Journal of Nursing, 87*(9), 1170–1172.

Benner, P. (1992). The role of narrative experience and community in ethical comportment. *Advances in Nursing Science, 14*(2), 1–21.

Benner, P. (1994). The tradition and skill of interpretive phenomenology in studying health, illness, and caring practices. In P. Benner (Ed.), *Interpretive phenomenology: Embodiment, caring, and ethics in health and illness* (pp. 99–126). Thousand Oaks, CA: Sage.

Benner, P. (1996a). Embodiment, caring and ethics: A nursing perspective: The 1995 Helen Nahm lecture. *The Science of Caring, 8*(2), 30–36.

Benner, P. (1996b). A response by P. Benner to K. Cash. Benner and expertise in nursing: a critique. *International Journal of Nursing Studies, 33*(6), 669–674.

Benner, P. (1999). Claiming the wisdom and worth of clinical practice. *Nursing and Health Care Perspectives, 20*(6), 312–319.

Benner, P. (2000). The quest for control and the possibilities of care. In M. A. Wrathall & J. Malpas (Eds.), *Heidegger, coping and cognitive science: Essays in honor of Hubert L. Dreyfus* (vol. 2, pp. 293–383). Cambridge, MA: MIT Press.

Benner, P. (2005). Using the Dreyfus Model of Skill Acquisition to describe and interpret skill acquisition and clinical judgment in nursing practice and education. *The Bulletin of Science, Technology and Society Special Issue: Human Expertise in the Age of the Computer, 24*(3), 188–199.

Benner, P. (2012). Educating nurses: A call for radical transformation—how far have we come? *Journal of Nursing Education, 51*(4), 183–184.

Benner, P. (2015). Pedagogical implications for the Carnegie Study. *Educating Nurses: A Call for Radical Transformation. Asian Nursing Research, 9*(1), 1–6.

Benner, P., & Benner, R. V. (1999). The clinical practice development model: Making the clinical judgment, caring and collaborative work of nurses visible. In B. Haag-Heitman (Ed.), *Clinical practice development: Using novice to expert theory* (pp. 17–42). Gaithersburg, MD: Aspen.

Benner, P., Hooper-Kyriakidis, P., & Stannard, D. (1999). *Clinical wisdom and interventions in critical care: A thinking-in-action approach*. Philadelphia: Saunders.

Benner, P., Hooper-Kyriakidis, P., & Stannard, D. (2011). *Clinical wisdom and interventions in acute and critical care: A thinking-in-action approach* (2nd ed.). New York: Springer.

Benner, P., Malloch, K., & Sheets, V. (Eds.). (2010). *Nursing pathways for patient safety: Expert panel on practice breakdown.* Philadelphia: Elsevier International Press.

Benner, P., Sheets, V., Uris, P., Malloch, K., Schwed, K., & Jamison, D. (2002). Individual, practice, and system causes of errors in nursing: A taxonomy. *Journal of Nursing Administration, 32*(10), 509–523.

Benner, P., Stannard, D., & Hooper-Kyriakidis, P. (2001). *Clinical wisdom and interventions in critical care: A thinking-in-action approach* (CD-ROM). Philadelphia: Saunders.

Benner, P., Sutphen, M., Leonard, V., & Day, L. (2010). *Educating nurses: A call for radical transformation.* Stanford, CA: The Carnegie Foundation for the Advancement of Teaching; San Francisco: Jossey-Bass.

Benner, P., & Tanner, C. (1987). Clinical judgment: How expert nurses use intuition. *American Journal of Nursing, 87*(1), 23–31.

Benner, P., Tanner, C., & Chesla, C. (1992). From beginner to expert: Gaining a differentiated clinical world in critical care nursing. *Advances in Nursing Science, 14*(3), 13–28.

Benner, P., Tanner, C., & Chesla, C. (1996). *Expertise in nursing practice: Caring, clinical judgment, and ethics.* New York: Springer.

Benner, P., Tanner, C., & Chesla, C. (2009). *Expertise in nursing practice: Caring, clinical judgment, and ethics* (2nd ed.). New York: Springer.

Benner, P., & Wrubel, J. (1982). Skilled clinical knowledge: The value of perceptual awareness. *Nurse Educator, 7*(3), 11–17.

Benner, P., & Wrubel, J. (1989). *The primacy of caring: Stress and coping in health and illness.* Menlo Park, CA: Addison-Wesley.

Brykczynski, K. A. (1985). *Exploring the clinical practice of nurse practitioners.* [Doctoral dissertation, University of California, San Francisco.] *Dissertation Abstracts International, 46,* 3789B. (University Microfilms No. DA8600592.)

Brykczynski, K. A. (1993–1995). Principal investigator. Developing a profile of expert nursing practice. Project of the UTMB Nursing Service Task Force studying expert nursing practice, supported by UTMB Joint Ventures. Galveston, TX: University of Texas Medical Branch.

Brykczynski, K., A. (1998). Clinical exemplars describing expert staff nursing practice. *Journal of Nursing Management, 6,* 351–359.

Brykczynski, K. A. (1999). An interpretive study describing the clinical judgment of nurse practitioners. *Scholarly Inquiry for Nursing Practice: An International Journal, 13*(2), 141–166.

Brykczynski, K., & Benner, P. (2010). The living tradition of interpretive phenomenology. In G. K. Chan, K. A. Brykczynski, R. E. Malone, & P. Benner (Eds.), *Interpretive phenomenology in health care research* (pp. 113–141). Indianapolis, IN: Sigma Theta Tau International.

Cash, K. (1995). Benner and expertise in nursing: A critique. *International Journal of Nursing Studies, 32*(6), 527–534.

Cathcart, E. B. (2010). The making of a nurse manager: The role of experiential learning in leadership development. *Journal of Nursing Management, 18*(4), 440–447.

Chan, G. K., Brykczynski, K. A., Malone, R. E., & Benner, P. (2010). (Eds.). *Interpretive phenomenology in health care research.* Indianapolis, IN: Sigma Theta Tau International.

Chesla, C. A. (1996). Reconciling technologic and family care in critical-care nursing. *Image: The Journal of Nursing Scholarship, 28*(3), 199–203.

Coyle, J. S. (2011). Development of a model home health nurse internship program for new graduates: Key lessons learned. *Journal of Continuing Education in Nursing, 42*(5), 201–214.

Crider, M. C., & McNiesh, S. G. (2011). Integrating a professional apprenticeship model with psychiatric clinical simulation. *Journal of Psychosocial Nursing & Mental Health Services, 49*(5), 42–49.

Crissman, S., & Jelsma, N. (1990). Cross-training: Practicing effectively on two levels. *Nursing Management, 21*(3), 64a–64h.

Darbyshire, P. (1994). Skilled expert practice: Is it "all in the mind"? A response to English's critique of Benner's novice to expert model. *Journal of Advanced Nursing, 19,* 755–761.

Day, L., & Benner, P. (2002). Ethics, ethical comportment, and etiquette. *American Journal of Critical Care, 11*(1), 76–79.

Day, L., & Benner, P. (2014). The hidden curriculum in nursing education. In F. W. Hafferty, J. F. O'Donnell, & D. W. C. Baldwin, Jr. (Eds.), *The hidden curriculum in health professional education* (pp. 140–149). Lebanon: NH: University Press of New England.

De Jong, M. J., Benner, R., Benner, P., Richard, M. L., Kenny, D. J., Kelley, P., et al. (2010). Mass casualty care in an expeditionary environment: Developing local knowledge and expertise in context. *Journal of Trauma Nursing, 17*(1), 45–58.

Dilthey, W. (1976). *Selected writings.* [H. P. Rickman, Trans. & Ed.] London: Cambridge University Press.

Dolan, K. (1984). Building bridges between education and practice. In P. Benner (Ed.), *From novice to expert: Excellence and power in clinical nursing practice* (pp. 275–284). Menlo Park, CA: Addison-Wesley.

Dreyfus, H. L. (1979). *What computers can't do.* New York: Harper & Row.

Dreyfus, H. L. (1991). *Being-in-the-world: A commentary on being and time dimension.* Cambridge, MA: MIT Press.

Dreyfus, H. L., & Dreyfus, S. E. (1986). *Mind over machine.* New York: The Free Press.

Dreyfus, H. L., & Dreyfus, S. E. (1996). The relationship of theory and practice in the acquisition of skill. In P. Benner, C. Tanner, & C. Chesla (Eds.), *Expertise in nursing practice: Caring, clinical judgment, and ethics* (pp. 29–47). New York: Springer.

Dreyfus, S. E., & Dreyfus, H. L. (1980). *A five-stage model of the mental activities involved in directed skill acquisition.* Unpublished report supported by the Air Force Office of Scientific Research, USAF (Contract F49620-79-c-0063). Berkeley, CA: University of California, Berkeley.

Dunlop, M. J. (1986). Is a science of caring possible? *Journal of Advanced Nursing, 11,* 661–670.

Dunne, J. (1993). *Back to the rough ground: Practical judgment and the lure of technique.* Notre Dame, IN: Indiana University Press.

Eckle, N. J. (1996). Family presence—where would you want to be? *Critical Care Nurse, 16*(1), 102.

English, I. (1993). Intuition as a function of the expert nurse: A critique of Benner's novice to expert model. *Journal of Advanced Nursing, 18,* 387–393.

Farrell, P., & Bramadat, I. J. (1990). Paradigm case analysis and stimulated recall: Strategies for developing clinical reasoning skills. *Clinical Nurse Specialist, 4*(3), 153–157.
Fenton, M. V. (1984). Identification of the skilled performance of master's prepared nurses as a method of curriculum planning and evaluation. In P. Benner (Ed.), *From novice to expert: Excellence and power in clinical nursing practice* (pp. 262–274). Menlo Park, CA: Addison-Wesley.
Fenton, M. V. (1985). Identifying competencies of clinical nurse specialists. *Journal of Nursing Administration, 15*(12), 31–37.
Fenton, M. V., & Brykczynski, K. A. (1993). Qualitative distinctions and similarities in the practice of clinical nurse specialists and nurse practitioners. *Journal of Professional Nursing, 9*(6), 313–326.
Gadamer, G. (1970). *Truth and method*. London: Sheer & Ward.
Gaston, C. (1989). Inservice education: Career development for South Australian nurses. *Australian Journal of Advanced Nursing, 6*(4), 5–9.
Glass, H. (1975). A guest in the house. In M. Z. Davis, M. Kramer, & A. I. Strauss (Eds.), *Nurses in practice: A perspective on work environments* (pp. 178–189). St Louis: Mosby.
Gordon, D. R. (1986). Models of clinical expertise in American nursing practice. *Social Science and Medicine, 22*(9), 953–961.
Hamric, A. B., Whitworth, T. R., & Greenfield, A. S. (1993). Implementing a clinically focused advancement system. *Journal of Nursing Administration, 23*(9), 20–28.
Hargreaves, L., Nichols, A., Shanks, S., & Halamak, L. P. (2010). A handoff report card for general nursing orientation. *Journal of Nursing Administration, 40*(10), 424–431.
Heidegger, M. (1962). *Being and time.* [J. MacQuarrie & E. Robinson, Trans.] New York: Harper & Row.
Huntsman, A., Lederer, J. R., & Peterman, E. M. (1984). Implementation of staff nurse III at El Camino Hospital. In P. Benner (Ed.), *From novice to expert: Excellence and power in clinical nursing practice* (pp. 244–257). Menlo Park, CA: Addison-Wesley.
Kelley, P. W., Kenny, D. J., Gordon, D. R., & Benner, P. (2015). The evolution of case management for service members injured in Iraq and Afghanistan. *Qualitative Health Research, 25*(3), 426–439.
Kierkegaard, S. (1962). *The present age.* [A. Dur, Trans.] New York: Harper & Row.
Kleinman, A., Eisenberg, L., & Good, B. (1978). Culture, illness, and care: Clinical lessons from anthropologic and cross-cultural research. *Annals of Internal Medicine, 88*, 251–258.
Kuhn, T. S. (1970). *The structure of scientific revolutions* (2nd ed.). Chicago: University of Chicago Press.
Lazarus, R. S. (1985). The trivialization of distress. In J. C. Rosen & L. J. Solomon (Eds.), *Preventing health risk behaviors and promoting coping with illness* (vol. 8, pp. 279–298). Hanover, NH: University Press of New England.
Lazarus, R. S., & Folkman, S. (1984). *Stress appraisals and coping.* New York: Springer.
Levy, K. (2004). Practices that facilitate critically burned children's healing. *Qualitative Health Research, 13*(10), 1–21.
Lindeke, L. L., Canedy, B. H., & Kay, M. M. (1997). A comparison of practice domains of clinical nurse specialists and nurse practitioners. *Journal of Professional Nursing, 13*(5), 281–287.
Lock, M., & Gordon, D. R. (Eds.). (1989). *Biomedicine examined.* Boston, MA: Kluwer Academic.
Løgstrup, K. E. (1995a). *Metaphysics* (Vol. I). [R. L. Dees, Trans.] Milwaukee, WI: Marquette University Press.
Løgstrup, K. E. (1995b). *Metaphysics* (Vol. II). [R. L. Dees, Trans.] Milwaukee, WI: Marquette University Press.
Løgstrup, K. E. (1997). *The ethical demand* (with introduction by A. Maclntyre & H. Fink). Notre Dame, IN: University of Notre Dame Press.
Maclntyre, A. (1981). *After virtue: A study in moral theory*. Notre Dame, IN: University of Notre Dame Press.
Maclntyre, A. (1999). *Dependent rational animals: Why human beings need the virtues.* Chicago: Open Court.
McNiesh, S., Benner, P., & Chesla, C. (2011). Learning formative skills of nursing practice in an accelerated program. *Qualitative Health Research, 21*(1), 51–61.
Martin, L. L. (1996). *Factors affecting performance of advanced nursing practice.* [Doctoral dissertation, Virginia Commonwealth University School of Nursing.] (University Microfilms No. 9627443.)
Mauleon, A. L., Palo-Bengtsson, L., & Ekman, S. (2005). Anesthesia care of older patients as experienced by nurse anesthetists. *Nursing Ethics, 12*(3), 263–272.
Merleau-Ponty, M. (1962). *Phenomenology of perception.* [C. Smith, Trans.] London: Routledge and Kegan Paul.
National Organization of Nurse Practitioner Faculties (NONPF). (1990). *Curriculum guidelines and program standards for nurse practitioner education.* Washington, DC: Author.
Neverveld, M. E. (1990). Preceptorship: One step beyond. *Journal of Nursing Staff Development, 6*(4), 186–189, 194.
Nuccio, S. A., Lingen, D., Burke, L. J., Kramer, A., Ladewig, N., Raum, J., et al. (1996). The clinical practice developmental model: The transition process. *Journal of Nursing Administration, 26*, 29–37.
O'Neill, O. (1996). *Towards justice and virtue: A constructive account of practical reasoning.* Cambridge, MA: Cambridge University Press.
Packer, M. J. (1985). Hermeneutic inquiry in the study of human conduct. *American Psychologist, 40*(10), 1081–1093.
Paley, J. (1996). Intuition and expertise: Comments on the Benner debate. *Journal of Advanced Nursing, 23*(4), 665–671.
Phillips, S., & Benner, P. (Eds.). (1994). *The crisis of care: Affirming and restoring caring practices in the helping professions.* Washington, DC: Georgetown University Press.
Polanyi, M. (1958). *Personal knowledge.* Chicago: University of Chicago Press.
Rubin, J. (1984). *Too much of nothing: Modern culture, the self and salvation in Kierkegaard's thought.* [Unpublished doctoral dissertation.] Berkeley, CA: University of California, Berkeley.
Schwartz, A. (2005). State of nursing education. *Science of Caring, 17*(1), 12–15.
Silver, M. (1986a). A program for career structure: from neophyte to expert. *The Australian Nurse, 16*(2), 38–41.
Silver, M. (1986b). A program for career structure: A vision becomes a reality. *The Australian Nurse, 16*(2), 44–47.

Taylor, C. (1971). Interpretation and the sciences of man. *The Review of Metaphysics, 25*, 3–34.

Taylor, C. (1982). *Theories of meaning.* Dawes Hicks Lecture. Proceedings of the British Academy (pp. 283–327). Oxford, UK: Oxford University Press.

Taylor, C. (1989). *Sources of the self: The making of modern identity*. Cambridge, MA: Harvard.

Taylor, C. (1991). *Ethics of authenticity*. Cambridge, MA: Harvard.

Taylor, C. (1993). Explanation and practical reason. In M. Nussbaum & A. Sen (Eds.), *The quality of life* (pp. 208–231). Oxford, UK: Clarendon.

Taylor, C. (1994). Philosophical reflections on caring practices. In S. S. Phillips & P. Benner (Eds.), *The crisis of care: Affirming and restoring caring practices in the helping professions* (pp. 174–187). Washington, DC: Georgetown University Press.

Uhrenfeldt, L. (2009). Caring for nursing staff among proficient first-line nurse leaders. *International Journal for Human Caring, 13*(2), 39–44.

Ullery, J. (1984). Focus on excellence. In P. Benner (Ed.), *From novice to expert: Excellence and power in clinical nursing practice* (pp. 258–261). Menlo Park, CA: Addison-Wesley.

Visintainer, M. (1988). [Book Review], *The primacy of caring: Stress and coping in health and illness. Image: The Journal of Nursing Scholarship, 20*(2), 113–114.

BIBLIOGRAPHY

Primary Sources

Books

Benner, P. (2001). *From novice to expert.* [Commemorative edition.] Upper Saddle River, NJ: Prentice Hall.

Benner, P. (2004). *The use of nursing narratives for reflecting on ethical and clinical judgment.* Tokyo, Japan: Shorinsha.

Gordon, S., Benner, P., & Noddings, N. (Eds.). (1996). *Caregiving readings in knowledge, practice, ethics, and politics.* Philadelphia: University of Pennsylvania Press.

Kyriakidis, P., Ahrens, T., Benner, P. (2016). *Adult health I and II, NovEx, novice to expert learning.* Saddleback, NJ: Pearson Publishers.

Book Chapters

Benner, P. (1997). A dialogue between virtue ethics and care ethics. In D. Thomasma (Ed.), *The moral philosophy of Edmund Pellegrino* (pp. 47–61). Dordrecht, Netherlands: Kluwer.

Benner, P. (1998). When health care becomes a commodity: The need for compassionate strangers. In J. F. Kilner, R. D. Orr, & J. A. Shelly (Eds.), *The changing face of health care* (pp. 119–135). Grand Rapids, MI: William B. Eerdmans.

Benner, P. (1999). Caring as a concept for the practice. (pp. 171–181). In A. Solari-Twaddell (Ed.), *Parish nursing.* Thousand Oaks, CA: Sage.

Benner, P. (2001). The phenomenon of care. In S. K. Tombs (Ed.), *Handbook of phenomenology and medicine* (pp. 351–369). Dordrecht, Netherlands: Kluwer.

Benner, P. (2002). Learning through experience and expression: Skillful ethical comportment in nursing practice. In E. D. Pellegrino, D. C. Thomasma, & J. L. Kissel (Eds.), *The healthcare professional as friend and healer: Building on the work of Edmund Pellegrino* (pp. 49–64). Washington, DC: Georgetown University Press.

Benner, P. (2003). Clinical reasoning articulating experiential learning in nursing practice. In O. Slevin & L. Basford (Eds.), *Theory and practice of nursing* (2nd ed., pp. 176–186). London: Nelson Thornes.

Benner, P. (2005). Stigma and personal responsibility: Moral dimensions of a chronic illness. In R. B. Purtillo, G. M. Jensen, & R. C. Brasic (Eds.), *Educating for moral action: A sourcebook in health and rehabilitation ethics.* Philadelphia: F. A. Davis.

Benner, P. (2007). Interpretive phenomenology. In L. M. Given (Ed.), *The Sage encyclopedia of qualitative methods.* Thousand Oaks, CA: Sage.

Benner, P. (2010). Experiential learning, skill acquisition and gaining clinical knowledge. In K. Obsborn, K. Wraa, A. Watson, & C. Wraa (Eds.), *Medical-surgical nursing* (pp. 32–44). Saddleback, NJ: Prentice-Hall.

Benner, P. (2013). *Celebrating the work of Kari Martinsen: Celebrating the centrality of care and a receptive ethic a festschrift in honor of Professor Kari Martinsen.* Oslo, Norway: Akribe AS.

Benner, P. (2013). Patricia Benner, five philosophical questions. In A. Forss, C. Ceci, & J. S. Drummod (Eds.), *Philosophy of nursing, five questions* (pp. 19–31). London: Automatic Press.

Benner, P., & Leonard, V. W. (2005). Patient concerns and choices and clinical judgment in EBP. In B. Melnyk & E. Fineout-Overholt (Eds.), *Evidence-based practice in nursing and healthcare: A guide to best practices.* Philadelphia: Lippincott.

Benner, P., & Gordon, S. (1996). Caring practice. In S. Gordon, P. Benner, & N. Noddings (Eds.), *Caregiving, readings in knowledge, practice, ethics and politics* (pp. 40–55). Philadelphia: University of Pennsylvania Press.

Benner, P., & Leonard, V. W. (2005). Patient concerns, choices, and clinical judgment in evidence-based practice. In B. M. Mszurek (Ed.), *Evidence-based practice in nursing & healthcare: A guide to best practice* (pp. 163–182). Philadelphia: Lippincott.

Benner P., & Sutphen, M. (2007). Clinical reasoning, decision-making in action: Thinking critically and clinically. In R. Hughes (Ed.), *Patient safety and quality for nursing center for primary care, prevention, & clinical partnerships.* Rockville, MD: Agency for Healthcare Research and Quality.

Benner, P., & Sutphen, M. (2010). Professional nursing education: Teaching for the complex practice of nursing. In P. Peterson, E. Baker, & B. McGaw (Eds.), *Elsevier international encyclopedia for education* (pp. 65–70). Philadelphia, PA: Elsevier.

Day, L., Benner, P., Sutphen, M., & Leonard, V. (2009). Reflections on clinical education: Insights from the Carnegie Study. In T. Valiga & N. Ard (Eds.), *Clinical nursing education: Current reflections* (pp. 71–88). New York: National League for Nursing.

Journal Articles

Benner, P. (1996). A dialogue between virtue ethics and care ethics. *Theoretical Medicine, 23*, 1–15.

Benner, P. (1996). A response by P. Benner to K. Cash, Benner expertise in nursing: A critique. *International Journal of Nursing Studies, 33*(6), 669–674.

Benner, P. (2000). The roles of embodiment, emotion and lifeworld for rationality and agency in nursing practice. *Nursing Philosophy, 1*, 5–19.

Benner, P. (2000). The wisdom of our practice. *American Journal of Nursing, 100*(10), 99–101, 103, 105.

Benner, P. (2001). Curing, caring, and healing in medicine: Symbiosis and synergy or syncretism? *Park Ridge Center Bulletin, 23*, 11–12.

Benner, P. (2003). [Book review] *From detached concern to empathy: Humanizing medical practice*, J. Halpern (Ed.). *The Cambridge Quarterly for Health Care Ethics, 12*(1), 134–136.

Benner, P. (2004). The dangers of geneticism. *Journal of Midwifery and Women's Press, 49*(3), 260–262.

Benner, P. (2011). Formation in professional education: An examination of the relationship between theories of meaning and theories of the self. *Journal of Medicine and Philosophy. Special Edition on the Influence of Charles Taylor on Medical Ethics, 36*, 342–353.

Benner, P., Brennan, M. R., Sr., Kessenich, C. R., & Letvak, S. A. (1996). Critique of Silva's philosophy, science and theory: Interrelationships and implications for nursing research. *Image: The Journal of Nursing Scholarship, 29*(3), 214–215.

Benner, P., Ekegren, K., Nelson, G., Tsolinas, T., & Ferguson-Dietz, L. (1997). The nurse as a wise, skillful and compassionate stranger. *American Journal of Nursing, 97*(11), 27–34.

Benner, P., Halpern, J., Gordon, D.R., & Kelley, P. (In Press). Beyond pathologizing harm: Understanding PTSD in the context of war experience. *Journal of Medicine and Humanities.*

Benner P., & Sutphen, M. (2007). Learning across the professions: The clergy, a case in point. *Journal of Nursing Education, 46*(3), 103–108.

Benner, P., Sutphen, M., Leonard, V., & Day, L. (2007). Learning to see and think like a nurse: Clinical reasoning and caring practices. *Journal of Japanese Society of Nursing Research, 30*(1), 20–24.

Benner, P., Sutphen, M., Leonard, V., & Day, L. (2008). Formation and ethical comportment in nursing. *American Journal of Critical Care, 17*(5), 173–176.

Benner, P., Stannard, D., & Hooper, P. L. (1996). "Thinking-in-action" approach to teaching clinical judgment: A classroom innovation for acute care advanced practice nurses. *Advanced Practice Nursing Quarterly, 1*, 70–77.

Benner, P., Tanner, C. A., & Chesla, C. A. (1996). Nurse practitioner extra: Becoming an expert nurse. Adapted with permission from Benner, Tanner, & Chesla (Eds.), *Expertise in nursing practice: Caring, clinical judgment, and ethics*. New York: Springer.

Benner, P., Tanner, C. A., & Chesla, C. A. (1996). The social fabric of nursing knowledge. Adapted with permission from Benner, Tanner, & Chesla (Eds.), *Expertise in nursing practice: Caring, clinical judgment, and ethics*. New York: Springer.

Brant, M., Rosen, L., & Benner, P. (1998). Nurses as skilled Samaritans: The nurse as wise, skillful, and compassionate stranger. *American Journal of Nursing, 98*(4), 22–23.

Cohen H., & Benner, P. (2002). Individual, practice, and system causes of errors in nursing: A taxonomy. *Journal of Nursing Administration, 32*(10), 509–523.

Dracup, K., Cronenwett, L., Meleis, A., & Benner, P. (2005). Reflections on the doctorate of nursing practice. *Nursing Outlook, 53*(4), 177–182.

Ekegren, K., Nelson, G., Tsolinas, A., Ferguson-Dietz, L., & Benner, P. (1997). The nurse as wise, skillful, and compassionate stranger. *American Journal of Nursing, 97*, 26–34.

Emami, A., Benner, P., & Ekman, S. L. (2001). A sociocultural health model for late-in-life immigrants. *Journal of Transcultural Nursing, 12*(1), 15–24.

Emami, A., Benner, P., Lipson, J. G., & Ekman, S. L. (2001). Health as continuity and balance in life. *Western Journal of Nursing Research, 22*, 812–825.

Fowler, M., & Benner, P. (2001). The new code of ethics for nurses: A dialogue with Marsha Fowler. *American Journal of Critical Care, 10*(6), 434–437.

Harrington, C., Crider, M. C., Benner, P., & Malone, R. (2005). Advanced nursing training in health policy: Designing and implementing a new program. *Policy, Politics & Nursing Practice, 6*(2), 99–108.

Massimo, L, Evans, L. K., & Benner, P. (2013). Caring for loved ones with frontotemporal degeneration: The lived experiences. *Geriatric Nursing, 34*(4), 302–306.

Puntillo, K. A., Benner, P., Drought, T., Drew, B., Stotts, N., Stannard, D., et al. (2001). End-of-life issues in intensive care units: A national random survey of nurses' knowledge and beliefs. *American Journal of Critical Care, 10*(4), 216–229.

Spichiger, E., Wallhagen, M., & Benner, P. (2005). Nursing as a caring practice from a phenomenological perspective. *Scandinavian Journal of Caring Sciences, 19*(4), 303–309.

Sullivan, W., & Benner, P. (2005). Challenges to professionalism: Work integrity and the call to renew and strengthen the social contract of the professions. *American Journal of Critical Care, 14*(1), 78–84.

Sunvisson, H., Haberman, B., Weiss, S., & Benner, P. (2009). Augmenting the Cartesian medical discourse with an understanding of the person's lifeworld, lived body, life story and social identity. *Nursing Philosophy, 10*, 241–252.

Weiss, S. M., Malone, R. E., Merighi, J. R., & Benner, P. (2002). Economism, efficiency, and the moral ecology of good nursing practice. *Canadian Journal of Nursing Research, 34*(2), 95–119.

Secondary Sources

Doctoral Dissertations

Boller, J. E. (2001). *The ecology of exercise: An interpretive phenomenological account of exercise in the lifeworld of persons on maintenance hemodialysis.* [Doctoral dissertation, University of California, San Francisco.] *Dissertation Abstracts International*, B62/12, 5638. (University Microfilms No. 3034743.)

Brykczynski, K. A. (1985). *Exploring the clinical practice of nurse practitioners.* [Doctoral dissertation, University of California, San Francisco.] *Dissertation Abstracts International,* 46, 3789B. (University Microfilms No. DA8600592.)

Chan, G. K. (2005). *E.R. = exit required. A philosophical, theoretical, and phenomenological investigation of care at the end-of-life in the emergency department.* [Doctoral dissertation, University of California, San Francisco.] *Dissertation*

Abstracts International, B66/06, 3054. (University Microfilms No. 3179943.)

Chesla, C. A. (1988). *Parents' caring practices and coping with schizophrenic offspring, an interpretive study.* [Doctoral dissertation, University of California, San Francisco.] *Dissertation Abstracts International,* 49-B, 2563. (University Microfilms No. AAD88-13331.)

Cho, A. (2001). *Understanding the lived experience of heart transplant recipients in North America and South Korea: An interpretive phenomenological cross-cultural study.* [Doctoral dissertation, University of California, San Francisco.] *Dissertation Abstracts International,* B62/12, 5639. (University Microfilms No. 3034721.)

Day, L. J. (1999). *Nursing care of potential organ donors: An articulation of ethics, etiquette and practice.* [Doctoral dissertation, University of California, San Francisco.] *Dissertation Abstracts International,* 60-B, 5431. (University Microfilms No. AADAA-19951464.)

Doolittle, N. (1990). *Life after stroke.* [Doctoral dissertation, University of California, San Francisco.] *Dissertation Abstracts International,* 51-B, 1742. (University Microfilms No. AAD90-24963.)

Dunlop, M. (1990). *Shaping nursing knowledge: An interpretive analysis of curriculum documents from NSW Australia.* [Doctoral dissertation, University of California, San Francisco.] *Dissertation Abstracts International,* 51-B, 659. (University Microfilms No. AAD90-16380.)

Hooper, P. L. (1995). *Expert titration of multiple vasoactive drugs in post-cardiac surgical patients: An interpretive study of clinical judgment and perceptual acuity.* [Doctoral dissertation, University of California, San Francisco.] *Dissertation Abstracts International,* 57-B, 238. (University Microfilms No. AAD85-19614338.)

Kesselring, A. (1990). *The experienced body, when taken-for-grantedness falters: A phenomenological study of living with breast cancer.* [Doctoral dissertation, University of California, San Francisco.] *Dissertation Abstracts International,* 52-B, 1955. (University Microfilms No. AAD91-19579.)

Kinavey, C. (2003). *Adolescents living with spina bifida: Moving from parental to self-care.* [Doctoral dissertation, University of California, San Francisco.] *Dissertation Abstracts International.* (University Microfilms No. 3051044.)

Leonard, V. W. (1993). *Stress and coping in the transition to parenthood of first time mothers with career commitments: An interpretive study.* [Doctoral dissertation, University of California, San Francisco.] *Dissertation Abstracts International,* 54-A, 3221. (University Microfilms No. AAD94-02354.)

MacIntyre, R. (1993). *Sex, drugs, and T-cell counts in the gay community: Symbolic meanings among gay men with asymptomatic HIV infections (immune deficiency).* [Doctoral dissertation, University of California, San Francisco.] *Dissertation Abstracts International,* 54-B, 4601. (University Microfilms No. AAD94-06617.)

Mahrer-Imhof, R. (2003). *Couples' daily experiences after the onset of cardiac disease: An interpretive phenomenological study.* [Doctoral dissertation, University of California, San Francisco.]

McNiesh, S. G. (2009). *Formation in an accelerated nursing program: Learning existential skills of nursing practice.* [Doctoral dissertation, University of California, San Francisco.] *Dissertation Abstracts International,* B69/9, 5320. (University Microfilms No. 3324573.)

Oakes-Greenspan, M. (2008). *Running toward: Reframing possibility and finitude through physicians' stories at the end of life.* [Doctoral dissertation, University of California, San Francisco.] *Dissertation Abstracts International,* A68/11. (University Microfilms No. 3289310.)

Orsolini-Hain, L. M. (2009). *An interpretive phenomenological study on the influences on associate degree prepared nurses to return to school to earn a higher degree in nursing.* [Doctoral dissertation, University of California, San Francisco.] *Dissertation Abstracts International,* B69/09, 5321. (University Microfilms No. 3324576.)

Prakke, H. (2004). *Articulating maternal caregivers' concerns, knowledge and needs.* [Doctoral dissertation, University of California, San Francisco.] *Dissertation Abstracts International.* (University Microfilms No. 3149700.)

Rodriguez, L. (2007). *Student and faculty experiences of practice breakdown and error in nursing school.* [Doctoral dissertation, University of California, San Francisco.] Dissertation Abstracts International. (University Microfilms No. 3289350.)

Spichiger, E. (2004). *Dying patients' and their families' experiences of hospital end-of-life care.* [Doctoral dissertation, University of California, San Francisco.] *Dissertation Abstracts International.* (University Microfilms No. 3136071.)

Weiss, S. M. (1996). *Possibility or despair: Biographies of aging.* [Doctoral dissertation, University of California, San Francisco.] *Dissertation Abstracts International,* 57-B, 3662. (University Microfilms No. AAD96-34295.)

10

Philosophy of Caring

Herdis Alvsvåg[†]

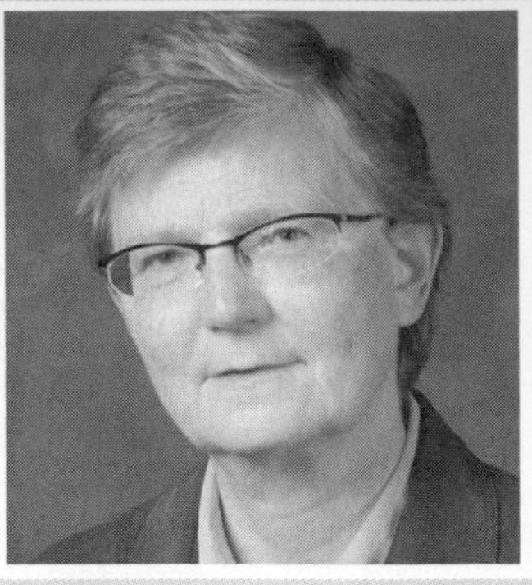

Kari Martinsen (1943–Present)

"Nursing is founded on caring for life, on neighbourly love. . . . At the same time it is necessary that the nurse is professionally educated."

(Martinsen, 2006, p. 78)

CREDENTIALS AND BACKGROUND OF THE THEORIST

Kari Marie Martinsen, a nurse and philosopher, was born in Oslo, Norway, in 1943, during the World War II German occupation of Norway. Her parents were engaged in the Resistance Movement. After the war, moral and sociopolitical discussions dominated home life, a home that consisted of three generations: a younger sister, parents, and a grandmother. Both parents were economists who had been educated at the University of Oslo. Her mother worked all of her adult life outside the home.

After high school, Martinsen began her studies at Ullevål College of Nursing in Oslo, graduating in 1964. She worked in clinical practice at Ullevål hospital for 1 year while doing preparatory studies for university entry. Before embarking upon a university degree, she specialized as a psychiatric nurse in 1966 and worked for 2 years at Dikemark Psychiatric Hospital near Oslo.

While practicing as a nurse, she became concerned about social inequalities in general and in the health service in particular. Health, illness, care, and treatment were obviously distributed unequally. She also became disturbed over perceived discrepancies between health care theories, ideals, and goals on the one hand, and practical results of nursing, medicine, and the health service on the other. She began to pose questions about how a society and a profession must be constituted to support and aid the ill and the unemployed. One particularly poignant question was how the nursing profession must operate to avoid letting down its weakest patients and those who need care the most. The obvious follow-up question was how the nurse might be able to care for the patient when medical science first and foremost relates to patients' diseases. In other words, Martinsen wanted to know how those who represent the health services provide adequate nursing for the subjects of their care, when they are so closely allied with a science that objectifies the patient. She posed questions about whether that same objectification would increase with emphasis on a scientific base for the discipline of nursing.

These fundamental questions urged Martinsen to take up additional studies, this time for a bachelor's degree in psychology at the University of Oslo in 1968, with the goal of obtaining a master's degree in psychology. As a prerequisite, she needed an intermediate examination in physiology and another free credit at the intermediate level; here she chose philosophy. This encounter with philosophy and phenomenology changed her thinking drastically. She realized that philosophy rather than psychology might better illuminate the existential questions with which she was concerned. The study of phenomenology attracted her to the University of Bergen, Norway's second largest city.

From 1972 to 1974, she attended the Department of Philosophy at the University of Bergen. In her work for the graduate degree in philosophy (Magister artium), Martinsen grappled philosophically with questions that had disturbed

Photo credit: Lars Jakob Løtvedt, Bergen, Norway.

[†]Translators: Vigdis Elisabeth Brekke, Bjørn Follevåg, and Kirsten Costain Schou.

her as a citizen, a professional, and a health care worker. Her dissertation *Philosophy and Nursing: A Marxist and Phenomenological Contribution* (Martinsen, 1975) created an instant debate and received much critical attention. The dissertation directed a critical gaze toward the nursing profession for its refusal to take seriously the consequences of the nursing discipline, uncritically adopting characteristics of a profession and embracing only a scientific basis for nursing. Such a development might contribute to distancing nurses from the patients who need them most. This dissertation, the first written by a nurse in Norway, analyzed the discipline of nursing from a critical philosophical and social perspective.

During the mid-1970s, Norway experienced a marked shortage of nursing teachers. The rectors of three nursing colleges in Bergen took the initiative to establish a temporary nursing teacher–training course to address this problem. The course was established jointly by the University of Bergen, the county authorities, and three nursing colleges. A nurse with university-level qualifications was needed to head the program. Martinsen was asked to be Dean of the Faculty of Nursing Teachers' Training in Bergen, which she accepted from 1976 to 1977.

Through her philosophical studies and the sociological issues she encountered in practical nursing and in nursing education, Martinsen developed an interest in nursing history. How did education of nurses in Norway begin, who was responsible for its inception, and what did they wish to achieve? To look more closely at some of these issues, Martinsen applied for and received a grant from the Norwegian Nurses' Association in 1976. She was affiliated with the Department of Hygiene and Social Medicine at the University of Bergen, where she lectured to students in the nursing teachers' training program and students in social medicine.

At that time, an intense debate over nursing education was raging in Norway. A public commission proposed retention of the traditional 3-year degree but eventually agreed to alter this to a system of stage-based qualification. This meant that after completion of 1 year, a student became a qualified care assistant, and after 2 additional years, a qualified nurse. This implied the end of the principle of a comprehensive 3-year degree. Nurses throughout the country, with the Norwegian Nurses' Association at the forefront, marched in protest to save the 3-year nursing degree. Sides in this debate remained rigidly opposed, and the tone of the political discourse on the issue of nursing education was heated. Martinsen threw herself into this debate. She suggested that nursing education be changed to a 4-year program, but also gave her approval to the principle of stage-based education. She sketched an educational model in which one is qualified as a care assistant after 2 years and as a nurse after 4 years (Martinsen, 1976). With the comprehensive 3-year degree as the stated goal for the nursing association, her suggestion was viewed as a provocation.

In 1978 Martinsen received a grant from Norway's General Science Research Council. At this time, she was attached to the history department at the University of Oslo, where she worked on her new project on the social history of nursing while lecturing master's degree students in sociopolitical history. From 1981 to 1985, she was a scientific assistant at the history department at the University of Bergen. In addition to conducting her own research, Martinsen lectured and supervised master's degree students in feminist history and developed a database of Norwegian feminist history.

The period from 1976 to 1986 can be described as a historical phase in Martinsen's work (Kirkevold, 2000). She published several historical articles (Martinsen, 1977, 1978, 1979a, 1979b). Close collaborators during this phase were Anne Lise Seip, professor of social history; Ida Blom, professor of feminist history; and Kari Wærness, professor of sociology. In 1979 Martinsen and Wærness published a book with the provocative title, *Caring Without Care?* (Martinsen & Wærness, 1979). In this book, the authors raised important questions:

- Were nurses "moving away" from the sickbed?
- Was caring for the ill and infirm disappearing with the advent of increasingly technical care and treatment?
- Were nurses becoming administrators and researchers who increasingly relinquished the concrete execution of care to other occupational groups?

Aiding ill and care-dependent people was considered women's work, and this view has long historical roots. However, the existence of the professionally trained nurse is not very old in Norway, originating in the late 1800s. The deaconesses (Christian lay sisters), who were educated at different deaconess houses in Germany, were the first trained health workers in Norway. Martinsen described how these first trained nurses built up a nursing education in Norway, and how they expanded and wrote textbooks and practiced nursing both in institutions and in homes. They were the forerunners of Norway's public health system. This pioneer period was described by Martinsen in her book, *History of Nursing: Frank and Engaged Deaconesses: A Caring Profession Emerges 1860–1905* (Martinsen, 1984). Based on this work, Martinsen attained her doctor of philosophy degree from the University of Bergen in 1984.

In defense of her dissertation, Martinsen had to prepare two lectures: "Health Policy Problems and Health Policy Thinking Behind the Hospital Law of 1969" (Martinsen, 1989a), and "The Doctors' Interest in Pregnancy—Part of

Perinatal Care: The Period ca. 1890–1940" (Martinsen, 1989b). This work emerged from her 10-year historical phase, beginning in the mid-1970s, when she wrote about nursing's social history and feminist history and the social history of medicine.

From 1986, Martinsen worked for 2 years as Associate Professor at the Department of Health and Social Medicine at the University of Bergen. She lectured and supervised master's degree students, in addition to writing a series of philosophical and historical papers, published in 1989 under the title *Caring, Nursing and Medicine: Historical-Philosophical Essays* (Martinsen, 1989c). With this book, the threads of Martinsen's historical phase were drawn together, marking the beginning of a more philosophical period (Kirkevold, 2000). The book has several editions, and the 2003 publication includes an interview with the author (Karlsson & Martinsen, 2003). Fundamental problems in caring and interpretations of the meaning of **discernment** are what preoccupied Martinsen from 1985 to 1990. In a Danish anthology published in 1990, she contributed a paper titled "Moral Practice and Documentation in Practical Nursing." Here she writes:

> *"Moral practice is based upon caring. Caring does not merely form the value foundation of nursing; it is a fundamental precondition of our life. . . . Discernment demands emotional involvement and the capacity for situational analysis in order to assess alternatives for action. . . . To learn moral practice in nursing is to learn how the moral is founded in concrete situations. It is accounted for through experiential objectivity or through discretion, in action or in speech. In both cases learning good nursing is of the essence."*
>
> ***(Martinsen, 1990, pp. 60, 64–65)***

In 1990 Martinsen moved to Denmark for a 5-year period. She was employed at the University of Århus to establish master's degree and PhD programs in nursing. Her philosophical foundation was further developed during these years mainly through encounters with Danish life philosophy (Martinsen, 2002a) and theological tradition. In *Caring, Nursing and Medicine: Historical-Philosophical Essays,* Martinsen (1989c, 2003b) had connected the concept of caring to the German philosopher Martin Heidegger (1889–1976). While she was living in Denmark, Heidegger's role as a Nazi sympathizer during World War II became public knowledge. At that time, a series of academic articles were published that proved that Heidegger was a member of the national Socialist Party in Germany and that he had betrayed his Jewish colleagues and friends such as Edmund Husserl (1859–1938) and Hannah Arendt (1906–1975). Heidegger was banned from teaching for several years after the war because of his involvement with the Nazis (Lubcke, 1983).

Martinsen confronted Heidegger and her own thinking about his philosophy in *From Marx to Løgstrup: On Morality, Social Criticism and Sensuousness in Nursing* (Martinsen, 1993b). Precisely because life and learning cannot be separated, it became important for Martinsen to go to sources other than Heidegger to illustrate the fundamental aspects of caring. Knud E. Løgstrup (1905–1981) was the Danish theologian and philosopher who became her alternative source, although the two never met. Martinsen knew him through his books and via his wife, Rosemarie Løgstrup, who was originally German. She met her husband in Germany, where both were studying philosophy. She later translated his books into German.

While Martinsen lived and worked in Denmark, she met with Patricia Benner on several occasions for public dialogues in Norway and Denmark, and again in 1996 in California. One of these dialogues was later published with the title, "Ethics and Vocation, Culture and the Body" (Martinsen, 1997b); it took place at a conference at the University of Tromsø.

Martinsen also had important dialogues with Katie Eriksson, the Finnish professor of nursing. They met in Norway, Denmark, Sweden, and Finland. In the beginning, their discussions were tense and strained, but over time, they developed into fruitful and enlightening conversations that later were published as *Phenomenology and Caring: Three Dialogues* (Martinsen, 1996). Martinsen's first chapter in this book is titled "Caring and Metaphysics—Has Nursing Science Got Room for This?"; the second, "The Body and Spirit in Practical Nursing"; and the third, "The Phenomenology of Creation—Ethics and Power: Løgstrup's Philosophy of Religion Meets Nursing Practice." These headings employ impressive language, similar to that of the dialogues that Martinsen conducted with Benner; in her preface to the book, she elaborates:

> *"The words about which we speak and write are compassion, hope, suffering, pain, sacrifice, shame, violation, doubt. These are 'big words.' But they are no bigger than their location in life, our everyday nursing situation. Mercy, writes the Danish theologian and philosopher Løgstrup, is the renewal of life, it is to afford others life. . . . What else is nursing but to release the patient's possibilities for living a meaningful life within the life cycle we inhabit between life and death? We must venture into life amongst our fellow humans in order to experience the actual meaning of these big words."*
>
> ***(Martinsen, 1996, p. 7)***

While Martinsen was teaching in Århus, she became Adjunct Professor at the Department of Nursing Science at the University of Tromsø in 1994. In 1997 she moved north and become a full-time professor. However, needing more time for her research and writings, she left after only 1 year in this position to become a freelancer in 1998.

In 2002 and for a 5-year period, Martinsen made her way back to the University of Bergen as professor at the Department of Public Health and Primary Health Care section for nursing science. Teaching master's and doctoral students was central. She arranged doctoral courses and was much in demand in the Nordic countries as supervisor and lecturer.

The period from 1990 is characterized by philosophical research. Fundamental philosophical and ontological questions and their meaning for nursing dominated Martinsen's thought. During this period, in addition to her own books, she worked on a variety of projects and published in several journals and anthologies. Books from this period have already been mentioned (Martinsen, 1993b, 1996). In 2000 *The Eye and the Call* (Martinsen, 2000b) was published. The chapter titles in this book ring more poetically than those in her earlier works: "To See with the Eye of the Heart," "Ethics, Culture and the Vulnerability of the Flesh," "The Calling—Can We Be Without It?" and "The Act of Love and the Call."

Martinsen also worked with ideas about space and architecture. According to her, space and architecture influence human dignity. She first wrote about this idea in the article "The House and the Song, the Tears and the Shame: Space and Architecture as Caretakers of Human Dignity" (Martinsen, 2001).

Martinsen has held positions at three nursing colleges. From 1989 to 1990, she was employed as a researcher at Bergen Deaconess University College, Bergen, and from 2006 as an Adjunct Professor. From 1999 to 2004, she was Adjunct Professor at Lovisenberg Deaconess University College in Oslo. In 2007 she became a full-time professor at Harstad University College in northern Norway.

Ideas and academic ventures sprouted and flourished easily around Martinsen, and she drew others into academic projects. She edited a collection of articles that several nursing college teachers contributed to, *The Thoughtful Nurse* (Martinsen, 1993a). Lovisenberg Deaconess University College in Oslo, with Martinsen's assistance, took the initiative to publish a new edition of the first Norwegian nursing textbook, which was originally published in 1877 (Nissen, 2000). In this edition, Martinsen (2000a) wrote an afterword, placing the text within a context of academic nursing. With a colleague in Oslo, Martinsen edited another collection of articles by the editors and college lecturers for the book *Ethics, Discipline and Refinement: Elizabeth Hagemann's Ethics Book—New Readings* (Martinsen & Wyller, 2003). This book provides an analysis of a text on ethics for nurses published in 1930 and was used as a textbook until 1965. When the ethics text was republished in 2003, it was interpreted in the light of two French philosophers, Pierre Bourdieu (1930–2002) and Michel Foucault (1926–1984), as well as the German sociologist Max Weber (1864–1920). In 2012, together with colleagues at Harstad University College, Martinsen published a book about narratives and ethics in nursing (Thorsen, Mæhre, & Martinsen, 2012).

Thus historical and philosophical threads are each present in different phases of Martinsen's thought, and they color her work differently during the different periods. In 2011 Martinsen was made Knight, First Class, of the Royal Norwegian Order of St. Olav for her very significant work, thought, and authorship in nursing science.

THEORETICAL SOURCES

In Martinsen's analysis of the profession of nursing in the early 1970s, she looked to three philosophers in particular: German philosopher, politician, and social theorist Karl Marx (1818–1883); German philosopher and founder of phenomenology Edmund Husserl (1859–1938); and French philosopher and phenomenologist of the body Maurice Merleau-Ponty (1908–1961). Later, she broadened her theoretical sources to include other philosophers, theologians, and sociologists.

Karl Marx: Critical Analysis—A Transformative Practice

Marxist philosophy gave Martinsen some analytical tools to describe the reality of the discipline of nursing and the social crisis in which it found itself. The crisis consisted of the failure of the discipline to examine and recognize its nature as fragmented, specialized, and technically calculating, as it pretends a holistic perspective on care. She found that the discipline was part of positivism and the capitalist system, without praxis of liberation. A "reversed care law" rules in such a way that those who need care most receive the least. Karl Marx criticized individualism and the satisfaction of the needs of the rich at the expense of the poor. Martinsen's view is that it is important to expose this phenomenon when it occurs in health service. Such exposure of this reality can be a force for change. She maintains that nurses must question the nature of nursing, its content and inner structure, its historical origins, and the genesis of the profession. This questioning results in a critical nursing practice as the practitioner views her occupation and profession in a historical and social context. Martinsen's historical interest has a critical and transformative intention.

Edmund Husserl: Phenomenology as the Natural Attitude

Edmund Husserl's phenomenology is important for Martinsen's critiques of science and positivism. Positivism's view of the self lies in its attitude of objectification and a dehumanizing and calculating attitude toward the person. Husserl viewed phenomenology as a strict science. The strict methodological processes of phenomenology produce an attitude of composed reflection over scientific reality, so that individuals may uncover structures and contexts within which they otherwise perform taken-for-granted and unconscious work. This practice is about making the taken-for-granted problematic. By problematizing taken-for-granted self-understanding, the individuals find opportunities to grasp "the thing itself," which will always reveal itself perspectively. Phenomenology works with the prescientific, what is encountered in the natural attitude, when people are directed toward something with the intent to recognize and understand it meaningfully. Phenomenology insists upon context, wholeness, involvement, engagement, the body, and the lived life. Humans live in contexts, in time and space, and live historically. The body cannot be divided into body and soul; it is a wholeness that relates to other bodies, to things in the world, and to nature.

Maurice Merleau-Ponty: The Body as the Natural Attitude

Maurice Merleau-Ponty (1908–1961) builds upon Husserl's thought, but focuses more than any other thinker on the human body in the world. Both Husserl and Merleau-Ponty criticized Descartes (1596–1650), who separates the person from the world in which one lives with other persons. The body is representing the natural attitude in the world. The nursing profession relates to the body in all of its aspects. Nurses use their own bodies in the performance of caring, and they relate to other bodies who are in need of nursing, treatment, and care. Nurses' bodies and those of their patients express themselves through actions, attitudes, words, tone of voice, and gestures. Phenomenology involves acts of interpretation, description, and recognition of lived life, the everyday life that people live together with others in a mutual natural world, including the professional contexts in which caring is performed.

Martin Heidegger: Existential Being as Caring

Martin Heidegger (1889–1976) was a German phenomenologist and a student of Husserl, among others. He investigated existential being, that is to say, that which is and how it is. Martinsen connects the concept of caring to Heidegger because he "has caring as a central concept in his thought. . . . The point is to try to elicit the fundamental qualities of caring, or what caring is and encompasses" (Martinsen, 1989c, p. 68). She continues: "An analysis of our practical life and an analysis of what caring is, are inseparable. To investigate the one is at the same time to investigate the other. Together, they form an inseparable unit. Caring is a fundamental concept in understanding the person" (Martinsen, 1989c, p. 69). With phenomenology and Heidegger as a backdrop, Martinsen gives content and substance to caring: caring will always have at least two parts as a precondition. One is concerned and anxious for the other. Caring involves how individuals relate to each other, and how they show concern for each other in their daily life. Caring is the most natural and the most fundamental aspect of human existence.

As mentioned earlier, Martinsen revised her perspective on Heidegger (Martinsen, 1993b). At the same time, she did not reject "Heidegger's original and acute thought" (Martinsen, 1993b, p. 17). She turns back to Heidegger when she explains what it means to dwell. Heidegger had examined precisely the concept that to dwell is always to live among things (Martinsen, 2001). Heidegger reinforces an idea also maintained by Merleau-Ponty: that the things individuals surround themselves with are not merely things for them, objectively speaking, but they actually participate in shaping their lives. People leave something of themselves within these things when they dwell amid them. It is the body that dwells, surrounded by an environment.

Knud Eiler Løgstrup: Ethics as a Primary Condition of Human Existence

Knud Eiler Løgstrup (1905–1981), the Danish philosopher and theologian, became important for Martinsen in the "void" left by Heidegger. Løgstrup can be summarized through two intellectual strands: phenomenology and creation theology, the latter containing his philosophy of religion (creation theology should not be confused with the more recent "creationism" in the United States). As a phenomenologist, he sought to reveal and analyze the essential phenomena of human existence. Through his phenomenological investigations, Løgstrup arrived at what he termed *sovereign* or *spontaneous life utterances:* trust, hope, compassion, and openness of speech. That these are essential is to say that they are precultural characteristics of existence. As characteristics, they provide conditions for culture, conditions for existence; they make human community possible (Lubcke, 1983). According to Heidegger, caring is such a characteristic. In Løgstrup's opinion, the sovereign life utterances were the necessary characteristics for human coexistence.

Martinsen maintains that for Løgstrup, metaphysics and ethics are interwoven in the concept of creation:

> *"They are characteristic phenomena which sustain us in such a way that caring for the other arises out of the condition of our having been created. Caring for the other reveals itself in human relationship through trust, open speech, hope and compassion. These phenomena, which Løgstrup also calls sovereign life utterances, are 'born ethical' which means that they are essentially ethical. Trust, open speech, hope and compassion are fundamentally good in themselves without requiring our justification. If we try to gain dominance over them, they will be destroyed. Metaphysics and ethics, or rather metaphysical ethics, is practical. It is linked to questions of life in which the person is stripped of omnipotence."*
>
> ***(Martinsen, 1993b, pp. 17–18)***

Humans must care for that which exists, not seek to control it: "Western culture is singular in its need to understand and control. It has moved away from the cradle of our culture and our religion in the narrative of creation from the Old Testament. In The Old Testament 'guarding,' 'watching,' and 'caring' on one side, and cultivating and using on the other, formed a unified opposition" (Martinsen, 1996, p. 79). That these are unified opposites is to say that they singularly and in themselves are opposites that separate and are insurmountable, but when they are adjusted to one another, they enter into an opposition that unifies and creates a sound whole. To care for, guide and guard, cultivate, and make use of, that is to say, cultivate and use in a caring manner as a unified opposition, means that individuals do not become domineering and exploitative, but restrained and considerate in their dealings with one another and with nature.

The ethical question is how a society combats suffering and takes care of those who need help. In a nursing context, Martinsen formulates this very question like this: "How do we as nurses take care of the person's eternal meaning, the individual's unending worth—independent of what the individual is capable of, can be useful for or can achieve? Can I bear to see the other as the other, and yet not as fundamentally different from myself?" (Martinsen, 1993b, p. 18).

Klim, the Danish publishing house, issues the works by and about Løgstrup under the label *The Løgstrup Library.* Here Martinsen has contributed the monograph *Løgstrup og sygepleien (Løgstup and Nursing),* (Martinsen, 2012a) subsequently published in Norwegian (Martinsen, 2012b).

Max Weber: Vocation as the Duty to Serve One's Neighbor Through One's Work

Max Weber (1864–1920) was a German sociologist who made a major impact on the philosophy of social science. Weber sought to understand the meaning of human action. He was also a critic of the society he saw emerging with the advent of industrialization. In Weber, Martinsen found a new alliance, in addition to Marx, in the criticism of both capitalism and science. Whereas Løgstrup was a philosopher of religion, Weber was a sociologist of religion. Weber also criticized the West for its boundless intervention and its boundless consumption. Science disenchants the created world precisely because it relates to what was created as objects in its objectification of all that exists (Martinsen, 2000b, 2001, 2002b).

To a great extent, Martinsen joins Weber in her explication of vocation (Martinsen, 2000b). Weber looked to Martin Luther (1483–1546), who discussed vocation in the secular sense, as follows:

> *"Vocation is work in the sense of a life's occupation or a restricted field of work, in which the individual will endow his fellow person. . . . The young Luther linked vocation to work, and understood it as an act of neighbourly love. Vocation is understood on the basis of the notion of creation, that we are created in order to care for one another through work."*
>
> ***(Martinsen, 2000b, pp. 94–95)***

In other words, vocation is in the service of creation. With reference to the young Luther, Martinsen wrote that vocation "means that we are placed in life contexts which demand something of us. It is a challenge that I, in this my vocation, meet and attend to my neighbour. It lies in Existence as a law of life" (Martinsen, 1996, p. 91).

Michel Foucault: The Effect of His Method Intensifying Phenomenologists' Phenomenology

Phenomenologists underscore the importance of history for our experience. Martinsen (1975) referred to Foucault in her dissertation in philosophy, but was especially concerned with this philosopher in connection with her historical works from 1976 (Martinsen 1978, 1989a, 2001, 2002b, 2003a). Foucault (1926–1984) was a French philosopher and historian of ideas. He was concerned with the notions of fracture and difference, rather than continuity and context. He claimed that some shared common structures, systems of terms, and forms of thought that shape societies reside within each historical epoch and within the different cultures. In this way, Foucault confronted subjective philosophy, which emphasizes the person as a private and independent individual. For example, Foucault asked which fundamental conditions were present during the historical epoch in which institutions for the insane were created. In later epochs, he defined the insane as mentally ill. Something new had happened; what did it depend on? Why did it happen and what was to be achieved in society? What actions were undertaken; were there alliances of power and did they involve establishing order and discipline? To question in this way is to dig through several layers of understanding, getting beyond the general conception to understand the meaning of history in a new and different way. Foucault elicits the basic social distinctions that make it possible to characterize people. They are dug out of tacit preconditions (Lubcke, 1983). In this way, Foucault's method intensified the phenomenological process. He encouraged thinking anew and differently from the existing mode of thinking within the epoch and within the contexts in which one lives. The gaze became not only descriptive, but also critical.

Martinsen stated that, in caring for the other, individuals relate to the other in a different way and look for things different from those that are looked for within natural science that objectify medicine using their "classification gaze" and "examining gaze" (Martinsen, 1989b, pp. 142–168, 2000a). Such gazes require special space; caring requires different types of space to develop different types of knowledge. Several questions affect caring in the health service: Which disciplinary characteristics or structures are found in practice today, in nursing practice and its spatial arrangements? What will it mean to think differently from those of a particular epoch? Is critical nursing found here, and, if so, what are the implications for today's health service and research?

Paul Ricoeur: The Bridge-Builder

Paul Ricoeur (1913–2005) was a French philosopher. His position is often designated as *critical hermeneutics* or *hermeneutic phenomenology.* He sought to build a bridge between natural science and human science, between phenomenology and structuralism and other opposing positions. He focused on topics such as time and narrative, language and history, discernment, and science. Ricoeur is concerned with human communication, on what it is to understand one another. He points to everyday language and its many meanings, in contrast to the language of science. Martinsen refers to parallels in the philosophy of language of Løgstrup and Ricoeur. Martinsen states:

> *"The culture of medicine is dominated by an abstract conceptual language in which words are embedded in different classifications, and in which they are not always in accordance with actual practical and concrete situations. . . . In everyday language of the caring tradition on the other hand, words are followed by the manner in which they unfold in different contexts of meaning within concrete caring—in the company of the patient and the professional community. When spoken in everyday language, the words are distinguished by their power of expression. They strike a tone."*
>
> ***(Martinsen, 1996, p. 103)***

MAJOR CONCEPTS & DEFINITIONS

Martinsen is reluctant to provide definitions of terms, because definitions have a tendency to close off concepts. Rather, she maintains, the content of concepts should be presented. It is important to circumscribe the meaningful content of a term, explain what the term means, but avoid having terms locked up in definitions.

Care

Care "forms not only the value base of nursing, but is a fundamental precondition for our lives. Care is the positive development of the person through the Good" (Martinsen, 1990, p. 60). Care is a trinity: relational, practical, and moral simultaneously (Alvsvåg, 2003; Martinsen, 2003b, 2012b). Caring is directed outward toward the situation of the other. In professional contexts, caring requires education and training. "Without professional knowledge, concern for the patient becomes mere sentimentality" (Martinsen, 1990, p. 63). She is clear that guardianship negligence and sentimentality are not expressions of care.

Professional Judgment and Discernment

These qualities are linked to the concrete. It is through the exercise of professional judgment in practical, living contexts that nurses learn clinical observation. It is "training not only to see, listen and touch clinically, but to see, listen and touch clinically in a good way" (Martinsen, 1993b, p. 147). The patient makes an impression on the nurse, who is moved bodily, and the impression is sensuous. "Because perception has an analogue character, it evokes variation and context in the situation" (Martinsen, 1993b, p. 146). One thing is reminiscent of another, and this recollection creates a connection between the impressions in the situation, professional knowledge, and previous experience. Discretion expresses professional knowledge through the natural senses and everyday language (Martinsen, 2005, 2006).

MAJOR CONCEPTS & DEFINITIONS—cont'd

Moral Practice Is Founded on Care

"**Moral practice** is when empathy and reflection work together in such a way that caring can be expressed in nursing" (Martinsen, 1990, p. 60). Morality is present in concrete situations and must be accounted for. Individual actions need to be accounted for; they are learned and justified through the objectivity of empathy, which consists of empathy and reflection. This means in concrete terms to discover how the other will best be helped, and the basic conditions are recognition and empathy. Sincerity and judgment enter into moral practice (Martinsen, 1990).

Person-Oriented Professionalism

Person-oriented professionalism is "to demand professional knowledge which affords the view of the patient as a suffering person, and which protects his integrity. It challenges professional competence and humanity in a benevolent reciprocation, gathered in a communal basic experience of the protection and care for life. . . . It demands an engagement in what we do, so that one wants to invest something of oneself in encounters with the other, and so that one is obligated to do one's best for the person one is to care for, watch over or nurse. It is about having an understanding of one's position within a life context that demands something from us, and about placing the other at the center, about the caring encounter's orientation toward the other" (Martinsen, 2000b, pp. 12, 14).

Sovereign Life Utterances

Sovereign life utterances are phenomena that accompany the Creation itself. They exist as precultural phenomena in all societies; they are present as potentials. They are beyond human control and influence, and are therefore sovereign. Sovereign life utterances are openness, mercy, trust, hope, and love. These are phenomena that humans are given in the same way that they are given time, space, air, water, and food (Alvsvåg, 2003). Unless they receive them, life disintegrates. Life is self-preservation through reception (Martinsen, 2000b, 2012b). Sovereign life utterances are preconditions for care simultaneously as caring actions are necessary conditions for the realization of sovereign life utterances in the concrete life. An individual can act in such a way that openness, trust, hope, mercy, and love are realized through interactions or can shut them out. Without their presence in an individual's actions, caring cannot be realized. At the same time, caring actions clear the way for the realization of sovereign life utterances in personal and professional lives. Caring can bring the patient to experience the meaning of love and mercy; caring can light hope or give it sustenance, and caring can be that which makes trust and openness foremost in relations with the nurse. In the same way, lack of care can block the other's experience of mercy; it can create mistrust and an attitude of restraint in relation to the health service.

The Untouchable Zone

The **untouchable zone** is an area that must not be interfered with in encounters with the other and encounters with nature. It refers to boundaries for which individuals must have respect. The untouchable zone creates a certain protective distance in the relation; it ensures impartiality and demands argumentation, theory, and professionalism. In caring, the untouchable zone is united with its opposite, which is openness, in which closeness, vulnerability, and motive have their correct place. Openness and the untouchable zone constitute a unifying contradiction in caring (Martinsen, 1990, 2006).

Vocation

Vocation "is a demand life makes to me in a completely human way to encounter and care for one's fellow person. Vocation is given as a law of life concerning neighborly love which is foundationally human" (Martinsen, 2000b, p. 87). It is an ethical demand to take care of one's neighbor. For this reason, nursing requires a personal refinement, in addition to professional knowledge (Malchau, 2000).

The Eye of the Heart

The concept of the **eye of the heart** stems from the parable of the Good Samaritan. The heart says something about the existence of the whole person, about being touched or moved by the suffering of the other and the situation the other experiences. In sensuousness and perception, we are moved before we understand, but we are also challenged by the afterthought of understanding. To see and be seen with the eye of the heart is a form of participatory attention based on a reciprocation that unifies perception and understanding, in which the eye's understanding is led by the senses (Martinsen, 2000b, 2006).

The Registering Eye

The **registering eye** is objectifying, and the perspective is that of the observer. It is concerned with finding connections, systematizing, ranking, classifying, and placing in a system. The registering eye represents an alliance between modern natural science, technology, and industrialization. If one as a patient is exposed to, or if one as a professional employs this gaze in a one-sided manner, compassion is lifted out of the situation, and the will to life is reduced (Martinsen, 2000b).

EMPIRICAL EVIDENCE

In Martinsen's philosophy of caring, language and reflection involved in professional judgment and narrative are ways of accounting convincingly for case conditions, situations, and phenomena (Martinsen, 1997a, 2002c, 2003c, 2004, 2005). She states that obvious perceptions must be accounted for convincingly. With reference to Husserl, she points to different forms of evidence: the undoubtable (apodictic), the exhaustive, and the partial. Each type represents different evidential requirements. Facts, themes, and situations provide different forms of evidence. For example, one cannot accept mathematical evidence that is undoubtable and transfer this to physical objects and persons. In the field of caring, it is discernment and narrative that can clarify the empirical facts of a case in an evidentiary, enlightening, or convincing manner (Martinsen 2003c, 2004, 2005, 2009, 2012). To exercise discretion is to interpret the impressions one gets of the patient. The professional knowledge and experience one has built up give one a horizon of understanding that is flexible in encounters with the patient's situation (Martinsen, 1990, 2002c). The narrative can both describe and prescribe action (Kjær, 2000; Martinsen, 1997a, 2012). "A good narrative tells existential morality into being, and makes practical action unavoidable" (Martinsen, 1993b, p. 161).

MAJOR ASSUMPTIONS

Nursing

Although care goes beyond nursing, caring is fundamental to nursing and to other work of a caring nature. Caring involves having consideration for, taking care of, and being concerned about the other. When speaking about caring, three things must be simultaneously present; they could be called the "trinity of caring": caring must be **relational, practical,** and **moral** (Alvsvåg, 2011).

- *Relational* means that caring requires at least two people. Martinsen describes it thus:

> *"The one has concern for the other. When the one suffers, the other will 'grieve' (in the sense of suffer with) and provide for the alleviation of pain. . . . Caring is the most natural and the most fundamental aspect of the person's existence. In caring, the relationship between people is the most essential element. . . . The essence of the person is that one is created for the sake of others—for one's own sake. . . . The point here is that caring always presupposes others. Further, that I can never understand myself or realise myself alone or independent of others."*
>
> ***(Martinsen, 1989c, p. 69)***

- Caring is *practical.* It is about concrete and practical action. Caring is trained and learned through its practice.
- Caring is also *moral:* "If caring is to be genuine, I must relate to the other from an attitude (mood, 'befindlichkeit') which acknowledges the other in light of his situation. . . . [We must] neither overestimate nor underestimate his ability to help himself" (Martinsen, 1989c, p. 71).

Caring requires a correct understanding of the situation, which presupposes a good evaluation of the goals inherent in the caring situation: "Performing nursing is essentially directed towards persons not capable of self-help, who are ill and in need of care. To encounter the ill person with caring through nursing involves a set of preconditions such as knowledge, skills, and organization" (Martinsen, 1989c, p. 75). Nurses need training in all types of caring work. They must practice and reflect alone and with others to develop professional judgment. Caring and professional judgment are integrated in nursing (Martinsen, 1990, 1997a, 2003c, 2004, 2005, 2006, 2012b).

Person

It is the meaning-bearing fellowship of tradition that turns the individual into a person. The person cannot be torn away from the social milieu and the community of persons (Martinsen, 1975). In one way, there is a parallel between the person and the body. It is as bodies that individuals relate to ourselves, to others, and to the world (Alvsvåg, 2000; Martinsen, 1997a). The body is a unit of soul and flesh, or spirit and flesh. The person is bodily, and as bodies we both perceive and understand.

Health

Health is discussed from a sociohistorical perspective. Two rival historical health ideals, the classical Greek and the modern one of intervention and expansion, form the background when Martinsen writes: "Health does not only reflect the condition of the organism, it is also an expression of the current level of competence in medicine. To put it pointedly, the tendencies of the modern concept of health are such that if one has an unnecessary 'defect' or an organ which 'could' be better, one is not completely healthy" (Martinsen, 1989c, p. 146). The modern reductionist health ideal on which modern medicine is built is both analytical and individualistic; it is oriented toward all that is not "good enough." Combined with medicine's autonomy and resources, it has yielded success in terms of treatment. Martinsen is concerned with the point that this ideology does not withstand critical examination. Medicine's sometimes damaging effects and insufficient service for people with chronic diseases and illnesses bring Martinsen to turn toward the conservative, classic health ideal. What is important is to cure sometimes, help often, and comfort always. This requires society to offer people the opportunity to live the best life possible and the individual to live sensibly; both requirements have environmental implications. The environment must not be changed at such a speed and to such an extent that the change exceeds the knowledge base; restraint and caution are required (Martinsen, 1989c, 2003b).

Environment: Space and Situation

The person is always in a particular situation in a particular space. In space are found time, ambience, and power (Martinsen, 2001, 2002b, 2002c). Martinsen asks what time, architecture, and knowledge do to the ambience of a space. Architecture, interactions among individuals, use of objects, words, knowledge, one's being-in-the-room—all set the tone and color the situation and the space. The person enters into universal space, natural space, but through dwelling creates cultural space. We build houses with rooms, and the activities of the health service take place in different rooms. "The sick-room is important as a physical, material and constructed place, but it is also a place we share with other people. . . . The room with its interior and objects makes visible the patient's and the nurse's interpretation of it" (Martinsen, 2001, pp. 175–176). The challenge for nurses is to give patients and each other dignity in these spaces. What is needed then is deliberate knowledge gathered in slowed down, deliberate spaces, "space in which to perceive—smell, listen, see and care" (Martinsen, 2001, p. 176).

THEORETICAL ASSERTIONS

People are created dependent and relational. Care is fundamental to human life. Humans live not merely in fellowship with one another, but also enter into relationships with animals and with nature and relate to a creative force that sustains the whole. The person is fundamentally dependent on community and the creation. To the created belong the sovereign life utterances, "These are first *given to* us, and second they are *sovereign.* That is to say it is impossible for the person to avoid their power. . . . These are phenomena which are present in the service of life. They create life, they release life's possibilities" (Martinsen, 1996, p. 80).

The body is created as a whole, that is to say that need and spirit, or body and spirit, enter into a benevolent interaction, in which sensing cannot be avoided. Martinsen writes the following:

> *"Sensing initiates interaction and maintains it. Care of the body becomes central. In this respect, nursing is secular vocational work which through professional care of the body protects and provides space for the life possibilities of the patient. The vocation is seen as a demand life makes on us to care for our neighbour, in this case the patient, through our work. It is work in the service of life processes. Vocation, the body and work are seen as a counterweight to the new (bodiless) spirituality in nursing."*
>
> ***(Martinsen, 1996, p. 72)***

Love of one's neighbor is coupled with a concrete, practical, professional, and moral discernment. Sensuous and experience-based knowledge is the most fundamental and essential for the practice of nursing. Caring is learned through practical experience in concrete situations under the supervision of expert and experienced nurses (Martinsen, 1993b, 2003b).

Metaphysics is not speculation about that of which one cannot know anything. It is an interpretation of phenomena all humans recognize through their senses and can experience. These phenomena are prescientific and foundational.

LOGICAL FORM

Martinsen's logical form can be described as inductive and analogous. The inductive aspect of her thought is based on the idea that experiences in life and in health service are the starting point for her theoretical works. She turns toward philosophy and history in the hope of gaining greater insight and understanding of the concrete work of nursing and the lived life. In her meeting with the philosophy of life and the phenomenology of creation, she encounters the ontological and metaphysical in a different way than that of traditional philosophy. Life utterances, the creation, time, and space are ontological and metaphysical facts. Analogy would say that humans think these facts and recognize them in their concrete experiences in their practical life. They come to expression in meetings between persons, in narratives, and in the exercise of discernment. "In this way, metaphysics pries at the empirical," writes Martinsen with reference to Løgstrup (Martinsen, 1996). Further, she states, "The narrative takes time, it is slow. It provides context through analogous forms of recognition, that is to say, it is relevant to us when we can recognize ourselves in the life phenomena it relates" (Martinsen, 2002b, p. 267).

Kirkevold writes the following:

> *"Martinsen does not mean to present a logically constructed theory. On the contrary, she distances herself from that view of knowledge that insists theory have a logical structure of terms, principles and rules. Martinsen's theory is an interpretive analysis of caring, upon which the author tries to shed light from several perspectives. Her treatment of this phenomenon must be said to be both extensive and thorough."*
>
> ***(Kirkevold, 1998, p. 180)***

ACCEPTANCE BY THE NURSING COMMUNITY

Practice

Martinsen herself is reluctant to provide concrete directions for practical nursing. However, she recommends that nurses "think along" and assess what she writes and speaks about in their own lives, their own practice and experience, and, against this background, imagine their own way to alternatives for action. This is how Kirkevold puts it:

> *"Martinsen's theory of caring is practically relevant as an overarching/general philosophy of nursing. It is clearly articulated and encompasses a precise formulation of how (one ought) to understand and approach patients and nursing. Its strength is the ability to promote reflection upon nursing practice in different contexts, in that it gives a clear picture of what the author believes must be present so that nursing may be considered caring or moral practice."*
>
> ***(Kirkevold, 1998, p. 181)***

Many of these texts have, she maintains:

> *"a normative character, and are intended to mobilize a counterculture in nursing, which does not only revolutionize the discipline of nursing and its practice, but which also stands as a resisting force against the societal tendency in opposition to the concept of care. . . . In recent years the personal, inspiring and poetic style has become more pronounced. It communicates Martinsen's normatively founded philosophy of caring in a gripping way, and has therefore had great impact on nurses and students."*
>
> ***(Kirkevold, 1998, p. 204)***

Martinsen herself addresses practicing nurses through their professional journal, *Sykepleien.* Kirkevold writes: "In choosing the journal *Nursing* as a main vehicle for communicating her academic work, she has underscored her roots in practical nursing rather than in science" (Kirkevold, 1998, p. 203).

Education

Most nursing colleges in Norway and Denmark make good use of Martinsen's texts, and her works form part of the curriculum at a variety of educational levels. Her books are reprinted regularly and have had considerable impact. Several prescribed texts for nursing education deal with her thought (Alvsvåg, 2011; Kirkevold, 1998; Kristoffersen, 2002; Mekki & Tollefsen, 2000; Nielsen, 2011). In addition, other books have been written for nursing education in which the aim is to make Martinsen's thinking relevant for both nursing generally and for specific professional issues. For example, several college lecturers in Norway and Denmark produced an article compilation in 2000, which gives an introduction to Martinsen's thought and for which the target group is students (Alvsvåg & Gjengedal, 2000). The book *The Philosophy of Caring in Practice: Thinking with Kari Martinsen in Nursing* was published in 2002 and republished in 2010 (Austgard, 2010).

In 2003 a Danish nurse wrote a textbook of spiritual care. Central to the book is Martinsen's thinking, in addition to that of Katie Eriksson and Joyce Travelbee (Overgaard, 2003). In the *Danish Encyclopedia of Nursing,* published in 2008, Kari Martinsen is portrayed in a separate article, and several other articles refer to her thinking on caring and judgment (Jørgensen & Lyngaa, 2008).

Research

In the same way as one in practical nursing can "think along" and assess what she writes, her writings can also be applied in research. Countless dissertations based on practical, concrete, and more theoretical issues discuss the relationship between empirical experience in light of Martinsen's terminology and philosophy. In one doctoral dissertation from 2006, the Norwegian pedagogue Pål Henning Walstad addresses Kari Martinsen's Grundtvig-Løgstrupian influence, calling it *Care for Life,* and discusses this in relation to practical work and professional education (Walstad, 2006). Moreover, nursing teacher Betty-Ann Solvoll's (2007) doctoral dissertation includes a field study of nursing education and discusses the data in relation to Martinsen's reflections on care. Two Danish doctoral dissertations (Dahlgard, 2007; Mark 2008) reflect Martinsen's theory applied to empirical material dealing with care for the dying, and with anorectic and diabetic patients, respectively. Similar applications are made with reference to bathing of patients (Jeanne Boge, 2008), dignified encounters in the final phase of life (Bøe, 2008), and the importance of space and architecture for psychiatric patients (Larsen, 2009). Else Foss is a preschool teacher who analyzes children's crying in kindergartens in her doctoral dissertation (Foss, 2009). These examples of applications of Martinsen's thought in research are even beyond those of traditional nursing.

FURTHER DEVELOPMENT

Caring can be understood on several levels: ontological, concrete, and practical, or at the level of system or organization. Nurses are encouraged to act in a professional and moral manner, so that caring and life utterances are given the space they need to emerge in nurse-patient encounters. Nurses are continuously challenged to reflect critically over whether this happens. It would involve the manifestation of a person-oriented professionalism, the manifestation of loving deeds in the profession, over and over (Martinsen, 1993b, 2000b).

It is important, moreover, to develop a mode of thinking about caring in nursing research. Science in nursing might face certain boundaries. The challenge is to develop a type of research that does not impoverish practice, but that upgrades the available knowledge and wisdom developed through practice—in other words to develop or create a practice-oriented research, a cooperation between researcher and practitioner (Martinsen, 1989c, 1993b). Kirkevold writes as follows:

> *"Martinsen's theory is especially important because it is one of the few existing Norwegian nursing theories, and because it is one of the first Nordic nursing theories that gives expression to a new understanding of reality and the need for new nursing theories based upon this."*
>
> ***(Kirkevold, 1998, p. 182)***

At the organizational and social levels, the concept of care is also highly relevant. It is important to develop social systems and organizations, such as the health service, so that a person-oriented professionalism can be facilitated. Martinsen writes about both a merciful and a political Samaritan (Martinsen, 1993b, 2000b, 2003b). What is important at both organizational and social levels is how the political Samaritans facilitate the work of the merciful Samaritans.

CRITIQUE

Clarity

Martinsen's theory clearly states that life has been created and given to us. Humans have been created in dependence on one another and on nature. Caring for one another and for nature is fundamental. The challenge for nurses is to meet patients and their families with person-oriented professionality, and that (patient encounter) is at the heart of person-oriented professionality.

Simplicity

At first glance, Martinsen's theory seems complex. But this may be because she turns so many familiar assumptions on their heads—for example, that we as human beings are free, independent, and boundless in our capacity for activity and interference with creation. Western societies live in a culture of individualism. Her view of humanity can be described as *collectivist*. She uses a poetic and philosophical rather than a scientific mode of speaking, which might also seem alien in a scientized society. She writes about general phenomena that affect us all, and that we can easily recognize in our personal lives, either occupationally or in daily life. Seen this way, the theory of caring is not hard to understand. Martinsen asks that we read slowly while imagining our own experiences in light of what she writes (Martinsen, 2000b).

Generality

Because Martinsen's nursing theory deals with essential phenomena of life and nursing, phenomena present in all human situations, it can be seen as relevant to patients in general (Martinsen, 2006). Her theory of care "seems to be relevant for all patients who, because of illness or other reasons, need help and assistance" (Kirkevold, 1998, p. 181).

Accessibility

The patient's and the nurse's worlds of experience are diverse, nuanced, and multifaceted. A nuanced and varied language is required to deal with a multifaceted reality, one that is on par with what is to be described. This language is close to philosophy and also to everyday language; it is a poetic language. The poetic language is perhaps the most precise in describing manifold phenomena and situations open to interpretation. Reflection on professional judgment and professional narratives creates the contexts of a community of nursing and the tradition of nursing; nurses recognize situations and thus find professional and moral insight. This enables nurses to perform situation-dependent, good nursing—a professional moral practice.

Importance

Martinsen's theory of caring is a critique of the prevailing system and at the same time an inspiration to individuals in concrete caring situations (Gjengedal, 2000). Gjengedal (2000) writes that Martinsen's motivation for theoretical work "has precisely a practical point of departure, a wish to understand and protect against devaluation of the aspect of care in nursing" (p. 38). Devaluation of caring might occur if one uncritically accepts "a scientific perspective blind to the lived life and all that gives meaning to being" (Gjengedal, 2000, p. 54).

Nurses, as all individuals, are challenged to live in a way that allows positive meaning to be expressed in their human relations, for example, in relations between patients and their family members. How they express this in a concrete way in a nursing context is for nurses as professionals to decide, and the philosophy on which Martinsen bases her thinking provides ideas for individual reflection in specific situations. Specific situations present themselves with both possibilities and limitations. Socially created structural arrangements such as lack of personnel, financial resources, and lack of institutional beds present serious limitations on a daily basis. Opportunities for caring become more accessible within a caring community and are shaped by politically aware people:

> *"A caring community is not dictatorial, nor is it society's passive extended arm. The caring community exists only to the extent that we struggle for its existence. We must form it ourselves: through solidarity, through morally responsible action, through the fight for greater equality and for community and social integration. Caring is an active and radical concept."*
> ***(Martinsen, 1989c, p. 62)***

It is important to create conditions for good and equitable health care and living standards for all, but in the fight over limited budgetary resources, the starting point should be those who are weakest, who most need help; it is about turning the inverted law of care around such that those who have the least receive the most.

SUMMARY

Martinsen has both personal and sociopolitical interest in the ill and in those who, for other reasons, fall outside of society. Her theoretical stance can be called critical and phenomenological. She takes as her starting point the idea that human beings are created and are beings for whom we may have administrative responsibility. We are relational and dependent on each other and on the creation. Therefore caring, solidarity, and moral practice are unavoidable realities.

On the subject of caring, Martinsen challenges society, the politics of health care, and health care workers themselves to realize the values inherent in caring through concrete policies and practical nursing. She deliberately gives few directives for action. Rather, she asks nurses to think themselves into the situations of patients and family members and to arrive at the best choices for action based on a rich situational understanding, professional insight, and a caring attitude.

Martinsen's thought has provoked, engaged, and created debate and professional development in nursing in the Nordic countries over the past 30 years. Her thought challenges nurses to both think and act well and correctly, critically, and differently in nursing, in education, and in research. Martinsen's "caring thought" contributes to the enlightenment of nursing and nursing research through its perspectives, concepts, and insights based on historical and philosophical scholarship and research.

CASE STUDY

As nurses, we meet patients and their family members in many different life situations. Patients may be of all age groups, acutely or chronically ill, might return to life and health, or are coming to the end of their lives and must face death as a reality. Nurses meet patients and family members in their homes, the hospital, the nursing home, the school health service, the local clinic, and so forth. Some meetings with patients and family members make a greater impression on us than others, and all meetings represent situations of learning.

Against this background, write a brief case study from your personal clinical experience using the critical thinking activities listed here and discuss how caring was expressed in that particular case situation.

CRITICAL THINKING ACTIVITIES

1. Center your thinking on a concrete nursing situation with which you had personal experience as an active participant or as an observer.
2. Consider the human caring aspects of the situation in the first item.
3. From the starting point of the situation in the first item, discuss what is meant by *person-oriented professionalism* and *moral practice.*

POINTS FOR FURTHER STUDY

- Martinsen, K. (2006). *Care and vulnerability.* Oslo: Akribe.
- Martinsen, K. (2009). *Å se og* å innse—Om ulike former for evidens [*To see and to realize—On various forms of evidence.* Oslo: Akribe.

REFERENCES*

Alvsvåg, H. (2000). Menneskesynet—Fra kroppsfenomenologi til skapelsesfenomenologi. I H. Alvsvåg & E. Gjengedal (red.), *Omsorgstenkning. En innføring i Kari Martinsens forfatterskap*. Bergen: Fagbokforlaget. [The view of the person—from the phenomenology of the body to creation phenomenology. In H. Alvsvåg & E. Gjengedal (Eds.), *Caring thought: An introduction to the writings of Kari Martinsen*. Bergen: Fagbokforlaget.]

Alvsvåg, H. (2011). Omsorg—Med utgangspunkt i Kari Martinsens omsorgstenkning. I B. K. Nielsen (red.), *Sygeplejebogen 3. Teori og metode*. 3. opplag. København: Gads Forlag. [Caring—From the starting point of Kari Martinsen's philosophy. In B. K. Nielsen (Ed.), *Nursing textbook 3. Theoretical-methodological basis of clinical nursing*. Copenhagen: Gads Forlag.]

Alvsvåg, H., & Gjengedal, E. (red.). (2000). *Omsorgstenkning. En innføring i Kari Martinsens forfatterskap*. Bergen: Fagbokforlaget. [*Caring thought: An introduction to the writings of Kari Martinsen*. Bergen: Fagbokforlaget.]

Austgard, K. (2010). *Omsorgsfilosofi i praksis. A tenke med Kari Martinsen i sykepleien*. Oslo: Cappelen Akademisk Forlag. [*Philosophy of caring in practice. Thinking with Kari Martinsen in nursing*. Oslo: Cappelen Akademisk Forlag.]

Bøe, K. G. (2008). *Verdige møter mellom helsepersonale og pasienter i livets sluttfase*. Avhandling for dr. art.-graden. Universitetet i Oslo. [*Dignified encounters between health workers and patients in the final phase of life*. Dissertation for the degree of philosophiae doctor (PhD). University of Oslo.]

Boge, J. (2008). *Kroppsvask i sjukepleia*. Avhandling for philosophiae doctor (PhD). Universitetet i Bergen. [*Bathing the patient*. Dissertation for the degree of philosophiae doctor (PhD). University of Bergen.]

Dalgaard, K. M. (2007). *At leve med uhelbredelig sygdom*. Det samfundsvidenskabelige Fakultet, (PhD). Aalborg Universitet. [*Living with incurable disease*. PhD. School of Social Sciences University of Aalborg.]

Foss, E. (2009). *Den omsorgsfulle væremåte*. Avhandling for philosophiae doctor (PhD). Universitetet i Bergen. [*The caring way of being*. Dissertation for the degree of philosophiae doctor (PhD). University of Bergen.]

Gjengedal, E. (2000). Omsorg og sykepleie. I H. Alvsvåg & E. Gjengedal (red.), *Omsorgstenkning: En innføring i Kari Martinsens forfatterskap*. Bergen: Fagbokforlaget. [Caring and nursing. In H. Alvsvåg & E. Gjengedal (Eds.), *Caring thought: An introduction to the writings of Kari Martinsen*. Bergen: Fagbokforlaget.]

Jørgensen, B. B., & Lyngaa, J. (Eds.). (2008). *Sygeplejeleksikon*. København: Munksgaard. [*Encyclopedia of Nursing*. Copenhagen: Munksgaard.]

*Norwegian titles are provided with approximate translation into English.

Karlsson, B., & Martinsen, K. (2003). Prolog. In K. Martinsen, *Omsorg, sykepleie og medisin*. 2. utgave. Oslo: Universitetsforlaget. [Prologue. In K. Martinsen. *Caring, nursing and medicine: Historical-philosophical essays* (2nd ed.). Oslo: Universitetsforlaget.]

Kirkevold, M. (1998). *Sykepleieteorier—Analyse og evaluering*. Oslo: ad Notam Gyldendal. 2. utgave. [*Nursing theories—Analysis and evaluation* (2nd ed.). Oslo: ad Notam Gyldendal.]

Kirkevold, M. (2000). Utviklingstrekk i Kari Martinsens forfatterskap. I H. Alvsvåg & E. Gjengedal (red.), *Omsorgstenkning—En innføring i Kari Martinsens forfatterskap*. Bergen: Fagbokforlaget. [Developmental characteristics in the writings of Kari Martinsen. In H. Alvsvåg & E. Gjengedal (Eds.), *Caring thought: An introduction to the writings of Kari Martinsen*. Bergen: Fagbokforlaget.]

Kjær, T. (2000). Fænomenologi, etikk og fortælling: I H. Alvsvåg & E. Gjengedal (red.), *Omsorgstenkning—En innføring i Kari Martinsens forfatterskap*. Bergen: Fagbokforlaget. [Phenomenology, ethics and narrative. In H. Alvsvåg & E. Gjengedal (Eds.), *Caring thought: An introduction to the writings of Kari Martinsen*. Bergen: Fagbokforlaget.]

Kristoffersen, N. J. (2002). *Generell sykepleie*. Oslo: Universitetsforlaget. [*Fundamental nursing*. Oslo: Universitetsforlaget.]

Larsen, I. B. (2009). *"Det sitter i veggene" Materialitet og mennesker i distriktspsykiatriske sentra*. Avhandling for philosophiae doctor (PhD). Universitetet i Bergen. [*"It's in the woodwork"—Materiality and people in Regional Psychiatric Centers*. Dissertation for the degree of philosophiae doctor (PhD). University of Bergen.]

Lubcke, P. (red.). (1983). *Politikens filosofiske leksikon*. København: Politikens Forlag. [*Politiken's philosophical lexicon*. Copenhagen: Politikens Forlag.]

Malchau, S. (2000). Kaldet. I H. Alvsvåg & E. Gjengedal (red.), *Omsorgstenkning—En innføring i Kari Martinsens forfatterskap*. Bergen: Fagbokforlaget. [The call. In H. Alvsvåg & E. Gjengedal (Eds.), *Caring thought: An introduction to the writings of Kari Martinsen*. Bergen: Fagbokforlaget.]

Mark, E. (2008). *Restriktiv spising i narrativ belysning. En fænomenologisk undersøgelse af børns oplevelser af spisning ved diabetes eller overvægt*. PhD. Det humanistiske fakultet. Aalborg Universitet. [*Restrictive eating in a narrative perspective. A phenomenological study of children's experience of eating in relation to diabetes or obesity*. PhD. School of Humanities, Aalborg University.]

Martinsen, K. (1975). *Filosofi og sykepleie. Et marxistisk og fenomenologisk bidrag*. Filosofisk institutes stensilserie nr. 34. Bergen: Universitetet i Bergen. [*Philosophy and nursing: A Marxist and phenomenological contribution* (Philosophical Institute's Stencil Series No. 34). Bergen: University of Bergen.]

Martinsen, K. (1976). Historie og sykepleie—Momenter til en utdanningsdebatt. *Kontrast, 7*, 430–446. [History and nursing—elements of an educational debate. *Contrast, 7*, 430–446.]

Martinsen, K. (1977). Nightingale—Ingen opprører bak myten. *Sykepleien, 18*(65), 1022–1025. [Nightingale—no rebel behind the myth. *Nursing,* 18(65), 1022–1025.]

Martinsen, K. (1978). Det 'kliniske blikk' i medisinen og i sykepleien. *Sykepleien, 20*(66), 1271–1272. [The "clinical gaze" in medicine and in nursing. *Nursing,* 20(66), 1271–1272.]

Martinsen, K. (1979a). Den engelske sanitation—Bevegelsen, hygiene og synet på sykdom. I Ø. Larsen (red.), *Synet på sykdom.* Oslo: Seksjon for medisinsk historie, Universitetet i Oslo. [The English sanitation movement, hygiene and the view of illness. In Ø. Larsen (Ed.), *The view of illness.* Oslo: University of Oslo (Section for medical history).]

Martinsen, K. (1979b). Diakonissesykepleiens framvekst. Fra vekkelser og kvinneforeninger til moderhus og fattigomsorg. I NAVF's sekretariat for kvinneforskning (red.), *Lønnet og ulønnet omsorg. En seminarrapport.* Arbeidsnotat nr. 5/79. Oslo: NAVF. [Development of the professional trained Christian nurses. From revival and woman's charitable groups to the mother house and care of the poor. In NAVF's Secretariat for Feminist Research (Ed.), *Paid and unpaid care: A seminar report.* Working paper no. 5/79. Oslo: NAVE]

Martinsen, K. (1984). *Sykepleiens historie. Freidige og uforsagte diakonisser. Et omsorgsyrke vokser fram 1860–1905.* Oslo: Aschehoug/Tanum-Norli. [*History of nursing: Frank and engaged deaconesses: A caring profession emerges 1860–1905.* Oslo: Aschehoug/Tanum-Norli.]

Martinsen, K. (1989a). Helsepolitiske problemer og helsepolitisk tenkning bak sykehusloven av 1969. I K. Martinsen, *Omsorg, sykepleie og medisin. Historisk-filosofiske essays.* Oslo: Tano Forlag. [Health policy problems and health policy thinking behind the hospital law of 1969. In K. Martinsen, *Caring, nursing and medicine: Historical-philosophical essays.* Oslo: Tano Forlag.]

Martinsen, K. (1989b). Legers interesse for svangerskapet—En del av den perinatale omsorg. Tidsrommet ca. 1890-1940. I K. Martinsen, *Omsorg, sykepleie og medisin. Historisk-filosofiske essays.* Oslo: Tano Forlag. [The doctor's interest in pregnancy—Part of perinatal care: The period ca. 1890–1940. In K. Martinsen, *Caring, nursing and medicine: Historical-philosophical essays.* Oslo: Tano Forlag.]

Martinsen, K. (1989c). *Omsorg, sykepleie og medisin. Historisk-filosofiske essays.* Oslo: Tano Forlag. [*Caring, nursing and medicine: Historical-philosophical essays.* Oslo: Tano Forlag.]

Martinsen, K. (1990). Moralsk praksis og dokumentasjon i praktisk sykepleie. I T. Jensen, L. U. Jensen, & W. C. Kim (red.), *Grundlagsproblemer i sygeplejen. Etik, videnskabsteori, ledelse & samfunn.* Aarhus: Philosophia. [Practice and documentation in practical nursing. In T. Jensen, L. U. Jensen, & W. C. Kim (Eds.), *Foundational problems in nursing: Ethics, theories of science, leadership and society.* Aarhus: Philosophia.]

Martinsen, K. (red.). (1993a). *Den omtenksomme sykepleier.* Oslo: Tano. [*The thoughtful nurse.* Oslo: Tano.]

Martinsen, K. (1993b). *Fra Marx til Løgstrup. Om moral, samfunnskritikk og sanselighet i sykepleien.* Oslo: Tano Forlag. [*From Marx to Løgstrup: On morality, social criticism and sensuousness in nursing.* Oslo: Tano Forlag.]

Martinsen, K. (1996). *Fenomenologi og omsorg. Tre dialoger.* Oslo: Tano-Aschehoug. [*Phenomenology and caring: Three dialogues.* Oslo: Tano-Aschehoug.]

Martinsen, K. (1997a). De etiske fortellinger. *Omsorg, 1*(14), 58–63. [The ethical narratives. *Caring, 1*(14), 58–63.]

Martinsen, K. (1997b). Etikk og kall, kultur og kropp—En dialog med Patricia Benner. I M. Sæther (red.), *Sykepleiekonferanse på Nordkalottens tak.* Tromsø: Universitetet i Tromsø. [Ethics and vocation, culture and the body—A dialogue with Patricia Benner. In M. Sæther (Ed.), *Nursing conference on the roof of Nordkalotten.* Tromsø: University of Tromsø.]

Martinsen, K. (2000a). Kjærlighetsgjerningen og kallet. Betraktninger omkring Rikke Nissens "Lærebog i Sygepleje for diakonisser". I R. Nissen, *Lærebog i Sygepleie. Med etterord av Kari Martinsen.* Oslo: Gyldendal Akademisk. [The loving act and the call. Reflections on Rikke Nissen's textbook of nursing for deaconesses. In R. Nissen, *Textbook of nursing. With afterword by Kari Martinsen.* Oslo: Gyldendal Akademisk.]

Martinsen, K. (2000b). *Øyet og kallet.* Bergen: Fagbokforlaget. [*The eye and the call.* Bergen: Fagbokforlaget.]

Martinsen, K. (2001). Huset og sangen, gråten og skammen. Rom og arkitektur som ivaretaker av menneskets verdighet. I T. Wyller (red.), *Skam. Perspektiver på skam, ære og skamløshet i det moderne.* Bergen: Fagbokforlaget. [The house and the song, the tears and the shame: Space and architecture as caretakers of human dignity. In T. Wyller (Ed.), *Shame. Perspectives on shame, honor and shamelessness in modernity.* Bergen: Fagbokforlaget.]

Martinsen, K. (2002a). Livsfilosofiske betraktninger. *Diakoninytt, 3*(118), 8–12. [Reflections on the philosophy of life. *Deaconry News, 3*(118), 8–12.]

Martinsen, K. (2002b). Rommets tid, den sykes tid, pleiens tid. I I. T. Bjørk, S. Helseth, & F. Nortvedt (red.), *Møte mellom pasient og sykepleier.* Oslo: Gyldendal Akademisk. [The room's time, the ill person's time, nursing time. In I. T. Bjørk, S. Helseth, & F. Nortvedt (Eds.), *The meeting between patient and nurse.* Oslo: Gyldendal Akademisk.]

Martinsen, K. (2002c). Samtalen, kommunikasjonen og sakligheten i omsorgsyrkene. *Omsorg, 1*(19), 14–22. [Conversation, communication and professionality in the caring professions. *Caring, 1*(19), 14–22.]

Martinsen, K. (2003a). Disiplin og rommelighet. I K. Martinsen & T. Wyller (red.), *Etikk, disiplin og dannelse. Elisabeth Hagemanns etikkbok—Nye lesinger.* Oslo: Gyldendal Akademisk. [Discipline and spaciousness. In K. Martinsen & T. Wyller (Eds.), *Ethics, discipline and refinement: Elizabeth Hagemann's ethics book—new readings.* Oslo: Gyldendal Akademisk.]

Martinsen, K. (2003b). *Omsorg, sykepleie og medisin. Historisk-filosofiske essays.* 2. utgave. Oslo: Universitetsforlaget. [*Caring, nursing and medicine: Historical-philosophical essays* (2nd ed.). Oslo: University Press.]

Martinsen, K. (2003c). Talens åpenhet og evidens—Dialog med Jens Bydam. *Klinisk Sygepleje, 4*(17), 36–46. [The openness of speech and evidence—Dialogue with Jens Bydam. *Clinical Nursing, 4*(17), 36–46.]

Martinsen, K. (2004). Skjønn—Språk og distanse—Dialog med Jens Bydam. *Klinisk Sygepleje, 2*(18), 50–56. [Discernment—language and distance—dialogue with Jens Bydam. *Clinical Nursing, 2*(18), 50–56.]

Martinsen, K. (2005). *Samtalen, skjønnet og evidensen.* Oslo: Akribe. [*Dialog, discernment and the evidence.* Oslo: Akribe.]

Martinsen, K. (2006). *Care and vulnerability.* Oslo: Akribe.

Martinsen, K. (2009). *Å se og å innse—Om ulike former for evidens.* Oslo: Akribe. [*To see and to realize—On various forms of evidence.* Oslo: Akribe.].

Martinsen, K. (2012a). *Løgstrup og sykepleien.* Århus: Klim Forlag. [*Løgstrup and nursing.* Aarhus: Klim.]

Martinsen, K. (2012b). *Løgstrup og sykepleien.* Oslo: Akribe. [*Løgstrup and nursing.* Oslo: Akribe.]

Martinsen, K., & Wærness, K. (1979). *Pleie uten omsorg?* Oslo: Pax Forlag A/S. [*Caring without care?* Oslo: Pax Forlag.]

Martinsen, K., & Wyller, T. (Ed.). (2003). *Etikk, disiplin og dannelse. Elisabeth Hagemanns etikkbok—Nye lesinger.* Oslo: Gyldendal Akademisk. [*Ethics, discipline and refinement: Elizabeth Hagemann's ethics book—new readings.* Oslo: Gyldendal Akademisk.]

Mekki, T. E., & Tollefsen, S. (2000). *På terskelen. Introduksjon til sykepleie som fag og yrke.* Oslo: Akribe. [*On the threshold: Introduction to nursing as discipline and profession.* Oslo: Akribe.]

Nielsen, B. K. (Ed.). (2011). *Sygeplejebogen 3. Teori og metode.* 3. utg. København: Gads Forlag. [*Nursing textbook 3. Theoretical-methodical basis of clinical nursing.* Copenhagen: Gads.]

Nissen, R. (2000). *Lærebog i Sygepleie. Med etterord av Kari Martinsen.* Oslo: Gyldendal Akademisk. [*Textbook of nursing. With an afterword by Kari Martinsen.* Oslo: Gyldendal Akademisk.]

Olsen, R. H. (1998). *Klok av erfaring? Om sansing og oppmerksomhet, kunnskap og refleksjon i praktisk sykepleie.* Oslo: Tano Aschehoug. [*Wise with experience? On sensation and attention, knowledge and reflection in practical nursing.* Oslo: Tano Aschehoug.]

Overgaard, A. E. (2003). *Åndelig omsorg—En lærebog.* København: Nytt Nordisk Forlag Arnold Busck. [*Spiritual care—Textbook.* Copenhagen: Nyt Nordisk Forlag Arnold Busck.]

Solvoll, B. A. (2007). *Omsorgsferdigheter som pedagogisk prosjekt—en feltstudie i sykepleieutdanningen.* Oslo: Universitetet i Oslo, Det medisinske fakultet, nr. 540. [*Caring skills as pedagogical project—A field study in nursing education.* Oslo: University of Oslo, Faculty of Medicine, Doctoral Dissertation No. 540.]

Thorsen, R., Mæhre, K. S., & Martinsen, K. (Eds.). (2012). *Fortellinger om etikk.* Bergen: Fagbokforlaget. [*Narratives on ethics.*]

Walstad, P. B. (2006). *Dannelse og Duelighed for livet. Dannelse og yrkesutdanning i den grundtvigske tradisjon.* Trondheim: Norges teknisk-naturvitenskapelige universitet, NTNU Doctoral dissertations 2006:88. [*Education and capability for life. Education and professional training in the Grundtvigian tradition.* Trondheim: Norges teknisk-naturvitenskapelige universitet, NTNU Doctoral Dissertation 2006:88.]

BIBLIOGRAPHY*

Primary Sources

Books

Kjær, T. A., & Martinsen, K. (Eds.). (2015). *Utenfor tellekantene. Essays om rom og rommelighet.* Bergen: Fagbokforlaget. [Beyond audits. Essays on space and spaciousness. Bergen: Fagbok forlaget.]

Martinsen K. (1975). *Filosofi og sykepleie. Et marxistisk og fenomenologisk bidrag.* Filosofisk institutts stensilserie nr. 34. Bergen: Universitetet i Bergen. [*Philosophy and nursing: A Marxist and phenomenological contribution.* Philosophical Institute's Stencil Series No. 34. Bergen: University of Bergen.]

Martinsen, K. (1979). *Medisin og sykepleie, historie og samfunn.* Oslo: Norsk Sykepleierforbund. [*Medicine and nursing, history and society.* Oslo: The Norwegian Nursing Association.]

Martinsen, K. (1984). *Sykepleiens historie. Freidige og uforsagte diakonisser. Et omsorgsyrke vokser fram 1860–1905.* Oslo: Aschehoug/Tanum-Norli. [*History of nursing: Frank and engaged deaconesses. A caring profession emerges 1860–1905.* Oslo: Aschehoug/Tanum-Norli.]

Martinsen, K. (1989). *Omsorg, sykepleie og medisin. Historisk-filosofiske essays.* Oslo: Tano Forlag. [*Caring, nursing and medicine. Historical-philosophical essays.* Oslo: Tano Forlag.]

Martinsen, K. (red.). (1993). *Den omtenksomme sykepleier.* Oslo: Tano. [*The thoughtful nurse.* Oslo: Tano.]

Martinsen, K. (1993). *Fra Marx til Løgstrup. Om moral, samfunnskritikk og sanselighet i sykepleien.* Oslo: Tano Forlag. [*From Marx to Løgstrup. On morality, social criticism and sensuousness in nursing.* Oslo: Tano Forlag.]

Martinsen, K. (1996). *Fenomenologi og omsorg. Tre dialoger.* Oslo: Tano-Aschehoug. [*Phenomenology and caring. Three dialogues.* Oslo: Tano-Aschehoug.]

Martinsen, K. (2000). *Øyet og kallet.* Bergen: Fagbokforlaget. [*The eye and the call.* Bergen: Fagbokforlaget.]

Martinsen, K. (2005). *Samtalen, skjønnet og evidensen.* Oslo: Akribe. [*Dialog, discernment and evidence.* Oslo: Akribe.]

Martinsen, K. (2006). *Care and vulnerability.* Oslo: Akribe.

Martinsen, K. (2008). *Å se og å innse—om ulike former for evidens.* Oslo: Akribe. [*To see and to realize—On various forms of evidence.* Oslo: Akribe.] (In process with Katie Ericsson).

Martinsen, K. (2012). *Løgstrup og sykepleien* [*Løgstrup and nursing*]. Århus: KLIM Forlag.

Martinsen, K. (2012). *Løgstrup og sykepleien* [*Løgstrup and nursing*]. Oslo: Akribe.

Martinsen, K., & Wærness, K. (1979). *Pleie uten omsorg?* Oslo: Pax Forlag A/S. [*Caring without care?* Oslo: Pax Forlag.]

Martinsen, K., & Wyller, T. (red.). (2003). *Etikk, disiplin og dannelse. Elisabeth Hagemanns etikkbok—Nye lesinger.* Oslo: Gyldendal Akademisk. [*Ethics, discipline and refinement.*

*Norwegian titles are provided with approximate translation into English.

Elizabeth Hagemann's ethics book—New readings. Oslo: Gyldendal Akademisk.]

Thorsen, R., Mæhre, K. S., & Martinsen, K. (red.). (2012). *Fortellinger om etikk.* Bergen: Fagbokforlaget. [*Narratives on ethics.* Bergen: Fagbok forlaget].

Book Chapters

Martinsen, K. (1972). Samfunnets krise og sykepleiernes oppgave. I I. K. Haugen, T. Malmin, S., Midtgaard, & K. Nicolaysen (red.), *Pedialogen* (s. 3–14). Oslo: Norsk Sykepleierforbund. [The crises of society and the nursing objectives. In I. K. Haugen, T. Malmin, S. Midtgaard, & K. Nicolaysen (Eds.), *Pedialog* (pp. 3–14). Oslo: Norwegian Nursing Association.]

Martinsen, K. (1972). Sykepleie som sosial-moralsk praksis. I I. K. Haugen, T. Malmin, S. Midtgaard, & K. Nicolaysen (red.), *Pedialogen* (s. 15–36). Oslo: Norsk Sykepleierforbund. [Nursing as social and moral practice. In I. K. Haugen, T. Malmin, S. Midtgaard, & K. Nicolaysen (Eds.), *Pedialog* (pp. 15–36). Oslo: Norwegian Nursing Association.]

Martinsen, K. (1978). Fra ufaglært fattigsykepleie til profesjonelt yrke—Konsekvenser for omsorg. I B. Persson, K. Ravn, & R. Truelsen (red.), *Fokus på sygeplejen-79. Årbok* (s. 128–157). København: Munksgaard. [From unskilled nursing the poor to professional occupation—Consequences for nursing. In B. Persson, K. Ravn, & R. Truelsen (Eds.), *Focus on nursing* (Annual 79, pp. 128–157). Copenhagen: Munksgaard.]

Martinsen, K. (1979). Den engelske sanitation-bevegelsen, hygiene og synet på sykdom. I Ø. Larsen (red.), *Synet på sykdom* (s. 78–87). Oslo: Seksjon for medisinsk historie, Universitetet i Oslo. [The English sanitation movement: Hygiene and the view of illness. In Ø. Larsen (Ed.), *The view of illness* (pp. 78–87). Oslo: University of Oslo, Section for Medical History.]

Martinsen, K. (1979). Diakonissesykepleiens framvekst. Fra vekkelser og kvinneforeninger til moderhus og fattigomsorg. I NAVF's sekretariat for kvinneforskning (red.), *Lønnet og ulønnet omsorg. En seminarrapport* (Arbeidsnotat nr. 5, s. 135–170). Oslo: NAVF. [Development of the professional trained Christian nurses: From revival and woman's charitable groups to the mother house and care of the poor. In NAVF's Secretariat for Feminist Research (Ed.), *Paid and unpaid care: A seminar report* (Working paper no. 5, pp. 135–170). Oslo: NAVE]

Martinsen, K. (1979). Diakonissene. I E. Mehlum (red.), *Bak maskinene, under fanene.* Utgitt i forbindelse med "Kristiania-utstillingen" om arbeidsfolk i byen for 100 år siden (s. 54–56). Oslo: Tiden. [Deconesses. In E. Mehlum (Ed.), *Behind the machines and the banners* (pp. 54–56). Oslo: Tiden. Published in connection with "The Christiania (Oslo) exhibition" on the condition of workers 100 years ago.]

Martinsen, K. (1979). Sykepleien, historien og den omvendte omsorgen. I R. Wendt (red.), *Utveckling av omvårdnadsarbete* (s. 90–102). Lund: Studentlitteratur. [Nursing, history and the converse caring. In R. Wendt (Ed.), *Development of health care* (pp. 90–102). Lund: Studentlitteratur.]

Martinsen, K. (1979). Sykepleien i historisk perspektiv: Fra omsorg mot egenomsorg. I M. S. Fagermoen & R. Nord (red.), *Sykepleie: Teori/praksis* (s. 5–23). Oslo: Norwegian Nursing Association. [Nursing in a historical perspective: From care to self caring. In M. S. Fagermoen & R. Nord (Eds.), *Nursing: Theory/practice* (pp. 5–23). Oslo: Norwegian Nursing Association.]

Martinsen, K. (1981). Diakonisser. I H. F. Dahl, J. Elster, I. Iversen, m.fl. (red.), *Pax leksikon.* Oslo: Pax Forlag (s. 89–90). [Deaconessses. In H. F. Dahl, J. Elster, I. Iversen, et al. (Eds.), *Pax lexicon* (pp. 89–90). Oslo: Pax Forlag.]

Martinsen, K. (1981). Guldberg, Cathinka. I H. F. Dahl, J. Elster, I. Iversen, m.fl. (red.), *Pax leksikon* (s. 553–554). Oslo: Pax forlag. [Guldberg, Cathinka. In H. F. Dahl, J. Elster, I. Iversen, et al. (Eds.), *Pax lexicon* (pp. 553–554). Oslo: Pax Forlag.]

Martinsen, K. (1981). Nightingale, Florence. I H. F. Dahl, J. Elster, I. Iversen, m.fl. (red.), *Pax leksikon* (s. 448–449). [Nightingale, Florence. In H. F. Dahl, J. Elster, I. Iversen, et al. (Eds.), *Pax lexicon* (pp. 448–449). Oslo: Pax Forlag.]

Martinsen, K. (1981). Omsorg i sykepleie. I E. Barnes & S. Solbak (red.), *Sykepleielære 1.* Lærebok for hjelpepleiere (Kap. 3). Oslo: Aschehoug. [Care in nursing. In E. Barnes & S. Solbak (Eds.), *Nursing textbook 1. Textbook for licensed practical nurses* (Chapter 3). Oslo: Aschehoug.]

Martinsen, K. (1981). Sykepleier. I H. F. Dahl, J. Elster, I. Iversen, m.fl. (red.), *Pax leksikon* (s. 179–180). Oslo: Pax forlag. [Nurse. In H. F. Dahl, J. Elster, I. Iversen, S. et al. (Eds.), *Pax lexicon* (pp. 179–180). Oslo: Pax Forlag.]

Martinsen, K. (1981). Sykepleieraksjonen 1972. I H. F. Dahl, J. Elster, I. Iversen, m.fl. (red.), *Pax leksikon* (s. 180–181). Oslo: Pax forlag. [Nurses on strike 1972. In H. F. Dahl, J. Elster, I. Iversen, et al. (Eds.), *Pax lexicon* (pp. 180–181). Oslo: Pax Forlag.]

Martinsen, K. (1981). Sykepleierforbund, Norsk (NSF). I H. F. Dahl, J. Elster, I. Iversen, m.fl. (red.), *Pax leksikon* (s. 181–183). Oslo: Pax Forlag. [Nursing association. In H. F. Dahl, J. Elster, I. Iversen, et al. (Eds.), *Pax lexicon* (pp. 181–183). Oslo: Pax Forlag.]

Martinsen, K. (1981). Trekk av hjelpepleiernes historie. I E. Barnes & S. Solbak (red.), *Sykepleielære 1. Lærebok for hjelpepleiere.* (Kap. 2). Oslo: Aschehoug. [Aspects of licensed practical nurse history. In E. Barnes & S. Solbak (Eds.), *Nursing textbook 1. Textbook for licensed practical nurses* (Chapter 2). Oslo: Aschehoug.]

Martinsen, K. (1985). Organisering av omsorg: diakonisser i Norge. I J. Bjørgum, K. Gundersen, S. Lie, & K. Vogt (red.), *Kvinnenes kulturhistorie* (s. 131–134). Oslo: Universitetsforlaget. [Organization of care: Deaconesses in Norway. In J. Bjørgum, K. Gundersen, S. Lie, & K. Vogt (Eds.), *Woman's cultural history* (pp. 131–134). Oslo: Universitetsforlaget.]

Martinsen, K. (1986). Sykepleierne—Helsemisjonerer, oppdragere og profesjonelle yrkeskvinner. I I. Fredriksen & H. Rømer (red.), *Kvinder, Mentalitet og arbejde. Kvindehistorisk forskning i Norden* (s. 151–156). Aarhus: Aarhus universitetsforlag. [Nurses—health missionaries, educators and professional working women. In I. Fredriksen & H. Rømer (Eds.), *Woman, mentality and work: Research on feminist history in Nordic countries* (pp. 151–156). Aarhus: Aarhus universitetsforlag.]

Martinsen, K. (1987). Ledelse og omsorgsrasjonalitet—Gir patriarkatbegrepet innsikt? I NAVFs sekretariat for kvinneforskning (red.), *Kjønn og makt: teoretiske perspektiver* (s. 18–26).

Arbeidsnotat nr. 2. Oslo: NAVE. [Leadership and rationality of care—does the concept of patriarchy yield insight? In *Gender and power: theoretical perspectives* (Working paper no. 2, pp. 18–26). Oslo: NAVF.]

Martinsen K. (1989). Omsorg i sykepleien—In moralsk utfordring. I B. Persson, J. Petersen, & R. Truelsen (red.), *Fokus på sygeplejen-90* (s. 181–200). København: Munksgaard. [Caring in nursing—a moral challenge. In B. Persson, J. Petersen, & R. Truelsen (Eds.), *Focus on Nursing—90* (pp. 181–200). Copenhagen: Munksgaard.]

Martinsen, K. (1990). Fra resultater til situasjoner: Omsorg, makt og solidaritet. I Samkvind (Center for samfundsvidenskabelig kvindeforskning). *Kvinder og kommuner i Norden* (s. 61–82), København: Samkvind. [From results to situations: Care, power and solidarity. In Samkvind (Center for Feminist Research), Woman and municipals in Nordic countries (pp. 61–82). Copenhagen: Samkvind.]

Martinsen, K. (1990). Moralsk praksis og dokumentasjon i praktisk sykepleie. I T. Jensen, L. U. Jensen, & W. C. Kim (red.), *Grundlagsproblemer i sygeplejen. Etik, videnskabsteori, ledelse & samfunn* (s. 60–84). Aarhus: Philosophia. [Moral practice and documentation in practical nursing. In T. Jensen, L. U. Jensen, & W. C. Kim, *Foundational problems in nursing: Ethics, theories of science, leadership and society* (pp. 60–84). Aarhus: Philosophia.]

Martinsen, K. (1993). Etikk og diakoni. I P. Frølich, J. Midtbø, & A. Tang, *Bergen Diakonissehjem 75 år* (s. 22–26). Bergen: Bergen Diakonissehjem. [Etichs and Diaconi. In P. Frølich, J. Midtbø, & A. Tang, *Bergen Diakonissehjem 75 years* (pp. 22–26). Bergen: Bergen Diakonissehjem.]

Martinsen, K. (1993). Omsorgens filosofi og dens praksis. I H. M. Dahl (red.), *Omsorg og kjærlighet i velfærdsstaten* (Samfundsvidenskabelig kvindeforskning/Cekvina, s. 7–23). Århus: Universitetet i Århus. [Caring philosophy and its practice. In H. M. Dahl (Ed.), *Care and love in the welfare state* (Social scientifically woman studies, pp. 7–23). Århus: The University of Århus.]

Martinsen, K. (1995). Omsorgsfeltet i den kliniske sygepleje. I I. Andersen & M. G. Erikstrup (red.), *Statens sundhedsvidenskabelige forskningsråds sygeplejeforskn-ingsinitiativ. Betydning for sygeplejepraksis* (s. 31–43). Århus: Århus Universitet. [Area for care in clinical nursing. In I. Andersen & M. G. Erikstrup (Eds.), *The state's initiative in nursing science. The significance for nursing practice* (pp. 31–43). Århus: Århus University.]

Martinsen, K. (1997). Etikk og kall, kultur og kropp—En dialog med Patricia Benner. I M. Sæther (red.), *Sykepleiekonferanse på Nordkalottens tak* (s. 111–157). Tromsø: Universitetet i Tromsø. [Ethics and vocation, culture and the body—A dialogue with Patricia Benner. In M. Sæther (Ed.), *Nursing conference on the roof of Nordkalotten* (pp. 111–157). Tromsø: University of Tromsø.]

Martinsen, K. (1999). Etikken og kulturen, og kroppens sårbarhet. I K. Christensen & L. J. Syltevik (red.), *Omsorgens forvitring? En antologi om utfordringer i velferdsstaten—Tilegnet Kari Wærness* (s. 241–269). Bergen: Fagbokforlaget. [Ethics and culture, and vulnerability of the body. In K. Christensen & L. J. Syltevik (Eds.), *Weathering of caring? An anthology about challenges in the welfare state—dedicated to Kari Wærness* (pp. 241–269). Bergen: Fagbokforlaget.]

Martinsen, K. (2000). Kjærlighetsgjerningen og kallet. Betraktninger omkring Rikke Nissens "Lærebog i Sygepleje for diakonisser". I R. Nissen, *Lærebog i Sygepleie. Med etterord av Kari Martinsen* (s. 245–300). Oslo: Gyldendal Akademisk. [The loving act and the call. Reflections on Rikke Nissen's *Textbook of nursing for deaconesses.* In R. Nissen, *Textbook of nursing. With afterword by Kari Martinsen* (pp. 245–300). Oslo: Gyldendal Akademisk.]

Martinsen, K. (2001). Huset og sangen, gråten og skammen. Rom og arkitektur som ivaretaker av menneskets verdighet. I T. Wyller (red.), *Skam: Perspektiver på skam, ære og skamløshet i det moderne* (s. 167–190). Bergen: Fagbokforlaget. [The house and the song, the tears and the shame: Space and architecture as caretakers of human dignity. In T. Wyller (Ed.), *Shame: Perspectives on shame, honor and shamelessness in modernity* (pp. 167–190). Bergen: Fagbokforlaget.]

Martinsen, K. (2002). Rikke Nissen. Kjærlighetsgjerningen og sykestuen. I R. Birkelund (red.), *Omsorg, kald og kamp. Personer og ideer i sygeplejens historie* (s. 305–328). København: Munksgaard forlag. [The loving act and the room for the sick. In R. Birkelund (Ed.), *Care, vocation and love in action and the sick-room. Persons and ideas in nursing history* (pp. 305–328). Copenhagen: Munksgaard.]

Martinsen, K. (2002). Rommets tid, den sykes tid, pleiens tid. I I. T. Bjørk, S. Helseth, & F. Nortvedt (red.), *Møte mellom pasient og sykepleier* (s. 250–271). Oslo: Gyldendal Akademisk. [The room's time, the ill person's time, nursing time. In I. T. Bjørk, S. Helseth, & F. Nortvedt (Eds.), *The meeting between patient and nurse* (pp. 250–271). Oslo: Gyldendal Akademisk.]

Martinsen, K. (2003). Disiplin og rommelighet. I K. Martinsen & T. Wyller (red.), *Etikk, disiplin og dannelse. Elisabeth Hagemanns etikkbok—Nye lesinger* (s. 51–85). Oslo: Gyldendal Akademisk. [Discipline and spaciousness. In K. Martinsen & T. Wyller (Eds.), *Ethics, discipline and refinement. Elizabeth Hagemann's ethics book—New readings* (pp. 51–85). Oslo: Gyldendal Akademisk.]

Martinsen, K. (2005). Å bo på sykehuset og erfare arkitektur. I K. Larsen (red.), *Arkitektur, kropp og læring.* København: Reitzels forlag. [To dwell in hospitals and experience architecture. In K. Larsen (Ed.), *Architecture, body and learning.* Copenhagen: Reitzels forlag.]

Martinsen, K. (2005). Sårbarheten og omveiene. Løgstrup og sykepleien. I D. Bugge, P. Bøvadt and P. Sørensen (red.). *Løgstrups mange ansikter* (s. 255–270). Fredriksberg: Anis. [Vulnerability and detours. Løgstrup and nursing. In D. Bugge, P. Bøvadt, and P. Sørensen (Eds.). *Løgstrup's many faces* (pp. 255–270). Fredriksberg: Anis.]

Martinsen, K. (2007). Angår du meg? Etisk fordring og disiplinert godhet. I H. Alvsvåg & O. Førland (red.). *Engasjement og læring* (s. 315–344). Oslo: Akribe. [Do you concern me? Ethical demand and disciplined goodness. In H. Alvsvåg & O. Førland (Eds.), *Commitment and learning* (pp 315–344) Oslo: Akribe.]

Martinsen, K., Beedholm, K., & Fredriksen, K. (2007). Metadebatten der forsvandt. I K. Fredriksen, K. Lomborg, & U. Zeitler (red.). *Perspektiver på forskning* (s. 43–55). Århus: JCVU udviklingsinitiativet for sygeplejerskeuddannelsen.

[The Meta debate that disappeared. In K. Fredriksen, K. Lomborg, & U. Zeitler (Eds.), *Perspectives on research* (pp. 43–55). Århus: JCVU udviklingsinitiativet for sygeplejerskeuddannelsen.]

Martinsen, K. (2008). Modernitet, avtrylling og skam. En måte å lese vestens medisin på i det moderne. In K. A. Petersen and M. Høyen (red.), *At sette spor på en vandring fra Aquinas til Bordieu—æresbog til Staf Callewaert.* Forlag@hexis.dk [Modernity, disenchantment and shame. A way of reading Western medicine in the modern. In K. A. Petersen & M. Høyen (Eds.), *Leaving a trail on the way from Aquinas to Bordieu—Honorary volume for Staf Callewaert.* Forlag@hexis.dk.]

Martinsen, K. (2012). Skammens to sider [The two faces of shame]. I Thorsen, R., Mæhre, K. S., & Martinsen, K. (red.), *Fortellinger om etikk.* Bergen: Fagbokforlaget. [The two faces of shame. In Thorsen, R., Mæhre, K. S., & Martinsen, K. (Eds.), *Narratives on ethics.* Bergen: Fagbok forlaget.]

Martinsen, K. (2012). Etikk i sykepleien—mellom spontanitet og ettertanke. I M. Pahuus & P. K. Telleus (red.), *Antologi—Anvendt etikk—problemer og arbejdsområder.* Aalborg: Aalborg Universitetsforlag. [Ethics in Nursing—between spontaneity and reflection. In M. Pahuus & P. K. Telleus (Eds.), *Anthology—Applied ethics—Problems and areas of application.* Aalborg: Aalborg University Press.]

Martinsen, K. (2014). «Vil du meg noe?» Om sårbarhet og travelhet i helsevesenets rom. I H. Alvsvåg, O. Førland & F. Jacobsen (red.), *Rom for omsorg?* (s. 225–245). Bergen: Fagbokforlaget. ["Do you want something of me?" On vulnerability and busyness in the health care rooms. In H. Alvsvåg, O. Førland, & F. Jacobsen (Eds.), *Room for caring?* (pp. 225–245). Bergen: Fagbok forlaget.]

Journal Articles

Eriksson, K., & Martinsen, K. (2012). The hidden and forgotten evidence. *Scandinavian Journal of Caring Sciences, 26*(4), 625–626.

Martinsen, K. (1981). Omsorgens filosofi og omsorg i praksis. *Sykepleien, 8*(69), 4–10. [The philosophy of caring—And the practice. *Nursing, 8*(69), 4–10.]

Martinsen, K. (1982). Den tvetydige veldedigheten. *Sosiologi i dag,* temanummer *Kvinner og omsorgsarbeid, 1*(12), 29–41. [The ambiguity of charity. *Sociology, 1*(12), 29–41.]

Martinsen, K. (1982). Diakonissene—De første faglærte sykepleiere. *Sykepleien, 7*(70), 6–9. [The deaconesses—The first professionally trained nurses. *Nursing, 7*(70), 6–9.]

Martinsen, K. (1985). Kallsarbeidere og yrkeskvinner: Diakonissene—Våre første sykepleiere. *Forskningsnytt,* temanummer: *Kvinner og arbeid, 1,* 18–23. [Women with a calling and a profession: The deaconesses—Our first nurses. *News in Science, 1,* 18–23.]

Martinsen, K. (1985). Sykepleiertradisjonen—Et nødvendig korrektiv til dagens sykepleieforskning. *Sykepleien, 15*(73), 6–14. [The nursing tradition—a necessary corrective to today's nursing science. *Nursing, 15*(73), 6–14.]

Martinsen, K. (1986). Omsorg og profesjonalisering—Med fagutviklingen i sykepleien som eksempel. *Nytt om kvinneforskning, 2*(10), 21–32. [Care and professionalism—An example from the development in nursing. *News in Woman Science, 2*(10), 21–32.]

Martinsen, K. (1987). Arbeidsdeling—Kjønn og makt. *Sykepleien, 1*(74), 18–23. [Division of labor—Gender and power. *Nursing, 1*(74), 18–23.]

Martinsen, K. (1987). Endret kunnskapsideal og to pleiegrupper. *Sykepleien, 4*(74), 20–25. [A changing paradigm and two types of nurses. *Nursing, 4*(74), 20–25.]

Martinsen, K. (1987). Helsepolitiske problemer og helsepolitisk tenkning bak sykehusloven av 1969. *Historisk tidsskrift, 3*(66), 357–372. [Health policy problems and health policy thinking underlying the new hospital law. *History, 3*(66), 357–372.]

Martinsen, K. (1987). Ledelse og omsorgsrasjonalitet—Gir patriarkatbegrepet innsikt? *Sykepleien, 1*(74), 18–23. [Management and caring rationality—Does the concept of patriarchate give insight? *Nursing, 1*(74), 18–23.]

Martinsen, K. (1987). Legers interesse for svangerskapet—En del av den perinatale omsorg. Tidsrommet ca. 1890-1940. *Historisk tidsskrift, 3*(66), 373–390. [Doctors' interests in pregnancy—a part of perinatal care. *History, 3*(66), 373–390.]

Martinsen, K. (1987). Norsk Sykepleierskeforbund på barrikadene for utdanning fra første stund. *Sykepleien, 3*(74), 6–12. [The Norwegian Nursing Association on the barricades from day one. *Nursing, 3*(74), 6–12.]

Martinsen, K. (1988). Ansvar og solidaritet. En moralfilosofisk og sosialpolitisk forståelse av omsorg. *Sykepleien, 12*(75), 17–21. [Responsibility and solidarity. A moral-philosophical and sociopolitical understanding of caring. *Nursing, 12*(75), 17–21.]

Martinsen, K. (1988). Etikk og omsorgsmoral. *Sykepleien, 13*(75), 16–20. [Ethics and the moral practice of caring. *Nursing, 13*(75), 16–20.]

Martinsen, K. (1990). Diakoni er fellesskap og samhørighet. *Under Ulriken, 5*(30), 6–10. [Diaconi is community and fellowship. *Under Ulrikken, 5*(30), 6–10.]

Martinsen, K. (1991). Omsorg og makt, ord og kropp i sykepleien. *Sykepleien, 2*(78), 2–11, 29. [Caring and power, word and body in nursing profession. *Nursing, 2*(78), 2–11, 29.]

Martinsen, K. (1991). Under kjærlig forskning. Fenomenologiens åpning for den levde erfaring i sykepleien. *Perspektiv—Sygeplejersken, 36*(91), 4–15. [Compassionate research. Phenomenology opening up for lived experience in nursing. *Perspective—Nursing* (Danish), *36*(91), 4–15.]

Martinsen, K. (1993). Grunnforskning—Trofast og troløs forskning—Noen fenomenologiske overveielser. *Tidsskrift for Sygeplejeforskning, 1*(9), 7–28. [Basic research—Faithful and faithless research—Some phenomenological considerations. *Nursing Research* (Danish), *1*(9), 7–28.]

Martinsen, K. (1997). De etiske fortellinger. *Omsorg, 1*(14), 58–63. [The ethical narratives. *Caring, 1*(14), 58–63.]

Martinsen, K. (1997). Kallet—Kan vi være det foruten? *Tidsskrift for sygeplejeforskning, 2*(13), 9–41. [The vocation—Can we do without it? *Nursing Science, 2*(13), 9–41.]

Martinsen, K. (1998). Det fremmede og vedkommende (I). *Klinisk Sygepleje, 1*(12), 13–19. [Strangeness and relevance (I). *Clinical Nursing, 1*(12), 13–19.]

Martinsen, K. (1998). Det fremmede og vedkommende (II). *Klinisk Sygepleje, 1-2*(12), 78–84. [Strangeness and relevance (II). *Clinical Nursing, 2*(12), 78–84.]

Martinsen, K. (2001). Er det mørketid for filosofien? Et svar til Marit Kirkevold. *Tidsskrift for sygeplejeforskning (dansk), 1*(17), 19–23. [Is philosophy in shadow? A reply to Marit Kirkevold. *Nursing Science* (Danish), *1*(17), 19–23.]

Martinsen, K. (2002). Livsfilosofiske betraktninger. I *Diakoninytt, 3*(118), 8–12. [Reflections on the philosophy of life. *Deaconry News, 3*(118), 8–12.]

Martinsen, K. (2002). Samtalen, kommunikasjonen og sakligheten i omsorgsyrkene. *Omsorg, 1*(19), 14–22. [Conversation, communication and professionality in the caring professions. *Caring, 1*(19), 14–22.]

Martinsen, K. (2003). Talens åpenhet og evidens—Dialog med Jens Bydam. *Klinisk Sygepleje, 4*(17), 3–46. [The openness of speech and evidence—Dialogue with Jens Bydam. *Clinical Nursing, 4*(17), 36–46.]

Martinsen, K. (2004). Skjønn—Språk og distanse: dialog med Jens Bydam. *Klinisk Sygepleje, 2*(18), 50–56. [Discernment—Language and distance: Dialogue with Jens Bydam. *Clinical Nursing, 2*(18), 50–56.]

Martinsen, K. (2008). Innfallet—og dets betydning i liv og arbeid. Metafysisk inspirerte overveielser over innfallets natur og måter å vise seg på. *Klinisk Sygepleje, 1*(22). [The Innfall (impulse)—and its significance in life and work. Metaphysically inspired reflections on the nature of the Innfall and its ways of showing itself. *Clinical Nursing, 1*(22).]

Martinsen, K. (2012). Filosofi og fortellinger om sårbarhet. *Klinisk Sygepleje, 2*(26), 30–37. [Philosophy and narratives of vulnerability. *Clinical Nursing, 2*(26), 30–37.]

Martinsen, K. (2013). Stedet. *Omsorg, 4*(30), 61–67. [The Place, *Caring, 4*(30), 61–67.]

Martinsen, K. (2015). Sykeværelset – sett fra sengen. *Klinisk Sygepleje, 4*(29), 4–19. [The patient's room—seen from the bed. *Clinical Nursing, 4*(29), 4–19.]

Martinsen, K. (2016). The articulation of impressions. An interview with Kari Martinsen. Interviewed by Christine Øye and Tone Elin Mekki, translated by Hilde Haaland-Kramer. *International Practice Development Journal, 6*(1), 1–6.

Martinsen, K., & Wærness, K. (1976). Sykepleierrollen—En undertrykt kvinnerolle i helsesektoren (I). *Sykepleien, 4*(64), 220–224. [The nursing role—An oppressed female role in National Health Service. *Nursing, 4*(64), 220–224.]

Martinsen, K., & Wærness, K. (1976). Sykepleierrollen—En undertrykt kvinnerolle i Helsesektoren (II). *Sykepleien, 5*(64), 274–275, 281–282. [The nursing role—An oppressed female role in National Health Service. *Nursing, 5*(64), 274–275, 281–282.]

Martinsen, K., & Wærness, K. (1980). Klientomsorg og profesjonalisering. *Sykepleien, 4*(68), 12–14. [Client care and the professionalization. *Nursing, 4*(68), 12–14.]

Sviland, R., Martinsen, K., & Råheim, M. (2007). Hvis ikke kropp og psyke—hva da? *Fysioterapeuten, 12*, 23–28. [If not body, not psyche—what then? *The Physiotherapeut, 12*, 23–28.]

Sviland, R., Martinsen, K., & Råheim, M. (2014). To be held and to hold one's own: Narratives of embodied transformation in the treatment of long lasting musculoskeletal problems. *Medicine, Health Care and Philosophy, 17*(4), 609–624.

Sviland, R., Råheim, M., & Martinsen, K. (2009). Å komme til seg selv – i bevegelse, sansing og forståelse. *Matrix, 2*, 257–275. [Coming to one's senses—In moving, sensing, understanding. *Matrix, 2*, 257–275.]

Sviland, R., Råheim, M., & Martinsen, K. (2010). Språk—uttrykk for inntrykk. *Matrix, 2*, 132–156. [Language—Expressing impressions. *Matrix, 2*, 132–156.]

Sviland, R., Råheim, M., & Martinsen, K. (2012). Touched in sensation—Moved by respiration. Embodied narrative identity—A treatment process. *Scandinavian Journal of Caring Sciences, 26*(4), 811–819.

Secondary Sources

Alvsvåg, H., Bergland Å., & Førland, O. (red.). (2013). Nødvendige omveier. En vitenskapelig antologi til Kari Martinsens 70-årsdag. Oslo: Cappelen Damm Akademisk. [Necessary De tours. A scientific anthology for Kari Martinsen on her 70th birthday. Oslo: Cappelen Damm Akademisk.]

Alvsvåg, H., & Gjengedal, E. (red.). (2000). *Omsorgstenkning. En innføring i Kari Martinsens forfatterskap*. Bergen: Fagbokforlaget. [*Caring thought: An introduction to the writings of Kari Martinsen.* Bergen: Fagbok forlaget.]

Austgard, K. (2010). Omsorgsfilosofi i praksis. Å tenke med filosofen Kari Martinsen i sykepleien. Oslo: Cappelen Akademisk Forlag. [*Philosophy of caring in practice: Thinking with philosopher Kari Martinsen in nursing.* Oslo: Cappelen Akademisk Forlag.]

Boge, J. (2011). *Kroppsvask i sjukepleie. Eit politisk og historisk perspektiv*. [*Bathing the patient. A political and historical perspective*]. Oslo: Akribe.

Forss, A. Ceci, C., & Drummond (Eds.). (2013). *Philosophy of nursing. 5 Questions*. Copenhagen Automatic Press/VIP.

Jørgensen, B. B., & Lyngaa, J. (red.). (2008). *Sygeplejeleksikon*. København: Munksgaard. [*Encyclopedia of nursing.* Copenhagen: Munksgaard.]

Mathisen, J. (2006). *Sykepleiehistorie [History of nursing]*. Oslo: Gyldendal Akademisk.

Mekki, T. E., & Tollefsen, S. (2000). *På terskelen. Introduksjon til sykepleie som fag og yrke*. Oslo: Akribe. [*On the threshold: An introduction to nursing as discipline and profession.* Oslo: Akribe.]

Olsen, R. (1998). *Klok av erfaring? Om sansing og opp-merksomhet, kunnskap og refleksjon i praktisk sykepleie*. Oslo: Tano Aschehoug. [*Wise with experience? On sensation and attention, knowledge and reflection in practical nursing.* Oslo: Tano Aschehoug.]

Overgaard, A. E. (2003). *Åndelig omsorg—En lærebog. Kari Martinsen, Katie Eriksson og Joyce Travelbee i nytt lys*. København: Nyt Nordisk Forlag Arnold Busck. [*Spiritual care—A textbook. Kari Martinsen, Katie Eriksson and Joyce Travelbee in a new light.* Copenhagen: Nyt Nordisk Forlag Arnold Busck.]

Walstad, P. B. (2006). *Dannelse og Duelighed for livet. Dannelse og yrkesutdanning i den grundtvigske tradisjon*. Trondheim: Norges teknisk-naturvitenskapelige universitet. Doctoral dissertation 2006:88. [*Education and capability for life. Education and professional training in the Grundtvigian tradition.* Trondheim: Norges teknisk-naturvitenskapelige universitet, NTNU Doctoral Dissertations 2006:88.]

11

Theory of Caritative Caring

Unni Å. Lindström, Lisbet Lindholm Nyström, and Joan E. Zetterlund

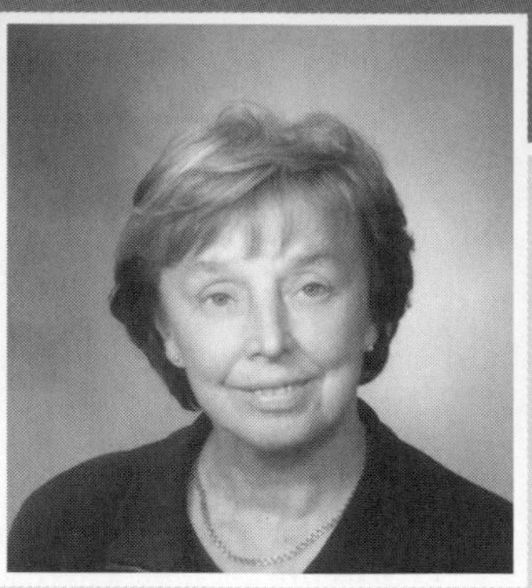

Katie Eriksson (1943–Present)

"Caritative caring means that we take 'caritas' into use when caring for the human being in health and suffering. . . . Caritative caring is a manifestation of the love that 'just exists.' . . . Caring communion, true caring, occurs when the one caring in a spirit of caritas alleviates the suffering of the patient."

(Eriksson, 1992c, pp. 204, 207)

CREDENTIALS AND BACKGROUND OF THE THEORIST

Katie Eriksson is one of the pioneers of caring science in the Nordic countries. When she started her career 30 years ago, she had to open the way for a new science. Those who followed her work and progress in Finland have noticed her ability from the beginning to design caring science as a discipline, while bringing to life the abstract substance of caring.

Eriksson was born on November 18, 1943, in Jakobstad, Finland. She belongs to the Finland-Swedish minority in Finland, and her native language is Swedish. She is a 1965 graduate of the Helsinki Swedish School of Nursing, and in 1967, she completed her public health nursing specialty education there. She graduated in 1970 from the nursing teacher education program at Helsinki Finnish School of Nursing. She continued her academic studies at the University of Helsinki, where she received her MA degree in philosophy in 1974 and her licentiate degree in 1976; she defended her doctoral dissertation in pedagogy *(The Patient Care Process—An Approach to Curriculum Construction Within Nursing Education: The Development of a Model for the Patient Care Process and an Approach for Curriculum Development Based on the Process of Patient Care)* in 1982 (Eriksson, 1974, 1976, 1981). In 1984 Eriksson was appointed Docent of Caring Science (part time) at University of Kuopio, the first docentship in caring science in the Nordic countries. She was appointed Professor of Caring Science at Åbo Akademi University in 1992. Between 1993 and 1999, she held a professorship in caring science at the University of Helsinki, Faculty of Medicine, where she has been a docent since 2001. Since 1996 she has served as Director of Nursing at Helsinki University Central Hospital, with responsibilities for research and development of caring science in connection with her professorship at Åbo Akademi University.

In the late 1960s and early 1970s, Eriksson worked in various fields of nursing practice and continued her studies. Her main area of work has been teaching and research. Since the 1970s, Eriksson has systematically deepened her thoughts about caring, partly through development of an ideal model for caring that formed the basis for the caritative caring theory, and partly through the development of an autonomous, humanistically oriented caring science. Eriksson, one of the few caring science researchers in the Nordic countries, is a forerunner of basic research in caring science.

Eriksson's scientific career and professional experience comprise two periods: the years 1970–1986 at the Helsinki Swedish School of Nursing, and the period from 1986, when she founded the Department of Caring Science at Åbo Akademi University, which she has directed since 1987.

In 1972, after teaching for 2 years at the nursing education unit at the Helsinki Swedish School of Nursing, Eriksson was assigned to start and develop an educational program to prepare nurse educators at that institution. Such a program taught in the Swedish language had not existed in Finland. This education program, in collaboration with the University of Helsinki, was the beginning of caring science didactics. Under Eriksson's leadership, Helsinki Swedish School of Nursing developed a leading educational program in caring science and nursing, the forerunner of education based on caring science and integration of research in education. Eriksson was in charge of the program for 2 years, until she became dean at the Helsinki Swedish School of Nursing in 1974. She remained the dean until 1986, when she was nominated to start academic education and research at Åbo Akademi University.

Toward the end of the 1980s, nursing science became a university subject in Finland, and professorial chairs were established at four Finnish universities and at Åbo Akademi University, the Finland-Swedish university. In 1986 Eriksson was asked to plan an education and research program in caring science at Åbo Akademi University's Faculty of Education in Vaasa, Finland. A fully developed education program for health care, with three focus options and a research program for caring science, became known as the Department of Caring Science in 1987. It was an autonomous department within the Faculty of Education of Åbo Akademi University until 1992, when a Faculty of Social and Caring Sciences was founded. Eriksson developed an academic education for Master's and Doctoral degrees in Caring Science. The doctoral program started in 1987 under Eriksson's direction, and many doctoral dissertations have since been published.

With her staff and researchers, Eriksson further developed the caritative theory of caring and caring science as a leading academic discipline in the Nordic countries. In addition to her work with teaching, research, and supervision, Eriksson has been the dean of the Department of Caring Science with a central task of developing Nordic and international contacts within caring science.

Eriksson has been a very popular guest and keynote speaker in Finland, in the Nordic countries, and at various international congresses. In 1977 she was guest speaker at the Symposium of Medical and Nursing Education in Istanbul, Turkey; in 1978 she participated in the Foundation of Medical Care teacher education in Reykjavik, Iceland; in 1982 she presented her nursing care didactic model at the First Open Conference of the Workgroup of European Nurse-Researchers in Uppsala, Sweden; and for several years, she participated in education and advanced education of nurses at the Statens Utdanningscenter for Helsopersonell in Oslo, Norway. In 1988 Eriksson taught "Basic Research in Nursing Care Science" at the University in Bergen, Norway, and "Nursing Care Science's Theory of Science and Research" at Umeå University in Sweden. She consulted at many educational institutions in Sweden; she has been a regular lecturer at Nordiska Hälsovårdsskolan in Gothenburg, Sweden. In 1991 she was a guest speaker at the 13th International Association for Human Caring (IAHC) Conference in Rochester, New York; in 1992 she presented her theory at the 14th IAHC Conference in Melbourne, Australia; and in 1993 she was the keynote speaker at the 15th IAHC Conference, Caring as Healing: Renewal Through Hope, in Portland, Oregon (Eriksson, 1994b).

Eriksson has been a yearly keynote speaker at the annual congresses for nurse managers and, since 1996, at the annual caring science symposia in Helsinki, Finland. In public dialogues with Kari Martinsen from Norway, Eriksson discussed basic questions about caring and caring science, some of which have been published (Martinsen, 1996; Martinsen & Eriksson, 2009).

Eriksson worked as a leader of many symposia: the 1975 Nordic Symposium about the Nursing Care Process (the first Nordic Nursing Care Science Symposium in Finland); the 1982 Symposium in Basic Research in Nursing Care Science; the 1985 Nordic Symposium in Nursing Care Science; the 1989 Nordic Humanistic Caring Symposium; the 1991 Nordic Caring Science Conference, "Caritas & Passio in Vaasa, Finland"; and the 1993 Nordic Caring Science Conference, "To Care or Not to Care—The Key Question" in Vaasa, Finland.

Eriksson's caritative theory of caring came into clearer focus internationally in 1997, when the IAHC for the first time arranged its conference in a European country. The Department of Caring Science served as the host of this conference, which was arranged in Helsinki, Finland, with the topic, "Human Caring: The Primacy of Love and Existential Suffering."

Eriksson is a member of editorial committees for international journals in nursing and caring science. She has been invited to many universities in Finland and other Nordic countries as a faculty opponent for doctoral students and an expert consultant in her field. She is an advisor for her own research students and for research students at Kuopio and Helsinki Universities, where she is an associate professor (docent). Eriksson served as chairperson of the Nordic Academy of Caring Science from 1999 to 2002.

Eriksson has produced an extensive list of textbooks, scientific reports, professional journal articles, and short papers. Her publications started in the 1970s and include about 400 titles. Some of her publications have been translated into other languages, mainly into Finnish. *Vårdandets Idé (The Idea of Caring)* has been published in Braille. Her first English translation, The *Suffering Human Being (Den Lidande Människan),* was published in 2006 by Nordic Studies Press in Chicago.

Eriksson has received many awards and honors for her professional and academic accomplishments. In 1975 she was nominated to receive the 3M–International Council of Nurses (ICN) Nursing Fellowship Award; in 1987 she received the Sophie Mannerheim Medal of the Swedish Nursing Association; and in 1998 she received the Caring Science Gold Mark for academic nursing care at Helsinki University Central Hospital and also received an Honorary Doctorate in Public Health from the Nordic School of Public Health in Gothenburg, Sweden. Other awards include the 2001 Åland Islands Medal for caring science and the 2003 Topelius Medal, instituted by Åbo Akademi University for excellent research. In 2003 she was honored nationally as a Knight, First Class, of the Order of the White Rose of Finland.

THEORETICAL SOURCES

Since the 1970s, Eriksson's leading thoughts have been not only to develop the substance of caring, but also to develop caring science as an independent discipline (Eriksson, 1988). From the beginning, Eriksson went back to the Greek classics by Plato, Socrates, and Aristotle, for inspiration for the development of both the substance and the discipline of caring science (Eriksson, 1987b). From her basic idea of caring science as a humanistic science, she developed a metatheory that she refers to as "the theory of science for caring science" (Eriksson, 1988, 2001).

When developing caring science as an academic discipline, Eriksson's most important sources of inspiration besides Plato and Aristotle were Swedish theologian Anders Nygren (1972) and Hans-Georg Gadamer (1960/1994). Nygren and later Tage Kurtén (1987) provided her with support for her division of caring science into systematic and clinical caring science. Eriksson introduces Nygren's concepts of motive research, context of meaning, and basic motive, which give the discipline structure. The aim of motive research is to find the essential context, the leading idea of caring. Motive research applied to caring science shows the characteristics of caring (Eriksson, 1992c).

The basic motive in caring science and caring for Eriksson is caritas, which constitutes the leading idea and keeps the various elements together. It gives both the substance and the discipline of caring science a distinctive character. In development of the basic motive, St. Augustine (1957) and Søren Kierkegaard (1843/1943) became important sources. In further development of the discipline, Eriksson's thinking was influenced by sources such as Thomas Kuhn (1971) and Karl Popper (1997), and later by American philosopher Susan Langer (1942) and Finnish philosophers Eino Kaila (1939) and Georg von Wright (1986), all of whom support the human science idea that science cannot exist without values.

For many years, Eriksson collaborated with Håkan Törnebohm (1978), holder of the first Nordic professorial chair in the theory of science at the University of Gothenburg, Sweden. Törnebohm's research in and development of paradigms related to various scientific cultures inspired Eriksson (Eriksson, 1989; Lindström, 1992).

The thought that concepts have both meaning and substance has been prominent in Eriksson's scientific work. This appears through a systematic analysis of fundamental concepts with the help of a semantic method of analysis rooted in the idea of hermeneutics, which professor Peep Koort (1975) developed. Koort was Eriksson's mentor and unmistakably the most important source of inspiration in her scientific conceptual work. Building on the foundation of his methodology, Eriksson subsequently developed a model for concept development that has been important to many researchers in their scientific work.

In her formulation of the caritas-based caring ethic, which Eriksson conceives as an ontological ethic, Emmanuel Lévinas' (1988) idea that ethics precedes ontology has been a guiding principle. Eriksson agrees especially with Lévinas' thought that the call to serve precedes dialogue, that ethics is always more important in relations with other human beings. The fundamental substance of ethics—caritas, love, and charity—is supported by Aristotle's (1993), Nygren's (1972), Kierkegaard's (1843/1943), and St. Augustine's (1957) ideas. In the formulation of caritative ethics, Eriksson was inspired by Kierkegaard's ideas of the innermost spirit of a human being as a synthesis of the eternal and temporal, and that acting ethically is to will absolutely or to will the eternal (Kierkegaard, 1843/1943). She stresses the importance of knowledge of history of ideas for the preservation of the whole of spiritual culture and finds support for this in Nikolaj Berdâev (1990), the Russian philosopher and historian. In intensifying the basic conception of the human being as body, soul, and spirit, Eriksson carries on an interesting dialogue with several theologians such as Gustaf Wingren (1960/1996), Antnio Barbosa da Silva (1993), and Tage Kurtén (1987), while developing the subdiscipline she refers to as *caring theology.* Perhaps the most prominent feature of Eriksson's thinking has been her clear formulation of the ontological, epistemological, and ethical basic assumptions with regard to the discipline of caring science.

MAJOR CONCEPTS & DEFINITIONS

Caritas

Caritas means "love and charity." In caritas, eros and agapé are united, and caritas is by nature unconditional love. Caritas, which is the fundamental motive of caring science, also constitutes the motive for all caring. It means that caring is an endeavor to mediate faith, hope, and love through tending, playing, and learning.

Caring Communion

Caring communion constitutes the context of the meaning of caring and is the structure that determines caring reality. Caring gets its distinctive character through caring communion (Eriksson, 1990). It is a form of intimate connection that characterizes caring. Caring communion requires meeting in time and space, an absolute, lasting presence (Eriksson, 1992c). Caring communion is characterized by intensity and vitality, and by warmth, closeness, rest, respect, honesty, and tolerance. It cannot be taken for granted but presupposes a conscious effort to be with the other. Caring communion is seen as the source of strength and meaning in caring. Eriksson (1990) writes in *Pro Caritate,* referring to Lévinas:

> *"Entering into communion implies creating opportunities for the other—to be able to step out of the enclosure of his/her own identity, out of that which belongs to one towards that which does not belong to one and is nevertheless one's own—it is one of the deepest forms of communion." (pp. 28–29)*

Joining in a communion means creating possibilities for the other. Lévinas suggests that considering someone as one's own son implies a relationship "beyond the possible" (1985, p. 71; 1988). In this relationship, the individual perceives the other person's possibilities as if they were his or her own. This requires the ability to move toward that which is no longer one's own but which belongs to oneself. It is one of the deepest forms of communion (Eriksson, 1992b). Caring communion is what unites and ties together and gives caring its significance (Eriksson, 1992a).

The Act of Caring

The **act of caring** contains the caring elements (faith, hope, love, tending, playing, and learning), involves the categories of *infinity* and *eternity,* and invites to deep communion. The act of caring is the art of making something very special out of something less special.

Caritative Caring Ethics

Caritative caring ethics comprises the ethics of caring, the core of which is determined by the caritas motive. Eriksson makes a distinction between caring ethics and nursing ethics. She also defines the foundations of ethics in care and its essential substance. Caring ethics deals with the basic relationship between the patient and the nurse—the way in which the nurse meets the patient in an ethical sense. It is about the approach the nurse has toward the patient. Nursing ethics deals with the ethical principles and rules that guide one's work or decisions. Caring ethics is the core of nursing ethics. The foundations of caritative ethics can be found not only in history, but also in the dividing line between theological and human ethics in general. Eriksson has been influenced by Nygren's (1966) human ethics and Lévinas' (1988) "face ethics," among others. Ethical caring is what nurses actually make explicit through their approach and the things they do for the patient in practice. An approach that is based on ethics in care means that nurses, without prejudice, see the human being with respect, and that they confirm his or her absolute dignity. It also means a willingness to sacrifice something of oneself. The ethical categories that emerge as basic in caritative caring ethics are human dignity, caring communion, invitation, responsibility, good and evil, and virtue and obligation. In an ethical act, good is brought out through ethical actions (Eriksson, 1995, 2003).

Dignity

Dignity constitutes one of the basic concepts of caritative caring ethics. Human dignity is partly absolute dignity, partly relative dignity. Absolute dignity is granted the human being through creation, whereas relative dignity is influenced and formed through culture and external contexts. A human being's absolute dignity involves the right to be confirmed as a unique human being (Eriksson, 1988, 1995, 1997a).

Invitation

Invitation refers to the act that occurs when the carer welcomes the patient to the caring communion. The concept of invitation finds room for a place where the human being is allowed to rest, a place that breathes genuine hospitality, and where the patient's appeal for charity meets with a response (Eriksson, 1995; Eriksson & Lindström, 2000).

Suffering

Suffering is an ontological concept described as a human being's struggle between good and evil in a state of becoming. Suffering implies in some sense dying away from

Continued

MAJOR CONCEPTS & DEFINITIONS—cont'd

something, and through reconciliation, the wholeness of body, soul, and spirit is re-created, when the human being's holiness and dignity appear. Suffering is a unique, isolated total experience and is not synonymous with pain (Eriksson, 1984, 1993).

Suffering Related to Illness, to Care, and to Life

There are three different forms of suffering: **suffering related to illness, to care, and to life**. Suffering related to illness is experienced in connection with illness and treatment. When the patient is exposed to suffering caused by care or absence of caring, the patient experiences suffering related to care, which is always a violation of the patient's dignity. Not to be taken seriously, not to be welcome, being blamed, and being subjected to the exercise of power are various forms of suffering related to care. In the situation of being a patient, the entire life of a human being may be experienced as suffering related to life (Eriksson, 1993, 1994a; Lindholm & Eriksson, 1993).

The Suffering Human Being

The **suffering human being** is the concept that Eriksson uses to describe the patient. The patient refers to the concept of *patiens* (Latin), which means "suffering." The patient is a suffering human being, or a human being who suffers and patiently endures (Eriksson, 1994a; Eriksson & Herberts, 1992).

Reconciliation

Reconciliation refers to the drama of suffering. Human beings who suffer want to be confirmed in their suffering and be given time and space to suffer and reach reconciliation. Reconciliation implies a change through which a new wholeness is formed of the life the human being has lost in suffering. In reconciliation, the importance of sacrifice emerges (Eriksson, 1994a). Having achieved reconciliation implies living with an imperfection with regard to oneself and others but seeing a way forward and meaning in one's suffering. Reconciliation is a prerequisite of caritas (Eriksson, 1990).

Caring Culture

Caring culture is the concept that Eriksson (1987b) uses instead of *environment*. It characterizes the total caring reality and is based on cultural elements such as traditions, rituals, and basic values. Caring culture transmits an inner order of value preferences or ethos, and the different constructions of culture have their basis in the changes of value that ethos undergoes. If communion arises based on the ethos, the culture becomes inviting. Respect for the human being, his or her dignity and holiness, forms the goal of communion and participation in a caring culture. The origin of the concept of culture is to be found in such dimensions as reverence, tending, cultivating, and caring; these dimensions are central to the basic motive of preserving and developing a caring culture (Eriksson, 1987b; Eriksson & Lindström, 2003).

USE OF EMPIRICAL EVIDENCE

From the beginning of developing her theory, Eriksson established it in empiricism by systematically employing a hermeneutical and hypothetical deductive approach. In conformity with a human science and hermeneutical way of thinking, Eriksson developed a caring science concept of evidence (Eriksson, Nordman, & Myllymäki, 1999). Her main argument for this is that the concept of evidence in natural science is too narrow to capture and reach the depth of the complex caring reality. Her concept of evidence is derived from Gadamer's concept of truth (Gadamer, 1960/1994), which encompasses the true, the beautiful, and the good. She points out, in accordance with Gadamer, that evidence cannot be connected solely with a method and empirical data. Evidence in a human science perspective contains two aspects: a conceptual, logical one, which she calls *ontological*, and an empirical one, each presupposing the other. The evidence concept developed by Eriksson has been shown to be empirically evident when tested in two comprehensive empirical studies in which the idea was to develop evidence-based caring cultures in seven caring units in the Hospital District of Helsinki and Uusimaa (Eriksson & Nordman, 2004). A further development of evidence resulted in caring scientific evidence concept and theory (Martinsen & Eriksson, 2009).

During the 1970s, Eriksson initially developed a nursing care process model (Eriksson, 1974), which later, in her doctoral dissertation (1981), was formulated as a theory. Since then, Eriksson, step by step, has deepened her conceptual and logical understanding of the basic concepts and phenomena that have emerged from the theory. She has tested their validity in empirical contexts, in which the concepts have assumed contextual and pragmatic attributes (Kärkkäinen & Eriksson, 2004). This logical way of working, a constant movement between logical and empirical evidence, has been summarized by Eriksson in her model of concept development (Eriksson, 1997b). The validity of this model has been tested in several doctoral dissertations since 1995 (Gustafsson,

2008; Hilli, 2007; Kasén, 2002; Lassenius, 2005; Lindwall, 2004; Nåden, 1998; Näsman, 2010; Rundqvist, 2004; Sivonen, 2000; von Post, 1999; Wallinvirta, 2011). She started more comprehensive systematic as well as clinical research programs on caring when she was appointed director of the Department of Caring Science at Åbo Akademi University. The 44 doctoral dissertations written at the Department of Caring Science between 1992 and 2012 in different ways test and validate her ideas and theory.

MAJOR ASSUMPTIONS

Eriksson distinguishes two kinds of major assumptions: axioms and theses. She regards axioms as fundamental truths in relation to the conception of the world; theses are fundamental statements concerning the general nature of caring science, and their validity is tested through basic research. Axioms and theses jointly constitute the ontology of caring science and therefore also are the foundation of its epistemology (Eriksson, 1988, 2001). The caritative theory of caring is based on the following axioms and theses, as modified and clarified from Eriksson's basic assumptions with her approval (Eriksson, 2002). The axioms are as follows:

- The human being is fundamentally an entity of body, soul, and spirit.
- The human being is fundamentally a religious being.
- The human being is fundamentally holy. Human dignity means accepting the human obligation of serving with love, of existing for the sake of others.
- Communion is the basis for all humanity. Human beings are fundamentally interrelated to an abstract and/or concrete other in a communion.
- Caring is something human by nature, a call to serve in love.
- Suffering is an inseparable part of life. Suffering and health are each other's prerequisites.
- Health is more than the absence of illness. Health implies wholeness and holiness.
- The human being lives in a reality that is characterized by mystery, infinity, and eternity.

The theses are as follows:

- Ethos confers ultimate meaning on the caring context.
- The basic motive of caring is the *caritas* motive.
- The basic category of caring is suffering.
- Caring communion forms the context of meaning of caring and derives its origin from the ethos of love, responsibility, and sacrifice, namely, caritative ethics.
- Health means a movement in becoming, being, and doing while striving for wholeness and holiness, which is compatible with endurable suffering.
- Caring implies alleviation of suffering in charity, love, faith, and hope. Natural basic caring is expressed through tending, playing, and learning in a sustained caring relationship, which is asymmetrical by nature.

The Human Being

The conception of the human being in Eriksson's theory is based on the axiom that the human being is an entity of body, soul, and spirit (Eriksson, 1987b, 1988). She emphasizes that the human being is fundamentally a religious being, but all human beings have not recognized this dimension. The human being is fundamentally holy, and this axiom is related to the idea of human dignity, which means accepting the human obligation of serving with love and existing for the sake of others. Eriksson stresses the necessity of understanding the ontological context of the human being. The human being is seen as in constant becoming, constantly in change and therefore never in a state of full completion. He is understood in terms of the dual tendencies that exist within him, engaged in a continued struggle and living in a tension between being and nonbeing. Eriksson sees the human being's conditional freedom as a dimension of becoming. She links her thinking with Kierkegaard's (1843/1943) ideas of free choice and decision in the human being's various stages—esthetic, ethical, and religious stages—and she believes that the human being's power of transcendency is the foundation of real freedom. The dual tendency of the human being also emerges in his effort to be unique, while he simultaneously longs for belonging in a larger communion.

The human being is fundamentally dependent on communion; he is dependent on another, and it is in the relationship between a concrete other (human being) and an abstract other (some form of God) that the human being constitutes himself and his being (Eriksson, 1987b). The human being seeks a communion where he can give and receive love, experience faith and hope, and be aware that his existence here and now has meaning. According to Eriksson (1987a), the human being we meet in care is creative and imaginative, has desires and wishes, and is able to experience phenomena; therefore a description of the human being only in terms of his needs is insufficient. When the human being is entering the caring context, he or she becomes a patient in the original sense of the concept—a suffering human being (Eriksson, 1994a).

Nursing

Love and charity, or *caritas,* as the basic motive of caring has been a principal idea from Eriksson's early works (1987a, 1990, 2001). The *caritas* motive can be traced through semantics, anthropology, and the history of ideas (Eriksson, 1992c). The history of ideas indicates that the foundation of the caring professions through the ages has been an inclination to help and minister to those who are suffering (Lanara, 1981).

Caritas constitutes the motive for caring, and it is through the caritas motive that caring gets its deepest formulation. This motive, according to Eriksson, is also the core of all teaching and fostering growth in all forms of human relations. In caritas, the two basic forms of love—eros and agapá (Nygren, 1966)—are combined. When the two forms of love combine, generosity becomes a human being's attitude toward life, and joy is its form of expression. The motive of caritas becomes visible in a special ethical attitude in caring, or what Eriksson calls a *caritative outlook,* which she formulates and specifies in caritative caring ethics (Eriksson, 1995). Caritas constitutes the inner force that is connected with the mission to care. A carer beams forth what Eriksson calls *claritas,* or the strength and light of beauty.

Caring is something natural and original. Eriksson thinks that the substance of caring can be understood only by a search for its origin. This origin is in the foundation of the concept and in the idea of natural caring. The fundamentals of natural *caring* are constituted by the idea of motherliness, which implies cleansing and nourishing, and spontaneous and unconditional love.

Natural basic caring is expressed through tending, playing, and learning in a spirit of love, faith, and hope. The characteristics of tending are warmth, closeness, and touch; playing is an expression of exercise, testing, creativity, and imagination, and desires and wishes; learning is aimed at growth and change. To tend, play, and learn implies sharing, and sharing, Eriksson (1987b) says, is "presence with the human being, life and God" (p. 38). True care therefore is "not a form of behavior, not a feeling or state. It is to be there—it is the way, the spirit in which it is done, and this spirit is caritative" (Eriksson, 1998, p. 4). Eriksson explains that caring through the ages can be seen as various expressions of love and charity, with a view toward alleviating suffering and serving life and health. In her later texts, she stresses that caring also can be seen as a search for truth, goodness, beauty, and the eternal, and for what is permanent in caring, and making it visible or evident (Eriksson, 2002). Eriksson emphasizes that caritative caring relates to the innermost core of nursing. She distinguishes between caring nursing and *nursing care.* She means that nursing care is based on the nursing care process, and it represents good care only when it is based on the innermost core of caring. Caring nursing represents a kind of caring without prejudice that emphasizes the patient and his or her suffering and desires (Eriksson, 1994a).

The core of the caring relationship, between nurse and patient as described by Eriksson (1993), is an open invitation that contains affirmation that the other is always welcome. The constant open invitation is involved in what Eriksson (2003) today calls the *act of caring.* The act of caring expresses the innermost spirit of caring and recreates the basic motive of caritas. The caring act expresses the deepest holy element, the safeguarding of the individual patient's dignity. In the caring act, the patient is invited to a genuine sharing, a communion, to make the caring fundamentals alive and active (Eriksson, 1987b) (i.e., appropriated to the patient). The appropriation has the consequence of somehow restoring the human being and making him or her more genuinely human. In an ontological sense, the ultimate goal of caring cannot be health only; it reaches further and includes human life in its entirety. Because the mission of the human being is to serve, to exist for the sake of others, the ultimate purpose of caring is to bring the human being back to this mission (Eriksson, 1994a).

Environment

Eriksson uses the concept of ethos in accordance with Aristotle's (1935, 1997) idea that ethics is derived from ethos. In Eriksson's sense, the ethos of caring science, as well as that of caring, consists of the idea of love and charity and respect and honor of the holiness and dignity of the human being. Ethos is the sounding board of all caring. Ethos is ontology in which there is an "inner ought to," a target of caring "that has its own language and its own key" (Eriksson, 2003, p. 23). Good caring and true knowledge become visible through ethos. Ethos originally refers to home, or to the place where a human being feels at home. It symbolizes a human being's innermost space, where he appears in his nakedness (Lévinas, 1989). Ethos and ethics belong together, and in the caring culture, they become one (Eriksson, 2003). Eriksson believes that ethos means that we feel called to serve a particular task. This ethos she sees as the core of caring culture. Ethos, which forms the basic force in caring culture, reflects the prevailing priority of values through which the basic foundations of ethics and ethical actions appear.

At the beginning of the 1990s, when Eriksson reintroduced the idea of suffering as a basic category of caring, she returned to the fundamental historical conditions of all caring, the idea of charity as the basis of alleviating suffering (Eriksson, 1984, 1993, 1994a, 1997a). This meant a change in the view of caring reality to a focus on the suffering human being. Her starting point is that suffering is an inseparable part of human life, and that it has no distinct reason or definition. Suffering as such has no meaning, but a human being can ascribe meaning to it by becoming reconciled to it. Eriksson makes a distinction between endurable and unendurable suffering and thinks that an unendurable suffering paralyzes the human being, preventing him or her from growing, whereas endurable suffering is compatible with health. Every human being's suffering is enacted in a drama of suffering. Alleviating a human being's suffering implies being a coactor in the drama and confirming his or her suffering. A human being who suffers wants to have the suffering confirmed and be given time and space to become reconciled to it. The ultimate purpose of caring is to alleviate suffering. Eriksson has described three different forms: suffering related to illness, suffering related to care, and suffering related to life (Eriksson, 1993, 1994a, 1997a).

Health

Eriksson considers health in many of her earlier writings in accordance with an analysis of the concept in which she defines health as soundness, freshness, and well-being. The subjective dimension, or well-being, is emphasized strongly (Eriksson, 1976). In the current axiom of health, *health* implies being whole in body, soul, and spirit. *Health* means as a pure concept wholeness and holiness (Eriksson, 1984). In accordance with her view of the human being, Eriksson developed various premises regarding the substance and laws of health, which have been summed up in an ontological health model. She sees health as both movement and integration. The health premise is a movement comprising various partial premises: health as movement implies a change; a human being is being formed or destroyed, but never completely; health is movement between actual and potential; health is movement in time and space; health as movement is dependent on vital force and on vitality of body, soul, and spirit; the direction of this movement is determined by the human being's needs and desires; the will to find meaning, life, and love constitutes the source of energy of the movement; and health as movement strives toward a realization of one's potential (Eriksson, 1984).

In the ontological conception, health is conceived as a becoming, a movement toward a deeper wholeness and holiness. As a human being's inner health potential is touched, a movement occurs that becomes visible in the different dimensions of health as *doing, being,* and *becoming* with a wholeness that is unique to human beings (Eriksson, Bondas-Salonen, Fagerström et al., 1990). In doing, the person's thoughts concerning health are focused on healthy life habits and preventing illness; in being, the person strives for balance and harmony; in becoming, the human being becomes whole on a deeper level of integration.

THEORETICAL ASSERTIONS

Eriksson's fundamental theoretical assertions connect four levels of knowledge: the metatheoretical, the theoretical, the technological, and caring as art. The generation of theory takes place through dialectical movement between these levels, but here deduction constitutes the basic epistemological idea (Eriksson, 1981). The theory of science for caring science, which contains the fundamental epistemological, logical, and ethical standpoints, is formed on the metatheoretical level. Eriksson (1988), in accordance with Nygren (1972), sees the basic motive as the element that permeates the formation of knowledge at all levels and gives scientific knowledge its unique characteristics. A clearly formulated ontology constitutes the foundation of both the caritative caring theory and caring science as a discipline. The caritas motive, the ethos of love and charity, and the respect and reverence for human holiness and dignity, which determine the nature of caring, give the caritative caring theory its feature. This ethos, which encircles caring as science and as art, permeates caring culture and creates the preconditions for caring. The ethos is reflected in the process of nursing care, in the documentation, and in various care planning models.

Caring communion constitutes the context of meaning from which the concepts in the theory are to be understood. Human suffering forms the basic category of caring and summons the carer to true caring (i.e., serving in love and charity). In the act of caring, the suffering human being, or patient, is invited and welcomed to the caring communion, where the patient's suffering can be alleviated through the act of caring in the drama of suffering that is unique to every human being. Alleviation of suffering implies that the carer is a coactor in the drama, confirms the patient's suffering, and gives time and space to suffer until reconciliation is reached. Reconciliation is the ultimate aim of health or being and signifies a reestablishment of wholeness and holiness (Eriksson, 1997a).

LOGICAL FORM

Metatheory has always had a fundamental place in Eriksson's thinking, and her epistemological work is anchored in Aristotle's theory of knowledge (Aristotle, 1935). Searching for knowledge, which is intrinsically hermeneutic and takes place within the scope of an articulated theoretical perspective, is understood as a search for the original text in a historical-hermeneutic tradition, that which in the old hermeneutic sense represents truth (Gadamer, 1960/1994). To achieve the depth in the development of knowledge and theory Eriksson has consistently striven for, she has used various logical models for the hypothetical deductive method and hermeneutics guiding principles.

Eriksson stresses the importance of the logical form being created on the basis of the substance of caring (i.e., caritas), not on the basis of method. It is thus deduction combined with abduction that formed the guiding logic. The language, words, and concepts carry the content of meaning, and Eriksson stresses the necessity of choosing words, concepts, and language that correspond to human science.

In the dynamic change between the natural world and the world of science, there has constantly occurred a striving toward the source of the true, the beautiful, and the good—that which is evident. Eriksson (1999) shapes her theory of scientific thought, as reflection moves between patterns at different levels and interpretation is subject to the theoretical perspective. The movement takes place distinctly between doxa (empirical-perceptive knowledge) and episteme (rational-conceptual knowledge) and "the infinite." Movement thus takes place between the two basic epistemological categories of the theory of knowledge: perception and conception.

Eriksson applied three forms of inference—deduction, induction, and abduction or retroduction (Eriksson & Lindström, 1997)—that give the theory a logical external structure. The substance of her caring theory has moved simultaneously by abductive leaps (Eriksson & Lindström, 1997; Peirce, 1990), which sometimes created a new chaos but also carried Eriksson's thinking toward new discoveries. Through abduction, the ideal model for caritative caring was shaped, proceeding from historical and self-evident suppositions (Nygren, 1972). Eriksson in this way made use of old original texts that testify to caritative caring as her research material. Through induction and deduction, the validity of the theory has been tested.

Theory as conceived by Eriksson is in accordance with the Greek concept of theory, theoria, in the sense of seeing the beautiful and the good, participating in the common, and dedicating it to others (Gadamer, 2000, p. 49). Theory and practice are different aspects of the same core. The convincing force and potential of the whole theory are found in its innermost core, caritas, around which the generation of theory takes place. The caring substance is formed in a dialectical movement between the potential and the actual, the abstract general and the concrete individual. With the help of logical abstract thinking combined with the logic of the heart (Pascal, 1971), the theory of caritative caring becomes perceptible through the art of caring.

ACCEPTANCE BY THE NURSING COMMUNITY

Practice

A characteristic feature of Eriksson's manner of working is her way of structuring abstract thinking as a natural and obvious precondition of clinical activity and an evidence-based form of caring that opens up a deeper insight. Several nursing units in the Nordic countries have based their practice and caring philosophy on Eriksson's ideas and her caritative theory of caring. These include the Hospital District of Helsinki and Uusimaa in Finland, Stiftelsen Hemmet in the Åland Islands of Finland, and Stora Sköndal in Sweden. Because Eriksson's thinking and process model of caring are general, the nursing care process model has proved to be applicable in all contexts of caring, from acute clinical caring and psychiatric care to health-promoting and preventive care.

Since the 1970s, Eriksson's nursing care process model was systematically used, tested, and developed as a basis of nursing care and documentation at Helsinki University Central Hospital. From the beginning of the 1990s, Eriksson served as director of the clinical research program "In the World of the Patient." In various studies, Eriksson's theory has been tested, and the results have been presented in doctoral and master's theses and published in professional and scientific journals. The study "In the Patient's World II: Alleviating the Patient's Suffering—Ethics and Evidence" led to recommendations for the care of patients and is an ongoing research project that will become a handbook for clinical caring science.

Eriksson's model has been subjected to more comprehensive academic research (Fagerström, 1999; Kärkkäinen & Eriksson, 2003, 2004; Lukander, 1995; Turtiainen, 1999). Eriksson's thinking has been influential in nursing leadership and nursing administration, where the caritative theory of nursing forms the core of the development of nursing leadership at various levels of the nursing organization. That Eriksson's ideas about caring and her nursing care process model work in practice has been verified by many essays and tests of learning in clinical practice and master's theses, licentiates' theses, and doctoral dissertations produced all over the Nordic countries.

Education

Since the 1970s, Eriksson's theory has been integrated into the education of nurses at various levels, and her books have been included continuously in the examination requirements in various forms of nursing education in the Nordic countries. The education for master's and doctoral degrees that started in 1986 at the Department of Caring Science, Åbo Akademi University, has been based entirely on Eriksson's ideas, and her caritative caring theory forms the core of the development of substance in education and research.

Development of the caring science–centered curriculum and caring didactics continued in the educational and research program in caring science didactics. Development of teachers within the education of nurses forms a part of the master's degree program and resulted in the first doctoral dissertation in the didactics of caring science (Ekebergh, 2001).

Eriksson realized at an early stage the importance of integrating academic courses in the education of nurses; nowadays, academic courses in caring science based on Eriksson's theory are offered as part of continuing education for those who work in clinical practice. Approximately 200 nurses take part annually in these academic courses.

Because Eriksson sees caring science not as profession oriented but as a "pure" academic discipline, it has aroused interest among students in other disciplines and other occupational groups, such as teachers, social workers, psychologists, and theologians. Eriksson stresses that it is necessary for doctors as well to study caring science, so that genuine interdisciplinary cooperation is achieved between caring science and medicine.

Research

Eriksson and her teaching and research colleagues at the Department of Caring Science designed a research program based on her caring science tradition. This program comprises systematic caring science, clinical caring science, didactic caring science, caring administration, and interdisciplinary research. Eriksson's caritative caring theory has been tested and further developed in various contexts with different methodological approaches, both within the department's own research projects and in doctoral dissertations that have been published at the department.

Eriksson has always emphasized the importance of basic research as necessary for clinical research, and her main thesis is that substance should direct the choice of research method. In her book *Pausen (The Pause)* (Eriksson, 1987a), she describes how the research object is structured, starting from the caritative theory of caring. In her book *Broar (Bridges)* (Eriksson, 1991), she describes the research paradigm and various methodological approaches based on a human science perspective. During the first few years, the emphasis lay on basic research, with the focus on development of the basic concepts and assumptions of the theory and on the fundamentals of history and the history of ideas. An especially strong point in Eriksson's research is the clearly formulated theoretical perspective that confers explicitness and greater depth to the generation of knowledge. Development of the theory and research have always moved hand in hand with the focus on various dimensions of the theory, and, in this connection, some central results of the research deserve illustration.

Eriksson has emphasized the necessity of an exhaustive and systematic analysis of basic concepts and developed her own model of concept development (Eriksson, 1991, 1997b), which proved fruitful and is used by many researchers, including Nåden (1998) in his study of the art of caring, von Post (1999) in her study of the concept of natural care, Sivonen (2000) in studies of the concepts of soul and spirit, and Kasén (2002) in her study of the concept of the caring relationship. Other studies focused on the concept of dignity (Edlund, 2002), the concepts of power and authority (Rundqvist, 2004), and the concept of the body in a perioperative context (Lindwall, 2004).

Continued development of Eriksson's concept of health took place in the research project Den Mångdimensionella Hälsan (Multidimensional Health) during the years 1987–1992 and resulted in the ontological health model (Eriksson, 1994a; Eriksson et al., 1990; Eriksson & Herberts, 1992). The project resulted in a number of master's theses. Of these, Lindholm's study of young people's conception of health (1998; Lindholm & Eriksson, 1998) and Bondas' study of women's health during the perinatal period (2000; Bondas & Eriksson, 2001) led to doctoral dissertations.

The ontological health model subsequently formed the basis for several studies. Wärnå (2002), in her study concerning the worker's health, related Aristotle's theory of virtue to Eriksson's ontological health model. The study opened a new line of thought in preventive health service in working environments; continued research and development are now in progress in a number of factories in the wood-processing industry in Finland.

Since the mid-1980s, when suffering as the basic category in caring was made explicit in Eriksson's theory, examples of research related to suffering have been legion. One is Wiklund's (2000) study of suffering as struggle and drama, among both patients who had undergone coronary bypass surgery and patients addicted to drugs. In several clinical studies, Råholm focused on suffering and alleviation of suffering in patients undergoing coronary bypass surgery (Råholm, 2003; Råholm, Lindholm, & Eriksson, 2002). The manifestation of suffering in a psychiatric context has been studied by Fredriksson, who illustrates the possibilities of the caring conversation in the alleviation of suffering (Fredriksson, 2003; Fredriksson & Eriksson, 2003; Fredriksson & Lindström, 2002). Nyback (2008) studied suffering in the Chinese culture, and Lindholm (2008) focused on suffering and its connection to domestic violence. In a Norwegian study, Nilsson (2004) studied suffering in patients in psychiatric noninstitutional care units with a high degree of ill health and found that the experience of loneliness is of basic importance. Caspari (2004) in her study illustrated the importance of esthetics for health and suffering.

In a cooperative project between researchers in Sweden and Finland, the suffering of women with breast cancer was studied. This project comprised intervention studies in which the importance of different forms of care for the alleviation of suffering was illustrated (Arman et al., 2002; Arman-Rehnsfeldt & Rehnsfeldt, 2003; Lindholm, Nieminen, Mäkelä, & Rantanen-Siljamäki, 2004). Arman-Rehnsfeldt, in her dissertation, illustrated how the drama of suffering is formed among these women (Arman, 2003).

Continuous research has been carried out since the 1970s, with a view toward developing caring science as an academic discipline, and a theory of science for caring science has been formulated (Eriksson, 1988, 2001; Eriksson & Lindström, 2000, 2003; Lindström, 1992). Eriksson has developed subdisciplines of caring science, which means that researchers of caring science and other scientific disciplines enter into dialogues with each other and constitute a research area. An example of this is the development of caritative caring ethics (Andersson, 1994; Eriksson, 1991, 1995; Fredriksson & Eriksson, 2001; Råholm & Lindholm, 1999; Råholm, Lindholm, & Eriksson, 2002). Another interesting subdiscipline that Eriksson has developed is caring theology, within which she has articulated spiritual and doctrinal questions in caring with a scientific group of themes, and in this respect has cleared the way for new thinking. Caring theology has aroused great interest among caregivers in clinical practice that can be studied in academic courses.

FURTHER DEVELOPMENT

Eriksson continues developing her thinking and the caritative caring theory with unabated energy and constantly finds new ways, re-creating and deepening what has been stated before. Systematic research and the development of caritative caring theory and the discipline of caring science take place chiefly within the scope of the research programs in her own department with her own staff and the postdoctoral group. The dissertation topics of doctoral candidates are connected with the research programs and form an important contribution of knowledge to the ongoing development of Eriksson's thinking.

During the past few years, Eriksson emphasized the necessity of basic research in clinical caring science, where she has especially stressed the understanding of the research object caring reality. She describes the object of research from three points of view: the experienced world, praxis as activity, and the real reality. In the real reality, which carries the attributes of mystery, one finds something of the deepest potential of caring, and it is a reality that can be understood in Gadamer's sense, in the old Greek meaning of *praxis,* as a way of living, a mode of being—that is, an ontology (Gadamer, 2000). The development of knowledge in caring science becomes fundamentally different depending on which object of knowledge constitutes the focus of research (Eriksson & Lindström, 2003). Another central area of interest for Eriksson (2003) is formed by the development of caritative caring ethics. Continued development of the caritative theory of caring occurs through continued implementation and testing in various clinical contexts.

CRITIQUE

Clarity

The strong point of Eriksson's theory is the overall logical structure of the theory, in which every new concept becomes a part of an ever more comprehensive whole in which an element of internal logic can be seen clearly. Her main thesis has always been that basic conceptual clarity is needed before developing the contextual features of the theory. Eriksson used concept analysis and analysis of ideas as central methods, which has led to semantic and structural clarity. It means the concepts may have assumed dimensions regarded as strange to those unfamiliar with the theoretical perspective of the development of the theory. Having had the opportunity to follow Eriksson's work, we realize that her way of thinking forms a logical whole, where the abstract scientific reveals the concrete in a new understanding (i.e., provides an experience of evidence and verifies the convincing force of the theory).

Simplicity

The theoretical clarity of Eriksson's theory reflects the simplicity of the theory by showing the general in a clear and logical conceptual entirety. The hermeneutic approach has deepened the understanding of the substance and thus contributed to the simplicity of the theory (Gadamer, 1960/1994). The simplicity also can be understood as an expression of Gadamer's concept of theory by making it comprehensible that theory and practice belong together and reflect two sides of the same reality. Eriksson agrees with Gadamer's thought that understanding includes application, and the theory opens the way to deeper participation and communion. Eriksson (2003) formulates this process by the statement that "ideals reach reality and reality reaches the ideals" (p. 26).

Generality

Eriksson's theory is general in the sense that it aims at creating an ontological and ethical basis of caring, and it constitutes the core of the discipline and involves epistemology as well. Eriksson's theory is general as a result of the wide convincing force it receives through its theoretical core concepts and its theoretical axioms and theses. Eriksson stressed the importance of describing the core concepts on an optimal level of abstraction to include the complex caring reality that simultaneously carries a wealth of signification that opens up understanding in various caring contexts.

Accessibility

Eriksson's thinking as a whole has reached an understanding that extends to other disciplines and professions. She developed a language and a rhetoric that reaches researchers and practitioners in the human scientific field. The empirical precision of Eriksson's theory demonstrated in multiple deductive testings manifests a combination of the clarity, simplicity, and generality combined with a rich substance and clearly formulated ethos.

Importance

Eriksson's work to develop her caritative caring theory has been successful for 30 years, and there is abundant evidence that her thinking is of importance to clinical practice, research, and education and to the development of the caring discipline. By her development of the caritative theory of care, Eriksson created her own caring science tradition, a tradition that has grown strong and set the tone for nursing advancement and caring science.

SUMMARY

Eriksson has been a guide and visionary who has gone before and "ploughed new furrows" in theory development for many years. Eriksson's *caritas*-based theory and her whole caring science thinking have developed over the course of 30 years. Although she is working at an abstract level developing concepts and theory, the theory is characteristically rooted in clinical reality and teaching, where the caritative theory and caring have distinctive character and deeper meaning. The ultimate goal of caring is to alleviate suffering and serve life and health.

Knowledge formation, which Eriksson sees as a hermeneutic spiral, starts from the thought that ethics precedes ontology. In a concrete sense, this implies that the thought of human holiness and dignity is always kept alive in all phases of the search for knowledge. Ethics precedes ontology in theory as well as in practice.

Eriksson's caring science tradition and discipline of caring science form a basis for the activity at the Department of Caring Science at Åbo Akademi University. Eriksson's caritative caring theory and the discipline of caring science have inspired many and are used as the basis for research, education, and clinical practice. Many of her original textbooks, published mainly in Swedish, have been translated into Finnish, Norwegian, and Danish.

CASE STUDY

The case presented is a philosophy of practice, by Ulf Donner, leader of the Foundation Home at the psychiatric nursing home in Finland that for 15 years has based its practice on Eriksson's caritative theory of caring.

Even at an early stage in our serving in caring science, we caregivers recognized ourselves in the caring science theory, which stresses the healing force of love and compassion in the form of tending, playing, and learning in faith, hope, and charity. The caritative culture is made visible with the help of rituals, symbols, and traditions, for instance, with the stone that burns with the light of the Trinity and the daily common time for spiritual reflection. In every meeting with the suffering human being, the attributes of love and charity are striven for, and the day involves discussions of reconciliation, forgiveness, and how we as caregivers can tend by nourishing and cleansing on the level of becoming, being, and doing. In the struggle in love and compassion to reach a fellow human being who, because of suffering, has withdrawn from the communion to find common horizons, the sacrifice of the caregiver is constantly available.

We work with people who often have the feeling that they do not deserve the love they encounter and who, in various ways, try to convince us caregivers of this. We experience patients' disappointment in their destructive acts, and we constantly have to remember that it may be broken promises that produce such dynamics. Sometimes, it may be difficult to recognize that suffering expressed in this way in an abstract sense seeks an embrace that does not give way but is strong enough to give shelter to this suffering, in a way that makes a becoming movement possible. In recognizing what is bad and what is difficult, horizons in the field of force are expanded, and the possibility of bringing in a ray of light and hope is opened.

As caregivers, we constantly ask ourselves whether the words, the language we use, bring promise, and how we can create linguistic footholds in the void by means of images and symbols. In our effort to nourish and cleanse, that which constitutes the basic movement of tending, we often recognize the importance of teaching the patient to be able to mourn disappointments and affirm the possibilities of forgiveness in the movement of reconciliation.

We also try to bring about the open invitation to the suffering human being to join a communion with the help of myths, legends, and tales concerned with human questions about evil versus good and about eternity and infinity. Reading aloud with common reflective periods often provides us caregivers a possibility of getting closer to patients without getting too close, and opens the door for the suffering the patient bears.

Continued

CASE STUDY—cont'd

In the act of caring, we strive for openness with regard to the patient's face and a confirmative attitude that responds to the appeal that we can recognize that the patient directs to us. When we as caregivers respond to the patient's appeal for charity, we are faced with the task of confirming the holiness of the other as a human being. Our constant effort is to make it possible for the patient to reestablish his or her dignity, accomplish his or her human mission, and enter true communion.

CRITICAL THINKING ACTIVITIES

1. Reflect on the meaning of caritas as the ethos of caring.
   a. How is caritas culture formed in a care setting?
   b. How do caritative elements appear in caring?
   c. What is the nature of nursing ethics based on caritas?
2. Health and suffering are each other's preconditions. Think of what this meant in the life of a patient you cared for recently.
3. How have you recognized the elements of caring—faith, hope, love and tending, playing, and learning—in a concrete caring situation? Give examples.
4. Suffering as a consequence of lack of caritative caring is a violation of a human being's dignity. Think about a situation in which you saw this occur, and consider what can be done to prevent suffering related to care.

POINTS FOR FURTHER STUDY

- Eriksson, K. (2007). The theory of caritative caring: A vision. *Nursing Science Quarterly, 20*(3), 201–202.
- Eriksson, K. (2006). *The suffering human being.* Chicago: Nordic Studies Press. [English translation of *Den Lidande Människan. Stockholm:* Liber Förlag, 1994.]
- Eriksson, K. (2010). Concept determination as part of the development of knowledge in caring science. *Scandinavian Journal of Caring Sciences, 24,* 2–11.
- Eriksson, K. (2010). Evidence—To see or not to see. *Nursing Science Quarterly, 23*(4), 275–279.
- For further literature and information visit our website at http://www.abo.fi/institution/vardvetenskap

REFERENCES

Andersson, M. (1994). *Integritet som begrepp och princip.* En studie av ett vårdetiskt ideal i utveckling. Doktorsavhandling, Turku, Finland: Åbo Akademis Förlag. [*Integrity as a concept and as a principle in health care ethics.* Doctoral dissertation, Turku, Finland: Åbo Akademi University Press.]

Aristotle. (1935). *Metaphysics, X-XIV oeconomica magna moralia.* (H. Tredennick & G. C. Armstrong, Trans.). Cambridge, MA: Harvard University Press.

Aristotle. (1993). *Den nikomachiska etiken.* Gothenburg, Sweden: Daidalos. [*The nicomachean ethics* (M. Ringbom, Trans. & Commentary). Gothenburg, Sweden: Daidalos.]

Aristotle. (1997). *Retoriikka.* Helsinki, Finland: Gaudeamus. [*Rhetoric* (P. Hohti, Trans.). Helsinki, Finland: Gaudeamus.]

Arman, M. (2003). *Lidande i existens i patientens värld—Kvinnors upplevelser av att leva med bröstcancer.* Doktorsavhandling, Turku, Finland: Åbo Akademis Förlag. [*Suffering and existence in the patient's world—Women's experiences of living with breast cancer.* Doctoral dissertation, Turku, Finland: Åbo Akademi University Press.]

Arman, M., Rehnsfeldt, A., Lindholm, L., & Hamrin, E. (2002). The face of suffering among women with breast cancer—being in a field of forces. *Cancer Nursing, 25*(2), 96–103.

Arman-Rehnsfeldt, M., & Rehnsfeldt, A. (2003). Vittnesbördet som etisk grund i vårdandet. I K. Eriksson & U. Å. Lindström (red.), *Gryning II. Klinisk vårdvetenskap* (s. 109–121), Vaasa, Finland: Institutionen för vårdvetenskap, Åbo Akademi. [Bearing witness as an ethical base in caring. In K. Eriksson & U. Å. Lindström (Eds.), *Dawn II. Clinical caring science* (pp. 109–121). Vaasa, Finland: Department of Caring Science, Åbo Akademi.]

Barbosa da Silva, A. (1993). *Vetenskap och männiksosyn i sjukvården: en introduktion till vetenskapsfilosofi och vårdetik.* Stockholm: Svenska hälso och sjukvårdens tjänstemannaförbund, (SHSTF). [*Science and view of human nature in nursing: An introduction to philosophy of science and caring ethics.* Stockholm: Svenska hälso och sjukvårdens tjänstemannaförbund, (SHSTF).]

Berdâev, N. A. (1990). *Historiens mening: ett försök till en filosofi om det mänskliga ödet.* Skellefteå, Sweden: Artos. [*The meaning of history: An attempt at philosophy of human fate.* Skellefteå, Sweden: Artos.]

Bondas, T. (2000). *Att vara med barn: en vårdvetenskaplig studie av kvinnors upplevelser under perinatal tid.* Doktorsavhandling, Turku, Finland: Åbo Akademis Förlag. [*To be with child: A study of women's lived experiences during the perinatal period from a caring science perspective.* Doctoral dissertation, Turku, Finland: Åbo Akademi University Press.]

Bondas, T., & Eriksson, K. (2001). Women's lived experiences of pregnancy: A tapestry of joy and suffering. *Qualitative Health Research, 11*(6), 824–840.

Caspari, S. (2004). Det Gyldne snitt. *Den estetiske dimensjon et etisk anliggende.* Doktorsavhandling, Turku, Finland: Åbo Academis Förlag. [*The golden section. The aesthetic dimension—A source of health.* Doctoral dissertation. Turku, Finland: Åbo Akademi University Press.]

Edlund, M. (2002). *Människans värdighet—Ett grundbegrepp inom vårdvetenskapen.* Doktorsavhandling, Turku, Finland: Åbo Akademis Förlag. [*Human dignity—A basic caring science concept.* Doctoral dissertation, Turku, Finland: Åbo Akademi University Press.]

Ekebergh, M. (2001). *Tillägnandet av vårdveteskaplig kunskap. Reflexionens betydelse för lärandet.* Doktorsavhandling, Turku, Finland: Åbo Akademis Förlag. [*Acquiring caring science knowledge—The importance of reflection for learning.* Doctoral dissertation, Turku, Finland: Åbo Akademi University Press.]

Eriksson, K. (1974). *Vårdprocessen (kompendium).* Helsinki, Finland: Helsingfors svenska sjukvårdsinstitut. [*The nursing care process (Compendium).* Helsinki, Finland: Helsingfors svenska sjukvårdsinstitut.]

Eriksson, K. (1976). *Hälsa. En teoretisk och begreppsanalytisk studie om hälsan och dess natur som mål för hälsovårdsedukation.* Licentiatavhandling, Helsinki, Finland: Institutionen för pedagogik, Helsingfors universitet. [*Health. A conceptual analysis and theoretical study of health and its nature as a goal for health care education.* Unpublished Licentiate thesis, Helsinki, Finland: Department of Education, University of Helsinki.]

Eriksson, K. (1981). *Vårdprocessen—En utgångspunkt för läroplanstänkande inom vårdutbildningen. Utvecklande av en vårdprocessmodell samt ett läroplanstänkande utgående från vårdprocessen,* n. 94. Helsinki, Finland: Helsingfors universitet, Pedagogiska Institutionen. [*The nursing care process—An approach to curriculum construction within nursing education. The development of a model for the nursing care process and an approach for curriculum development based on the process of nursing care* (No. 94). Helsinki, Finland: Department of Education, University of Helsinki.]

Eriksson, K. (1984). *Hälsans idé.* Stockholm: Almqvist & Wiksell. [*The idea of health.* Stockholm: Almqvist & Wiksell.]

Eriksson, K. (1987a). *Pausen. En beskrivning av vårdvetenskapens kunskapsobjekt.* Stockholm: Almqvist & Wiksell. [*The pause: A description of the knowledge object of caring science.* Stockholm: Almqvist & Wiksell.]

Eriksson, K. (1987b). *Vårdandets idé.* Stockholm: Almqvist & Wiksell. [*The idea of caring.* Stockholm: Almqvist & Wiksell.]

Eriksson, K. (1988). *Vårdvetenskap som disciplin, forsknings—och tillämpningsområde* (Vårdforskningar 1/1988). Vaasa, Finland: Institutionen för vårdvetenskap, Åbo Akademi. [*Caring science as a discipline, field of research and application* (Caring research 1/1988). Vaasa, Finland: Department of Caring Science, Åbo Akademi.]

Eriksson, K. (1989). Caring paradigms. A study of the origins and the development of caring paradigms among nursing students. *Scandinavian Journal of Caring Sciences, 3*(4), 169–176.

Eriksson, K. (1990). *Pro Caritate. En lägesbestämning av caritativ vård.* Vårdforskningar 2/1990. Vaasa, Finland: Institutionen för vårdvetenskap, Åbo Akademi. [*Caritative caring—A positional analysis.* Vaasa, Finland: Department of Caring Science, Åbo Akademi.]

Eriksson, K. (1991). *Broar. Introduktion i vårdvetenskaplig metod.* Vaasa, Finland: Institutionen för vårdvetenskap, Åbo Akademi. [*Bridges. Introduction to the methods of caring science* (test ed.). Vaasa, Finland: Department of Caring Science, Åbo Akademi.]

Eriksson, K. (1992a). The alleviation of suffering—The idea of caring. *Scandinavian Journal of Caring Sciences, 6*(2), 119–123.

Eriksson, K. (1992b). Different forms of caring communion. *Nursing Science Quarterly, 5,* 93.

Eriksson, K. (1992c). Nursing: The caring practice "being there." In D. Gaut (Ed.), *The practice of caring in nursing* (pp. 201–210). New York: National League for Nursing Press.

Eriksson, K. (1993). Lidandets idé. I K. Eriksson (red.), *Möten med lidanden.* Vårdforskning 4/1993 (s. 1–27). Vaasa, Finland: Institutionen för vårdvetenskap, Åbo Akademi. [The idea of suffering. In K. Eriksson (Ed.), *Encounters with suffering* (pp. 1–27). Vaasa, Finland: Department of Caring Science, Åbo Akademi.]

Eriksson, K. (1994a). *Den lidande människan.* Stockholm: Liber Förlag. [*The suffering human being.* Stockholm: Liber Förlag.] [English translation published in 2006 by Nordic Studies Press, Chicago.]

Eriksson, K. (1994b). Theories of caring as health. In D. Gaut & A. Boykin (Eds.), *Caring as healing: Renewal through hope* (pp. 3–20). New York: National League for Nursing Press.

Eriksson, K. (Ed.). (1995). *Mot en caritativ vårdetik* (Vårdforskning 5/1995). Vaasa, Finland: Institutionen för vårdvetenskap, Åbo Akademi. [*Toward a caritative caring ethic* (Caring research 5/1995). Vaasa, Finland: Department of Caring Science, Åbo Akademi.]

Eriksson, K. (1997a). Caring, spirituality and suffering. In M. S. Roach (Ed.), *Caring from the heart: The convergence between caring and spirituality* (pp. 68–84). New York: Paulist Press.

Eriksson, K. (1997b). Perustutkimus ja käsiteanalyysi. I M. Paunonen & J. Vehviläinen-Julkunen, *Hoitotieteen tutkimusmetodiikka* (s. 50–75). Helsinki Porvoo, Finland: WSOY. [Basic research and concept analysis. In M. Paunonen & J. Vehviläinen-Julkunen, *The research methodology of caring science* (pp. 50–75). Helsinki Porvoo, Finland: WSOY.]

Eriksson, K. (1998). Understanding the world of the patient, the suffering human being: The new clinical paradigm from nursing to caring. In C. E. Guzzetta (Ed.), *Essential readings in holistic nursing* (pp. 3–9). Gaithersburg, MD: Aspen.

Eriksson, K. (1999, November). *Teoriutveckling inom vårdvetenskapen. Human vetenskaplig angreppspunkt.* Stockholm: Nordisk Akademi för Sykepleievitenskap, Kongress i Stockholm. [*Theory development in caring science. A humanistic approach.* Stockholm: Nordisk Akademi for Sykepleievitenskap, Kongress i Stockholm.]

Eriksson, K. (2001). *Vårdvetenskap som akademisk disciplin* (Vårdforskning 7/2001). Vaasa, Finland: Institutionen för vårdvetenskap, Åbo Akademi. [*Caring science as an academic discipline* (Caring research 7/2001). Vaasa, Finland: Department of Caring Science, Åbo Akademi.]

Eriksson, K. (2002). Caring science in a new key. *Nursing Science Quarterly, 15*(1), 61–65.

Eriksson, K. (2003). Ethos. I K. Eriksson & U. Å. Lindström (red.), *Gryning II. Klinisk vårdvetenskap* (s. 21–34). Vaasa, Finland: Institutionen för vårdvetenskap, Åbo Akademi. [Ethos. In K. Eriksson & U. Å. Lindström (Eds.), *Dawn II. Clinical caring science* (pp. 21–34). Vaasa, Finland: Department of Caring Science, Åbo Akademi.]

Eriksson, K., Bondas-Salonen, T., Fagerström, L., et al. (1990). *Den mångdimensionella hälsan—En pilotstudie över uppfattningar bland patienter, skolungdomar och lärare (Projektrapport).* Vaasa, Finland: Vasa Sjukvårdsdistrikt kf. och Institutionen för vårdvetenskap, Åbo Akademi. [*Multidimensional health—A pilot study of how patients, school students, and teachers experience health (Project Rep. 1).* Vaasa, Finland: Vasa Sjukvårdsdistrikt kf. och Institutionen för vårdvetenskap, Åbo Akademi.]

Eriksson, K., & Herberts, S. (1992). *Den mångdimensionella hälsan. En studie av hälsobilden hos sjukvårdsledare och sjukvårdspersonal (Projektrapport 2).* Vaasa, Finland: Vasa sjukvårdsdistrikt kf. och Institutionen för vårdvetenskap, Åbo Akademi. [*The multidimensional health. A study of the view of health among health care leaders and health care personnel (Project Rep. 2).* Vaasa, Finland: Vasa sjukvårdsdistrikt kf. och Institutionen för vårdvetenskap, Åbo Akademi.]

Eriksson, K., & Lindström, U. Å. (1997). Abduction—A way to deeper understanding of the world of caring. *Scandinavian Journal of Caring Sciences, 11*(4), 195–198.

Eriksson, K., & Lindström, U. Å. (2000). Siktet, sökandet, slutandet—Om den vårdvetenskapliga kunskapen. I K. Eriksson & U. Å. Lindström (red.), *Gryning—En vårdvetenskaplig antologi* (s. 5–18). Vaasa, Finland: Institutionen för vårdvetenskap, Åbo Akademi. [In the prospect of, searching for, and ending of—The caring science knowledge. In K. Eriksson & U. Å. Lindström (Eds.), *Dawn. An anthology of caring science* (pp. 5–18). Vaasa, Finland: Department of Caring Science, Åbo Akademi.]

Eriksson, K., & Lindström, U. Å. (2003). Klinisk vårdvetenskap. I K. Eriksson & U. Å. Lindström (red.), *Gryning II. Klinisk vårdvetenskap* (s. 3–20). Vaasa, Finland: Institutionen för vårdvetenskap, Åbo Akademi. [Clinical caring science. In K. Eriksson & U. Å. Lindström (Eds.), *Dawn II. Clinical caring science* (pp. 3–20). Vaasa, Finland: Department of Caring Science, Åbo Akademi.]

Eriksson, K., & Nordman, T. (2004). *Trojanska hästen II. Utvecklande av evidensbaserade vårdande kulturer.* Vaasa, Finland: Institutionen för vårdvetenskap, Åbo Akademi. [*Trojan Horse II. The development of evidence-based caring cultures.* Vaasa, Finland: Department of Caring Science, Åbo Akademi University.]

Eriksson K., Nordman T., & Myllymäki, I. (1999). *Den trojanska hästen. Evidensbaserat vårdande och vårdarbete ur ett vårdvetenskapligt perspektiv* (Rapport 1). Institutionen för vårdvetenskap. Vaasa, Finland: Åbo Akademi; Helsingfors universitetscentralsjukhus & Vasa sjukvårdsdistrikt. [*The Trojan horse. Evidence-based caring and nursing care in a caring science perspective.* (Report). Department of Caring Science. Vaasa, Finland: Åbo Akademi; Helsingfors universitetscentralsjukhus & Vasa sjukvårdsdistrikt.]

Fagerström, L. (1999). *The patients' caring needs.* To understand and measure the unmeasurable. Doctoral dissertation. (Turku, Finland: Åbo Akademi University Press.)

Fredriksson, L. (2003). *Det vårdande samtalet.* Turku, Finland: Doktorsavhandling, Åbo Akademis Förlag. [*The caring conversation.* Doctoral dissertation, Turku, Finland: Åbo Akademi University Press.]

Fredriksson, L., & Eriksson, K. (2001). The patient's narrative of suffering—A path to health? An interpretative research synthesis on narrative understanding. *Scandinavian Journal of Caring Sciences, 15*(1), 3–11.

Fredriksson, L., & Eriksson, K. (2003). The ethics of the caring conversation. *Nursing Ethics, 10*(2), 138–148.

Fredriksson, L., & Lindström, U. Å. (2002). Caring conversations—Psychiatric patients' narratives about suffering. *Journal of Advanced Nursing, 40*(4), 396–404.

Gadamer, H-G. (1994). *Truth and method* (2nd rev. ed., J. Weinsheimer & D. G. Marshall, Trans.). New York: Continuum.

Gadamer, H-G. (2000). *Teoriens lovprisning.* Århus: Systeme. [*Praise the theory.* New Haven: Yale University Press, 1998.] [German orig: Lob der Theorie, 3. Auflage, 1991.]

Gustafsson, L-K. (2008). *Försoning ur ett vårdvetenskapligt perspektiv.* Doktorsavhandling, Turku, Finland: Åbo Akademis förlag. [*Reconciliation—From a caring perspective.* Doctoral dissertation, Turku, Finland: Åbo Akademi University Press.]

Hilli, Y. (2007). *Hemmet som ethos. En idéhistorisk studie av hur hemmet som ethos blev evident i hälsosysterns vårdande under 1900-talets första hälft.* Doktorsavhandling, Turku, Finland: Åbo Akademis Förlag. [*The home as ethos. A history of ideas study of how the home as ethos became evident in public health nurses' caring during the first half of the 20th century.* Doctoral dissertation, Turku, Finland: Åbo Akademi University Press.]

Kaila, E. (1939). *Den mänskliga kunskapen: vad den är och vad den icke är.* Helsinki, Finland: Söderström. [*Human knowledge: What it is and what it is not* (G. H. von Wright, Trans.). Helsinki, Finland: Söderström.]

Kasén, A. (2002). *Den vårdande relationen.* Doktorsavhandling, Turku, Finland: Åbo Akademis Förlag. [*The caring relationship.* Doctoral dissertation, Turku, Finland: Åbo Akademi University Press.]

Kierkegaard, S. (1943). *Antingen—Eller* [Orig. 1843. Enten—Eller.]. Utgiver under pseudonymen Victor Eremita. Köpenhamn: Meyer. [*Either/or.* Princeton, NJ: Princeton University Press, 1987.]

Koort, P. (1975). *Semantisk analys och konfigurationsanalys.* Lund, Sweden: Studentlitteratur. [*Semantic analysis and analysis of configuration.* Lund, Sweden: Studentlitteratur.]

Kuhn, T. (1971). *The structure of scientific revolutions*. Chicago: University of Chicago Press.
Kurtén, T. (1987). *Grunder för en kontextuell teologi: ett wittgensteinskt sätt att närma sig teologin I diskussion med Anders Jeffner*. Turku, Finland: Åbo Akademis Förlag. [*Bases for a contextual theology: A Wittgensteinian way of approaching theology in a discussion with Anders Jeffner*. Turku, Finland: Åbo Akademi University Press.]
Kärkkäinen, O., & Eriksson, K. (2003). Evaluation of patient records as a part of developing a nursing care classification. *Journal of Clinical Nursing, 12*(2), 198–205.
Kärkkäinen, O., & Eriksson, K. (2004). Structuring the documentation of nursing care on the basis of a theoretical process model. *Scandinavian Journal of Caring Sciences, 18*(2), 229–236.
Lanara, V. (1981). *Heroism as a nursing value*. Athens, Greece: Sisterhood Evniki.
Langer, S. K. (1942). *Filosofi i en ny tonart*. Stockholm: Geber. [*Philosophy in a new key*. Stockholm: Geber.]
Lassenius, E. (2005). *Rummet i vårdandets värld*. Doktorsavhandling, Turku, Finland: Åbo Akademis Förlag. [*The space in the world of caring*. Doctoral dissertation, Turku, Finland: Åbo Akademi University Press.]
Lévinas, E. (1985). *Ethics and infinity*. Pittsburgh, PA: Duquesne University Press.
Lévinas, E. (1988). *Etik och oändlighet*. Stockholm-Lund: Symposion. [*Ethics and infinity*. Stockholm-Lund: Symposium.]
Lévinas, E. (1989). *The Lévinas reader* (S. Hand, Ed.). Oxford: Blackwell.
Lindholm, L. (1998). *Den unga människans hälsa och lidande*. Doktorsavhandling, Vaasa, Finland: Institutionen för vårdvetenskap, Åbo Akademi. [*The young person's health and suffering*. Doctoral dissertation, Vaasa, Finland: Åbo Akademi, Department of Caring Science.]
Lindholm, L., & Eriksson, K. (1993). To understand and to alleviate suffering in a caring culture. *Journal of Advanced Nursing, 18*, 1354–1361.
Lindholm, L., & Eriksson, K. (1998). The dialectic of health and suffering: An ontological perspective on young people's health. *Qualitative Health Research, 8*(4), 513–525.
Lindholm, L., Nieminen, A-L., Määkelää, C., & Rantanen-Siljamäki, S. (2004). *Significant others—A source of strength in the care of women with breast cancer*. Unpublished paper.
Lindholm, T. (2008). *Kaikki se kärsii? Parisuhdeväkivalta, kärsimys ja sen lievittäminen naisten ja miesten näkökulmasta*. Doktorsavhandling, Turku, Finland: Åbo Akademis förlag. [*Love endures all things? Violence between spouses, suffering and alleviation of suffering from the viewpoint of women and men*. Doctoral dissertation, Turku, Finland: Åbo Akademi University Press.]
Lindström, U. Å. (1992). *De psykiatriska specialsjukskötarnas yrkesparadigm*. Doktorsavhandling, Turku, Finland: Åbo Akademis Förlag. [*The professional paradigm of the qualified psychiatric nurses*. Doctoral dissertation, Turku, Finland: Åbo Akademi University Press.]
Lindwall, L. (2004). *Kroppen som bärare av hälsa och lidande*. Doktorsavhandling, Turku, Finland: Åbo Akademis Förlag. [*The body as a carrier of health and suffering*. Doctoral dissertation, Turku, Finland: Åbo Akademi University Press.]
Lukander, E. (1995). *Developing and testing a method: Nursing audit, for evaluation of nursing care*. Kuopio, Finland: Licentiate thesis, Kuopion yliopisto.
Martinsen, K. (Ed.). (1996). *Fenomenologi og omsorg*. Oslo, Norway: TANO. [*Phenomenology and care*. Oslo, Norway: TANO.]
Martinsen, K., & Eriksson, K. (2009). *Å se og Å innse*. Oslo: Akribi.
Nåden, D. (1998). *Når sykepleie er kunstutøvelse. En undersøkelse av noen nødvendige forutsetninger for sykepleie som kunst*. Doktorsavhandling, Vaasa, Finland: Institutionen för vårdvetenskap, Åbo Akademi. [*When caring is an exercise of art. An examination of some necessary preconditions of nursing as art*. Doctoral dissertation, Department of Caring Science, Åbo Akademi, Vaasa, Finland.]
Näsman, Y. (2010). *Hjärtats vanor, tankens välvilja och handens gärning—dygd som vårdetiskt grundbegrepp*. Doktorsavhandling, Turku, Finland: Åbo Akademis förlag. [*Habits of the heart, benevolence of the mind, and deeds of the hand—Virtue as a basic concept in caring ethics*. Doctoral dissertation, Turku, Finland: Åbo Akademi University Press.]
Nilsson, B. (2004). *Savnets tone i ensomhetens melodi*. Ensomhet hos aleneboende personer med alvorlig psykisk lidelse. Doktorsavhandling, Turku, Finland: Åbo Akademis Förlag. [*The tune of want in the loneliness melody*. Doctoral dissertation, Turku, Finland: Åbo Akademi University Press.]
Nyback, M-H. (2008). *Generic and professional caring in a Chinese setting—An ethnographic study*. Doctoral dissertation, Turku, Finland: Åbo Akademi University Press.
Nygren, A. (1966). *Eros och agapé*. Stockholm: Aldus Bonniers. [*Eros and agapé*. Stockholm: Aldus Bonniers.]
Nygren, A. (1972). *Meaning and method: Prolegomena to a scientific philosophy of religion and a scientific theology*. London: Epworth Press.
Pascal, B. (1971). *Tankar*. Uddevalla, Sweden: Bohusläningens AB. [*Thoughts*. Uddevalla, Sweden: Bohusläningens AB.]
Peirce, C. S. (1990). *Pragmatism och kosmologi*. Valda uppsatser. Gothenburg, Sweden: Daidalos. [*Pragmatism and cosmology (Chosen essays)*. Gothenburg, Sweden: Daidalos.]
Popper, K. R. (1997). *Popper i urval av Miller. Kunskapsteori, vetenskapsteori*. Stockholm: Thales. [*Popper in selection of Miller. Theory of knowledge and theory of science*. Stockholm: Thales.]
Råholm, M-B. (2003). *I kampens och modets dialektik*. Doktorsavhandling, Turku, Finland: Åbo Akademis Förlag. [*In the dialectic of struggle and courage*. Dissertation, Turku, Finland: Åbo Akademi University Press.]
Råholm, M-B., & Lindholm, L. (1999). Being in the world of the suffering patient: A challenge to nursing ethics. *Nursing Ethics, 6*, 528–539.
Råholm, M-B., Lindholm, L., & Eriksson, K. (2002). Grasping the essence of the spiritual dimension reflected through the horizon of suffering—An interpretative research synthesis. *Australian Journal of Holistic Nursing, 9*, 4–12.
Rundqvist, E. (2004). *Makt som fullmakt. Ett vårdvetenskapligt perspektiv*. Doktorsavhandling, Turku, Finland: Åbo Akademis

Förlag. [*Power as authority. A caring science perspective.* Doctoral dissertation, Turku, Finland: Åbo Akademi University Press.]

Sivonen, K. (2000). *Vården och det andliga. En bestämning av begreppet 'andlig' ur ett vårdvetenskapligt perspektiv.* Doktorsavhandling, Turku, Finland: Åbo Akademis Förlag. [*Care and the spiritual dimension. A definition of the concept of "spiritual" in a caring science perspective.* Doctoral dissertation, Turku, Finland: Åbo Akademi University Press.]

St. Augustine, A. (1957). *Bekännelser.* Stockholm: Söderström. [*Confessions.* Stockholm: Söderström.]

Törnebohm, H. (1978). *Paradigm i vetenskapsteorin (Del 2.* Rapport nr. 100). Gothenburg, Sweden: Institutionen för vetenskapsteori, Göteborgs universitet. [*Paradigms in the theory of science (Part 2 Report nr. 100).* Gothenburg, Sweden: Institutionen för vetenskapsteori, Göteborgs universitet.]

Turtiainen, A-M. (1999). *Hoitotyön käytännön kuvaamisen yhtenäistäminen: Belgialaisen hoitotyön minimitiedoston (BeNMDS) kulttuurinen adaptio Suomeen.* Kuopio, Finland: Doktorsavhandling, Väitöskirja, Kuopion yliopisto. [*Methods to describe nursing with uniform language: The cross-cultural adaptation process of the Belgium Nursing Minimum Data Set in Finland.* Doctoral dissertation, Kuopio University, Kuopio, Finland.]

von Post, I. (1999). *Professionell naturlig vård ur anestesi och operationassjuksköterskors perspektiv.* Doktorsavhandling, Turku, Finland: Åbo Akademis Förlag. [*Professional natural care from the perspective of nurse anesthetists and operating room nurses.* Doctoral dissertation, Turku, Finland: Åbo Akademi University Press.]

von Wright, G. H. (1986). *Vetenskapen och förnuftet.* Helsinki, Finland: Söderström. [*Science and reason.* Helsinki, Finland: Söderström.]

Wallinvirta, E. (2011). *Ansvar som klangbotten i vårdandets meningssammanhang.* Doktorsavhandling, Turku, Finland: Åbo Akademis förlag. [*Responsibility as sounding board in the caring's context of meaning.* Doctoral dissertation, Turku, Finland: Åbo Akademi University Press.]

Wärnå, C. (2002). *Dygd och hälsa.* Doktorsavhandling, Turku, Finland: Åbo Akademis Förlag. [*Virtue and health.* Doctoral dissertation, Turku, Finland: Åbo Akademi University Press.]

Wiklund, L. (2000). *Lidandet som kamp och drama.* Doktorsavhandling, Turku, Finland: Åbo Akademis Förlag. [*Suffering as struggle and as drama.* Doctoral dissertation, Turku, Finland: Åbo Akademi University Press.]

Wingren, G. (1996). *Predikan: en principiell studie.* Lund, Sweden: Gleerup. [*The sermon: A study based on principles.* Lund, Sweden: Gleerup.]

BIBLIOGRAPHY

Primary Sources

Articles in Scientific Journals With Referee Practice

Arman, M., Rehnsfeldt, A., Lindholm, L., Hamrin, E., & Eriksson, K. (2004). Suffering related to health care: A study of breast cancer patients' experiences. *International Journal of Nursing Practice, 10*(6), 248–256.

Blegen, N., Eriksson, K., & Bondas, T. (2014). Through the depths and heights of darkness; mothers as patients in psychiatric care. *Scandinavian Journal of Caring Sciences, 28*(4), 852–860.

Caspari, S., Eriksson, K., & Nåden, D. (2011). The importance of aesthetic surroundings: A study interviewing experts within different aesthetic fields. *Scandinavian Journal of Caring Sciences, 25*(1), 134–142.

Caspari, S., Nåden, D., & Eriksson, K. (2006). The aesthetic dimension in hospitals—An investigation into strategic plans. *International Journal of Nursing Studies, 43,* 851–859.

Caspari, S., Nåden, D., & Eriksson, K. (2007). Why not ask the patient? An evaluation of the aesthetic surroundings in hospital by patients. *Quality Management in Health Care, 16*(3), 280–292.

Eriksson, K. (1976). Nursing—Skilled work or a profession? *International Nursing Review, 23*(4), 118–120.

Eriksson, K. (1980). Hoitotieteen loogiset ja tieteenteoreettiset perusteet. *Sosiaalinen aikakauskirja, 14*(5), 6–10. [The theory of science and logical basics of caring science. *Sosiaalinen aikakauskirja, 14*(5), 6–10.

Eriksson, K. (1980). Hoitotieteen teoreettisista malleista, käsitejärjestelmistä ja niiden merkityksestä alan kehittämisessä. *Sosiaalilääketieteellinen aikakauslehti, 17*(2), 66–70. [The importance of caring scientific theoretical models and concept systems for the development of the science. *Sosiaalilääketieteellinen aikakauslehti, 17*(2), 66–70.]

Eriksson, K. (1982). Sjukskötarnas strävan efter högskoleutbildning. *Kasvatus, 13*(3), 192–194. [The nurses strive for a university education. *Kasvatus, 13*(3), 192–194.]

Eriksson, K. (1989). Det finns en gemensam substans i allt vårdandet. *Vård i Norden, 15*(2), 27–28. [There is a common substance in all caring. *Nordic Journal of Nursing Research and Clinical Studies, 15*(2), 27–28.]

Eriksson, K. (1989). Motivforskning inom vårdvetenskapen. En beskrivning av vårdvetenskapens grundmotiv. *Hoitotiede, 1*(2), 61–67. [Motive research within caring science. A description of the basic motive in caring science. *Journal of Nursing Science, 1*(2), 61–67.]

Eriksson, K. (1990). Nursing science in a Nordic perspective. Systematic and contextual caring science. A study of the basic motive of caring and context. *Scandinavian Journal of Caring Sciences, 4*(1), 3–5.

Eriksson, K. (1994). Hälsovårdskandidatutbildningen vid Helsingfors universitet—Historisk tillbakablick och visioner. *Hoitotiede, 3,* 122–126. [The bachelor's degree in health care at Helsinki University—A historical retrospect and visions. *Journal of Nursing Science, 3,* 122–126.]

Eriksson, K. (1995). Teologi og bioetik. *Vård i Norden, 1,* 33. [Theology and bio-ethics. *Nordic Journal of Nursing Research and Clinical Studies, 1,* 33.]

Eriksson, K. (1997). Understanding the world of the patient, the suffering human being—The new clinical paradigm from nursing to caring. *Advanced Practice Nursing Quarterly, 3*(1), 8–13.

Eriksson, K. (1998). Hälsans tragedy. *Finsk tidskrift, 10,* 590–599. [The tragedy of health. *Finsk tidskrift, 10,* 590–599.]

Eriksson, K. (2007). Becoming through suffering—The path to health and holiness. *International Journal for Human Caring, 11*(2), 8–16.

Eriksson, K. (2007). The theory of caritative caring: A vision. *Nursing Science Quarterly*, *20*(3), 201–202.

Eriksson, K. (2010). Concept determination as part of the development of knowledge in caring science. *Scandinavian Journal of Caring Sciences*, *24*, 2–11.

Eriksson, K. (2010). Evidence—To see or not to see. *Nursing Science Quarterly*, *23*(4), 275–279.

Eriksson, K., Bondas, T., Lindholm, L., Kasén, A., & Matilainen, D. (2002). Den vårdvetenskapliga forskningstraditionen vid Institutionen för vårdvetenskap, Åbo Akademi. *Hoitotiede*, *14*(6), 307–315. [The tradition of research at the Department of Caring Science, Åbo Akademi University. *Journal of Nursing Science*, *14*(6), 307–315.]

Eriksson, K., Herberts, S., & Lindholm, L. (1994). Bilder av lidande—Lidande i belysning av aktuell vårdvetenskaplig forskning. *Hoitotiede*, *4*, 155–162. [Views of suffering—Suffering in the light of current research within caring science. *Journal of Nursing Science*, *4*, 155–162.]

Eriksson, K., & Lindström, U. Å. (1999). Abduktion och pragmatism—Två vägar till framsteg inom vårdvetenskapen. *Hoitotiede*, *11*(5), 292–299. [Abduction and pragmatism—Two ways to progress within caring science. *Journal of Nursing Science*, *11*(5), 292–299.]

Eriksson, K., & Lindström, U. Å. (1999). En vetenskapsteori för vårdvetenskapen. *Hoitotiede*, *11*(6), 358–364. [A theory of science for caring science. *Journal of Nursing Science*, *11*(6), 358–364.]

Eriksson, K., & Lindström, U. Å. (1999). The fundamental idea of quality assurance. *International Journal for Human Caring*, *3*(3), 21–27.

Eriksson, K., & von Post, I. (1999). A hermeneutic textual analysis of suffering and caring in the peri-operative context. *Journal of Advanced Nursing*, *30*(4), 983–989.

Fagerström, L., Eriksson, K., & Bergbom Engberg, I. (1998). The patient's perceived caring needs as a message of suffering. *Journal of Advanced Nursing*, *28*(5), 978–987.

Fagerström, L., Eriksson, K., & Bergbom Engberg, I. (1999). The patient's perceived caring needs—Measuring the unmeasurable. *International Journal of Nursing Practice*, *5*(4), 199–208.

Foss, B., Nåden, D., & Eriksson, K. (2014). Toward a new leadership model: To serve in responsibility and love. *International Journal for Human Caring*, *18*(3), 43–51.

Fredriksson, L., & Eriksson, K. (2001). The patient's narrative of suffering—A path to health? An interpretative research synthesis on narrative understanding. *Scandinavian Journal of Caring Sciences*, *15*(1), 3–11.

Fredriksson, L., & Eriksson, K. (2003). The ethics of the caring conversation. *Nursing Ethics*, *10*(2), 138–148.

Herberts, S., & Eriksson, K. (1995). Nursing leaders' and nurses' view of health. *Journal of Advanced Nursing*, *22*, 868–878.

Kärkkäinen, O., Bondas, T., & Eriksson, K. (2005). Documentation of individualized patient care: a qualitative metasynthesis. *Nursing Ethics*, *12*(2), 123–132.

Kärkkäinen, O., & Eriksson, K. (2003). Evaluation of patient records as a part of developing a nursing care classification. *Journal of Clinical Nursing*, *12*(2), 198–205.

Kärkkäinen, O., & Eriksson, K. (2004). A theoretical approach to documentation of care. *Nursing Science Quarterly*, *17*(3), 2–6.

Kärkkäinen, O., & Eriksson, K. (2004). Structuring the documentation on nursing care on the basis of a theoretical caring process model. *Scandinavian Journal of Caring Sciences*, *18*(2), 229–236.

Kärkkäinen, O., & Eriksson, K. (2005). Recording the content of the caring process. *Journal of Nursing Management*, *13*, 202–208.

Korhonen, E.-S., Nordman, T., & Eriksson, K. (2014). Determination of concept technology—the ontology of the concept as a component in caring science. *Scandinavian Journal of Caring Sciences*, *28*(4), 867–877.

Levy-Malmberg, R., & Eriksson, K. (2010). Legitimizing basic research by evaluating quality. *Nursing Ethics*, *17*(1), 107–116.

Levy-Malmberg, R., Eriksson, K., & Lindholm, L. (2008). Caritas—Caring as an ethical conduct. *Scandinavian Journal of Caring Sciences*, *22*(4), 662–667.

Lindholm, L., & Eriksson, K. (1993). To understand and to alleviate suffering in a caring culture. *Journal of Advanced Nursing*, *18*, 1354–1361.

Lindholm, L., & Eriksson, K. (1998). The dialectic of health and suffering: An ontological perspective on young people's health. *Qualitative Health Research*, *8*(4), 513–525.

Lindholm, T., & Eriksson, K. (2011). Caring of the patients suffering from violence between spouses—Intersectional encounters. *International Journal for Human Caring*, *15*(3), 72.

Lindwall, I., von Post, I., & Eriksson, K. (2010). Clinical research with a hermeneutical design and an element of application. *International Journal of Qualitative Methods*, *9*(2), 172–186.

Nåden, D., & Eriksson, K. (2000). The phenomenon of confirmation—An aspect of nursing as an art. *International Journal for Human Caring*, *4*(3), 23–28.

Nåden, D., & Eriksson, K. (2002). Encounter: A fundamental category of nursing as an art. *International Journal for Human Caring*, *6*(1), 34–40.

Nåden, D., & Eriksson, K. (2003). Semantisk begrepsanalyse—Et grunnleggende aspekt i en disiplins teoriutvikling. *Vård i Norden*, *23*(1), 21–26. [Semantic concept analysis—A fundamental aspect in the theory development of a discipline. *Nordic Journal of Nursing Research and Clinical Studies*, *23*(1), 21–26.]

Nåden, D., & Eriksson, K. (2004). Understanding the importance of values and moral attitudes in nursing care in preserving human dignity. *Nursing Science Quarterly*, *17*(1), 86–91.

Nåden, D., & Eriksson, K. (2004). Values and moral attitudes in nursing care. Understanding the patient perspective. *Norsk Tidskrift for Sygepleieforskning*, *6*(1), 3–17.

Näsman, Y., Nyström, L., & Eriksson, K. (2011). Virtue, ethics and quality of care. *International Journal for Human Caring*, *15*(3), 74.

Nordman, T., Santavirta, N., & Eriksson, K. (2008). Developing an instrument to evaluate suffering related to care. *Scandinavian Journal of Caring Sciences*, *22*(4), 608–615.

Råholm, M-B., & Eriksson, K. (2001). Call to life: Exploring the spiritual dimension as a dialectic between suffering and desire experienced by coronary bypass patients. *International Journal for Human Caring*, *5*(1), 14–20.

Råholm, M-B., Lindholm, L., & Eriksson, K. (2002). Grasping the essence of the spiritual dimension reflected through the horizon of suffering: An interpretative research synthesis. *The Australian Journal of Holistic Nursing, 9*(1), 4–13.

Rehnsfeldt, A., & Eriksson, K. (2004). The progression of suffering implies alleviated suffering. *Scandinavian Journal of Caring Sciences, 18*(3), 264–272.

Roxberg, Å., Rehnsfeldt, A., Fridlund, B., & Eriksson, K. (2008). The meaning of consolation as experienced by nurses in a home-care setting. *Journal of Clinical Nursing, 17*(8), 1079–1087.

Rudolfsson, G., von Post, I., & Eriksson, K. (2007). The development of caring in the perioperative culture—Nurse leaders' perspective on the struggle to retain sight of the patient. *Nursing Administration Quarterly, 31*(4), 312–324.

Rudolfsson, G., von Post, I., & Eriksson, K. (2007). The expression of caring within the perioperative dialogue: A hermeneutic study. *International Journal of Nursing Studies, 44*, 905–915.

Rykkje, L., Eriksson, K., & Råholm, M-B. (2011). A qualitative metasynthesis of spirituality from a caring science perspective. *International Journal for Human Caring, 15*(4), 40–53.

Sivonen, K., Kasén, A., & Eriksson, K. (2010). Semantic analysis according to Peep Koort—A substance-oriented research methodology. *Scandinavian Journal of Caring Sciences, 24*, 12–20.

Thorkildsen, K. M., Eriksson, K., & Råholm, M.-B. (2014). Kierkegaard's works of love reflected through the lens of caring. *International Journal for Human Caring, 18*(3), 36–41.

Thorkildsen, K. M., Eriksson, K., & Råholm, M.-B. (2015). The core of love when caring for patients suffering from addiction. *Scandinavian Journal of Caring Sciences, 29*(2), 353–360.

von Post, I., & Eriksson, K. (2000). The ideal and practice concepts of "professional nursing care." *International Journal for Human Caring, 4*(1), 14–22.

Wärnå, C., Lindholm, L., & Eriksson, K. (2007). Virtue and health—Finding meaning and joy in working life. *Scandinavian Journal of Caring Sciences, 21*(2), 191–198.

Wärnå, C., Lindholm, L., & Eriksson, K. (2008). Virtue and health—Describing virtue as a path to the inner domain of health. *International Journal for Human Caring, 12*(1), 17–24.

Wikberg, A., & Eriksson, K. (2008). Intercultural caring—An abductive model. *Scandinavian Journal of Caring Sciences, 22*(3), 485–496.

Wiklund-Gustin, L., & Eriksson, K. (2009). The drama of suffering as narrated by patients who have undergone coronary bypass surgery. *International Journal for Human Caring, 13*(4), 17–25.

Wikström-Grotell, C., Lindholm, L., & Eriksson, K. (2002). Det mångdimensionella rörelsebegreppet i fysioterapin—En kontextuell analys. *Nordisk Fysioterapi, 6*, 146–184. [The multidimensional concept of movement in physiotherapy—A contextual analysis. *Nordisk Fysioterapi, 6*, 146–184.]

Articles in Compilation Works and Proceedings With Referee Practice

Compilation Works

Eriksson, K. (1971). En analys av sjuksköterskeutbildningen utgående från en utbildningsteknologisk model. I *Sairaanhoidon vuosikirja VIII* (s. 54–77). Helsinki, Finland: Sairaanhoitajien Koulutussäätiö. [An analysis of nursing education from an educational-technological model. In *Health care yearbook VIII* (pp. 54–77). Helsinki, Finland: Sairaanhoitajien Koulutussäätiö.]

Eriksson, K. (1974). Sairaanhoidon kehittäminen oppiaineena. I *Sairaanhoidon vuosikirja XI* (s. 9–21). Helsinki, Finland: Sairaanhoitajien Koulutussäätiö. [The development of health care as a subject. In *Health care yearbook XI* (pp. 9–21). Helsinki, Finland: Sairaanhoitajien Koulutussäätiö.]

Eriksson, K. (1977). Hälsa—En teoretisk och begreppsanalytisk studie om hälsa och dess nature. I *Sairaanhoidon vuosikirja XIV* (s. 55–195). [Health—A conceptual analysis and theoretical study of health and its nature. In *Health care yearbook XIV* (pp. 155–195). Helsinki, Finland: Sairaanhoitajien Koulutussäätiö.]

Eriksson, K. (1978). Modellen—Ett sätt att beskriva vårdskeendet. I *Sairaanhoidon vuosikirja XV* (s. 189–225). Helsinki, Finland: Sairaanhoitajien Koulutussäätiö. [The model—A way of describing the act of nursing care. In *Health care yearbook XV* (pp. 189–225). Helsinki, Finland: Sairaanhoitajien Koulutussäätiö.]

Eriksson, K. (1982). Den vårdvetenskapscentrerade läroplanen—Ett alternativ för dagens vårdutbildning. I *Sairaanhoidon vuosikirja XIX* (s. 173–187). Helsinki, Finland: Sairaanhoitajien Koulutussäätiö. [The caring science centered curriculum—An alternative for health education today. In *Health care yearbook XIX* (pp. 173–187). Helsinki, Finland: Sairaanhoitajien Koulutussäätiö.]

Eriksson, K. (1983). Den fullvuxna insulindiabetikern i hälsovårdens vårdprocess. I *Sairaanhoidon vuosikirja XIX* (s. 428–430). Helsinki, Finland: Sairaanhoitajien Koulutussäätiö. [The adult insulin-dependent diabetic in the health care nursing process. In *Health care yearbook XIX* (pp. 428–430). Helsinki, Finland: Sairaanhoitajien Koulutussäätiö.]

Eriksson, K. (1983). Vårdområdet finner sin profil—Den vårdvetenskapliga eran har inlets. I *Epione, Jubileumsskrift 1898–1983* (s. 12–17). [The area of caring finds its profile—The caring science era has begun. In *Epione, Jubileescript 1898–1983* (pp. 12–17). Helsinki, Finland: SSY-Sjuksköterskeföreningen i Finland.]

Eriksson, K. (1986). Hoito, Caring—Hoitotyön primaari substanssi. Puheenvuoro 2. I T. Martikainen & K. Manninen (red.), *Hoitotyö ja koulutus* (s. 17–41). Hämeenlinna, Finland: Sairaanhoitajien Koulutussäätiö. [Caring—The primary substance of nursing. Speech 2. In T. Martikainen & K. Manninen (Eds.), *Nursing and education* (pp. 17–41). Hämeenlinna, Finland: Sairaanhoitajien Koulutussäätiö.]

Eriksson, K. (1987). Vårdvetenskapen som humanistisk vetenskap. I *Hoitotiede vuosikirja*, 68–77. [Caring science as a humanistic science. *Journal of Nursing Science Yearbook*, 68–77.]

Eriksson, K. (1988). Vårdandets idé och ursprung. I *Panakeia. Vårdvetenskaplig årsbok* (s. 17–35). Stockholm: Almqvist & Wiksell. [The origin and idea of caring. In *Panakeia. Caring science yearbook* (pp. 17–35). Stockholm: Almqvist & Wiksell.]

Eriksson, K. (1989). Ammatillisuus hoitamisessa. I *Hoitoopin perusteet* (2: 2 yppl., s. 125–129). Vaasa, Finland: Sairaanhoitajien Koulutussäätiö. [Professionalism in caring. In *The basics of nursing science* (2nd ed., pp. 125–129). Vaasa, Finland: Sairaanhoitajien Koulutussäätiö.]

Eriksson, K. (1990). Framtidsvisioner—om utvecklingen av sjukskötarens arbete. I *Epione, Jubileumsskrift 1898–1988* (s. 28–38). Helsinki, Finland: SSY-sjukskötersksföreningen i Finland r.f. [Future visions of the development of the nurse's work. *In Epione, Jubilee-script 1898–1988* (pp. 28–38). Helsinki, Finland: SSY-sjuksköterske-föreningen i Finlandr.f.]

Eriksson, K. (1991). Hälsa är mera än frånvaro av sjukdom. I *Centrum för vårdvetenskap, Vård—Utbildning—Utveckling—Forskning* (s. 1–2, 29–35). Stockholm: Karolinska Institutet. [Health is more than the absence of illness. In *Centrum för vårdvetenskap, Vård—Utbildning—Utveckling—Forskning* (pp. 1–2, 29–35). Stockholm: Karolinska Institute.]

Eriksson, K. (1993). De första åren—Några reflektioner kring den vårdvetenskapliga eran. I *Epione, Jubileumsskrift 1898–1993* (s. 7–15). Helsinki, Finland: SSY-Sjuksköterskeföreningen. [The first years—Reflections upon the era of caring science. In *Epione, Jubilee-script 1898–1993* (pp. 7–15). Helsinki, Finland: SSY-Sjuksköterskeföreningen.]

Eriksson, K. (1994). Vårdvetenskapen som autonom discipline. I H. Willman (red.), *Hygieia. Hoitotyön vuosikirja 1994* (s. 87–91). Helsinki, Finland: Kirjayhtymä. [Caring science as an autonomous discipline. In H. Willman (Ed.), *Hygieia. Nursing yearbook 1994* (pp. 87–91). Helsinki, Finland: Kirjayhtymä.]

Eriksson, K. (1996). Efterskrift—Om vårdvetenskapens möjligheter och gränser. I K. Martinsen (red.), *Fenomenologi og omsorg* (s. 140–150). Oslo, Norway: TANO. [Postscript—About the possibilities and boundaries of caring science. In K. Martinsen (Ed.), *Phenomenology and caring* (pp. 140–150). Oslo, Norway: TANO.]

Eriksson, K. (1996). Om dokumentation—Vad den är och inte är. I K. Dahlberg (red.), *Konsten att dokumentera omvårdnad* (s. 9–13). Lund, Sweden: Studentlitteratur. [On documentation—What it is and what it is not. In K. Dahlberg (Ed.), *The art of documenting care* (pp. 9–13). Lund, Sweden: Studentlitteratur.]

Eriksson, K. (1996). Om människans värdighet. I T. Bjerkreim, J. Mathinsen, & R. Nord (red.), *Visjon, viten og virke. Festskrift till sykepleieren Kjellaug Lerheim, 70 år* (s. 79–86). Oslo, Norway: Universitetsförlaget. [On human dignity. In T. Bjerkreim, J. Mathinsen, & R. Nord (Eds.), *Vision, knowledge and influence. Jubilee-script for the nurse Kjellaug Lerheim, 70 years* (pp. 79–86). Oslo, Norway: Universitetsförlaget.]

Eriksson, K. (1997). Mot en vårdetisk teori. I *Hoitotyön vuosikirja 1997. Pro Nursing RY:n vuosikirja, Hygieia* (s. 9–23). Helsinki, Finland: Kirjayhtymä. [Toward an ethical caring theory. In *Nursing yearbook 1997. Pro Nursing RY:s yearbook, Hygieia* (pp. 9–23). Helsinki, Finland: Kirjayhtymä.]

Eriksson, K. (1998). Epione—Vårdandets ethos. I *Epione, Jubileumsskrift 1898–1998.* Helsinki, Finland: SSY-Sjuksköterskeföreningen. [Epione—The ethos of caring. In *Epione, Jubilee-script 1898–1998.* Helsinki, Finland: SSY-Sjuksköterskeföreningen.]

Eriksson, K. (1998). Människans värdighet, lidande och lidandets ethos. I *Suomen Mielenterveysseura, Tuhkaa ja linnunrata. Henkisyys mielenterveystyössä* (s. 67–82). Helsinki: Suomen Mielenterveysseura, SMS-julkaisut. [Human dignity, suffering and the ethos of suffering. In *Ashes and the Milky Way: Spirituality in mental health care nursing* (pp. 67–82). Helsinki: Suomen Mielenterveysseura, SMS-julkaisut.]

Eriksson, K. (1999). Tillbaka till Popper och Kuhn—En evolutionär epistemologi för vårdvetenskapen. I J. Kinnunen, P. Meriläinen, K. Vehviläinen-Julkunen, & T. Nyberg (red.), *Terveystieteiden monialainen tutkimus ja yliopistokoulutus. Suunnistuspoluilta tiedon valtatielle. Professor Sirkka Sinkkoselle omistettu juhlakirja* (s. 21–35). Kuopio, Finland: Kuopion yliopiston julkaisuja E, Yhteiskuntatieteet 74. [Back to Popper and Kuhn—An evolutionary epistemology for caring science. In J. Kinnunen, P. Meriläinen, K. Vehviläinen-Julkunen, & T. Nyberg (Eds.), *The multiscientific health science university education and research. Paths to the highway of science. A jubilee book dedicated to Professor Sirkka Sikkonen* (pp. 21–35). Kuopio, Finland: Kuopion yliopiston julkaisuja E, Yhteiskuntatieteet 74.]

Eriksson, K. (1999). Vårdvetenskapen—En akademisk disciplin. I S. Janhonen, I. Lepola, M. Nikkonen, & M. Toljamo (red.), *Suomalainen hoitotiede uudelle vuosituhannelle. Professori Maija Hentisen juhlakirja* (s. 59–64). Oulu, Finland: Oulun yliopiston hoitotieteen ja terveyshallinnon laitoksen julkaisuja 2. [Caring science—An academic discipline. In S. Janhonen, I. Lepola, M. Nikkonen, & M. Toljamo (Eds.), *The Finnish caring science in the new millennium. A jubilee-script dedicated to Professor Maija Hentinen* (pp. 59–64). Oulu, Finland: Oulun yliopiston hoitotieteen ja terveyshallinnon laitoksen julkaisuja 2.]

Eriksson, K. (2000). Caritas et passio—Liebe und leiden—Als grundkategorien der pflegewissenschaft. I T. Strom, *Diakonie an der Schwelle zum neuen Jahrtausend*. Heidelberg, Germany: Diakoniewissenschaftlichen Instituts, Universität Heidelberg. [Caritas et passio—Love and suffering as basic categories in caring science. In T. Strom, *The diaconate on the threshold of the new millennium.* Heidelberg, Germany: Diakoniewissenschaftlichen Instituts, Universität Heidelberg.]

Eriksson, K. (2002). Rakkaus—Diakoniatieteen ydin ja ethos? I M. Lahtinen & T. Toikkanen (red.), *Anno Domini. Diakoniatieteen vuosikirja 2002* (s. 155–164). Tampere, Finland: Tammerpaino. [Love—The core and ethos of deacony? In M. Lahtinen & T. Toikkanen (Eds.), *Anno Domini. Diakonic yearbook 2002* (pp. 155–164). Tampere, Finland: Tammerpaino.]

Eriksson, K. (2003). Diakonian erityisyys hoitotyössä. I M. Lahtinen & T. Toikkanen (red.), *Anno domini. Diakoniatieteen vuosikirja 2003* (s. 120–126). Tampere, Finland: Tammerpaino. [The uniqueness of deacony in nursing. In M. Lahtinen & T. Toikkanen (Eds.), *Anno Domini. Diakonic yearbook 2003* (pp. 120–126). Tampere, Finland: Tammerpaino.]

Eriksson, K. (2009). Evidens—Det sanna, det sköna, det goda och det eviga. I K. Martinsen & K. Eriksson, *Å se og innse. Om ulike former for evidens* (s. 35–80). Oslo, Norge: Akribe. [Evidence—The true, the beautiful, the good and the eternal. In K. Martinsen & K. Eriksson, *To see and to understand. About different forms of evidence* (pp. 35–80). Oslo, Norway: Akribe.]

Eriksson, K., & Hamrin, E. (1988). Vårdvetenskapen formas—En tillbakablick och ett framtidsperspektiv. I *Panakeia*, *vårdvetenskaplig årsbok* (s. 9–16). Stockholm: Almqvist & Wiksell. [Caring science is formed—A historical and futuristic perspective. In *Panakeia, caring science yearbook* (pp. 9–16). Stockholm: Almqvist & Wiksell.]

Eriksson, K., & Lindholm T. (2010). "Love endures all things?" Violence between spouses, suffering, and alleviation of suffering—developing a theory model. *International Journal for Human Caring, 14*(3), 72.

Books and Monographs

Eriksson, K. (1976). *Hoitotapahtuma. Hoito-oppi 2.* Helsinki, Finland: Sairaanhoitajien Koulutussäätiö. [*The nursing care process. Nursing science 2.* Helsinki, Finland: Sairaanhoitajien Koulutussäätiö.]

Eriksson, K. (1981). *Vårdprocessen—En utgångspunkt för läroplanstänkande inom vårdutbildningen. Utvecklande av en vårdprocessmodell samt ett läroplanstänkande utgående från vårdprocessen* (Nr. 94). Helsinki, Finland: Helsingfors universitet, Pedagogiska Institutionen. [*The nursing care process—An approach to curriculum construction within nursing education. The development of a model for the nursing care process and an approach for curriculum development based on the process of nursing care* (No. 94). Helsinki, Finland: Department of Education University of Helsinki.]

Eriksson, K. (1982). *Vårdprocessen* (2:a uppl.). Stockholm: Almqvist & Wiksell. [*The nursing care process* (2nd ed.). Stockholm: Almqvist & Wiksell.]

Eriksson, K. (1985). *Vårdprocessen* (3: e uppl.). Stockholm: Almqvist & Wiksell. [*The nursing care process* (3rd ed.). Stockholm: Almqvist & Wiksell.]

Eriksson, K. (1986). *Hoito-opin didaktiikka.* Helsinki, Finland: Sairaanhoitajien Koulutussäätiö. [*The didactics of caring science.* Helsinki, Finland: Sairaanhoitajien Koulutussäätiö.]

Eriksson, K. (1986). *Introduktion till vårdvetenskap* (2:a uppl.). Stockholm: Almqvist & Wiksell. [*An introduction to caring science* (2nd ed.). Stockholm: Almqvist & Wiksell.]

Eriksson, K. (1987). *Hoitamisen idea.* Forssa, Finland: Sairaanhoitajien Koulutussäätiö. [*The idea of caring.* Forssa, Finland: Sairaanhoitajien Koulutussäätiö.]

Eriksson, K. (1987). *Vårdandets idé.* Stockholm: Almqvist & Wiksell. [*The idea of caring.* Stockholm: Almqvist & Wiksell.]

Eriksson, K. (1988). *Hoito tieteenä.* Forssa, Sweden: Sairaanhoitajien Koulutussäätiö. [*Caring as a science.* Forssa, Sweden: Sairaanhoitajien Koulutussäätiö.]

Eriksson, K. (1989). *Caritas-idea.* Helsinki, Finland: Sairaanhoitajien Koulutussäätiö. [*The idea of caritas.* Helsinki, Finland: Sairaanhoitajien Koulutussäätiö.]

Eriksson, K. (1989). *Hälsans idé* (2:a uppl.). Stockholm: Almqvist & Wiksell. [*The idea of health* (2nd ed.). Stockholm: Almqvist & Wiksell.]

Eriksson, K. (1989). *Terveyden idea.* Helsinki, Finland: Sairaanhoitajien Koulutussäätiö. [*The idea of health.* Helsinki, Finland: Sairaanhoitajien Koulutussäätiö.]

Eriksson, K. (1995). *Det lidende menneske* (Danish translation). Copenhagen: Munksgaard. [*The suffering human being* (Danish translation). Copenhagen: Munksgaard.]

Eriksson, K. (1995). *Den lidende menneske* (Norwegian translation). Oslo: TANO. [*The suffering human being* (Norwegian translation). Oslo: TANO.]

Eriksson, K. (1996). *Omsorgens idé* (Danish translation). Copenhagen: Munksgaard. [*The idea of caring* (Danish translation). Copenhagen: Munksgaard.]

Eriksson, K. (1997). *Vårdandets idé (Kassettband). Talboksoch punktskriftsbiblioteket.* Stockholm: Almqvist & Wiksell. [*The idea of caring (Audiotape). Talboksoch punktskriftsbiblioteket.* Stockholm: Almqvist & Wiksell.]

Eriksson, K. (2001). *Gesundheit. Ein Schlüsselbegriff der Pflegetheorie.* (German translation). Bern, Germany: Verlag Hans Huber. [*The idea of health* (German translation). Bern, Germany: Verlag Hans Huber.]

Eriksson, K. (2006). *The suffering human being.* Chicago: Nordic Studies Press. [English translation of: *Den lidande människan.* Stockholm, Sweden: Liber Förlag.]

Eriksson, K., & Barbosa da Silva, A. (Eds.). (1994). *Usko ja terveys—johdatus hoitoteologiaan.* (Finnish translation). Helsinki, Finland: Sairaanhoitajien Koulutussäätiö. [*Caring theology* (Finnish translation). Helsinki, Finland: Sairaanhoitajien Koulutussäätiö.]

Eriksson, K., Byfält, H., Leijonqvist, G-B., Nyberg, K., & Uuspää, B. (1986). *Vårdteknologi.* Stockholm: Almqvist & Wiksell. [*Caring technology.* Stockholm: Almqvist & Wiksell.]

University and Department Publications

Eriksson, K. (1991). Att lindra lidande. I K. Eriksson & A. Barbosa da Silva (red.), *Vårdteologi. Vårdforskningar 3/1991* (s. 204–221). Vaasa, Finland: Institutionen för vårdvetenskap, Åbo Akademi. [To alleviate suffering. In K. Eriksson & A. Barbosa da Silva (Eds.), *Caring theology* (pp. 204–221). Vaasa, Finland: Department of Caring Science, Åbo Akademi.]

Eriksson, K. (1991). Vårdteologins framväxt. I K. Eriksson & A. Barbosa da Silva (red.). *Vårdteologi. Vårdforskningar 3/1991* (s. 1–25). [The growth of caring theology. In K. Eriksson & A. Barbosa da Silva (Eds.), *Caring theology* (pp. 1–25). Vaasa, Finland: Department of Caring Science, Åbo Akademi.]

Eriksson, K. (red.). (1993). *Möten med lidanden.* Vårdforskning 4/1993. Vaasa, Finland: Institutionen för vårdvetenskap, Åbo Akademi. [*Encounters with suffering.* Vaasa, Finland: Department of Caring Science, Åbo Akademi.]

Eriksson, K. (red.). (1995). *Den mångdimensionella hälsan—Verklighet och visioner.* Slutrapport. Vaasa, Finland: Vasa sjukvårdsdistrikt kf. och Institutionen för vårdvetenskap, Åbo Akademi. [*Multidimensional health—Visions and reality. Final report.* Vaasa, Finland: Vasa sjukvårdsdistrikt kf. och Institutionen för vårdvetenskap, Åbo Akademi.]

Eriksson, K. (1995). Vad är vårdetik? I K. Eriksson (red.), *Mot en caritativ vårdetik.* Vårdforskning 5/1995 (s. 1–8). Vaasa, Finland: Institutionen för vårdvetenskap, Åbo Akademi. [What is caring ethic? In K. Eriksson (Ed.), *Toward a caritative caring ethic* Caring research 5/1995. (pp. 1–8). Vaasa, Finland: Department of Caring Science, Åbo Akademi.].

Eriksson, K. (1997). Att insjukna i demens—Ett tungt lidande för patient och anhöriga. I B. Beck-Friis & G. Grahn (red.), *Leva med demenshandikapp.* Lund, Sweden: Lunds universitet: Stiftelsen Silviahemmet. [Becoming ill with dementia—A burdensome suffering for the patient and his/her family. In B. Beck-Friis & G. Grahn (Eds.), *Living with the handicap of dementia (Action in favor of people suffering from neurodegenerative diseases)*. Lund, Sweden: Lunds universitet, Stiftelsen Silviahemmet.]

Eriksson, K. (1998). Vårdvetenskapens framväxt som akademisk disciplin—Ett finlandssvenskt perspektiv. I K. Eriksson (red.), *Jubileumsskrift 1987–1997* (s. 1–7). Vaasa, Finland: Institutionen för vårdvetenskap, Åbo Akademi. [The growth of caring science as an academic discipline—A Finland-Swedish perspective. In K. Eriksson (Ed.), *Jubilee-script 1987–1997* (pp. 1–7). Vaasa, Finland: Department of Caring Science, Åbo Akademi.]

Eriksson, K. (2002). *Den trojanske hest. Evidensbasering og sygepleje.* (Danish translation). Copenhagen: Gads Förlag. [*The Trojan horse. Evidence-based nursing and caring through a caring science perspective* (Danish translation). Copenhagen: Gads Förlag.]

Eriksson, K. (2002). Idéhistoria som deldisciplin inom vårdvetenskapen. I K. Eriksson & D. Matilainen (red.), *Vårdandets och vårdvetenskapens idéhistoria. Strövtåg i spårandet av "caritas originalis."* Vårdforskning 8/2002 (s. 1–14). Vaasa, Finland: Institutionen för vårdvetenskap, Åbo Akademi. [The history of ideas as a sub-discipline within caring science. In K. Eriksson & D. Matilainen (Eds.), *The history of ideas of caring and caring science. Wanderings in search of "caritas originalis."* Caring research 8/2002 (pp. 1–14). Vaasa, Finland: Department of Caring Science, Åbo Akademi.]

Eriksson, K. (2002). Vårdandets idéhistoria. I K. Eriksson & D. Matilainen (red.), *Vårdandets och vårdvetenskapens idéhistoria. Strövtåg i spårandet av "caritas originalis."* Vårdforskning 8/2002 (s. 15–34). Vaasa, Finland: Institutionen för vårdvetenskap, Åbo Akademi. [The history of ideas of caring. In K. Eriksson & D. Matilainen (Eds.), *The history of ideas of caring and caring science. Wanderings in search of "caritas originalis."* Caring research 8/2002 (pp. 15–34). Vaasa, Finland: Department of Caring Science, Åbo Akademi.]

Eriksson, K., & Barbosa da Silva, A. (1991). Vååardteologi som vårdvetenskapens deldisciplin. I K. Eriksson & A. Barbosa da Silva (red.), *Vårdteologi. Vårdforskningar 3/1991* (s. 26–64). Vaasa, Finland: Institutionen för vårdvetenskap, Åbo Akademi. [Caring theology as a sub-discipline of caring science. In K. Eriksson & A. Barbosa da Silva (Eds.), *Caring theology.* Caring research 3/1991 (pp. 26–64). Vaasa, Finland: Department of Caring Science, Åbo Akademi.]

Eriksson, K., & Herberts, S. (1991). Tron i hälsans tjänst. I K. Eriksson & A. Barbosa da Silva (red.), *Vårdteologi. Vårdforskningar 3/1991* (s. 222–258). Vaasa, Finland: Institutionen för vårdvetenskap, Åbo Akademi. [Faith in the service of health. In K. Eriksson & A. Barbosa da Silva (Eds.), *Caring theology. Caring research 3/1991* (pp. 222–258). Vaasa, Finland: Department of Caring Science, Åbo Akademi.]

Eriksson, K., & Herberts, S. (1993). Lidande—En begreppsanalytisk studie. I K. Eriksson (red.), *Möten med lidanden. Vårdforskningar 4/1993* (s. 29–54). Vaasa, Finland: Institutionen för vårdvetenskap, Åbo Akademi. [A study of suffering—A concept analysis. In K. Eriksson (Ed.), *Encounters with suffering. Caring research 4/1993* (pp. 29–54). Vaasa, Finland: Department of Caring Science, Åbo Akademi.]

Eriksson, K., Herberts, S., & Lindholm, L. (1993). Bilder av lidande—Lidande i belysning av aktuell vårdvetenskaplig forskning. I K. Eriksson (red.), *Möten med lidanden. Vårdforskningar 4/1993 suffering* (s. 55–78). Vaasa, Finland: Institutionen för vårdvetenskap, Åbo Akademi. [Views of suffering—Suffering in the light of current caring science research. In K. Eriksson (Ed.), *Encounters with suffering. Caring research 4/1993* (pp. 55–78). Vaasa, Finland: Department of Caring Science, Åbo Akademi.]

Eriksson, K., & Koort, P. (1973). *Sjukvårdspedagogik (Kompendium).* Helsinki, Finland: Helsingfors svenska sjukvårdsinstitut. [*The pedagogy of nursing care (Compendium).* Helsinki, Finland: Helsingfors svenska sjukvårdsinstitut.]

Eriksson, K., & Lindholm, L. (1993). Lidande och kärlek ur ett psykiatriskt vårdperspektiv—En casestudie av mötet mellan mänskligt lidande och kärlek. I K. Eriksson (red.), *Möten med lidanden. Vårdforskningar 4/1993 suffering* (s. 79–137). Vaasa, Finland: Institutionen för vårdvetenskap, Åbo Akademi. [Love and suffering through a psychiatric caring perspective—A case study of the encounters with human love and suffering. In K. Eriksson (Ed.), *Encounters with suffering. Caring research 4/1993* (pp. 79–137). Vaasa, Finland: Department of Caring Science, Åbo Akademi.]

Eriksson, K., & Lindström, U. Å. (2000). *Gryning. En vårdvetenskaplig antologi.* Vaasa, Finland: Institutionen för vårdvetenskap, Åbo Akademi. [*Dawn. An anthology of caring science.* Vaasa, Finland: Department of Caring Science, Åbo Akademi.]

Eriksson, K., & Lindström, U. Å. (2000). Siktet, Sökandet, slutandet. I K. Eriksson & U. Å. Lindström (red.), *Gryning. En vårdvetenskaplig antologi* (s. 5–18). Vaasa, Finland: Institutionen för vårdvetenskap, Åbo Akademi. [Envisioning, seeking and ending. In K. Eriksson & U. Å. Lindström (eds.), *Dawn. An anthology of caring science* (pp. 5–18). Vaasa, Finland: Department of Caring Science, Åbo Akademi.]

Eriksson, K., & Lindström, U. Å. (2003). Klinisk vårdvetenskap. I K. Eriksson & U. Å. Lindström (red.), *Gryning II. Klinisk vårdvetenskap* (s. 3–20). Vaasa, Finland: Institutionen för vårdvetenskap, Åbo Akademi. [Clinical caring science. In K. Eriksson & U. Å. Lindström (Eds.), *Dawn II. Clinical caring science* (pp. 3–20). Vaasa, Finland: Department of Caring Science, Åbo Akademi.]

Eriksson, K., & Lindström, U. Å. (2007). Vårdvetenskapens vetenskapsteori på hermeneutisk grund—några grunddrag. I K. Eriksson, U. Å. Lindström, D. Matilainen & L. Lindholm (red.), *Gryning III. Vårdvetenskap och hermeneutik* (s. 5–20). Vaasa, Finland: Enheten för vårdvetenskap, Åbo Akademi. [The theory of science for caring science on a hermeneutic foundation—some basic features. In K. Eriksson, U. Å. Lindström, D. Matilainen, & L. Lindholm (Eds.), *Dawn III. Caring science and hermeneutics* (pp. 5–20). Vaasa, Finland: Department of Caring Science, Åbo Akademi.]

Eriksson, K., & Matilainen, D. (red.). (2002). *Vårdandets och vårdvetenskapens idéhistoria. Strövtåg i spårandet av "caritas originalis." Vårdforskning 8/2002.* Vaasa, Finland: Institutionen för vårdvetenskap, Åbo Akademi. [Eriksson, K., & Matilainen, D. (eds.). *The history of ideas of caring and caring science. Wanderings* in search of "caritas originalis." Caring research 8/2002. Vaasa, Finland: Department of Caring Science, Åbo Akademi.]

Eriksson, K., & Matilainen, D. (red.). (2004). *Vårdvetenskapens didaktik. Caritativ didaktik i vårdandets tjänst. Vårdforskningar 9/2004*. Vaasa, Finland: Institutionen för vårdvetenskap, Åbo Akademi. [*The didactics of caring science. Caritative didactics in the service of caring*. Vaasa, Finland: Department of Caring Science, Åbo Akademi.]

Eriksson, K., Nordman, T., & Myllymäki, I. (1999). *Den trojanska hästen. Evidensbaserat vårdande och vårdarbete ur ett vårdvetenskapligt perspektiv cultures (Rap. 1)*. Vaasa, Finland: Institutionen för vårdvetenskap, Åbo Akademi; Helsingfors universitetscentralsjukhus & Vasa sjukvårdsdistrikt. [*The Trojan horse II—Development of evidence-based caring cultures (Rap. 1)*. Vaasa, Finland: Institutionen för vårdvetenskap, Åbo Akademi; Helsingfors universitetscentralsjukhus & Vasa sjukvårdsdistrikt.]

Herberts, S., & Eriksson, K. (1995). Vårdarnas etiska profil. I K. Eriksson (red.), *Mot en caritativ vårdetik. Vårdforskning 5/1995* (s. 41–62). Vaasa, Finland: Institutionen för vårdvetenskap, Åbo Akademi. [The ethical profile of the carers. In K. Eriksson (Ed.), *Toward a caritative caring ethic. Caring research 5/1995* (pp. 41–62). Vaasa, Finland: Department of Caring Science, Åbo Akademi.]

Secondary Sources

Doctoral Dissertations

Blegen, N. (2015). *Kallet til livets embete: mødre i helse og lidelse*. Doktorsavhandling, Turku, Finland: Åbo Akademis Förlag. [*The call to the ministry of life. Mothers in the health and suffering*. Doctoral dissertation, Turku, Finland: Åbo Akademi University Press.]

Frilund, M. (2013). *En vårdvetenskaplig syntes mellan vårdandets ethos och vårdintensitet*. Doktorsavhandling, Turku, Finland: Åbo Akademis Förlag. [*A synthesizer of caring science and nursing intensity*. Doctoral dissertation, Turku, Finland: Åbo Akademi University Press.]

Foss, B. (2012). *Ledelse—en bevegelse i ansvar og kjærlighet*. Doktorsavhandling, Turku, Finland: Åbo Akademis förlag. [*Leadership—A movement in responsibility and love*. Doctoral dissertation, Turku, Finland: Åbo Akademi University Press.]

Gabrielsen, E. (2014). *Det hjemløse menneske. En studie av sykdom og lidelse*. Doktorsavhandling, Turku, Finland: Åbo Akademis Förlag. [*The homeless human being—a study of disease, illness and suffering*. Doctoral dissertation, Turku, Finland: Åbo Akademi University Press.]

Helin, K. (2011). *Den vårdande och helande bilden—möten med bildkonst i vårdandets värld*. Doktorsavhandling, Turku, Finland: Åbo Akademis förlag. [*The caring and healing image—Encountering works of visual art in the caring context*. Doctoral dissertation, Turku, Finland: Åbo Akademi University Press.]

Hemberg, J. (2015). *Livets källa kärleken: hälsans urkraft*. Doktorsavhandling, Turku, Finland: Åbo Akademis Förlag. [*The source of life, love—Health's primordial wellspring of strength*. Doctoral dissertation, Turku, Finland: Åbo Akademi University Press.]

Högström, M. (2016). *Den Äldsta—Livet är ett tillägnande. En vårdvetenskaplig explorativ studie av ett meningsbärande budskap och innerlig visdom*. Doktorsavhandling, Turku, Finland: Åbo Akademis Förlag. [*The Eldest—Life is acquiring. An explorative study in caring science of a meaningful message and an innermost wisdom*. Doctoral dissertation, Turku, Finland: Åbo Akademi University Press.]

Honkavuo, L. (2014). *Serva ad ministrare. Tjänandets ethos i vårdledarskap*. Doktorsavhandling, Turku, Finland: Åbo Akademis Förlag. [*Serva ad ministrare. The ethos of serving in nursing leadership*. Doctoral dissertation, Turku, Finland: Åbo Akademi University Press.]

Karlsson, M. (2013). *Bry sig om—ett vårdvetenskapligt praxisbegrepp*. Doktorsavhandling, Turku, Finland: Åbo Akademis Förlag. [*To care for—A caring science praxis concept*. Doctoral dissertation, Turku, Finland: Åbo Akademi University Press.]

Koskinen, C. (2011). *Lyssnande—en vårdvetenskaplig betraktelse*. Doktorsavhandlin, Turku, Finland: Åbo Akademis förlag. [*Listening—A caring science reflection*. Doctoral dissertation, Turku, Finland: Åbo Akademi University Press.]

Koslander, T. (2011). *Ljusets gemenskap—en gestaltning av den andliga dimensionen i vårdandet*. Doktorsavhandling, Turku, Finland: Åbo Akademis förlag. [*The Communion of the Light—Shaping of spiritual dimension in the caritative caring*. Doctoral dissertation, Turku, Finland: Åbo Akademi University Press.]

Levy-Malmberg, R. (2010). *Interpretive dialogical evaluation. Evaluating caring science basic research*. Doctoral dissertation, Turku, Finland: Åbo Akademi University Press.

Lindberg, S. (2013). *I hälsans spelrum: lek på vårdandets scen*. Doktorsavhandling, Turku, Finland: Åbo Akademis Förlag. [*In the playhouse of health—Play on the stage of caring*. Doctoral dissertation, Turku, Finland: Åbo Akademi University Press.]

Melheim, A. (2014). *Bevegelsens lindring - lindringens bevegelse. Omsorgssamtale med barn*. Doktorsavhandling, Turku, Finland: Åbo Akademis Förlag. [*The alleviation of movement—The movement of alleviation. Caring conversations with children*. Doctoral dissertation, Turku, Finland: Åbo Akademi University Press.]

Nyback, M-H. (2008). *Generic and professional caring in a Chinese setting—an ethnographic study*. Doctoral dissertation, Turku, Finland: Åbo Akademi University Press.

Nyholm, L. (2015). *Urvilja: när livet är människans hem*. Doktorsavhandling, Turku, Finland: Åbo Akademis Förlag. [*Will—When life is the home of the human being*. Doctoral dissertation, Turku, Finland: Åbo Akademi University Press.]

Rydenlund, K. (2012). *Vårdandets imperativ i de yttersta livsrummen. Hermeneutiska vårdande samtal inom den rättspsykiatriska vården*. Doktorsavhandling, Turku, Finland: Åbo Akademis förlag. [*The imperative of caring in extreme living-spaces—Hermeneutical caring conversations in forensic psychiatric care*. Doctoral dissertation, Turku, Finland: Åbo Akademi University Press.]

Rykkje, L. (2014). *Kjærlighet i forbundethet—en kraft i gamle menneskers åndelighet og verdighet*. Doktorsavhandling, Turku,

Finland: Åbo Akademis Förlag. [*Love in connectedness—A force in older people's spirituality and dignity.* Doctoral dissertation, Turku, Finland: Åbo Akademi University Press.]

Salmela, S. (2012). *Leda förändring genom relationer, processer och kulturer.* Doktorsavhandling, Turku, Finland: Åbo Akademis Förlag. [*Leading change by leading relationships, processes and cultures.* Doctoral dissertation, Turku, Finland: Åbo Akademi University Press.]

Sandvik, A-H. (2015). *Att bli en 'caring' sjukskötare—kärnan i vårdutbildningen.* Doktorsavhandling, Turku, Finland: Åbo Akademis Förlag. [*Becoming a caring nurse—The heart of the matter in nurse education.* Doctoral dissertation, Turku, Finland: Åbo Akademi University Press.]

Selander, G. (2014). *Glädje i vårdandets värld.* Doktorsavhandling, Turku, Finland: Åbo Akademis Förlag. [*Joy in the world of Caring.* Doctoral dissertation, Turku, Finland: Åbo Akademi University Press.]

Ueland, V. (2013). *Lengsel—en kraft til helse.* Doktorsavhandling, Turku, Finland: Åbo Akademis Förlag. [*Longing—A force to health.* Doctoral dissertation, Turku, Finland: Åbo Akademi University Press.]

Wikberg, A. (2014). *En vårdvetenskaplig teori om interkulturellt vårdande—att föda barn i en annan kultur.* Doktorsavhandling, Turku, Finland: Åbo Akademis Förlag. [*A caring science theory on intercultural caring—Giving birth in another culture.* Doctoral dissertation, Turku, Finland: Åbo Akademi University Press.]

UNIT III

Nursing Conceptual Models

- Nursing conceptual models are concepts and their relationships that specify a perspective and produce evidence among phenomenon specific to the discipline.
- Conceptual models address broad metaparadigm concepts (human beings, health, nursing and environment) that are central to their meaning in the context of a particular framework and the discipline of nursing.
- Nursing conceptual models provide perspectives with different foci for critical thinking about persons, families, and communities and for making knowledgeable nursing decisions.
- Nursing conceptual models provide a nursing perspective for theory development at various levels of abstraction.

Philosophy
sets forth the meaning of nursing phenomena through analysis, reasoning and logical presentation of concepts and ideas.

Conceptual Models
are sets of concepts that address phenomena central to nursing in propositions that explain the relationship among them.

Grand Theory
concepts that derive from a conceptual model and propose a testable proposition that tests the major premise of the model.

Nursing Theory
testable propositions from philosophies, conceptual models, grand theories, abstract nursing theories, or theories from other disciplines. Theories are less abstract than grand theory and less specific than middle-range theory.

Middle-Range Theory
concepts most specific to practice that propose precise testable nursing practice questions and include details such as patient age group, family situation, health condition, location of the patient, and action of the nurse.

The Future of Nursing Theory
Nursing theoretical systems give direction and create understanding in practice, research, administration, and education.

Metaparadigm

The broad conceptual boundaries of the discipline of nursing: Human beings, environment, health, and nursing

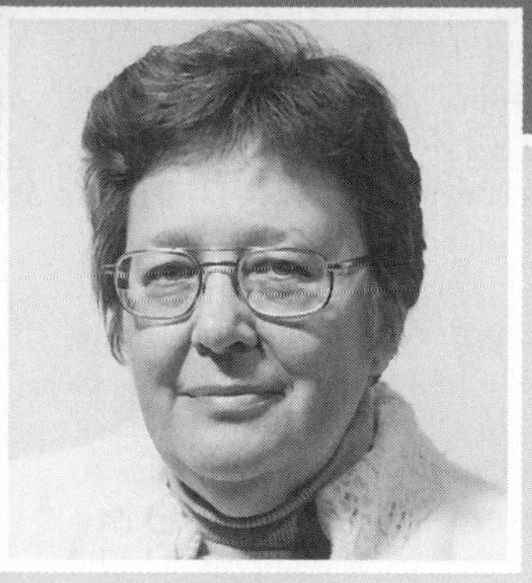

Myra Estrin Levine
(1921–1996)

The Conservation Model

Linda C. Mefford

"For a nurse to apply the four conservation principles, it is essential that she identify the specific patterns of adaptation of every patient. Truly patient-centered plans for nursing care are then possible. Understanding the message and responding to it accurately constitute the substance of nursing science."
(Levine, 1967b, p. 47)

"The goal of all nursing care should be to promote wholeness, realizing that for every individual that requires a unique and separate cluster of activities. The individual's integrity—his one-ness, his identity as an individual, his wholeness—is his abiding concern, and it is the nurse's responsibility to assist him to defend and to seek its realization."
(Levine, 1971a, p. 258)

CREDENTIALS AND BACKGROUND OF THE THEORIST*

Myra Estrin Levine enjoyed a varied career. She was a private duty nurse (1944), a civilian nurse in the U.S. Army (1945), a preclinical instructor in the physical sciences at Cook County School of Nursing (1947–1950), director of nursing at Drexel Home in Chicago (1950–1951), and surgical supervisor at both the University of Chicago Clinics (1951–1952) and the Henry Ford Hospital in Detroit (1956–1962). Levine worked her way up the academic ranks at Bryan Memorial Hospital in Lincoln, Nebraska (1951), Cook County School of Nursing (1963–1967), Loyola University (1967–1973), Rush University (1974–1977), and the University of Illinois (1962–1963, 1977–1987). She chaired the Department of Clinical Nursing at Cook County School of Nursing (1963–1967) and coordinated the graduate nursing program in oncology at Rush University (1974–1977). Levine was director of the Department of Continuing Education at Evanston Hospital (March to June 1974) and consultant to the department (July 1974–1976). She was adjunct associate professor of Humanistic Studies at the University of Illinois (1981–1987). In 1987 she became a Professor Emerita, Medical Surgical Nursing, at the University of Illinois at Chicago. In 1974 Levine went to Tel-Aviv University, Israel, as a visiting associate professor and returned as a visiting professor in 1982. She also was a visiting professor at Recanati School of Nursing, Ben Gurion University of the Negev, at Beer Sheva, Israel (March to April 1982).

Levine received numerous honors, including charter fellow of the American Academy of Nursing (1973), honorary member of the American Mental Health Aid to Israel (1976), and honorary recognition from the Illinois Nurses Association (1977). She was the first recipient of the Elizabeth Russell Belford Award for excellence in teaching from Sigma

*Previous authors: Karen Moore Schaefer, Gloria S. Artigue, Karen J. Foil, Tamara Johnson, Ann Marriner Tomey, Mary Carolyn Poat, LaDema Poppa, Roberta Woeste, and Susan T. Zoretich.

*The information in this section is informed by Levine's autobiographical chapter (1988a), her curriculum vitae, and the program from the 1992 Mid-Year Convocation, Loyola University, Chicago.

Theta Tau (1977). Both the first and second editions of her book *Introduction to Clinical Nursing* (Levine, 1969a, 1973) received *American Journal of Nursing* Book of the Year awards, and her book *Renewal for Nursing* was translated into Hebrew (Levine, 1971c). Levine was listed in *Who's Who in American Women* (1977–1988) and in *Who's Who in American Nursing* (1987). She was elected fellow of the Institute of Medicine of Chicago (1987–1991). The Alpha Lambda Chapter of Sigma Theta Tau recognized Levine for her outstanding contributions to nursing in 1990. In January 1992, she was awarded an honorary doctorate of humane letters from Loyola University, Chicago, at the Mid-Year Convocation. Levine was an active leader in the American Nurses Association and the Illinois Nurses Association. After her retirement in 1987, she remained active in theory development and encouraged questions and research about her theory (Levine, 1996).

A dynamic speaker, Levine was a frequent presenter of programs, workshops, seminars, and panels and a prolific writer regarding nursing and education. She also served as a consultant to hospitals and schools of nursing. Although she never intended to develop theory, she developed a conceptual organizational structure for teaching medical-surgical nursing that stimulated theory development (Stafford, 1996). "The Four Conservation Principles of Nursing" was the first statement of the conservation principles (Levine, 1967b). Other preliminary work included "Adaptation and Assessment: A Rationale for Nursing Intervention," "For Lack of Love Alone," and "The Pursuit of Wholeness" (Levine, 1966a, 1967a, 1969b). The first edition of Levine's book using the conservation principles, *Introduction to Clinical Nursing*, was published in 1969 (1969a). Levine addressed the goal of the four conservation principles (wholeness, or health) in *Holistic Nursing* (Levine, 1971a). The second edition of *Introduction to Clinical Nursing* was published in 1973 (Levine, 1973). After that, Levine (1984) presented the conservation principles at nurse theory conferences, some of which have been audiorecorded, and at the Allentown College of St. Francis de Sales (now DeSales University) Conference.

Levine (1989) published a substantial enhancement and clarification of her theory in "The Four Conservation Principles: Twenty Years Later." She elaborated on how redundancy maximizes availability of adaptive responses when stability is threatened. This redundancy of adaptive processes establishes a body economy to safeguard individual integrity. The product of adaptation is conservation of wholeness and integrity (Levine, 1989). Levine explicitly linked health to the process of conservation to clarify that the Conservation Model views health as one of its essential components (Levine, 1991). The essence of nursing care is the use of the Conservation Principles to promote health, which conserves wholeness and integrity.

Levine died on March 20, 1996, at 75 years of age. She leaves a legacy as an administrator, educator, friend, mother, nurse, scholar, student of humanities, and wife (Pond, 1996). Dr. Baumhart, President of Loyola University, said the following of Levine (Mid-Year Convocation, Loyola University, 1992):

> *"Mrs. Levine is a renaissance woman . . . who uses knowledge from several disciplines to expand the vision of health needs of persons that can be met by modern nursing. In the Talmudic tradition of her ancestors, [she] has been a forthright spokesperson for social justice and the inherent dignity of [the] human person as a child of God." (p. 6)*

THEORETICAL SOURCES

From Beland's (1971) presentation of the theory of specific causation and multiple factors, Levine learned historical viewpoints of diseases and learned that the way people think about disease changes over time. Beland directed Levine's attention to numerous authors who became influential in her thinking, including Goldstein (1963), Hall (1966), Sherrington (1906), and Dubos (1961, 1965). Levine uses Gibson's (1966) definition of perceptual systems, Erikson's (1964, 1968) differentiation between total and whole, Selye's (1956) stress theory, and Bates' (1967) model of external environment. Levine was proud that Rogers (1970) edited her first publication (Levine, 1965). She also acknowledged Nightingale's contribution to her thinking about the "guardian activity" of observation used by nurses to "save lives and increase health and comfort" (Levine, 1992, p. 42).

MAJOR CONCEPTS & DEFINITIONS

Fig. 12.1 provides a conceptual diagram of Levine's Conservation Model.

Wholeness/Health/Integrity (Holism)

The word "health" comes from the Anglo-Saxon word *hāl.* The translation of *hāl* is *whole.* Human life must be described in the language of "wholes" (Levine, 1971a, p. 255). Levine's use of "integrity" reflects this same concept of holism: "I use the word 'integrity' to encompass the wholeness of the individual and the sense of independence and selfhood that is implied in that term. Conserving the integrity of the individual is the hallmark

MAJOR CONCEPTS & DEFINITIONS—cont'd

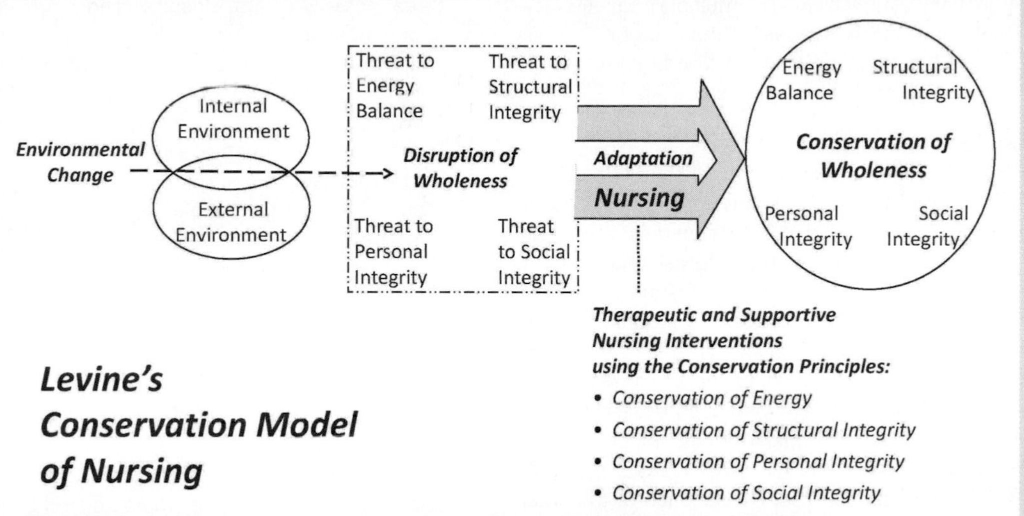

FIG. 12.1 Levine's Conservation Model of nursing. (From Mefford, L. C. (1999). The Relationship of Nursing Care to Health Outcomes of Preterm Infants: Testing a Theory of Health Promotion for Preterm Infants Based on Levine's Conservation Model of Nursing, *Dissertation Abstracts International, 60(09B), 4522.* Copyright 1999 by L.C. Mefford. Adapted and reprinted with permission.)

of nursing intervention" (Levine, 1996, p. 40). Levine builds upon Erikson's (1964, 1968) description of wholeness as an open system. Levine (1996) quotes Erikson as stating: "Wholeness emphasizes a sound, organic, progressive mutuality between diversified functions and parts within an entirety, the boundaries of which are open and fluid" (p. 39).

In Levine's view: "Healing is the defense of wholeness" (1996, p. 40). Regarding the process of healing, Levine (1991) stated:

"The word *healing* also shares the same root as *whole* and *health.* Healing is the avenue of return to the daily activities compromised by ill health. It is not only the insult or injury that is repaired *but the person himself or herself.* . . . It is not merely the healing of an affected part. It is, rather, a return to selfhood, where the encroachment of the disability can be set aside entirely, and the individual is free to pursue once more his or her own interests without constraint" (p. 4).

Adaptation

Adaptation is critical for conserving wholeness in the midst of constant environmental change:

"There must be a bridge that allows ready movement from one environmental reality to another. Adaptation is the bridge. Adaptation is the process by which individuals 'fit' the environments in which they live." (Levine, 1996, p. 38).

"Change is characteristic of life, and adaptation is the method of change. The organism retains its integrity in both the internal and external environment through its adaptive capability. Adaptation is the process of change whereby the individual retains his integrity within the realities of his environments. Adaptation is basic to survival, and it is an expression of the integration of the entire organism. The measure of effective adaptation is compatibility with life. A poor adaptation may threaten life itself, but at the same time the degree of adaptive potential available to the individual may be sufficient to maintain life at a *different level of effectiveness.* Adaptation is not "all-or-none." It is susceptible to an infinite range within the limits of life compatibility. Within that range, there are numerous possible degrees of adaptation" (Levine, 1973, pp. 11–12). "Health and disease are patterns of adaptive change" (Levine, 1966a, p. 2452).

The goal of adaptive change is the conservation of wholeness (health) and integrity. Levine (1991, 1996) identifies three characteristics of adaptation: historicity (patterned responses passed on through genetics), specificity (unique adaptive responses to specific environmental challenges),

Continued

MAJOR CONCEPTS & DEFINITIONS—cont'd

and redundancy (availability of multiple adaptive responses). Levine (1991) suggests "the possibility exists that aging itself is a consequence of failed redundancy of physiological and psychological processes" (p. 6).

Environment

The environment consists of an internal environment (the physiological and pathophysiological processes) and an external environment; both are in constant interaction (Levine, 1973). In discussing the internal environment, Levine uses the conceptualization by Claude Bernard in the 19th century of the *milieu interne:* "Bernard identified the primordial seas, captured within the integument of the human body and providing the organism with a tightly regulated solution of substances essential to its continued well-being. . . . Man carried the essentials with him, safely packaged inside his skin" (1969a, pp. 6–7). Levine (1973) uses Bates' (1967) description of the external environment as having three components:

1. Perceptual: aspects of the world that individuals intercept and interpret with their sense organs
2. Operational: environmental components that physically affect individuals, although they cannot directly perceive them, such as microorganisms
3. Conceptual: characterized by cultural patterns, spirituality, and aspects mediated through the symbols of language, thought, and history

Organismic Response (Integrated or Holistic Response)

"The human being responds to forces in his environment in a singular yet integrated fashion . . . in a way which is peculiar to him and to him alone" (Levine, 1966a, p. 2452). The term "organismic" reflects the language of the biology of living organisms, with multiple components working together to generate a whole, integrated organismic response. Levine (1967b) noted that "every response is an organismic one—no other kind is possible—and every adaptive change is accomplished by the entire individual" (p. 46). Levine (1969b) identifies "at least four levels of protective organismic response, each physiologically predetermined, and each used to protect the organism so that it may make a viable adaptation to its environment" (p. 95). Nursing care focuses on the management of these integrated organismic (holistic) responses (Levine, 1969a, 1969b), which include:

1. Response to fear (fight or flight)

   The most primitive response, these adrenocortical-sympathetic reactions are activated whenever individuals perceive that they are threatened, whether or not a threat actually exists. Hospitalization, illness, and new experiences elicit this response. Individuals respond by being on the alert to gather more information and ensure their safety and well-being (Levine, 1969b, 1973, 1989).
2. Inflammatory-immune response

   The mechanism that protects the organism from environmental irritants and pathogens, the inflammatory-immune response is a way of healing; however, it drains energy reserves. Many nursing interventions focus on supporting the reparative components of the inflammatory-immune process while minimizing tissue damage. Environmental control to minimize exposure to irritants and pathogens is also an important focus of nursing care (Levine, 1969b, 1973, 1989).
3. Response to stress

   Levine (1969b) built on Selye's (1956) model of the adaptive stress response, characterized by predictable behavioral and biological responses (particularly adrenocortical hormones) to various nonspecific stressors of life. Selye referred to the "adaptive energy" expended over time to respond to stressors and noted that long-term stress can take a toll on the individual, sometimes leading to a state of exhaustion when adaptive energy is depleted. Irreversible stress-induced structural tissue changes can also occur (Levine, 1969b).
4. Sensory response

   This response is generated through perceptual awareness as individuals experience the world around them through sensory stimuli. Individuals are constantly immersed in an environmental background of sensory input that never ceases, even during sleep. Responsiveness to this sensory input prompts individuals to maintain safety and seek wholeness (Levine, 1967b, 1969b).

Nursing

Nursing has a conservative function, seeking to actively support the patient's adaptive efforts to achieve the best available environmental fit (Levine, 1989), thus conserving wholeness and integrity. Both the nurse and the patient have active roles in this conservation of wholeness. "Nursing intervention must be founded not only on scientific knowledge, but specifically on recognition of the individual's behavioral responses which *indicate the nature of the adaptation taking place"* (Levine, 1966a, p. 2452). The goal of nursing care is to support adaptation and the strong drive of the individual to seek wholeness. Because of the uniqueness of each individual, nursing care for

MAJOR CONCEPTS & DEFINITIONS—cont'd

each patient must be highly individualized (Levine, 1971a). Levine specifically viewed the individual receiving nursing care as a patient, not as a client, to emphasize the nursing goal of returning the patient to a state of wholeness and health, restoring as much independence as possible (Levine, 1996).

Nursing interventions are both therapeutic and supportive in nature. Therapeutic nursing care focuses on enhancing adaptation and improving well-being. Supportive interventions are used when nursing care is unable to improve the adaptive response or "fail to halt a downhill course" (Levine, 1966a, p. 2452), including nursing care for the dying patient.

Conservation

"Conservation" is from the Latin word *conservatio,* which means "to keep together" (Levine, 1973). Conservation is a natural law which "describes the way complex systems are able to continue to function even when severely challenged" (Levine, 1990, p. 192). Through conservation, individuals are able to confront challenges, adapt accordingly, and maintain their uniqueness (Levine, 1990).

The Four Conservation Principles

"Nursing principles are fundamental assumptions which provide a unifying structure for understanding a wide variety of nursing activities" (Levine, 1967b, p. 45). Levine proposed four "conservation principles" to guide nursing care which "have as a postulate the unity and integrity of the individual" (1967b, p. 46).

Conservation of Energy

"All of life's processes are fundamentally dependent upon the production and expenditure of energy" (Levine, 1967b, p. 47). This fundamental concept of energy balance is drawn from the first law of thermodynamics (from the adjunctive discipline of physics), which applies to everything in the universe, including people (Levine, 1973, 1989). The individual requires a balance of energy and a constant renewal of energy to maintain life activities. Pathophysiological processes challenge the balance of energy, as do the normal physiological processes of healing and aging.

"Conservation of energy is typical of the natural defense against disease processes. The lethargy and withdrawal that accompany many acute disease conditions decrease the general demand on the organism for energy expenditure and indicate that the physiological function is mobilized in the interests of the healing mechanisms. . . . Energy conservation during acute illness demands nursing intervention which cautiously balances the individual's resource with the expenditure he can safely afford (Levine, 1967b, p. 48).

Energy balance is a critical focus of nursing care for patients with chronic illness as well as acute illnesses. "Chronic disease represents an alteration in the individual's ability to adapt to the environment, and this alteration, too, involves a realignment of the energy resource available to the individual. The development of chronic disease is always accompanied by a period during which relearning and readjustment must take place" (Levine, 1967b, p. 49). Conservation of energy applies equally for health promotion as during times of illness. Environmental change is constant, and the individual must continually adapt to stressors.

Conservation of Structural Integrity

Structure and function are strongly interrelated complementary aspects of the human organism. Therefore nursing interventions to ensure adequate energy to support life processes (function) must be balanced by interventions to conserve the normal structure of the body (Levine, 1967b). Under optimal conditions, tissue healing occurs with minimal structural change; however, sequelae of the healing process can preserve continuity of tissue but at the expense of normal structural organization, leading to disturbance of function (Levine, 1967b). In some cases, structural disturbance leads to a permanent disability. Then the focus of nursing care shifts to guiding the disabled person to a new level of adaptation (Levine, 1996). All nursing care should maintain a continual rehabilitative focus to minimize structural damage and prevent disability (Levine, 1967b). Levine noted that "all varieties of surgical intervention are designed to restore or redesign structural integrity" (1967b, p. 51) and "every infection is an assault on structural integrity" (1967b, p. 51).

Conservation of Personal Integrity

Conservation of personal integrity is based in a valuing of self-identity, self-worth, and self-respect, also reflecting the understanding that "the body does not exist separately from the mind, emotions, and soul" (Levine, 1967b, pp. 53–54). Nursing interventions to conserve integrity include interventions to teach patients; promote patient participation in decision making and consent to treatment; and protect patient privacy, personal possessions, and support of cultural practices. The patient's quest to preserve personal integrity can also be seen through the patient's unique psychological and behavioral responses to health challenges (Levine, 1967b). The goal of the

Continued

MAJOR CONCEPTS & DEFINITIONS—cont'd

nurse is to support the patient's individual adaptive response such that "personal integrity is fortified" (Levine, 1967b, p. 55) and "to impart knowledge and strength so that the individual can resume a private life—no longer a patient, no longer dependent" (Levine, 1990, p. 199). The spiritual nature of life is embedded within the concepts of wholeness and personal integrity. Levine (1996) stated: "The wholeness of the human being is also holiness, and the sanctity of life is manifested in everyone. It never seemed necessary to me to pursue spirituality as a separate path since the holiness of life itself testified to its spiritual reality. The Conservation of Personal Integrity includes recognition of the holiness of each person" (p. 40).

Conservation of Social Integrity

Social integrity is reflected in dynamic relationships among human beings (Levine, 1967b). Family is a critical social unit and the life of each individual is "woven in the fabric" (Levine, 1967b, p. 58) of family, with the constitution of the social group that is "family" defined by each individual patient. Nursing care to conserve social integrity encompasses care of the family as well as care for the patient and "lays the groundwork" (Levine, 1967b, p. 59) to transition care from the nurse to the patient and family. Nursing care to conserve social integrity also includes interventions to assist the patient with maintaining "ethnic and subcultural affiliations" of community (Levine, 1967b, p.57), and supporting any socially connected religious needs. When matched to the patient's level of tolerance, the appropriate use of external sources of news and social connectedness (e.g., social media, phones, television, etc.) contribute to social convalescence (Levine, 1967b). Nursing interventions to promote social connectedness can be very basic, such as the simple nursing act of positioning the patient in a manner that facilitates communication with others and minimizes sensory deprivation (Levine, 1967b). The nurse-patient interaction is also a social relationship in which the patient "can see his integrity mirrored in that of the nurse" (Levine, 1967b, p. 59).

USE OF EMPIRICAL EVIDENCE

Levine (1973) based much of her work on accepted scientific principles that were well researched. She believed that specific nursing activities could be deduced from scientific principles.

MAJOR ASSUMPTIONS

Introduction to Clinical Nursing is a text for beginning nursing students that uses the conservation principles as an organizing framework (Levine, 1969a, 1973). Although she did not state them specifically as assumptions, Levine (1973) valued "a holistic approach to care of all people, well or sick" (p. 151) and respect for the individuality of each person:

> *"Ultimately, decisions for nursing interventions must be based on the unique behavior of the individual patient. . . . Patient centered nursing care means individualized nursing care . . . and as such he requires a unique constellation of skills, techniques, and ideas designed specifically for him."*
>
> **(Levine, 1973, p. 6)**

Schaefer (1996) identified the following statements as assumptions about the model:

- The person can be understood only in the context of the environment (Levine, 1973).
- "Every self-sustaining system monitors its own behavior by conserving the use of the resources required to define its unique identity" (Levine, 1991, p. 4).
- Human beings respond in a singular, yet integrated, fashion (Levine, 1971c).

Nursing

Levine viewed nursing as both a profession and scientific discipline. Nursing practice is based on nursing's unique knowledge and the scientific knowledge of other disciplines adjunctive to nursing knowledge (Levine, 1988a).

> *"Nursing is a human interaction."*
>
> **(Levine, 1973, p. 1)**

> *"Nursing is a profession as well as an academic discipline, always practiced and studied in concert with all of the disciplines that together form the health sciences."*
>
> **(Levine, 1988a, p. 17)**

> *"Professional nursing should be reserved for those few who can complete a graduate program as demanding as that expected of professionals in any other discipline. . . . There will be very few professional nurses."*
>
> **(Levine, 1965, p. 214)**

> *"There are no magic scales which allow nurses to weight the multiplicity of factors operating in a single individual. Ultimately, decisions for nursing intervention must be based on the unique behavior of the individual*

patient. It is the nurse's task to bring a body of scientific principles on which decisions depend into the precise situation that she shares with the patient. Sensitive observation and the selection of relevant data form the basis for her assessment of his nursing requirements. A theory of nursing must recognize the importance of unique detail of care for a single patient within an empiric framework which successfully describes the requirements of all patients."

(Levine, 1969a, p. 6)

The essence of *nursing* in Levine's model is as follows:

1. "The goal of nursing is to promote adaptation and maintain wholeness" (1971a, p. 258).
2. "The nurse participates actively in every patient's environment and much of what she does supports his adjustments as he struggles in the predicament of illness" (Levine, 1966a, p. 2452).
3. "[W]hen nursing intervention influences adaptation favorably, or toward renewed social well-being, then the nurse is acting in a therapeutic sense; when the response is unfavorable, the nurse provides supportive care" (1966a, p. 2450).
4. "Nursing principles are all 'conservation' principles" (1973, p. 13).

The four conservation principles are:

1. The conservation of energy of the individual.
2. The conservation of structural integrity of the individual.
3. The conservation of personal integrity of the individual.
4. The conservation of social integrity of the individual (1989, p. 331).

Levine (1966a, 1966b) proposed the use of the term *trophicognosis* (referring to the use of the scientific method to develop a nursing care judgment) as an alternative to nursing diagnosis.

Levine's major theoretical writings do not develop this concept; therefore it does not appear that she considered it as a component of her conservation model of nursing.

Person

Person is described as a holistic being; wholeness is integrity (Levine, 1991). Integrity means the person has freedom of choice and movement. The person has a sense of identity and self-worth. Levine also described person as a "system of systems, and in its wholeness expresses the organization of all the contributing parts" (pp. 8–9). Persons experience life as change through adaptation; the goal of adaptation is the conservation of wholeness. According to Levine (1989), "The life process is the process of change" (p. 326). Levine intentionally refers to the person receiving nursing care as a *patient:*

"The word patient comes from the Latin 'to suffer' while the word client comes from the Latin 'to follow' . . . Any individual who enters into the dependency of health care is a patient. The nurse provides whatever service is needed—even if it is only health counseling—but only for as long as the nurse's professional services are required. Then the dependency must be ended. I want the patient to walk away from me. As participants in their care, individuals need to retain whatever portion of their independence they can and they should not be defined as followers."

(1996, p. 40)

Health

Health is socially determined by the ability to function in a reasonably normal manner (Levine, 1969b). Health is not just an absence of pathological conditions. Health is the return to self; individuals are free and able to pursue their own interests within the context of their own resources. Even for a single individual, the definition of *health* will change over time. Levine stressed the following:

"It is important to keep in mind that health is also culturally determined—it is not an entity on its own, but rather a definition imparted by the ethos and beliefs of the groups to which individuals belong."

(M. Levine, personal communication, February 21, 1995)

Environment

Environment is the context in which individuals live their lives. It is not a passive backdrop. "The individual actively participates in his environment" (Levine, 1973, p. 443). "All adaptations represent the accommodation that is possible between the internal and external environment" (1973, p. 12). Complex biochemical processes mediate the interface of the internal environment (the physiological and pathophysiological processes) with the external environment, composed of perceptual, operational, and conceptual components (1973, 1989). "The *process* of the interaction is *adaptation*" (1989, p. 326).

THEORETICAL ASSERTIONS

Although many theoretical assertions can be generated from Levine's work, the four major assertions follow:

1. "Nursing intervention is based on the conservation of the individual patient's energy" (Levine, 1967b, p. 49).
2. "Nursing intervention is based on the conservation of the individual patient's structural integrity" (Levine, 1967b, p. 56).

3. "Nursing intervention is based on the conservation of the individual patient's personal integrity" (Levine, 1967b, p. 56).
4. "Nursing intervention is based on the conservation of the individual patient's social integrity" (Levine, 1967a, p. 179).

Levine (1991) provided some thoughts about two theories in their early stages of development. The **theory of therapeutic intention** is intended to provide the basis of nursing interventions that focus on biological realities of the patient. The theory naturally flows from the conservation principles. The **theory of redundancy** expands the redundancy domain of adaptation and offers explanations for redundant options such as those found in aging and the physiological adaptation of a failing heart.

LOGICAL FORM

Levine primarily uses deductive logic. In developing her model, Levine integrates theories and concepts from the humanities and the sciences of nursing, physiology, psychology, and sociology. She uses the information to analyze nursing practice situations and describe nursing skills and activities. With the assistance of many of her students and colleagues, and through her own personal health encounters, Levine experienced the conservation model and its principles operating in practice.

APPLICATIONS TO THE NURSING COMMUNITY

Practice

Conservation principles and other concepts within the model can be used in numerous contexts (Fawcett, 2000; Levine, 1990, 1991; Schaefer & Pond, 1991, 1994). Levine's model has been applied to nursing practice with many patient types:

- Neonates (Langer, 1990; Mefford, 2004; Newport, 1984; Tribotti, 1990)
- Children (Dever, 1991; Savage & Culbert, 1989)
- Women in labor (Roberts, Fleming, & Yeates-Giese, 1991)
- Women with chronic illness (Schaefer, 1996)
- African American women with fibromyalgia (Schaefer, 2005)
- Older adults (Abumaria, Hastings-Tolsma, & Sakraida, 2015; Hirschfeld, 1976)
- Patients with cancer (O'Laughlin, 1986; Webb, 1993)
- Patients with neurological dysfunction (Taylor & Ballenger, 1980)
- Patients with sepsis (Chang, Lai, Liu, & Huang, 2013)
- The homeless (Pond, 1990)
- Fatigue in heart failure (Schaefer, 1990; Schaefer & Shober-Potylycki, 1993)
- Sleep disturbance following coronary artery bypass surgery (Schaefer et al., 1996)
- Testing respiratory capacity (Roberts et al., 1994; Roberts, Brittin, & deClifford, 1995)
- Critical care and cardiac care (Brunner, 1985; Delmore, 2006; Lynn-McHale & Smith, 1991; Molchany, 1992)
- Wound care and enterostomal therapy nursing (Cooper, 1990; Leach, 2006; Neswick, 1997)
- Perioperative nursing (Crawford-Gamble, 1986)
- Life transitions in serious illness (Fawcett, Tulman, & Samarel, 1995)
- Management of nursing staff, outcomes management, and quality improvement (Fawcett, 2014; Jost, 2000; Taylor, 1974)

Education

Levine (1969a, 1973) wrote her textbook *Introduction to Clinical Nursing* as an organizational structure for teaching medical-surgical nursing to beginning students. It introduced new material into the curricula and presented an early discussion of death and dying. The teachers' manual that accompanies the text remains a timely source of educational principles that may be helpful to both beginning and seasoned teachers (Levine, 1971b). Although the text is labeled as an introduction, beginning students would have benefited from a background in physical and social sciences to use it. An emphasis of scientific principles in the second edition bridged this gap. Evidence supporting the model has been integrated successfully into undergraduate and graduate curricula (Grindley & Paradowski, 1991; Schaefer, 1991a). Levine also authored *Renewal for Nursing* (1971c), a text for nurses returning to active practice after a period of inactivity. Interest in applying the conservation model as a guide for teaching undergraduates continues (Diniz & Avelar, 2009).

Research

Fawcett (1995) challenged researchers to perform research in various clinical settings and to design "studies that test conceptual-theoretical-empirical structures directly derived from or linked with the conservation principles" (p. 208). Many research questions can be generated from Levine's model (Fawcett, 2000; Radwin & Fawcett, 2002; Schaefer, 1991b). Researchers have used the conservation principles as a framework to guide research in wide-ranging clinical situations:

- Confusion in hospitalized older adults (Foreman, 1989)
- Critical care (Ballard et al., 2006)

- Use of music therapy in acute care (Gagner-Tjellesen, Yurkovich, & Gragert, 2001)
- Neonatal nursing (Mefford & Alligood, 2011a, 2011b)
- Fatigue in cancer patients (Mock et al., 2007)
- Patients adjusting to an ostomy (Gomes et al., 2011)
- Perioperative nursing (Basso & Piccoli, 2004; Florio & Galvao, 2003; Piccoli & Galvao, 2001, 2005)
- Low back pain (Melancon & Miller, 2005)
- Effects of exercise (Hanna, 2008)
- Violence against women (Netto et al., 2014)

FURTHER DEVELOPMENT

Levine and others have worked on using the conservation principles as the basis for a nursing diagnosis taxonomy (Stafford, 1996; Taylor, 1974, 1989). Middle range theories can be drawn from the conservation model for various nursing situations to develop specific research hypotheses, then theoretical propositions, and tested. Mefford (2004) developed a middle range theory of health promotion for preterm infants based on Levine's conservation model that was tested by Mefford and Alligood (2011a, 2011b). A primary test of the theory using structural equation modeling revealed that the effect of the physiological integrity of preterm infants at birth on age at which health was attained was completely mediated by the degree of consistency of nursing caregivers (2011a). Testing of subsidiary research questions indicated that consistency of nursing caregivers also served as a partial mediator of the effects of physiological integrity at birth on the use of clinical resources by preterm infants in the neonatal intensive care unit (2011b).

The Conservation Model is increasingly attracting global interest, with several recent reports using the model to guide practice and research published in Portuguese, Spanish, and Chinese. In 2001 Schaefer addressed the potential of the conservation model as a guide for the future of nursing. The continued use of the model in the United States combined with this global interest validates Schaefer's prediction.

CRITIQUE

Clarity

Levine's model possesses clarity. Fawcett (2000) states, "Levine's Conservation Model provides nursing with a logically congruent, holistic view of the person" (p. 189). George (2002) affirms, "this theory directs nursing actions that lead to favorable outcomes" (p. 237). The model has numerous terms; however, Levine adequately defines them for clarity.

Simplicity

Although the four conservation principles appear simple initially, they contain subconcepts and multiple variables. Nevertheless, this model is still one of the simpler ones to understand.

Generality

The four conservation principles can be used in all nursing contexts.

Accessibility

Levine used deductive logic to develop her model, which has been used to generate research questions. As she lived her conservation model, she verified the use of inductive reasoning to further develop and inform her model (Levine, personal communication, May 17, 1989).

Importance

Levine's conservation model is recognized as one of the earliest nursing models to organize and clarify elements of patient care for nursing practice. Furthermore, the model continues to demonstrate powerful evidence of its utility for nursing practice and research and is receiving increased recognition in this 21st century.

SUMMARY

Levine developed her Conservation Model to provide a framework to teach beginning nursing students. In the first chapter of her book, she introduces her assumptions about holism and her view that the conservation principles support a holistic approach to patient care (Levine, 1969a, 1973). The model is logically congruent, is externally and internally consistent, has breadth as well as depth, and can be understood by both professionals and consumers of health care. Nurses use the conservation model to guide nursing care and to anticipate, explain, and predict patient care needs. However, continued testing to learn how the use of conservation model influences outcomes of care is indicated. The conservation model of nursing is just as applicable to nursing practice and nursing science now as when it was initially developed, because as Levine (1990) said, "everywhere that nursing is essential, the rules of conservation and integrity hold" (p. 195).

CASE STUDY*

Yolanda is a 55-year-old married African American mother of two adult children who has a history of breast cancer. She was diagnosed with fibromyalgia 2 years ago, after years of unexplained muscle aches and what she thought was arthritis. The diagnosis was a relief for her; she was able to read about it and learn how to care for herself. Over the past 2 months, Yolanda stopped taking all of her medicine, because she was seeing a new primary care provider and wanted to start her care at "ground zero." In addition to her family responsibilities, she is completing her degree as an English major. At the time of her clinic appointment, she told the nurse practitioner that she was having the worst pain possible.

Using Levine's conservation model, the nurse practitioner completes a comprehensive assessment in preparation for developing a plan of care. A thorough assessment of characteristics of the internal and external environments is performed, with assessment of the adequacy of the adaptive fit that Yolanda has achieved in response to the changing environmental conditions produced by this health challenge. Nursing care is planned using the conservation principles. Yolanda's diagnosis of fibromyalgia was based on the cluster of presenting symptoms (pain, fatigue, and sleeplessness) and the exclusion of other illnesses.

The assessment of the *internal environment* (physiological and pathophysiological processes) was performed by a thorough physical examination and various laboratory and diagnostic tests. Yolanda's tests results were within normal limits.

The **external environment** includes perceptual, operational, and conceptual factors. Perceptual factors are perceived through sensory input. Yolanda reported a history of unexplained fatigue and sensations of pain for years. She recently stopped her medications "to clean my body out." However, she reported that the pain became unbearable and was making it difficult for her to sleep. She noted that when she sleeps at least 6 hours a night, her pain is less intense. With the current insomnia, her pain is very intense.

Operational factors are threats within the environment that the patient cannot perceive through the senses. Yolanda reported severe pain in response to both the cold weather and changes in barometric pressure.

The **conceptual environment** includes cultural and personal values about health care, the meaning of health and illness, knowledge about health care, education, language use, and spiritual beliefs. In response to breast cancer, Yolanda developed her spirituality through prayer and reading the Bible. She believes this is how she is getting through the painful moments of her current illness.

Conservation of energy focuses on the balance of energy input and output to prevent excessive fatigue. Yolanda complains of a fatigue that just "comes over me." She has difficulty doing housework. A day of work usually means 1 day in bed because of extreme fatigue. Her hemoglobin level and hematocrit are normal; her oxygen saturation is also within normal limits. These normal physiological assessments are typical in patients with fibromyalgia.

Conservation of structural integrity involves maintaining the structure of the body to promote normal functioning. Fibromyalgia treatment focuses on reducing symptoms. Yolanda's symptoms could not be traced to any physical or structural alteration, yet she reports severe pain and fatigue. It is important to acknowledge the reality of the symptoms and work with the patient to determine whether activities of daily living result in changes in the pattern of illness. In addition, Yolanda thinks she is going through menopause (a normal physiological change in body structure), and she is having trouble determining whether her symptoms are menopause or fibromyalgia.

With continued questioning, Yolanda revealed that she was diagnosed with irritable bowel syndrome several years earlier. This condition presents further risks to structural integrity. She is not worried about constipation but is concerned about sudden diarrhea. She is afraid to go to school, fearing embarrassment because she might have an "accident." Interventions to conserve structural integrity include interventions to promote normal bowel function and optimize Yolanda's nutritional status.

Personal integrity involves the maintenance of one's sense of personal worth and self-esteem. Yolanda reported that she "lost control" when she was diagnosed with breast cancer. A dear friend convinced her to go to church and encouraged her to use prayer. When feeling sorry for herself, she would go into her bedroom and read her Bible, cry by herself, and pray. She believes that prayer and Bible reading helped her heal. She continues to pray and read her Bible to gain the strength she needs to live with her illness. She also believes that she needs to be able to laugh at aspects of her situation; humor helps her feel better. She actively seeks health information, as indicated by her quest to learn about her diagnosis of fibromyalgia. She is most upset about not being able to walk as she used to walk. One of her favorite pastimes was shopping for shoes at the mall, which now is difficult for her.

Social integrity acknowledges that the patient is a social being. Yolanda is a married mother of two grown children. She conceals many of her feelings from her children but does share with her husband, who is supportive. Among the ways that he cares for her are to take her places she needs to go (such as grocery shopping) and to make sure she gets to her health care appointments on time.

CASE STUDY—cont'd

An initial plan of care for Yolanda includes interventions based on the four conservation principles:

- *Conservation of energy:* (1) Discuss strategies to balance rest and activity; (2) discuss strategies to help her achieve restful sleep; (3) discuss both nonpharmacological and pharmacological approaches to manage pain; and (4) assess her nutritional intake to ensure adequate energy stores.
- *Conservation of structural integrity:* (1) Discuss any needed modifications of activities to prevent injury; (2) assess diet to identify whether any foods exacerbate gastrointestinal symptoms; (3) discuss the normal physiological process of menopause, including associated symptoms; and (4) consider additional laboratory work or referrals to evaluate hormone levels and assess whether additional treatment is indicated to relieve menopause symptoms.
- *Conservation of personal integrity:* (1) Validate the illness experience; (2) encourage continued use of prayer, Bible reading, and humor to help her feel better; and (3) discuss strategies to help her manage her anxiety related to the irritable bowel syndrome, including both nonpharmacological and pharmacological approaches.
- *Conservation of social integrity:* (1) Praise Yolanda for the strong family relationships that she has built and encourage her to continue to work together with her family to optimize her health; (2) with Yolanda's permission, talk with her husband to answer his questions about her condition and discuss how they can continue to work together to improve her health; and (3) praise Yolanda for continuing to seek achievement of her goal of completing her English degree and discuss strategies to manage the irritable bowel syndrome and manage problems to help her feel more confident about going to school.

In Yolanda's follow-up care, these outcomes suggest effective adaptation that is conserving wholeness and integrity:

- Feels rested, with 6 hours of uninterrupted sleep
- Reduction in pain and fatigue
- Distinguishes symptoms of menopause from symptoms of fibromyalgia
- Collaborates with health care providers to manage symptoms of menopause
- Reports comfort as a result of prayer, Bible reading, and humor
- Minimal adverse bowel symptoms and adequate nutritional intake
- Healthy relationships with family and friends.
- Attends school and participates in other social activities with minimal limitations.

*This case study was developed from a fibromyalgia study (Schaefer, 2005). A fictitious name was used to protect privacy and anonymity.

CRITICAL THINKING ACTIVITIES

1. Are there any aspects of Yolanda's care that you would add to the plan as you consider nursing care with the conservation principles?
2. Keep a reflective journal about a personal health or illness experience and apply the conservation model to that experience.
3. As you consider application of the conservation principles in question 2, what aspects of care are assessed that previously were not included in your plans of care?
4. Use the perspective of the conservation model to identify what may be missed in simulation experiences of nursing practice. What does it capture that other perspectives miss?
5. Suggest how you might begin to develop your style of nursing practice using the conservation model.

POINTS FOR FURTHER STUDY

- Cardinal Stitch University Library, Nursing Theorist Myra Levine, at https://www.stritch.edu/Library/Doing-Research/Research-by-Subject/Health-Sciences-Nursing-Theorists/Nursing-Theorists/
- Hahn School of Nursing and Health Science, University of San Diego, at http://www.sandiego.edu/nursing/research/nursing-theory-research.php/
- Schaefer, K. (2014). Levine's conservation nursing model in nursing practice (pp. 181–199). In M. R. Alligood, *Nursing theory: Utilization & application,* 5th ed. St Louis: Mosby-Elsevier
- *The nursing theorist: Portraits of excellence.* "Myra Levine" (video, CD, or electronically). Oakland: Studio III, Oakland, CA. Available at Fitne, Inc., 5 Depot Street, Athens, Ohio 45701 or https://www.fitne.net/nurse_theorists1.jsp

REFERENCES

Abumaria, I. M., Hastings-Tolsma, M., & Sakraida, T. J. (2015). Levine's conservation model: A framework for advanced gerontology nursing practice. *Nursing Forum, 50*(3), 179–188.

Ballard, N., Robley, L., Barrett, D., Fraser, D., & Mendoza, I. (2006). Patients' recollections of therapeutic paralysis in the intensive care unit. *American Journal of Critical Care, 15*(1), 86–94.

Basso, R. S., & Piccoli, M. (2004). Post-anesthesic [sic] recuperation unit: Nursing diagnosis based in Levine's conceptual frame (Portuguese with English abstract). *Revista Electronica de Enfermagem, 6*(3), 309–323.

Bates, M. (1967). A naturalist at large. *Natural History, 76*(6), 8–16.

Beland, I. (1971). *Clinical nursing: Pathophysiological and psychosocial implications* (2nd ed.). New York: Macmillan.

Brunner, M. (1985). A conceptual approach to critical care nursing using Levine's model. *Focus on Critical Care, 12*(2), 39–40.

Chang, N. Y., Lai, T. Y., Liu, Y. J., & Huang, T. Y. (2013). A nursing case experience using Levine's conservation model to provide sepsis care (Chinese with English abstract). *Journal of Nursing, 60*(2), 103–110.

Cooper, D. H. (1990). Optimizing wound healing: A practice within nursing domains. *Nursing Clinics of North America, 25*(1), 165–180.

Crawford-Gamble, P. E. (1986). An application of Levine's conceptual model. *Perioperative Nursing Quarterly, 2*(1), 64–70.

Delmore, B. A. (2006). Levine's framework in long-term ventilated patients during the weaning course. *Nursing Science Quarterly, 19*(3), 247–258.

Dever, M. (1991). Care of children. In K. M. Schaefer & J. B. Pond (Eds.), *The Conservation Model: A framework for nursing practice* (pp. 71–82). Philadelphia: F. A. Davis.

Diniz, S. N., & Avelar, M. C. Q. (2009). Teaching nurses from health institutions in a private university (Portugese with English abstract). *Ciencia, Cuidado e Saude, 8*(2), 176–183.

Dubos, R. (1961). *Mirage of health*. Garden City, NY: Doubleday.

Dubos, R. (1965). *Man adapting*. New Haven, CT: Yale University Press.

Erikson, E. H. (1964). *Insight and responsibility*. New York: W. W. Norton.

Erikson, E. H. (1968). *Identity: Youth and crisis*. New York: W. W. Norton.

Fawcett, J. (1995). Levine's conservation model. In J. Fawcett (Ed.), *Analysis and evaluation of conceptual models of nursing* (pp. 165–215). Philadelphia: F. A. Davis.

Fawcett, J. (2000). Levine's conservation model. In J. Fawcett (Ed.), *Analysis and evaluation of contemporary nursing knowledge: Nursing models and theories* (pp. 151–193). Philadelphia: F. A. Davis.

Fawcett, J. (2014). Thoughts about conceptual models, theories, and quality improvement projects. *Nursing Science Quarterly, 27*(4), 336–339.

Fawcett, J., Tulman, L., & Samarel, N. (1995). Enhancing function in life transitions and serious illness. *Advanced Practice Nursing Quarterly, 1*, 50–57.

Florio, M. C. S., & Galvao, C. M. (2003). Surgery in out-patient units: Identification of nursing diagnoses in the perioperative period. *Revista Latino-Americana de Enfermagem, 11*(5), 630–637.

Foreman, M. D. (1989). Confusion in the hospitalized elderly: Incidence, onset, and associated factors. *Research in Nursing and Health, 12*(1), 21–29.

Gagner-Tjellesen, D., Yurkovich, E. E., & Gragert, M. (2001). Use of music therapy and other ITNIs in acute care. *Journal of Psychosocial Nursing and Mental Health Services, 39*(10), 26–37.

George, J. B. (2002). The conservation principles: A model for health. In J. George (Ed.), *Nursing theories: The base for professional nursing practice* (pp. 225–240). Upper Saddle River, NJ: Prentice Hall.

Gibson, J. E. (1966). *The senses considered as perceptual systems*. Boston: Houghton Mifflin.

Goldstein, K. (1963). *The organism*. Boston: Beacon Press.

Gomes, A. M. S., Vasconcelos, M. A., da Silva, R. C. C., & Neto, F. R. G. X. (2011). Feelings and expectations of subject with ostomy in light of the conceptual model of Levine (Spanish with English abstract). *Enfermeria Comunitaria, 7*(1), 7.

Grindley, J., & Paradowski, M. B. (1991). Developing an undergraduate program using Levine's model. In K. M. Schaefer & J. B. Pond (Eds.), *Levine's conservation model: A framework for nursing practice* (pp. 199–208). Philadelphia: F. A. Davis.

Hall, E. T. (1966). *The hidden dimension*. Garden City, NY: Doubleday.

Hanna, L. R., Avila, P. F., Meteer, J. D., Nicholas, D. R., & Kaminsky, L. A. (2008). The effects of a comprehensive exercise program on physical function, fatigue, and mood in patients with various types of cancer. *Oncology Nursing Forum, 35*(3), 461–469.

Hirschfeld, M. J. (1976). The cognitively impaired older adult. *American Journal of Nursing, 76*(12), 1981–1984.

Jost, S. G. (2000). An assessment and intervention strategy for managing. *Journal of Nursing Administration, 30*(1), 34–40.

Langer, V. S. (1990). Minimal handling protocol for the intensive care nursery. *Neonatal Network, 9*(3), 23–27.

Leach, M. J. (2006). Using Levine's conservation model to guide practice. *Ostomy Wound Management, 52*(8), 74–80.

Levine, M. E. (1965, June). The professional nurse and graduate education. *Nursing Science, 3*(3), 206.

Levine, M. E. (1966a). Adaptation and assessment: A rationale for nursing intervention. *American Journal of Nursing, 66*(11), 2450–2454.

Levine, M. E. (1966b). Trophicognosis: An alternative to nursing diagnosis. *American Nurses Association Regional Clinical Conferences, 2*, 55–70.

Levine, M. E. (1967a, Dec.). For lack of love alone. *Minnesota Nursing Accent, 39*, 179.

Levine, M. E. (1967b). The four conservation principles of nursing. *Nursing Forum, 6*(1), 45–59.

Levine, M. E. (1969a). *Introduction to clinical nursing*. Philadelphia: F. A. Davis.

Levine, M. E. (1969b). The pursuit of wholeness. *American Journal of Nursing, 69*(1), 93.

Levine, M. E. (1971a). Holistic nursing. *Nursing Clinics of North America*, *6*(2), 253–263.

Levine, M. E. (1971b). *Instructor's guide to introduction to clinical nursing*. Philadelphia: F. A. Davis.

Levine, M. E. (1971c). *Renewal for nursing*. Philadelphia: F. A. Davis. [Translated into Hebrew, Am Oved, Jerusalem, 1978.]

Levine, M. E. (1973). *Introduction to clinical nursing* (2nd ed.). Philadelphia: F. A. Davis.

Levine, M. E. (1984, April). *A conceptual model for nursing: The four conservation principles*. Proceedings from Allentown College of St. Francis Conference, Philadelphia.

Levine, M. E. (1988a). Antecedents from adjunctive disciplines: Creation of nursing theory. *Nursing Science Quarterly*, *1*(1), 16–21.

Levine, M. E. (1989). The four conservation principles: Twenty years later. In J. Riehl-Sisca (Ed.), *Conceptual models for nursing practice* (3rd ed., pp. 325–337). New York: Appleton-Century-Crofts.

Levine, M. E. (1990). Conservation and integrity. In M. Parker (Ed.), *Nursing theories in practice* (pp. 189–201). New York: National League for Nursing.

Levine, M. E. (1991). The conservation principles: A model for health. In K. Schaefer & J. Pond (Eds.), *Levine's conservation model: A framework for nursing practice* (pp. 1–11). Philadelphia: F. A. Davis.

Levine, M. E. (1992). Nightingale redux. In B. S. Barnum (Ed.), *Nightingale's notes on nursing* (pp. 39–43). Philadelphia: Lippincott.

Levine, M. E. (1996). The conservation principles: A retrospective. *Nursing Science Quarterly*, *9*(1), 38–41.

Lynn-McHale, D. J., & Smith, A. (1991). Comprehensive assessment of families of the critically ill. *AACN clinical Issues in Critical Care Nursing*, *2*(2), 195–209.

Mefford, L. C. (1999). *The relationships of nursing care to health outcomes of preterm infants: Testing a theory of health promotion for preterm infants based on Levine's Conservation Model*. Doctoral Dissertation, University of Tennessee, Knoxville, Dissertation Abstracts International, 60(09B), 4522.

Mefford, L. C. (2004). A theory of health promotion for preterm infants based on Levine's conservation model of nursing. *Nursing Science Quarterly*, *17*(3), 260–266.

Mefford, L. C., & Alligood, M. R. (2011a). Testing a theory of health promotion for preterm infants based on Levine's conservation model of nursing. *Journal of Theory Construction and Testing*, *15*(2), 41–47.

Mefford, L. C., & Alligood, M. R. (2011b). Evaluating nurse staffing patterns and neonatal intensive care unit outcomes using Levine's conservation model of nursing. *Journal of Nursing Management*, *19*(11), 998–1011.

Melancon, B., & Miller, L. H. (2005). Massage therapy versus traditional therapy for low back pain relief. *Holistic Nursing Practice*, *19*(3), 116–121.

Mid-Year Convocation: Loyola University, Chicago. (1992). The Conferring of Honorary Degrees by R. C. Baumhart, Candidate for the degree of Doctor and Humane Letters, p. 6.

Mock, V., St. Ours, C., Hall, S., Bositis, A., Tillery, M., Belcher, A., et al. (2007). Using a conceptual model in nursing research—mitigating fatigue in cancer patients. *Journal of Advanced Nursing*, *58*(5), 503–512.

Molchany, C. B. (1992). Ventricular septal and free wall rupture complicating acute MI. *Journal of Cardiovascular Nursing*, *6*(4), 38–45.

Neswick, R. S. (1997). Myra E. Levine: A theoretical basis for ET nursing. *Journal of Wound, Ostomy and Continence Nursing*, *24*(1), 6–9.

Netto, L. D., Moura, M. A. V., Queiroz, A. B. A., Tyrrell, M. A. R., & Bravo, M. D. (2014). Violence against women and its consequences (Published in both English and Portuguese). *Acta Paulista de Enfermagem*, *27*(5), 458–464.

Newport, M. A. (1984). Conserving thermal energy and social integrity in the newborn. *Western Journal of Nursing Research*, *6*(2), 175–197.

O'Laughlin, K. M. (1986). Change in bladder function in the woman undergoing radical hysterectomy for cervical cancer. *Journal of Obstetrical, Gynecological and Neonatal Nursing*, *15*(5), 380–385.

Piccoli, M., & Galvao, C. M. (2001). Perioperative nursing: Identification of the nursing diagnosis infection risk based on Levine's conceptual model (Portuguese with English abstract). *Revista Latino-Americana de Enfermagem*, *9*(4), 37–43.

Piccoli, M., & Galvao, C. M. (2005). Pre-operative nursing visit: Methodological proposal based on Levine's conservation model. (Portuguese with English abstract). *Revista Electronica de Enfermagem*, *7*(3), 365–371.

Pond, J. B. (1990). Application of Levine's conservation model to nursing the homeless community. In M. E. Parker (Ed.), *Nursing theories in practice* (pp. 203–215). New York: National League for Nursing.

Pond, J. B. (1996). Myra Levine, nurse educator and scholar dies. *Nursing Spectrum*, *5*(8), 8.

Radwin, L., & Fawcett, J. (2002). A conceptual model based programme of nursing research: Retrospective and prospective applications. *Journal of Advanced Nursing*, *40*(3), 355–360.

Roberts, J. E., Fleming, N., & Yeates-Giese, D. (1991). Perineal integrity. In K. M. Schaefer & J. B. Pond (Eds.), *The conservation model: A framework for nursing practice* (pp. 61–70). Philadelphia: F. A. Davis.

Roberts, K. L., Brittin, M., Cook, M., & deClifford, J. (1994). Boomerang pillows and respiratory capacity. *Clinical Nursing Research*, *3*(2), 157–165.

Roberts, K. L., Brittin, M., & deClifford, J. (1995). Boomerang pillows and respiratory capacity in frail elderly women. *Clinical Nursing Research*, *4*(4), 465–471.

Rogers, M. E. (1970). *An introduction to the theoretical basis of nursing*. Philadelphia: F. A. Davis.

Savage, T. A., & Culbert, C. (1989). Early intervention: The unique role of nursing. *Journal of Pediatric Nursing*, *4*(5), 339–345.

Schaefer, K. M. (1990). A description of fatigue associated with congestive heart failure: Use of Levine's conservation model. In M. E. Parker (Ed.), *Nursing theories in practice* (pp. 217–237). New York: National League for Nursing.

Schaefer, K. M. (1991a). Developing a graduate program in nursing: Integrating Levine's philosophy. In K. M. Schaefer & J. B. Pond (Eds.), *Levine's conservation model: A framework for nursing practice* (pp. 209–218). Philadelphia: F. A. Davis.

Schaefer, K. M. (1991b). Levine's conservation principles and research. In K. M. Schaefer & J. B. Pond (Eds.), *Levine's conservation model: A framework for nursing practice* (pp. 45–60). Philadelphia: F. A. Davis.

Schaefer, K. M. (1996). Levine's conservation model: Caring for women with chronic illness. In P. H. Walker & B. Neuman (Eds.), *Blueprint for use of nursing models: Education, research, practice and administration* (pp. 187–228). New York: National League for Nursing Press.

Shaefer, K. M. (2005). The lived experience of fibromyalgia in African American women. *Holistic Journal of Nursing, 19*(1), 17–25.

Schaefer, K. M. (2014). Levine's conservation model in nursing practice. In M. R. Alligood (Ed.), *Nursing theory: Utilization & application* (5th ed., pp. 181–199) St Louis: Mosby-Elsevier.

Schaefer, K. M., & Pond, J. B. (Eds.). (1991). *Levine's conservation model: A framework for nursing practice.* Philadelphia: F. A. Davis.

Schaefer, K. M., & Pond, J. (1994). Levine's conservation model as a guide to nursing practice. *Nursing Science Quarterly, 7*(2), 53–54.

Schaefer, K. M., & Shober Potylycki, M. J. (1993). Fatigue in congestive heart failure: Use of Levine's conservation model. *Journal of Advanced Nursing, 18*(2), 260–268.

Schaefer, K. M., Swavely, D., Rothenberger, C., Hess, S., & Willistin, D. (1996). Sleep disturbances post coronary artery bypass surgery. *Progress in Cardiovascular Nursing, 11*(1), 5–14.

Selye, H. (1956). *The stress of life.* New York: McGraw-Hill.

Sherrington, A. (1906). *Integrative function of the nervous system.* New York: Charles Scribner's Sons.

Stafford, M. J. (1996). In tribute: Myra Estrin Levine, Professor Emerita, MSN, RN, FAAN. *Chart, 93*(3), 5–6.

Taylor, J. W. (1974). Measuring the outcomes of nursing care. *Nursing Clinics of North America, 9*, 337–348.

Taylor, J. W. (1989). Levine's conservation principles: Using the model for nursing diagnosis in a neurological setting. In J. P. Riehl-Sisca (Ed.), *Conceptual models for nursing practice* (3rd ed., pp. 349–358). Norwalk, CT: Appleton & Lange.

Taylor, J. W., & Ballenger, S. (1980). *Neurological dysfunction and nursing interventions.* New York: McGraw-Hill.

Tribotti, S. (1990). Admission to the neonatal intensive care unit: Reducing the risks. *Neonatal Network, 8*(4), 17–22.

Webb, H. (1993). Holistic care following a palliative Hartmann's procedure. *British Journal of Nursing, 2*(2), 128–132.

BIBLIOGRAPHY

Additional Primary Sources

Book Chapters

Levine, M. E. (1992). Nightingale redux. In B. S. Barnum (Ed.), *Nightingale's notes on nursing: Commemorative edition with commentaries by nursing theorists.* Philadelphia: Lippincott.

Levine, M. E. (1994). Some further thoughts on nursing rhetoric. In J. F. Kikuchi & H. Simmons (Eds.), *Developing a philosophy of nursing* (pp. 104–109). Thousand Oaks, CA: Sage.

Journal Articles

Levine, M. E. (1963). Florence Nightingale: The legend that lives. *Nursing Forum, 2*(4), 24–35.

Levine, M. E. (1964). Not to startle, though the way were steep. *Nursing Science, 2*(1), 58–67.

Levine, M. E. (1964). There need be no anonymity. *First, 18*(9), 4.

Levine, M. E. (1967). Medicine-nursing dialogue belongs at patient's bedside. *Chart, 64*(5), 136–137.

Levine, M. E. (1967). This I believe: About patient-centered care. *Nursing Outlook, 15*(2), 53–55.

Levine, M. E. (1968). Knock before entering personal space bubbles (part 1). *Chart, 65*(2), 58–62.

Levine, M. E. (1968). Knock before entering personal space bubbles (part 2). *Chart, 65*(3), 82–84.

Levine, M. E. (1968). The pharmacist in the clinical setting: A nurse's viewpoint. *American Journal of Hospital Pharmacy, 25*(4), 168–171. [Also translated into Japanese and published in *Kyushu National Hospital Magazine* for Western Japan.]

Levine, M. E. (1969, Feb.). Constructive student power. *Chart, 66*(2), 42FF.

Levine, M. E. (1969). Small hospital—Big nursing. *Chart, 66*(10), 265–269.

Levine, M. E. (1969). Small hospital—Big nursing. *Chart, 66*(11), 310–315.

Levine, M. E. (1970). Breaking through the medications mystique. *American Journal of Hospital Pharmacy, 27*(4), 294–299; *American Journal of Nursing, 70*(4), 799–803.

Levine, M. E. (1970). Dilemma. *ANA Clinical Conferences*, 338–342.

Levine, M. E. (1970). Symposium on a drug compendium: View of a nursing educator. *Drug Information Journal, 4*, 133–135.

Levine, M. E. (1970). The intransigent patient. *American Journal of Nursing, 70*(10), 2106–2111.

Levine, M. E. (1971). Consider implications for nursing in the use of physician's assistant. *Hospital Topics, 49*, 60–63.

Levine, M. E. (1971). The time has come to speak of health care. *AORN Journal, 13*(1), 37–43.

Levine, M. E. (1972). Benoni. *American Journal of Nursing, 72*(3), 466–468.

Levine, M. E. (1972). Nursing educators—An alienating elite? *Chart, 69*(2), 56–61.

Levine, M. E. (1973). On creativity in nursing. *Image: The Journal of Nursing Scholarship, 3*(3), 15–19.

Levine, M. E. (1974). The pharmacist's clinical role in interdisciplinary care: A nurse's viewpoint. *Hospital Formulary Management, 9*(1), 47.

Levine, M. E. (1975). On creativity in nursing. *Nursing Digest, 3*(3), 38–40.

Levine, M. E. (1977). Nursing ethics and the ethical nurse. *American Journal of Nursing, 77*(5), 845–849.

Levine, M. E. (1978). Cancer chemotherapy: A nursing model. *Nursing Clinics of North America, 13*(2), 271–280.

Levine, M. E. (1978). Does continuing education improve nursing practice? *Hospitals, 52*(21), 138–140.

Levine, M. E. (1978). Kapklavoo and nursing, too (Editorial). *Research in Nursing and Health, 1*(2), 51.

Levine, M. E. (1979). Knowledge base required by generalized and specialized nursing practice. *ANA Publications*, (G-127), 57–69.

Levine, M. E. (1980). The ethics of computer technology in health care. *Nursing Forum, 19*(2), 193–198.
Levine, M. E. (1982). Bioethics of cancer nursing. *Rehabilitation Nursing, 7*(2), 27–31, 41.
Levine, M. E. (1982). The bioethics of cancer nursing. *Journal of Enterostomal Therapy, 9*(1), 11–13.
Levine, M. E. (1988). What does the future hold for nursing? 25th Anniversary Address, 18th District. *Illinois Nurses Association Newsletter, 24*(6), 1–4.
Levine, M. E. (1989). Beyond dilemma. *Seminars in Oncology Nursing, 5*(2), 124–128.
Levine, M. E. (1989). The ethics of nursing rhetoric. *Image: The Journal of Nursing Scholarship, 21*(1), 4–5.
Levine, M. E. (1989). Ration or rescue: The elderly in critical care. *Critical Care Nursing, 12*(1), 82–89.
Levine, M. E. (1995). The rhetoric of nursing theory. *Image: The Journal of Nursing Scholarship, 27*(1), 11–14.
Levine, M. E. (1996). On the humanities in nursing. *Canadian Journal of Nursing Research, 27*(2), 19–23.
Levine, M. E. (1997). On creativity in nursing. *Image: The Journal of Nursing Scholarship, 29*(3), 216–217.
Levine, M. E., Hallberg, C., Kathrein, M., & Cox, R. (1972). Nursing grand rounds: Congestive failure. *Nursing '72, 2*(10), 18–23.
Levine, M. E., Line, L., Boyle, A., & Kopacewski, E. (1972). Nursing grand rounds: Insulin reactions in a brittle diabetic. *Nursing '72, 2*(5), 6–11.
Levine, M. E., Moschel, P., Taylor, J., & Ferguson, G. (1972). Nursing grand rounds: Complicated case of CVA. *Nursing '72, 2*(3), 3–34.
Levine, M. E., Zoellner, J., Ozmon, B., & Simunek, E. (1972). Nursing grand rounds: Severe trauma. *Nursing '72, 2*(9), 33–38.

13

Unitary Human Beings

*Mary E. Gunther**

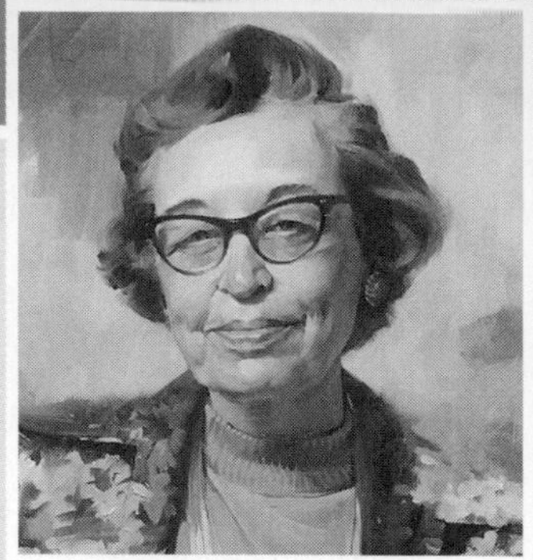

Martha E. Rogers (1914–1994)[†]

"Professional practice in nursing seeks to promote symphonic interaction between man and environment, to strengthen the coherence and integrity of the human field, and to direct and redirect patterning of the human and environmental fields for realization of maximum health potential."

(Rogers, 1970, p. 122)

CREDENTIALS AND BACKGROUND OF THE THEORIST

Martha Elizabeth Rogers, the eldest of four children of Bruce Taylor Rogers and Lucy Mulholland Keener Rogers, was born May 12, 1914, in Dallas, Texas. Soon after her birth, her family returned to Knoxville, Tennessee. She began her college education (1931–1933) studying science at the University of Tennessee. After receiving her nursing diploma from Knoxville General Hospital School of Nursing (1936), she quickly obtained a bachelor of science degree from George Peabody College in Nashville, Tennessee (1937). Her other degrees included a master's of arts degree in public health nursing supervision from Teachers College, Columbia University, New York (1945), and a master's of public arts degree (1952) and doctor of science degree (1954) from Johns Hopkins University in Baltimore.

Rogers' early nursing practice was in rural public health nursing in Michigan and in visiting nurse supervision, education, and practice in Connecticut. Rogers subsequently established the Visiting Nurse Service of Phoenix, Arizona. For 21 years (from 1954–1975), she was professor and head of the Division of Nursing at New York University. After 1975, she continued her duties as professor until she became Professor Emerita in 1979. She held this title until her death on March 13, 1994, at 79 years of age.

Rogers' publications include three books and more than 200 articles. She lectured in 46 states, the District of Columbia, Puerto Rico, Mexico, the Netherlands, China, Newfoundland, Colombia, Brazil, and other countries (M. Rogers, personal communication, March 1988). Rogers received honorary doctorates from such renowned institutions as Duquesne University, University of San Diego, Iona College, Fairfield University, Emory University, Adelphi University, Mercy College, and Washburn University of Topeka. The numerous awards for her contributions and leadership in nursing include citations for Inspiring Leadership in the Field of Intergroup Relations by Chi Eta Phi Sorority, In Recognition of Your Outstanding Contribution to Nursing by New York University, and For Distinguished Service to Nursing by Teachers College. In addition, New York University houses the Martha E. Rogers Center for the Study of Nursing Science. In 1996 Rogers was inducted posthumously into the American Nurses Association Hall of Fame.

In 1988, colleagues and students joined her in forming the Society of Rogerian Scholars (SRS) and immediately

*Previous authors: Kaye Bultemeier, Mary Gunther, Joann Sebastian Daily, Judy Sporleder Maupin, Cathy A. Murray, Martha Carole Satterly, Denise L. Schnell, and Therese L. Wallace. Earlier editions of this chapter were critiqued by Dr. Lois Meier and Dr. Martha Rogers.
[†]Photo credit: Kathleen Leininger, Shiner, TX.

began to publish *Rogerian Nursing Science News,* a members' newsletter, to disseminate theory developments and research studies (Malinski, 2009). In 1993 the SRS began to publish a refereed journal, *Visions: The Journal of Rogerian Nursing Science.* The society includes a foundation that maintains and administers the Martha E. Rogers Fund. In 1995 New York University established the Martha E. Rogers Center to provide a structure for continuation of Rogerian research and practice.

A verbal portrait of Rogers includes such descriptive terms as *stimulating, challenging, controversial, idealistic, visionary, prophetic, philosophical, academic, outspoken, humorous, blunt,* and *ethical.* Rogers remains a widely recognized scholar honored for her contributions and leadership in nursing. Butcher (1999) noted, "Rogers, like Nightingale, was extremely independent, a determined, perfectionist individual who trusted her vision despite skepticism" (p. 114). Colleagues consider her one of the most original thinkers in nursing for the way she synthesized and resynthesized knowledge into "an entirely new system of thought" (Butcher, 1999, p. 111). Today she is thought of as "ahead of her time, in and out of this world" (Ireland, 2000, p. 59).

THEORETICAL SOURCES

Rogers' grounding in the liberal arts and sciences is apparent in both the origin and the development of her conceptual model, published in 1970 as *An Introduction to the Theoretical Basis of Nursing* (Rogers, 1970). Aware of the interrelatedness of knowledge, Rogers credited scientists from multiple disciplines with influencing the development of the Science of Unitary Human Beings (SUBH). Rogerian science emerged from the knowledge bases of anthropology, psychology, sociology, astronomy, religion, philosophy, history, biology, physics, mathematics, and literature to create a model of unitary human beings and the environment as energy fields integral to the life process. Within nursing, the origins of Rogerian science can be traced to Nightingale's proposals and statistical data, placing the human being within the framework of the natural world. This "foundation for the scope of modern nursing" began nursing's investigation of the relationship between human beings and the environment (Rogers, 1970, p. 30). Newman (1997) describes the Science of Unitary Human Beings as "the study of the moving, intuitive experience of nurses in mutual process with those they serve" (p. 9).

MAJOR CONCEPTS & DEFINITIONS

In 1970, Rogers' conceptual model of nursing rested on a set of basic assumptions that described the life process in human beings: wholeness, openness, unidirectionality, pattern and organization, sentience, and thought characterized the life process (Rogers, 1970).

Rogers postulates that human beings are dynamic energy fields that are integral with environmental fields. Both human and environmental fields are identified by pattern and characterized by a universe of open systems. In her 1983 paradigm, Rogers postulated four building blocks for her model: *energy field, a universe of open systems, pattern,* and *four-dimensionality.*

Rogers consistently updated the conceptual model through revision of the homeodynamic principles. Such changes corresponded with scientific and technological advances. In 1983 Rogers changed her wording from that of *unitary man* to *unitary human being,* to remove the concept of gender. Additional clarification of unitary human beings as separate and different from the term *holistic* stressed the unique contribution of nursing to health care. In 1992 *four-dimensionality* evolved into *pandimensionality.* Rogers' fundamental postulates have remained consistent since their introduction; her subsequent writings served to clarify her original ideas.

Energy Field

An *energy field* constitutes the fundamental unit of both the living and the nonliving. *Field* is a unifying concept, and *energy* signifies the dynamic nature of the field. Energy fields are infinite and pandimensional. Two fields are identified: the human field and the environmental field. "Specifically human beings and environment are energy fields" (Rogers, 1986b, p. 2). The **unitary human being (human field)** is defined as an irreducible, indivisible, pandimensional energy field identified by pattern and manifesting characteristics that are specific to the whole and that cannot be predicted from knowledge of the parts. The **environmental field** is defined as an irreducible, pandimensional energy field identified by pattern and integral with the human field. Each environmental field is specific to its given human field. Although not necessarily quantifiable, an energy field has the inherent ability to create change (Todaro-Franceschi, 2008). In this case both human and environmental fields change continuously, creatively, and integrally (Rogers, 1994a).

Universe of Open Systems

The concept of the **universe of open systems** holds that energy fields are infinite, open, and integral with one another (Rogers, 1983). The human and environmental fields are in continuous process and are open systems.

Continued

MAJOR CONCEPTS & DEFINITIONS—cont'd

Pattern

Pattern identifies energy fields. It is the distinguishing characteristic of an energy field and is perceived as a single wave. The nature of the pattern changes continuously and innovatively, and these changes give identity to the energy field. Each human field pattern is unique and is integral with the environmental field (Rogers, 1983). Manifestations emerge as a human–environmental mutual process. Musker (2012) notes, "the phenomenon of unitary pattern is the configuration of inherent wholeness" (p. 253). Pattern is an abstraction; it reveals itself through manifestation. A sense of self is a field manifestation, the nature of which is unique to each individual. Some variations in pattern manifestations have been described in phrases such as "longer *versus* shorter rhythms," "pragmatic versus imaginative," and time experienced as "fast" or "slow." Pattern is changing continually and may manifest disease, illness, or well-being. Pattern change is continuous, innovative, and relative.

Pandimensionality

Rogers defines **pandimensionality** as a nonlinear domain without spatial or temporal attributes, or as Phillips (2010) notes: "essentially a spaceless and timeless reality" (p. 56). The term *pandimensional* provides for an infinite domain without limit. It best expresses the idea of a unitary whole.

USE OF EMPIRICAL EVIDENCE

Being an abstract conceptual system, the Science of Unitary Human Beings does not directly identify testable empirical indicators. Rather, it specifies a worldview and philosophy used to identify the phenomena of concern to the discipline of nursing. As was mentioned previously, Rogers' model emerged from multiple knowledge sources; the most readily apparent of these are the nonlinear dynamics of quantum physics and general system theory.

Evident in her model are the influence of Einstein's (1961) theory of relativity in relation to space-time and Burr and Northrop's (1935) electrodynamic theory relating to electrical fields. By the time von Bertalanffy (1960) introduced the general system theory, theories regarding a universe of open systems were beginning to affect the development of knowledge within all disciplines. With the general system theory, the term **negentropy** was brought into use to signify increasing order, complexity, and heterogeneity in direct contrast to the previously held belief that the universe was winding down. Rogers, however, refined and purified the general system theory by denying hierarchical subsystems, the concept of single causation, and the predictability of a system's behavior through investigations of its parts.

Introducing quantum theory and the theories of relativity and probability fundamentally challenged the prevailing absolutism. As new knowledge escalated, the traditional meanings of *homeostasis, steady state, adaptation,* and *equilibrium* were questioned seriously. The closed-system, entropic model of the universe was no longer adequate to explain phenomena, and evidence accumulated in support of a universe of open systems (Rogers, 1994b). Continuing development within other disciplines of the acausal, nonlinear dynamics of life validated Rogers' model. Most notable of this development is that of chaos theory, quantum physics' contribution to the science of complexity (or wholeness), which blurs the boundaries between the disciplines, allowing exploration and deepening of the understanding of the totality of human experience.

MAJOR ASSUMPTIONS

Nursing

Nursing is a learned profession and is both a science and an art. It is an empirical science and, like other sciences, it lies in the phenomenon central to its focus. Rogerian nursing focuses on concern with people and the world in which they live—a natural fit for nursing care, as it encompasses people and their environments. The integrality of people and their environments, operating from a pandimensional universe of open systems, points to a new paradigm and initiates the identity of nursing as a science. The purpose of nursing is to promote health and well-being for all persons. The art of nursing is the creative use of the science of nursing for human betterment (Rogers, 1994b). "Professional practice in nursing seeks to promote symphonic interaction between human and environmental fields, to strengthen the integrity of the human field, and to direct and redirect patterning of the human and environmental fields for realization of maximum health potential" (Rogers, 1970, p. 122). Nursing exists for the care of people and the life process of humans.

Person

Rogers defines **person** as an open system in continuous process with the open system that is the environment (integrality). She defines **unitary human being** as an "irreducible, indivisible, pandimensional energy field identified by pattern and manifesting characteristics that are specific to the whole" (Rogers, 1992, p. 29). Human beings "are not disembodied entities, nor are they mechanical aggregates.... Man is a unified whole possessing his own integrity and manifesting characteristics that are more than and different from the sum of his parts" (Rogers, 1970, pp. 46–47). As such, "body exists merely as an expression of the underlying energy patterns within an energy field" (Daly, 2012, p. 13). Within a conceptual model specific to nursing's concern, people and their environment are perceived as irreducible energy fields integral with one another and continuously creative in their evolution.

Health

Rogers uses the term **health** in many of her earlier writings without clearly defining the term. She uses the term **passive health** to symbolize wellness and the absence of disease and major illness (Rogers, 1970). Her promotion of positive health connotes direction in helping people with opportunities for rhythmic consistency (Rogers, 1970). Later, she wrote that wellness "is a much better term... because the term *health* is very ambiguous" (Rogers, 1994b, p. 34).

Rogers uses *health* as a value term defined by the culture or the individual. Health and illness are manifestations of pattern and are considered "to denote behaviors that are of high value and low value" (Rogers, 1980). Events manifested in the life process indicate the extent to which a human being achieves maximum health according to some value system. In Rogerian science, the phenomenon central to nursing's conceptual system is the human life process. The life process has its own dynamic and creative unity that is inseparable from the environment and is characterized by the whole (Rogers, 1970). Using this definition as a foundation for their research, Gueldner and colleagues (2005) postulate that a human being's sense of well-being (wellness) manifests itself by higher frequency and increasing pattern diversity.

In "Dimensions of Health: A View from Space," Rogers (1986b) reaffirms the original theoretical assertions, adding philosophical challenges to the prevailing perception of health. Stressing a new worldview that focuses on people and their environment, she lists iatrogenesis, nosocomial conditions, and hypochrondriasis as the major health problems in the United States. Rogers (1986b) writes, "A new world view compatible with the most progressive knowledge available is a necessary prelude to studying human health and to determining modalities for its promotion whether on this planet or in the outer reaches of space" (p. 2).

Environment

Rogers (1994a) defines environment as "an irreducible, pandimensional energy field identified by pattern and manifesting characteristics different from those of the parts. Each environmental field is specific to its given human field. Both change continuously and creatively" (p. 3). Environmental fields are infinite, and change is continuously innovative, unpredictable, and characterized by increasing diversity. Environmental and human fields are identified by wave patterns manifesting continuous mutual change.

THEORETICAL ASSERTIONS

The principles of homeodynamics postulate a way of perceiving unitary human beings. The evolution of these principles from 1970 to 1994 is depicted in Table 13.1. Rogers (1970) wrote, "The life process is homeodynamic... these principles postulate the way the life process is and predict the nature of its evolving" (p. 96). Rogers identified the principles of change as **helicy, resonancy,** and **integrality**. The helicy principle describes spiral development in continuous, nonrepeating, and innovative patterning. Rogers' articulation of the principle of helicy describing the nature of change evolved from probabilistic to unpredictable, while remaining continuous and innovative. According to the principle of resonancy, patterning changes with the development from lower to higher frequency, that is, with varying degrees of intensity. Resonancy embodies wave frequency and energy field pattern evolution. Integrality, the third principle of homeodynamics, "reflects the unity or wholeness of humans and their environment" (Jarrin, 2012, p. 14). The principles of homeodynamics (nature, process, and context of change) support and exemplify the assertion that "the universe is energy that is always becoming more diverse through changing, continuous wave frequencies" (Phillips, 2010, p. 57). In addition, Todaro-Franceschi (2008) reminds us that this changing nature is intrinsic *to,* not *outside of,* fields.

In 1970 Rogers identified the following five assumptions that are also theoretical assertions supporting her model derived from literature on human beings, physics, mathematics, and behavioral science:

1. "Man is a unified whole possessing his own integrity and manifesting characteristics more than and different from the sum of his parts" (energy field) (p. 47).
2. "Man and environment are continuously exchanging matter and energy with one another" (openness) (p. 54).
3. "The life process evolves irreversibly and unidirectionally along the space-time continuum" (helicy) (p. 59).

TABLE 13.1 Evolution of Principles of Homeodynamics

An Introduction to the Theoretical Basis of Nursing, 1970	Nursing: A Science of Unitary Man, 1980	Science of Unitary Human Beings: A Paradigm for Nursing, 1983	Dimensions of Health: A View From Space, 1986	Nursing Science and the Space Age, 1992
Resonancy				
Continuously propagating series of waves between man and environment	Continuous change from lower- to higher-frequency wave patterns in the human and environmental fields	Continuous change from lower- to higher-frequency wave patterns in the human and environmental fields	Continuous change from lower- to higher-frequency wave patterns in the human and environmental fields	Continuous change from lower- to higher-frequency wave patterns in the human and environmental fields
Helicy				
Continuous, innovative change growing out of mutual interaction of man and environment along a spiraling longitudinal axis bound in space-time	Nature of change between human and environmental fields is continuously innovative, probabilistic, and increasingly diverse, manifesting nonrepeating rhythmicities	Continuous innovative, probabilistic, increasing diversity of human and environmental field patterns, characterized by nonrepeating rhythmicities	Continuous, innovative, probabilistic, increasing, and environmental diversity characterized by nonrepeating rhythmicities	Continuous, innovative, unpredictable, increasing diversity of human and environmental field patterns
Reciprocy				
Continuous mutual interaction between the human and environmental fields	—	—	—	—
Synchrony				
Change in the human field and simultaneous state of environmental field at any given point in space-time	Continuous, mutual, simultaneous interaction between human and environmental fields	Continuous, mutual human field and environmental field process	Continuous, mutual human field and environmental field process	Continuous, mutual human field and environmental field process

Conceptualized by J. S. Daily; revised by D. Schnell & T. Wallace; updated by C. Murray.

4. "Pattern and organization identify man and reflect his innovative wholeness" (pattern and organization) (p. 65).
5. "Man is characterized by the capacity for abstraction and imagery, language and thought, sensation, and emotion" (sentient, thinking being) (p. 73).

LOGICAL FORM

Rogers uses a dialectic method as opposed to a logistical, problematic, or operational method; that is, Rogers explains nursing by referring to broader principles that explain human beings. She explains human beings through principles that characterize the universe, based on the perspective of a whole that organizes the parts.

Rogers' model of unitary human beings is deductive and logical. The theory of relativity, the general system theory, the electrodynamic theory of life, and many other theories contributed ideas for Rogers' model. Unitary human beings and environment, the central components of the model, are integral with each other. The basic building blocks of her model are energy field, openness, pattern, and pandimensionality providing a new worldview. These concepts form the basis of an abstract conceptual system defining nursing and health. From the abstract conceptual system, Rogers derived the principles of homeodynamics, which postulate the nature and direction of human beings' evolution. Although Rogers coined the terms **homeodynamics** (similar state of change and growth), **helicy** (evolution), **resonancy** (intensity of change), and **integrality** (wholeness), all definitions are etymologically consistent and logical.

ACCEPTANCE BY THE NURSING COMMUNITY

Practice

The Rogerian model is an abstract system of ideas from which to approach the practice of nursing. Rogers' model, stressing the totality of experience and existence, is relevant in today's health care system, where a continuum of care is more important than episodic illness and hospitalization. This model provides the abstract philosophical framework from which to view the unitary human–environmental field phenomenon. Within the Rogerian framework, nursing is based on theoretical knowledge that guides nursing practice. The professional practice of nursing is creative and imaginative and exists to serve people. It is rooted in intellectual judgment, abstract knowledge, and human compassion.

Historically, nursing has equated practice with the practical and theory with the impractical. More appropriately, theory and practice are two related components in a unified nursing practice. Alligood (1994) articulates how theory and practice direct and guide each other as they expand and increase unitary nursing knowledge. Nursing knowledge provides the framework for the emergent artistic application of nursing care (Rogers, 1970). In other words, it is the "translation of knowledge into a way of being" (Alligood & Fawcett, 2012, p. 70).

Within Rogers' model, the critical thinking process directing practice can be divided into three components: pattern appraisal, mutual patterning, and evaluation. Cowling (2000) states that pattern appraisal is meant to avoid, if not transcend, reductionistic categories of physical, mental, spiritual, emotional, cultural, and social assessment frameworks. Through observation and participation, the nurse focuses on human expressions of reflection, experience, and perception to form a profile of the patient. Mutual exploration of emergent patterns allows identification of unitary themes predominant in the pandimensional human–environmental field process. Mutual understanding implies knowing participation but does not lead to the nurse prescribing change or predicting outcomes. As Cowling (2000) explains, "A critical feature of the unitary pattern appreciation process, and also of healing through appreciating wholeness, is a willingness on the part of the scientist or practitioner to let go of expectations about change" (p. 31). Evaluation centers on the perceptions emerging during mutual patterning.

Noninvasive patterning modalities used within Rogerian practice include, but are not limited to, acupuncture, aromatherapy, touch and massage, guided imagery, meditation, self-reflection, guided reminiscence, humor, hypnosis, dietary manipulation, transcendent presence, and music (Alligood, 1991a; Jonas-Simpson, 2010; Larkin, 2007; Levin, 2006; Lewandowski et al., 2005; Malinski & Todaro-Franceschi, 2011; Siedliecki & Good, 2006; Smith et al., 2002; Smith & Kyle, 2008; Walling, 2006; Yarcheski, Mahon, & Yarcheski, 2002). Barrett (1998) notes that integral to these modalities are "meaningful dialogue, centering, and pandimensional authenticity (genuineness, trustworthiness, acceptance, and knowledgeable caring)" (p. 138). Nurses participate in the lived experience of health in a multitude of roles, including "facilitators and educators, advocates, assessors, planners, coordinators, and collaborators," by accepting diversity, recognizing patterns, viewing change as positive, and accepting the connectedness of life (Malinski, 1986, p. 27) These roles may require the nurse to "let go of traditional ideas of time, space, and outcome" (Malinski, 1997, p. 115).

The Rogerian model provides a challenging and innovative framework from which to plan and implement nursing practice, which Barrett (1998) defines as the "continuous process (of voluntary mutual patterning) whereby the nurse assists clients to freely choose with awareness ways to participate in their well-being" (p. 136).

Education

Rogers clearly articulated guidelines for the education of nurses within the Science of Unitary Human Beings. Rogers discusses structuring nursing education programs to teach nursing as a science and as a learned profession. Barrett (1990b) calls Rogers a "consistent voice crying out against antieducationalism and dependency" (p. 306). Rogers' model clearly articulates values and beliefs about human beings, health, nursing, and the educational process. As such, it has been used to guide curriculum development in all levels of nursing education (Barrett, 1990b; DeSimone, 2006; Hellwig & Ferrante, 1993; Mathwig, Young, & Pepper, 1990). Rogers (1990) stated that nurses must commit to lifelong learning and noted, "The nature of the practice of nursing (is) the use of knowledge for human betterment" (p. 111).

Rogers advocated separate licensure for nurses prepared with an associate's degree and those with a baccalaureate degree, recognizing that there is a difference between the technically oriented and the professional nurse. In her view, the professional nurse must be well rounded and educated in the humanities, sciences, and nursing. Such a program would include a basic education in language, mathematics, logic, philosophy, psychology, sociology, music, art, biology, microbiology, physics, and chemistry; elective courses could include economics, ethics, political science, anthropology, and computer science (Barrett, 1990b). With regard to the research component of the curriculum, Rogers stated the following:

> *"Undergraduate students need to be able to identify problems, to have tools of investigation and to do studies that will allow them to use knowledge for the improvement of practice, and they should be able to read the literature intelligently. People with master's degrees ought to be able to do applied research. . . . The theoretical research, the fundamental basic research is going to come out of doctoral programs of stature that focus on nursing as a learned field of endeavor."*
>
> ***(1994a, p. 34)***

Barrett (1990b) notes that with increasing use of technology and increasing severity of illness of hospitalized patients, students may be limited to observational experiences in these institutions. Therefore the acquisition of manipulative technical skills must be accomplished in practice laboratories and at alternative sites, such as clinics and home health agencies. Other sites for education include health promotion programs, managed care programs, homeless shelters, and senior centers.

Research

Rogers' conceptual model provides a stimulus and direction for research and theory development in nursing science. Fawcett (2000), who insists that the level of abstraction affects direct empirical observation and testing, endorses the designation of the Science of Unitary Human Beings as a conceptual model rather than a grand theory. She states clearly that the purpose of the work determines its category. Conceptual models "identify the purpose and scope of nursing and provide frameworks for objective records of the effects of nursing" (Fawcett, 2005, p. 18).

Emerging from Rogers' model are theories that explain human phenomena and direct nursing practice. The Rogerian model, with its implicit assumptions, provides broad principles that conceptually direct theory development. The conceptual model provides a stimulus and direction for scientific activity. Relationships among identified phenomena generate both grand (further development of one aspect of the model) and middle-range (description, explanation, or prediction of concrete aspects) theories (Fawcett, 1995).

Three prominent grand theories are grounded in Rogers' conceptual model: Newman's theory of health as expanding consciousness, Parse's theory of human-becoming, and Fitzpatrick's life perspective rhythm model (Fawcett, 2015). Numerous middle-range theories have emerged from Rogers' three homeodynamic principles, (1) helicy, (2) resonancy, and (3) integrality (Fig. 13.1). Exemplars of middle-range theories derived from homeodynamic principles include power as knowing participation in change (helicy) (Barrett, 2010), the theory of perceived dissonance (resonancy) (Bultemeier, 2002), and the theory of interactive rhythms (integrality) (Floyd, 1983). In her overview of Rogerian science–based theories, Malinski (2009) identifies work within specific concepts: (1) self-transcendence (Reed, 2003), enlightenment (Hills & Hanchett, 2001), and spirituality (Malinski, 1994; Smith, 1994); (2) turbulence (Butcher, 1993) and dissonance (Bultemeier, 2002); (3) aging (Alligood & McGuire, 2000; Butcher, 2003); (4) intentionality (Ugarizza, 2002; Zahourek, 2005); and (5) unitary caring (Watson & Smith, 2002). Other middle-range theories encompass the phenomena of human field motion (Ference, 1986), as well as creativity, actualization, and empathy (Alligood, 1991b). Fawcett (2015) expanded the list to include middle-range theories of health empowerment (Shearer, 2009), diversity of human field pattern (Hastings-Tolsma, 2006), and health as wholeness and harmony (Carboni, 1995). Recently, a situation-specific theory has been derived from the Science of Unitary Human Beings by Willis, DeSanto-Madeya, and Fawcett (2015): the theory of men's healing from childhood maltreatment.

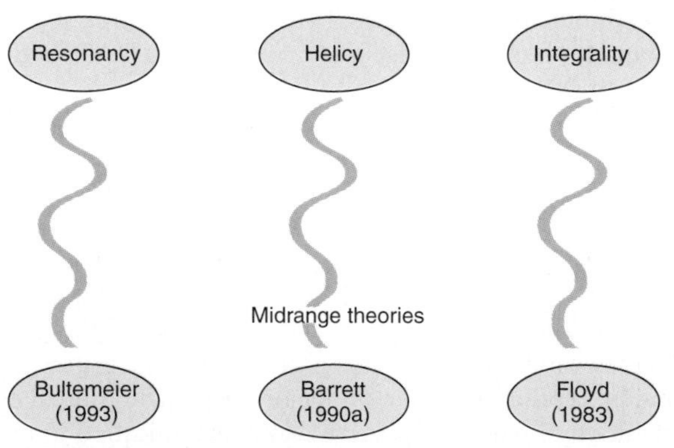

FIG. 13.1 Theory development within the Science of Unitary Human Beings.

Rogers (1986a) maintains that research in nursing must examine unitary human beings as integral with their environment. Therefore the intent of nursing research is to examine and understand a phenomenon and, from this understanding, design patterning activities that promote healing. To obtain a clearer understanding of lived experiences, the person's perception and sentient awareness of what is occurring are imperative. The variety of events associated with human phenomena provides the experiential data for research that is directed toward capturing the dynamic, ever-changing life experiences of human beings. Selecting the correct method for examining the person and the environment as health-related phenomena is the challenge of the Rogerian researcher. Both quantitative and qualitative approaches have been used in the Science of Unitary Human Beings research, although not all researchers agree that both are appropriate. Researchers do agree that ontological and epistemological congruence between the model and the approach must be considered and reflected by the research question (Barrett et al., 1997). Quantitative experimental and quasi-experimental designs are not appropriate, because their purpose is to reveal causal relationships. Descriptive, explanatory, and correlational designs are more appropriate, because they acknowledge diversity, universality, and patterned change.

Specific research methods emerging from middle-range theories based on the Rogerian model capture the human–environmental phenomena. As a means of capturing the unitary human being, Cowling (1998) describes the process of pattern appreciation using the combined research and practice case study method. Case study attends to the whole person (irreducibility), aims at comprehending the essence (pattern), and respects the inherent interconnectedness of phenomena. A pattern profile is composed through a synopsis and synthesis of the data (Barrett et al., 1997). Other innovative methods of recording and entering the human–environmental field phenomenon include photo-disclosure (Bultemeier, 1997), descriptive phenomenology (Willis & Griffith, 2010), hermeneutic text interpretation (Alligood & Fawcett, 1999), and measurement of the effect of dialogue combined with noninvasive modalities (Leddy & Fawcett, 1997).

Rogerian instrument development is extensive and ever-evolving. A wide range of instruments for measuring human–environmental field phenomena have emerged (Table 13.2). The continual emergence of middle-range theories, research approaches, and instruments demonstrates recognition of the importance of Rogerian science to nursing.

TABLE 13.2 Research Instruments and Practice Tools Derived from the Science of Unitary Human Beings

Practice Tool and Citation	Description
Human Field Motion Test (HFMT) (Ferenco, 1986)	Measures human field motion by means of semantic differential ratings of the concepts "my motor is running" and "my field expansion"
Perceived Field Motion Scale (PFM) (Yarcheski & Mahon, 1991)	Measures the perceived experience of motion by means of semantic differential ratings of the concept "my field motion"
Human Field Rhythms (HFR) (Yarcheski & Mahon, 1991)	Measures the frequency of rhythms in the human–environmental energy field mutual process by means of a one-item visual analog scale
The Well-Being Picture Scale (Gueldner et al., 2005; Terwilliger, Gueldner, & Bronstein, 2012)	A non–language-based pictorial scale that measures concepts of frequency, awareness, action, and power of energy field (general well-being) in adults; evaluated in children in 2012
Power as Knowing Participation in Change Tool (PKPCT) (Barrett, 1990a, 2010)	Measures the person's capacity to participate knowingly in change by means of semantic differential ratings of the concepts of awareness, choices, freedom to act intentionally, and involvement in creating changes
Diversity of Human Field Pattern Scale (DHFPS) (Hastings-Tolsma, 1993)	Measures diversity of human field pattern, or degree of change in the evolution of human potential throughout the life process, by means of Likert scale ratings of 16 items
Human Field Image Metaphor Scale (HFIMS) (Johnston, 1993, 1994)	Measures the individual's awareness of the infinite wholeness of the human field by means of Likert scale ratings of 14 metaphors that represent perceived potential and 11 metaphors that represent perceived field integrality

Continued

TABLE 13.2 Research Instruments and Practice Tools Derived from the Science of Unitary Human Beings—cont'd

Practice Tool and Citation	Description
Temporal Experience Scale (TES) (Paletta, 1990)	Measures subjective experience of temporal awareness by means of Likert scale ratings of 24 metaphors representing the factors of time dragging, time racing, and timelessness
Assessment of Dream Experience (ADE) (Watson, 1999)	Measures dreaming as a beyond waking experience by means of Likert scale ratings of the extent to which 20 items describe what the individual's dreams have been like during the past 2 weeks
Person-Environment Participation Scale (PEPS) (Leddy, 1995, 1999)	Measures the person's experience of continuous human-environment mutual process by means of semantic differential ratings of 15 bipolar adjectives representing the content areas of comfort, influence, continuity, ease, and energy
Leddy Heartiness Scale (LHS) (Leddy, 1996)	Measures the person's perceived purpose and power to achieve goals by means of Likert scale ratings of 26 items representing meaningfulness, ends, choice, challenge, confidence, control, capability to function, and connections
McCanse Readiness for Death Instrument (MRDI) (McCanse, 1995)	Measures physiological, psychological, sociological, and spiritual aspects of healthy field pattern, as death is developmentally approached by means of a 26-item structured interview questionnaire
Mutual Exploration of the Healing Human–Environmental Field Relationship (Carboni, 1992)	Measures nurses' and clients' experiences and expressions of changing configurations of energy field patterns of the healing human–environmental field relationship using semistructured and open-ended items; forms for a nurse and a single client and for a nurse and two or more clients are available
Nursing Process Format (Falco & Lobo, 1995)	Guides use of a Rogerian nursing process, including nursing assessment, nursing diagnosis, nursing planning for implementation, and nursing evaluation, according to the homeodynamic principles of integrality, resonancy, and helicy
Assessment Tool (Smith et al., 1991)	Guides use of a Rogerian nursing process, including assessment, diagnosis, implementation, and evaluation, according to the homeodynamic principles of complementarity (i.e., integrality), resonancy, and helicy, for patients hospitalized in a critical care unit and their family members, using open-ended questions
Critical Thinking for Pattern Appraisal, Mutual Patterning, and Evaluation Tool (Bultemeier, 2002)	Provides guidance for the nurse's application of pattern appraisal, mutual patterning, and evaluation, as well as areas for the client's self-reflection, patterning activities, and personal appraisal
Nursing Assessment of Patterns Indicative of Health (Madrid & Winstead-Fry, 1986)	Guides assessment of patterns, including relative present, communication, sense of rhythm, connection to environment, personal myth, and system integrity
Assessment Tool for Postpartum Mothers (Tettero et al., 1993)	Guides assessment of mothers experiencing the challenges of their first child during the postpartum period
Assessment Criteria for Nursing Evaluation of the Older Adult (Decker, 1989)	Guides assessment of the functional status of older adults living in their own homes, including demographic data, client prioritization of problems, sequential patterning (e.g., family of origin culture, past illnesses), rhythmical patterning (e.g., health care usage, medication usage, social contacts, acute illnesses), and cross-sectional patterning (e.g., current living arrangements and health concerns, cognitive and emotional status)

TABLE 13.2 Research Instruments and Practice Tools Derived from the Science of Unitary Human Beings—cont'd

Practice Tool and Citation	Description
Holistic Assessment of the Chronic Pain Client (Garon, 1991)	Guides holistic assessment of clients living in their own homes and experiencing chronic pain, including the environmental field, the community, and all systems in contact with the client; the home environment; client needs and expectations; client and family strengths; the client's pain experience—location, intensity, cause, meaning, effects on activities, life, and relationships, relief measures, and goals; and client and family feelings about illness and pain
Human Energy Field Assessment Form (Wright, 1991)	Used to record findings related to human energy field assessment as practiced in therapeutic touch, including location of field disturbance on a body diagram and strength of the overall field and intensity of the field disturbance on visual analog scales
Family Assessment Tool (Whall, 1981)	Guides assessment of families in terms of individual subsystem considerations, interactional patterns, unique characteristics of the whole family system, and environmental interface synchrony
An Assessment Guideline for Work with Families (Johnston, 1986)	Guides assessment of the family unit, in terms of definition of family, family organization, belief system, family developmental needs, economic factors, family field and environmental field complementarity, communication patterns, and supplemental data, including health assessment of individual family members, developmental factors, member interactions, and relationships
Nursing Process Format for Families (Reed, 1986)	Guides the use of a developmentally oriented nursing process for families
Community Health Assessment (Hanchett, 1988)	Guides assessment of a community in areas of diversity; rhythms, including frequencies of colors, rhythms of light, and patterns of sound; motion; experience of time; pragmatic-imaginative-visionary worldviews; and sleep-wake beyond waking rhythms

Adapted from Fawcett, J. (2005). *Contemporary nursing knowledge: Analysis and evaluation of nursing models and theories* (pp. 337–339). Philadelphia: F. A. Davis. Used with permission.

FURTHER DEVELOPMENT

Rogers (1986a) believed that knowledge development within her model was a "never-ending process" using "a multiplicity of knowledge from many sources . . . to create a kaleidoscope of possibilities" (p. 4). Explorations by Rogerian scholars into transcendence and universality exemplify this belief in a unifying wholeness (Phillips, 2010).

Fawcett (2005) identified the following three rudimentary theories developed by Rogers from the Science of Unitary Human Beings:

1. Theory of accelerating evolution
2. Theory of rhythmical correlates of change
3. Theory of paranormal phenomena

Continued explication and testing of these theories and the homeodynamic principles by nurse researchers contributes to nursing science knowledge.

CRITIQUE

Clarity

There were early criticisms of the model with comments such as difficult-to-understand principles, lack of operational definitions, and inadequate tools for measurement (Butterfield, 1983). However, the model has passed the test of time for the development of nursing science as nursing matured as a science. Rogers' ideas continue to demonstrate clarity for nursing research with human beings of all ages (Terwilliger, Gueldner, & Bronstein, 2012).

Simplicity

Ongoing studies and work within the model have served to simplify and clarify some of the concepts and relationships. However, when the model is examined in total perspective, some still classify it as complex. With its continued use in practice, research, and education, nurses will come to appreciate the model's elegant simplicity. As Whall (1987) noted, "With only three principles, a few major concepts, and five assumptions, Rogers has explained the nature of man and the life process" (p. 154).

Generality

Rogers' conceptual model is abstract and therefore generalizable and powerful. It is broad in scope, providing a framework for the development of nursing knowledge through the generation of grand and middle-range theories.

Accessibility

Drawing on knowledge from a multitude of scientific fields, Rogers' conceptual model is deductive in logic with an inherent lack of immediate empirical support (Barrett, 1990b). As Fawcett (1995) points out, failure to properly categorize the work as a conceptual model rather than as a theory leads to "considerable misunderstandings and inappropriate expectations" (p. 29), which can result in the work being labeled inadequate.

As noted earlier, the development of the model by Rogerian scientists has resulted in the generation of testable theories accompanied by tools of measurement.

Importance

Rogers' science has the fundamental intent of understanding human evolution and its potential for human betterment. The science "coordinates a universe of open systems to identify the focus of a new paradigm and initiate nursing's identity as a science" (Rogers, 1989, p. 182).

Although all the metaparadigm concepts have been explored, the emphasis is on the integrality of human–environmental field phenomena. Rogers suggested many ideas for future studies; on the basis of this and the research of others, it can be said that the conceptual model is useful. Such utility has been proven in the arenas of practice, education, administration, and research.

SUMMARY

The Rogerian model emerged from a broad historical base and has moved to the forefront as scientific knowledge has evolved. Understanding the concepts and principles of the Science of Unitary Human Beings requires a foundation in general education, a willingness to let go of the traditional, and an ability to perceive the world in a new and creative way. Emerging from a strong educational base, this model provides a challenging framework from which to provide nursing care. The abstract ideas expounded in the Rogerian model and their congruence with modern scientific knowledge spur new and challenging theories that further the understanding of the unitary human being.

CASE STUDY

Charlie Dee is a 56-year-old male client with a 30-year history of smoking two packs of cigarettes per day. He is seeing nurse practitioner Sandra Gee for the first time after being diagnosed with chronic obstructive pulmonary disease. Pattern appraisal begins with eliciting the client's description of his experience with this disease, his perceptions of his health, and how the disease is expressed (symptoms). Mr. Dee states that he has a productive cough that is worse in the morning, gets short of breath whenever he is physically active, and always feels tired. Through specific questions, the nurse practitioner discovers that Mr. Dee has experienced a change in his sleep patterns and nutritional intake. He is sleeping for shorter periods and eating less. She also learns that Mr. Dee's wife smokes, and that they have indoor cats for pets. He does not think that his wife will be amenable to changing her habits or getting rid of the cats. During this appraisal, the nurse seeks to discover what is important to Mr. Dee and how he defines *healthy.*

Mutual patterning involves sharing knowledge and offering choices. Upon completion of the appraisal, the nurse summarizes what she has been told and how she understands it. In this way, the nurse and the client can reach consensus about what activities would be acceptable to Mr. Dee. Ms. Gee provides information about the disease and suggestions that will increase his comfort. Noninvasive interventions include breathing retraining, recommendations for a high-protein high-calorie diet, eating smaller meals more frequently, sleeping with the head elevated, and using progressive relaxation exercises at bedtime. The nurse recommends that the Dees buy a high-efficiency particulate air (HEPA) filter and humidifier to assist in removing environmental pollutants and maintaining proper humidity in the home.

Because Mr. Gee has expressed a desire to quit smoking, the nurse suggests that he use forms of centering, such as guided imagery and meditation, to supplement the nicotine patches prescribed by his physician. She also provides him with written material about the disease that he can share with his wife. At the end of the visit, Mr. Dee states that he feels better knowing that he has the power to change some things about his life.

CRITICAL THINKING ACTIVITIES

1. Review two published research articles with Rogerian science as the framework guiding the research process. Identify the middle-range theory that was developed or guided the research process in each of the articles.
2. What is the nature of the evidence generated by research of the middle-range theory in critical thinking activity 1?
3. What philosophical tenets from Nightingale contributed to the basis for development of the Rogerian conceptual model?
4. Locate three publications and discuss how the authors used Rogerian science in nursing education.
5. Analyze your clinical practice, and identify areas in which practice based on Rogerian science would improve nursing care. Enumerate the changes and the anticipated positive outcomes.

POINTS FOR FURTHER STUDY

Publications

- *Visions: The Journal of Rogerian Nursing Science*
- Bultemeier, K. (2014). Rogers' science of unitary human beings in nursing practice (pp. 245–262). In M. R. Alligood, *Nursing theory: Utilization & application*, 5th ed. St Louis: Mosby-Elsevier.

Websites

- American Nurses Association Hall of Fame Inductee Page at www.nursingworld.org/MarthaElizabethRogers
- Martha E. Rogers Gravesite at http://www.aahn.org/gravesites/rogers.html
- New York University, Martha E. Rogers Center at http://www.foundationnysnurses.org/media/courier/Fall2007-MERogers.pdf
- Rogerian Nursing Science Wiki at http://rogeriannursingscience.wikispaces.com/. Created by H. K. Butcher, RN, PhD, University of Iowa College of Nursing. The intended purpose is twofold: (1) to bring together a collaborative participative community to cocreate a definitive comprehensive explication of the Science of Unitary Human Beings; (2) to create an online resource that anyone can access to learn how Rogerian nursing science serves as a foundation for nursing research, practice, education, and administration.
- Society of Rogerian Scholars at http://www.societyofrogerianscholars.org/
- Society of Rogerian Scholars Newsletter at http://www.societyofrogerianscholars.org/vol_1_2.html

REFERENCES

Alligood, M. R. (1991a). Guided reminiscence: A Rogerian based intervention. *Rogerian Nursing Science News, 3*(3), 1–3.

Alligood, M. R. (1991b). Testing Rogers' theory of accelerating change: The relationship among creativity, actualization, and empathy in persons 18 to 92 years of age. *Western Journal of Nursing Research, 13*, 84–96.

Alligood, M. R. (1994). Toward a unitary view of nursing practice. In M. Madrid & E. A. M. Barrett (Eds.), *Rogers' scientific art of nursing practice* (pp. 223–240). New York: National League for Nursing.

Alligood, M. R., & Fawcett, J. (1999). Acceptance of an invitation to dialogue: Examination of an interpretive approach for the science of unitary human beings. *Visions: Journal of Rogerian Nursing Science, 7*(1), 5–13.

Alligood, M. R., & Fawcett, J. (2012). Rogers' Science of Unitary Human Beings and praxis: An ontological review. *Visions, 19*(1), 65–74.

Alligood, M. R., & McGuire, S. L. (2000). Perception of time, sleep patterns and activity in senior citizens: A test of the Rogerian theory of aging. *Visions: The Journal of Rogerian Nursing Science, 8*(1), 6–14.

Barrett, E. A. M. (1990a). An instrument to measure power-as-knowing-participation-in-change. In O. Strickland & C. Waltz (Eds.), *The measurement of nursing outcomes: Measuring client self-care and coping skills* (Vol. 4, pp. 159–180). New York: Springer.

Barrett, E. A. M. (1990b). *Visions of Rogers' science-based nursing*. New York: National League for Nursing.

Barrett, E. A. M. (1998). A Rogerian practice methodology for health patterning. *Nursing Science Quarterly, 11*(4), 136–138.

Barrett, E. A. M. (2010). Power as knowing participation in change: What's new and what's next. *Nursing Science Quarterly, 23*(1), 47–54.

Barrett, E. A. M., Cowling, W. R., Carboni, J. T., & Butcher, H. K. (1997). Unitary perspectives on methodological practices. In M. Madrid (Ed.), *Patterns of Rogerian knowing* (pp. 47–62). New York: National League for Nursing.

Bultemeier, K. (1997). Photo-disclosure: A research methodology for investigating the unitary human being. In M. Madrid (Ed.), *Patterns of Rogerian knowing*. New York: National League for Nursing.

Bultemeier, K. (2002). Rogers' science of unitary human beings in nursing practice. In M. R. Alligood & A. Marriner Tomey (Eds.),

Nursing theory: Utilization and application (2nd ed., pp. 267–288). St Louis: Mosby.

Bultemeier, K. (2014). Rogers' science of unitary human beings in nursing practice. In M. R. Alligood (Ed.), *Nursing theory: Utilization & application* (5th ed., pp. 245–262). St Louis: Mosby-Elsevier.

Burr, H. S., & Northrup, F. S. C. (1935). The electrodynamic theory of life. *Quarterly Review of Biology*, *10*(4), 322–323.

Butcher, H. K. (1993). Kaleidoscoping in life's turbulence: From Seurat's art to Rogers' nursing science. In M. E. Parker (Ed.), *Patterns of nursing theories in practice* (pp. 183–198). New York: National League for Nursing.

Butcher, H. K. (1999). Rogerian ethics: An ethical inquiry into Rogers' life and science. *Nursing Science Quarterly*, *12*(2), 111 118.

Butcher, H. K. (2003). Aging as emerging brilliance: Advancing Rogers' unitary theory of aging. *Visions: The Journal of Rogerian Nursing Science*, *11*(1), 55–66.

Butterfield, S. E. (1983). In search of commonalties: Analysis of two theoretical frameworks. *International Journal of Nursing Studies*, *20*(1), 15–22.

Carboni, J. T. (1992). Instrument development and the measurement of unitary constructs. *Nursing Science Quarterly*, *5*(3), 134–142.

Carboni, J. T. (1995). Enfolding health-as-wholeness-and-harmony: A theory of Rogerian nursing practice. *Nursing Science Quarterly*, *8*(2), 71–78.

Cowling, W. R. (1998). Unitary case inquiry. *Nursing Science Quarterly*, *11*(4), 139–141.

Cowling, W. R. (2000). Healing as appreciating wholeness. *Advances in Nursing Science*, *22*(3), 16–32.

Daly, L.D. (2012). Slaves immersed in a liberal ideology. *Nursing Philosophy*, *13*(1), 69–77.

Decker, K. (1989). Theory in action: The geriatric assessment team. *Journal of Gerontological Nursing*, *15*(10), 25–28.

DeSimone, B. B. (2006). Curriculum design to promote the critical thinking of accelerated bachelor's degree nursing students. *Nurse Educator*, *31*(5), 213–217.

Einstein, A. (1961). *Relativity*. New York: Crown.

Falco, S. M., & Lobo, M. L. (1995). Martha E. Rogers. In J. B. George (Ed.), *Nursing theories. The base for professional nursing practice* (4th ed., pp. 229–248). Norwalk, CT: Appleton & Lange.

Fawcett, J. (1995). *Analysis and evaluation of conceptual models of nursing* (3rd ed.). Philadelphia: F. A. Davis.

Fawcett, J. (2000). *Analysis and evaluation of contemporary nursing knowledge: Nursing models and theories*. Philadelphia: F. A. Davis.

Fawcett, J. (2005). *Contemporary nursing knowledge: Analysis and evaluation of nursing models and theories*. Philadelphia: F. A. Davis.

Fawcett, J. (2015). Evolution of the Science of Human Beings: The conceptual system, theory development, and research and practice methodologies. *Visions*, *21*(1), 10–16.

Ference, H. M. (1986). The relationship of time experience, creativity traits, differentiation, and human field motion. In V. M. Malinski (Ed.), *Explorations in Martha Rogers' science of unitary human beings* (pp. 95–106). Norwalk, CT: Appleton-Century-Crofts.

Floyd, J. A. (1983). Research using Rogers' conceptual system: Development of a testable theorem. *Advances in Nursing Science*, *5*(2), 37–48.

Garon, M. (1991). Assessment and management of pain in the home care setting: Application of Rogers' science of unitary human beings. *Holistic Nursing Practice*, *6*(1), 47–57.

Gueldner, S. H., Michel, Y., Bramlett, M. H., Liu, C., Johnston, L. W., Endo, E., et al. (2005). The Well-Being Picture Scale: A revision of the Index of Field Energy. *Nursing Science Quarterly*, *18*(1), 42–50.

Hanchett, E. S. (1988). *Nursing frameworks and community as client: Bridging the gap*. Norwalk, CT: Appleton & Lange.

Hastings-Tolsma, M. T. (1993). The relationship of diversity of human field pattern to risk-taking and time experience: An investigation of Rogers' principles of homeodynamics (Doctoral dissertation, New York University, 1992). *Dissertation Abstracts International*, *53*, 4029B.

Hastings-Tolsma, M. (2006). Toward a theory of diversity of human field pattern. *Visions: The Journal of Rogerian Science*, *14*(2), 34–47.

Hellwig, S. D., & Ferrante, S. (1993). Martha Rogers' model in associate degree education. *Nurse Educator*, *18*(5), 25–27.

Hills, R. G. S., & Hanchett, E. (2001). Human change and individuation in pivotal life situations: Development and testing the theory of enlightenment. *Visions: The Journal of Rogerian Nursing Science*, *9*(1), 6–19.

Ireland, M. (2000). Martha Rogers' odyssey. *American Journal of Nursing*, *100*(10), 59.

Jarrin, O. F. (2012). The integrality of situated caring in nursing and the environment. *Advances in Nursing Science*, *35*(1), 14–24.

Johnston, L. W. (1993). The development of the human field image metaphor scale. *Visions: The Journal of Rogerian Nursing Science*, *1*, 55–56.

Johnston, L. W. (1994). Psychometric analysis of Johnston's human field image metaphor scale. *Visions: The Journal of Rogerian Nursing Science*, *2*(1), 7–11.

Johnston, R. L. (1986). Approaching family intervention through Rogers' conceptual model. In A. L. Whall (Ed.), *Family therapy theory for nursing. Four approaches* (pp. 11–32). Norwalk, CT: Appleton-Century-Crofts.

Jonas-Simpson, C. (2010). Awakening to space consciousness and timeless transcendent presence. *Nursing Science Quarterly*, *23*(3), 195–200.

Larkin, D. M. (2007). Ericksonian hypnosis in chronic care support groups: A Rogerian exploration of power and self-defined health-promoting goals. *Nursing Science Quarterly*, *20*(4), 357–369.

Leddy, S. K. (1995). Measuring mutual process: Development and psychometric testing of the person-environment participation scale. *Visions: The Journal of Rogerian Nursing Science*, *3*(1), 20–31.

Leddy, S. K. (1996). Development and psychometric testing of the Leddy healthiness scale. *Research in Nursing and Health*, *19*(5), 431–440.

Leddy, S. K. (1999). Further exploration of the psychometric properties of the Person-Environment Participation Scale: Differentiating instrument reliability and construct validity. *Visions: The Journal of Rogerian Nursing Science, 7*, 55–57.

Leddy, S. K., & Fawcett, J. (1997). Testing the theory of healthiness: Conceptual and methodological issues. In M. Madrid (Ed.), *Patterns of Rogerian knowing* (pp. 75–86). New York: National League for Nursing.

Levin, J. D. (2006). Unitary transformative practice: Using metaphor and imagery for self-reflection and theory informed practice. *Visions: The Journal of Rogerian Nursing Science, 14*(1), 27–35.

Lewandowski, W., Good, M., & Drauker, C. B. (2005). Changes in the meaning of pain with the use of guided imagery. *Pain Management Nursing, 6*(2), 58–67.

Madrid, M., & Winstead-Fry, P. (1986). Rogers' conceptual model. In P. Winstead-Fry (Ed.), *Case studies in nursing theory* (pp. 73–102). New York: National League for Nursing.

Malinski, V. M. (Ed.), (1986). *Explorations on Martha Rogers' science of unitary human beings*. New York: Appleton-Century-Crofts.

Malinski, V. M. (1994). Spirituality: A pattern manifestation of the human/environment mutual process. *Visions: The Journal of Rogerian Nursing Science, 2*, 12–18.

Malinski, V. M. (1997). Rogerian health patterning: Evolving into the 21st century. *Nursing Science Quarterly, 10*(3), 115–116.

Malinski, V. M. (2009). Evolving paths of transformative change in Rogerian nursing science. *Visions: The Journal of Rogerian Nursing Science, 9*, 8–18.

Malinski, V. M., & Todaro-Franceschi, V. (2011). Exploring co-meditation as a means of reducing anxiety and facilitating relaxation in a nursing school setting. *Journal of Holistic Nursing, 29*(4), 242–248.

Mathwig, G. M., Young, A. A., & Pepper, J. M. (1990). Using Rogerian science in undergraduate and graduate nursing education. In E. A. M. Barrett (Ed.), *Visions of Rogers' science-based nursing* (pp. 319–334). New York: National League for Nursing.

McCanse, R. L. (1995). The McCanse Readiness for Death Instrument (MRDI): A reliable and valid measure for hospice care. *Hospice Journal: Physical, Psychosocial, and Pastoral Care of the Dying, 10*(1), 15–26.

Musker, K. M. (2012). Unitary pattern: A review of theoretical literature. *Nursing Science Quarterly, 25*(3), 253–260.

Newman, M. A. (1997). A dialogue with Martha Rogers and David Bohm about the science of unitary human beings. In M. Madrid (Ed.), *Patterns of Rogerian knowing* (pp. 3–10). New York: National League for Nursing.

Paletta, J. L. (1990). The relationship of temporal experience to human time. In E. A. M. Barrett (Ed.), *Visions of Rogers' science-based nursing* (pp. 239–254). New York: National League for Nursing.

Phillips, J. R. (2010). The universality of Rogers' science of unitary human beings. *Nursing Science Quarterly, 23*(1), 55–59.

Reed, P. G. (1986). The developmental conceptual framework: Nursing reformulations and applications for family therapy. In A. L. Whall (Ed.), *Family therapy for nursing. Four approaches* (pp. 69–91). Norwalk, CT: Appleton-Century-Crofts.

Reed, P. G. (2003). The theory of self-transcendence. In M. J. Smith & P. R. Liehr (Eds.), *Middle range theory for nursing* (pp. 145–166). New York: Springer.

Rogers, M. E. (1970). *An introduction to the theoretical basis of nursing*. Philadelphia: F. A. Davis.

Rogers, M. E. (1980). *The science of unitary man. Tape V: Health and illness* (Audiotape). New York: Media for Nursing.

Rogers, M. E. (1983). Science of unitary human beings: A paradigm for nursing. In I. W. Clements & F. B. Roberts (Eds.), *Family health: A theoretical approach to nursing care* (pp. 219–227). New York: Wiley.

Rogers, M. E. (1986a). Science of unitary human beings. In V. M. Malinski (Ed.), *Explorations in Martha Rogers' science of unitary human beings* (pp. 3–8). Norwalk, CT: Appleton-Century-Crofts.

Rogers, M. E. (1986b). Dimensions of health: A view from space. Paper presented at the conference on "Law and Life in Space," September 12, 1986. Center for Aerospace Sciences, University of North Dakota.

Rogers, M. E. (1989). Nursing: A science of unitary human beings. In J. P. Riehl-Sisca (Ed.), *Conceptual models for nursing practice* (3rd ed., pp. 181–188). Norwalk, CT: Appleton-Century-Crofts.

Rogers, M. E. (1990). Space-age paradigm for new frontiers in nursing. In M. E. Parker (Ed.), *Nursing theories in practice* (pp. 105–114). New York: National League for Nursing.

Rogers, M. E. (1992). Nursing science and the space age. *Nursing Science Quarterly, 5*(1), 27–34.

Rogers, M. E. (1994a). Nursing science evolves. In M. Madrid & E. A. M. Barrett (Eds.), *Rogers' scientific art of nursing practice* (pp. 3–9). New York: National League for Nursing.

Rogers, M. E. (1994b). The science of unitary human beings: Current perspectives. *Nursing Science Quarterly, 7*(1), 33–35.

Shearer, N. B. (2009). Health empowerment theory as a guide for practice. *Geriatric Nursing, 30*(2), 4–10.

Siedliecki, S. L., & Good, M. (2006). Effect of music on power, pain, depression and disability. *Journal of Advanced Nursing, 54*(5), 553–562.

Smith, D. W. (1994). Toward developing a theory of spirituality. *Visions: The Journal of Rogerian Nursing Science, 2*(1), 35–43.

Smith, K., Kupferschmid, B. J., Dawson, C., & Briones, T. L. (1991). A family-centered critical care unit. *AACN Clinical Issues in Critical Care Nursing, 2*(2), 258–268.

Smith, M. C., Kemp, J., Hemphill, L., & Vojir, C. P. (2002). Outcomes of therapeutic massage for hospitalized cancer patients. *Journal of Nursing Scholarship, 34*(3), 257–262.

Smith, M. C., & Kyle, L. (2008). Holistic foundations of aromatherapy for nursing. *Holistic Nursing Practice, 22*(1), 3–11.

Terwilliger, S., Gueldner, S., & Bronstein, L. (2012). A preliminary evaluation of the Well-being Picture Scale–Children's Version (WBPS-CV) in a sample of fourth and fifth graders. *Nursing Science Quarterly, 25*(2), 160–166.

Tettero, I., Jackson, S., & Wilson, S. (1993). Theory to practice: Developing a Rogerian-based assessment tool. *Journal of Advanced Nursing, 18*(5), 776–782.

Todaro-Franceschi, V. (2008). Clarifying the enigma of energy, philosophically speaking. *Nursing Science Quarterly, 21*(4), 285–290.

Ugarizza, D. N. (2002). Intentionality: Applications within selected theories of nursing. *Holistic Nursing Practice, 16*(4), 41–50.

von Bertalanffy, L. (1960). *General system theory: Foundations, developments, application.* New York: George Braziller.

Walling, A. (2006). Therapeutic modulation of the psychoneuro-immune system by medical acupuncture creates enhanced feelings of well-being. *Journal of the American Academy of Nurse Practitioners, 18*(4), 135–143.

Watson, J. (1999). Measuring dreaming as a beyond waking experience in Rogers' conceptual model. *Nursing Science Quarterly, 12,* 245–250.

Watson, J., & Smith, M. C. (2002). Caring science and the science of unitary human beings: A trans-theoretical discourse for nursing knowledge development. *Journal of Advanced Nursing, 37*(5), 452–461.

Whall, A. L. (1981). Nursing theory and the assessment of families. *Journal of Psychiatric Nursing and Mental Health Services, 19*(1), 30–36.

Whall, A. L. (1987). A critique of Rogers' framework. In R. R. Parse (Ed.), *Nursing science: Major paradigms, theories, and critiques* (pp. 147–158). Philadelphia: Saunders.

Willis, D. G., DeSanto-Madeya, S., Ross, R., Sheehan, D. L., & Fawcett, J. (2015). Spiritual healing in the aftermath of childhood maltreatment. *Advances in Nursing Science, 38*(3), 162–174.

Willis, D. G., & Griffith, C.A. (2010). Healing patterns revealed in middle school boys' experiences of being bullied using Roger's [sic] science of unitary human beings (SUHB). *Journal of Child and Adolescent Psychiatric Nursing, 23*(3), 125–132.

Wright, S. M. (1991). Validity of the human energy field assessment form. *Western Journal of Nursing Research, 13*(5), 635–647.

Yarcheski, A., & Mahon, N. E. (1991). An empirical test of Rogers' original and revised theory of correlates in adolescents. *Research in Nursing and Health, 14*(6), 447–455.

Yarcheski, A., Mahon, N. E., & Yarcheski, T. J. (2002). Humor and health in early adolescents: Perceived field motion as a mediating variable. *Nursing Science Quarterly, 15*(2), 150–155.

Zahourek, R. P. (2005). Intentionality: Evolutionary development in healing: A grounded theory study for holistic nursing. *Journal of Holistic Nursing, 23*(1), 89–109.

BIBLIOGRAPHY

Primary Sources

Books

Rogers, M. E. (1961). *Educational revolution in nursing.* New York: Macmillan.

Rogers, M. E. (1964). *Reveille in nursing.* Philadelphia: F. A. Davis.

Rogers, M. E. (1970). *An introduction to the theoretical basis of nursing.* Philadelphia: F. A. Davis.

Book Chapters

Rogers, M. E. (1977). Nursing: To be or not to be. In B. Bullough & V. Bullough (Eds.), *Expanding horizons for nursing.* New York: Springer.

Rogers, M. E. (1978). Emerging patterns in nursing education. In *Current perspectives in nursing education* (Vol. II, pp. 1–8). St Louis: Mosby.

Rogers, M. E. (1980). Nursing: A science of unitary man. In J. P. Riehl & C. Roy (Eds.), *Conceptual models for nursing practice* (2nd ed., pp. 329–337). New York: Appleton-Century-Crofts.

Rogers, M. E. (1981). Science of unitary man: A paradigm for nursing. In G. E. Laskar (Ed.), *Applied systems and cybernetics* (Vol. IV, pp. 1719–1722). New York: Pergamon.

Rogers, M. E. (1983). Beyond the horizon. In N. L. Chaska (Ed.), *The nursing profession: A time to speak.* New York: McGraw-Hill.

Rogers, M. E. (1983). The family coping with a surgical crisis: Analysis and application of Rogers' theory to nursing care. (Rogers' response). In I. W. Clements & F. B. Roberts (Eds.), *Family health: A theoretical approach to nursing care.* New York: Wiley.

Rogers, M. E. (1985). High touch in a high-tech future. In *National League for Nursing, Perspectives in nursing—1985–1987* (pp. 25–31). New York: National League for Nursing.

Rogers, M. E. (1985). Nursing education: Preparing for the future. In *National League for Nursing, Patterns of education: The unfolding of nursing* (pp. 11–14). New York: National League for Nursing.

Rogers, M. E. (1985). Science of unitary human beings: A paradigm for nursing. In R. Wood & J. Kekhababh (Eds.), *Examining the cultural implications of Martha E. Rogers' science of unitary human beings* (pp. 13–23). Lecompton, KS: Wood-Kekhababh.

Rogers, M. E. (1986). Science of unitary human beings. In V. M. Malinski (Ed.), *Explorations on Martha Rogers: Science of unitary human beings* (pp. 3–8). Norwalk, CT: Appleton-Century-Crofts.

Rogers, M. E. (1987). Nursing research in the future. In J. Roode (Ed.), *Changing patterns in nursing education* (pp. 121–123). New York: National League for Nursing.

Rogers, M. E. (1987). Rogers' science of unitary human beings. In R. R. Parse (Ed.), *Nursing science: Major paradigms, theories, and critiques* (pp. 139–146). Philadelphia: Saunders.

Rogers, M. E. (1989). Nursing: A science of unitary human beings. In J. P. Riehl-Sisca (Ed.), *Conceptual models for nursing practice* (3rd ed., pp. 181–188). Norwalk, CT: Appleton & Lange.

Rogers, M. E. (1990). Nursing: Science of unitary, irreducible, human beings: Update 1990. In E. A. M. Barrett (Ed.), *Visions of Rogers' science-based nursing* (p. 5–25). New York: National League for Nursing.

Rogers, M. E. (1992). Nightingale's notes on nursing: Prelude to the 21st century. In F. Nightingale (Ed.), *Notes on nursing; What it is and what it is not* (Commemorative edition, pp. 58–62). Philadelphia: Lippincott.

Rogers, M. E., Doyle, M. B., Racolin, A., & Walsh, P. C. (1990). A conversation with Martha Rogers on nursing in space. In E. A. M. Barrett (Ed.), *Visions of Rogers' science-based nursing* (pp. 375–386). New York: National League for Nursing.

Journal Articles

Rogers, M. E. (1963). Building a strong educational foundation. *American Journal of Nursing, 63*(6), 94–95.

Rogers, M. E. (1963). Some comments on the theoretical basis of nursing practice. *Nursing Science, 1*(1), 11–13, 60–61.

Rogers, M. E. (1963). The clarion call. *Nursing Science, 1*(1), 134–135.

Rogers, M. E. (1964). Professional standards: Whose responsibility? *Nursing Science, 2*(1), 71–73.

Rogers, M. E. (1965). Collegiate education in nursing (Editorial). *Nursing Science, 3*(5), 362–365.

Rogers, M. E. (1965). Higher education in nursing (Editorial). *Nursing Science, 3*(6), 443–445.

Rogers, M. E. (1965). Legislative and licensing problems in health care. *Nursing Administration Quarterly, 2*(3), 71–78.

Rogers, M. E. (1965). What the public demands of nursing today. *RN, 28*, 80.

Rogers, M. E. (1966). Doctoral education in nursing. *Nursing Forum, 5*(2), 75–82.

Rogers, M. E. (1968). Nursing science: Research and researchers. *Teachers College Record, 69*, 469.

Rogers, M. E. (1969). Nursing education for professional practice. *Catholic Nurse, 18*(1), 28–37, 63–64.

Rogers, M. E. (1969). Preparation of the baccalaureate degree graduate. *New Jersey State Nurses Association Newsletter, 25*(5), 32–37.

Rogers, M. E. (1970). Yesterday a nurse, tomorrow a manager: What now? *Journal of New York State Nurses Association, 1*(1), 15–21.

Rogers, M. E. (1972). Nursing's expanded role . . . and other euphemisms. *Journal of New York State Nurses Association, 3*(4), 5–10.

Rogers, M. E. (1972). Nursing: To be or not to be? *Nursing Outlook, 20*(1), 42–46.

Rogers, M. E. (1975). Euphemisms and nursing's future. *Image: The Journal of Nursing Scholarship, 7*(2), 3–9.

Rogers, M. E. (1975). Forum: Professional commitment in nursing. *Image: The Journal of Nursing Scholarship, 2*(1), 12–13.

Rogers, M. E. (1975). Nursing is coming of age. *American Journal of Nursing, 75*(10), 1834–1843, 1859.

Rogers, M. E. (1975). Yesterday a nurse, today a manager: What now? *Image: The Journal of Nursing Scholarship, 2*(1), 12–13.

Rogers, M. E. (1977). Legislative and licensing problems in health care. *Nursing Administration Quarterly, 2*(3), 71–78.

Rogers, M. E. (1978). A 1985 dissent (Peer review). *Health/PAC Bulletin, 80*(1), 32–35.

Rogers, M. E. (1979). Contemporary American leaders in nursing: An oral history. An interview with Martha E. Rogers. *Kango Tenbo, 4*(12), 1126–1138.

Rogers, M. E. (1985). The nature and characteristics of professional education for nursing. *Journal of Professional Nursing, 1*(6), 381–383.

Rogers, M. E. (1985). The need for legislation for licensure to practice professional nursing. *Journal of Professional Nursing, 1*(6), 384.

Rogers, M. E. (1988). Nursing science and art: A prospective. *Nursing Science Quarterly, 1*(3), 99–102.

Rogers, M. E. (1989). Creating a climate for the implementation of a nursing conceptual framework. *Journal of Continuing Education in Nursing, 20*(3), 112–116.

Rogers, M. E. (1990). AIDS: Reason for optimism. *Philippine Journal of Nursing, 60*(2), 2–3.

Rogers, M. E. (1994). The science of unitary human beings: Current perspectives. *Nursing Science Quarterly, 7*(1), 33–35.

Rogers, M. E., & Malinski, V. (1989). Vital signs in the science of unitary human beings. *Rogerian Nursing Science News, 1*(3), 6.

Audiotapes

Rogers, M. E. (1980). *The science of unitary man. Tape I: Unitary man and his world: A paradigm for nursing* (Audiotape). New York: Media for Nursing.

Rogers, M. E. (1980). *The science of unitary man. Tape II: Developing an organized abstract system* (Audiotape). New York: Media for Nursing.

Rogers, M. E. (1980). *The science of unitary man. Tape III: Principles and theories* (Audiotape). New York: Media for Nursing.

Rogers, M. E. (1980). *The science of unitary man. Tape IV: Theories of accelerating change, paranormal phenomenon, and other events* (Audiotape). New York: Media for Nursing.

Rogers, M. E. (1980). *The science of unitary man. Tape V: Health and illness* (Audiotape). New York: Media for Nursing.

Rogers, M. E. (1980). *The science of unitary man. Tape VI: Interventive modalities: Translating theories into practice* (Audiotape). New York: Media for Nursing.

Rogers, M. E. (1987). *Rogers' framework* (Audiotape). Nurse Theorist Conference held in Pittsburgh, PA. Available through Meetings International, 1200 Delor Avenue, Louisville, KY 40217.

Videotapes

Distinguished leaders in nursing—Martha Rogers (Videotape). (1982). Capitol Heights, MD: The National Audiovisual Center. Available from the National Institutes of Health, National Library of Medicine, Bethesda, MD 20894, and from Sigma Theta Tau International, 550 West North Street, Indianapolis, IN 46202.

The nurse theorist: Portraits of excellence—Martha Rogers (Videotape/DVD). (1988). Produced by Fuld Video Project, Oakland, CA: Studio III, available from Fitne, Inc., Athens, Ohio.

Dissertation

Rogers, M. E. (1954). *The association of maternal and fetal factors with the development of behavior problems among elementary school children.* Doctoral dissertation, Johns Hopkins University, Baltimore, MD.

Secondary Sources

Books

Barrett, E. A. M. (1990). *Visions of Rogers' science-based nursing.* New York: National League for Nursing.

Barrett, E. A. M., & Malinski, V. M. (1994). *Martha E. Rogers: 80 years of excellence.* New York: Society of Rogerian Scholars.

Madrid, M. (1997). *Patterns of Rogerian knowing.* New York: National League for Nursing.

Madrid, M., & Barrett, E. A. M. (1994). *Rogers' scientific art of nursing practice.* New York: National League for Nursing.

Malinski, V. M. (Ed.). (1986). *Explorations on Martha Rogers' science of unitary human beings*. Norwalk, CT: Appleton-Century-Crofts.

Malinski, V. M., & Barrett, E. A. M. (1994). *Martha E. Rogers: Her life and her work*. Philadelphia: F. A. Davis.

Sarter, B. (1988). *The stream of becoming: A study of Martha Rogers' theory*. New York: National League for Nursing.

Book Chapters

Garon, M. (2011). Science of Unitary Human Beings: Martha E. Rogers. In J. B. George (Ed.), *Nursing theories: The base for professional practice* (6th ed.) (p. 265–290). Upper Saddle River, NJ: Prentice Hall.

Gunther, M. (2010). Rogers' Science of Unitary Human Beings in nursing practice. In M. R. Alligood & A. Marriner Tomey (Eds.), *Nursing theory: Utilization and application* (4th ed., pp. 287–308). St Louis: Mosby Elsevier.

Hemphill, J. C., & Quillen, S. I. (2005). Martha Rogers' model: Science of unitary beings. In J. J. Fitzpatrick & A. L. Whall (Eds.), *Conceptual models of nursing: Analysis and application* (4th ed.). Upper Saddle River, NJ: Pearson Prentice Hall.

Sitzman, K., & Eichenberger, L. W. (2011). Martha Rogers' Unitary Human Beings. In K. Sitzman & L. W. Eichenberger (Eds.), *Understanding the work of nurse theorists: A creative beginning* (2nd ed., pp. 179–186). Boston: Jones & Bartlett.

Wills, E. (2014). Grand nursing theories based on unitary process. In M. McEwen & E. M. Wills (Eds.), *Theoretical basis for nursing* (4th ed., pp. 192–212). Philadelphia: Lippincott Williams & Wilkin.

Journal Articles

Alligood, M. R. (2002). A theory of the art of nursing discovered in Rogers' science of unitary human beings. *International Journal of Human Caring, 6*(2), 55–60.

Alligood, M. R., & Fawcett, J. (2004). An interpretive study of Martha Rogers' conception of pattern. *Visions: The Journal of Rogerian Science, 12*(1), 8–13.

Barrett, E. A. M. (2006). The theoretical matrix for a Rogerian nursing practice. *Theoria: Journal of Nursing Theory, 15*(4), 11–15.

Baumann, S. L., Wright, S. G., & Settecase-Wu, C. (2014). A Science of Unitary Human Beings perspective of global health nursing. *Nursing Science Quarterly, 27*(4), 324–328.

Biley, F. C. (2000). Nursing for the new millennium: Martha Rogers and the science of unitary human beings. *Theoria: Journal of Nursing Theory, 9*(3), 19–22.

Biley, A., & Biley, F. C. (2006). Nursing models and theories: More than just passing fads. *Theoria: Journal of Nursing Theory, 15*(4), 16–22.

Blumenschein, L. (2009). Analysis and application of Rogers' science of unitary human beings. *Visions: The Journal of Rogerian Science, 16*(1), 55–61.

Butcher, H. K. (2000). Rogerian-praxis: A synthesis of Rogerian practice models and theories. *Rogerian Nursing Science News, 12*(1), 2.

Butcher, H. K. (2005). The unitary field pattern portrait research method: Facets, processes, and findings. *Nursing Science Quarterly, 18*(4), 293–297.

Butcher, H. K. (2006). Unitary pattern-based praxis: A nexus of Rogerian cosmology, philosophy, and science. *Visions: The Journal of Rogerian Science, 14*(2), 8–33.

Caratao-Mojica, R. (2015). The Science of Unitary Human Beings in a creative perspective. *Nursing Science Quarterly, 28*(4), 297–299.

Caroselli, C. (2010). Evolutionary emergent: Chief nurse executive as chief vision officer. *Nursing Science Quarterly, 23*(1), 72–76.

Cowling, W. R. (2001). Unitary appreciative inquiry. *Advances in Nursing Science, 23*(4), 32–48.

Cowling, W. R. (2004). Pattern, participation, praxis, and power in unitary appreciative inquiry. *Advances in Nursing Science, 27*(3), 202–214.

Cowling, W. R. (2007). A unitary participatory vision of nursing knowledge. *Advances in Nursing Science, 30*(1), 61–70.

Cowling, W. R., & Taliaferro, D. (2004). Emergence of a healing-caring perspective: Contemporary conceptual and theoretical directions. *Journal of Theory Construction & Testing, 8*(2), 54–59.

Dunn, D. J. (2009). A way of knowing, being, valuing and living with compassion energy: A unitary science and nursing as caring perspective. *Visions: The Journal of Rogerian Science, 16*(1), 40–47.

Fawcett, J. (2003). The science of unitary human beings: Analysis of qualitative research approaches. *Visions: The Journal of Rogerian Science, 11*(1), 7–20.

Fawcett, J., & Alligood, M. R. (2001). SUHB instruments: An overview of research instruments and clinical tools derived from the science of unitary human beings. *Theoria: Journal of Nursing Theory, 10*(3), 5–12.

Kim, T. S. (2008). Science of unitary human beings: An update on research. *Nursing Science Quarterly, 21*(4), 294–299.

Kim, T. S. (2009). The theory of power as knowing participation in change: A literature review update. *Visions: The Journal of Rogerian Science, 16*(1), 19–25.

Kim, T. S., Kim, C., Park, K. M., Park, Y. S., & Lee, B. S. (2008). The relation of power and well-being in Korean adults. *Nursing Science Quarterly, 21*(3), 247–254.

Kim, T. S., Park, J. S., Kim, M. A. (2008). The relation of meditation to power and well being. *Nursing Science Quarterly, 21*(1), 49–58.

Love, K. L. (2008). Interconnectedness in nursing: A concept analysis. *Journal of Holistic Nursing, 26*(4), 255–265.

Malinski, V. M. (2008). Research diversity from the perspective of the science of unitary human beings. *Nursing Science Quarterly, 21*(4), 291–293.

Malinski, V. M. (2012). Meditations on the unitary rhythm of dying-grieving. *Nursing Science Quarterly, 25*(3), 239–244.

Onieva-Zafra, M. D., Garcia, L. H., & Del Valle, M. G. (2015). Effectiveness of guided imagery relaxation on levels of pain and depression in patients diagnosed with fibromyalgia. *Holistic Nursing Practice, 29*(1), 13–21.

Phillips, J. R. (2016). Rogers' Science of Unitary Human Beings: Beyond the frontier of science. *Nursing Science Quarterly, 29*(1), 38–46.

Reis, P. J. (2014). Prenatal yoga practice in late pregnancy and patterning of change in optimism, power, and well-being. *Nursing Science Quarterly, 27*(1), 30–36.

Repede, E. J. (2009). Participatory dreaming: A conceptual exploration from a unitary appreciative inquiry perspective. *Nursing Science Quarterly, 22*(4), 360–368.

Ring, M. E. (2009). An exploration of the perception of time from the perspective of the science of unitary human beings. *Nursing Science Quarterly, 22*(1), 8–12.

Ring, M. E. (2009). Reiki and changes in pattern manifestations. *Nursing Science Quarterly, 22*(3), 250–258.

Shearer, N. B. C., & Reed, P. G. (2009). The rhythm of health in older women with chronic illness. *Research and Theory for Nursing Practice: An International Journal, 23*(2), 148–160.

Todaro-Franceschi, V. (2001). Energy: A bridging concept for nursing science. *Nursing Science Quarterly, 14*(2), 132–140.

Willis, D. G., DeSanto-Madeya, S., & Fawcett, J. (2015). Moving beyond dwelling in suffering: A situation-specific theory of men's healing from childhood maltreatment. *Nursing Science Quarterly, 28*(1), 57–63.

Wright, B. W. (2010). Power, trust, and science of unitary human beings influence political leadership. *Nursing Science Quarterly, 23*(1), 60–62.

Doctoral Dissertations

Alligood, R. R. (2007). *The life pattern of people with spinal cord injury*. Unpublished doctoral dissertation, Virginia Commonwealth University, Richmond, VA.

Coroneos-Shannon, D. L. (2014). *The relationship between belief, experience, and use of Reiki by registered nurses*. Unpublished doctoral dissertation, Walden University, Minneapolis, MN.

England, T. P. (2008). *Feeling overwhelmed: The lived experience of nurse managers*. Unpublished doctoral dissertation, East Tennessee State University, Johnson City, TN.

Fuller, J. M. (2011). *A family unitary field pattern portrait of power as knowing participation in change among adult substance users in rehabilitation*. Unpublished doctoral dissertation, Hampton University, Hampton, VA.

Grantham, C. A. (2005). *Individual and maternal factors influential with male adolescent physical sexual intimacy*. Unpublished doctoral dissertation, University of Michigan, Ann Arbor, MI.

Heelan, L. (2015). *Exploring the relationships of power, attitudes regarding intermittent fetal monitoring, and perceived barriers to research utilization with a labor and delivery nurse's attitude toward patient advocacy*. Unpublished doctoral dissertation, Seton Hall University, South Orange, NJ.

Hoke, T. M. (2014). *Improving outcomes through patient empowerment at transition of care: A fall prevention program for stroke survivors*. Unpublished doctoral dissertation, University of Arizona, Tucson, AZ.

Larson, K. M. (2008). *Understanding the lived experience of patients who suffer from medically unexplained physical symptoms using a Rogerian perspective*. Unpublished doctoral dissertation, Boston College, Boston, MA.

Musker, K. M. (2005). *Life patterns of women transitioning through menopause*. Unpublished doctoral dissertation, Loyola University, Chicago, IL.

Nelson, P. T. (2008). *Sound as a gateway to a personal relationship with nature*. Unpublished doctoral dissertation, Pacifica Graduate Institute, Carpinteria, CA.

Reis, P. J. (2011). *Prenatal yoga practice in late pregnancy and patterning of change in optimism, power, and well-being*. Unpublished doctoral dissertation, East Carolina University, Greeneville, NC.

Repede, E. J. (2009). *Women abused as children and participatory dreaming: A study of unitary healing*. Unpublished doctoral dissertation, University of North Carolina, Greensboro, NC.

Ring, M. E. (2006). *Reiki and changes in pattern manifestations: A Unitary Field Pattern Portrait research study*. Unpublished doctoral dissertation, The Catholic University of America, Washington, DC.

Rushing, A. M. (2005). *The unitary life pattern of a group of people experiencing serenity in recovery from addiction to alcohol/drugs in 12-step programs*. Unpublished doctoral dissertation, Virginia Commonwealth University, Richmond, VA.

Sarno, L. (2010). *Incidence of advance directives for the elderly admitted to the hospital*. Unpublished doctoral dissertation, Northern Kentucky University, Highland Heights, KY.

Schneider, M. A. (2015). *An investigation of the relationships between and among power, trust, and job satisfaction of nurse managers in acute care hospitals using Rogers' Science of Unitary Human Beings*. Unpublished doctoral dissertation, Seton Hall University, South Orange, NJ.

Scroggs, N. H. (2010). *Life patterning of women experiencing midlife transition*. Unpublished doctoral dissertation, University of North Carolina, Greensboro, NC.

Siedlecki, S. L. (2005). *The effect of music on power, pain, depression, and disability: A clinical trial*. Unpublished doctoral dissertation, Case Western Reserve University, Cleveland, OH.

Stiles, K. A. (2007). *Complex holism: New worldview for nursing as lived in nursing practice*. Unpublished doctoral dissertation, California Institute of Integral Studies, San Francisco, CA.

Waters, P. J. (2008). *Characteristics of a healing environment as described by expert nurses who practice within the conceptual framework of Rogers' Science of Unitary Human Beings: A qualitative study*. Unpublished doctoral dissertation, University of Texas Medical Branch Graduate School of Biomedical Sciences, Galveston, TX.

14

Self-Care Deficit Theory of Nursing

*Violeta A. Berbiglia and Barbara Banfield**

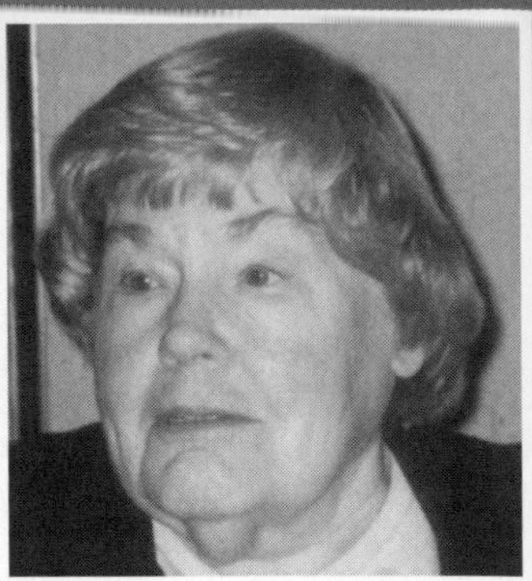

Dorothea E. Orem (1914–2007)[†]

"Nursing is practical endeavor, but it is practical endeavor engaged in by persons who have specialized theoretic nursing knowledge with developed capabilities to put this knowledge to work in concrete situations of nursing practice."

(Orem, 2001, p. 161)

CREDENTIALS AND BACKGROUND OF THE THEORIST

Dorothea Elizabeth Orem was born in Baltimore, Maryland, in 1914. She began her nursing career at Providence Hospital School of Nursing in Washington, DC, where she received a diploma of nursing in the early 1930s. Orem received a bachelor of science degree in Nursing Education from Catholic University of America (CUA) in 1939, and she received a master's of science degree in Nursing Education from the same university in 1946.

Orem's early nursing experiences included operating room nursing, private duty nursing (home and hospital), hospital staff nursing on pediatric and adult medical and surgical units, evening supervisor in the emergency room, and biological science teaching. Orem held the directorship of both the nursing school and the Department of Nursing at Providence Hospital, Detroit, from 1940 to 1949. After leaving Detroit, she spent 8 years (1949–1957) in Indiana working at the Division of Hospital and Institutional Services of the Indiana State Board of Health. Her goal was to upgrade the quality of nursing in general hospitals throughout the state. During this time, Orem developed her definition of nursing practice (Orem, 1956).

In 1957, Orem moved to Washington, DC, to take a position at the Office of Education, U.S. Department of Health, Education, and Welfare, as a curriculum consultant. From 1958 to 1960, she worked on a project to upgrade practical nurse training. That project stimulated a need to address the question: What is the subject matter of nursing? As a result, *Guides for Developing Curricula for the Education of Practical Nurses* was developed (Orem, 1959). Later that year, Orem became an assistant professor of nursing education at CUA. She subsequently served as acting dean of the School of Nursing and as associate professor of nursing education. She continued to develop her concepts of nursing and self-care at CUA. Formalization of concepts sometimes was accomplished alone and sometimes with others. Members of the Nursing Models Committee at CUA and the Improvement in Nursing Group, which later became the Nursing Development Conference Group (NDCG), contributed to the development of the theory. Orem provided intellectual leadership throughout these collaborative endeavors.

In 1970, Orem left CUA and began her consulting firm. Orem's first published book was *Nursing: Concepts of Practice* (Orem, 1971). She was editor for the NDCG as they prepared and later revised *Concept Formalization in Nursing: Process and Product* (NDCG, 1973, 1979). In 2004 a reprint of the second edition was produced and distributed by the International Orem Society for Nursing Science and Scholarship (IOS). Subsequent editions of *Nursing: Concepts of Practice* were published in 1980, 1985, 1991, 1995, and 2001. Orem retired in 1984 and continued developing the self-care deficit nursing theory (SCDNT).

*Previous authors: Susan G. Taylor, Angela Compton, Jeanne Donohue Eben, Sarah Emerson, Nergess N. Gashti, Ann Marriner Tomey, Margaret J. Nation, and Sherry B. Nordmeyer. Sang-arun Isaramalai is acknowledged for research and editorial assistance in a previous edition.

[†]Photo credit: Gerd Bekel Archives, Cloppenburg, Germany.

Georgetown University conferred the honorary degree of Doctor of Science on Orem in 1976. She received the CUA Alumni Association Award for Nursing Theory in 1980. Other honors included Honorary Doctor of Science, Incarnate Word College, 1980; Doctor of Humane Letters, Illinois Wesleyan University, 1988; Linda Richards Award, National League for Nursing, 1991; and Honorary Fellow of the American Academy of Nursing, 1992. She was awarded the Doctor of Nursing from the University of Missouri in 1998.

At age 92, Dorothea Orem's life ended after a period of being bedridden. She died Friday, June 22, 2007, at her residence on Skidaway Island, Georgia. Survivors were her lifelong friend, Walene Shields of Savannah, Georgia, and her cousin, Martin Conover of Minneapolis, Minnesota. Tributes by Orem's close colleagues were featured in the IOS official journal, *Self-Care, Dependent-Care & Nursing (SCDCN).*

Orem's many papers and presentations provide insight into her views on nursing practice, nursing education, and nursing science. Some of these papers are available to nursing scholars in a compilation edited by Renpenning and Taylor (2003). Other papers of Orem, and scholars who worked with her in developing the theory, are in the Orem Archives at the Alan Mason Chesney Medical Archives of the Johns Hopkins Medical Institutions.

THEORETICAL SOURCES

Orem (2001) stated, "Nursing belongs to the family of health services that are organized to provide direct care to persons who have legitimate needs for different forms of direct care because of their health states or the nature of their health care requirements" (p. 3). Like other direct health services, nursing has social features and interpersonal features that characterize the helping relations between those who need care and those who provide the required care. What distinguishes these health services from one another is the nature of the helping service that each provides. Orem's SCDNT provides a conceptualization of the distinct helping service that nursing provides.

Early on, Orem recognized that if nursing was to advance as a field of knowledge and as a field of practice, a structured, organized body of nursing knowledge was needed. From the mid-1950s, when she first put forth a definition of nursing, until shortly before her death in 2007, Orem pursued the development of a theoretical structure that would serve as an organizing framework for such a body of knowledge.

The primary source for Orem's ideas about nursing was her experiences in nursing. Through reflection on nursing practice situations, she was able to identify the proper object, or focus, of nursing. The question that directed Orem's (2001) thinking was, "What condition exists in a person when judgments are made that a nurse(s) should be brought into the situation?" (p. 20). The condition that indicates the need for nursing assistance is "the inability of persons to provide continuously for themselves the amount and quality of required self-care because of situations of personal health" (Orem, 2001, p. 20). It is the proper object or focus that determines the domain and boundaries of nursing, both as a field of knowledge and as a field of practice. The specification of the proper object of nursing marks the beginning of Orem's theoretical work. The efforts of Orem, working independently as well as with colleagues, resulted in the development and refinement of the SCDNT. Consisting of a number of conceptual elements and theories that specify the relationships among these concepts, the SCDNT is a general theory, "one that is descriptively explanatory of nursing in all types of practice situations" (Orem, 2001, p. 22). Originally, three specific theories were articulated: the theory of nursing systems, the theory of self-care deficits, and the theory of self-care. An additional theory, the theory of dependent-care, has been articulated. This theory is regarded as being parallel with the theory of self-care and serves to illustrate the ongoing development of the SCDNT.

In addition to her experiences in nursing practice situations, Orem was well versed in contemporary nursing literature and thought. Her association with nurses over the years provided many learning experiences, and she viewed her work with graduate students and her collaborative work with colleagues as valuable endeavors. Orem cited other nurses' works in terms of their contributions to nursing, including, but not limited to, Abdellah, Henderson, Johnson, King, Levine, Nightingale, Orlando, Peplau, Riehl, Rogers, Roy, Travelbee, and Wiedenbach.

Orem's familiarity with literature was not limited to nursing literature. In her discussion of various topics related to nursing, Orem cited authors from a number of other disciplines. The influence of scholars such as Allport (1955), Arnold (1960a, 1960b), Barnard (1962), Fromm (1962), Harre (1970), Macmurray (1957, 1961), Maritain (1959), Parsons (1949, 1951), Plattel (1965), and Wallace (1979, 1996) can be seen in Orem's ideas and positions. Familiarity with these sources helps promote a comprehensive understanding of Orem's work.

Foundational to Orem's SCDNT is the philosophical system of moderate realism. Banfield (1998, 2008, 2011) conducted philosophical inquiries to explicate the metaphysical and epistemological underpinnings of Orem's work. These inquiries revealed consistency between Orem's views regarding the nature of reality, human beings, the environment, and nursing as a science–ideas and positions associated with the philosophy of moderate realism. Taylor et al. (2000) have also explored the philosophical foundations of the SCDNT.

According to the moderate realist position, there is a world that exists independent of the thoughts of the knower. The nature of the world is not determined by the thoughts of the knower, although it is possible to obtain knowledge about the world.

Orem did not specifically address the nature of reality; however, statements and phrases that she uses reflect a moderate realist position. Four categories of postulated entities are identified as establishing the ontology of the SCDNT (Orem, 2001, p. 141). These four categories are (1) persons in space-time localizations, (2) attributes or properties of these persons, (3) motion or change, and (4) products brought into being.

With regard to the nature of human beings, "the view of human beings as dynamic, unitary beings who exist in their environments, who are in the process of becoming, and who possess free-will as well as other essential human qualities" is foundational to the SCDNT (Banfield, 1998, p. 204). This position, which reflects the philosophy of moderate realism, is seen throughout Orem's work.

Orem (1997) identified "five broad views of human beings that are necessary for developing understanding of the conceptual constructs of the SCDNT and for understanding the interpersonal and societal aspects of nursing systems" (p. 28). These are the view of **person, agent, user of symbols, organism,** and **object.** The view of human beings as person reflects the philosophical position of moderate realism; this position regarding the nature of human beings is foundational to Orem's work. She made the point that taking a particular view for some practical purpose does not negate the position that human beings are unitary beings (Orem, 1997, p. 31).

The view of person-as-agent is central to the SCDNT. Self-care, which refers to those actions in which a person engages for the purpose of promoting and maintaining life, health, and well-being, is conceptualized as a form of deliberate action. "Deliberate action refers to actions performed by individual human beings who have intentions and are conscious of their intentions to bring about, through their actions, conditions or states of affairs that do not at present exist" (Orem, 2001, pp. 62–63). When engaging in deliberate action, the person acts as an agent. The view of person-as-agent is also reflected in the SCDNT's conceptual elements of the nursing care and dependent-care. In relation to the view of person-as-agent and the idea of deliberate action, Orem cited a number of scholars, including Arnold, Parsons, and Wallace. She identified seven assumptions regarding human beings that pertain to deliberate action (Orem, 2001, p. 65). These explicit assumptions, which address deliberate action, rest upon the implicit assumption that human beings have free will.

The SCDNT represents Orem's work regarding the substance of nursing as a field of knowledge and as a field of practice. She also put forth a position regarding the form of nursing as a science, identifying it as a practical science. In relation to her ideas about the form of nursing science, Orem cites the work of Maritain (1959) and Wallace (1979), philosophers associated with the moderate realist tradition. In practical sciences, knowledge is developed for the sake of the work to be done. In the case of nursing, knowledge is developed for the sake of nursing practice. Two components make up the practical science: the speculative and the practical. The speculatively practical component is theoretical in nature, whereas the practically practical component is directive of action. The SCDNT with its concepts and theories is speculatively practical knowledge. The theory of dependent-care reflects further development of the speculatively practical knowledge. Practically practical nursing science is made up of models of practice, standards of practice, and technologies.

Orem (2001) identified two sets of speculatively practical nursing science: nursing practice sciences and foundational nursing sciences. The set of nursing practice sciences includes (1) wholly compensatory nursing science, (2) partly compensatory nursing science, and (3) supportive developmental nursing science. The foundational nursing sciences are (1) the science of self-care, (2) the science of the development and exercise of the self-care agency in the absence or presence of limitations for deliberate action, and (3) the science of human assistance for persons with health-associated self-care deficits. In relation to this proposed structure of nursing sciences, Orem (2001) stated, "the isolation, naming, and description of the two sets of sciences are based on my understanding of the nature of the practical sciences, on my knowledge of the organization of subject matter in other practice fields, and on my understanding of components of curricula for education for the professions" (pp. 174–175). In their text *Self-Care Science, Nursing Theory, and Evidence-Based Practice,* Taylor and Renpenning (2011) address the foundational nursing sciences, the nursing practice sciences, and evidence-based practice.

In addition to the two types of practical science, scientific knowledge necessary for nursing practice includes sets of applied sciences and basic nonnursing sciences. In the development of applied sciences, theories from other fields are used to solve problems in the practice field. These applied nursing sciences have yet to be identified and developed. Box 14.1 describes the structure of nursing science.

Orem's articulation of the form of nursing science provides the framework for the development of a body of knowledge for the education of nurses and for the provision of nursing care in concrete situations of nursing practice. The SCDNT with its conceptual elements and four theories identifies the substance or content of nursing science.

BOX 14.1 Speculatively Practical Nursing Science

Nursing Practice Sciences
Wholly compensatory nursing
Partly compensatory nursing
Supportive-developmental nursing

Foundational Nursing Sciences
The science of self-care
The science of the development and exercise of self-care agency in the absence or presence of limitations for deliberate action
The science of human assistance for persons with health-associated self-care deficits

Applied Nursing Sciences
Basic Nonnursing Sciences
Biological
Medical
Human
Environmental

From Orem, D. E. (2001). *Nursing: Concepts of practice* (6th ed.). St Louis: Mosby.

MAJOR CONCEPTS & DEFINITIONS

The self-care deficit nursing theory is a general theory composed of the following four related theories:

1. The theory of self-care, which describes why and how people care for themselves
2. The theory of dependent-care, which explains how family members and/or friends provide dependent-care for a person who is socially dependent
3. The theory of self-care deficit, which describes and explains why people can be helped through nursing
4. The theory of nursing systems, which describes and explains relationships that must be brought about and maintained for nursing to be produced

The major concepts of these theories are identified here and discussed more fully in Orem (2001), *Nursing: Concepts of Practice* (Fig. 14.1).

Self-Care

Self-care comprises the practice of activities that maturing and mature persons initiate and perform, within time frames, on their own behalf in the interest of maintaining life, healthful functioning, continuing personal development, and well-being by meeting known requisites for functional and developmental regulations (Orem, 2001, p. 522).

Dependent-Care

Dependent-care refers to the care that is provided to a person who, because of age or related factors, is unable to perform the self-care needed to maintain life, healthful functioning, continuing personal development, and well-being.

Self-Care Requisites

A self-care requisite is a formulated and expressed insight about actions to be performed that are known or hypothesized to be necessary in the regulation of an aspect of human functioning and development, continuously or under specified conditions and circumstances. A formulated self-care requisite names the following two elements:

1. The factor to be controlled or managed to keep an aspect of human functioning and development within the norms compatible with life, health, and personal well-being
2. The nature of the required action

Formulated and expressed self-care requisites constitute the formalized purposes of self-care. They are the reasons for which self-care is undertaken; they express the intended or desired result—the goal of self-care (Orem, 2001, p. 522).

Universal Self-Care Requisites

Universally required goals are to be met through self-care or dependent care, and they have their origins in what is known and what is validated, or what is in the process of being validated, about human structural and functional integrity at various stages of the life cycle. Eight self-care requisites common to men, women, and children are suggested:

1. Maintenance of a sufficient intake of air
2. Maintenance of a sufficient intake of food
3. Maintenance of a sufficient intake of water
4. Provision of care associated with elimination processes and excrements
5. Maintenance of balance between activity and rest
6. Maintenance of balance between solitude and social interaction
7. Prevention of hazards to human life, human functioning, and human well-being
8. Promotion of human functioning and development within social groups in accordance with human potential, known human limitations, and the human desire to be normal; normalcy is used in the sense of that which is essentially human and that which is in accordance with the genetic and constitutional characteristics and talents of individuals (Orem, 2001, p. 225)

Continued

MAJOR CONCEPTS & DEFINITIONS—cont'd

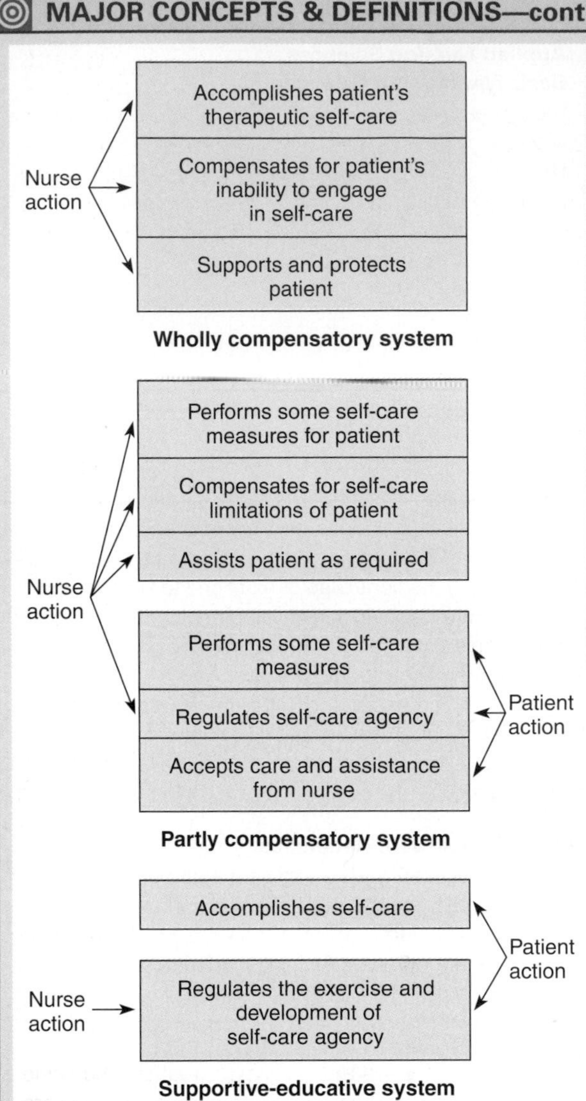

FIG. 14.1 Basic nursing systems. (From Orem, D. E. [2001]. *Nursing: Concepts of practice* [6th ed., p. 351]. St Louis: Mosby.)

Developmental Self-Care Requisites

Developmental self-care requisites (DSCRs) were separated from universal self-care requisites in the second edition of *Nursing: Concepts of Practice* (Orem, 1980). Three sets of DSCRs have been identified:

1. Provision of conditions that promote development
2. Engagement in self-development
3. Prevention of or overcoming effects of human conditions and life situations that can adversely affect human development (Orem, 1980, p. 231)

Health Deviation Self-Care Requisites

Health deviation self-care requisites exist for persons who are ill or injured, who have specific forms of pathological conditions or disorders, including defects and disabilities, and who are under medical diagnosis and treatment. The characteristics of health deviation as conditions extending over time determine the types of care demands that individuals experience as they live with the effects of pathological conditions and live through their durations.

Disease or injury affects not only specific structures and physiological or psychological mechanisms, but also integrated human functioning. When integrated functioning is affected seriously (severe mental retardation and comatose states), the individual's developing or developed powers of agency are seriously impaired, either permanently or temporarily. In abnormal states of health, self-care requisites arise from both the disease state and the measures used in its diagnosis or treatment.

Care measures to meet existent health deviation self-care requisites must be made action components of an individual's systems of self-care or dependent-care. The complexity of self-care or dependent-care systems is increased by the number of health deviation requisites that must be met within specific time frames.

Therapeutic Self-Care Demand

Therapeutic self-care demand consists of the summation of care measures necessary at specific times or over a duration of time to meet all of an individual's known self-care requisites, particularized for existent conditions and circumstances by methods appropriate for the following:

- Controlling or managing factors identified in the requisites, the values of which are regulatory of human functioning (sufficiency of air, water, and food)
- Fulfilling the activity element of the requisites (maintenance, promotion, prevention, and provision) (Orem, 2001, p. 523)

Therapeutic self-care demand at any time (1) describes factors in the patient or the environment that must be held steady within a range of values or brought within and held within such a range for the sake of the patient's life, health, or well-being, and (2) has a known degree of instrumental effectiveness derived from the choice of technologies and specific techniques for using, changing, or in some way controlling patient or environmental factors.

MAJOR CONCEPTS & DEFINITIONS—cont'd

Dependent-Care Demand

Dependent-care demand is the summation of care measures at a specific point in time or over a duration of time for meeting the dependent's therapeutic self-care demand when his or her self-care agency is not adequate or operational (Taylor et al., 2001, p. 40).

Self-Care Agency

The **self-care agency** is a complex acquired ability of mature and maturing persons to know and meet their continuing requirements for deliberate, purposive action to regulate their own human functioning and development (Orem, 2001, p. 522).

Dependent-Care Agency

Dependent-care agency refers to the acquired ability of a person to know and meet the therapeutic self-care demand of the dependent person and/or regulate the development and exercise of the dependent's self-care agency.

Self-Care Deficit

Self-care deficit is the relationship between an individual's therapeutic self-care demand and his or her powers of self-care agency in which the constituent-developed self-care capabilities within self-care agency are inoperable or inadequate for knowing and meeting some or all components of the existent or projected therapeutic self-care demand (Orem, 2001, p. 522).

Dependent-Care Deficit

Dependent-care deficit is a relationship that exists when the dependent-care provider's agency is not adequate to meet the therapeutic self-care demand of the person receiving dependent-care.

Nursing Agency

Nursing agency comprises developed capabilities of persons educated as nurses that empower them to represent themselves as nurses and within the frame of a legitimate interpersonal relationship to act, to know, and to help persons in such relationships to meet their therapeutic self-care demands and to regulate the development or exercise of their self-care agency (Orem, 2001, p. 518). Nursing agency also incorporates the capabilities of nurses to assist persons who provide dependent-care to regulate the development or exercise of their dependent-care agency.

Nursing Design

Nursing design, a professional function performed both before and after nursing diagnosis and prescription, allows nurses, on the basis of reflective practical judgments about existent conditions, to synthesize concrete situational elements into orderly relations to structure operational units. The purpose of nursing design is to provide guides for achieving needed and foreseen results in the production of nursing toward the achievement of nursing goals; these units taken together constitute the pattern that guides the production of nursing (Orem, 2001, p. 519).

Nursing Systems

Nursing systems are series and sequences of deliberate practical actions of nurses performed at times in coordination with the actions of their patients to know and meet components of patients' therapeutic self-care demands and to protect and regulate the exercise or development of patients' self-care agency (Orem, 2001, p. 519).

Helping Methods

A helping method from a nursing perspective is a sequential series of actions that, if performed, will overcome or compensate for the health-associated limitations of individuals to engage in actions to regulate their own functioning and development or that of their dependents. Nurses use all methods, selecting and combining them in relation to the action demands on individuals under nursing care and their health-associated action limitations, as follows:

- Acting for or doing for another
- Guiding and directing
- Providing physical or psychological support
- Providing and maintaining an environment that supports personal development
- Teaching (Orem, 2001, pp. 55–56)

Basic Conditioning Factors

Basic conditioning factors condition or affect the value of the therapeutic self-care demand and/or the self-care agency of an individual at particular times and under specific circumstances. Ten factors have been identified:

- Age
- Gender
- Developmental state
- Health state
- Pattern of living
- Health care system factors
- Family system factors
- Sociocultural factors
- Availability of resources
- External environmental factors

USE OF EMPIRICAL EVIDENCE

As a practical science, nursing knowledge is developed to inform nursing practice. Orem (2001) stated that "nursing is practical endeavor, but it is practical endeavor engaged in by persons who have specialized theoretic nursing knowledge with developed capabilities to put this knowledge to work in concrete situations of nursing practice" (p. 161). The provision of nursing care occurs in concrete situations. As nurses enter into nursing practice situations, they use knowledge of nursing science to assign meaning to the features of the situation, to make judgments about what can and should be done, and to design and implement systems of nursing care. From the perspective of the SCDNT, desired nursing outcomes include meeting the patient's therapeutic self-care demand and/or regulating and developing the patient's self-care agency.

The conceptual elements and the specific theories of the SCDNT are abstractions about the features common to all nursing practice situations. The SCDNT was developed and refined through the use of intellectual processes that focused on nursing practice situations. For example, Orem reflected on her nursing practice experiences to identify the proper object of nursing. In their work related to the SCDNT, the Nursing Development Conference Group (1979) engaged in analysis of nursing cases and in processes of analogical reasoning. In a tribute to Orem, Allison (2008) talks about the Nursing Development Conference Group, saying that "these nurses came together because they were interested in and willing to commit themselves to examining nursing situations to formalize ways of thinking about nursing that they felt were descriptive of nursing and would contribute to nursing knowledge" (p. 50). Since the SCDNT was first published, extensive empirical evidence has contributed to the development of theoretical knowledge. Much of this is incorporated into continuing refinement of the theory; however, the basics of the theory remain unchanged. The theory of dependent-care represents a major advancement in terms of the development of the SCDNT. "The increased need in societies for dependent-care indicates the importance for nurses of understanding dependent-care and their relationships to dependent-care agents" (Orem, 2001, p. 286).

In addition to the development of the theory of dependent-care, there have been other theoretical advances. Hartwig and Pickens (2016) used a conceptual analysis approach to explicate the meaning of normalcy. Six defining attributes of normalcy were identified: (1) having adequate resources to provide for the basic necessities of life, (2) being able to perform activities of daily living and those activities consistent with personal interests, (3) accepting and adjusting to a new normal, (4) maintaining one's health through making decisions about and implementing care for oneself, (5) engaging in fulfilling interpersonal relationships, and (6) being safe—not harming or being harmed by self or others (pp. 8–9). The literature analyzed in the conceptual analysis process supported the four categories of actions proposed by Orem to promote normalcy.

White, Peters, and Schim (2011) examined and analyzed the concept of spirituality and its relationship with the SCDNT. The authors proposed "that spirituality be conceptualized as a foundational disposition" (p. 51). Foundational capabilities and dispositions are components of the concepts of self-care agency, dependent-care agency, and nursing agency (Orem, 2001, pp. 260–264). These capabilities and dispositions are foundational to the person's abilities to engage in deliberate action.

White et al. (2011) also identify spiritual self-care as a form of self-care related to the meeting of developmental self-care requisites. "Spiritual self-care is defined as the set of spiritually based activities that a person engages in to maintain or promote continued person development and well-being in health and illness" (White et al., p. 53). The authors discuss a number of practices that can be regarded as self-care. In addition, they claim that religious affiliation is an element of the basic conditioning factor, sociocultural orientation.

MAJOR ASSUMPTIONS

Assumptions basic to the general theory were formalized during the early 1970s and were first presented at Marquette University School of Nursing in 1973. Orem (2001) identifies five premises underlying the general theory of nursing:

1. Human beings require continuous, deliberate inputs to themselves and their environments to remain alive and function in accordance with natural human endowments.
2. Human agency, the power to act deliberately, is exercised in the form of care for self and others in identifying needs and making needed inputs.
3. Mature human beings experience privations in the form of limitations for action in care for self and others involving making of life-sustaining and function-regulating inputs.
4. Human agency is exercised in discovering, developing, and transmitting ways and means to identify needs and make inputs to self and others.
5. Groups of human beings with structured relationships cluster tasks and allocate responsibilities for providing care to group members who experience privations for making required, deliberate input to self and others (p. 140).

Orem stated presuppositions and propositions for the theory of nursing systems, the theory of self-care deficit, and the theory of self-care. These constitute the expression of the theories and are summarized in the following sections.

THEORETICAL ASSERTIONS

Presented as a general theory of nursing that represents a complete picture of nursing, the SCDNT is expressed in the following three theories:

1. Theory of nursing systems
2. Theory of self-care deficit
3. Theory of self-care

The three constituent theories, taken together in relationship, constitute the SCDNT. The theory of nursing systems is the unifying theory and includes all the essential elements. It subsumes the theory of self-care deficit and the theory of self-care. The theory of self-care deficit addresses the reason why a person may benefit from nursing. The theory of self-care, foundational to the others, expresses the purpose, method, and outcome of taking care of self. The theory of dependent-care was initially introduced as a corollary to the theory of self-care (Taylor & Renpenning, 2011, p. 107). Work to further develop the conceptual elements and relationships related to this theory is ongoing.

Theory of Nursing Systems

The theory of nursing systems proposes that nursing is human action; nursing systems are action systems formed (designed and produced) by nurses through the exercise of their nursing agency for persons with health-derived or health-associated limitations in self-care or dependent-care. Nursing agency includes concepts of deliberate action, including intentionality, and the operations of diagnosis, prescription, and regulation. Fig. 14.1 shows the basic nursing systems categorized according to the relationship between patient and nurse actions. Nursing systems may be produced for individuals, for persons who constitute a dependent-care unit, for groups whose members have therapeutic self-care demands with similar components or who have similar limitations for engagement in self-care or dependent-care, and for families or other multiperson units.

Theory of Self-Care Deficit

The central idea of the theory of self-care deficit is that the requirements of persons for nursing are associated with the subjectivity of mature and maturing persons to health-related or health care–related action limitations. These limitations render them completely or partially unable to know existent and emerging requisites for regulatory care for themselves or their dependents. They also limit the ability to engage in the continuing performance of care measures to control or in some way manage factors that are regulatory of their own or their dependent's functioning and development.

Self-care deficit is a term that expresses the relationship between the action capabilities of individuals and their demands for care. Self-care deficit is an abstract concept that, when expressed in terms of action limitations, provides guides for the selection of methods for helping and understanding patient roles in self-care.

Theory of Self-Care

Self-care is a human regulatory function that individuals must, with deliberation, perform themselves or must have performed for them to maintain life, health, development, and well-being. Self-care is an action system. Elaboration of the concepts of self-care, self-care demand, and self-care agency provides the foundation for understanding the action requirements and action limitations of persons who may benefit from nursing. Self-care, as a human regulatory function, is distinct from other types of regulation of human functioning and development, such as neuro-endocrine regulation. Self-care must be learned, and it must be performed deliberately and continuously in time and in conformity with the regulatory requirements of individuals. These requirements are associated with their stages of growth and development, states of health, specific features of health or developmental states, levels of energy expenditure, and environmental factors.

Theory of Dependent-Care

The theory of dependent-care "explains how the self-care system is modified when it is directed toward a person who is socially dependent and needs assistance in meeting his or her self-care requisites" (Taylor & Renpenning, 2011, p. 24). For persons who are socially dependent and unable to meet their therapeutic self-care demand, assistance from other persons is necessary. In many ways self-care and dependent-care are parallel; the main difference is that when providing dependent-care, the person is meeting the self-care needs of another person. For the dependent-care agent, the demands of providing dependent-care can influence or condition the agent's therapeutic self-care demand and self-care agency. The need for dependent-care is expected to grow with the increasing age of the population and the number of persons living with chronic and/or disabling conditions.

LOGICAL FORM

Orem's insight led to her initial formalization and subsequent expression of a general concept of nursing. This generalization then made possible inductive and deductive thinking about nursing. The form of the theory is shown in the many models that Orem and others have developed, such as those shown in Fig. 14.1 and Fig. 14.2. Orem described the models and their importance to the development and understanding of the reality of the entities. These

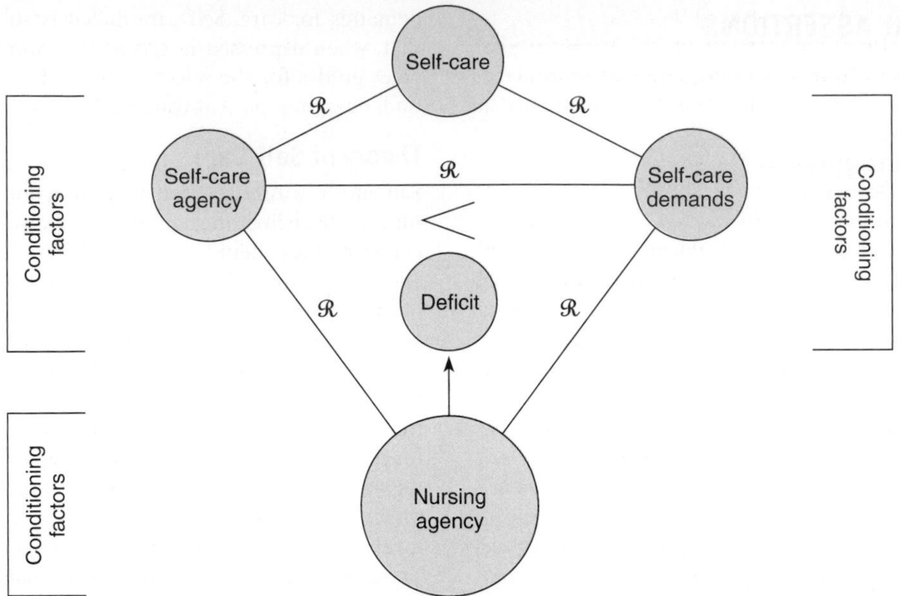

FIG. 14.2 A conceptual framework for nursing. *R,* Relationship; <, deficit relationship, current or projected. (From Orem, D. E. [2001]. *Nursing: Concepts of practice* [6th ed., p. 491]. St Louis: Mosby.)

models are "directed toward knowing the structure of the processes that are operational or become operational in the production of nursing systems, systems of care for individuals or for dependent-care units or multiperson units served by nurses" (Orem, 1997, p. 31). The overall theory is logically congruent.

ACCEPTANCE BY THE NURSING COMMUNITY

Orem's SCDNT has achieved a significant level of acceptance by the international nursing community, as evidenced by the magnitude of published material and presentations at the International Orem Society World Congresses (2008, 2011, and 2012). In research using the SCDNT or components, Biggs (2008) found more than 800 references. Berbiglia (2014) identified selected practice settings and SCDNT conceptual foci from a review of more than 3 decades of use of the SCDNT in practice and research and publicized selected international SCDNT practice models for the 21st century.

The SCDNT was introduced as the basic structure for nursing management in German hospitals implementing DRG (diagnosis-related group) pricing (G. Bekel, personal communication, 2004). The movement toward SCDNT-based nursing management in Germany is credited to Bekel's leadership, scholarship (1997, 2014, 2015), and futuristic thinking. A Nursing Therapeutic Center, oriented on new definitions in German nursing law and offering SCDNT-framed nursing therapy, is in the planning stages (G. Bekel, personal communication, April 23, 2016). Although it is difficult to fully assess the international application of the SCDNT, it is clear that, over time, Germany and Thailand have been landmark examples of the recent use of the SCDNT (Bekel, 2002, 2015; Harnucharunkul, 2012). A review of the World Health Organization website references to the global application of the concept of self-care featured 326 examples (http://www.who.int/en/, April 24, 2016). Although this finding is not based only on the SCDNT, it is what Orem envisioned as a final outcome of her theory—that the concept *self-care* would become commonplace.

The following U.S. schools' BSN programs offer SCDNT-based curricula (Berbiglia, 2011, 2012):

- Illinois Wesleyan University
- University of Tennessee at Chattanooga
- College of Saint Benedict
- Anderson College
- University of Toledo
- Alcorn State University
- Southern University Baton Rouge

The influence of Orem's SCDNT has continued at the international level through the translation of *Nursing*

Concepts of Practice into several languages (Spanish in 1993, German in 1997, and Japanese in 2005) and the proliferation of SCDNT-based practice, education, and research worldwide.

FURTHER DEVELOPMENT

From the time of publication of the first edition of *Nursing: Concepts of Practice* in 1971, Orem was engaged in continual development of her conceptualizations. She worked by herself and with colleagues. The sixth and final edition was published in 2001. Her work with a group of scholars, known as the Orem Study Group, further developed the various conceptualizations and structured nursing knowledge using elements of the theory. This work led to the expression of a theory of dependent-care (Taylor et al., 2001) and the foundational science of self-care (Denyes, Orem, & Bekel, 2001).

Nursing: Concepts of Practice (Orem, 2001) is organized with two foci: nursing as a unique field of knowledge and nursing as practical science. The text includes an expansion, from earlier editions, of content on nursing science and the theory of nursing systems. Important work has been done on the nature of person and interpersonal features of nursing. Orem identified many areas for further development in her descriptions of the stages of theory development. She also described the development of the foundational science of self-care (Denyes, Orem, & Bekel, 2001).

The IOS was established in 1993 for the purpose of advancing nursing science and scholarship through the use of Orem's nursing conceptualizations in nursing education, practice, and research. In 2015 the official name of the organization became Orem International Society of Nursing Science and Scholarship (OIS) (IOS conference call minutes).

The OIS publishes *Self-Care, Dependent-Care & Nursing,* an open-access online journal found on the OIS website (http://www.oreminternationalsociety.org). Since its inception, the OIS has sponsored international conferences and maintains a record of the content of these conferences.

CRITIQUE

Clarity

The terms Orem used are defined precisely. The language of the theory is consistent with the 21st-century language used in action theory and philosophy. The terminology of the theory is congruent throughout. The term *self-care* has multiple meanings across disciplines; Orem defined the term and elaborated the substantive structure of the concept in a way that is unique but also congruent with other interpretations. References made to the difficulty of Orem's language early on seem to no longer apply as more nurses become familiar with the work. Once a basic familiarity with the terminology of the SCDNT is achieved, further reading and studying of Orem's work fosters a comprehensive understanding of her view of nursing as a field of knowledge and as a field of practice.

Simplicity

Orem's theory is expressed in a limited number of terms. These terms are defined and used consistently in the expression of the theory. Orem's general theory, the SCDNT, comprises four constituent theories: **self-care, dependent-care, self-care deficit,** and **nursing systems.** The SCDNT is a synthesis of knowledge about eight entities, which include *self-care* (and *dependent-care*), *self-care agency* (and *dependent-care agency*), *therapeutic self-care demand, self-care deficit, nursing agency,* and *nursing system.* Development of the theory using these entities is parsimonious. The relationship between and among these entities is presented in a simple diagram. The substantive structure of the theory is seen in the development of these entities. The depth of development of the concepts gives the theory the complexity necessary to describe and understand a human practice discipline.

Generality

Orem commented on the generality, or universality, of the theory as follows:

> *"The self-care deficit theory of nursing is not an explanation of the individuality of a particular concrete nursing practice situation, but rather the expression of a singular combination of conceptualized properties or features common to all instances of nursing. As a general theory, it serves nurses engaged in nursing practice, in development and validation of nursing knowledge, and in teaching and learning nursing."*
>
> ***(1995, pp. 166–167)***

A review of the research and other literature attests to the generality of the theory.

Accessibility

As a general theory, the SCDNT provides a descriptive explanation of why persons require nursing and what processes are needed for the production of required nursing care. The concepts of the theory are abstractions of the entities that represent the proper object of nurses in concrete nursing practice situations. Self-care, dependent-care, and nursing care all are forms of deliberate action engaged in to achieve a particular purpose. The concepts of *therapeutic self-care demand, self-care agency, dependent-care agency,* and *nursing agency* refer to properties of persons. *Self-care deficit* and *dependent-care deficit* refer to relationships between properties of persons. *Self-care system, dependent-care system,* and *nursing system* are systems of care that are designed and implemented to achieve desired outcomes. *Basic conditioning factors* refer to factors that condition or influence the variables of persons. These factors may be internal to the person, such as developmental level, or external, such as available resources. In nursing practice situations, the data collected by nurses can readily be categorized according to the concepts of the SCDNT.

For research purposes, both quantitative and qualitative research methods are appropriate for the development of knowledge related to the SCDNT. Specific research methods to be used in any investigation are selected on the basis of the questions being asked. Examples of various approaches can be found in this publication's companion text summary of recent SCDNT-based research (Berbiglia, 2014). Although the concepts of the SCDNT refer to real entities, they are complex in nature. Operationalization of these concepts requires a comprehensive understanding of Orem's work. Instruments to measure some of these concepts have been developed.

The current emphasis in the SCDNT is on building a body of knowledge-related nursing practice, rather than engaging in theory-testing research. Instrument development has an important role in building nursing knowledge as well as other types of scholarly work. A great deal of work is needed with regard to the structuring of existent knowledge around the practice sciences and the foundational nursing sciences identified by Orem. Therefore comprehensive descriptive studies of various populations in terms of their self-care requisites and self-care practices are needed. The structuring of existent knowledge and the findings from descriptive studies will provide a solid base for the development of instruments to measure the concepts of the SCDNT.

Importance

The SCDNT differentiates the focus of nursing from other disciplines. Although other disciplines find the theory of self-care helpful and contribute to its development, the theory of nursing systems provides a unique focus for nursing. The significance of Orem's work extends far beyond the development of the SCDNT. In her works, she provided expression of the form of nursing science as practical science, along with a structure for ongoing development of nursing knowledge in the stages of theory development. Orem presented a visionary view of contemporary nursing practice, education, and knowledge development expressed through the general theory.

SUMMARY

The critical question—What is the condition that indicates that a person needs nursing care?—was the starting point for the development of the SCDNT. Orem noted that it was the inability of persons to maintain on a continuous basis their own care or the care of dependents. From this observation, she began the process of formalizing knowledge about what persons need to do or have done for themselves to maintain health and well-being. When a person needs assistance, what are the appropriate nursing assistive actions? The theory of self-care describes what a person requires and what actions need to be taken to meet those requirements. The theory of dependent-care is complex. It parallels Orem's theory of self-care. The theory of self-care deficits describes the limitations involved in meeting requirements for ongoing care and the effects they have on the health and well-being of the person or dependent. The theory of nursing systems provides the structure for examining the actions and antecedent knowledge required to assist the person. These theories also are descriptive of situations involving families and communities.

Orem's work related to nursing as a practical science and the identification of three practice sciences and three foundational nursing sciences provides direction for the development of nursing science. This work offers a structure for the organization of existing nursing knowledge, as well as for the generation of new knowledge.

In an interview with Jacqueline Fawcett (2001), Orem identified factors essential for the development of nursing science. They included the following: (1) a model of practice science; (2) a valid, reliable, general theory of nursing; (3) models of the operations of nursing practice; (4) development of the conceptual structure of the general theory; and (5) integration of the conceptual elements of the theory with the practice operations (p. 36). Orem's work related to the SCDNT and the form of nursing science as a practical science provides a foundation for the development of a body of knowledge. The efforts of nurse scholars and nurse researchers to build on this foundation will result in a body of knowledge that serves nurses in their provision of care to persons requiring nursing.

CASE STUDY

Theory of Dependent-Care

This case study documents an ongoing interaction between a wife and her husband who live in a spacious home in a gated community.

When Dan (now 80) and Jane (now 65) began dating more than 15 years ago, both were emotionally charged to begin their lives anew. Well-educated and financially secure, they had a lot in common. Dan was a protestant minister, and Jane's deceased husband had been a protestant minister. Both had lost their spouses. Jane's first husband had suffered a catastrophic cerebral aneurysm 2 years earlier. Dan had conducted the funeral service for Jane's husband. Dan's wife had died of terminal cancer a little over a year earlier. Dan's first wife had been a school counselor; Jane was a school teacher. Both had children in college. They shared a love for travel. Dan was retired but continued part-time employment, and Jane planned to continue teaching to qualify for retirement. Both were in great health and had more than adequate health benefits. Within the year they were married. Summer vacations were spent snorkeling in Hawaii, mountain climbing in national parks, and boating with family. After 7 years, Dan experienced major health problems: a quadruple cardiac bypass surgery, followed by surgery for pancreatic cancer. Jane's plans to continue working were dropped so she could assist Dan to recover and then continue to travel with him and enjoy their remaining time together. Dan did recover—only to begin to exhibit the early signs and symptoms of Alzheimer's disease. One of the early signs appeared the previous Christmas as they were hanging outdoor lights. To Jane's dismay, she noted that Dan could not follow the sequential directions she gave him. As time passed, other signs appeared, such as some memory loss and confusion, frequent repeating of favorite phrases, sudden outbursts of anger, and decreased social involvement. Assessments resulted in the diagnosis of early Alzheimer's disease. Dan was prescribed Aricept, and Jane began to prepare herself to face this new stage of their married life. She read literature about Alzheimer's disease avidly and organized their home for physical and psychological safety. A kitchen blackboard displayed phone numbers and the daily schedule. Car keys were appropriately stowed. It was noted that she began to savor her time with Dan. Just sitting together with him on the sofa brought gentle expressions to her face. They continued to attend church services and functions but stopped their regular swims at their exercise facility when Dan left the dressing room naked one day. Within the year, Jane's retired sister and brother-in-law relocated to a home a short walk from Jane's. Their intent was to be on call to assist Jane in caring for Dan. Dan and Jane's children did not live nearby so could only assist occasionally. As Dan's symptoms intensified, a neighbor friend, Helen, began to relieve Jane for a few hours each week. At this time, Jane is still the primary dependent-care agent. She prides herself in mastering a dual shower; she showers Dan in his shower chair first, and then, while she showers, he sits on the nearby toilet seat drying himself. Her girlfriends suggested that this was material for an entertaining home video! Although Jane is cautious in her care for Dan, she often drives a short distance to her neighborhood tennis court for brief games with friends or spends time tending the lovely gardens she and Dan planted. During these times, she locks the house doors and leaves Dan seated in front of the television with a glass of juice. She watches the time and returns home midway through the hour to check on Dan. On one occasion when she forgot to lock the door while she was gardening, Dan made his way to the street, lost his balance, reclined face-first in the flower bed, and was discovered by a neighbor. Jane has given up evenings out and increased her favorite pastime of reading. Her days are filled with assisting Dan in all of his activities of daily living. And, often, her sleep is interrupted by Dan's wandering throughout their home. At times, when the phone rings, Dan answers and tells callers Jane is not there. Jane, only in the next room, informs him "Dan, I am Jane." Friends are saddened by Dan's decline and concerned with the burdens and limitations Jane has assumed as a result of Dan's dependency.

CRITICAL THINKING ACTIVITIES

1. Examine this case study through the dependency cycle model (Fig. 14.3). The outer arrows show a progression through varying stages of dependency. The inner circle represents who can be involved in the dependency cycle. Where are Jane and Dan in this cycle?
2. Using the basic dependent-care system model (Fig. 14.4), assess Dan and Jane. Identify the basic conditioning factors (BCFs) for each. What is the effect of Dan's BCFs on his self-care agency? Is he able to meet his therapeutic self-care demands? Continue

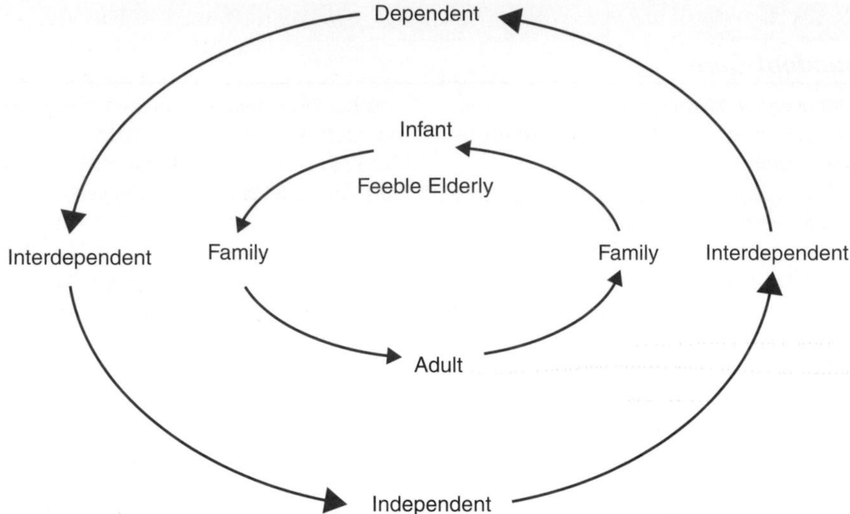

FIG. 14.3 Dependency cycle. (From Taylor, S. G., Renpenning, K. E., Geden, E. A., Neuman, B. M., & Hart, M. A. [2001]. The theory of dependent-care: A corollary to Orem's theory of self-care. *Nursing Science Quarterly, 14*[1], 39–47.)

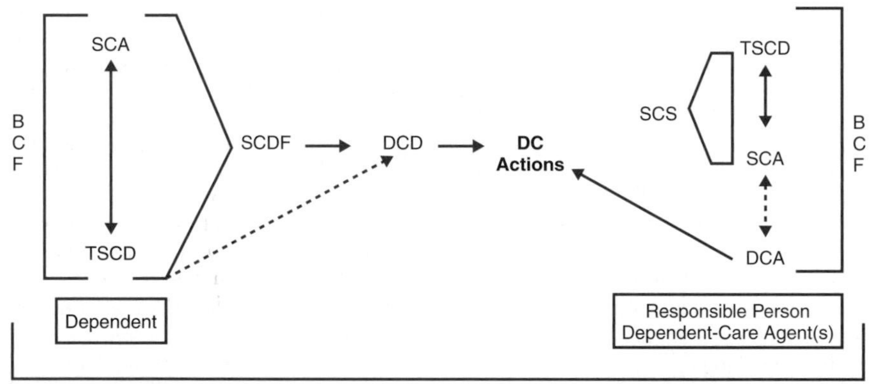

FIG. 14.4 Basic dependent-care system. *BCF,* Basic conditioning factors; *DCA,* dependent-care agency; *DCD,* dependent-care demand; *SCA,* self-care agency; *SCDF,* self-care deficit; *SCS,* self-care system; *TSCD,* therapeutic self-care demand. (From Taylor, S. G., Renpenning, K. E., Geden, E. A., Neuman, B. M., & Hart, M. A. [2001]. The theory of dependent-care: A corollary to Orem's theory of self-care. *Nursing Science Quarterly, 14*[1], 39–47.)

on to diagnose Dan's self-care deficit and resulting dependent-care deficit. Now assess Jane's self-care system.

3. Design a nursing system that addresses Jane's self-care system as she increases her role as dependent-care agent for Dan.

POINTS FOR FURTHER STUDY

- Berbiglia, V. A. (2014). Orem's self-care deficit nursing theory in practice. In M. R. Alligood (Ed.), *Nursing theory: Utilization & application* (5th ed., pp. 222–244). St Louis: Mosby Elsevier.

- Fawcett, J. (1988). *The nurse theorists. Portraits of excellence: Dorothea Orem* (Video/DVD). Athens, OH: Fitne, Inc.
- Fawcett, J. (1992). *Excellence in action: Dorothea Orem* (Video/DVD). Athens, OH: Fitne, Inc.
- The Orem International Society (OIS) at http://www.oreminternationalsociety.org
- The Johns Hopkins Archives house the Dorothea Orem Collection at http://www.medicalarchives.jhmi.edu
- The official OIS online journal, *Self-Care, Dependent-Care & Nursing,* is archived at OremInternational society.org.

REFERENCES

Allison, S. E. (2008). Some early efforts to conceptualize nursing: A tribute to Dorothea E. Orem (Electronic version). *Self-care, Dependent-Care & Nursing, 16*(1), 49–50.

Allport, G. W. (1955). *Becoming.* New Haven: Yale University Press.

Arnold, M. B. (1960a). *Emotion and personality* (Vol. 1). New York: Columbia University Press.

Arnold, M. B. (1960b). *Emotion and personality* (Vol. 2). New York: Columbia University Press.

Banfield, B. E. (1998). *A philosophical inquiry of Orem's self-care deficit nursing theory.* (Unpublished doctoral dissertation). Wayne State University, Detroit, MI.

Banfield, B. E. (2008). Philosophic position on nature of human beings foundational to Orem's self-care deficit nursing theory. *Self-Care, Dependent-Care, & Nursing, 16*(1), 33–40.

Banfield, B. E. (2011). Environment: A perspective of the self-care deficit nursing theory. *Nursing Science Quarterly, 24*(2), 96–100.

Barnard, C. I. (1962). *The functions of the executive.* Cambridge: Harvard University Press. *Society Newsletter, 7*(1), 1–3.

Bekel, G. (2002). Development of therapeutic self-care demand for nursing practice situations (Abstract). 7th International Self-Care Deficit Nursing Theory Conference November 1-3, 2002, Atlanta, GA.

Bekel, G. (2014). *Strukturmodelle und Methoden selbstpflegeorientierter Pflegediagnostik (Structural models and methods of self-care oriented nursing diagnostic).* Stuttgart: Thieme CNE-Fortbildung, 04-2014, Pflegewissenschaft. S. 2-9.

Bekel, G. (2015). Die Selbstpflegedefizit-Theorie: Ein Erkenntnisprogramm für diePflege als Praxiswissenschaft (SCDNT—A scientific program for nursing as a practice science) (pp. 185–214). In H. Brandenburg, S. Dorschner (Hrsg.), Pflegewissenschaft I. Ein Arbeitsbuch. 3. überarb. u. erw. Aufl. Bern, Hans Huber.

Berbiglia, V. A. (2011). The self-care deficit nursing theory as a curriculum conceptual framework in baccalaureate education. *Nursing Science Quarterly, 24*(2), 137–145.

Berbiglia, V. A. (2012). 2012 update on the self-care deficit nursing theory as a curriculum conceptual framework in baccalaureate education. (Abstract). 12th IOS World Congress, May, 2012, Luxembourg.

Berbiglia, V. A. (2014). Orem's self-care deficit theory in nursing practice. In M. R. Alligood (Ed.), *Nursing theory: Utilization & application* (5th ed., pp. 222–244). St Louis: Mosby.

Biggs, A. (2008). Orem's Self-Care Deficit Nursing theory: Update on the state of the art and science. *Nursing Science Quarterly, 21*(3), 200–206.

Denyes, M. J., Orem, D. E., & Bekel, G. (2001). Self-care: A foundational science. *Nursing Science Quarterly, 14*(1), 48–54.

Fawcett, J. (2001). The nurse theorists: 21st-century updates—Dorothea E. Orem 2001. *Nursing Science Quarterly, 14*(1), 34–38.

Fromm, E. (1962). *The art of loving.* New York: Harper Colophon Books.

Harnucharunkul, S. (2012, May). Keynote. 12th IOS World Congress, Luxembourg.

Harre, R. (1970). *The principles of scientific thinking.* Chicago: University of Chicago Press.

Hartweg, D., & Pickens, J. (2016). A concept analysis of normalcy within Orem's self-care deficit nursing theory. *Self-Care, Dependent-Care & Nursing, 22*(1), 12–15.

Macmurray, J. (1957). *The self as agent.* London: Faber and Faber.

Macmurray, J. (1961). *Persons in relation.* New York: Harper.

Maritain, J. (1959). *The degrees of knowledge.* New York: Charles Scribner's Sons.

Nursing Development Conference Group; Orem, D. E. (Ed.), (1973). *Concept formalization in nursing: Process and product.* Boston: Little Brown.

Nursing Development Conference Group; Orem, D. E. (Ed.), (1979). *Concept formalization in nursing: Process and product* (2nd ed.). Boston: Little Brown.

OIS (Orem International Society). (2015, Dec.). Conference call minutes.

Orem, D. E. (1956). *Hospital nursing service: An analysis.* Report to the Division of Hospital and Institutional Services of the Indiana State Board of Health. Indianapolis: Division of Hospital and Institutional Services.

Orem, D. E. (1959). *Guides for developing curricula for the education of practical nurses.* Washington, DC: U.S. Department of Health, Education, and Welfare.

Orem, D. E. (1971). *Nursing: Concepts of practice.* New York: McGraw-Hill.

Orem, D. E. (1980). *Nursing: Concepts of practice* (2nd ed.). New York: McGraw-Hill.

Orem, D. E. (1995). *Nursing: Concepts of practice* (5th ed.). St Louis: Mosby.

Orem, D. E. (1997a) *Strukturkonzepte der Pflegepraxis (Nursing concepts of practice).* (G. Bekel, Trans.). Berlin: Ullstein Mosby.

Orem, D. E. (1997b). Views of human beings specific to nursing. *Nursing Science Quarterly, 10*(1), 26–31.

Orem, D. E. (2001). *Nursing: Concepts of practice* (6th ed.). St Louis: Mosby.

Parsons, T. (1949). *Essays in sociological theory*. New York: Free Press.
Parsons, T. (1951). *The social system*. New York: Free Press.
Plattel, M. G. (1965). *Social philosophy*. Pittsburgh: Duquesne University Press, *13*(3), 158–163.
Renpenning, K., & Taylor, S. G. (Eds.). (2003). *Self-care theory in nursing: Selected papers of Dorothea Orem*. New York: Springer.
Taylor, S., Geden, E., Isaramalai, S., & Wongvatunyu, S. (2000). Orem's self-care deficit nursing theory: Its philosophical foundation and the state of the science. *Nursing Science Quarterly*, *13*(2), 104–109.
Taylor, S. G., & Renpenning, K. (2011). *Self-care science, nursing theory and evidence based practice*. New York: Springer.
Taylor, S. G., Renpenning, K., Geden, E., Neuman, B., & Hart, M. (2001). A theory of dependent care. *Nursing Science Quarterly*, *14*(3), 39–47.
Wallace, W. A. (1979). *From a realist point of view*. Washington, DC: University Press of America.
Wallace, W. A. (1996). *The modeling of nature, philosophy of science and philosophy of nature in synthesis*. Washington, DC: Catholic University of America Press.
Wesleyan University School of Nursing Curriculum. (n.d.). Retrieved from http://www2.iwu.edu/nursing/curriculum/index.shtml.
White, M. L., Peters, R., & Schim, S. M. (2011). Spirituality and spiritual self-care: Expanding self-care deficit nursing theory. *Nursing Science Quarterly*, *24*(1), 48–56.

BIBLIOGRAPHY

Primary Sources

Books

Nursing Development Conference Group; Orem, D. E. (Ed.). (1972). *Concept formalization in nursing: Process and product*. Boston: Little Brown.
Nursing Development Conference Group; Orem, D. E. (Ed.). (1979). *Concept formalization in nursing: Process and product* (2nd ed.). Boston: Little Brown.
Orem, D. E. (Ed.). (1959). *Guides for developing curricula for the education of practical nurses*. Vocational Division #274. Trade and Industrial Education #68. Washington, DC: U.S. Department of Health, Education, and Welfare.
Orem, D. E., & Parker, K. S. (Eds.). (1963). *Nurse practice education workshop proceedings*. Washington, DC: The Catholic University of America.
Orem, D. E., & Parker, K. S. (Eds.). (1964). *Nursing content in preservice nursing curriculum*. Washington, DC: The Catholic University of America Press.
Orem, D. E. (1985). *Nursing: Concepts of practice* (3rd ed.). New York: McGraw-Hill.
Orem, D. E. (1991). *Nursing: Concepts of practice* (4th ed.). St Louis: Mosby.

Book Chapters

Orem, D. E. (1966). Discussion of paper—Another view of nursing care and quality. In K. M. Straub & K. S. Parker (Eds.), *Continuity of patient care: The role of nursing*. Washington, DC: The Catholic University of America Press.
Orem, D. E. (1969). Inservice education and nursing practice forces effecting nursing practice. In D. K. Petrowski & K. M. Staub (Eds.), *School of nursing education*. Washington, DC: The Catholic University of America Press.
Orem, D. E. (1981). Nursing: A triad of action systems. In G. E. Lasker (Ed.), *Applied systems and cybernetics. Systems research in health care, biocybernetics, and ecology* (Vol. IV). New York: Pergamon Press.
Orem, D. E. (1982). Nursing: A dilemma for higher education. In Sr. A. Power (Ed.), *Words commemorated: Essays celebrating the centennial of Incarnate Word College*. San Antonio, TX: Incarnate Word College.
Orem, D. E. (1983). The self-care deficit theory of nursing: A general theory. In I. Clements & F. Roberts (Eds.), *Family health: A theoretical approach to nursing care*. New York: Wiley Medical.
Orem, D. E. (1984). Orem's conceptual model and community health nursing. In M. K. Asay & C. C. Ossler (Eds.), *Proceedings of the Eighth Annual Community Health Nursing Conference: Conceptual models of nursing applications in community health nursing*. Chapel Hill, NC: University of North Carolina, Department of Public Health Nursing, School of Public Health.
Orem, D. E. (1988). Nursing administration: A theoretical approach. In B. Henry, C. Arndt, M. DiVincenti, & A. M. Tomey (Eds.), *Dimensions of nursing administration*. Boston: Blackwell Scientific.
Orem, D. E. (1990). A nursing practice theory in three parts, 1956–1989. In M. E. Parker (Ed.), *Nursing theories in practice*. New York: National League for Nursing.
Orem, D. E., & Taylor, S. (1986). Orem's general theory of nursing. In P. Winstead-Fry (Ed.), *Case studies in nursing theory* (pp. 37–71; Pub. No. 15–2152). New York: National League for Nursing.

Journal Articles

Orem, D. E. (1962). The hope of nursing. *Journal of Nursing Education*, *1*(1), 5.
Orem, D. E. (1979). Levels of nursing education and practice. *Alumnae Magazine*, *68*(1), 2–6.
Orem, D. E. (1985). Concepts of self-care for the rehabilitation client. *Rehabilitation Nursing*, *10*(3), 33–36.
Orem, D. E. (1988, May). The form of nursing science. *Nursing Science Quarterly*, *1*(2), 75–79.
Orem, D. E. (1997). Views of human beings specific to nursing. *Nursing Science Quarterly*, *10*(1), 26–31.
Orem, D. E., & O'Malley, M. (1952, Aug.). Diagnosis of hospital nursing problems. *Hospitals*, *26*(8), 63–65.
Orem, D. E., & Vardiman, E. (1995). Orem's nursing theory and positive mental health: Practical considerations. *Nursing Science Quarterly*, *8*(4), 165–173.

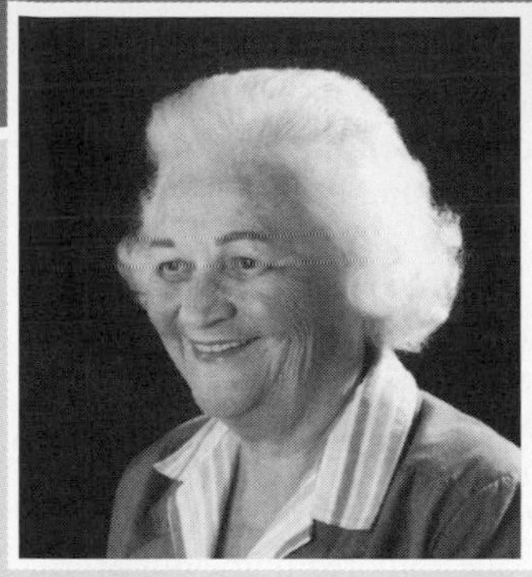

Imogene M. King, EdD, RN, FAAN†
(1923–2007)

Conceptual System and Middle-Range Theory of Goal Attainment

Christina L. Sieloff and Patricia R. Messmer

"Theory is an abstraction that implies prediction based in research. Theory without research and research without some theoretical basis will not build scientific knowledge for a discipline."
(King, 1977, p. 23)

CREDENTIALS AND BACKGROUND OF THE THEORIST

The Nightingale Tribute to Imogene King

Imogene M. King was born on January 30, 1923, in West Point, Iowa. She died December 24, 2007, in St. Petersburg, Florida, and is buried in Fort Madison, Iowa. In 1945 King received a diploma in nursing from St. John's Hospital School of Nursing in St. Louis, Missouri. While working in a variety of staff nurse roles, King began course work toward a bachelor's of science in nursing education, which she received from St. Louis University in 1948. In 1957 she received a master's of science in nursing from St. Louis University. From 1947 to 1958, King worked as an instructor in medical-surgical nursing and was an assistant director at St. John's Hospital School of Nursing. King went on to study with Mildred Montag as her dissertation chair at Teachers College, Columbia University, New York, and received her EdD in 1961.

From 1961 to 1966 at Loyola University in Chicago, King developed a master's degree program in nursing based on a nursing conceptual framework. Her first theory article appeared in 1964 in the journal *Nursing Science,* which nurse theorist Martha Rogers edited.

Between 1966 and 1968, King served under Jessie Scott as Assistant Chief of Research Grants Branch, Division of Nursing at the U.S. Department of Health, Education, and Welfare. While King was in Washington, DC, her article "A Conceptual Frame of Reference for Nursing" was published in *Nursing Research* (1968).

From 1968 to 1972, King was the director of the School of Nursing at Ohio State University in Columbus. While at Ohio State, her book *Toward a Theory for Nursing: General Concepts of Human Behavior* (1971) was published. In this early work, King concluded, "a systematic representation of nursing is required ultimately for developing a science to accompany a century or more of art in the everyday world of nursing" (1971, p. 129). Her book received the *American Journal of Nursing* Book of the Year Award in 1973 (King, 1995a).

King then returned to Chicago in 1972 as a professor in the Loyola University graduate program. She also served from 1978 to 1980 as Coordinator of Research in Clinical Nursing at the Loyola Medical Center Department of Nursing. In 1980 King was awarded an honorary PhD from Southern Illinois University (Messmer, 2000). In May 1998 she received an honorary doctorate from Loyola University,

*Previous authors: C. L. Sieloff, M. L. Ackermann, S. A. Brink, J. A. Clanton, C. G. Jones, A. Marriner-Tomey, S. L. Moody, G. L. Perlich, D. L. Price, and B. B. Prusinski. The authors encourage all readers to read Dr. King's original materials in conjunction with this chapter.

†Photo courtesy of Patricia R. Messmer, PhD, RN-BC, FAAN.

where her "Nursing Collection" is housed. From 1972 to 1975, King was a member of the Defense Advisory Committee on Women in the Services for the U.S. Department of Defense. She also was elected alderman for a 4-year term (1975–1979) in Ward 2 of Wood Dale, Illinois.

In 1980 King was appointed professor at the University of South Florida College of Nursing in Tampa (Houser & Player, 2007). In 1981 her second book, *A Theory for Nursing: Systems, Concepts, Process,* was published. In addition to her first two books, she authored multiple book chapters and articles in professional journals, and a third book, *Curriculum and Instruction in Nursing: Concepts and Process,* was published in 1986. King retired in 1990 and was named professor emeritus at the University of South Florida.

King continued to provide community service and helped plan care through her conceptual system and theory at various health care organizations, including Tampa General Hospital (Messmer, 1995). King never really retired; she was always there for students, faculty, and colleagues who were using her theory and even went "round the clock" to implement her theory at Tampa General Hospital. She also served on the nursing advisory board and guest lectured at the University of Tampa.

King was a long-time member of the American Nurses Association (ANA), first with the Missouri Nurses Association, and she was also active in Illinois and Ohio. Upon her move to Tampa, Florida, she became a member in the Florida Nurses' Association (FNA) and FNA District 4, Tampa. King held offices such as president of the Florida Nurses Foundation, served on the FNA and the FNA District 4 boards, and was a delegate from the FNA to the ANA House of Delegates. In 1997 King received a gold medallion from Governor Chiles for advancing the nursing profession in the state of Florida. She was inducted into the FNA Hall of Fame and the ANA Hall of Fame in 2004. In 1994 King was inducted as a fellow in the American Academy of Nursing (AAN) and served on the AAN Theory Expert Panel. In 2005 she was named a Living Legend. In 1996 King received the Jessie M. Scott Award and was thrilled that Jessie Scott was present. King was in the ANA House of Delegates to hear President Bill Clinton's congratulations on the ANA's 100th anniversary and his admiration of his mother as a nurse anesthetist.

In 2000 King was keynote speaker for the 37th Annual Isabel Maitland Stewart Conference in Research in Nursing at Teachers College, Columbia University (Messmer & Fawcett, 2008) and was pleased that Mildred Montag was present. In 1999 King was inducted into the Teachers College, Columbia University of Hall of Fame. The King International Nursing Group (KING) was created to facilitate the dissemination and use of King's conceptual system, the Theory of Goal Attainment, and related theories. King consulted with members of the organization on an individual basis regarding her theory.

King was one of the original Sigma Theta Tau International (STTI) Virginia Henderson Fellows, and she received the STTI Elizabeth Russell Belford Founders Award for Excellence in Education in 1989 (Messmer, 2007). King was keynote speaker at two STTI theory conferences in 1992 and presented application of her theory at multiple regional, national, and international STTI conferences. King communicated regularly with students who were learning about theories within her conceptual system.

King (1971, 1981) was recognized as one of the early nurse theorists through her publications, which were translated into Japanese, Spanish, and German. She authored numerous articles and served on the editorial board of *Nursing Science Quarterly.* King authored chapters in several books, including Frey and Sieloff's *Advancing King's Systems Framework and Theory of Nursing* (1995) and Sieloff and Frey's *Middle Range Theories for Nursing Practice Using King's Conceptual System* (2007), which highlighted her studies by other authors.

THEORETICAL SOURCES

King described the purpose of her first book as follows:

> *"[P]ropos[ing] a conceptual frame of reference for nursing... intended to be utilized specifically by students and teachers, and also by researchers and practitioners, to identify and analyze events in specific nursing situations. The conceptual system suggests that the essential characteristics of nursing are those properties that have persisted in spite of environmental changes."*
>
> ***(1971, p. ix)***

> *"It is a way of thinking about the real world of nursing; ... an approach for selecting concepts perceived to be fundamental for the practice of professional nursing; [and] shows a process for developing concepts that symbolize experiences within the physical, psychological, and social environment in nursing."*
>
> ***(1971, p. 125)***

King's (1981) concepts are presented in the Major Concepts & Definitions box.

USE OF EMPIRICAL EVIDENCE

King (1971) spoke of concepts as "abstract ideas that give meaning to our sense perceptions, permit generalizations, and tend to be stored in our memory for recall and use at a later time in new and different situations" (pp. 11–12). King (1984) defined theory as "a set of concepts, that, when defined, are interrelated and observable in the world of nursing practice" (p. 11). Theory serves to build "scientific knowledge for nursing" (King, 1995b, p. 24).

MAJOR CONCEPTS & DEFINITIONS

"Concepts give meaning to our sense perceptions and permit generalizations about persons, objects, and things" (King, 1995a, p. 16). A limited number of definitions based on the systems framework are listed here, and additional definitions can be found in King's 1981 book, *A Theory for Nursing: Systems, Concepts, Process.*

Health

"Health is defined as dynamic life experiences of a human being, which implies continuous adjustment to stressors in the internal and external environment through optimum use of one's resources to achieve maximum potential for daily living" (King, 1981, p. 5).

Nursing

"Nursing is defined as a process of action, reaction, and interaction whereby nurse and client share information about their perceptions in the nursing situation" (King, 1981, p. 2).

Self

"The self is a composite of thoughts and feelings which constitute a person's awareness of his [or her] individual existence, his [or her] conception of who and what he [or she] is. A person's self is the sum total of all he [or she] can call his [or hers]. The self includes, among other things, a system of ideas, attitudes, values, and commitments. The self is a person's total subjective environment. It is a distinctive center of experience and significance. The self-constitutes a person's inner world as distinguished from the outer world consisting of all other people and things. The self is the individual as known to the individual. It is that to which we refer when we say, 'I'" (Jersild, 1952, p. 10).

King (1975b) identified two methods for developing theory: (1) a theory can be developed and then tested in research, and (2) research provides data from which theory may be developed. King (1978) believed that building knowledge for a complex profession such as nursing required these two strategies.

King cited research studies in her 1981 book, *A Theory for Nursing: Systems, Concepts, Process.* Within the personal system, King examined studies related to perception by Allport (1955), Kelley and Hammond (1964), Ittleson and Cantril (1954), and others. For her definition of *space,* King cited studies from Sommer (1969), Ardrey (1966), and Minckley (1968). For the concept of time, she acknowledged Orme's (1969) work.

Within the interpersonal system, King cited the studies of Watzlawick, Beavin, and Jackson (1967) and Krieger (1975). She examined studies by Whiting (1955), Orlando (1961), and Diers and Schmidt (1977) for interaction. King noted Dewey and Bentley's (1949) theory of knowledge, which addressed self-action, interaction, and transaction in *Knowing and the Known,* and Kuhn's (1975) work on transactions.

Commenting on research existing at that time, particularly operations research regarding patient care, King (1975a) noted that "most studies have centered on technical aspects of patient care and of the health care systems rather than on patient aspects directly. . . . Few problems have been stated that begin with what the patient's condition demands or what the patient wants" (p. 9). King (1981) noted "several theoretical formulations about interpersonal relations and nursing process have been described in nursing situations" (pp. 151–152) and cited Peplau (1952), Orlando (1961), Paterson and Zderad (1976), and Yura and Walsh (1978) supporting the transactional process in her theory of goal attainment.

Developing the Conceptual System

King posed the following questions in preparation for the 1971 book, *Toward a Theory for Nursing: General Concepts of Human Behavior:*

- What is the goal of nursing?
- What are the functions of nurses?
- How can nurses continue to expand their knowledge to provide quality care? (pp. 30, 39)

Fig. 15.1 demonstrates the conceptual system that provided "one approach to studying systems as a whole rather than as isolated parts of a system" (King, 1995a, p. 18) and was "designed to explain (the) organized wholes within which nurses are expected to function" (1995b, p. 23).

King (1981) used a systems approach in the development of her conceptual systems and her middle-range theory of goal attainment. King noted that "some scientists who have been studying systems have noted that the only way to study human beings interacting with the environment is to design a conceptual framework of interdependent variables and interrelated concepts" (King, 1981, p. 10). King (1995a) believed that her "framework differs from other conceptual schema in that it is concerned not with fragmenting human beings and the environment but with human transactions in different kinds of environments" (p. 21).

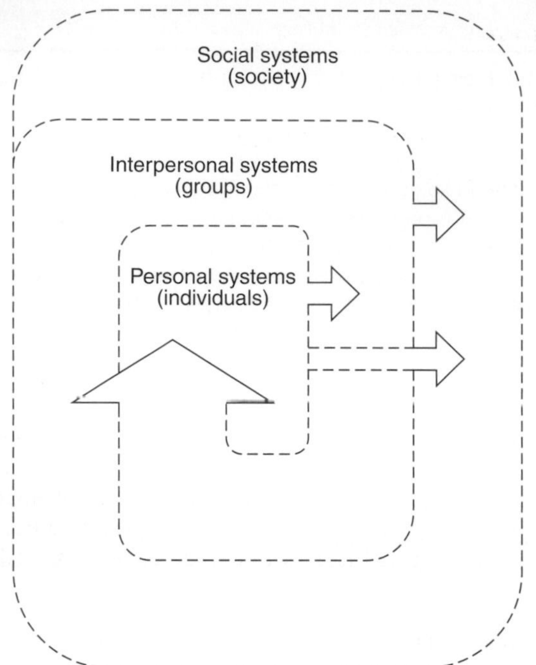

FIG. 15.1 Dynamic conceptual systems. (From King, I. [1981]. *A theory for nursing: Systems, concepts, process* [p. 11]. New York: Delmar. Used with permission from I. King.)

"An awareness of the complex dynamics of human behavior in nursing situations prompted [King's] formulation of a conceptual framework that represented personal, interpersonal, and social systems as the domain of nursing" (King, 1981, p. 130). Each system identifies human beings as the basic element in the system, thus "the unit of analysis in [the] framework [was] human behavior in a variety of social environments" (King, 1995a, p. 18). King designated an example of a personal system as a patient or a nurse. King specified the concepts of body image, growth and development, perception, self, space, and time to comprehend human beings as persons.

Interpersonal systems form when two or more individuals interact, forming dyads (two people) or triads (three people). The dyad of a nurse and a patient is one type of interpersonal system. Families, when acting as small groups, also can be considered interpersonal systems. Understanding the interpersonal system requires the concepts of communication, interaction, role, stress, and transaction.

A more comprehensive interacting system consists of groups that make up society, referred to as the **social system.** Religious, educational, and health care systems are examples of social systems. The influential behavior of an extended family on an individual's growth and development is another social system example. Within a social system, the concepts of authority, decision making, organization, power, and status guide system understanding. Thus concepts in the framework are organizing dimensions and represent knowledge to understand interactions among the three systems (King, 1995a).

King's Middle-Range Theory of Goal Attainment

In 1981, King derived her middle-range Theory of Goal Attainment from her conceptual system. The question that motivated King to develop this theory was, "What is the nature of nursing?" (King, 1995b, p. 25). She noted the answer to be: "the way in which nurses, in their role, do with and for individuals that differentiates nursing from other health professionals" (King, 1995b, p. 26). This thinking guided her development of the theory of goal attainment using the following theory development process:

- What are the philosophical assumptions?
- Are the concepts clearly identified and defined?
- Are the concepts related in propositional statements or models?
- Does the theory generate questions to be answered or hypotheses to be tested in research to generate knowledge and affirm the theory?

"The human process of interactions formed the basis for designing a model of transactions that depicted theoretical knowledge used by nurses to help individuals and groups attain goals" (King, 1995b, p. 27) (Fig. 15.2).

King stated the following:

> *"Mutual goal setting [between a nurse and a client] is based on (a) nurses' assessment of a client's concerns, problems, and disturbances in health; (b) nurses' and clients' perceptions of the interference; and (c) their sharing of information whereby each functions to help the client attain the goals identified. In addition, nurses interact with family members when clients cannot verbally participate in the goal setting."*
>
> ***(1995b, p. 28)***

To test her theory, King (1981) conducted research, identifying that her study varied from previous studies in that it "described the nurse-patient interaction process that leads to goal attainment" (p. 153) and determines whether nurses made transactions. King used a method of nonparticipant observation to collect information about nurse-patient interactions on a patient care unit in a hospital setting with patients and nurses volunteering to participate in the study. King trained graduate students in nonparticipant observation technique to collect data. She examined multiple interactions and recorded verbal and nonverbal behaviors data. King further tested her Criterion-Reference Measure of Goal Attainment Tool, a measure of functional abilities and goal attainment in the University of Maryland

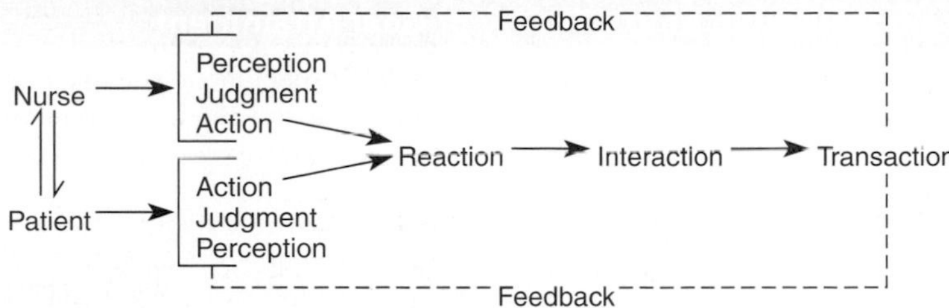

FIG. 15.2 A process of human interactions that lead to transactions: a model of transaction. (From King, I. [1981]. *A theory for nursing: Systems, concepts, process* [p. 61]. New York: Delmar. Used with permission.)

Measurement of Nursing Outcomes project. She reported the instrument to have a Content Validity Index (CVI) of 0.88 and reliability of 0.99 for assessing functional abilities of patients in making decisions about goal setting with and for patients to measure goal attainment (King, 1988, 2003).

MAJOR ASSUMPTIONS

King's personal philosophy about human beings and life influenced her assumptions related to environment, health, nursing, individuals, and nurse-patient interactions. King's conceptual system and theory of goal attainment were "based on an overall assumption that the focus of nursing is human beings interacting with their environment, leading to a state of health for individuals, which is an ability to function in social roles" (King, 1981, p. 143).

Nursing

"Nursing is an observable behavior found in the health care systems in society" (King, 1971, p. 125). The goal of nursing "is to help individuals maintain their health so they can function in their roles" (King, 1981, pp. 3–4). Nursing is an interpersonal process of action, reaction, interaction, and transaction. Perceptions of a nurse and a patient influence the interpersonal process.

Person

King detailed specific assumptions related to persons in 1981 and in subsequent works:

- Individuals are spiritual beings (I. King, personal communication, July 11, 1996).
- Individuals have the ability through their language and other symbols to record their history and preserve their culture (King, 1986).
- Individuals are unique and holistic, of intrinsic worth, and capable of rational thinking and decision making in most situations (King, 1995b).
- Individuals differ in their needs, wants, and goals (King, 1995b).

Health

Health is a dynamic state in the life cycle, whereas illness interferes with that process. Health "implies continuous adjustment to stress in the internal and external environment through the optimum use of one's resources to achieve the maximum potential for daily living" (King, 1981, p. 5).

Environment

King (1981) believed that "an understanding of the ways that human beings interact with their environment to maintain health was essential for nurses" (p. 2). Open systems imply that interactions occur constantly between the system and the system's environment. Furthermore, "adjustments to life and health are influenced by [an] individual's interaction with environment. . . . Each human being perceives the world as a total person in making transactions with individuals and things in the environment" (King, 1981, p. 141).

THEORETICAL ASSERTIONS

King's theory of goal attainment (1981) focuses on the interpersonal system and the interactions that take place between individuals, specifically in the nurse-patient relationship. In the nursing process, each member of the dyad perceives the other, makes judgments, and takes actions. Together, these activities culminate in reaction. Interactions result and, if perceptual congruence exists and disturbances are conquered, transactions will occur. The system is open to permit feedback because each phase of the activity potentially influences perception.

King (1981) developed eight propositions in her theory of goal attainment that describe the relationships among the concepts detailed in Box 15.1. Diagrams follow each proposition. When the propositions were analyzed, 23 relationships were not specified, 22 relationships were positive, and no relationship was negative (Austin & Champion, 1983) (Fig. 15.3). King (1981, p. 156) derived

BOX 15.1 Propositions Within King's Theory of Goal Attainment

1. If perceptual congruence (PC) is present in nurse-client interactions (I), transactions (T) will occur.

   $PC(I) \xrightarrow{+} T$

2. If nurse and client make transactions (T), goals will be attained (GA).

   $T \xrightarrow{+} GA$

3. If goals are attained (GA), satisfaction (S) will occur.

   $GA \xrightarrow{+} S$

4. If goals are attained (GA), effective nursing care (NC_e) will occur.

   $GA \xrightarrow{+} NC_e$

5. If transactions (T) are made in nurse-client interactions (I), growth and development (GD) will be enhanced.

   $(I)T \xrightarrow{+} GD$

6. If role expectations and role performance as perceived by nurse and client are congruent (RCN), transactions (T) will occur.

   $RCN \xrightarrow{+} T$

7. If role conflict (RC) is experienced by nurse or client or both, stress (ST) in nurse-client interactions (I) will occur.

   $RC(I) \xrightarrow{+} ST$

8. If nurses with special knowledge and skills communicate (CM) appropriate information to clients, mutual goal setting (T) and goal attainment (GA) will occur. (Mutual goal setting is a step in transaction and thus has been diagrammed as a transaction.)

   $CM \xrightarrow{+} T \xrightarrow{+} GA$

From Austin, J. K., & Champion, V. L. (1983). King's theory of nursing: Explication and evaluation. In P. L. Chinn (Ed.), *Advances in nursing theory development* (p. 55). Rockville, MD: Aspen.

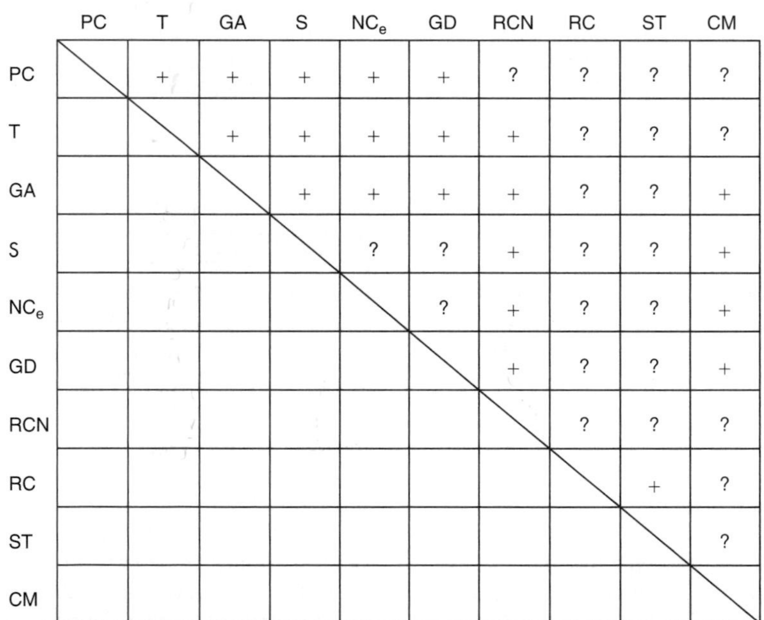

	PC	T	GA	S	NC_e	GD	RCN	RC	ST	CM
PC		+	+	+	+	+	?	?	?	?
T			+	+	+	+	+	?	?	?
GA				+	+	+	+	?	?	+
S					?	?	+	?	?	+
NC_e						?	+	?	?	+
GD							+	?	?	+
RCN								?	?	?
RC									+	?
ST										?
CM										

FIG. 15.3 Relationship table. *CM,* Communicate; *GA,* goals attained; *GD,* growth and development; *NC_e*, effective nursing care; *PC,* perceptional congruence; *RC,* role conflict; *RCN,* role congruency; *S,* satisfactions; *ST,* stress; *T,* transactions. (From Austin, J. K., & Champion, V. L. [1983]. King's theory for nursing: Explication and evaluation. In P. L. Chinn [Ed.], *Advances in theory development* [p. 58]. Rockville, MD: Aspen.)

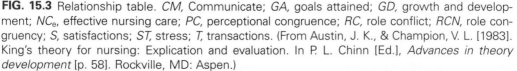

BOX 15.2 Hypotheses from the Theory of Goal Attainment

1. Perceptual accuracy in nurse-patient interactions increases mutual goal setting.
2. Communication increases mutual goal setting between nurses and patients and leads to satisfaction.
3. Satisfactions in nurses and patients increase goal attainments.
4. Goal attainment decreases stress and anxiety in nursing situations.
5. Goal attainment increases patient learning and coping ability in nursing situations.
6. Role conflict experienced by patients, nurses, or both decreases transactions in nurse-patient interactions.
7. Congruence in role expectations and role performance increases transactions in nurse-patient interactions.

From King, I. M. (1981). *A theory for nursing: Systems, concepts, process.* New York: Wiley.

seven hypotheses from the theory of goal attainment listed in Box 15-2.

LOGICAL FORM

In her 1968 article, King set forth her first conceptual frame of reference with four concepts that center on human beings:

1. Health
2. Interpersonal relationships
3. Perceptions
4. Social systems

Although King's original framework was abstract and dealt with "only a few elements of concrete situations" (King, 1981, p. 128), she maintained that her four "universal ideas (social systems, health, perception, and interpersonal relations) were relevant in every nursing situation" (King, 1981, p. 128). King (1981) began further development of her conceptual system and proposed her middle-range theory of goal attainment to describe "the nature of nurse-client interactions that lead to achievement of goals" (p. 142) as follows:

> *"Nurses purposely interact with clients to mutually establish goals, and to explore and agree on means to achieve goals. Mutual goal setting is based on nurses' assessment of clients' concerns, problems, and disturbances in health, their perceptions of problems, and their sharing information to move toward goal attainment."*
>
> ***(1981, pp. 142–143)***

A logical progression of development occurred in the conceptual system from 1971 to 1981, with King deriving her middle-range theory of goal attainment from her conceptual system. The theory of goal attainment "organize[s] elements in the process of nurse-client interactions that result in outcomes, that is, goals attained" (King, 1981, p. 143).

King initially had stated the following:

> *"[I]f nurses are to assume the roles and responsibilities expected of them, . . . the discovery of knowledge must be disseminated in such a way that they are able to use it in their practice. . . . Descriptive data collected systematically provide cues for generating hypotheses for research in human behavior in nursing situations."*
>
> ***(1971, p. 128)***

In 1981 King spoke of fewer dichotomies between health and illness, referring to illness as interference in the life cycle. Through reformulation, King provided a more open system relationship between person and environment. King also revised her terminology, using **adjustment** instead of *adaptation,* and **person, human being,** and **individual** rather than *man.*

ACCEPTANCE BY THE NURSING COMMUNITY

Practice

King's (1971) early publication led to nursing curriculum development and practice application at Ohio State University and other universities. Professionals in most nursing specialty areas have used the concepts of King's (1981) theory of goal attainment in nursing practice. Its relationship to practice is obvious, because nurses function primarily through interactions with individuals and groups within the environment. King (1984) proposed "nurses, who have knowledge of the concepts of this Theory of Goal Attainment, are able to perceive what is happening to patients and family members and are able to suggest approaches for coping with the situations" (p. 12).

King developed a documentation system, the goal-oriented nursing record (GONR), to accompany her middle-range theory of goal attainment and to record goals and outcomes. The GONR was a method of collecting data, identifying problems, and implementing and evaluating care that has been effective in patient settings. Nurses can use the GONR approach to document the effectiveness of nursing care. "The major elements in this record system are: (a) data base, (b) nursing diagnosis, (c) goal list, (d) nursing orders, (e) flow sheets, (f) progress notes, and (g) discharge summary" (King, 1995b, pp. 30–31).

Health care professionals have implemented King's (1981) conceptual system and middle-range theory of goal attainment in various national and international practice settings (King, 2006, 2007). This section identifies some settings, and references additional settings. Batson and Yoder (2012) used the conceptual systems framework and the theory of goal attainment to conduct a concept analysis of managerial coaching within health care organizations to determine what skills and attributes were necessary to establish effective managerial coaching relationships with staff nurses. King's work provided a useful lens for nurses to assess the functional status of clients (Caceres, 2015). Ketcham (2013) and Sullivan (2013) applied King's work in emergency nursing. Chaves, Araujo, and Lopes (2007) clarified the use of social system in Brazil. Abraham (2009) explored planned teaching programs in environmental health. D'Souza, Somayaji, and Subrahmanya Nairy (2011) examined "determinants of reproductive health and related quality of life among Indian women in mining communities" (p. 1963).

Khowaja (2006) described the use of King's conceptual system and theory of goal attainment in the development of a clinical pathway. Lane-Tillerson et al. (2007) emphasized that "the idea of continuous advancement is central to Imogene King's (1981) conceptual framework" (p. 141), imagining nursing practice in 2050. Killeen and King (2007) provided additional support and addressed the use of King's conceptual system with nursing informatics and nursing classification systems for global communications. Clarke et al. (2009) described King's influence on nursing science. Bond and colleagues (2011) analyzed the use of King's theory of goal attainment over 5 years of publications. Messmer and Cooper (2011) described the application of King's theory of goal attainment for understanding a pediatric fall prevention and fall injury risk program.

Education

Nursing faculty at several universities used King's concepts to design nursing curricula, such as King and Daubenmire (1973) at Ohio State University; Gold, Haas, and King (2000) at Loyola University in Chicago; and Gulitz and King (1988) at the University of South Florida. In 1980 Brown and Lee reported that King's concepts were useful in developing a framework for "use in nursing education, nursing practice, and for generating hypotheses for research. . . . [They] provide a systematic means of viewing the nursing profession, organizing a body of knowledge for nursing, and clarifying nursing as a discipline" (p. 468). Other studies report use of King's conceptual system to improve educational strategies (Ward, 2010). King's conceptual system and theory have nursing applications internationally as described by Rooke (1995b) for a Swedish educational setting, Bello (2000) in research with Portuguese undergraduate students, Costa and colleagues (2007) in regard to a model of care for families at risk, and Bist and Tomar (2015) in their examination of the "effectiveness of self-instructional guidelines on child trafficking in . . . selected rural schools of Bisrakh, Greater Noida" (p. 34).

Research

Many researchers have used King's work as a theoretical basis, as cited here and listed in the bibliography. Langford (2008) incorporated the concept of transactions in research with "nurse practitioners and weight loss in obese adolescents." Bezerra et al. (2010) used personal and interpersonal concepts for research with patients experiencing hypertension. Joseph, Laughon, and Bogue (2011) used interpretative phenomenology, with an interview protocol, to examine the adoption and movement toward a culture of whole-person care (WPC). De Leon-Demare et al. (2015) used King's theory of goal attainment to describe the interactions between nurse practitioners and patients in the primary care setting.

Others have used King's (1981) conceptual system in either quantitative or qualitative research:

- Khowaja (2006) used King's conceptual system and theory of goal attainment to develop a clinical pathway.
- Greeff and colleagues (2009) qualitatively explored "students' community health service delivery through the experiences of the involved parties" (p. 33).
- George, Roach, and Andrade (2011) examined the view of nursing held by consumers, surgeons, and nurses.
- Draaistra et al. (2012) qualitatively explored "patients' perceptions of their roles in goal setting in a spinal cord injury regional rehabilitation program" (p. 22).
- Shanta and Connolly (2013) linked emotional intelligence and nursing practice using King's conceptual systems model.

Researchers have developed many middle-range theories using King's conceptual system (King, 1978; Sieloff & Frey, 2007). These theories include Frey's (1995) theory of families, children, and chronic illness; Killeen's (2007) theory of patient satisfaction with professional nursing care; Sieloff's theory of work team/group power empowerment within organizations (2010; Sieloff & Bularzik, 2011; Sieloff & Dunn, 2008); Wicks' theory of family health (Wicks, Rice, & Talley, 2007), Doornbos' (2007) theory of family health; and the advance directive decision-making model of Goodwin, Kiehl, and Peterson (2002). Fairfax (2007) derived a theory of quality of life of stroke survivors. Nwinee (2011) used King's work to develop the Nwinee Socio-Behavioral Self-Care Management Nurse Model.

Alligood (2010) examined exemplars of King-based research in family health care. Bond and colleagues (2011) conducted a "univariate descriptive analysis of five years' research articles" (p. 404). Caceres (2015) explored the concept of functional health status. Huan and Cao (2012) applied King's theory of goal attainment to care in China.

FURTHER DEVELOPMENT

Over the years, King consistently demonstrated her belief in the need for further testing of the theory of goal attainment. "Any profession that has as its primary mission the delivery of social services requires continuous research to discover new knowledge that can be applied to improve practice" (King, 1971, p. 112).

In 1995 Fawcett and Whall identified five major areas in which further development of King's work would be helpful. Recent research in these areas is identified here:

1. The concept of environment would benefit from additional definition and clarification (work is in progress as a result of the 2015 conference of the KING).
2. King's views of illness, health, and wellness would benefit from additional clarification and discussion (Caceres, 2015).
3. Future linkages between King's (1981) conceptual system and other existing middle-range theories should continue in a manner that ensures congruency between the conceptual system and the specific middle-range theory.
4. Empirical testing should continue for the theory of goal attainment (King, 1981) and other middle-range theories developed within King's conceptual system (Fawcett & Whall, 1995) (e.g., Sieloff & Dunn, 2008; Sieloff & Bularzik, 2011).
5. Middle-range theories that are implied rather than explicit, such as those of Rooke (1995b), would benefit from development into formal theories (e.g., Nwinee, 2011).

In 2007, Sieloff and Frey reported the status of middle-range theory development from within King's conceptual system. Fawcett (2007) again examined the development of middle-range theory, from within King's conceptual system, and made recommendations. Recent research is again identified in relation to each recommendation:

1. The credibility of King's conceptual system could be further supported through "a meta-analysis or other integrative review of the results obtained from empirical tests of . . . the middle range theory propositions" (Fawcett, 2007, p. 301).
2. "Additional metatheoretical research is needed to specify the relations between the concepts within the personal, interpersonal, and social systems" (Fawcett, 2007, p. 301).
3. Continued empirical testing of all middle-range theories is also needed.
4. Additional research instruments need to be developed to measure middle-range theory concepts. The utility of those instruments then needs to be evaluated in terms of their utility for practice (Fawcett, 2007).

Since the previous edition, graduate students continue to use King's conceptual system and theory of goal attainment for their research, including nine master's students (Anyaoha, 2013; Chung, 2012; Conerly, 2013; Houston, 2015; Kangkolo, 2012; Laney, 2013; Ongoco, 2012; Scott, 2011; Swain, 2012) and 34 doctoral students (Ali, 2015; Burks, 2015; Carmack, 2014; Cheng, 2012; D'Alessandro, 2012; Dickman, 2014; Doyle, 2015; Echevarria, 2015; Fleischer, 2015; Fuson, 2012; Grandinetti, 2013; Hand, 2015; Heid, 2014; Herm-Barabasz, 2015; Hutchison, 2013; Johnson, 2013; Ketcham, 2013; Kim, 2013; Krmpotic, 2015; Lauck, 2013; Lazarus, 2013; Miller, 2014; Moore, 2015; Mwangi, 2013; Quarshie, 2014; Sanko, 2015; Sullivan, 2013; Teeter, 2014; Thakral, 2015; Thomas, 2016; Tolson, 2013; Vincent, 2015; Warren, 2014; Wetter, 2014).

CRITIQUE

Clarity

A major strong point of King's conceptual system and theory of goal attainment is the ease with which it can be understood by nurses. Concepts are concretely defined and illustrated.

Simplicity

King's definitions are clear and are conceptually derived from research literature. King's 1978 theory of goal attainment presents 10 major concepts, which are also easily understood and derived from research literature.

Generality

King's 1981 theory of goal attainment has been criticized for having limited application in areas of nursing in which patients are unable to interact competently with the nurse. King maintained the broad use of the theory in most nursing situations. In support of King's perspective, health care professionals have documented examples of the application of the theory of goal attainment with patients with diabetes (Maloni, 2007) and surgical patients (Bruns et al., 2009; Sivaramalingam, 2008). Wang and Yang (2006) applied King's theory to the care of patients with psychosis. Kameoka, Funashima, and Sugimori (2007) tested a proposition of the theory and explored "the characteristics of nurses whose degree of goal attainment and satisfactions in interactions with patients were both high" (p. 261). Smithgall (2010) examined the relationships between maternal stress and neonatal patient outcomes in private rooms versus neonatal intensive care units. D'Alessandro and Malcolm (2012) explored the use of a low-dose medication to manage disruptive behaviors with children experiencing autism spectrum disorders. In 2015 Houston explored the use of multisensory stimulation environments to reduce negative behaviors in patients experiencing dementia.

Accessibility

King gathered empirical data on nurse-patient interaction that led to goal attainment. A descriptive study was conducted to identify the characteristics of transaction and whether nurses made transactions with patients. With a sample of 17 patients, goals were attained in 12 cases, or 70% of the sample. King (1981) believed that if nursing students were taught the transactional process in the theory of goal attainment and used it in nursing practice, goal attainment could be measured and evidence of the effectiveness of nursing care demonstrated.

The theory of goal attainment guided Karlin's (2011) intrapartum nurses' perspective of King's theory of goal attainment. Draaistra et al. (2012) used King's theory to examine *Patients' perceptions of their roles in goal setting in a spinal cord injury regional rehabilitation program.* Cho's (2013) research focused on the effects of health contracts on patient outcomes with patients experiencing renal dialysis in Korea.

Importance

King's (1981) middle-range theory of goal attainment focused on all aspects of the nursing process: assessment, planning, goal setting, implementation, and evaluation. The body of literature clearly establishes King's work as important for knowledge building in the discipline of nursing.

In the United States and Canada and in many countries of the world, health care professionals continue to use King's conceptual system and middle-range theory of goal attainment. Theory-based practice is reported in Asia (Chugh, 2005; Li, Li, & Xu, 2010; Park & Oh, 2012), Australia (Khowaja, 2006), Brazil (Marziale & de Jesus, 2008), China (Huan & Cao, 2012), India (Abraham, 2009; George, Roach, & Andrade, 2011), Japan (Kameoka, Funashima, & Sugimori, 2007), Korea (Cho, 2013), Portugal (Chaves & de Araujo, 2006; Costa et al., 2007; Firmino et al., 2010), Slovenia (Harih & Pajnkihar, 2009), Sweden (Rooke, 1995a, 1995b), and West Africa (Nwinee, 2011). King's work has structured curriculum development at various educational levels.

SUMMARY

Imogene King contributed to the advancement of nursing knowledge through the development of her conceptual system and middle-range theory of goal attainment. By focusing on the attainment of goals, or outcomes, by nurse-patient partnerships, King provided a conceptual system and middle-range theory that has demonstrated its usefulness to nurses. Nurses working in a variety of settings with patients from around the world continue to use King's work to improve the quality of patient care.

CASE STUDY

Upon receiving an assignment at the start of the shift, Colin Jennings, RN, makes initial rounds of the patients. One patient, Amed Kyzeel, as reported by nurses on the previous shift, has been difficult to work with, demanding the attention of staff throughout the shift.

Mr. Jennings visits Mr. Kyzeel last during rounds so that additional time is available for an assessment. Upon entering Mr. Kyzeel's room, Mr. Jennings asks him how he is feeling about going home. Mr. Kyzeel complains about a variety of minor concerns about his pending discharge. Accepting that Mr. Kyzeel's perceptions are unique and valid to him, Mr. Jennings spends a few minutes just listening.

Because Mr. Jennings knows that Mr. Kyzeel is to be discharged today, he asks the patient what he knows about his pending discharge and his goals for leaving today. Mr. Kyzeel admits that he is concerned about leaving the hospital because he does not know what to expect during the first 24 hours at home. Mr. Jennings talks with the patient and asks him what goals he wants to achieve while in the hospital and upon returning home. Mr. Kyzeel identifies two to three goals that he would like to achieve in the hospital and says that he would like to have someone stay with him at his home for the first night because he is not sure that his wife will be able to take care of him like the nurses do in the hospital.

Of the goals identified, Mr. Jennings and Mr. Kyzeel identify the most important ones and the order in which Mr. Kyzeel would like to achieve them. Then Mr. Jennings and Mr. Kyzeel identify activities that can be done by the patient and the staff to achieve these goals. Before leaving the room, they agree on the goals, their priority, and the specific activities to be done, and they arrange for Mr. Kyzeel's wife to be involved in the discharge planning.

Having established times when Mr. Jennings and Mr. Kyzeel will briefly talk to evaluate achievement of the goals, Mr. Jennings leaves the room and Mr. Kyzeel calls his wife to begin work on the activities he needs to accomplish.

CRITICAL THINKING ACTIVITIES

1. Analyze an interaction you had recently with a patient. Was a transaction achieved? If so, identify why you were successful; if not, reflect to consider why and what you might have done differently.
2. Does your health care agency's philosophy encourage involvement of patients in their care? If so, does mutual goal setting occur?
3. Use King's theory of goal attainment to illustrate how and why you actively involve patients in their care.
4. Analyze the action, reaction, and interaction in the goal-setting process in your own nursing practice.
5. Describe goal setting in the relationship between the nursing staff and nursing administration in the health care agency where you practice.

POINTS FOR FURTHER STUDY

Publications

- Gunther, M. (2014). King's conceptual system and theory of goal attainment in nursing practice. In M. R. Alligood, *Nursing theory: Utilization & application* (5th ed., pp. 160-180). St Louis: Mosby-Elsevier.
- King, I. M. (1996). The theory of goal attainment in research and practice. *Nursing Science Quarterly*, *9*(2), 61–66.
- King, I. M. (1997). King's theory of goal attainment in practice. *Nursing Science Quarterly*, *70*(4), 180–185.
- King, I. M. (1999). A theory of goal attainment: Philosophical and ethical implications. *Nursing Science Quarterly*, *12*(4), 292–296.

Websites

- Imogene King at http://nursing-theory.org/nursing-theorists/Imogene-King.php
- Imogene King's Theory of Goal Attainment at http://currentnursing.com/nursing_theory/goal_attainment_theory.html
- *King International Nursing Group* at http://king.clubexpress.com
- *Nurses.info* at http://www.nurses.info/nursing_theory_person_king_imogene.htm
- Reflections on Nursing Leadership at http://www.reflectionsonnursingleadership.org/Pages/Vol34_1_Messmer_Palmer.aspx

Videos

- *Imogene King Nursing Theorist: Portraits of Excellence.* Fitne, Inc., Athens, OH.

REFERENCES

Abraham, L. (2009). Planned teaching programme on environmental health. *Nursing Journal of India*, *100*(6), 2.

Ali, S. (2015). *Nurses' use of power to standardize nursing terminology in electronic patient records.* (DNP project). ProQuest Dissertations & Theses. (Order No. 10027560).

Alligood, M. R. (2010). Family healthcare with King's theory of goal attainment. *Nursing Science Quarterly*, *23*(2), 99–104.

Allport, F. H. (1955). *Theories of perception and the concept of structure.* New York: Wiley.

Anyaoha, A. L. (2013). *Surgical time-out: A nursing team training approach.* (Master's thesis). Retrieved from ProQuest Dissertations & Theses (Order No. 522616).

Ardrey, R. (1966). *The territorial imperative.* New York: Atheneum.

Austin, J. K., & Champion, V. L. (1983). King's theory for nursing: Explication and evaluation. In P. Chinn (Ed.), *Advances in nursing theory development* (pp. 49–61). Rockville, MD: Aspen.

Batson, V. D., & Yoder, L. H. (2012). Managerial coaching: A concept analysis. *Journal of Advanced Nursing*, *68*(7), 1658–1669.

Bello, I. T. R. (2000). Imogene King's theory as the foundation for the set of a teaching-learning process with undergraduation [sic] students [Portuguese]. *Texto & Contexto Enfermagem*, *9*(2 Part 2), 646–657.

Bezerra, S. T. F., Silva, L. D. F. D., Guedes, M. V. C., & Freitas, M. C. D. (2010). Perceptions of people about hypertension and concepts of Imogene King. *Revista Gaúcha de Enfermagem*, *31*(3), 499–507.

Bist, L. S., & Tomar, N. (2015). Effectiveness of self instructional guidelines on child trafficking in terms of knowledge and attitude of students studying in selected rural school of Bisrakh, Greater Noida. *International Journal of Nursing Education*, *7*(2), 34–37.

Bond, A. E., Eshah, N. F., Bani-Khaled, M., Hamad, A. O., Habashneh, S., Kataua', H., et al. (2011). Who uses nursing theory? A univariate descriptive analysis of five years' research articles. *Scandinavian Journal of Caring Sciences*, *25*(2), 404–409.

Brown, S. T., & Lee, B. T. (1980). Imogene King's conceptual framework: A proposed model for continuing nursing education. *Journal of Advanced Nursing*, *5*(5), 467–473.

Burks, K. S. (2015). *Intravenous acetaminophen reduces opioid use for postoperative pain in obese patients undergoing laparoscopic cholecystectomy.* (DNP project). Retrieved from ProQuest Dissertations & Theses. (Order No. 3731844).

Caceres, B. A. (2015). King's theory of goal attainment: Exploring functional status. *Nursing Science Quarterly*, *28*(2), 151–155.

Carmack, J. K. (2014). *Simulation collaboration: Will screen capture change attitudes?* (DNP project). Retrieved from ProQuest Dissertations & Theses. (Order No. 3642202).

Chaves, E. S., Araujo, T. L., & Lopes, M. V. O. (2007). Clarity in the use of the social systems from the theory of goal attainment [Portuguese]. *Revista da Escola de Enfermagem da USP, 41*(4), 698–704.

Cheng, L. S. W. (2012). *The effects of mutual goal setting on the outcomes of care of the patients in the community.* (Doctoral dissertation). Retrieved from ProQuest Dissertations & Theses. (Order No. 3569041).

Cho, M. (2013). Effect of health contract intervention on renal dialysis patients in Korea. *Nursing & Health Sciences, 15*(1), 86–93.

Chung, S. M. (2012). *An overview of collaborative work: The student experience.* (Master's thesis). Retrieved from ProQuest Dissertations & Theses. (Order No. 1541862).

Clarke, P., Killeen, M., Messmer, P., & Sieloff, C. (2009). Imogene M. King's scholars reflect on her wisdom and influence on nursing science. *Nursing Science Quarterly, 22*(2), 128–133.

Clements, I. W., & Roberts, F. B. (1983). *Family health: A theoretical approach to nursing care.* New York: Wiley.

Conerly, T. (2013). *Guidelines for conducting peer support groups of HIV patients in southwest Mississippi.* (Master's thesis). Retrieved from ProQuest Dissertations & Theses. (Order No. EP69089).

Costa, M., Santos, M., Martinho, N., Barroso, M., & Vieira, N. (2007). Family at-risk situation: Model of care emphasizing health education [Portuguese]. *Revista Gaucha De Enfermagem, 28*(1), 45–51.

D'Alessandro, T., Malcolm, M. (2012). *Low-dose Abilify and the treatment of disruptive behaviors in children with autism spectrum disorders.* (Doctoral dissertation). Retrieved from ProQuest Dissertations & Theses. (Order No. 3569569).

Dewey, J., & Bentley, A. (1949). *Knowing and the known.* Boston: Beacon Press.

Dickman, J. (2014). *A quality improvement project using technology to improve caregiver com-munication.* (DNP project). Retrieved from ProQuest Dissertations & Theses. (Order No. 3617688).

Diers, D., & Schmidt, R. (1977). Interaction analysis in nursing research. In P. Verhonick (Ed.), *Nursing research II* (pp. 77–132). Boston: Little, Brown.

Doornbos, M. M. (2007). King's conceptual system and family health theory in the families of adults with persistent mental illness—An evolving conceptualization. In C. L. Sieloff & M. A. Frey (Eds.), *Middle range theory development using King's conceptual system* (pp. 31–49). New York: Springer.

Doyle, M. L. (2015). *Personality traits found in a sample of nurse CEOs and CNOs utilizing the NEO five-factor inventory 3.* Retrieved from ProQuest Dissertations & Theses. (Order No. 3664652).

Draaistra, H., Singh, M. O., Ireland, S., & Harper, T. (2012). Patients' perceptions of their roles in goal setting in a spinal cord injury regional rehabilitation program. *Canadian Journal of Neuroscience Nursing, 34*(3), 22–30.

D'Souza, M. S., Somayaji, G., & Subrahmanya Nairy, K. (2011). Determinants of reproductive health and related quality of life among Indian women in mining communities. *Journal of Advanced Nursing, 67*(9), 1963–1975.

Echevarria, I. M. (2015). *The relationships among education, leadership experience, emotional intelligence, and transformational leadership of nurse managers.* Retrieved from ProQuest Dissertations & Theses. (Order No. 3739273).

Fairfax, J. (2007). Development of a middle range theory of quality of life of stroke survivors derived from King's conceptual system. In C. L. Sieloff & M. A. Frey (Eds.), *Middle range theory development using King's conceptual system* (pp. 124–137). New York: Springer.

Fawcett, J. (2007). Development of middle range theories based on King's conceptual system: A commentary on progress and future directions. In C. L. Sieloff & M. A. Frey (Eds.), *Middle range theory development using King's conceptual system* (pp. 297–307). New York: Springer.

Fawcett, J. M., & Whall, A. L. (1995). State of the science and future directions. In M. A. Frey & C. L. Sieloff (Eds.), *Advancing King's systems framework and theory of nursing* (pp. 327–334). Thousand Oaks, CA: Sage.

Fleischer, E. (2015). *Quality improvement to increase nurse knowledge on nursing informatics project management standards.* Retrieved from ProQuest Dissertations & Theses. (Order No. 3706088).

Frey, M. A. (1995). Toward a theory of families, children, and chronic illness. In M. A. Frey & C. L. Sieloff (Eds.). *Advancing King's systems framework and theory of nursing* (pp. 109–125). Thousand Oaks, CA: Sage.

Frey, M. A., & Sieloff, C. L. (Eds.). (1995). *Advancing King's framework and theory for nursing.* Thousand Oaks, CA: Sage.

Fuson, J. K. (2012). *The use of music to reduce test anxiety in nursing students.* (DNP project). Retrieved from ProQuest Dissertations & Theses. (Order No. 1520139).

George, A., Roach, E. J., & Andrade, M. (2011). Nursing education: Opportunities and challenges. *Nursing Journal of India, 102*(6), 136–139.

Gold, C., Haas, S., & King, I. (2000). Conceptual frameworks: Putting the nursing focus into core curricula. *Nurse Educator, 25*(2), 95–98.

Goodwin, Z., Kiehl, E. M., & Peterson, J. Z. (2002). King's theory as foundation for an advance directive decision-making model. *Nursing Science Quarterly, 15*(3), 237–241.

Grandinetti, M. (2013). *Motivation to learn, learner independence, intellectual curiosity and self-directed learning readiness of prelicensure sophomore baccalaureate nursing students.* (Doctoral dissertation). Retrieved from ProQuest Dissertations & Theses. (Order No. 3579581).

Gulitz, E., & King, I. (1988). King's general system model: Application to curriculum development. *Nursing Science Quarterly, 3*(2), 128–132.

Hand, M. C. (2015). *Job satisfaction and intent to leave of nursing assistants in the hospital setting.* (Doctoral dissertation). Retrieved from ProQuest Dissertations & Theses. (Order No. 3705602).

Harih, M., & Pajnkihar, M. (2009). Application of Imogene M. King's nursing model in the treatment of elderly diabetes patients. *Slovenian Nursing Review, 43*(3), 201–208.

Heid, C. L. (2014). *Motivation and persistence among BSN1964 students in northeast Ohio: A correlational study.* (Doctoral dissertation). Retrieved from ProQuest Dissertations & Theses. (Order No. 3691440).

Herm-Barabasz, R. (2015). *Intraprofessional nursing communication and collaboration: APN-RN-patient bedside rounding* (DNP project). Retrieved from ProQuest Dissertations & Theses. (Order No. 3715072).

Houser, B. P., & Player, K. N. (2007). Imogene M. King. In *Pivotal moments in nursing* (Vol. 2, pp. 106–131). Indianapolis, IN: Sigma Theta Tau International.

Houston, M. (2015). *Multi-sensory stimulation environments for use with dementia patients: Staff perspectives on reduction of agitation and negative behaviors.* (Master's thesis). Retrieved from ProQuest Dissertations & Theses. (Order No. 1570838).

Huan, Y., & Cao, M. (2012). King's theory of goal attainment and its application to care [Chinese]. *Chinese Nursing Research, 26*(10C), 2785–2787.

Hutchison, B. E. (2013). *Critical thinking skill acquisition in accelerated LVN to RN nursing programs: An evaluative case study.* (Doctoral dissertation). Retrieved from ProQuest Dissertations & Theses. (Order No. 3577938).

Ittleson, W., & Cantril, H. (1954). *Perception: A transactional approach.* Garden City, NY: Doubleday.

Jersild, A. T. (1952). *In search of self.* New York: Teachers College Press.

Johnson, G. J. (2013). *The nursing process and allegations of malpractice against perinatal registered nurses in Florida.* (Doctoral dissertation). Retrieved from ProQuest Dissertations & Theses. (Order No. 3577284).

Joseph, M., Laughon, D., & Bogue, R. J. (2011). An examination of the sustainable adoption of whole-person care (WPC). *Journal of Nursing Management, 19*(8), 989–997.

Kameoka, T., Funashima, N., & Sugimori, M. (2007). If goals are attained, satisfaction will occur in nurse-patient interaction: An empirical test. In C. L. Sieloff & M. A. Frey (Eds.), *Middle range theory development using King's conceptual system* (pp. 261–272). New York: Springer.

Kangkolo, M. (2012). *The relationship of frequent visitation and pressure ulcer development.* (Master's thesis). Retrieved from ProQuest Dissertations & Theses. (Order No. 1516270).

Kelley, K. J., & Hammond, K. R. (1964). An approach to the study of clinical inference. *Nursing Research, 13*(4), 314–322.

Khowaja, D. (2006). Utilization of King's interacting systems framework and theory of goal attainment with new multidisciplinary model: Clinical pathway. *Australian Journal of Advanced Nursing, 24*(2), 44–50.

Killeen, M. B. (2007). Development and initial testing of a theory of patient satisfaction with nursing care. In C. L. Sieloff & M. A. Frey (Eds.), *Middle range theory development using King's conceptual system* (pp. 138–163). New York: Springer.

Killeen, M. B., & King, I. M. (2007). Use of King's conceptual system, nursing informatics, and nursing classification systems for global communication. *International Journal of Nursing Terminologies and Classifications, 18*(2), 51–57.

Kim, J. A. G. (2013). *The relationship between the perception of nurse caring, and the phase II cardiac rehabilitation patients' depression, anxiety, and adherence.* (Doctoral dissertation). Retrieved from ProQuest Dissertations & Theses. (Order No. 3562992).

King, I. M. (1968). A conceptual frame of reference for nursing. *Nursing Research, 17*(1), 27–31.

King, I. M. (1971). *Toward a theory for nursing: General concepts of human behavior.* New York: Wiley.

King, I. M. (1975a). Patient aspects. In L. J. Schumann, R. D. Spears, Jr., & J. P. Young (Eds.), *Operations research in health care: A critical analysis.* Baltimore: Johns Hopkins University Press.

King, I. M. (1975b). A process for developing concepts for nursing through research. In P. Verhonick (Ed.), *Nursing research.* Boston: Little, Brown.

King, I. M. (1977). Knowledge development in nursing: A process. In I. M. King & J. Fawcett (Eds.), *The language of nursing theory and metatheory* (pp. 19–25). Indianapolis: Sigma Theta Tau International.

King, I. M. (Speaker). (1978). *Speech presented at 2nd Annual Nurse Educators' Conference.* Chicago: Teach 'Em.

King, I. M. (1981). *A theory for nursing: Systems, concepts, process.* New York: Wiley.

King, I. M. (1984). Effectiveness of nursing care: Use of a goal oriented nursing record in end stage renal disease. *American Association of Nephrology Nurses and Technicians Journal, 11*(2), 11–17, 60.

King, I. M. (1986). *Curriculum and instruction in nursing: Concepts and process.* Norwalk, CT: Appleton-Century-Crofts.

King, I. M. (1988). Measuring health goal attainment in patients. In C. F. Waltz & O. L. Strickland (Eds.), *Measurement of nursing outcomes Volume one: Measuring client outcomes* (pp. 109–127). New York: Springer.

King, I. M. (1995a). A systems framework for nursing. In M. A. Frey & C. L. Sieloff (Eds.), *Advancing King's systems framework and theory of nursing* (pp. 14–22). Thousand Oaks, CA: Sage.

King, I. M. (1995b). The theory of goal attainment. In M. A. Frey & C. L. Sieloff (Eds.), *Advancing King's systems framework and theory of nursing* (pp. 23–32). Thousand Oaks, CA: Sage.

King, I. M. (2000). Evidence-based nursing practice. *Theoria: Journal of Nursing Theory, 9*(2), 4–9.

King, I. M. (2003). Assessment of functional abilities and goal attainment scales: A criterion-reference measure. In O. L. Strickland & C. Dilorio (Eds.), *Measurement of nursing outcomes: Client outcomes and quality of care* (2nd ed., pp. 3–20). New York: Springer.

King, I. M. (2006). A system approach in nursing administration: Structure, process and outcome. *Journal of Nursing Administration, 30*(2), 100–104.

King, I. M. (2007). King's conceptual system, theory of goal attainment, and transaction process in the 21st century. *Nursing Science Quarterly, 20*(2), 109–116.

King, I., & Daubenmire, J. (1973). Nursing process models: A systems approach. *Nursing Outlook, 13*(19), 50–51.

Krieger, D. (1975). Therapeutic touch: The imprimatur of nursing. *American Journal of Nursing, 75*(5), 784–787.

Krmpotic, J. (2015). *Transitional care: The time is now.* (DNP project). Retrieved from ProQuest Dissertations & Theses. (Order No. 3718713).

Kuhn, A. (1975). *Unified social science.* Homewood, IL: Dorsey.

Lane-Tillerson, C. (2007). Imaging practice in 2050. King's conceptual framework. *Nursing Science Quarterly, 20*(2), 140–143.

Lane-Tillerson, C., Davis, B. L., Killion, C. M., & Baker, S. (2005). Evaluating nursing outcomes: A mixed-methods approach. *Journal of National Black Nurses Association, 16*(2), 20–26.

Laney, I. (2013). *Registered nurses' perceptions of patient advocacy behaviors in the clinical setting.* (Master's thesis). Retrieved from ProQuest Dissertations & Theses. (Order No. 1542581).

Langford, R. (2008). Perceptions of transactions with nurse practitioners and weight loss in obese adolescents. *Southern Online Journal of Nursing Research, 8*(2), 1.

Lauck, K. J. (2013). *Patients lived experience of information shared between one's family and service providers.* (Doctoral dissertation). Retrieved from ProQuest Dissertations & Theses. (Order No. 3589452).

Lazarus, E. M. C. (2013). *College health: Meeting the health care needs of international students.* (DNP project). Retrieved from ProQuest Dissertations & Theses. (Order No. 3605253).

Li, H., Li, C., & Xu, C. (2010). Review of the development of the concept of holistic nursing. *Zhonghua Yi Shi Za Zhi, 40*(1), 33–37.

Marziale, M., & de Jesus, L. (2008). Explanative and intervention models in workers' health promotion. *Acta Paulista De Enfermagem, 21*(4), 654–659.

Messmer, P. R. (1995). Implementation of theory-based nursing practice. In M. A. Frey & C. L. Sieloff (Eds.), *Advancing King's systems framework and theory of nursing* (pp. 294–304). Thousand Oaks, CA: Sage.

Messmer, P. R. (2000). Imogene M. King. In V. L. Bullough & L. Sentz (Eds.), *American nursing: A biographical dictionary* (Vol. 3, pp. 164–166). New York: Springer.

Messmer, P. R. (2007). Tribute to the theorists: Imogene M. King over the years. *Nursing Science Quarterly, 20*(3), 198.

Messmer, P. R., & Cooper, C. (2011). *Symposium: Pediatric falls based on King's theory of goal attainment.* King's Theory Conference, Bozeman, Montana, April 7–8, 2011.

Messmer, P. R., & Fawcett, J. (2008). In memoriam: Imogene M. King 1923–2007. *Nursing Science Quarterly, 21*(2), 102–103.

Miller, T. (2014). *A qualitative phenomenological study: Hiring nurses re-entering the workforce after chemical dependence.* (Doctoral dissertation). Retrieved from ProQuest Dissertations & Theses. (Order No. 3583325).

Minckley, B. B. (1968). Space and place in patient care. *American Journal of Nursing, 68*(3), 510–516.

Moore, B. W. (2015). *The innovation of simulation laboratories and the novice nurse in the clinical setting.* (DNP project). Retrieved from PsycINFO. (Order No. AAI3665865).

Nwinee, J. (2011). Nwinee socio-behavioural self-care management nursing model. *West African Journal of Nursing, 22*(1), 91–98.

Ongoco, E. K. P. (2012). *Comparison of attitudes and beliefs toward obesity of student nurse practitioners and non-nursing students.* (Master's thesis). Retrieved from ProQuest Dissertations & Theses. (Order No. 1511377).

Orlando, I. J. (1961). *The dynamic nurse-patient relationship: Functions, process, principles.* New York: Putnam.

Orme, J. E. (1969). *Time, experience and behavior.* New York: American Elsevier.

Paterson, J., & Zderad, L. (1976). *Humanistic nursing.* New York: Wiley.

Peplau, H. E. (1952). *Interpersonal relations in nursing.* New York: Putnam.

Quarshie, J. L. (2014). *An inpatient process to improve nurse-physician communication.* (DNP project). Retrieved from ProQuest Dissertations & Theses. (Order No. 3606628).

Rooke, L. (1995a). The concept of space in King's systems framework: Its implications for nursing. In M. A. Frey & C. L. Sieloff (Eds.). *Advancing King's systems framework and theory of nursing* (79–96). Thousand Oaks, CA: Sage.

Rooke, L. (1995b). Focusing on King's theory and systems framework in education by using an experiential learning model: A challenge to improve the quality of nursing care. In M. A. Frey & C. L. Sieloff (Eds.), *Advancing King's systems framework and theory of nursing* (pp. 278–293). Thousand Oaks, CA: Sage.

Sanko, J. S. (2015). *Exploring the cohesion—performance relationship in inter-professional healthcare teams.* (Doctoral dissertation). Retrieved from ProQuest Dissertations & Theses. (Order No. 3704959).

Scott, F. (2011). *Adolescents' perception of early pregnancy and role expectations.* (Master's thesis). Retrieved from ProQuest Dissertations & Theses. (Order No. 1513899).

Shanta, L. L., & Connolly, M. (2013). Using King's interacting systems theory to link emotional intelligence and nursing practice. *Journal of Professional Nursing, 29*(3), 174–180.

Sieloff, C. L. (2010). Improving the work environment through the use of research instruments: An example. *Nursing Administration Quarterly, 34*(1), 56–60.

Sieloff, C. L., & Bularzik, A. M. (2011). Group power through the lens of the 21st century and beyond: Further validation of the Sieloff-King Assessment of Group Power within Organizations. *Journal of Nursing Management, 19*(8), 1020–1027.

Sieloff, C., & Dunn, K. (2008). Factor validation of an instrument measuring group power. *Journal of Nursing Measurement, 16*(2), 113–124.

Sieloff, C. L., & Frey, M. (2007). *Middle range theories for nursing practice using King's conceptual system.* New York: Springer.

Sommer, R. (1969). *Personal space.* Englewood Cliffs, NJ: Prentice-Hall.

Sullivan, T. (2013). *Emergency department nurses' perceptions of the benefits and challenges of hourly rounding.* (Doctoral dissertation). Retrieved from ProQuest Dissertations & Theses. (Order No. 3557522).

Swain, Z. (2012). *Older adult perceptions on the role of the primary care nurse practitioner.* (Master's thesis). Retrieved from ProQuest Dissertations & Theses. (Order No. 1509896).

Teeter, K. (2014). *Relationship between job satisfaction and nurse to patient ratio with nurse burnout.* (Doctoral dissertation). Retrieved from ProQuest Dissertations & Theses. (Order No. 1567760).

Thakral, M. (2015). *Pain qualities and their persistence in the elder population.* (Doctoral dissertation). Retrieved from ProQuest Dissertations & Theses. (Order No. 10010647).

Thomas, B. (2016). *The use of women to educate men: A Nontraditional strategy for prostate cancer awareness.* (DNP project). Retrieved from ProQuest Dissertations & Theses. (Order No. 10012946).

Tolson, D. (2013). *Minority graduates' perceptions on national council licensure examination at a historically black college and university.* (Doctoral dissertation). Retrieved from ProQuest Dissertations & Theses. (Order No. 3578031).

Vincent, A. (2015). *The effect of breastfeeding self-efficacy on breastfeeding initiation, exclusivity, and duration.* (DNP project). Retrieved from ProQuest Dissertations & Theses. (Order No. 3734306).

Wang, S., & Yang, T. (2006). Applying King's theory to establish psychotic patients' awareness of illness [Chinese]. *Tzu Chi Nursing Journal, 5*(1), 120–130.

Ward, D. (2010). Infection control in clinical placements: Experiences of nursing and midwifery students. *Journal of Advanced Nursing, 66*(7), 1533–1542.

Warren, H. (2014). *A proposal comparing a clinician-guided patient information module to standard patient information evaluating treatment expectations of dermal fillers.* (DNP project). Retrieved from ProQuest Dissertations & Theses. (Order No. 3617761).

Watzlawick, P., Beavin, J. W., & Jackson, D. D. (1967). *Pragmatics of human communication.* New York: Norton.

Wetter, V. (2014). *A proposal to reduce hostility in nursing.* (DNP project). Retrieved from ProQuest Dissertations & Theses. (Order No. 3646709).

Whiting, J. F. (1955). Q-sort technique for evaluating perceptions of interpersonal relationship. *Nursing Research, 4*(2), 71–73.

Wicks, M. N., Rice, M. C., & Talley, C. H. (2007). Further exploration of family health within the context of chronic obstructive pulmonary disease. In C. L. Sieloff & M. A. Frey (Eds.), *Middle range theory development using King's conceptual system* (pp. 215–236). New York: Springer.

Yura, H., & Walsh, M. (1978). *The nursing process.* New York: Appleton-Century-Crofts.

BIBLIOGRAPHY

Additional Primary Sources

Books

Fawcett, J., & King, I. (Eds.), (1997). *The language of nursing theory and metatheory*. Indianapolis: Sigma Theta Tau International.

King, I. M., & Fawcett, J. (1997). *The language of nursing theory and metatheory*. Indianapolis: Sigma Theta Tau International.

Journal Articles

Daubenmire, M. J., & King, I. M. (1973). Nursing process models: A systems approach. *Nursing Outlook, 21*(8), 512–517.

King, I. M. (1964). Nursing theory—Problems and prospect. *Nursing Science, 2*(5), 394–403.

King, I. M. (1970). A conceptual frame of reference for nursing. *Japanese Journal of Nursing Research, 3*, 199–204.

King, I. M. (1987). Translating nursing research into practice. *Journal of Neuroscience Nursing, 19*(1), 44–48.

King, I. M. (1990). Health as the goal for nursing. *Nursing Science Quarterly, 3*(3), 123–128.

King, I. M. (1992). King's theory of goal attainment. *Nursing Science Quarterly, 5*(1), 19–26.

King, I. M. (1994). Quality of life and goal attainment. *Nursing Science Quarterly, 7*(1), 29–32.

King, I. M. (1998). The Bioethics Focus Group Report. *Florida Nurse, 46*(8), 24.

Olsson, H., & Forsdahl, T. (1996). Expectations and opportunities of newly employed nurses at the University Hospital, Tromso, Norway. *Social Sciences in Health: International Journal of Research and Practice, 2*(1), 14–22.

Quigley, P., Janzen, S. K., King, I, M., & Goucher, E. (1999). Nurse staffing patient outcomes from one acute care setting within the Department of Veteran's Affairs. *Florida Nurse, 47*(2), 34.

Secondary Sources

Book Chapters

Alligood, M. R. (1995). Theory of goal attainment: Application to adult orthopedic nursing. In M. A. Frey & C. L. Sieloff (Eds.), *Advancing King's systems framework and theory of nursing* (pp. 209–222). Thousand Oaks, CA: Sage.

Alligood, M. R. (2007). Rethinking empathy in nursing education: Shifting to a developmental view. In C. L. Sieloff & M. A. Frey (Eds.), *Middle range theory development using King's conceptual system* (pp. 287–296). New York: Springer.

Alligood, M. R., Evans, G. W., & Wilt, D. L. (1995). King's interacting system and empathy. In M. A. Frey & C. L. Sieloff (Eds.), *Advancing King's systems framework and theory of nursing* (pp. 66–78). Thousand Oaks, CA: Sage.

Benedict, M., & Frey, M. A. (1995). Theory-based practice in the emergency department. In M. A. Frey & C. L. Sieloff (Eds.), *Advancing King's systems framework and theory of nursing* (pp. 317–324). Thousand Oaks, CA: Sage.

Coker, E., Fridley, T., Harris, J., Tomarchio, D., Chan, V., & Caron, C. (1995). Implementing nursing diagnoses within the context of King's conceptual framework. In M. A. Frey & C. L. Sieloff (Eds.), *Advancing King's systems framework and theory of nursing* (pp. 161–175). Thousand Oaks, CA: Sage.

Doornbos, M. M. (1995). Using King's systems framework to explore family health in the families of the young chronically mentally ill. In M. A. Frey & C. L. Sieloff (Eds.), *Advancing King's systems framework and theory of nursing* (pp. 192–205). Thousand Oaks, CA: Sage.

duMont, P. (2007). A theory of asynchronous development: A mid-level theory derived from a synthesis of King and Peplau. In C. L. Sieloff & M. A. Frey (Eds.), *Middle range theory development using King's conceptual system* (pp. 50–74). New York: Springer.

Ehrenberger, H. E., Alligood, M. R., Thomas, S. P., Wallace, D. C., & Licavoli, C. M. (2007). Testing a theory of decision making derived from King's systems framework in women eligible for a cancer clinical trial. In C. L. Sieloff & M. A. Frey (Eds.), *Middle range theory development using King's conceptual system* (pp. 75–91). New York: Springer.

Fawcett, J. (1995). *King's open systems model. In Analysis and evaluation of conceptual models of nursing* (3rd ed., pp. 109–163). Philadelphia: F. A. Davis.

Fawcett, J. M., Vaillancourt, V. M., & Watson, C. A. (1995). Integration of King's framework into nursing practice. In M. A. Frey & C. L. Sieloff (Eds.), *Advancing King's systems framework and theory of nursing* (pp. 176–191). Thousand Oaks, CA: Sage.

Frey, M. A. (1995). From conceptual framework to nursing knowledge. In M. A. Frey & C. L. Sieloff (Eds.), *Advancing King's system framework and theory of nursing* (pp. 3–13). Thousand Oaks, CA: Sage.

Frey, M. A., Ellis, D. A., & Naar-King, S. (2007). Testing nursing theory with intervention research: The congruency between King's conceptual system and multisystemic therapy. In C. L. Sieloff & M. A. Frey (Eds.), *Middle range theory development using King's conceptual system* (pp. 273–286). New York: Springer.

Frey, M. A., & Norris, D. (1997). King's systems framework and theory in nursing practice. In M. R. Alligood & A. Marriner Tomey (Eds.), *Nursing theory: Utilization & application* (pp. 71–88). St Louis: Mosby.

Froman, D. (1995). Perceptual congruency between clients and nurses: Testing King's theory of goal attainment. In M. A. Frey & C. L. Sieloff (Eds.), *Advancing King's systems framework and theory of nursing* (pp. 223–238). Thousand Oaks, CA: Sage.

Hanna, K. M. (1995). Use of King's theory of goal attainment to promote adolescents' health behavior. In M. A. Frey & C. L. Sieloff (Eds.), *Advancing King's systems framework and theory of nursing* (pp. 239–250). Thousand Oaks, CA: Sage.

Hernandez, C. A. (2007). The theory of integration: Congruency with King's conceptual system. In C. L. Sieloff & M. A. Frey (Eds.), *Middle range theory development using King's conceptual system* (pp. 105–124). New York: Springer.

Hobdell, E. F. (1995). Using King's interacting systems framework for research on parents of children with neural tube defects. In M. A. Frey & C. L. Sieloff (Eds.), *Advancing King's systems framework and theory of nursing* (pp. 126–136). Thousand Oaks, CA: Sage.

Jolly, M. L., & Winker, C. K. (1995). Theory of goal attainment in the context of organizational structure. In M. A. Frey & C. L. Sieloff (Eds.), *Advancing King's systems framework and theory of nursing* (pp. 305–316). Thousand Oaks, CA: Sage.

Kameoka, T. (1995). Analyzing nurse-patient interactions in Japan. In M. A. Frey & C. L. Sieloff (Eds.), *Advancing King's systems framework and theory of nursing* (pp. 251–260). Thousand Oaks, CA: Sage.

Killeen, M. B. (2007). Development and initial testing of a theory of patient satisfaction with nursing care. In C. L. Sieloff & M. A. Frey (Eds.), *Middle range theory development using King's conceptual system* (pp. 164–177). New York: Springer.

Laben, J. K., Sneed, L. D., & Seidel, S. L. (1995). Goal attainment in short-term group psychotherapy settings: Clinical implications for practice. In M. A. Frey & C. L. Sieloff (Eds.), *Advancing King's systems framework and theory of nursing* (pp. 261–277). Thousand Oaks, CA: Sage.

May, B. A. (2007). Relationships among basic empathy, self-awareness, and learning styles of baccalaureate pre-nursing students within King's personal system. *Dissertation Abstracts International, 61*(06b), 2991.

Reed, J. E. F. (2007). Social support and health of older adults. In C. L. Sieloff & M. A. Frey (Eds.), *Middle range theory development using King's conceptual system* (pp. 92–104). New York: Springer.

Rooke, L. (1995). The concept of space in King's systems framework: Its implications for nursing. In M. A. Frey & C. L. Sieloff (Eds.), *Advancing King's systems framework and theory of nursing* (pp. 79–96). Thousand Oaks, CA: Sage.

Sharts-Hopko, N. C. (1995). Using health, personal, and interpersonal system concepts within the King's systems framework to explore perceived health status during the menopause transition. In M. A. Frey & C. L. Sieloff (Eds.), *Advancing King's systems framework and theory of nursing* (pp. 147–160). Thousand Oaks, CA: Sage.

Sharts-Hopko, N. C. (2007). A theory of health perception: Understanding the menopause transition. In C. L. Sieloff & M. A. Frey (Eds.), *Middle range theory development using King's conceptual system* (pp. 178–195). New York: Springer.

Sieloff, C. L. (1995). Defining the health of a social system within Imogene King's framework. In M. A. Frey & C. L. Sieloff (Eds.), *Advancing King's systems framework and theory of nursing* (pp. 137–146). Thousand Oaks, CA: Sage.

Sieloff, C. L. (1995). Imogene King: A conceptual framework for nursing. In C. Metzger McQuiston & A. Webb (Eds.), *Foundations of nursing theory: Contributions of 12 key theorists* (pp. 37–87). Thousand Oaks, CA: Sage.

Sieloff, C. L. (1998). Imogene King: Systems framework and theory of goal attainment. In A. Marriner-Tomey & M. R. Alligood (Eds.), *Nursing theorists and their work* (4th ed., pp. 300–319). St Louis: Mosby.

Sieloff, C. L. (2002). Imogene King: Systems framework and theory of goal attainment. In A. Marriner-Tomey & M. R. Alligood (Eds.), *Nursing theorists and their work* (5th ed., pp. 336–360). St Louis: Mosby.

Sieloff, C. L. (2006). Imogene King: Systems framework and theory of goal attainment. In A. Marriner-Tomey & M. R. Alligood (Eds.), *Nursing theorists and their work* (6th ed., pp. 336–360). St Louis: Mosby.

Sieloff, C. L. (2007). The theory of group power within organizations—Evolving conceptualization within King's conceptual system. In C. L. Sieloff & M. A. Frey (Eds.), *Middle range theory development using King's conceptual system* (pp. 196–214). New York: Springer.

Sieloff, C. L., Frey, M., & Killeen, M. (2006). Application of King's interacting systems framework. In M. Parker (Ed.), *Nursing theorists and their application in practice* (2nd ed., pp. 244–267). Philadelphia: F. A. Davis.

Whelton, B. J. B. (2007). The nursing act is an excellent human act: A philosophical analysis derived from classical philosophy and the conceptual system and theory of Imogene King. In C. L. Sieloff & M. A. Frey (Eds.), *Middle range theory development using King's conceptual system* (pp. 12–28). New York: Springer.

Wicks, M. N. (1995). Family health as derived from King's framework. In M. A. Frey & C. L. Sieloff (Eds.), *Advancing King's systems framework and theory of nursing* (pp. 97–108). Thousand Oaks, CA: Sage.

Winker, C. K. (1995). A systems view of health. In M. A. Frey & C. L. Sieloff (Eds.), *Advancing King's systems framework and theory of nursing* (pp. 35–45). Thousand Oaks, CA: Sage.

Zurakowski, T. L. (2007). Theory of social and interpersonal influences on health. In C. L. Sieloff & M. A. Frey (Eds.), *Middle range theory development using King's conceptual system* (pp. 237–257). New York: Springer.

Journal Articles

Alligood, M. R., & May, B. A. (2000). A nursing theory of personal system empathy: Interpreting a conceptualization of empathy in King's interacting systems. *Nursing Science Quarterly, 13*(3), 243–247.

Baumann, S. L. (2000). Research issues: Family nursing: Theory-anemic, nursing theory-deprived. *Nursing Science Quarterly, 13*(4), 285–290.

Brooks, E. M., & Thomas, S. (1997). The perception and judgment of senior baccalaureate student nurses in clinical decision making. *Advances in Nursing Science, 19*(3), 50–69.

Bruns, A., Norwood, B., Bosworth, G., & Hill, L. (2009). The cerebral oximeter: What is the efficacy? *AANA Journal, 77*(2), 137–144.

Calladine, M. L. (1996). Nursing process for health promotion using King's theory. *Journal of Community Health Nursing, 13*(1), 51–57.

Campbell-Begg, T. (2000). A case study using animal-assisted therapy to promote abstinence in a group of individuals who are recovering from chemical addictions. *Journal of Addictions Nursing, 12*(1), 31–35.

Caris-Verhallen, W. M., Kerkstra, A., van der Heijden, P. G., & Bensing, J. M. (1998). Nurse-elderly patient communication in home care and institutional care: An explorative study. *International Journal of Nursing Studies, 35*(1–2), 95–108.

Carter, K. F., & Dufour, L. T. (1994). King's theory: A critique of the critiques. *Nursing Science Quarterly, 7*(3), 128–133.

Chaves, E. S., & de Araujo, T. L. (2006). Nursing care for an adolescent with cardiovascular risk [Portuguese]. *Ciencia, Cuidado e Saude, 5*(1), 82–87.

Cheng, M. (2006). Using King's goal attainment theory to facilitate drug compliance in a psychiatric patient [Chinese]. *Journal of Nursing, 53*(3), 90–97.

Chugh, D. (2005). Care analysis using goal attainment model. *Asian Journal of Cardiovascular Nursing, 13*(2), 2–6.

Crossan, F., & Robb, A. (1998). Role of the nurse: Introducing theories and concepts. *British Journal of Nursing, 7*(10), 608–612.

Daniel, J. M. (2002). Young adults' perceptions of living with chronic inflammatory bowel disease. *Gastroenterology Nursing, 25*(3), 83–94.

David, G. L. B. (2000). Ethics in the relationship between nursing and AIDS-afflicted families [Portuguese]. *Texto & Contexto Enfermagem, 9*(2), 590–599.

Doornbos, M. M. (2000). King's systems framework and family health: The derivation and testing of a theory. *Journal of Theory Construction & Testing, 4*(1), 20–26.

Doornbos, M. M. (2002). Predicting family health in families with young adults with severe mental illness. *Journal of Family Nursing, 8*(3), 241–263.

Fawcett, J. (2001). Scholarly dialogue. The nurse theorists: 21st-century updates—Imogene M. King. *Nursing Science Quarterly, 14*(4), 311–315.

Frey, M. A. (1996). Behavioral correlates of health and illness in youths with chronic illness. *Advanced Nursing Research, 9*(4), 167–176.

Frey, M. A. (1997). Health promotion in youth with chronic illness: Are we on the right track? *Quality Nursing, 3*(5), 13–18.

Frey, M., Rooke, L., Sieloff, C., Messmer, P., Kameoka, T. (1995). Implementing King's conceptual framework and theory of goal attainment in Japan, Sweden and United States. *Image, 27*(2), 127–130.

Frey, M. A., Sieloff, C. L., & Norris, D. M. (2002). King's conceptual system and theory of goal attainment: Past, present, and future. *Nursing Science Quarterly, 15*(2), 107–112.

Gill, J., Hopwood-Jones, L., Tyndall, J., Gregoroff, S., LeBlanc, P., Lovett, C., et al. (1995). Incorporating nursing diagnosis and King's theory in the O. R. documentation. *Canadian Operating Room Nursing Journal, 13*(1), 10–14.

Hanucharurnkui, S., & Vinya-nguag, P. (1991). Effects of promoting patients' participation in self-care on postoperative recovery and satisfaction with care. *Nursing Science Quarterly, 4*(1), 14–20.

Husting, P. M. (1997). A transcultural critique of Imogene King's theory of goal attainment. *Journal of Multicultural Nursing & Health, 3*(3), 15–20.

Jones, S., Clark, V. B., Merker, A., & Palau, D. (1995). Changing behaviors: Nurse educators and clinical nurse specialists design a discharge planning program. *Journal of Nursing Staff Development, 11*(6), 291–295.

Kemppainen, J. K. (1990). Imogene King's theory: A nursing case study of a psychotic client with human immunodeficiency virus infection. *Archives of Psychiatric Nursing, 4*(6), 384–388.

Kline, K. S., Scott, L. D., & Britton, A. S. (2007). The use of supportive-educative and mutual goal setting strategies to improve self-management for patients with heart failure. *Home Healthcare News, 25*(8), 502–510.

Kobayashi, F. T. (1970). A conceptual frame of reference for nursing. *Japanese Journal of Nursing Research, 3*(3), 199–204.

Kusaka, T. (1991). Application to the King's goal attainment theory in Japanese clinical setting. *Journal of the Japanese Academy of Nursing Education, 1*(1), 30–31.

Laramee, A. (1999). The building blocks of successful relationships. *Journal of Care Management, 5*(4), 40, 42, 44–45.

Lawler, J., Dowswell, G., Hearn, J., Forster, A., & Young, J. (1999). Recovering from stroke: A qualitative investigation of the role of goal setting in late stroke recovery. *Journal of Advanced Nursing, 30*(2), 401–409.

Lewinson, S. B. (2000). Professionally speaking: Interview with Imogene King. *Nursing Leadership Forum, 4*(3), 91–95.

Lockhart, J. S. (2000). Nurses' perceptions of head and neck oncology patients after surgery: Severity of facial disfigurement and patient gender. *Plastic Surgical Nursing, 20*(2), 68 80.

Long, J. M., Kee, C. C., Graham, M. V., Saethan, T. B., & Dames, F. D. (1998). Medication compliance and the older hemodialysis patient. *American Nephrology Nurses Association Journal, 25*(1), 43–49.

Mayer, B. W. (2000). Female domestic violence victims: Perspectives on emergency care. *Nursing Science Quarterly, 13*(4), 340–346.

McKinney, N., & Frank, D. I. (1998). Nursing assessment of adult females who are alcohol dependent and victims of sexual abuse. *Clinical Excellence for Nurse Practitioners, 2*(3), 152–158.

McKinney, N. L., & Dean, P. R. (2000). Application of King's theory of dynamic interacting systems to the study of child abuse and the development of alcohol use/dependence in adult females. *Journal of Addictions Nursing, 12*(2), 73–82.

Messmer, P. R. (2006). Professional model of care: Using King's theory of goal attainment. *Nursing Science Quarterly, 19*(3), 227–228.

Messmer, P. R., & Cooper, C. (2011). *Symposium: Pediatric falls based on King's theory of goal attainment.* King's Theory Conference, Bozeman, Montana, April 7–8, 2011.

Milne, J. (2000). The impact of information on health behaviors of older adults with urinary incontinence. *Clinical Nursing Research, 9*(2), 161–176.

Moreira, T. M. M., & Arajo, T. L. (2002). The conceptual model of interactive open systems and the theory of goal attainment by Imogene King [Portuguese]. *Revista Latino-Americana deEnfermagem, 10*(1), 97–103.

Murray, R. L. E., & Baier, M. (1996). King's conceptual framework applied to a transitional living program. *Perspectives in Psychiatric Care, 32*(1), 15–19.

Nagano, M., & Funashima, N. (1995). Analysis of nursing situations in Japan: Using King's goal attainment theory. *Quality Nursing, 1*(1), 74–78.

Ng, B. F. L., & Tsang, H. W. H. (2002). A program to assist people with severe mental illness in formulating realistic life goals. *Journal of Rehabilitation, 68*(4), 59–66.

Norgan, G. H., Ettipio, A. M., & Lasome, C. E. M. (1995). A program plan addressing carpal tunnel syndrome: The utility of King's goal attainment theory. *American Association of Occupational Health Nurses Journal, 43*(8), 407–411.

Palmer, J. A. (2006). Nursing implications for older adult patient education. *Plastic Surgical Nursing, 26*(4), 189–194.

Petrich, B. (2000). Medical and nursing students' perceptions of obesity. *Journal of Addictions Nursing, 12*(10), 3–16.

Richard-Hughes, S. (1997). Attitudes and beliefs of Afro-Americans related to organ and tissue donation. *International Journal of Trauma Nursing, 3*(4), 119–123.

Riggs, C. J. (2001). A model of staff-support to improve retention in long-term care. *Nursing Administration Quarterly, 25*(2), 43–54.

Scott, L. D. (1998). Perceived needs of parents of critically ill children. *Journal of the Society of Pediatric Nurses, 3*(1), 4–12.

Secrest, J., Iorio, D. H., & Martz, W. (2005). The meaning of work for nursing assistants who stay in long-term care. *International Journal of Older People Nursing, 14*(8b), 90–97.

Sieloff, C. L. (2003). Measuring nursing power within organizations. *Journal of Nursing Scholarship, 35*(2), 183–187.

Sredl, D. (2006). The triangle technique: A new evidence-based educational tool for pediatric medication calculations. *Nursing Education Perspectives, 27*(2), 84–88.

Stevens, K. R., & Messmer, P. R. (2008). In remembrance of Imogene M. King. January 30, 1923–December 24, 2007: Imogene, a pioneer and dear colleague. *Nursing Outlook, 56*(3), 100–101.

Suslick, D., Secrest, J., Holweger, J., & Myhan, G. (2007). The perianesthesia experience from the patient's perspective. *Journal of PeriAnesthesia Nursing, 22*(1), 10–20.

Tripp-Reimer, T., Woodworth, G., McCloskey, J. C., & Bulechek, G. (1996). The dimensional structure of nursing interventions. *Nursing Research, 45*(1), 10–17.

Tritsch, J. M. (1996). Application of King's theory of goal attainment and the Carondelet St. Mary's case management model. *Nursing Science Quarterly, 11*(2), 69–73.

Ugarriza, D. N. (2002). Intentionality: Applications within selected theories of nursing. *Holistic Nursing Practice, 16*(4), 41–50.

Viera, C. S., & Rossi, L. (2000). Nursing diagnoses from NANDA's taxonomy in women with a hospitalized preterm child and King's Conceptual System [Portuguese]. *Revista Latin-Americana de Enfermagem, 8*(6), 110–116.

Wadensten, B., & Carlsson, M. (2003). Nursing theory views on how to support the process of aging. *Journal of Advanced Nursing, 42*(2), 118–124.

Walker, K. M., & Alligood, M. R. (2001). Empathy from a nursing perspective: Moving beyond borrowed theory. *Archives of Psychiatric Nursing, 15*(3), 140–147.

Wilkinson, C. R., & Williams, M. (2002). Strengthening patient-provider relationships. *Lippincott's Case Management, 7*(3), 86–102.

16

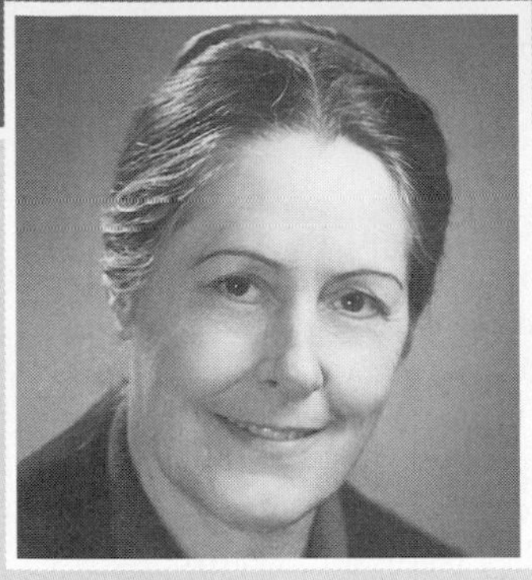

Betty Neuman*
(1924–Present)

Systems Model

*Theresa Gunter Lawson**

"I believe that theory is vital to the development of an autonomous and accountable nursing profession. . . . I believe that the model is relevant for the future because of its dynamic and systemic nature; its concepts and propositions are timeless."
(Neuman, 2011, p. 318)

CREDENTIALS AND BACKGROUND OF THE THEORIST

Betty Neuman was born in 1924 and grew up on a farm in Ohio. Her rural background helped her develop a compassion for people in need, which has been evident throughout her career. She completed her initial nursing education with double honors at Peoples Hospital School of Nursing (now General Hospital), Akron, Ohio, in 1947. As a young nurse, Neuman moved to California and worked in a variety of roles that included hospital nurse, school nurse, industrial nurse, and clinical instructor at the University of Southern California Medical Center. She earned a baccalaureate degree in public health and psychology with honors (1957) and a master's degree in mental health, public health consultation (1966), from the University of California, Los Angeles (UCLA). Neuman completed a doctoral degree in clinical psychology at Pacific Western University in 1985 (B. Neuman, personal communication, June 3, 1984).

Neuman was a pioneer of nursing involvement in mental health. She and Donna Aquilina were the first two nurses to develop the nurse counselor role within community crisis centers in Los Angeles (B. Neuman, personal communication, June 21, 1992). She developed, taught, and refined a community mental health program for post–master's level nurses at UCLA. She developed and published her first explicit teaching and practice model for mental health consultation in the late 1960s, before the creation of her systems model (Neuman, Deloughery, & Gebbie, 1971). Neuman designed a nursing conceptual model for students at UCLA in 1970 to expand their understanding of client variables beyond the medical model (Neuman & Young, 1972). Neuman first published her model during the early 1970s (Neuman, 1974; Neuman & Young, 1972). The first edition of *The Neuman Systems Model: Application to Nursing Education and Practice* was published in 1982; further development and revisions of the model are illustrated in subsequent editions (Neuman, 1989, 1995, 2002b, 2011b).

Since developing the Neuman systems model, Neuman has been involved in numerous publications, paper presentations, consultations, lectures, and conferences on application and use of the model. She is a Fellow of the American Association of Marriage and Family Therapy and of the American Academy of Nursing. She taught nurse continuing education at UCLA and in community agencies for 14 years and was in private practice as a licensed clinical marriage and family therapist, with an emphasis on pastoral counseling. Neuman lives in Seattle and maintains a leadership role in the Neuman Systems Model Trustees Group. She serves as a consultant nationally and internationally regarding implementation of the model for nursing education programs and for clinical practice agencies.

*Previous authors: Barbara T. Freese, Sarah J. Beckman, Sanna Boxley-Harges, Cheryl Bruick-Sorge, Susan Matthews Harris, Mary E. Hermiz, Mary Meininger, and Sandra E. Steinkeler.
Photo credit: www.neumansystemmodel.org

THEORETICAL SOURCES

The Neuman systems model is based on general system theory and reflects the nature of living organisms as open systems (Bertalanffy, 1968) in interaction with each other and with the environment (Neuman, 1982). Within this model, Neuman synthesizes knowledge from several disciplines and incorporates her own philosophical beliefs and clinical nursing expertise, particularly in mental health nursing.

The model draws from Gestalt theory (Perls, 1973), which describes homeostasis as the process by which an organism maintains its equilibrium, and consequently its health, under varying conditions. Neuman describes adjustment as the process by which the organism satisfies its needs. Many needs exist, and each may disrupt client balance or stability; therefore the adjustment process is dynamic and continuous. All life is characterized by this ongoing interplay of balance and imbalance within the organism. When the stabilizing process fails to some degree, or when the organism remains in a state of disharmony for too long, illness may develop. If the organism is unable to compensate through the illness, death may result (Neuman & Young, 1972).

The model is also derived from the philosophical views of de Chardin and Marx (Neuman, 1982). Marxist philosophy suggests that the properties of parts are determined partly by the larger wholes within dynamically organized systems. With this view, Neuman (1982) confirms that the patterns of the whole influence awareness of the part, which is drawn from de Chardin's philosophy of the wholeness of life.

Neuman used Selye's definition of stress, which is the nonspecific response of the body to any demand made on it. Stress increases the demand for readjustment. This demand is nonspecific; it requires adaptation to a problem, irrespective of the nature of the problem. Therefore the essence of stress is the nonspecific demand for activity (Selye, 1974). Stressors are the tension-producing stimuli that result in stress; they may be positive or negative.

Neuman adapts the concept of levels of prevention from Caplan's conceptual model (1964) and relates these prevention levels to nursing. Primary prevention is used to protect the organism before it encounters a harmful stressor. Primary prevention involves reducing the possibility of encountering the stressor or strengthening the client's normal line of defense to decrease the reaction to the stressor. Secondary and tertiary prevention are used after the client's encounter with a harmful stressor. Secondary prevention attempts to reduce the effect or possible effect of stressors through early diagnosis and effective treatment of illness symptoms; Neuman describes this as strengthening the internal lines of resistance. Tertiary prevention attempts to reduce the residual stressor effects and return the client to wellness after treatment (Capers, 1996; Neuman, 2002b).

MAJOR CONCEPTS & DEFINITIONS

Betty Neuman (2011b) describes the Neuman systems model as follows: "The Neuman systems model is a unique, open-systems-based perspective that provides a unifying focus for approaching a wide range of concerns. A system acts as a boundary for a single client, a group, or even a number of groups; it can also be defined as a social issue. A client system in interaction with the environment delineates the domain of nursing concerns" (p. 3).

Major concepts identified in the model (Fig. 16.1) are wholistic approach, open system, environment, client system, normal line of defense, flexible line of defense, health, stressors, degree of reaction, prevention as intervention, and reconstitution (Neuman, 2011c, pp. 327–329; see also Neuman, 1982, 1989, 1995, 2002b).

Wholistic Approach

The Neuman systems model is a dynamic, open, systems approach to client care originally developed to provide a unifying focus for defining nursing problems and for understanding the client in interaction with the environment. The client as a system may be defined as a person, family, group, community, or social issue (Neuman, 2011c).

Clients are viewed as wholes whose parts are in dynamic interaction. The model considers all variables simultaneously affecting the client system: physiological, psychological, sociocultural, developmental, and spiritual. Neuman included the spiritual variable in the second edition (1989). She changed the spelling of the term *holistic* to *wholistic* in the second edition to enhance understanding of the term as referring to the whole person (B. Neuman, personal communication, June 20, 1988).

Open System

A system is open when "there is a continuous flow of input and process, output, and feedback." "Stress and reaction to stress are basic components" of an open system (Neuman, 2011c, p. 328; see also Neuman, 1982, 1989, 1995, 2002b).

MAJOR CONCEPTS & DEFINITIONS—cont'd

Function or Process

The client as a system exchanges "energy, information, and matter with the environment as well as other parts and subparts of the system" as it uses available energy resources "to move toward stability and wholeness" (Neuman, 2011c, p. 328; see also Neuman, 1982, 1989, 1995, 2002b).

Input and Output

For the client as a system, input and output are "the matter, energy, and information that are exchanged between the client and the environment" (Neuman, 2011c, p. 328).

Feedback

System output in the form of "matter, energy, and information serves as feedback for future input "for corrective action to change, enhance, or stabilize the system" (Neuman, 2011c, p. 327).

Negentropy

"A process of energy conservation that increases organization and complexity, moving the system toward stability at a higher degree of wellness" (Neuman, 2011c, p. 328; see also Neuman, 1982, 1989, 1995, 2002b).

Stability

Stability is a dynamic and "desirable state of balance in which energy exchanges can take place without disruption of the character of the system," which points toward optimal health. (Neuman, 2011c, p. 328; see also Neuman, 1982, 1989, 1995, 2002b).

Environment

As defined by Neuman, "the environment consists of both internal and external forces surrounding the client, influencing and being influenced by the client, at any point in time" (Neuman, 2011c, p. 327; see also Neuman, 1982, 1989, 1995, 2002b).

Created Environment

The created environment is developed unconsciously by the client to express system wholeness symbolically. "Its purpose is to provide perceptual protection for client system functioning and to maintain system stability" (Neuman, 2011c, p. 327; see also Neuman, 1982, 1989, 1995, 2002a).

Client System

The client system is "a composite of five variables (physiological, psychological, sociocultural, developmental, and spiritual) in interaction with the environment" (Neuman, 2011c, p. 327). "The physiological variable refers to body structure and function. The psychological variable refers to mental processes in interaction with the environment. The sociocultural variable refers to the effects and influences of social and cultural conditions. The developmental variable refers to age-related processes and activities. The spiritual variable refers to spiritual beliefs and influences" (Neuman 2011c p. 16); see also Neuman, 1982, 1989, 1995, 2002a).

Basic Structure

The client as a system is composed of a central core surrounded by concentric rings. The inner circle of the diagram (see Fig. 16.1) represents the basic survival factors or energy resources of the client. This core structure "consists of basic survival factors common to human beings," such as innate or genetic features (Neuman, 2011c, p. 327; see also Neuman, 1982, 1989, 1995, 2002a).

Lines of Resistance

A series of broken rings surrounding the basic core structure are called the **lines of resistance.** These rings represent resource factors that help the client defend against a stressor (see Fig. 16.1). "Lines of resistance serve as protection factors that are activated by stressors penetrating the normal line of defense" (Neuman, 2011c, p. 328).

Normal Line of Defense

The normal line of defense is the model's outer solid circle (see Fig. 16.1). It represents the "adaptational level of health developed over the course of time and serves as the standard by which to measure wellness deviation determination" (Neuman, 2011c, p. 328; see also Neuman, 1982, 1989, 1995). "Expansion of the normal line of defense reflects an enhanced wellness state, and contraction indicates a diminished wellness state" (Neuman, 2011c, p. 327).

Flexible Line of Defense

The model's outer broken ring is called the **flexible line of defense** (see Fig. 16.1). It is perceived as serving as a protective buffer for preventing stressors from breaking through the usual wellness state as represented by the normal line of defense. Situational factors can affect the degree of protection afforded by the flexible line of defense, both positively and negatively (Neuman, 2011c, p. 327; see also Neuman, 1982, 1989, 1995, 2002a).

Neuman describes the flexible line of defense as the client system's first protective mechanism. "When the flexible line of defense expands, it provides greater short-term protection against stressor invasion; when it contracts, it provides less protection" (Neuman, 2011c, p. 327).

Continued

MAJOR CONCEPTS & DEFINITIONS—cont'd

Health

"Health is a continuum of wellness to illness that is dynamic in nature. Optimal wellness exists when the total system needs are being completely met" (Neuman, 2011c, p. 328).

Wellness

"Wellness exists when all system subparts interact in harmony with the whole system and all system needs are being met" (Neuman, 2011c, p. 329; see also Neuman, 1982, 1989, 1995, 2002b).

Illness

"Illness exists at the opposite end of the continuum from wellness and represents a state of instability and energy depletion" (Neuman, 2011c, p. 329; see also Neuman, 1982, 1989, 1995, 2002b).

Stressors

Stressors are tension-producing stimuli "that have the potential to disrupt system stability, leading to an outcome that may be positive or negative." They may arise from the following:

- Intrapersonal forces occurring within the individual, "such as conditioned responses"
- Interpersonal forces occurring "between one or more individuals, such as role expectations"
- "Extrapersonal forces occurring outside the individual, such as financial circumstances" (Neuman, 2011c, p. 22; see also Neuman, 1982, 1989, 1995).

Degree of Reaction

"The degree of reaction represents system instability that occurs when stressors invade the normal line of defense" (Neuman, 2011c, p. 327; see also Neuman, 1982, 1989, 1995, 2002a).

Prevention as Intervention

Interventions are purposeful actions to help the client retain, attain, or maintain system stability. They can occur before or after protective lines of defense and resistance are penetrated. Neuman supports beginning intervention when a stressor is suspected or identified. Interventions are based on possible or actual degree of reaction, resources, goals, and anticipated outcomes. Neuman identifies three levels of intervention: (1) primary, (2) secondary, and (3) tertiary (Neuman, 2011c; see also Neuman, 1982, 1989, 1995).

Primary Prevention

Primary prevention is used when a stressor is suspected or identified. "A reaction has not yet occurred," but the degree of risk is known. The purpose is to reduce the possibility of encounter with the stressor or to decrease the possibility of a reaction (Neuman, 2011c, p. 328).

Secondary Prevention

"Secondary prevention involves interventions or treatment initiated after symptoms from stress have occurred." The client's internal and external resources are used to strengthen internal lines of resistance, reduce the reaction, and increase resistance factors (Neuman, 2011c, p. 328).

Tertiary Prevention

"Tertiary prevention occurs after the active treatment or secondary prevention stage. It focuses on readjustment toward optimal client system stability." The goal is to maintain optimal wellness by preventing recurrence of reaction or regression. Tertiary prevention leads back in a circular fashion toward primary prevention (Neuman, 2011c, p. 328; see also Neuman, 1982).

Reconstitution

Reconstitution occurs after treatment for stressor reactions. "It represents return of the system to stability," which may be at a higher or lower level of wellness than before stressor invasion (Neuman, 2011c, p. 328).

USE OF EMPIRICAL EVIDENCE

Neuman conceptualized the model from sound theories before nursing research was begun on the model. She initially evaluated the utility of the model by submitting a tool to graduate nursing students at UCLA and published the outcome data in *Nursing Research* (Neuman & Young, 1972). Subsequent nursing research has produced sound empirical evidence in support of the Neuman systems model (see Fig. 16.1).

MAJOR ASSUMPTIONS

Nursing

Neuman (1982) believes that nursing is concerned with the whole person. She views nursing as a "unique profession in that it is concerned with all of the variables affecting an individual's response to stress" (p. 14). The nurse's perception influences the care given; therefore Neuman (1995) states that the perceptual field of the caregiver and the client must be assessed.

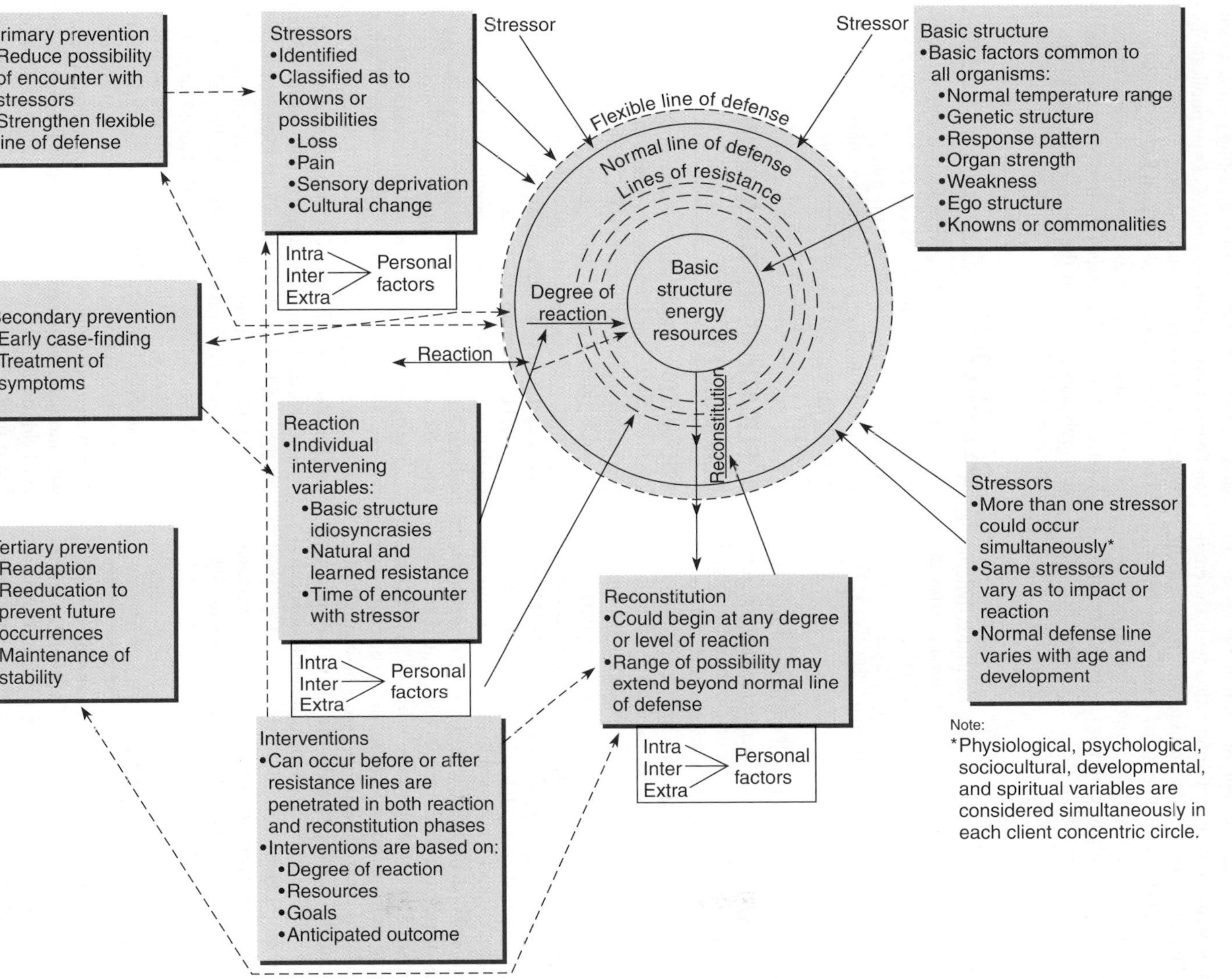

FIG. 16.1 **The Neuman systems model.** (Original copyright 1970 by Betty Neuman. Used with permission.)

Human Beings

"Neuman presents the concept of human beings as an open client system in reciprocal interaction with the environment. The client may be an individual, family, group, community, or social issue." The client system is a dynamic composite of interrelationships among physiological, psychological, sociocultural, developmental, and spiritual factors (Neuman, 2011b, p. 15).

Health

Neuman considers her work a wellness model. She views health as a continuum of wellness to illness that is dynamic in nature and is constantly changing. Neuman states that "Optimal wellness or stability indicates that total system needs are being met. A reduced state of wellness is the result of unmet systemic needs" (Neuman, 2011c, p. 328).

Environment

Neuman defines "**environment** as all the internal and external factors that surround and influence the client system." Stressors (intrapersonal, interpersonal, and extrapersonal) are significant to the concept of environment and are described as environmental forces that interact with and potentially alter system stability (Neuman, 2011b, p. 19).

Neuman (1995) identifies three relevant environments: (1) internal, (2) external, and (3) created. The internal environment is intrapersonal, with all interaction contained within the client. The external environment is interpersonal or extrapersonal, with all factors arising from outside the client. The created environment is unconsciously developed and is used by the client to support protective coping. It is primarily intrapersonal. The created environment is dynamic in nature and mobilizes all system variables to create an insulating effect that helps the client cope with the threat of environmental stressors by changing the self or the situation. Examples are the use of denial (psychological variable) and life cycle continuation of survival patterns (developmental variable). The created environment perpetually influences and is influenced by changes in the client's perceived state of wellness (Neuman, 1995, 2011b).

THEORETICAL ASSERTIONS

Theoretical assertions are the relationships among the essential concepts of a model (Torres, 1986). The Neuman model depicts the nurse as an active participant with the client and as "concerned with all the variables affecting an individual's response to stressors" (Neuman, 1982, p. 14). The client is in a reciprocal relationship with the environment in that "he interacts with this environment by adjusting himself to it or adjusting it to himself" (Neuman, 1982, p. 14). Neuman links the four essential concepts of person, environment, health, and nursing in her statements regarding primary, secondary, and tertiary prevention. Neuman's earlier publications stated basic assumptions that linked essential concepts of the model. These statements have been recognized as propositions and serve to define, describe, and link the concepts of the model. Numerous theoretical assertions have been proposed, tested, and published, as noted throughout the works of Neuman and Fawcett (2011).

LOGICAL FORM

Neuman used deductive and inductive logic in developing her model. As previously discussed, Neuman derived her model from other theories and disciplines. The model is also a product of her philosophy and of observations made in teaching mental health nursing and clinical counseling (Fawcett et al., 1982).

APPLICATIONS BY THE NURSING COMMUNITY

Alligood (2014) clarifies that a conceptual model provides a frame of reference, whereas a grand theory proposes direction or action that is testable. The Neuman systems model is both a model and a grand nursing theory. As a model, it provides a conceptual framework for nursing practice, research, and education (Freese et al., 2011; Louis et al., 2011; Newman, Lowry, & Fawcett, 2011). As a grand theory, it proposes ways of viewing nursing phenomena and nursing actions that are assumed to be true and form propositions for testing (Neuman, 2002a).

The model serves equally well for all levels of nursing education and for a wide variety of practice areas. It adapts well transculturally and is commonly used for public health nursing in other countries. The model is used extensively in the United States, Canada, Holland, and Belgium. It has been used throughout the world (Australia, Brazil, Costa Rica, Denmark, Egypt, Finland, Ghana, Hong Kong, Iceland, Japan, Korea, Kuwait, New Zealand, Portugal, Puerto Rico, the People's Republic of China, Spain, Sweden, Taiwan, and the United Kingdom).

The ongoing development and universal appeal of the model are reflected in the international Biennial Neuman Systems Model Symposia, which provide a forum across cultures for clinicians, educators, researchers, and students to share information about their use of the model. The first symposium was held in 1986 at Neumann College in Aston, Pennsylvania. Subsequent symposia have been held in Kansas City, Missouri (1988); Dayton, Ohio (1990); Rochester, New York (1993); Orlando, Florida (1995); Boston, Massachusetts (1997); Vancouver, British Columbia (1999); Salt Lake City,

Utah (2001); Willow Grove, Pennsylvania (2003); Akron, Ohio (2005); Ft. Lauderdale, Florida (2007); Las Vegas, Nevada (2009); Allentown, Pennsylvania (2011); Vancouver, British Columbia (2013); and Philadelphia, Pennsylvania (2015). Each symposium has attracted participation from countries throughout the world and from disciplines beyond nursing.

Practice

Use of the Neuman systems model for nursing practice facilitates goal-directed, unified, wholistic approaches to client care, yet the model is also appropriate for multidisciplinary use to prevent fragmentation of client care. The model delineates a client system and classification of stressors that can be understood and used by all members of the health care team (Mirenda, 1986). Guidelines have been published for use of the model in clinical nursing practice (Freese et al., 2011) and for the administration of health care services (Shambaugh, Neuman, & Fawcett, 2011).

Several instruments have been published to facilitate use of the model. These instruments include an assessment and intervention tool to assist nurses in collecting and synthesizing client data, a format for prevention as intervention, and a format for application of the nursing process within the framework of the Neuman systems model (Neuman, 2011a; Russell, 2002).

The Neuman Nursing Process Format consists of three steps: (1) nursing diagnosis, (2) nursing goals, and (3) nursing outcomes. (When used by other disciplines, the term *nursing* is changed accordingly.) Diagnosis involves obtaining a broad, comprehensive database from which variances from wellness can be determined. Goals are established by negotiation between client and caregiver for desired prescriptive changes to correct variances from wellness. Outcomes are established in relation to the goal for one or more of the three prevention-as-intervention modes. Evaluation then is used to confirm that the desired outcomes have been achieved or to reformulate the goals or outcomes. Neuman (2011a) outlines her nursing process format, clarifying the steps in the process for use of her model in Appendix C in Neuman and Fawcett (2011, pp. 338–350). Russell (2002) provides a review of clinical tools using the model to guide nursing practice with individuals, families, communities, and organizations.

The breadth of the Neuman model has resulted in its application and adaptation in a variety of nursing practice settings, including hospitals, nursing homes, rehabilitation centers, hospices, mental health units, childbirth centers, and community-based services such as congregational nurse practices. Numerous examples are cited in Neuman's books (Neuman, 1982, 1989, 1995; Newman & Fawcett, 2002, 2011). The model's wholistic approach makes it particularly applicable for clients who are experiencing complex stressors that affect multiple client variables such as chemotherapy-induced nausea and vomiting in women with breast cancer (Bourdeanu & Dee, 2013). The model has been used to guide nursing practice in countries throughout the world. As an example, it is used in Holland to guide Emergis, a comprehensive program of mental health that provides psychiatric care for children, adolescents, adults, and elderly and addiction care and social services (Merks et al., 2012).

Neuman's model provides a systems perspective for use with individuals and families, for community-based practice with groups, and in public health nursing, because its wholistic principles assist nurses to achieve high-quality care through evidence-based practices (Ume-Nwagbo, Dewan, & Lowry, 2006). Anderson, McFarland, and Helton (1986) used the model for a community health needs assessment in which they identified violence toward women as a major community health concern. Smith-Johnson and colleagues (2015) explored the utility of the model as a framework for assessing stress in the caregivers of stroke survivors. This model has been used as a framework to explore adolescent wellness (Spurr et al., 2012) and as a framework for advanced psychiatric nursing practice (Groesbeck, 2011).

Similarly, the model is functional in the acute care setting. For example, Allegiance Health in Michigan adopted the Neuman systems model to be implemented as the nursing conceptual model at their institution. As part of the implementation process, various documents were revised or created to reflect nursing care using concepts of the model, such as the use of the "six Neuman systems model questions" that were incorporated into the admission assessment (Burnett & Crisanti, 2011). The model also works well for multidisciplinary use. Black and colleagues (2011) developed a nurse-facilitated family participation intervention for psychological care of critically ill patients. Recently Aronowitz has been exploring the use of the model and its applicability for evaluating health policy issues (Aronowitz & Fawcett, 2015, 2016). Further research continues to validate its applicability in and beyond nursing.

Education

The model is well accepted in academia and is used widely as a curriculum guide. It has been used throughout the United States and in other countries, including Australia, Canada, Denmark, Holland, Japan, Korea, Kuwait, Portugal, Taiwan, and the United Kingdom (Beckman et al., 1994; Lowry, 2002). In an integrative review of use of the model in educational programs at all levels, Lowry (2002) reported that "the Neuman Systems Model has served many programs well . . . and frequently is selected in other countries to facilitate student learning" (p. 231). Guidelines have been published for use of the model in education for the health professions (Newman, Lowry, & Fawcett, 2002; Newman et al., 2011).

The model's wholistic perspective provides an effective framework for nursing education at all levels. Lowry and Newsome (1995) reported on a study of 12 associate degree programs that used the model as a conceptual framework for curriculum development. Results indicate that graduates use the model most often in the roles of teacher and care provider, and that they tend to continue practice from a Neuman systems model–based perspective after graduation. Neuman's model has been selected for baccalaureate programs on the basis of its theoretical and comprehensive perspectives for a wholistic curriculum and because of its potential for use with individuals, families, small groups, and the community. Neumann College Division of Nursing was the first school to select the Neuman systems model as its conceptual base for its curriculum and approach to client care in 1976. Neuman, Lowry, and Fawcett (2011) report that the Neuman systems model continues to serve as the conceptual framework for more than 25 nursing education programs both in the United States and abroad, including Loma Linda University (Burns, 2011), Anna Maria College (Cammuso, Audrey Silveri, & Remijan, 2011), Indiana University/Purdue University Fort Wayne (Beckman, Lowry, & Boxley-Harges, 2011), and Douglas College (Tarko & Helewka, 2011).

The model works equally well to guide clinical learning. For example, it is used with nursing students at a community nursing center (Newman, 2005) and to teach nursing students to promote the health of communities (Falk-Rafael et al., 2004). It is used as a comprehensive framework to organize data collected from maternity patients by undergraduate nursing students at the University of South Florida (Lowry, 2002). McClure and Gigliotti (2012) reported on a novel use of the model for debriefing after clinical simulation experiences. The Neuman systems model is used to guide learning in classroom and clinical settings for multiple levels of nursing and health-related curricula around the world. Acceptance by the nursing education community is clearly evident. As online nursing education increases, it will be imperative that nurse educators find novel approaches for presenting this information to all levels of students.

A new focus emerged when researchers using the model conceptualized the student and faculty relationship rather than the focus of the client and nurse in several publications. The use of stress-reducing techniques in nursing education (Bauer, 2014) as well as enhancing resilience and empowerment in nursing students (Pines et al., 2014) have been examined. Conversely, Couper's (2015) dissertation work focused on the relationships between and among role strain, faculty stress, and organizational support for clinical nursing faculty faced with assigning a failing clinical grade.

Research

A significant amount of research has been conducted over the past decade on the components of the model to generate nursing theory and use of the model as a conceptual framework to advance nursing as a scientific discipline. Rules for Neuman systems model–based nursing research as specified by Fawcett, a Neuman model trustee, are based on the content of the model and related literature (Fawcett & Gigliotti, 2001). Other guidelines have been published to guide the use of the model for nursing research (Louis et al., 2011).

In the fourth edition of *The Neuman Systems Model,* Fawcett and Giangrande (2002) present an integrated review of 200 research reports of model use that were published through 1997. Skalski, DiGerolamo, and Gigliotti (2006) reported a literature review of 87 Neuman systems model–based studies to identify and categorize client system stressors. The Neuman systems model is often used by nurse researchers as a conceptual framework, because it lends itself to both quantitative and qualitative methods. Recent examples of quantitative studies include explorations of the working conditions of third-party works in a public university in Brazil (Greco et al., 2016), the efficacy of virtual reality–based stress management programs on stress-related variables in patients with mood disorders (Shah et al., 2015), and the effect of healing touch on various indices during vaso-occlusive crisis in patients with sickle cell anemia (Thomas et al., 2013). Recent examples of qualitative studies include a study to explore the meaning of spirituality as described by aging adults in various states of health (Lowry, 2012) and spiritual healing after childhood maltreatment (Willis et al., 2015).

Graduate students commonly use the model for dissertations and theses. Recent examples include the lived experience of being a home hospice nurse (Williams, 2015); establishing risk for patients with medical device–related hospital-acquired pressure ulcers in intensive care (Rondinelli, 2014); roles stress, eating behavior, and obesity among clergy (Manister, 2012; Manister & Gigliotti, 2016); and prevalence of prehypertension among adults in Burkina Faso (Talato, 2014).

Earlier research studies using the Neuman systems model were reported in previous editions of this book, some of which are listed in the bibliography at the end of the chapter.

The Biennial Neuman Systems Model Symposium provides a rich forum for the presentation of research, both completed and in progress. At the 14th (2013) and 15th (2015) symposia, nurses from the United States, Canada, Holland, Brazil, and Mexico reported on numerous studies that used the model. Research presented at the 14th symposium included Hispanic nurses' perception of pain assessment and management (Bloch, 2013b), cultural competency intervention programs for health care workers (Bloch, 2013a), role stress and eating behaviors in clergy (Manister, 2013), and caregiver support during transition from hospital to nursing home (Green-Laughlin et al., 2013). Research presented at the 15th symposium included exploration of variables related to chronic obstructive pulmonary disease (Randazzo, Fongwa, & Van Dover, 2015), identification of human immunodeficiency virus (HIV)-risk behaviors among minority college students (Lyttle et al., 2015), analysis of "worries" between two professional college major groups (McDowell, Cox-Davenport, & Wharton, 2015), and factors influencing misuse and abuse of prescription stimulant medication among student nurses (Martin, 2015). Research projects that were reported at previous symposia (1993–2007) are cited in the Neuman chapter in previous editions of this book.

The Neuman systems model is used extensively to provide the conceptual framework for research projects in the United States and in other countries. Acceptance by the nursing community is clearly evident.

FURTHER DEVELOPMENT

When published initially, the Neuman systems model was described as being at a very early stage of theory development (Walker & Avant, 1983). Although the diagram itself has remained unchanged, the model has been refined based on its use and further developed in subsequent publications (Fawcett, 2001). At least two components have been supported and further developed since 2000. Major developments include spirituality (Beckman et al., 2007; DiJoseph & Cavendish, 2005; Lee, 2005; Lowry, 2002, 2012) and the concept of created environment (Hemphill, 2006).

Establishing full credibility of the model depends on extending the development and testing of middle-range theory from it. Neuman and Koertvelyessy identified two theories generated from the model: (1) the theory of optimal client system stability and (2) the theory of prevention as intervention (Fawcett, 1995b). Gigliotti (2011) points out additional middle-range theories derived from the Neuman systems model, including the theory of adolescent vulnerability to risk behaviors, theory of well-being, theory of maternal role stress, and the theory of dialysis decision making. Research based on the Neuman systems model is needed to validate the relationship between model concepts and research outcomes (Fawcett & Giangrande, 2002; Gigliotti, 2011).

The Neuman Systems Model Trustee Group was established in 1988 to preserve, protect, and perpetuate the integrity of the model for the future of nursing (Neuman, 2011d). The Neuman Systems Model Research Institute has been organized to generate and test middle-range theories derived from the model. Preliminary work that has been completed includes assembling resources, identifying concepts and the relationships among them, and synthesizing existing research based on Neuman systems model concepts (Gigliotti, 2003). The Research Institute offers grants and fellowships to deserving researchers in an effort to promote the use of the model and work in generating middle-range theories from the model and also offers consultation services regarding the use of the model in nursing research (Gigliotti, 2011).

CRITIQUE

Neuman developed a comprehensive conceptual model that operationalizes systems concepts that are relevant to the breadth of nursing phenomena. The model's wholistic perspective allows for a wide range of creativity in its use. It remains relevant for use by nurses and by other health care professions.

Clarity

Neuman presents abstract concepts that are familiar to nurses. The model's essential concepts of client, environment, health, and nursing are congruent with traditional understanding of the nursing metaparadigm. Concepts defined by Neuman and those borrowed from other disciplines are used consistently throughout the model. However, some authors have criticized lack of clarity, calling for concepts to be defined more completely (August-Brady, 2000; Heyman & Wolfe, 2000).

Simplicity

The model concepts are organized in a complex yet systematically logical manner. Multiple interrelationships exist among concepts, and variables overlap to some degree. Distinctions between concepts tend to blur at several points, but loss of theoretical meaning would occur if they were separated completely. Neuman states that the concepts can be separated for analysis, specific goal setting, and interventions (B. Neuman, personal communication, June 21, 1992). This model can be used to explain the client's dynamic state of equilibrium and the reaction or possible reaction to stressors. The concept of prevention as intervention can be used to describe or predict nursing phenomena. The model is complex; therefore it cannot be described as being simple, yet nurses using the model describe it as easy to understand, and it is used across cultures and in a wide variety of practice settings.

Generality

The Neuman systems model has been used in a wide variety of nursing situations; it is both comprehensive and adaptable. Some concepts are broad and represent the phenomenon of "client," which may be one person or a larger system. Other concepts are more definitive and identify specific modes of action, such as primary prevention. The model's systematic broad scope allows it to be useful to nurses and to other health care professionals working with individuals, families, groups, or communities in health care settings.

Health professionals beyond nursing use the model as a framework for care, because its wholistic perspective accommodates varied approaches to client assessment and care. Its systems approach and emphasis on involving the client as an active participant fit well with contemporary health care values such as prevention and interdisciplinary care management.

Accessibility

The model has been tested and is used extensively to guide nursing research. Early work (Hoffman, 1982; Louis & Koertvelyessy, 1989) provided initial documentation of empirical support. Continued testing and refinement through the work of the Research Institute and independent nurse researchers increase the model's empirical precision as research continues and findings from multiple studies are synthesized (Gigliotti, 1999, 2003, 2007, 2011; Skalski, DiGerolamo, & Gigliotti, 2006).

Importance

Neuman's conceptual model includes guidelines for the professional nurse for assessment of the client system, use of the nursing process, and implementation of preventive interventions, which are all important to delivery of care. The focus on primary prevention and interdisciplinary care is futuristic and serves to improve quality of care. The Neuman nursing process fulfills current health mandates by involving the client actively in negotiating the goals of nursing care (Neuman, 2011b).

A major feature of the model is its potential to generate nursing theory—for example, the theories of optimal client stability and prevention as intervention (Fawcett, 1995a). The model concepts are highly relevant for use by health professionals in the 21st century. According to Fawcett (1989, 1995b), the model meets social considerations of congruence, significance, and utility. The model is broad and systems based. It lends itself well to a comprehensive approach for nurses to evaluate evidence and respond to the world's rapidly changing health care needs.

SUMMARY

The Neuman systems model derives from general system theory, focusing on the client as a system, as an individual, family, group, or community, and on the client's responses to stressors. The client system includes five variables—physiological, psychological, sociocultural, developmental, and spiritual—and is conceptualized as an inner core (basic energy resources) surrounded by concentric circles that include lines of resistance, a normal line of defense, and a flexible line of defense. Each of the five variables is considered in each of the concentric circles. Stressors are tension-producing stimuli that may be intrapersonal, interpersonal, or extrapersonal.

The model proposes three levels of nursing intervention (primary prevention, secondary prevention, tertiary prevention) based on Caplan's (1964) concept of levels of prevention. The purpose of prevention as intervention is to achieve the maximum possible level of client system stability. Neuman suggests a nursing process format in which the client, as recipient of care, participates actively with the nurse as caregiver to set goals and select interventions.

This model has been well accepted by the nursing community and is used in administration, practice, education, and research. The Neuman Systems Model Trustees Group is actively involved in protecting the integrity of the model and advancing its development. The Neuman Systems Model Research Institute has been established and is working to generate and test middle-range theories based on the model.

CASE STUDY

Individuals and a Family as a Client

Mila Jefferies is a recently widowed 36-year-old mother of two children and the daughter of two aging parents in the southeastern United States. She and her children have recently relocated from an urban neighborhood to a rural town to care for her parents, Robert and Susan. The move involved a job change for Elizabeth, a change in schools for the children, and an increased distance from the family of the children's deceased father. Mila's older child is a 5-year-old daughter, recently diagnosed with autism spectrum disorder and dyslexia. The younger of the two children is a 3-year-old boy with asthma that has been difficult to control since the move. Robert is a 72-year-old

CASE STUDY—cont'd

Methodist minister who recently suffered a stroke, leaving him with diminished motor function on his left side and difficulty swallowing. Susan is 68 years old and suffers from fibromyalgia, limiting her ability to assist with the daily care of her husband. She has experienced an increase in generalized pain, difficulty sleeping, and worsening fatigue since her husband's stroke.

Use the Neuman systems model as a conceptual framework to respond to the following:

- Describe the Jefferies family as a client system using each of the five variables.
- What actual and potential stressors threaten the family? Which stressors are positive, and which are negative? Separate the actual and potential stressors that threaten the individual members of the family. Which of the stressors are positive, and which are negative?
- What additional nursing assessment data are needed considering Robert's medical diagnoses? What additional data would be helpful for Susan's medical diagnoses? What about each of the children?
- What levels of prevention intervention(s) are appropriate for the Jefferies family? Propose potential prevention intervention(s) for each member of the family.
- Identify your nursing priorities if you were providing care to this family.

CRITICAL THINKING ACTIVITIES

Community as Client

Select one organization with which you are familiar that would be considered a community, based on it having face-to-face interaction and a shared set of interests or values. This could be a group at church, an employing organization, or a civic group. Use the Neuman systems model as a framework to analyze the organization as a community-client and to support organizational planning, as follows:

1. What is the basic structure (core)? What factors in the lines of resistance support the status quo? What factors in the lines of defense support healthy organizational functioning?
2. What stressors, actual or potential, may disrupt the organization as a system and result in change?
3. If the perceptions of goals by the members and the leaders differ, how can the differences be resolved for mutual goal setting that will be beneficial for the organization?
4. What prevention as intervention strategies would support the organization in making changes successful?

POINTS FOR FURTHER STUDY

- Flaherty, K. (2014). Neuman System's Model in nursing practice. In M. R. Alligood (Ed.), *Nursing theory: Utilization and application* (5th ed., pp. 200–221). St Louis, MO: Mosby-Elsevier.
- www.neumansystemsmodel.org
- Neuman, B., & Fawcett, J. (2011). *The Neuman systems model* (5th ed.). Upper Saddle River, NJ: Pearson.
- Neuman, B., & Fawcett, J. (2012). Thoughts about the Neuman systems model: A dialogue. *Nursing Science Quarterly, 25*(4), 374–376.
- Neuman research publications at http://www.neumansystemsmodel.org/NSMdocs/archives.htm
- The Neuman Archives preserves and protects works related to the model. Housed in the Neumann College Library in Aston, PA.
- Neuman, Betty. *Nursing Theorists: Portraits of Excellence,* Vol. I. Fitne, Inc., Athens, OH.

REFERENCES

Alligood, M. R. (2014). Introduction to nursing theory: History, terminology and analysis. In M. R. Alligood (Ed.), *Nursing theorists and their work* (8th ed., pp. 2–13). St Louis, MO: Mosby.

Anderson, E., McFarland, J., & Helton, A. (1986). Community-as-client: A model for practice. *Nursing Outlook, 34*(5), 220–224.

Aronowitz, T., & Fawcett, F. (2015). Thoughts about conceptual models of nursing and health policies. *Nursing Science Quarterly, 28*(1), 88–91.

Aronowitz, T., & Fawcett, J. (2016). Thoughts about social issues. *Nursing Science Quarterly, 29*(2), 173–176.

August-Brady, M. (2000). Prevention as intervention. *Journal of Advanced Nursing, 31*(6), 1304–1308.

Bauer, J. S. (2014). The use of stress-reducing techniques in nursing education. *Western Journal of Nursing Research, 36*(10), 1386.

Beckman, S. J., Boxley-Harges, S., Bruick-Sorge, C., Harris, S. M., Hermiz, M. E., Meininger, M., et al. (1994). Betty Neuman systems model. In A. Marriner Tomey (Ed.), *Nursing theorists and their work* (3rd ed., pp. 269–304). St Louis: Mosby.

Beckman, S., Boxley-Harges, S., Bruick-Sorge, C., & Salmon, B. (2007). Five strategies that heighten nurses' awareness of spirituality to impact client care. *Holistic Nursing Practice, 21*(3), 135–139.

Beckman, S., Lowry, L., & Boxley-Harges, S. (2011). Nursing education at Indiana University/Purdue University Fort Wayne. In B. Neuman & J. Fawcett, 5th ed. (Eds.), *The Neuman systems model*, 5th ed. (pp. 194–215). Upper Saddle River, NJ: Pearson.

Bertalanffy, L. (1968). *General system theory*. New York: George Braziller.

Black, P., Boore, J., & Parahoo, K. (2011). The effect of nurse-facilitated family participation in the physiological care of the critically ill patient. *Journal of Advanced Nursing, 67*(5), 1091–1101.

Bloch, C. (2013a). *Cultural competency intervention program for healthcare workers.* Paper presented at the Fourteenth Biennial Neuman Systems Model Symposium, Vancouver, British Columbia.

Bloch, C. (2013b). *Hispanic nurses' perception of pain assessment and management.* Paper presented at the Fourteenth Biennial Neuman Systems Model Symposium, Vancouver, British Columbia.

Bourdeanu, L., & Dee, V. (2013). Assessment of chemotherapy induced nausea and vomiting in women with breast cancer: A Neuman systems model framework. *Research & Theory for Nursing Practice, 27*(4), 296–304.

Burnett, H. M., & Crisanti, K. J. (2011). Nursing services at Allegiance Health. In B. Neuman & J. Fawcett (Eds.), *The Neuman systems model* (pp. 267–275). Upper Saddle River, NJ: Pearson.

Burns, M. A. (2011). Nursing education at Loma Linda University. In B. Neuman & J. Fawcett (Eds.), *The Neuman systems model* (pp. 177–181). Upper Saddle River, NJ: Pearson.

Capers, C. F. (1996). The Neuman systems model: A culturally relevant perspective. *ABNF Journal, 7*(5), 113–117.

Caplan, G. (1964). *Principles of preventive psychiatry*. New York: Basic Books.

Cammuso, B., Audrey Silveri, A., & Remijan, P. (2011). Nursing education at Anna Maria College. In B. Neuman & J. Fawcett (Eds.), *The Neuman systems model* (pp. 182–193). Upper Saddle River, NJ: Pearson.

Couper, J. (2015). *Exploration of the relationship between and among role strain, faculty stress, and organizational support for clinical nurse faculty faced with a decision to assign a failing grade.* (Doctoral dissertation). Retrieved from ProQuest. (Order No. 3689898).

DiJoseph, J., & Cavendish, R. (2005). Expanding the dialog on prayer relevant to holistic care. *Holistic Nursing Practice, 19*(4), 147–154.

Falk-Rafael, A. R., Ward-Griffin, C., Laforet-Fliesser, Y., & Beynon, C. (2004). Teaching nursing students to promote the health of communities; a partnership approach. *Nurse Educator, 29*(2), 63–67.

Fawcett, J. (1989). *Analysis and evaluation of conceptual models of nursing* (2nd ed., pp. 172–177). Philadelphia: F.A. Davis.

Fawcett, J. (1995a). Constructing conceptual-theoretical-empirical structures for research. In B. Neuman (Ed.), *The Neuman systems model* (3rd ed., pp. 459–471). Norwalk, CT: Appleton & Lange.

Fawcett, J. (1995b). *Neuman's systems model: Analysis and evaluation of conceptual models of nursing* (3rd ed., pp. 217–275). Philadelphia: F. A. Davis.

Fawcett, J. (2001). Scholarly dialogue. The nurse theorists: 21st-century updates—Betty Neuman. *Nursing Science Quarterly, 14*(3), 211–214.

Fawcett, J., Carpenito, L. J., Efinger, J., Goldblum-Graff, D., Groesbeck, M., Lowry, L. W., et al. (1982). A framework for analysis and evaluation of conceptual models of nursing with an analysis of the Neuman systems model. In B. Neuman (Ed.), *The Neuman systems model: Application to nursing education and practice* (pp. 30–43). Norwalk, CT: Appleton-Century-Crofts.

Fawcett, J., & Giangrande, S. (2002). The Neuman systems model and research: An integrative review. In B. Neuman & J. Fawcett (Eds.), *The Neuman systems model* (4th ed., pp. 120–149). Upper Saddle River, NJ: Pearson.

Fawcett, J., & Gigliotti, E. (2001). Using conceptual models to guide nursing research: The case of the Neuman systems' model. *Nursing Science Quarterly, 14*(3), 339–345.

Freese, B. T., Russell, J., Neuman, B., & Fawcett, J. (2011). Neuman systems model-based practice: Guidelines and practice tools. In B. Neuman & J. Fawcett (Eds.), *The Neuman systems model* (pp. 136–152). Upper Saddle River, NJ: Pearson.

Gigliotti, E. (1999). Women's multiple role stress: Testing Neuman's flexible line of defense. *Nursing Science Quarterly, 12*(1), 36–44.

Gigliotti, E. (2003). The Neuman systems model institute: Testing middle-range theories. *Nursing Science Quarterly, 16*(3), 201–206.

Gigliotti, E. (2004). Etiology of maternal-student role stress. *Nursing Science Quarterly, 17*(2), 156–164.

Gigliotti, E. (2007). Improving external and internal validity of a model of midlife women's maternal-student role stress. *Nursing Science Quarterly, 20*(2), 161–170.

Gigliotti, E. (2011). Deriving middle-range theories from the Neuman systems model. In B. Neuman & J. Fawcett (Eds.), *The Neuman systems model* (pp. 283–298). Upper Saddle River, NJ: Pearson.

Greco, R. M., Alves de Moura, D. C., Arreguy-Sena, C., Alvarenga Martins, N., & da Silva Alves, M. (2016). Labour conditions and the theory of Betty Neuman: Third-party workers of a public university. *Journal of Nursing UPFE, 10*(2), 727–735.

Green-Laughlin, D., Davis, B., Montgomery, A., Magee, Z., & Cross, B. (2013). *Caregivers and nurses' support of family members in transition from hospital to nursing home.* Paper presented at the Fourteenth Biennial Neuman Systems Model Symposium, Vancouver, British Columbia.

Groesbeck, M. J. (2011). Reflections on Neuman systems model-based advanced psychiatric nursing practice. In B. Neuman & J. Fawcett (Eds.), *The Neuman systems model* (pp. 237–244). Upper Saddle River, NJ: Pearson.

Hemphill, J. C. (2006). Discovering strengths of homeless abused women. *Dissertation Abstracts International, 66*(7), 3635B. (UMI No. 3180908).

Heyman, P., & Wolfe, S. (2000). Neuman systems model. University of Florida. Retrieved from http://www.patheyman.com/essays/neuman/criticisms.htm.

Hoffman, M. K. (1982). From model to theory construction: An analysis of the Neuman health-care system model. In B. Neuman (Ed.), *The Neuman systems model: Application to nursing education and practice* (pp. 44–54). Norwalk, CT: Appleton-Century-Crofts.

Lee, F-P. (2005). The relationship of comfort and spirituality to quality of life among long-term care facility residents in southern Taiwan. *Dissertation Abstracts International, 66*(2), 815B. (UMI No. 3163392).

Louis, M., Gigliotti, E., Neuman, B., & Fawcett, J. (2011). Neuman systems model-based research: Guidelines and research instruments. In B. Neuman & J. Fawcett (Eds.), *The Neuman systems model* (pp. 160–174). Upper Saddle River, NJ: Pearson.

Louis, M., & Koertvelyessy, A. (1989). The Neuman model in research. In B. Neuman (Ed.), *The Neuman systems model* (2nd ed., pp. 93–114). Norwalk, CT: Appleton & Lange.

Lowry, L. W. (2002). The Neuman systems model and education: An integrative review. In B. Neuman & J. Fawcett (Eds.), *The Neuman systems model* (4th ed., pp. 216–237). Upper Saddle River, NJ: Pearson.

Lowry, L. W. (2012). A qualitative descriptive study of spirituality guided by the Neuman Systems Model. *Nursing Science Quarterly, 25*(4), 356–361.

Lowry, L. W., & Newsome, G. G. (1995). Neuman-based associate degree programs: Past, present, and future. In B. Neuman (Ed.), *The Neuman systems model* (3rd ed., pp. 197–214). Norwalk, CT: Appleton & Lange.

Lyttle, D., Montgomery, A. J., Davis, B. L., Burns, D. P., McGee, Z. T., & Fogel, J. (2015). *The identification of HIV-risk behaviors among minority college students using the Neuman Systems Model.* Poster presented at the Fifteenth Biennial Neuman Systems Model Symposium, Philadelphia, PA.

Manister, N. N. (2012). *Role stress, eating behaviors, and obesity in clergy.* (Doctoral dissertation). Retrieved from ProQuest. (Order No. 3508841).

Manister, N. N. (2013). *Role stress, eating behavior, and obesity in clergy.* Paper presented at the Fourteenth Biennial Neuman Systems Model Symposium, Vancouver, BC.

Manister, N., & Gigliotti, E. (2016). Emotional eating mediates the relationship between role stress and obesity in clergy. *Nursing Science Quarterly, 29*(2), 136–145.

Martin, C. (2015). *Factors influencing nursing students use, misuse & abuse of prescription stimulant medications.* Poster presented at the Fifteenth Biennial Neuman Systems Model Symposium, Philadelphia, PA.

McClure, M., & Gigliotti, E. (2012). A medieval metaphor to aid in the use of the Neuman systems model in simulation debriefing. *Nursing Science Quarterly, 25*(4), 318–324.

McDowell, L., Cox-Daveport, R., & Wharton, H. (2015). *Posting worries, a comparative analysis of stressors between professional education majors.* Poster presented at the Fifteenth Biennial Neuman Systems Model Symposium, Philadelphia, PA.

Merks, A., Verberk, F., de Kuiper, M., & Lowry, L. (2012). Neuman systems model in Holland: An update. *Nursing Science Quarterly, 25*(4), 364–368.

Mirenda, R. M. (1986). The Neuman systems model: Description and application. In P. Winstead-Fry (Ed.), *Case studies in nursing theory* (pp. 127–167). New York: National League for Nursing.

Neuman, B. (1974). The Betty Neuman health care systems model: A total person approach to patient problems. In J. P. Riehl & C. Roy (Eds.), *Conceptual models for nursing practice* (2nd ed., pp. 119–134). New York: Appleton-Century-Crofts.

Neuman, B. (1982). *The Neuman systems model: Application to nursing education and practice.* Norwalk, CT: Appleton-Century-Crofts.

Neuman, B. (1989). *The Neuman systems model* (2nd ed.). Norwalk, CT: Appleton & Lange.

Neuman, B. (1995). *The Neuman systems model* (3rd ed.). Norwalk, CT: Appleton & Lange.

Neuman, B. (2002a). The Neuman systems model. In B. Neuman & J. Fawcett (Eds.), *The Neuman systems model* (4th ed., pp. 3–34). Upper Saddle River, NJ: Prentice-Hall.

Neuman, B. (2002b). The Neuman systems model definitions. In B. Neuman & J. Fawcett (Eds.), *The Neuman systems model* (4th ed., pp. 322–324). Upper Saddle River, NJ: Prentice-Hall.

Neuman, B. (2011a). Assessment and intervention based on the Neuman systems model. In B. Neuman & J. Fawcett (Eds.), *The Neuman systems model* (pp. 338–350). Upper Saddle River, NJ: Pearson.

Neuman, B. (2011b). The Neuman systems model. In B. Neuman & J. Fawcett (Eds.), *The Neuman systems model* (pp. 1–33). Upper Saddle River, NJ: Pearson.

Neuman, B. (2011c). The Neuman systems model definitions. In B. Neuman & J. Fawcett (Eds.), *The Neuman systems model* (pp. 327–329). Upper Saddle River, NJ: Pearson.

Neuman, B. (2011d). Trustees of Neuman Systems Model International. In B. Neuman & J. Fawcett (Eds.), *The Neuman systems model* (pp. 355–358). Upper Saddle River, NJ: Pearson.

Neuman, B., & Fawcett, J. (2002). *The Neuman systems model* (4th ed.). Upper Saddle River, NJ: Prentice-Hall.

Neuman, B., & Fawcett, J. (2011). *The Neuman systems model* (5th ed.). Upper Saddle River, NJ: Pearson.

Neuman, B., Deloughery, G. W., & Gebbie, M. (1971). *Consultation and community organization in community mental health nursing.* Baltimore: Williams & Wilkins.

Neuman, B., Lowry, L., & Fawcett, J. (2011). Use of the Neuman systems model as a guide for nursing education. In B. Neuman & J. Fawcett (Eds.), *The Neuman systems model* (pp. 359–369). Upper Saddle River, NJ: Pearson.

Neuman, B. M., & Young, R. J. (1972). A model for teaching total person approach to patient problems. *Nursing Research, 21*(3), 264–269.

Newman, D. M. L. (2005). A community nursing center for the health promotion of senior citizens based on the Neuman systems model. *Nursing Education Perspectives, 26*(4), 221–223.

Newman, D. M. L., Gehrling, K. R., Lowry, L., Taylor, R., Neuman, B., & Fawcett, J. (2011). Neuman systems model-based education for the health professions: Guidelines and educational tools. In B. Neuman & J. Fawcett (Eds.), *The Neuman systems model* (5th ed., pp. 117–135). Upper Saddle River, NJ: Pearson.

Perls, F. (1973). *The gestalt approach: Eye witness to therapy*. Palo Alto, CA: Science and Behavior Books.

Pines, E. W., Rauschuber, M. L., Cook, J. D., Norgan, G. H., Canchosa, L., Richardson, C., & Jones, M. E. (2014). Enhancing resilience, empowerment, and conflict management among baccalaureate students: Outcomes of a pilot study. *Nurse Educator, 39*(2), 85–90.

Randazzo, V. P., Fongwa, M., & Van Dover, L. (2015). *Application of the Neuman systems model to chronic obstructive pulmonary disease*. Paper presented at the Fifteenth Biennial Neuman Systems Model Symposium. Philadelphia, PA.

Rondinelli, J. L. (2014). *Establishing risk for patients with medical device related hospital acquired pressure ulcers in intensive care: A multi-site study.* (Doctoral dissertation). Retrieved from ProQuest. (Order No. 3619292).

Russell, J. (2002). The Neuman systems model and clinical tools. In B. Neuman & J. Fawcett (Eds.), *The Neuman systems model* (4th ed., pp. 61–73). Upper Saddle River, NJ: Prentice-Hall.

Selye, H. (1974). *Stress without distress.* Philadelphia: Lippincott.

Shah, L. B. I., Torres, S., Kannusamy, P., Mui Lee Chng, C., Hong-Gu, H., Klainin-Yobas, P. (2015). Efficacy of the virtual reality-based stress management program on stress-related variables in people with mood disorders: The feasibility study. *Archives of Psychiatric Nursing, 29*(1), 6–13.

Shambaugh, B. F., Neuman, B., & Fawcett, J. (2011). Guidelines for Neuman systems model-based administration of health care services. In B. Neuman & J. Fawcett (Eds.), *The Neuman systems model* (pp. 153–159). Upper Saddle River, NJ: Pearson.

Skalski, C. A., DiGerolamo, L., Gigliotti, E. (2006). Stressors in five client populations: Neuman systems model-based literature review. *Journal of Advanced Nursing, 56*(1), 69–78.

Smith-Johnson, B., Davis, B. L., Burns, D., Montgomery, A. J., & McGee, Z. T. (2015). African American wives and perceived stressful experiences: Providing care for stroke survivor spouses. *ABNF Journal, 26*(2), 39–42.

Spurr, S., Bally, J., Ogenchuk, M., & Walker, K. (2012). A framework for exploring adolescent wellness. *Pediatric Nursing, 38*(6), 320–326.

Talato, K. (2014). *Prevalence and risk factors for pre-hypertension among adults in Burkina Faso.* (Doctoral dissertation). Retrieved from ProQuest. (Order No. 3614164).

Tarko, M., & Helewka, A. (2011). Psychiatric nursing education at Douglas College. In B. Neuman & J. Fawcett (Eds.), *The Neuman systems model* (pp. 216–220). Upper Saddle River, NJ: Pearson.

Thomas, L. S., Stephenson, N., Swanson, M., Jesse, D. E., & Brown, S. (2013). A pilot study: The effect of healing touch on anxiety, stress, pain, pain medication usage, and physiologic measures in hospitalized sickle cell disease adults experiencing a vaso-occlusive pain episode. *Journal of Holistic Nursing, 31*(4), 234–247.

Torres, G. (1986). *Theoretical foundations of nursing*. Norwalk, CT: Appleton-Century-Crofts.

Ume-Nwagbo, P. N., Dewan, S. A., & Lowry, L.W. (2006). Using the Neuman systems model for best practices. *Nursing Science Quarterly, 19*(1), 31–35.

Walker, L. O., & Avant, K. (1983). *Strategies for theory construction in nursing*. Norwalk, CT: Appleton-Century-Crofts.

Williams, J. B. (2015). *Gift and grievances: A hermeneutic phenomenological exploration of the lived experience of being a home hospice nurse.* (Doctoral dissertation). Retrieved from ProQuest. (Order No. 3691998).

Willis, D. G., DeSanto-Madeya, S., Ross, R., Sheehan, D. L., & Fawcett, J. (2015). Spiritual healing in the aftermath of childhood maltreatment: Translating men's lived experiences utilizing nursing conceptual models and theory. *Advances in Nursing Science, 38*(3), 162–174.

BIBLIOGRAPHY

Primary Sources

Books

Hinton Walker, P., & Neuman, B. (Eds.). (1996). *Blueprint for use of nursing models*. New York: National League for Nursing.

Neuman, B. M., & Walker, P. H. (1996). *Blueprint for use of nursing models: Education, research, practice, and administration.* New York: National League for Nursing.

Book Chapters

Freese, B. T., Neuman, B., & Fawcett, J. (2002). Guidelines for Neuman systems model-based clinical practice. In B. Neuman & J. Fawcett (Eds.), *The Neuman systems model* (4th ed., pp. 37–42). Upper Saddle River, NJ: Pearson.

Louis, M., Neuman, B., & Fawcett, J. (2002). Guidelines for Neuman systems model-based nursing research. In B. Neuman & J. Fawcett (Eds.), *The Neuman systems model* (4th ed., pp. 113–119). Upper Saddle River, NJ: Pearson.

Neuman, B. (1980). The Betty Neuman health care systems model: A total person approach to patient problems. In J. P. Riehl & C. Roy (Eds.), *Conceptual models for nursing practice* (2nd ed., pp. 119–134). New York: Appleton-Century-Crofts.

Neuman, B. (1983). Analysis and application of Neuman's health care model. In I. W. Clements & F. B. Roberts (Eds.), *Family health: A theoretical approach to nursing care* (pp. 239–254, 353–367). New York: Wiley.

Neuman, B. (1986). The Neuman systems model explanation: Its relevance to emerging trends toward wholism in nursing. In I. B. Engberg & K. Kuld (Eds.), *Omvårdnad 1986* [Nursing care book]. Mullsjö: Sweden: Omvårdnad's Forum HB.

Neuman, B. (1989). The Neuman nursing process format adapted to a family case study. In J. P. Riehl & C. Roy (Eds.), *Conceptual models for nursing practice* (pp. 49–62). Norwalk, CT: Appleton & Lange.

Neuman, B. (1990). The Neuman systems model: A theory for practice. In M. E. Parker (Ed.), *Nursing theories in practice* (pp. 24–26). New York: National League for Nursing.

Neuman, B. (1995). In conclusion—Toward new beginnings. In B. Neuman (Ed.), *The Neuman systems model* (3rd ed., pp. 671–703). Norwalk, CT: Appleton & Lange.

Neuman, B. (1995). The Neuman systems model. In B. Neuman (Ed.), *The Neuman systems model* (3rd ed., pp. 3–62). Norwalk, CT: Appleton & Lange.

Neuman, B. (2001). The Neuman systems model: A futuristic care perspective. In N. L Chaska (Ed.), *The nursing profession: Tomorrow and beyond* (pp. 321–329). Thousand Oaks, CA: Sage.

Neuman, B. (2002). Assessment and intervention based on the Neuman systems model. In B. Neuman & J. Fawcett (Eds.), *The Neuman systems model* (4th ed., pp. 347–359). Upper Saddle River, NJ: Pearson.

Neuman, B. (2002). Betty Neuman's autobiography and chronology of the development and utilization of the Neuman systems model. In B. Neuman & J. Fawcett (Eds.), *The Neuman systems model* (4th ed., pp. 325–346). Upper Saddle River, NJ: Pearson.

Neuman, B. (2002). The future and the Neuman systems model. In B. Neuman & J. Fawcett (Eds.), *The Neuman systems model* (4th ed., pp. 319–321). Upper Saddle River, NJ: Pearson.

Neuman, B. (2002). The Neuman Systems Model Trustees Group. In B. Neuman & J. Fawcett (Eds.), *The Neuman systems model* (4th ed., pp. 360–363). Upper Saddle River, NJ: Pearson.

Neuman, B. (2011). The Neuman systems model. In B. Neuman & J. Fawcett (Eds.), *The Neuman systems model* (pp. 1–33). Upper Saddle River, NJ: Pearson.

Neuman, B., & Lowry, L. (2011). The Neuman systems model and the future. In B. Neuman & J. Fawcett (Eds.), *The Neuman systems model* (pp. 317–324). Upper Saddle River, NJ: Pearson.

Neuman, B., & Wyatt, M. (1980). The Neuman stress/adaptation systems approach to education for nurse administrators. In J. P. Riehl & C. Roy (Eds.), *Conceptual models for nursing practice* (2nd ed., pp. 142–150). New York: Appleton-Century-Crofts.

Newman, D. M. L., Neuman, B., & Fawcett, J. (2002). Guidelines for Neuman systems model-based education for the health professions. In B. Neuman & J. Fawcett (Eds.), *The Neuman systems model* (4th ed., pp. 193–215). Upper Saddle River, NJ: Pearson.

Journal Articles

Neuman, B. (1985, Sept.). The Neuman systems model: Its importance for nursing. *Senior Nurse, 5*(3), 20–23.

Neuman, B. (1990). Health: A continuum based on the Neuman systems model. *Nursing Science Quarterly, 3*(3), 129–135.

Neuman, B. (1996). The Neuman systems model in research and practice. *Nursing Science Quarterly, 9*(2), 67–70.

Neuman, B. (1998). NDs should be future coordinators of health care (Letter to the Editor). *Image: The Journal of Nursing Scholarship, 30*, 106.

Neuman, B. (2000). Leadership-scholarship integration: Using the Neuman systems model for 21st century professional nursing practice. *Nursing Science Quarterly, 13*(1), 60–63.

Neuman, B., Chadwick, P. L., Beynon, C. E., Craig, D. M., Fawcett, J., Chang, N. J., et al. (1997). The Neuman systems model: Reflections and projections. *Nursing Science Quarterly, 10*(1), 18–21.

Neuman, B., Deloughery, G. W., & Gebbie, K. M. (1974). Teaching organizational concepts to nurses in community mental health. *Journal of Nursing Education, 13*(1), 8–14.

Neuman, B. M., Deloughery, G. W., & Gebbie, K. M. (1970). Changes in problem solving ability among nurses receiving mental health consultation: A pilot study. *Communicating Nursing Research, 3*, 41–52.

Neuman, B. M., Deloughery, G. W., & Gebbie, K. M. (1970). Levels of utilization: Nursing specialists in community mental health. *Journal of Psychiatric Nursing and Mental Health Services, 8*(1), 37–39.

Neuman, B. M., Deloughery, G. W., & Gebbie, K. M. (1972). Mental health consultation as a means of improving problem solving ability in work groups: A pilot study. *Comparative Group Studies, 3*(1), 81–97.

Neuman, B., & Fawcett, J. (2012). Thoughts about the Neuman systems model: A dialogue. *Nursing Science Quarterly, 25*(4), 372–376.

Neuman, B. M., & Martin, K. S. (1998). Neuman systems model and the Omaha system. *Image: The Journal of Nursing Scholarship, 30*(1), 8.

Neuman, B., Newman, D. M. L., & Holder, P. (2000). Leadership-scholarship integration: Using the Neuman systems model for 21st-century professional nursing practice. *Nursing Science Quarterly, 13*(1), 60–63.

Neuman, B., & Reed, K. S. (2007). A Neuman systems model perspective on nursing in 2050. *Nursing Science Quarterly, 20*(2), 111–113.

Neuman, B., & Wyatt, M. A. (1981). Prospects for change: Some evaluative reflections by faculty members from one articulated baccalaureate program. *Journal of Nursing Education, 20*(1), 40–46.

Secondary Sources

Books

Fawcett, J. (1989). *Analysis and evaluation of conceptual models of nursing.* Philadelphia: F. A. Davis.

Fawcett, J. (1999). *The relationship of theory and research* (3rd ed.). Philadelphia: F. A. Davis.

Fawcett, J. (2000). *Analysis and evaluation of contemporary nursing knowledge: Nursing models and theories.* Philadelphia: F. A. Davis.

Lowry, L. W. (1998). *The Neuman systems model and nursing education: Teaching strategies and outcomes.* Indianapolis: Sigma Theta Tau International. Indianapolis, Center Nursing Press.

Meleis, A. I. (1997). *Theoretical nursing: Development and progress* (3rd ed.). Philadelphia: Lippincott.

Reed, K. S. (1993). *Betty Neuman: The Neuman systems model.* Newbury Park, CA: Sage.

Book Chapters

Alyward, P. D. (2010). Betty Neuman's systems model. In M. E. Parker & M. C. Smith (Eds.), *Nursing theories and nursing practice* (3rd ed., pp. 182–201). Philadelphia: F.A. Davis.

Amaya, M. A. (2002). The Neuman systems model and clinical practice: An integrative review 1974–2000. In B. Neuman & J. Fawcett (Eds.), *The Neuman systems model* (4th ed., pp. 43–60). Upper Saddle River, NJ: Pearson.

Beckman, S. J., Boxley-Harges, S., Bruick-Sorge, C., & Eichenaur, J. (1998). Critical thinking, the Neuman systems model, and associate degree education. In L. Lowry (Ed.), *The Neuman systems model and nursing education: Teaching strategies and outcomes* (pp. 53–58). Indianapolis: Center Nursing Press.

Beckman, S. J., Boxley-Harges, S., Bruick-Sorge, C, & Eichenaur, J. (1998). Evaluation modalities for assessing student and program outcomes. In L. Lowry (Ed.), *The Neuman systems model and nursing education: Teaching strategies and outcomes* (pp. 149–160). Indianapolis: Center Nursing Press.

Breckenridge, D. M. (2011). The Neuman systems model and evidence-based nursing practice. In B. Neuman & J. Fawcett (Eds.), *The Neuman systems model* (pp. 245–252). Upper Saddle River, NJ: Pearson.

Breckenridge, D. M. (2002). Using the Neuman systems model to guide nursing research in the United States. In B. Neuman & J. Fawcett (Eds.), *The Neuman systems model* (4th ed., pp. 176–182). Upper Saddle River, NJ: Pearson.

Busch, P., & Lynch, M. (1998). Creative teaching strategies in a Neuman-based baccalaureate curriculum. In L. Lowry (Ed.), *The Neuman systems model and nursing education: Teaching strategies and outcomes* (pp. 59–70). Indianapolis: Center Nursing Press.

Cammuso, B. S., & Wallen, A. J. (2002). Using the Neuman systems model to guide nursing education in the United States. In B. Neuman & J. Fawcett (Eds.), *The Neuman systems model* (4th ed., pp. 244–253). Upper Saddle River, NJ: Pearson.

Chang, N. J., & Freese, B. T. (1998). Teaching culturally competent care: A Korean-American experience. In L. Lowry (Ed.), *The Neuman systems model and nursing education: Teaching strategies and outcomes* (pp. 85–90). Indianapolis: Center Nursing Press.

Chaponniere, P. A. (2010). Acculturation, pregnancy-related stress and birth outcomes in Mexican and Mexican-American women. *Dissertation Abstracts International, 71B*(04).

Crawford, J. A., & Tarko, M. (2002). Using the Neuman systems model to guide nursing practice in Canada. In B. Neuman & J. Fawcett (Eds.), *The Neuman systems model* (4th ed., pp. 90–110). Upper Saddle River, NJ: Pearson.

de Kuiper, M. (2002). Using the Neuman systems model to guide nursing education in Holland. In B. Neuman & J. Fawcett (Eds.), *The Neuman systems model* (4th ed., pp. 254–262). Upper Saddle River, NJ: Pearson.

de Kuiper, M. (2011). The created environment. In B. Neuman & J. Fawcett (Eds.), *The Neuman systems model* (5th ed., pp. 100–104). Upper Saddle River, NJ: Pearson.

Evans, B. (1998). Fourth-generation evaluation and the Neuman systems model. In L. Lowry (Ed.), *The Neuman systems model and nursing education: Teaching strategies and outcomes* (pp. 117–128). Indianapolis: Center Nursing Press.

Fashinpaur, D. (2002). Using the Neuman systems model to guide nursing practice in the United States: Nursing prevention interventions for postpartum mood disorders. In B. Neuman & J. Fawcett (Eds.), *The Neuman systems model* (4th ed., pp. 74–89). Upper Saddle River, NJ: Pearson.

Fawcett, J. (2002). Neuman systems model bibliography. In B. Neuman & J. Fawcett (Eds.), *The Neuman systems model* (4th ed., pp. 364–400). Upper Saddle River, NJ: Pearson.

Fawcett, J., & Giangrande, S. K. (2002). The Neuman systems model and research: An integrative review. In B. Neuman & J. Fawcett (Eds.), *The Neuman systems model* (4th ed., pp. 120–149). Upper Saddle River, NJ: Pearson.

Freese, B. T., & Lawson, T. G. (2011). Betty Neuman: Systems model. In M. R. Alligood & A. Marriner Tomey (Eds.), *Nursing theorists and their work* (7th ed., pp. 309–334). St Louis: Mosby Elsevier.

Freese, B. T., & Scales, C. J. (1998). NSM-based care as an NLN program evaluation outcome. In L. Lowry (Ed.), *The Neuman systems model and nursing education: Teaching strategies and outcomes* (pp. 135–139). Indianapolis: Center Nursing Press.

Frieburger, O. A. (1998). The Neuman systems model, critical thinking, and cooperative learning in a nursing issues course. In L. Lowry (Ed.), *The Neuman systems model and nursing education: Teaching strategies and outcomes* (pp. 79–84). Indianapolis: Center Nursing Press.

Frieburger, O. A. (1998). Overview of strategies that integrate the Neuman systems model, critical thinking, and cooperative learning. In L. Lowry (Ed.), *The Neuman systems model and nursing education: Teaching strategies and outcomes* (pp. 31–36). Indianapolis: Center Nursing Press.

Freiburger, O. A. (2011). Critical thinking. In B. Neuman & J. Fawcett (Eds.), *The Neuman systems model* (pp. 105–114). Upper Saddle River, NJ: Pearson.

Gehrling, K. R. (2011). Reconstitution. In B. Neuman & J. Fawcett (Eds.), *The Neuman systems model* (pp. 89–99). Upper Saddle River, NJ: Pearson.

Geib, K. (2010). Neuman system's model in nursing practice. In M. R. Alligood (Ed.), *Nursing theory: Utilization & application* (4th ed., pp. 235–260). St Louis, MO: Mosby-Elsevier.

Gigliotti, E., & Fawcett, J. (2002). The Neuman systems model and research instruments. In B. Neuman & J. Fawcett (Eds.), *The Neuman systems model* (4th ed., pp. 150–175). Upper Saddle River, NJ: Pearson.

Hassell, J. S. (1998). Critical thinking strategies for family and community client systems. In L. Lowry (Ed.), *The Neuman systems model and nursing education: Teaching strategies and outcomes* (pp. 71–78). Indianapolis: Center Nursing Press.

Jajic, A., Andrews, H., & Winson Jones, C. (2011). The client system as family, group, or community. In B. Neuman & J. Fawcett (Eds.), *The Neuman systems model* (pp. 70–88). Upper Saddle River, NJ: Pearson.

Kinder, L., Napier, D., Rubertino, M., Surace, A., & Burkholder, J. (2011). Utilizing the Neuman systems model to maintain and enhance the health of a nursing service: Riverside Methodist Hospital. In B. Neuman & J. Fawcett (Eds.), *The Neuman systems model* (pp. 276–280). Upper Saddle River, NJ: Pearson.

Kolcaba, K., & Kolcaba, R. (2011). Linking middle-range theories with the Neuman systems model. In B. Neuman & J. Fawcett (Eds.), *The Neuman systems model* (pp. 299–313). Upper Saddle River, NJ: Pearson.

Lowry, L. W. (1998). Creative teaching and effective evaluation. In L. Lowry (Ed.), *The Neuman systems model and nursing education: Teaching strategies and outcomes* (pp. 17–30). Indianapolis: Center Nursing Press.

Lowry, L. W. (1998). Efficacy of the Neuman systems model as a curriculum framework: A longitudinal study. In L. Lowry (Ed.), *The Neuman systems model and nursing education: Teaching strategies and outcomes* (pp. 139–148). Indianapolis: Center Nursing Press.

Lowry, L. W. (1998). Vision, values, and verities. In L. Lowry (Ed.), *The Neuman systems model and nursing education: Teaching strategies and outcomes* (pp. 167–174). Indianapolis: Center Nursing Press.

Lowry, L. W., Bruick-Sorge, C., Freese, B. T., & Sutherland, R. (1998). Development and renewal of faculty for Neuman-based teaching. In L. Lowry (Ed.), *The Neuman systems model and nursing education: Teaching strategies and outcomes* (pp. 161–166). Indianapolis: Center Nursing Press.

McDowell, B. (2011). Using the Neuman systems model to guide pediatric nursing practice. In B. Neuman & J. Fawcett (Eds.), *The Neuman systems model* (pp. 223–236). Upper Saddle River, NJ: Pearson.

Merks, A., van Tilburg, C., & Lowry, L. (2011). Excellence in practice. In B. Neuman & J. Fawcett (Eds.), *The Neuman systems model* (pp. 253–264). Upper Saddle River, NJ: Pearson.

Munck, C. K., & Merks, A. (2002). Using the Neuman systems model to guide administration of nursing services in Holland: The case of Emergis, institute for mental health care. In B. Neuman & J. Fawcett (Eds.), *The Neuman systems model* (4th ed., pp. 300–316). Upper Saddle River, NJ: Pearson.

Newsome, G. G., & Lowry, L. W. (1998). Evaluation in nursing: History, models, and Neuman's framework. In L. Lowry (Ed.), *The Neuman systems model and nursing education: Teaching strategies and outcomes* (pp. 37–52). Indianapolis: Center Nursing Press.

Nuttall, P. R., Stittich, E. M., & Flores, F. C. (1998). The Neuman systems model in advanced practice nursing. In L. Lowry (Ed.), *The Neuman systems model and nursing education: Teaching strategies and outcomes* (pp. 109–116). Indianapolis: Center Nursing Press.

Pothiban, L. (2002). Using the Neuman systems model to guide nursing research in Thailand. In B. Neuman & J. Fawcett (Eds.), *The Neuman systems model* (4th ed., pp. 183–190). Upper Saddle River, NJ: Pearson.

Reed, K. S. (2002). The Neuman systems model and educational tools. In B. Neuman & J. Fawcett (Eds.), *The Neuman systems model* (4th ed., pp. 238–243). Upper Saddle River, NJ: Pearson.

Sanders, N. F., & Kelley, J. A. (2002). The Neuman systems model and administration of nursing services: An integrative review. In B. Neuman & J. Fawcett (Eds.), *The Neuman systems model* (4th ed., pp. 271–287). Upper Saddle River, NJ: Pearson.

Seng, V. S. (1998). Clinical evaluation: The heart of clinical performance. In L. Lowry (Ed.), *The Neuman systems model and nursing education: Teaching strategies and outcomes* (pp. 129–134). Indianapolis: Center Nursing Press.

Strickland-Seng, V. (1998). Clinical evaluation: The heart of clinical performance. In L. Lowry (Ed.), *The Neuman systems model and nursing education: Teaching strategies and outcomes* (pp. 129–134). Indianapolis: Sigma Theta Tau International. Indianapolis, Center Nursing Press.

Sutherland, R., & Forrest, D. L. (1998). Primary prevention in an associate of science curriculum. In L. Lowry (Ed.), *The Neuman systems model and nursing education: Teaching strategies and outcomes* (pp. 99–108). Indianapolis: Center Nursing Press.

Tarko, M., & Helewka, A. (2011). The client system as an individual. In B. Neuman & J. Fawcett (Eds.), *The Neuman systems model* (pp. 37–69). Upper Saddle River, NJ: Pearson.

Torakis, M. L. (2002). Using the Neuman systems model to guide administration of nursing services in the United States: Redirecting nursing practice in a freestanding pediatric hospital. In B. Neuman & J. Fawcett (Eds.), *The Neuman systems model* (4th ed., pp. 288–299). Upper Saddle River, NJ: Pearson.

Weitzel, A. R., & Wood, K. C. (1998). Community health nursing: Keystone of baccalaureate education. In L. Lowry (Ed.), *The Neuman systems model and nursing education: Teaching strategies and outcomes* (pp. 91–98). Indianapolis: Center Nursing Press.

Journal Articles

Angosta, A. D., Ceria-Ulep, C. D., & Tse, A. M. (2014). Care delivery for Filipino Americans using the Neuman systems model. *Nursing Science Quarterly, 27*(2), 142–148.

Bachman, A. O., Danuser, B., & Morin, D. (2015). Developing a theoretical framework using a nursing perspective to investigate perceived health in the "sandwich generation" group. *Nursing Science Quarterly, 28*(4), 308–318.

Baldacchino, D., Torskenaes, K., Kalfoss, M., Borg, J., Tonna, A., Debattisata, C., et al. (2013). Spiritual coping in rehabilitation—a comparative study: Part 1. *British Journal of Nursing, 22*(4), 228–232.

Baldacchino, D., Torskenaes, K., Kalfoss, M., Borg, J., Tonna, A., Debattisata, C., Decelis, N., et al. (2013). Spiritual coping in rehabilitation—a comparative study: Part 2. *British Journal of Nursing, 22*(7), 402–408.

Baumann, S. L. (2012). What's wrong with the concept self-management? *Nursing Science Quarterly, 25*(4), 362–363.

Beckman, S. J., Boxley-Harges, S. L., & Kaskel, B. L. (2012). Experience informs: Spanning three decades with the Neuman systems model. *Nursing Science Quarterly, 25*(4), 341–346.

Bourdeanu, L., & Dee, V. (2013). Assessment of chemotherapy-induced nausea and vomiting in women with breast cancer: A Neuman systems model framework. *Research & Theory for Nursing Practice, 27*(4), 296–304.

Clarke, P. N., & Lowry, L. (2012). Dialogue with Lois Lowry: Development of the Neuman systems model. *Nursing Science Quarterly, 25*(4), 332–335.

Cobb, R. K. (2012). How well does spirituality predict health status in adults living with HIV-disease: A Neuman systems model study. *Nursing Science Quarterly, 25*(4), 347–355.

DaG, H., Kavlak, O., & Sirin, A. (2014). Neuman systems model and infertility stressors: Review. *Turkiye Klinikleri Hemsirelik Bilimleri, 6*(2), 121–128.

Florczak, K., Poradzisz, M., & Hampson, S. (2012). Nursing in a complex world: A case for grand theory. *Nursing Science Quarterly, 25*(4), 307–312.

Gigliotti, E. (2012). New advances in the use of Neuman's lines of defense and resistance in quantitative research. *Nursing Science Quarterly, 25*(4), 336–340.

Hammonds, L. S. (2012). Implementing a distress screening instrument in a university breast cancer clinic. *Clinical Journal of Oncology Nursing, 16*(5), 491–496.

Huth, J. J., Eliades, A., Handwork, C., Englehart, J. L., & Messenger, J. (2013). Shift worked, quality of sleep, and elevated body mass index in pediatric nurses. *Journal of Pediatric Nursing, 28*(6), e64–e73.

Kuar, S., & Kuar, B. (2012). A descriptive study to assess the awareness of the women regarding cervical cancer. *International Journal of Nursing Education, 4*(1), 66–68.

Lee, Q. (2014). Application of Neuman's system model on the management of a patient with asthma. *Singapore Nursing Journal, 41*(1), 20–25.

Manister, N., & Gigliotti, E. (2016). Emotional eating mediates the relationship between role stress and obesity in clergy. *Nursing Science Quarterly, 29*(2), 136–145.

McClure, M., & Gigliotti, E. (2012). A medieval metaphor to aid use of the Neuman systems model in simulation debriefing. *Nursing Science Quarterly, 25*(4), 318–324.

Morrow, M. R. (2012). Organizational stressors. *Nursing Science Quarterly, 25*(4), 377.

Olowokere, A. E., & Okanlawon, F. A. (2015). Application of Neuman systems model to psychosocial support of vulnerable school children. *West African Journal of Nursing, 26*(1), 14–25.

Piacentine, L. B. (2013). Spirituality, religiosity, depression, anxiety, and drug-use consequences during methadone maintenance therapy. *Western Journal of Nursing Research, 35*(6), 795–814.

Shah, L. B. I., Torres, S., Kannusamy, P., Mui Lee Chng, C., Hong-Gu, H., & Klainin-Yobas, P. (2015). Efficacy of the virtual reality-based stressed management program on stress-related variables in people with mood disorders: The feasibility study. *Archives of Psychiatric Nursing, 29*(1), 6–13.

Thomas, L. S., Stephenson, N., Swanson, M., Jesse, D. E., & Brown, S. (2013). A pilot study: The effect of healing touch on anxiety, stress, pain, pain medication usage, and physiologic measures in hospitalized sickle cell disease adults experiencing a vaso-occlusive pain episode. *Journal of Holistic Nursing, 31*(4), 234–247.

Turner, S. B., & Kaylor, S. D. (2015). Neuman systems model as a conceptual framework for nurse resilience. *Nursing Science Quarterly, 28*(3), 213–217.

Dissertations and Theses

Bynum, D. (2012). *The development and testing of the codependency-overeating model in undergraduate social science students in a Mississippi college.* (Doctoral dissertation). Retrieved from ProQuest. (Order No. 3529677).

Davis, P. A. (2012). *The relationship of sensory impairment and risk factors for falls in long term care elders.* (Doctoral dissertation). Retrieved from ProQuest. (Order No. 3587476).

Huggins, S. E. (2012). *Promoting successful nursing retention using orientation programs.* (Doctoral dissertation). Retrieved from ProQuest. (Order No. 3508892).

Ioli, J. G. (2015). *Basic social processes of primary care outpatient staff registered nurses.* (Doctoral dissertation). Retrieved from ProQuest. (Order No. 3701054).

Lyttle, D. (2014). *The identification of HIV-risk behaviors among minority college students using the Neuman systems model.* (Doctoral dissertation). Retrieved from ProQuest. (Order No. 3672349).

Manister, N. (2012). *Role stress, eating behaviors, and obesity in clergy.* (Doctoral dissertation). Retrieved from ProQuest. (Order No. 3508841).

Monahan, J. C. (2012). *Perioperative experiences of adolescents.* (Doctoral dissertation). Retrieved from ProQuest. (Order No. 3517560).

Ngangana, P. C. (2014). *Intra-family stressors among adult siblings sharing caregiving for parents.* (Doctoral dissertation). Retrieved from ProQuest. (Order No. 3672353).

Njoku, G. U. (2015). *The impact of caring for seniors on the caregiver's stress level.* (Doctoral dissertation). Retrieved from ProQuest. (Order No. 3687251).

Owens, A. (2014). *Comparing nurse job satisfaction between different work environments.* (Doctoral dissertation). Retrieved from ProQuest. (Order No. 3646160).

Rideout, L. C. (2012). *Nurses' perceptions of barriers and facilitators affecting the shaken baby syndrome education initiative: An exploratory study of a Massachusetts public policy.* (Doctoral dissertation). Retrieved from ProQuest. (Order No. 3539211).

Roojanavech, S. (2012). *Spirituality and early sexual initiation among Thai adolescents.* (Doctoral dissertation). Retrieved from ProQuest. (Order No. 3523206).

Smith-Johnson, B. A. (2013). *Perceived stress of African American family caregivers of stroke survivors.* (Doctoral dissertation). Retrieved from ProQuest. (Order No. 3561679).

Yau, C. Y. (2013). *The effects of nurse-initiated early pain management program (NIEPMP) for acute back pain in emergency medicine ward: A randomized controlled trial.* (Doctoral dissertation). Retrieved from ProQuest. (Order No. 3586798).

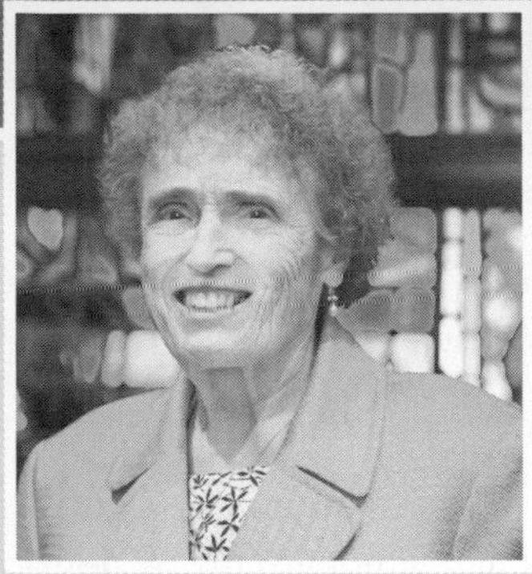

Sister Callista Roy
(1939–Present)

17

Adaptation Model

*Kenneth D. Phillips and Robin Harris**

"God is intimately revealed in the diversity of creation and is the common destiny of creation; persons use human creative abilities of awareness, enlightenment, and faith; and persons are accountable for the process of deriving, sustaining, and transforming the universe."
(Roy, 2000, p. 127)

CREDENTIALS AND BACKGROUND OF THE THEORIST

Sister Callista Roy, a member of the Sisters of Saint Joseph of Carondelet, was born on October 14, 1939, in Los Angeles, California. She received a bachelor's degree in nursing in 1963 from Mount Saint Mary's College in Los Angeles and a master's degree in nursing from the University of California, Los Angeles, in 1966. After earning her nursing degrees, Roy began her education in sociology, receiving both a master's degree in sociology in 1973 and a doctorate degree in sociology in 1977 from the University of California.

While working toward her master's degree, Roy was challenged in a seminar with Dorothy E. Johnson to develop a conceptual model for nursing. While working as a pediatric staff nurse, Roy had noticed the great resiliency of children and their ability to adapt in response to major physical and psychological changes. Roy was impressed by adaptation as an appropriate conceptual framework for nursing. Roy developed the basic concepts of the model while she was a graduate student at the University of California, Los Angeles, from 1964 to 1966. Roy began operationalizing her model in 1968 when Mount Saint Mary's College adopted the adaptation framework as the philosophical foundation of the nursing curriculum. The Roy adaptation model was first presented in the literature in an article published in *Nursing Outlook* in 1970 titled "Adaptation: A Conceptual Framework for Nursing" (Roy, 1970).

Roy was an associate professor and chairperson of the Department of Nursing at Mount Saint Mary's College until 1982. She was promoted to the rank of professor in 1983 at both Mount Saint Mary's College and the University of Portland, Oregon. She helped initiate and taught in a summer master's program at the University of Portland. From 1983 to 1985, she was a Robert Wood Johnson postdoctoral fellow at the University of California, San Francisco, as a clinical nurse scholar in neuroscience. During this time, she conducted research on nursing interventions for cognitive recovery in head injuries and on the influence of nursing models on clinical decision making. In 1987 Roy began the newly created position of nurse theorist at Boston College School of Nursing.

Roy has published many books, chapters, and periodical articles and has presented numerous lectures and workshops focusing on her nursing adaptation theory (Roy & Andrews, 1991). The refinement and restatement of the Roy adaptation model is published in her 1999 book, *The Roy Adaptation Model* (Roy & Andrews, 1999).

Roy is a member of Sigma Theta Tau, and she received the National Founder's Award for Excellence in Fostering

*Previous authors: Robin F. Harris, Kenneth D. Phillips, Carolyn L. Blue, Karen M. Brubaker, Julia M. B. Fine, Martha J. Kirsch, Katherine R. Papazian, Cynthia M. Riester, and Mary Ann Sobiech. The authors wish to express appreciation to Sister Callista Roy for critiquing the chapter.

Professional Nursing Standards in 1981. Her achievements include an Honorary Doctorate of Humane Letters from Alverno College (1984), honorary doctorates from Eastern Michigan University (1985) and St. Joseph's College in Maine (1999), and an *American Journal of Nursing* Book of the Year Award for *Essentials of the Roy Adaptation Model* (Andrews & Roy, 1986). Roy has been recognized as the World Who's Who of Women (1979); Personalities of America (1978); fellow of the American Academy of Nursing (1978); recipient of a Fulbright Senior Scholar Award from the Australian-American Educational Foundation (1989), and recipient of the Martha Rogers Award for Advancing Nursing Science from the National League for Nursing (1991). Roy received the Outstanding Alumna award and the prestigious Carondelet Medal from her alma mater, Mount Saint Mary's. The American Academy of Nursing honored Roy for her extraordinary life achievements by recognizing her as a Living Legend (2007).

THEORETICAL SOURCES

Derivation of the Roy adaptation model for nursing included a citation of Harry Helson's work in psychophysics that extended to social and behavioral sciences (Roy, 1984). In Helson's adaptation theory, adaptive responses are a function of the incoming stimulus and the adaptive level (Roy, 1984). A stimulus is any factor that provokes a response. Stimuli may arise from the internal or the external environment (Roy, 1984). The adaptation level is made up of the pooled effect of three classes of stimuli:

1. **Focal stimuli** immediately confront the individual.
2. **Contextual stimuli** are all other stimuli present that contribute to the effect of the focal stimulus.
3. **Residual stimuli** are environmental factors of which the effects are unclear in a given situation.

Helson's work developed the concept of the adaptation level zone, which determines whether a stimulus will elicit a positive or negative response. According to Helson's theory, adaptation is the process of responding positively to environmental changes (Roy & Roberts, 1981).

Roy (Roy & Roberts, 1981) combined Helson's work with Rapoport's definition of system to view the person as an adaptive system. With Helson's adaptation theory as a foundation, Roy (1970) developed and further refined the model with concepts and theory from Dohrenwend, Lazarus, Mechanic, and Selye. Roy gave special credit to coauthors Driever, for outlining subdivisions of self-integrity, and Martinez and Sato, for identifying common and primary stimuli affecting the modes. Other co-workers also elaborated the concepts. Poush-Tedrow and Van Landingham made contributions to the interdependence mode, and Randell made contributions to the role function mode.

After the development of her model, Roy presented it as a framework for nursing practice, research, and education. Roy (1971) acknowledged that more than 1500 faculty and students contributed to the theoretical development of the adaptation model. She presented the model as a curriculum framework to a large audience at the 1977 Nurse Educator Conference in Chicago (Roy, 1979). By 1987 it was estimated that more than 100,000 nurses in the United States and Canada had been prepared to practice using the Roy model.

In *Introduction to Nursing: An Adaptation Model,* Roy (1976a) discussed self-concept and group identity mode. She and her collaborators cited the work of Coombs and Snygg regarding self-consistency and major influencing factors of self-concept (Roy, 1984). Social interaction theories are cited to provide a theoretical basis. For example, Roy (1984) notes that Cooley (1902) theorizes that self-perception is influenced by perceptions of others' responses, termed the "looking glass self." She points out that Mead expands the idea by hypothesizing that self-appraisal uses the generalized other. Roy builds on Sullivan's suggestion that self arises from social interaction (Roy, 1984). Gardner and Erickson support Roy's developmental approaches (Roy, 1984). The other modes—physiological-physical, role function, and interdependence—were drawn similarly from biological and behavioral sciences for an understanding of the person.

Additional development of the model occurred during the later 1900s and into the 21st century. These developments included updated scientific and philosophical assumptions; a redefinition of adaptation and adaptation levels; extension of the adaptive modes to group-level knowledge development; and analysis, critique, and synthesis of the first 25 years of research based on the Roy adaptation model. Roy agrees with other theorists who believe that changes in the person-environment systems of the earth are so extensive that a major epoch is ending (Davies, 1988; De Chardin, 1966). During the 67 million years of the Cenozoic era, the Age of Mammals and an era of great creativity, human life appeared on Earth. During this era, humankind has had little or no influence on the universe (Roy, 1997). "As the era closes, humankind has taken extensive control of the life systems of the earth. Roy claims that we are now in the position of deciding what kind of universe we will inhabit" (Roy, 1997, p. 42). Roy "has made the foci of assumptions of the twenty-first century mutual complex person and environment self-organization and a meaningful destiny of convergence of the universe, persons, and environment in what can be considered a supreme being or God" (Roy & Andrews, 1999, p. 395). According to Roy (1997), "persons are coextensive with their physical and social environments" (p. 43) and they

MAJOR CONCEPTS & DEFINITIONS

System

A **system** is "a set of parts connected to function as a whole for some purpose and that does so by virtue of the interdependence of its parts" (Roy & Andrews, 1999, p. 32). In addition to having wholeness and related parts, "systems also have inputs, outputs, and control and feedback processes" (Andrews & Roy, 1991, p. 7).

Adaptation Level

"**Adaptation level** represents the condition of the life processes described on three levels as integrated, compensatory, and compromised" (Roy & Andrews, 1999, p. 30). A person's adaptation level is "a constantly changing point, made up of focal, contextual, and residual stimuli, which represent the person's own standard of the range of stimuli to which one can respond with ordinary adaptive responses" (Roy, 1984, pp. 27–28).

Adaptation Problems

Adaptation problems are "broad areas of concern related to adaptation. These describe the difficulties related to the indicators of positive adaptation" (Roy & Andrews, 1999, p. 65). Roy (1984) states the following: "It can be noted at this point that the distinction being made between adaptation problems and nursing diagnoses is based on the developing work in both of these fields. At this point, adaptation problems are seen not as nursing diagnoses, but as areas of concern for the nurse related to adapting person or group (within each adaptive mode)" (pp. 89–90).

"share a destiny with the universe and are responsible for mutual transformations" (Roy & Andrews, 1999, p. 395). Developments of the model that were related to the integral relationship between person and environment have been influenced by Pierre Teilhard De Chardin's law of progressive complexity and increasing consciousness (De Chardin, 1959, 1965, 1966, 1969) and the work of Swimme and Berry (1992).

Focal Stimulus

The **focal stimulus** is "the internal or external stimulus most immediately confronting the human system" (Roy & Andrews, 1999, p. 31).

Contextual Stimuli

Contextual stimuli "are all other stimuli present in the situation that contribute to the effect of the focal stimulus" (Roy & Andrews, 1999, p. 31); that is, "contextual stimuli are all the environmental factors that present to the person from within or without but which are not the center of the person's attention and/or energy" (Andrews & Roy, 1991, p. 9).

Residual Stimuli

Residual stimuli "are environmental factors within or without the human system with effects in the current situation that are unclear" (Roy & Andrews, 1999, p. 32).

Coping Processes

Coping processes "are innate or acquired ways of interacting with the changing environment" (Roy & Andrews, 1999, p. 31).

Innate Coping Mechanisms

Innate coping mechanisms "are genetically determined or common to the species and are generally viewed as automatic processes; humans do not have to think about them" (Roy & Andrews, 1999, p. 46).

Acquired Coping Mechanisms

Acquired coping mechanisms "are developed through strategies such as learning. The experiences encountered throughout life contribute to customary responses to particular stimuli" (Roy & Andrews, 1999, p. 46).

Regulator Subsystem

Regulator Subsystem is "a major coping process involving the neural, chemical, and endocrine systems" (Roy & Andrews, 1999, p. 32).

Cognator Subsystem

Cognator Subsystem is "a major coping process involving four cognitive-emotive channels: perceptual and information processing, learning, judgment, and emotion" (Roy & Andrews, 1999, p. 31).

Adaptive Responses

Adaptive responses are those "that promote integrity in terms of the goals of human systems" (Roy & Andrews, 1999, p. 31).

Ineffective Responses

Ineffective responses are those "that do not contribute to integrity in terms of the goals of the human system" (Roy & Andrews, 1999, p. 31).

Integrated Life Process

Integrated life process refers to the "adaptation level at which the structures and functions of a life process are working as a whole to meet human needs" (Roy & Andrews, 1999, p. 31).

Physiological-Physical Mode

The **physiological-physical mode** "is associated with the physical and chemical processes involved in the function and activities of living organisms" (Roy & Andrews, 1999, p. 102). Five needs are identified in the physiological-physical mode relative to the basic need of physiological integrity: (1) oxygenation, (2) nutrition, (3) elimination, (4) activity and rest, and (5) protection. Complex processes that include the senses; fluid, electrolyte, and acid-base balance; neurological function; and endocrine function contribute to physiological adaptation. The basic need of the physiological-physical mode is physiological integrity (Roy & Andrews, 1999). The physical mode is "the manner in which the collective human adaptive system manifests adaptation relative to basic operating resources, participants, physical facilities, and fiscal resources" (Roy & Andrews, 1999, p. 104). The basic need of the physical mode is operating integrity.

Self-Concept–Group Identity Mode

The **self-concept–group identity mode** is one of the three psychosocial modes; "it focuses specifically on the psychological and spiritual aspects of the human system. The basic need underlying the individual self-concept mode has been identified as psychic and spiritual integrity, or the need to know who one is so that one can be or exist with a sense of unity, meaning, and purposefulness in the universe" (Roy & Andrews, 1999, p. 107). "Self-concept is defined as the composite of beliefs and feelings about oneself at a given time and is formed from internal perceptions and perceptions of others' reactions" (Roy & Andrews, 1999, p. 107). Its components include (1) the physical self, which involves sensation and body image, and (2) the personal self, which is made up of self-consistency, self-ideal or expectancy, and the moral-ethical-spiritual self. The group identity mode "reflects how people in groups perceive themselves based on environmental feedback. The group identity mode [is composed] of interpersonal relationships, group self-image, social milieu, and culture" (Roy & Andrews, 1999, p. 108). The basic need of the group identity mode is identity integrity (Roy & Andrews, 1999).

Role Function Mode

The **role function mode** "is one of two social modes and focuses on the roles the person occupies in society. A role, as the functioning unit of society, is defined as a set of expectations about how a person occupying one position behaves toward a person occupying another position. The basic need underlying the role function mode has been identified as social integrity—the need to know who one is in relation to others so that one can act" (Hill & Roberts, 1981, pp. 109–110). Persons perform primary, secondary, and tertiary roles. These roles are carried out with both instrumental and expressive behaviors. Instrumental behavior is "the actual physical performance of a behavior" (Andrews, 1991, p. 348). Expressive behaviors are "the feelings, attitudes, likes or dislikes that a person has about a role or about the performance of a role" (Andrews, 1991, p. 348).

> *"The primary role determines the majority of behavior engaged in by the person during a particular period of life. It is determined by age, sex, and developmental stage."*
>
> ***(Andrews, 1991, p. 349)***

> *"Secondary roles are those that a person assumes to complete the task associated with a developmental stage and primary role."*
>
> ***(Andrews, 1991, p. 349)***

> *"Tertiary roles are related primarily to secondary roles and represent ways in which individuals meet their role associated obligations. . . . Tertiary roles are normally temporary in nature, freely chosen by the individual, and may include activities such as clubs or hobbies."*
>
> ***(Andrews, 1991, p. 349)***

The major roles that one plays can be analyzed by imagining a tree formation. The trunk of the tree is one's primary role, or developmental level, such as a generative adult female. Secondary roles branch off from this—for example, wife, mother, and teacher. Finally, tertiary roles branch off from secondary roles—for example, the mother role might involve the role of parent-teacher association president for a given period. Each of these roles is seen as occurring in a dyadic relationship, that is, with a reciprocal role (Roy & Andrews, 1999).

Interdependence Mode

> *"The interdependence mode focuses on close relationships of people (individually and collectively) and their purpose, structure, and development. . . . Interdependent relationships involve the willingness and ability to give to others and accept from them aspects of all that one has to offer such as love, respect, value, nurturing, knowledge, skills, commitments, material possessions, time, and talents."*
>
> ***(Roy & Andrews, 1999, p. 111)***

The basic need of this mode is termed *relational integrity* (Roy & Andrews, 1999).

> *"Two specific relationships are the focus of the interdependence mode as it applies to individuals. The first is with significant others, persons who are the most important to the individual. The second is with support systems, that is, others contributing to meeting interdependence needs."*
>
> ***(Roy & Andrews, 1999, p. 112)***

Two major areas of interdependence behaviors have been identified: receptive behavior and contributive behavior. These behaviors apply, respectively, to the "receiving and giving of love, respect and value in interdependent relationships" (Roy & Andrews, 1999, p. 112).

Perception

"Perception is the interpretation of a stimulus and the conscious appreciation of it" (Pollock, 1993, p. 169). Perception links the regulator with the cognator and connects the adaptive modes (Rambo, 1983).

USE OF EMPIRICAL EVIDENCE

From this beginning, the Roy adaptation model has been supported through research in practice and in education (Brower & Baker, 1976; Farkas, 1981; Mastal & Hammond, 1980; Meleis, 1985, 2007; Roy, 1980; Roy & Obloy, 1978; Wagner, 1976). In 1999 (Roy & Andrews, 1999) a group of seven scholars working with Roy conducted a meta-analysis, critique, and synthesis of 163 studies based on the Roy adaptation model that had been published in 44 English language journals on five continents and dissertations and theses from the United States. Of these 163 studies, 116 met the criteria established for testing propositions from the model. Twelve generic propositions based on Roy's earlier work were derived. To synthesize the research, findings of each study were used to state ancillary and practice propositions, and support for the propositions was examined. Of 265 propositions tested, 216 (82%) were supported. Roy (2011a) presented a comprehensive review of research based on the adaptation model for the past 25 years in *Nursing Science Quarterly*. The entire issue is dedicated to honoring Callista Roy and her life work.

MAJOR ASSUMPTIONS

Assumptions from systems theory and assumptions from adaptation level theory have been combined into a single set of scientific assumptions. From systems theory, human adaptive systems are viewed as interactive parts that act in unity for some purpose. Human adaptive systems are complex and multifaceted and respond to myriad environmental stimuli to achieve adaptation. With their ability to adapt to environmental stimuli, humans have the capacity to create changes in the environment (Roy & Andrews, 1999). Drawing on characteristics of creation spirituality by Swimme and Berry (1992), Roy combined the assumptions of humanism and veritivity into a single set of philosophical assumptions. Humanism asserts that the person and human experiences are essential to knowing and valuing, and that they share in creative power. Veritivity affirms the belief in the purpose, value, and meaning of all human life. These scientific and philosophical assumptions have been refined for use of the model in the 21st century (Box 17.1).

BOX 17.1 Assumption Revision Basic to Concepts for the Twenty-First Century

Scientific Assumptions

- Systems of matter and energy progress to higher levels of complex self-organization.
- Consciousness and meaning are constitutive of person and environment integration.
- Awareness of self and environment is rooted in thinking and feeling.
- Humans, by their decisions, are accountable for the integration of creative processes.
- Thinking and feeling mediate human action.
- System relationships include acceptance, protection, and fostering of interdependence.
- Persons and the earth have common patterns and integral relationships.
- Persons and environment transformations are created in human consciousness.
- Integration of human and environment meanings results in adaptation.

Philosophical Assumptions

- Persons have mutual relationships with the world and God.
- Human meaning is rooted in an omega point convergence of the universe.
- God is ultimately revealed in the diversity of creation and is the common destiny of creation.
- Persons use human creative abilities of awareness, enlightenment, and faith.
- Persons are accountable for the processes of deriving, sustaining, and transforming the universe.

Adaptation

Roy has further defined adaptation for use in the 21st century (Roy & Andrews, 1999). According to Roy, **adaptation** refers to "the process and outcome whereby thinking and feeling persons, as individuals or in groups, use conscious awareness and choice to create human and environmental integration" (Roy & Andrews, 1999, p. 30). Rather than being a human system that simply strives to respond to environmental stimuli to maintain integrity, every human life is purposeful in a universe that is creative, and persons are inseparable from their environment.

NURSING

Roy defines **nursing** broadly as a "health care profession that focuses on human life processes and patterns and emphasizes promotion of health for individuals, families, groups, and society as a whole" (Roy & Andrews, 1999, p. 4). Specifically, Roy defines nursing according to her model as the science and practice that expands adaptive abilities and enhances person and environmental transformation. She identifies nursing activities as the assessment of behavior and the stimuli that influence adaptation. Nursing judgments are based on this assessment, and interventions are planned to manage the stimuli (Roy & Andrews, 1999). Roy differentiates nursing as a science from nursing as a practice discipline. Nursing science is "a developing system of knowledge about persons that observes, classifies, and relates the processes by which persons positively affect their health status" (Roy, 1984, pp. 3–4). "Nursing as a practice discipline [is] nursing's scientific body of knowledge used for the purpose of providing an essential service to people, that is, promoting ability to affect health positively" (Roy, 1984). "Nursing acts to enhance the interaction of the person with the environment—to promote adaptation" (Andrews & Roy, 1991, p. 20).

Roy's goal of nursing is "the promotion of adaptation for individuals and groups in each of the four adaptive modes, thus contributing to health, quality of life, and dying with dignity" (Roy & Andrews, 1999, p. 19). Nursing fills a unique role as a facilitator of adaptation by assessing behavior in each of these four adaptive modes and factors influencing adaptation and by intervening to promote adaptive abilities and to enhance environment interactions (Roy & Andrews, 1999).

Person

According to Roy, humans are holistic, adaptive systems. "As an adaptive system, the human system is described as a whole with parts that function as unity for some purpose. Human systems include people as individuals or in groups, including families, organizations, communities, and society as a whole" (Roy & Andrews, 1999, p. 31). Despite their great diversity, all persons are united in a common destiny (Roy & Andrews, 1999). "Human systems have thinking and feeling capacities, rooted in consciousness and meaning, by which they adjust effectively to changes in the environment and, in turn, affect the environment" (Roy & Andrews, 1999, p. 36). Persons and the earth have common patterns and mutuality of relationships and meaning (Roy & Andrews, 1999). Roy (Roy & Andrews, 1999) defined the person as the main focus of nursing, the recipient of nursing care, a living, complex, adaptive system with internal processes (cognator and regulator) acting to maintain adaptation in the four adaptive modes (physiological, self-concept, role function, and interdependence).

Health

"Health is a state and a process of being and becoming integrated and a whole person. It is a reflection of adaptation, that is, the interaction of the person and the environment" (Andrews & Roy, 1991, p. 21). Roy (1984) derived this definition from the thought that adaptation is a process of promoting physiological, psychological, and social integrity, and that integrity implies an unimpaired condition leading to completeness or unity. In her earlier work, Roy viewed health along a continuum flowing from death and extreme poor health to high-level and peak wellness (Brower & Baker, 1976). During the late 1990s, Roy's writings focused more on health as a process in which health and illness can coexist (Roy & Andrews, 1999). Drawing on the writings of Illich (1974, 1976), Roy wrote, "health is not freedom from the inevitability of death, disease, unhappiness, and stress, but the ability to cope with them in a competent way" (Roy & Andrews, 1999, p. 52).

Health and illness is one inevitable, coexistent dimensions of the person's total life experience (Riehl & Roy, 1980). Nursing is concerned with this dimension. When mechanisms for coping are ineffective, illness is the result. Health ensues when humans continually adapt. As people adapt to stimuli, they are free to respond to other stimuli. The freeing of energy from ineffective coping attempts can promote healing and enhance health (Roy, 1984).

Environment

According to Roy, environment is "all the conditions, circumstances, and influences surrounding and affecting the development and behavior of persons or groups, with particular consideration of the mutuality of person and earth resources that includes focal, contextual, and residual stimuli" (Roy & Andrews, 1999, p. 81). "It is the changing environment [that] stimulates the person to make adaptive responses" (Andrews & Roy, 1991, p. 18). Environment is the input into the person as an adaptive system involving both internal and external factors. These factors may be slight or large, negative or positive. However, any environmental change demands increasing energy to adapt to the situation. Factors in the environment that affect the person are categorized as focal, contextual, and residual stimuli.

THEORETICAL ASSERTIONS

Roy's model focuses on the concept of adaptation of the person. Her concepts of nursing, person, health, and environment are all interrelated to this central concept. The person continually experiences environmental stimuli. Ultimately, a response is made and adaptation occurs. This response may be either an adaptive or an ineffective response. Adaptive responses promote integrity and help the person to achieve the goals of adaptation; that is, they achieve survival, growth, reproduction, mastery, and person and environmental transformations. Ineffective responses fail to achieve or threaten the goals of adaptation. Nursing has a unique goal to assist the person's adaptation effort by managing the environment. The result is attainment of an optimal level of wellness by the person (Andrews & Roy, 1986; Randell, Tedrow, & Van Landingham, 1982; Roy, 1970, 1971, 1980, 1984; Roy & Roberts, 1981).

As an open living system, the person receives inputs or stimuli from both the environment and the self. The adaptation level is determined by the combined effect of focal, contextual, and residual stimuli. Adaptation occurs when the person responds positively to environmental changes. This adaptive response promotes the integrity of the person, which leads to health. Ineffective responses to stimuli lead to disruption of the integrity of the person (Andrews & Roy, 1986; Randell, Tedrow, & Van Landingham, 1982; Roy, 1970, 1971, 1980; Roy & McLeod, 1981).

There are two interrelated subsystems in Roy's model (Fig. 17.1). The primary, functional, or control processes subsystem consists of the regulator and the cognator. The secondary, effector subsystem consists of four adaptive modes: (1) physiological needs, (2) self-concept, (3) role function, and (4) interdependence (Andrews & Roy, 1986; Limandri, 1986; Mastal, Hammond, & Roberts, 1982; Meleis, 1985, 2007; Riehl & Roy, 1980; Roy, 1971, 1975).

Roy views the regulator and the cognator as methods of coping. The regulator coping subsystem, by way of the physiological adaptive mode, "responds automatically through neural, chemical, and endocrine coping processes" (Andrews & Roy, 1991, p. 14). The cognator coping subsystem, by way of the self-concept, interdependence, and role function adaptive modes, "responds through four cognitive-emotive channels: perceptual information processing, learning, judgment, and emotion" (Andrews & Roy, 1991, p. 14). Perception is the interpretation of a stimulus, and perception links the regulator with the cognator in that "input into the regulator is transformed into perceptions. Perception is a process of the cognator. The responses following perception are feedback into both the cognator and the regulator" (Galligan, 1979, p. 67).

The four adaptive modes of the two subsystems in Roy's model provide form or manifestations of cognator and regulator activity. Responses to stimuli are carried out through four adaptive modes. The physiological-physical adaptive mode is concerned with the way humans interact with the environment through physiological processes to meet the basic needs of oxygenation, nutrition, elimination, activity and rest, and protection. The self-concept group identity adaptive mode is concerned with the need to know who one is and how to act in society. An individual's self-concept is defined by Roy as "the composite of beliefs or feelings that an individual holds about him- or herself at any given time" (Roy & Andrews, 1999, p. 49). An individual's self-concept is composed of the physical self (body sensation and body image) and the personal self (self-consistency, self-ideal, and moral-ethical-spiritual self). The role function adaptive mode describes the primary, secondary, and tertiary roles that an individual performs in society. A role describes the

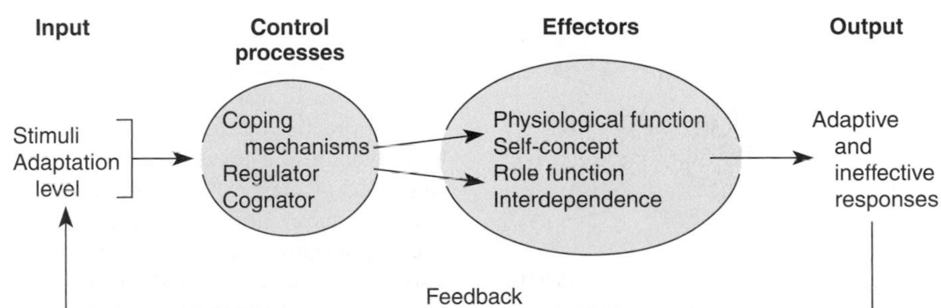

FIG. 17.1 Person as an adaptive system. (From Roy, C. [1984]. *Introduction to nursing: An adaptation model* [2nd ed., p. 30]. Englewood Cliffs, NJ: Prentice Hall.)

expectations about how one person behaves toward another person. The interdependence adaptive mode describes the interactions of people in society. The major task of the interdependence adaptive mode is for persons to give and receive love, respect, and value. The most important components of the interdependence adaptive mode are a person's significant other (spouse, child, friend, or God) and his or her social support system. The purpose of the four adaptive modes is to achieve physiological, psychological, and social integrity. The four adaptive modes are interrelated through perception (Roy & Andrews, 1999) (Fig. 17.2).

The person as a whole is made up of six subsystems. These subsystems (the regulator, the cognator, and the four adaptive modes) are interrelated to form a complex system for the purpose of adaptation. Relationships among the four adaptive modes occur when internal and external stimuli affect more than one mode, when disruptive behavior occurs in more than one mode, or when one mode becomes the focal, contextual, or residual stimulus for another mode (Brower & Baker, 1976; Chinn & Kramer, 2008; Mastal & Hammond, 1980).

With regard to human social systems, Roy broadly categorizes the control processes into the stabilizer and innovator subsystems. The stabilizer subsystem is analogous to the regulator subsystem of the individual and is concerned with stability. To maintain the system, the stabilizer subsystem involves organizational structure, cultural values, and regulation of daily activities of the system. The innovator subsystem is associated with the cognator subsystem of the individual and is concerned with creativity, change, and growth (Roy & Andrews, 1999).

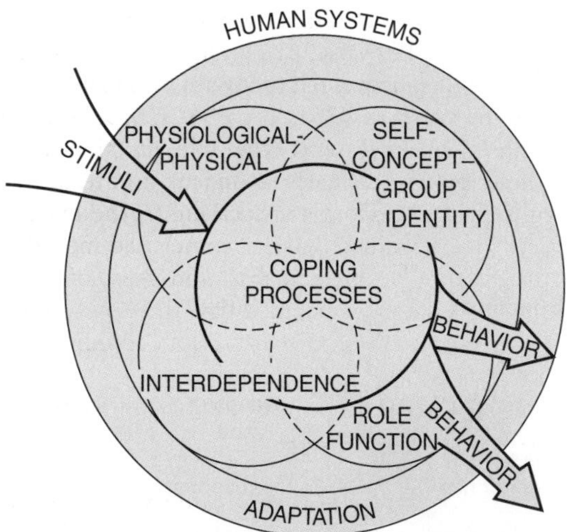

FIG. 17.2 Human adaptive systems. (Roy, Sister Callista; Andrews, Heather A., THE ROY ADAPTATION MODEL, 2nd Ed., ©1998. Reprinted by permission of Pearson Education, Inc., New York, New York.)

LOGICAL FORM

The Roy adaptation model of nursing is both deductive and inductive. It is deductive in that much of Roy's theory is derived from Helson's psychophysics theory. Helson developed the concepts of focal, contextual, and residual stimuli, which Roy (1971) redefined within nursing to form a typology of factors related to adaptation levels of persons. Roy also uses other concepts and theory outside the discipline of nursing and synthesizes these within her adaptation theory.

Roy's adaptation theory is inductive in that she developed the four adaptive modes from research and nursing practice experiences of herself, her colleagues, and her students. Roy built on the conceptual framework of adaptation and developed a step-by-step model by which nurses use the nursing process to administer nursing care to promote adaptation in situations of health and illness (Roy, 1976a, 1980, 1984).

ACCEPTANCE BY THE NURSING COMMUNITY

Practice

The Roy adaptation model is deeply rooted in nursing practice, and this, in part, contributes to its continued success (Fawcett, 2002). It remains one of the most frequently used conceptual frameworks to guide nursing practice, and it is used nationally and internationally (Roy & Andrews, 1999; Fawcett, 2005).

Roy's model is useful for nursing practice, because it outlines the features of the discipline and provides direction for practice, education, and research. The model considers goals, values, the patient, and practitioner interventions. Roy's nursing process is well developed. The two-level assessment assists in identification of nursing goals and diagnoses (Brower & Baker, 1976).

Early on, it was recognized as a valuable theory for nursing practice because of the goal that specified its aim for activity and a prescription for activities to realize the goal (Dickoff, James, & Wiedenbach, 1968a, 1968b). The goal of nursing and of the model is adaptation in four adaptive modes in a person's health and illness. The prescriptive interventions are when the nurse manages stimuli by removing, increasing, decreasing, or altering them. These prescriptions may be found in the list of practice-related hypotheses generated by the model (Roy, 1984).

When using Roy's six-step nursing process, the nurse performs six functions:

1. Assesses the behaviors manifested from the four adaptive modes
2. Assesses the stimuli for those behaviors and categorizes them as focal, contextual, or residual stimuli
3. Makes a statement or nursing diagnosis of the person's adaptive state
4. Sets goals to promote adaptation
5. Implements interventions aimed at managing the stimuli to promote adaptation
6. Evaluates whether the adaptive goals have been met

By manipulating the stimuli and not the patient, the nurse enhances "the interaction of the person with their environment, thereby promoting health" (Andrews & Roy, 1986, p. 51). The nursing process is well suited for use in a practice setting. The two-level assessment is unique to this model and leads to the identification of adaptation problems or nursing diagnoses.

Roy and colleagues have developed a typology of nursing diagnoses from the perspective of the Roy adaptation model (Roy, 1984; Roy & Roberts, 1981). In this typology, commonly recurring problems have been related to the basic needs of the four adaptive modes (Andrews & Roy, 1991).

Intervention is based specifically on the model, but there is a need to develop an organization of categories of nursing interventions (Roy & Roberts, 1981). Nurses provide interventions that alter, increase, decrease, remove, or maintain stimuli (Roy & Andrews, 1999). Roy recommends the nursing judgment model outlined by McDonald and Harms (1966) to guide selection of the best intervention for modifying a particular stimulus. According to this model, a number of alternative interventions are generated that may be appropriate for modifying the stimulus. Each possible intervention is judged for the expected consequences of modifying a stimulus, the probability that a consequence will occur (high, moderate, or low), and the value of the change (desirable or undesirable).

Senesac (2003) reviewed the literature for evidence that the Roy adaptation model is being implemented in nursing practice. She reported that the Roy adaptation model has been used to the greatest extent by individual nurses to understand, plan, and direct nursing practice in the care of individual patients. Although fewer examples of implementation of the adaptation model are found in institutional practice settings, such examples do exist. She concluded that if the model is to be implemented successfully as a practice philosophy, it should be reflected in the mission and vision statements of the institution, recruitment tools, assessment tools, nursing care plans, and other documents related to patient care.

The Roy adaptation model is useful in guiding nursing practice in institutional settings. It has been implemented in a neonatal intensive care unit, an acute surgical ward, a rehabilitation unit, two general hospital units, an orthopedic hospital, a neurosurgical unit, and a 145-bed hospital, among others (Roy & Andrews, 1999).

Weiland (2010) described use of the Roy adaptation model in the critical care setting by advanced practice nurses to incorporate spiritual care into nursing care of patients and families. Spiritual care is an important, but often overlooked, aspect of nursing care for patients in the critical care setting.

The Roy adaptation model has been applied to the nursing care of individual groups of patients. Examples of the wide range of applications of the Roy adaptation model are found in the literature. Villareal (2003) applied the model to the care of young women who were contemplating smoking cessation. The author provides a comprehensive discussion of the use of Roy's six-step nursing process to guide nursing care for women in their mid-20s who smoked and were members of a closed support group. The researcher performed a two-level assessment. In the first level, stimuli were identified for each of the four adaptive modes. In the second level, the nurse made a judgment about the focal (nicotine addiction), contextual (belief that smoking is enjoyable, makes them feel good, relaxes them, brings them a sense of comfort, and is part of their routine), and residual stimuli (beliefs and attitudes about their body image and that smoking cessation causes weight gain). The nurse made the nursing diagnosis that for this group, a lack of motivation to quit smoking was related to dependency. The women in the support group and the nurse mutually established short-term goals to change behaviors, rather than the long-term goal of smoking cessation. The intervention focused on discussion of the effects of smoking on the body, reasons and beliefs about smoking and smoking cessation, stress management, nutrition, physical activity, and self-esteem. During the evaluation phase, it was determined that the women had moved from precontemplation to the contemplation phase of smoking cessation. The author concluded that the Roy adaptation model provided a useful framework for providing care to women who smoke.

Samarel, Tulman, and Fawcett (2002) examined the effects of two types of social support (telephone and group social support) and education on adaptation to early-stage breast cancer in a sample of 125 women. Women in the experimental group received both types of social support and education ($n = 34$); women in the first control group received only telephone support and education, and women in the second control group received only education. Mood disturbance and loneliness were reduced significantly for the experimental group and for the first control group but were not reduced for the second control group. No differences were observed among the groups in terms of cancer-related worry or well-being. This study provides an excellent example of how the Roy adaptation model can be used to guide the conceptualization, literature review, theory construction, and development of an intervention.

Zeigler, Smith, and Fawcett (2004) described the use of the Roy adaptation model to develop a community-based breast cancer support group, the Common Journey Breast Cancer Support Group. A qualitative study design was used to evaluate the program from both participant and facilitator perspectives. Responses from participants were categorized using the Roy adaptation model. Findings from this study showed that the program was effective in providing support for women with various stages of breast cancer.

Newman (1997b) applied the Roy adaptation model to caregivers of chronically ill family members. With a thorough review of the literature, Newman demonstrated how the Roy adaptation model was used to provide care for this population. Newman views the chronically ill family member as the focal stimulus. Contextual stimuli include the caregiver's age, gender, and relationship to the chronically ill family member. The caregiver's physical health status is a manifestation of the physiological adaptive mode. The caregiver's emotional responses to caregiving (i.e., shock, fear, anger, guilt, increased anxiety) are effective or ineffective responses of the self-concept mode. Relationships with significant others and support indicate adaptive responses in the interdependence mode. Caregivers' primary, secondary, and tertiary roles are strained by the addition of the caregiving role. Practice and research implications illuminate the applicability of the Roy adaptation model for providing care to caregivers of chronically ill family members.

The Roy adaptation model has been applied to adult patients with various medical conditions, including post-traumatic stress disorder (Nayback, 2009), women in menopause (Cunningham, 2002), and the assessment of an elderly man undergoing a below-the-knee amputation. The model has been used to evaluate the care of needs of adolescents with cancer (Ramini, Brown, & Buckner, 2008), asthma (Buckner et al., 2007), high-normal or hypertensive blood pressure readings (Starnes & Peters, 2004), and death and dying (Dobratz, 2011).

Kan (2009) used the Roy adaptation model to study perceptions of recovery after coronary artery bypass surgery for patients who had undergone this surgery for the first time. Findings revealed a positive relationship between perception of recovery and role function. Knowledge of adaptive responses after cardiac surgery has important implications for discharge planning and discharge teaching.

Education

The Roy adaptation model defines the distinct purpose of nursing for students, which is to promote the adaptation of persons in each of the adaptive modes in situations of health and illness. This model distinguishes nursing science from medical science by having the content of these areas taught in separate courses. She stresses collaboration but delineates separate goals for nurses and physicians. According to Roy (1971), it is the nurse's goal to help the patient put his or her energy into getting well, whereas the medical student focuses on the patient's position on the health–illness continuum with the goal of causing movement along the continuum. She views the model as a valuable tool for analyzing the distinctions between the two professions of nursing and medicine. Roy (1979) believes that curricula based on this model support students' understanding of theory development as they learn about testing theories and experience theoretical insights. Roy (1971, 1979) noted early on that the model clarified objectives, identified content, and specified patterns for teaching and learning.

The Roy adaptation model has been used in the educational setting and has guided nursing education at Mount Saint Mary's College Department of Nursing in Los Angeles since 1970. As early as 1987, more than 100,000 student nurses had been educated in nursing programs based on the Roy adaptation model in the United States and abroad. The Roy adaptation model provides educators with a systematic way of teaching students to assess and care for patients within the context of their lives rather than just as victims of illness.

Dobratz (2003) evaluated the learning outcomes of a nursing research course designed from the perspective of the Roy adaptation model and described in detail how to teach the theoretical content to students in a senior nursing research course. The evaluation tool was a Likert-type scale that contained seven statements. Students were asked to disagree, agree, or strongly agree with seven statements. Four open-ended questions were included to elicit information from students about the most helpful learning activity, the least helpful learning activity, methods used by the instructor that enhanced learning and grasp of research, and what the instructor could have done to increase learning. The researcher concluded that a research course based on the Roy adaptation model helped students put the pieces of the research puzzle together.

Research

If research is to affect practitioners' behaviors, it must be directed toward testing and retesting theories derived from conceptual models for nursing practice. Roy (1984) has stated that theory development and the testing of developed theories are the highest priorities for nursing. The model continues to generate many testable hypotheses to be researched.

Roy's theory has generated a number of general propositions. From these general propositions, specific hypotheses can be developed and tested. Hill and Roberts (1981) have demonstrated the development of testable hypotheses from the model, as has Roy. Data to validate or support the model are created by the testing of such hypotheses; the model continues to generate more of this type of research. The Roy adaptation model has been used extensively to guide knowledge development through nursing research (Frederickson, 2000).

Roy (1970) has identified a set of concepts that form a model from which the process of observation and classification of facts would lead to postulates. These postulates concern the occurrence of adaptation problems, coping mechanisms, and interventions based on laws derived from factors that make up the response potential of focal, contextual, and residual stimuli. Roy and colleagues have outlined a typology of adaptation problems or nursing diagnoses (Roy, 1973, 1975, 1976b). Research and testing continue in the areas of typology and categories of interventions that have been derived from the model. General propositions also have been developed and tested (Roy & McLeod, 1981).

Practice-Based Research

DiMattio and Tulman (2003) described changes in functional status and correlates of functional status of 61 women during the 6-week postoperative period after a coronary artery bypass graft. Functional status was measured at 2, 4, and 6 weeks after surgery, using the Inventory of Functional Status in the Elderly and the Sickness Impact Profile. Significant increases were found in all dimensions of functional status except personal at the three measurement points. The greatest increases in functional status occurred at a time between 2 and 4 weeks after surgery. However, none of the dimensions of functional status had returned to baseline values at the 6-week point. This information will help women who have undergone coronary artery bypass graft surgery to better understand the recovery period and to set more realistic goals.

Young-McCaughan and colleagues (2003) studied the effects of a structured aerobic exercise program on exercise tolerance, sleep patterns, and quality of life in patients with cancer from the perspective of the Roy adaptation model. Subjects exercised for 20 minutes, twice a week, for 12 weeks. Significant improvements in exercise tolerance, subjective sleep quality, and psychological and physiological quality of life were demonstrated.

Yeh (2002) tested the Roy adaptation model in a sample of 116 Taiwanese boys and girls with cancer (7–18 years of age at the time of diagnosis). Two Roy propositions were tested. The first proposition is that environmental stimuli (severity of illness, age, gender, understanding of illness, and communication with others) influence biopsychosocial responses (health-related quality of life [HRQOL]). The second proposition is that the four adaptive modes are interrelated. Using structural equation modeling, the researcher found that severity of illness provided an excellent fit with stage of illness, laboratory values (white blood cell count, hemoglobin, platelets, absolute neutrophil count), and total number of hospitalizations. Although it is not altogether clear how the focal and contextual stimuli were defined, this study showed that environmental stimuli (severity of illness, age, gender, understanding of illness, and communication with others) influence the biopsychosocial adaptive responses of children to cancer. Finally, this study demonstrated the interrelatedness of the physiological (physical HRQOL), self-concept (disease and symptoms HRQOL), interdependence (social HRQOL), and role function (cognitive HRQOL) adaptive modes.

Woods and Isenberg (2001) provide an example of theory synthesis. In their study of intimate abuse and traumatic stress in battered women, they developed a middle-range theory by synthesizing the Roy adaptation model with the current literature reporting on intimate abuse and posttraumatic stress disorder. A predictive correlational model was used to examine adaptation as a mediator of intimate abuse and posttraumatic stress disorder. The focal stimulus of this study was the severity of intimate abuse, emotional abuse, and risk of homicide by an intimate partner. Adaptation was operationalized within the four adaptive modes and was tested as a mediator between intimate abuse and posttraumatic stress disorder. Direct relationships were reported between the focal stimulus and intimate abuse, and adaptation in each of the four modes mediated relationships between the focal stimulus and traumatic stress.

Chiou (2000) conducted a meta-analysis of the interrelationships among Roy's four adaptive modes. Using well-defined inclusion and exclusion criteria, a literature search of the *Cumulative Index to Nursing and Allied Health Literature* yielded eight research reports with diverse samples. One in-press report was included. Convenience samples for the nine studies included only adults, and some were elderly. The meta-analysis revealed small to medium correlations between each two-mode set and a nonsignificant association between the interdependence and physiological modes. Zhan (2000) found support for Roy's proposition about cognitive adaptive processes in relation to maintaining self-consistency. Using Roy's Cognitive Adaptation Processing

Scale (Roy & Zhan, 2001) to measure cognitive adaptation and the Self-Consistency Scale (Zhan & Shen, 1994), Zhan found that cognitive adaptation plays an important role in helping older adults maintain self-consistency in the face of hearing loss. Self-consistency was higher for hearing-impaired men than for hearing-impaired women, but it did not vary for age, educational level, race, marital status, or income.

Nuamah et al. (1999) studied quality of life in 515 patients with cancer. These researchers clearly established theoretical linkages among the concepts of the Roy adaptation model, middle-range theory concepts, and empirical indicators. Focal and contextual stimuli were identified. Variables in each of the adaptive modes were operationalized. Using structural equation modeling, the researchers found that two of the environmental stimuli (adjuvant cancer treatment and severity of the disease) explained 59% of the variance in biopsychosocial indicators of the latent variable HRQOL. Their findings supported the proposition of the Roy adaptation model that environmental stimuli influence biopsychosocial responses.

Samarel and colleagues (1998, 1999) used the Roy adaptation model to study women's perceptions of adaptation to breast cancer in a sample of 70 women who were participating in an experimental support and education group. The experimental group received coaching; the control group received no coaching. Using quantitative content analysis of structured telephone interviews, the researchers found that 51 of 70 women (72.9%) experienced a positive change toward their breast cancer over the study period, which was indicative of adaptation to the breast cancer. The researchers report qualitative indicators of adaptation for each of Roy's four adaptive modes.

Modrcin-Talbott and colleagues studied self-esteem from the perspective of the Roy adaptation model in 140 well adolescents (Modrcin-Talbott, Pullen, Ehrenberger, et al., 1998) and 77 adolescents in an outpatient mental health setting (Modrcin-Talbott, Pullen, Zandstra, et al., 1998). Well adolescents were grouped in terms of early (12–14 years), middle (15–16 years), or late adolescence (17–19 years). Well adolescents were recruited conveniently from a large, southeastern church. Self-esteem in well adolescents did not differ by age group, gender, or whether or not they smoked tobacco. Well adolescents who exercised regularly did score higher on self-esteem. Significant negative relationships were found between self-esteem and depression, state anger, trait anger, anger-in, anger-out, anger control, and anger expression. In the second study, adolescents were sampled from participants of regularly scheduled group sessions as part of an outpatient psychiatric treatment program. Self-esteem significantly differed by age group, with older adolescents scoring lowest on self-esteem. Self-esteem did not differ by gender or whether or not they smoked tobacco. A significant negative relationship was observed between self-esteem and depression. Unlike their study in well adolescents, no statistically significant relationship was found between self-esteem and the dimensions of anger. Self-esteem was not significantly related to parental alcohol use in either group.

Modrcin-Talbott et al. (2003) tested the effects of gentle human touch on the biobehavioral adaptation of preterm infants based on the Roy adaptation model. According to Roy, infants are born with two adaptive modes: the physiological and interdependence modes. Premature infants often are deprived of human touch, and an environment filled with machines, noxious stimuli, and invasive procedures surrounds them. These researchers found that gentle human touch (focal stimulus) promotes physiological adaptation for premature infants. Heart rate, oxygen saturation stability, increased quiet sleep, less active sleep and drowsiness, decreased motor activity, increased time not moving, and decreased behavioral distress cues were identified as effective responses in the physiological adaptive mode. This study supports Roy's conceptualization of adaptation in infants.

Weiss, Fawcett, and Aber (2009) used the Roy adaptation model to study adaptation in postpartum women after cesarean delivery. Findings showed fewer adaptive responses in women with unplanned cesarean delivery. Cultural differences in adaptive responses were found among African American and Hispanic women compared with Caucasian women. Implications for nursing practice include early assessment of adaptive responses and learning needs for patients who have had cesarean delivery to develop a discharge teaching plan to facilitate adaptive responses after discharge.

The University of Montreal Research Team in Nursing Science (Ducharme et al., 1998; Levesque et al., 1998) is studying adaptation to a variety of environmental stimuli. Four groups of individuals were included in their studies as follows: (1) informal family caregivers of a demented relative at home, (2) informal family caregivers of a psychiatrically ill relative at home, (3) nurses as professional caregivers in geriatric institutions, and (4) aged spouses in the community. Using linear structural relations (LISREL), perceived stress (focal stimulus), social support (contextual stimulus), and passive and avoidance coping (coping mechanism) were directly or indirectly linked to psychological distress. This finding supports Roy's proposition that coping promotes adaptation.

DeSanto-Madeya (2009) studied adaptation in individuals with spinal cord injury and their family members using the Roy adaptation model. This study included 15 patient and family member dyads. Of the 15 dyads, 7 dyads were 1 year postinjury, and 8 dyads were 3 years postinjury. Telephone interviews using the Adaptation to Spinal Cord Injury Interview Schedule (ASCIIS) were conducted. Findings showed that both individuals and families had moderate adaptation scores at both 1 year and 3 years. Study findings have important implications for nurses who must care for spinal cord injury patients in both acute and outpatient care settings.

Development of Adaptation Research Instruments

The Roy adaptation model has provided the theoretical basis for the development of a number of research instruments. Newman (1997a) developed the Inventory of Functional Status–Caregiver of a Child in a Body Cast to measure the extent to which parental caregivers continue their usual activities while a child is in a body cast. Reliability testing indicates that the subscales for household, social, and community child care of the child in a body cast, child care of other children, and personal care (rather than the total score) are reliable measures of these constructs. Modrcin-McCarthy, McCue, and Walker (1997) used the Roy adaptation model to develop a clinical tool that may be used to identify actual and potential stressors of fragile premature infants and to implement care for them. This tool measures signs of stress, touch interventions, reduction of pain, environmental considerations, state, and stability (STRESS).

Development of Middle-Range Theories of Adaptation

Silva (1986) pointed out early on that merely using a conceptual framework to structure a research study is not theory testing. Many researchers have used Roy's model but did not actually test propositions or hypotheses of her model. They have provided face validity of its usefulness as a framework to guide their studies. How theory derives from a conceptual framework must be made explicit; therefore development and testing of middle-range theories derived from the Roy adaptation model are needed. Some research of this nature has been conducted with the model, but more is needed for further validation and development of new areas. The model does generate many testable hypotheses related to both practice and nursing theory. The success of a conceptual framework is evaluated, in part, by the number and quality of middle-range theories it generates. The Roy adaptation model has been the theoretical source of a number of middle-range theories (Roy, 2011a). The utility of those theories in practice sustains the life of the model.

Dunn (2004) reports the use of theoretical substruction to derive a middle-range theory of adaptation for chronic pain from the Roy Adaptation Model. In Dunn's model of adaptation to chronic pain, pain intensity is specified as the focal stimulus. Contextual stimuli include age, race, and gender. Religious and nonreligious coping is a function of the cognator subsystem. Manifestations of adaptation to chronic pain are its effects on functional ability and psychological and spiritual well-being.

Frame, Kelly, and Bayley (2003) developed the Frame theory of adolescent empowerment by synthesizing the Roy adaptation model, Murrell-Armstrong's empowerment matrix, and Harter's developmental perspective. The theory of adolescent empowerment was tested using a quasi-experimental design in which children diagnosed with attention-deficit–hyperactivity disorder (ADHD) were randomly assigned to a treatment or a control group. Ninety-two fifth- and sixth-grade students were assigned to the treatment or the control group. Children in the treatment group attended an eight-session, school nurse–led support group intervention (twice weekly for 4 weeks). The treatment was designed to teach the children about ADHD; the gifts of having ADHD; powerlessness versus empowerment; empowerment with one's feelings, teachers, family, and classmates; and how to learn to relax. Children in the control group received no intervention. Using analysis of covariance, children in the treatment group reported significantly higher perceived social acceptance, perceived athletic competence, perceived physical appearance, and perceived global self-worth.

Jirovec et al. (1999) have proposed a middle-range urine control theory derived from the Roy adaptation model, intended to explicate the phenomenon of urine control and to decrease urinary incontinence. According to the theory of urine control, the focal stimulus for urine control is bladder distention. Contextual stimuli include accessible facilities and mobility skills. A residual stimulus is the intense socialization about bladder and sanitary habits that begin in childhood. This theory takes into account physiological coping mechanisms, regulator (spinal reflex mediated by S2 to S4, and coordinated detrusor muscle contraction and sphincter relaxation) and cognator (perception, learning judgment, and awareness of urgency or dribbling). Adaptive responses to prevent urinary incontinence are described for the four adaptive modes. Effective adaptation is defined as continence, and ineffective adaptation is defined as incontinence. The authors provide limited support for the theory of urine control through case studies. The theory of urine control illuminates the complexity, multidimensionality, and holistic nature of adaptation.

Researchers at the University of Montreal have proposed a middle-range theory of adaptation to caregiving that is based on the Roy adaptation model. This middle-range theory has been tested in a number of published studies of informal caregivers of demented relatives at home, informal caregivers of psychiatrically ill relatives at home, professional caregivers of elderly institutionalized patients, and aged spouses in the community. Perceived stress is conceptualized as the focal stimulus. Contextual stimuli include gender, conflicts, and social support. Coping mechanisms include active, passive, and avoidant coping strategies. In this middle-range theory, the adaptive (nonadaptive) response (psychological distress) is manifested in the self-concept mode. LISREL analyses have provided support for many of the propositions of this middle-range theory of adaptation to caregiving and for the Roy adaptation model (Ducharme et al., 1998; Levesque et al., 1998).

Tsai and colleagues (2003) derived a middle-range theory of pain from the Roy adaptation model. In the theory of chronic pain, chronic pain is the focal stimulus, disability and social support are contextual stimuli, and age and gender are residual stimuli. Perceived daily stress is a coping process. Depression is an outcome variable manifested in all four adaptive modes. Path analysis provided partial support for the theory of chronic pain. Greater chronic pain and disability were associated with more daily stress, and greater social support was associated with less daily stress. These three variables accounted for 35% of the variance in daily stress. Greater daily stress explained 35% of the variance in depression.

Other middle-range theories derived from the Roy adaptation model have been proposed. Tsai (2003) has proposed a middle-range theory of caregiver stress. Whittemore and Roy (2002) developed a middle-range theory of adapting to diabetes mellitus using theory synthesis. Based on an analysis of Pollock's (1993) middle-range theory of chronic illness and a thorough review of the literature, reconceptualization of the chronic illness model and the addition of concepts such as self-management, integration, and health-within-illness more specifically extend the Roy adaptation model to diabetes mellitus. Pollock's (1993) research on adaptation to chronic illness theory included patients with insulin-dependent diabetes, multiple sclerosis, hypertension, and rheumatoid arthritis. Adaptation to chronic illness theory was further tested in the study by Harris (2012) to examine the effects of a home-based exercise program on perception of illness in patients with chronic heart failure.

FURTHER DEVELOPMENT

The Roy adaptation model is an approach to nursing that has made and continues to make a significant contribution to the body of nursing knowledge; however, areas remain for future development as health care progresses. A thoroughly defined typology of nursing diagnoses and an organization of categories of interventions would facilitate its use in nursing practice. Scientists who do research from the perspective of the Roy adaptation model continue to note overlap in the psychosocial categories of self-concept, role function, and interdependence. Roy recently has redefined *health*, deemphasizing the concept of a health–illness continuum and conceptualizing health as integration and wholeness of the person. This approach more clearly incorporates the adaptive mechanisms of the comatose patient in response to tactile and verbal stimuli. However, because health was not conceptualized in this manner in the earlier work, this opens up a new area for research. Based on her integrative review of the literature, Frederickson (2000) concluded that there is good empirical support for Roy's conceptualization of person and health. She made the following recommendations for future research: First, there is a need to design studies to test propositions related to environment and nursing. Second, although interventions based on previously supported concepts and propositions have been tested, others remain to be tested to document evidence.

CRITIQUE

Clarity

The metaparadigm concepts of the Roy adaptation model (person, environment, nursing, and health) are clearly defined and consistent. Roy clearly defines the four adaptive modes (physiological, self-concept, interdependence, and role function). A challenge of the model that was identified is Roy's espousal of a holistic view of the person and environment, whereas the model views adaptation as occurring in four adaptive modes, and person and environment are conceptualized as two separate entities, with one affecting the other (Malinski, 2000). An answer to this challenge is that Roy's adaptation model is holistic, because change in the internal or external environment (stimulus) leads to response (adapts) as a whole. In fact, Roy's perspective is consistent with other holistic theories, such as psychoneuroimmunology and psychoneuroendocrinology. As one example, psychoneuroimmunology is a theory that proposes a bidirectional relationship between the mind and the immune system. Roy's model is broader than psychoneuroimmunology and provides a theoretical foundation for research about, and nursing care of, the person as a whole.

In more recent writings, Roy has acknowledged the holistic nature of persons who live in a universe that is "progressing in structure, organization, and complexity. Rather than a system acting to maintain itself, the emphasis shifts to the purposefulness of human existence in a universe that is creative" (Roy & Andrews, 1999, p. 35).

Roy has written that other disciplines focus on an aspect of the person, and that nursing views the person as a whole (Roy & Andrews, 1999). "Based on the philosophic assumptions of the nursing model, persons are seen as coextensive with their physical and social environments. The nurse takes a values-based stance, focusing on awareness, enlightenment and faith" (Roy & Andrews, 1999, p. 539). Roy contends that persons have mutual, integral, and simultaneous relationships with the universe and God, and that as humans they "use their creative abilities of awareness, enlightenment, and faith in the processes of deriving, sustaining, and transforming the universe" (Roy & Andrews, 1999, p. 35). Using these creative abilities, persons (sick or well) are active participants in their care and are able to achieve a higher level of adaptation (health).

Mastal and Hammond (1980) discussed difficulties with Roy's model in classifying certain behaviors because concept definitions overlapped. The problem dealt with theory conceptualization and the need for mutually exclusive categories to classify human behavior. Conceptualizing a person's position on the health–illness continuum is no longer a problem because Roy redefined health as personal integration. Other researchers have referred to difficulty in classifying behavior exclusively in one adaptive mode (Bradley & Williams, 1990; Limandri, 1986; Nyqvist & Sjoden, 1993; Silva, 1987). However, this observation supports Roy's proposition that behavior in one adaptive mode affects and is affected by the other modes.

Simplicity

The Roy model includes the concepts of nursing, person, health-illness, environment, adaptation, and nursing activities. It also includes two subconcepts (regulator and cognator) and four modes (physiological, self-concept, role function, and interdependence). This model has several major concepts and subconcepts, so the relational statements are complex until the model is learned.

Generality

The broad scope of Roy's model is an advantage because it may be used for theory building and for deriving middle-range theories for testing in studies of smaller ranges of phenomena (Reynolds, 1971). Roy's model (Roy & Corliss, 1993) is generalizable to all settings in nursing practice but is limited in scope, because it primarily addresses the person-environment adaptation of the patient, and information about the nurse is implied.

Accessibility

Roy's broad concepts stem from theory in physiological psychology, psychology, sociology, and nursing; empirical data indicate that this general theory base has substance. Roy's model offers direction for researchers who want to incorporate physiological phenomena in their studies. Roy (1980) studied and analyzed 500 samples of patient behaviors collected by nursing students. From this analysis, Roy proposed her four adaptive modes in humans.

Roy (Roy & McLeod, 1981; Roy & Roberts, 1981) has identified many propositions in relation to the regulator and cognator mechanisms and the self-concept, role function, and interdependence modes. These propositions have received varying degrees of support from general theory and empirical data. Most of the propositions are relational statements and can be tested (Tiedeman, 1983). Over the years, many testable hypotheses have been derived from the model (Hill & Roberts, 1981).

Despite the progress made over the past 25 years, the greatest need to increase the empirical precision of the Roy adaptation model is for researchers to develop middle-range theory based on the model with empirical referents specifically designed to measure concepts proposed in the derived theory. Roy has explicated a significant number of propositions, theorems, and axioms to serve in the development of middle-range theory. The holistic nature of the model serves nurse researchers worldwide who are interested in the complex nature of physiological and psychosocial adaptive processes (Roy, 2011a, 2011b).

Importance

The Roy adaptation model has a clearly defined nursing process and is useful in guiding clinical practice. The utility of the model has been demonstrated globally by nurses. This model provides direction for quality nursing care that addresses the holistic needs of the patient. The model is also capable of generating new information through the testing of hypotheses that have been derived from it (Roy, 2011a; Roy & Corliss, 1993; Smith, Garvis, & Martinson, 1983).

SUMMARY

The Roy adaptation model has greatly influenced the profession of nursing. It is one of the most commonly used models to guide nursing research, education, and practice. The model is taught as part of the curriculum of most baccalaureate, master's, and doctoral programs of nursing. The influence of the Roy adaptation model on nursing research is evidenced by the vast number of qualitative and quantitative research studies it has guided. The model has inspired the development of many middle-range nursing theories and of adaptation instruments. Sister Callista Roy continues to refine the adaptation model for nursing research, education, and practice.

According to Roy, persons are holistic adaptive systems and the focus of nursing. The internal and external environment consists of all phenomena that surround the human adaptive system and affect their development and behavior. Persons are in constant interaction with the environment and exchange information, matter, and energy; that is, persons affect and are affected by the environment. The environment is the source of stimuli that either threaten or promote a person's existence. For survival, the human adaptive system must respond positively to environmental stimuli. Humans make effective or ineffective adaptive responses to environmental stimuli. Adaptation promotes survival, growth, reproduction, mastery, and transformation of persons and the environment. Roy defines *health* as a state of becoming an integrated and whole human being.

Three types of environmental stimuli are described in the Roy adaptation model. The focal stimulus is that which most immediately confronts the individual and demands the most attention and adaptive energy. Contextual stimuli are all other stimuli present in the situation that contribute positively or negatively to the strength of the focal stimulus. Residual stimuli affect the focal stimulus, but their effects are not readily known. These three types of stimuli together form the adaptation level. A person's adaptation level may be integrated, compensatory, or compromised.

Coping mechanisms refer to innate or acquired processes that a person uses to deal with environmental stimuli. Coping mechanisms may be categorized broadly as the regulator or cognator subsystem. The regulator subsystem responds automatically through innate neural, chemical, and endocrine coping processes. The cognator subsystem responds through innate and acquired cognitive-emotive processes that include perceptual and information processing, learning, judgment, and emotion.

Behaviors that manifest adaptation can be observed in four adaptive modes. The physiological mode refers to the person's physical responses to the environment, and the underlying need is physiological integrity. The self-concept mode refers to a person's thoughts, beliefs, or feelings about himself or herself at any given time. The basic need of the self-concept mode is psychic or spiritual integrity. The self-concept is a composite belief about self that is formed from internal perceptions and the perceptions of others. The self-concept mode is composed of the physical self (body sensation and body image) and the personal self (self-consistency, self-ideal, and the moral-ethical-spiritual self). The role function mode refers to the primary, secondary, and tertiary roles a person performs in society.

The basic need of the role function adaptive mode is social integrity, or for one to know how to behave and what is expected of him or her in society. The interdependence adaptive mode refers to relationships among people. The basic need of the interdependence adaptive mode is social integrity or to give and receive love, respect, and value from significant others and social support systems (Table 17.1).

The goal of nursing is to promote adaptive responses. This is accomplished through a six-step nursing process: assessment of behavior, assessment of stimuli, nursing diagnosis, goal setting, intervention, and evaluation. Nursing interventions focus on managing environmental stimuli by "altering, increasing, decreasing, removing, or maintaining them" (Roy & Andrews, 1999, p. 86).

Meleis (1985) proposed that the focus of nursing theorist works is one of three types:

1. Those who focus on needs
2. Those who focus on interaction
3. Those who focus on outcome

Meleis (1985, 2007) classifies the Roy adaptation model as an outcome theory. In applying the concepts of system and adaptation to person as the patient of nursing, Roy has presented her articulation of the person for nurses to use as a tool in practice, education, and research. Her conceptions of person and of the nursing process contribute to the science and the art of nursing. The Roy adaptation model deserves further study and development by nurse educators, researchers, and practitioners.

CASE STUDY

A 23-year-old male patient is admitted with a fracture of C6 and C7 that has resulted in quadriplegia. He was injured during a football game at the university where he is currently a senior. His career as a quarterback had been very promising. At the time of the injury, contract negotiations were in progress with a leading professional football team.

1. Use Roy's criteria to identify focal and contextual stimuli for each of the four adaptive modes.
2. Consider what adaptations would be necessary in each of the following four adaptive modes: (1) physiological, (2) self-concept, (3) interdependence, and (4) role function.
3. Create a nursing intervention for each of the adaptive modes to promote adaptation.

TABLE 17.1 **Overview of the Adaptive Modes**

Subsystem	Adaptive Mode	Coping Need
Regulator	**Physiological** The physiological adaptive mode refers to the way a person, as a physical being, responds to and interacts with the internal and external environment. **Basic need:** Physiological integrity	**Oxygenation:** To maintain appropriate oxygenation through ventilation, gas exchange, and gas transport **Nutrition:** To maintain function, to promote growth, and to replace tissue through ingestion and assimilation of food **Elimination:** To excrete metabolic wastes primarily through the intestines and kidney **Activity and rest:** To maintain balance between physical activity and rest **Protection:** To defend the body against infection, trauma, and temperature changes primarily by way of integumentary structures and innate and acquired immunity **Senses:** To enable persons to interact with their environment by sight, hearing, touch, taste, and smell **Fluid and electrolyte and acid-base balance:** To maintain homeostatic fluid, electrolyte, and acid-base balance to promote cellular, extracellular, and systemic function **Neurological function:** To coordinate and control body movements, consciousness, and cognitive-emotional processes **Endocrine function:** To integrate and coordinate body functions
Cognator	**Self-concept** The self-concept adaptive mode refers to the psychological and spiritual characteristics of a person. The self-concept consists of the composite of a person's feelings about himself or herself at any given time. The self-concept is formed from internal perceptions and the perceptions of others' reactions. The self-concept has two major dimensions: the physical self and the personal self. **Basic need:** Psychic and spiritual integrity	**Physical Self** **Body sensation:** To maintain a positive feeling about one's physical being (i.e., physical functioning, sexuality, or health) **Body image:** To maintain a positive view of one's physical body and physical appearance **Personal Self** **Self-consistency:** To maintain consistent self-organization and to avoid disequilibrium **Self-ideal or self-expectancy:** To maintain a positive or hopeful view of what one is, what one expects to be, and what one hopes to do **Moral-spiritual-ethical self:** To maintain a positive evaluation of who one is
	Interdependence **Basic need:** Relational integrity or security in nurturing relationships	To maintain close, nurturing relationships with people who are willing to give and receive love, respect, and value
	Role Function **Basic need:** Social integrity	To know who one is and what society's expectations are so that one can act appropriately within society

CRITICAL THINKING ACTIVITIES

1. Karen, a recent graduate from a nursing program based on the Roy adaptation model, is performing her morning assessments. She enters Mr. Shadeed's room. Mr. Shadeed is awaiting preoperative preparation for a laparotomy to explore an unknown mass. Mr. Shadeed is very irritable this morning. He says that he is thirsty. Karen continues her assessment of Mr. Shadeed.
   a. What additional data will she need from each of the four adaptive modes before implementing nursing interventions?
   b. What are the focal stimuli, contextual stimuli, and residual stimuli?
   c. What are possible interventions?
   d. What process can Karen use to select the best nursing intervention?
2. Although it would be easy to assume that Mr. Shadeed's nursing care needs stem from anxiety during the preoperative period, this assumption may or may not be true. Assessment of stimuli in each of the four adaptive modes will enable Karen to assess focal, contextual, and residual stimuli and come to the correct diagnosis. Identify the additional assessment data that Karen will need to collect for each of the following adaptive modes:
   - Physiological adaptive mode
   - Self-concept adaptive mode
   - Role function adaptive mode
   - Interdependence adaptive mode

POINTS FOR FURTHER STUDY

- *Nursing Science Quarterly* (2011). *24*(4); entire issue honoring Roy and her work.
- Phillips, K. D. (2014). Roy's adaptation model in nursing practice. In M. R. Alligood (Ed.), *Nursing theory: Utilization & application* (5th ed., pp. 263–284). St Louis, MO: Mosby-Elsevier.
- Roy, C., & Jones, D. (Eds.). (2007). *Nursing knowledge development and clinical practice.* New York: Springer.
- Roy, C. (2007). Update from the future: Thinking of theorist Sr. Callista Roy. *Nursing Science Quarterly, 20*(2), 113–116.
- Sr. Callista Roy. *Portraits of excellence: The nurse theorists* video/DVD series, vol 1. Athens, OH: Fitne, Inc.
- Sr. Callista Roy. *Adaptation: Excellence in action* video/DVD. Athens, OH: Fitne, Inc.

REFERENCES

Andrews, H. (1991). Overview of the role function mode. In C. Roy & H. Andrews (Eds.), *The Roy adaptation model: The definitive statement* (pp. 347–361). Norwalk, CT: Appleton & Lange.

Andrews, H., & Roy, C. (1986). *Essentials of the Roy adaptation model.* Norwalk, CT: Appleton-Century-Crofts.

Andrews, H., & Roy, C. (1991). Essentials of the Roy adaptation model. In C. Roy & H. Andrews (Eds.), *The Roy adaptation model: The definitive statement* (pp. 3–25). Norwalk, CT: Appleton & Lange.

Bradley, K. M., & Williams, D. M. (1990). A comparison of the preoperative concerns of open heart surgery patients and their significant others. *Journal of Cardiovascular Nursing, 5*(1), 43–53.

Brower, H. T., & Baker, B. J. (1976). The Roy adaptation model. Using the adaptation model in a practitioner curriculum. *Nursing Outlook, 24,* 686–689.

Buckner, E. B., Simmons, S., Brakefield, J. A., Hawkins, A. K., Feeley, C., Kilgore, L. A. F., et al. (2007). Maturing responsibility in young teens participating in an asthma camp: Adaptive mechanisms and outcomes. *Journal for Specialists in Pediatric Nursing, 12,* 24–36.

Chinn, P., & Kramer, M. (2008). *Integrated theory and knowledge development in nursing.* St Louis: Mosby-Elsevier.

Chiou, C. P. (2000). A meta-analysis of the interrelationships between the modes in Roy's adaptation model. *Nursing Science Quarterly, 13,* 252–258.

Cooley, C. H. (1902). *Human nature and the social order.* New York: Scribner.

Cunningham, D. A. (2002). Application of Roy's adaptation model when caring for a group of women coping with menopause. *Journal of Community Health Nursing, 19,* 49–60.

Davies, P. (1988). *The cosmic blueprint.* New York: Simon & Schuster.

De Chardin, P. T. (1959). *The phenomenon of man.* New York: Harper & Row.

De Chardin, P. T. (1965). *Hymn of the universe.* New York: Harper & Row.

De Chardin, P. T. (1966). *Man's place in nature.* New York: Harper & Row.

De Chardin, P. T. (1969). *Human energy.* New York: Harper & Row.

DeSanto-Madeya, S. (2009). Adaptation to spinal cord injury for families post-injury. *Nursing Science Quarterly, 22,* 57–66.

Dickoff, J., James, P., & Wiedenbach, E. (1968a). Theory in a practice discipline. I. Practice oriented discipline. *Nursing Research, 17,* 415–435.

Dickoff, J., James, P., & Wiedenbach, E. (1968b). Theory in a practice discipline. II. Practice oriented research. *Nursing Research, 17*, 545–554.

DiMattio, M. J., & Tulman, L. (2003). A longitudinal study of functional status and correlates following coronary artery bypass graft surgery in women. *Nursing Research, 52*, 98–107.

Dobratz, M. C. (2003). Putting the pieces together: Teaching undergraduate research from a theoretical perspective. *Journal of Advanced Nursing, 41*, 383–392.

Dobratz, M. C. (2011). Toward development of a middle-range theory of psychological adaptation in death and dying. *Nursing Science Quarterly, 24*(4), 370–376.

Ducharme, E., Ricard, N., Duquette, A., Levesque, L., & Lachance, L. (1998). Empirical testing of a longitudinal model derived from the Roy adaptation model. *Nursing Science Quarterly, 11*, 149–159.

Dunn, K. S. (2004). Toward a middle-range theory of adaptation to chronic pain. *Nursing Science Quarterly, 77*, 78–84.

Farkas, L. (1981). Adaptation problems with nursing home application for elderly persons: An application of the Roy adaptation nursing model. *Journal of Advanced Nursing, 6*, 363–368.

Fawcett, J. (2002). The nurse theorists: 21st-century updates—Callista Roy. *Nursing Science Quarterly, 15*, 308–310.

Fawcett, J. (2005). Roy's adaptation model. In J. Fawcett (Ed.), *Analysis and evaluation of contemporary nursing knowledge: Nursing models and theories* (2nd ed., pp. 364–437). Philadelphia: F. A. Davis.

Frame, K., Kelly, L., & Bayley, E. (2003). Increasing perceptions of self-worth in preadolescents diagnosed with ADHD. *Journal of Nursing Scholarship, 35*, 225–229.

Frederickson, K. (2000). Nursing knowledge development through research: Using the Roy adaptation model. *Nursing Science Quarterly, 13*, 12–16.

Galligan, A. C. (1979). Addressing small children. Using Roy's concept of adaptation to care for young children. *American Journal of Maternal Child Nursing, 4*, 24–28.

Harris, R. F. (2012). *Effects of a home-based exercise program on perception of illness and adaptation in heart failure patients.* PhD diss., University of Tennessee, 2012. http://trace.tennessee.edu/utk_graddiss/1475.

Hill, B. J., & Roberts, C. S. (1981). Formal theory construction: An example of the process. In C. Roy & S. L. Roberts (Eds.), *Theory construction in nursing: An adaptation model.* Englewood Cliffs, NJ: Prentice-Hall.

Illich, I. (1974). Medical nemesis. *Lancet, 1*, 918–921.

Illich, I. (1976). *Limits to medicine: Medical nemesis, the expropriation of health.* London: Boyars.

Jirovec, M. M., Jenkins, J., Isenberg, M., & Baiardi, J. (1999). Urine control theory derived from Roy's conceptual framework. *Nursing Science Quarterly, 12*, 251–255.

Kan, E. Z. (2009). Perceptions of recovery, physical health, personal meaning, role function, and social support after first-time coronary artery bypass surgery. *Dimensions of Critical Care Nursing, 28*, 189–195.

Levesque, L., Ricard, N., Ducharme, F., Duquette, A., & Bonin, J. P. (1998). Empirical verification of a theoretical model derived from the Roy adaptation model: Findings from five studies. *Nursing Science Quarterly, 11*(1), 31–39.

Limandri, B. J. (1986). Research and practice with abused women—Use of the Roy adaptation model as an explanatory framework. *Advances in Nursing Science, 8*, 52–61.

Malinski, V. M. (2000). Commentary. *Nursing Science Quarterly, 13*(1), 16–17.

Mastal, M. F., & Hammond, H. (1980). Analysis and expansion of the Roy adaptation model: A contribution to holistic nursing. *Advances in Nursing Science, 2*, 71–81.

Mastal, M. F., Hammond, H., & Roberts, M. P. (1982). Theory into hospital practice: A pilot implementation. *Journal of Nursing Administration, 12*, 9–15.

McDonald, F. J., & Harms, M. (1966). Theoretical model for an experimental curriculum. *Nursing Outlook, 14*, 48–51.

Meleis, A. I. (1985). *Theoretical nursing development and progress.* Philadelphia: Lippincott.

Meleis, A. I. (2007). *Theoretical nursing development and progress* (4th ed.). Philadelphia: Lippincott.

Modrcin-McCarthy, M. A., McCue, S., & Walker, J. (1997). Preterm infants and STRESS: A tool for the neonatal nurse. *Journal of Perinatal & Neonatal Nursing, 10*, 62–71.

Modrcin-Talbott, M. A., Harrison, L. L., Groer, M. W., & Younger, M. S. (2003). The biobehavioral effects of gentle human touch on preterm infants. *Nursing Science Quarterly, 16*, 60–67.

Modrcin-Talbott, M. A., Pullen, L., Ehrenberger, H., Zandstra, K., & Muenchen, B. (1998). Self esteem in adolescents treated in an outpatient mental health setting. *Issues in Comprehensive Pediatric Nursing, 21*, 159–171.

Modrcin-Talbott, M. A., Pullen, L., Zandstra, K., Ehrenberger, H., & Muenchen, B. (1998). A study of self-esteem among well adolescents: Seeking a new direction. *Issues in Comprehensive Pediatric Nursing, 21*, 229–241.

Nayback, A. M. (2009). PTSD in the combat veteran: Using Roy's adaptation model to examine the combat veteran as a human adaptive system. *Issues in Mental Health Nursing, 30*, 304–310.

Newman, D. M. (1997a). The inventory of functional status—Caregiver of a child in a body cast. *Journal of Pediatric Nursing, 12*, 142–147.

Newman, D. M. (1997b). Responses to caregiving: A reconceptualization using the Roy adaptation model. *Holistic Nursing Practice, 12*, 80–88.

Nuamah, I. F., Cooley, M. E., Fawcett, J., & McCorkle, R. (1999). Testing a theory for health-related quality of life in cancer patients: A structural equation approach. *Research in Nursing & Health, 22*, 231–242.

Nyqvist, K. H., & Sjoden, P. O. (1993). Advice concerning breastfeeding from mothers of infants admitted to a neonatal intensive-care unit—The Roy adaptation model as a conceptual structure. *Journal of Advanced Nursing, 18*, 54–63.

Pollock, S. E. (1993). Adaptation to chronic illness: A program of research for testing nursing theory. *Nursing Science Quarterly, 6*(2), 86–92.

Rambo, B. (1983). *Adaptation nursing: Assessment and intervention.* Philadelphia: Saunders.

Ramini, S. K., Brown, R., & Buckner, E. B. (2008). Embracing changes: Adaptation by adolescents with cancer. *Pediatric Nursing, 34*, 72–79.

Randell, B., Tedrow, M. P., & Van Landingham, J. (1982). *Adaptation nursing: The Roy conceptual model applied.* St Louis: Mosby.

Reynolds, P. D. (1971). *A primer in theory construction.* Indianapolis: Bobbs-Merrill.

Riehl, J. P., & Roy, C. (1980). *Conceptual models for nursing practice* (2nd ed.). New York: Appleton-Century-Crofts.

Roy, C. (1970). Adaptation: A conceptual framework for nursing. *Nursing Outlook, 18*, 42–45.

Roy, C. (1971). Adaptation: A basis for nursing practice. *Nursing Outlook, 19*, 254–257.

Roy, C. (1973). Adaptation: Implications for curriculum change. *Nursing Outlook, 21*, 163–168.

Roy, C. (1975). A diagnostic classification system for nursing. *Nursing Outlook, 23*, 90–94.

Roy, C. (1976a). *Introduction to nursing: An adaptation model.* Englewood Cliffs, NJ: Prentice-Hall.

Roy, C. (1976b). The impact of nursing diagnosis. *Nursing Digest, 4*, 67–69.

Roy, C. (1979). Relating nursing theory to nursing education: A new era. *Nurse Educator, 4*, 16–21.

Roy, C. (1980). The Roy adaptation model. In J. P. Riehl & C. Roy (Eds.), *Conceptual models for nursing practice* (2nd ed., pp. 179–188). New York: Appleton-Century-Crofts.

Roy, C. (1984). *Introduction to nursing: An adaptation model* (2nd ed.). Englewood Cliffs, NJ: Prentice-Hall.

Roy, C. (1997). Future of the Roy model: Challenge to redefine adaptation. *Nursing Science Quarterly, 10*(1), 42–48.

Roy, C. (2000). The visible and invisible fields that shape the future of the nursing care system. *Nursing Administration Quarterly, 25*(1), 119–131.

Roy, C. (2011a). Research based on the Roy adaptation model: Last 25 years. *Nursing Science Quarterly, 24*(4), 312–320.

Roy, C. (2011b). Extending the Roy adaptation model to meet changing global needs. *Nursing Science Quarterly, 24*(4), 345–351.

Roy, C., & Andrews, H. (1991). *The Roy adaptation model: The definitive statement.* Norwalk, CT: Appleton & Lange.

Roy, C., & Andrews, H. (1999). *The Roy adaptation model* (2nd ed.). Upper Saddle River, NJ: Pearson.

Roy, C., & McLeod, D. (1981). Theory of the person as an adaptive system. In C. Roy & S. Roberts (Eds.), *Theory construction in nursing: Art adaptation model* (pp. 49–69). Englewood Cliffs, NJ: Prentice-Hall.

Roy, C., & Obloy, M. (1978). The practitioner movement. *American Journal of Nursing, 78*, 1698–1702.

Roy, C., & Roberts, S. (1981). *Theory construction in nursing: An adaptation model.* Englewood Cliffs, NJ: Prentice-Hall.

Roy, C., & Zhan, L. (2001). The Roy adaptation model: Theoretical update and knowledge for practice. In M. E. Parker (Ed.), *Nursing theories and nursing practice* (pp. 315–342). Philadelphia: F. A. Davis.

Roy, S. C., & Corliss, C. P. (1993). The Roy adaptation model: Theoretical update and knowledge for practice. In M. E. Parker (Ed.), *Patterns of nursing theories in practice.* (NLN Pub. 15–2548). New York: National League for Nursing.

Samarel, N., Tulman, L., & Fawcett, J. (2002). Effects of two types of social support and education on adaptation to early-stage breast cancer. *Research in Nursing & Health, 25*, 459–470.

Samarel, N., Fawcett, J., Krippendorf, K., Piacentino, J. C., Eliasof, B., Hughes, P., et al. (1998). Women's perception of group support and adaptation to breast cancer. *Journal of Advanced Nursing, 28*(6), 1259–1268.

Samarel, N., Fawcett, J., Tulman, L., Rothman, H., Spector, L., Spillane, P. A., et al. (1999). A resource kit for women with breast cancer: Development and evaluation. *Oncology Nursing Forum, 26*(3), 611–618.

Senesac, P., Chestnut Hill, MA (2003). Implementing the Roy adaptation model: From theory to practice. *Roy Adaptation Review, 4*(2).

Silva, M. C. (1986). Research testing nursing theory: State of the art. *Advances in Nursing Science, 9*, 1–11.

Silva, M. C. (1987). Needs of spouses of surgical patients: A conceptualization within the Roy adaptation model. *Scholarly Inquiry for Nursing Practice, 1*, 29–44.

Smith, C. E., Garvis, M. S., & Martinson, I. M. (1983). Content analysis of interviews using a nursing model: A look at parents adapting to the impact of childhood cancer. *Cancer Nursing, 6*, 269–275.

Starnes, T. M., & Peters, R. M. (2004). Anger, expression, and blood pressure in adolescents. *Journal of School Nursing, 20*, 335–342.

Swimme, B., & Berry, T. (1992). *The universe story.* San Francisco: Harper.

Tiedeman, M. E. (1983). The Roy adaptation model. In J. Fitzpatrick & A. Whall (Eds.), *The Roy adaptation model* (pp. 157–180). Bowie, MD: Brady.

Tsai, P. F. (2003). Middle-range theory of caregiver stress. *Nursing Science Quarterly, 16*(2), 137–145.

Tsai, P. F., Tak, S., Moore, C., & Palencia, I. (2003). Testing a theory of chronic pain. *Journal of Advanced Nursing, 43*, 158–169.

Villareal, E. (2003). Using Roy's adaptation model when caring for a group of young women contemplating quitting smoking. *Public Health Nursing, 20*, 377–384.

Wagner, P. (1976). The Roy adaptation model. Testing the adaptation model in practice. *Nursing Outlook, 24*, 682–685.

Weiland, S. (2010). Integrating spirituality into critical care: An APN perspective using Roy's adaptation model. *Critical Care Nursing Quarterly, 33*, 282–291.

Weiss, M., Fawcett, J., & Aber, C. (2009). Adaptation, postpartum concerns, and learning needs in the first two weeks after caesarean birth. *Journal of Clinical Nursing, 18*, 2938–2948.

Whittemore, R., & Roy, C. (2002). Adapting to diabetes mellitus: A theory synthesis. *Nursing Science Quarterly, 15*, 311–317.

Woods, S. J., & Isenberg, M. A. (2001). Adaptation as a mediator of intimate abuse and traumatic stress in battered women. *Nursing Science Quarterly, 14*(3), 215–221.

Yeh, C. H. (2002). Health-related quality of life in pediatric patients with cancer—A structural equation approach with the Roy adaptation model. *Cancer Nursing, 25*, 74–80.

Young-McCaughan, S., Mays, M. Z., Arzola, S. M., Yoder, L. H., Dramiga, S. A., Leclerc, K. M., et al. (2003). Research and commentary: Change in exercise tolerance, activity and sleep patterns, and quality of life in patients with cancer participating in a structured exercise program. *Oncology Nursing Forum, 30*, 441–454.

Zeigler, L., Smith, P. A., & Fawcett, J. (2004). Breast cancer: Evaluation of Common Journey Breast Cancer Support Group. *Journal of Clinical Nursing, 13*, 467–478.

Zhan, L. (2000). Cognitive adaptation and self-consistency in hearing-impaired older persons: Testing Roy's adaptation model. *Nursing Science Quarterly, 13*(2), 158–165.

Zhan, L., & Shen, C. (1994). The development of an instrument to measure self-consistency. *Journal of Advanced Nursing, 20*, 509–516.

BIBLIOGRAPHY

Primary Sources

Books

Andrews, H., & Roy, C. (1986). *Essentials of the Roy adaptation model*. Norwalk, CT: Appleton-Century-Crofts.

Boston-Based Adaptation Research in Nursing Society. (1999). *Roy adaptation model–based research: 25 years of contributions to nursing science*. Indianapolis: Sigma Theta Tau International.

Riehl, J. P., & Roy, C. (Eds.). (1974). *Conceptual models for nursing practice*. Englewood Cliffs, NJ: Prentice-Hall.

Riehl, J. P., & Roy, C. (Eds.). (1980). *Conceptual models for nursing practice* (2nd ed.). New York: Appleton-Century-Crofts.

Roy, C. (1976). *Introduction to nursing: An adaptation model*. Englewood Cliffs, NJ: Prentice-Hall.

Roy, C. (1982). *Introduction to nursing: An adaptation model* (Japanese translation by Yuriko Kanematsu). Tokyo, Japan: UNI Agency.

Roy, C. (1984). *Introduction to nursing: An adaptation model* (2nd ed.). Englewood Cliffs, NJ: Prentice-Hall.

Roy, C., & Andrews, H. A. (1991). *The Roy adaptation model: The definitive statement*. Norwalk, CT: Appleton & Lange.

Roy, C., & Andrews, H. A. (1999). *The Roy adaptation model* (2nd ed.). Stamford, CT: Appleton & Lange.

Roy, C., & Roberts, S. (1981). *Theory construction in nursing: An adaptation model*. Englewood Cliffs, NJ: Prentice-Hall.

Roy, C., & Jones, D. (Eds.). (2007). *Nursing knowledge development and clinical practice*. New York: Springer.

Book Chapters

Barone, S. H., & Roy, C. (1996). The Roy adaptation model in research: Rehabilitation nursing. In P. H. Walker & B. Neuman (Eds.), *Blueprint for use of nursing models: Education, research, practice, and administration* (pp. 64–87). New York: National League for Nursing.

Morgillo-Freeman, S., & Roy, C. (2005). Cognitive behavior therapy and the Roy adaptation model: A discussion of theoretical integration. In S. M. Freeman & A. Freeman (Eds.), *Cognitive behavior therapy in nursing practice* (pp. 3–27). New York: Springer.

Roy, C. (1974). The Roy adaptation model. In J. P. Riehl & C. Roy (Eds.), *Conceptual models for nursing practice* (pp. 135–144). New York: Appleton-Century-Crofts.

Roy, C. (1980). The Roy adaptation model. In J. P. Riehl & C. Roy (Eds.), *Conceptual models for nursing practice* (2nd ed., pp. 179–188). New York: Appleton-Century-Crofts.

Roy, C. (1981). A systems model of nursing care and its effect on the quality of human life. In G. E. Lasker (Ed.), *Applied systems and cybernetics. Vol. 4. Systems research in health care, biocybernetics, and ecology* (pp. 1705–1714). New York: Pergamon.

Roy, C. (1983). A conceptual framework for clinical specialist practice. In A. B. Hamrick & J. Spross (Eds.), *The clinical nurse specialist in theory and practice* (pp. 3–20). New York: Grune & Stratton.

Roy, C. (1983). The expectant family: Analysis and application of the Roy adaptation model, and the family in primary care—Analysis and application of the Roy adaptation model. In I. W. Clements & F. B. Roberts (Eds.), *Family health: A theoretical approach to nursing care* (pp. 298–303). New York: Wiley.

Roy, C. (1983). Roy adaptation model. In I. Clements & F. Roberts (Eds.), *Family health: A theoretical approach to family health* (pp. 255–278). New York: Wiley.

Roy, C. (1983). Theory development in nursing: A proposal for direction. In N. Chaska (Ed.), *The nursing profession: A time to speak* (pp. 453–467). New York: McGraw-Hill.

Roy, C. (1987). The influence of nursing models on clinical decision making II. In K. J. Hannah, M. Reimer, W. C. Mills, & S. Letourneau (Eds.), *Clinical judgment and decision making. The future of nursing diagnosis* (pp. 42–47). New York: Wiley.

Roy, C. (1987). Roy's adaptation model. In R. R. Parse (Ed.), *Nursing science: Major paradigms, theories, and critiques* (pp. 35–45). Philadelphia: Saunders.

Roy, C. (1988). Sister Callista Roy. In T. M. Schorr & A. Zimmerman (Eds.), *Making choices: Taking chances* (pp. 291–298). St Louis: Mosby.

Roy, C. (1989). The Roy adaptation model. In J. P. Riehl (Ed.), *Conceptual models for nursing practice* (3rd ed., pp. 105–114). Norwalk, CT: Appleton & Lange.

Roy, C. (1991). Altered cognition: An information processing approach. In P. H. Mitchell, L. C. Hodges, M. Muwaswes, & C. A. Walleck (Eds.), *AANN's neuroscience nursing: Phenomenon and practice: Human responses to neurological health problems* (pp. 185–211). Norwalk, CT: Appleton & Lange.

Roy, C. (1991). Structure of knowledge: Paradigm, model, and research specifications for differentiated practice. In I. E. Goertzen (Ed.), *Differentiating nursing practice: Into the twenty-first century* (pp. 31–39). Kansas City, MO: American Academy of Nursing.

Roy, C. (1992). Vigor, variables, and vision: Commentary of Florence Nightingale. In F. Nightingale (Ed.), *Notes on nursing: What it is, and what it is not* (Commemorative edition, pp. 63–71). Philadelphia: Lippincott.

Roy, C. (2000). Alteration in cognitive processing. In C. Stewart-Amidei, J. Kunkel, & K. Bronstein (Eds.), *AANN's neuroscience nursing: Human responses to neurologic dysfunction* (2nd ed., pp. 275–323). Philadelphia: Saunders.

Roy, C. (2000). NANDA and the nurse theorists: The truth of nursing theory. In North American Nursing Diagnosis Association, *Classification of nursing diagnoses* (pp. 59–57). St Louis: Mosby.

Roy, C. (2001). Alterations in cognitive processing. In C. Stewart-Amidei & J. A. Kunkel (Eds.), *AANN's neuroscience nursing: Human responses to neurologic dysfunction* (2nd ed.). Philadelphia: Saunders.

Roy, C. (2007). The Roy adaptation model: Historical and philosophical foundations. In Maria Elisa Moreno, et al. (Eds.), *Application del model adaptacion en el ciclo vital humano* (2nd ed.). Chia, Colombia: Universidad de La Sabana.

Roy, C., & Anway, J. (1989). Roy's adaptation model: Theories and hypotheses for nursing administration. In B. Henry, M. DiVincenti, C. Arndt, & A. Marriner Tomey (Eds.), *Dimensions of nursing administration: Theory, research, education, and practice* (pp. 75–88). Boston: Blackwell Scientific.

Roy, C., & Corliss, C. P. (1993). The Roy adaptation model. Theoretical update and knowledge for practice. In M. E. Parker (Ed.), *Patterns of nursing theories in practice* (pp. 215–229). New York: National League for Nursing.

Roy, C., & McLeod, D. (1981). Theory of the person as an adaptive system. In C. Roy & S. L. Roberts (Eds.), *Theory construction in nursing: An adaptation model* (pp. 49–69). Englewood Cliffs, NJ: Prentice-Hall.

Roy, C., & Zhan, L. (2001). The Roy adaptation model: A basis for developing knowledge for practice with the elderly. In M. Parker (Ed.), *Nursing theories and nursing practice* (pp. 315–342). Philadelphia: F. A. Davis.

Journal Articles

Artinian, N. T., & Roy, C. (1990). Strengthening the Roy adaptation model through conceptual clarification. Commentary (Artinian) and response (Roy). *Nursing Science Quarterly, 3*(2), 60–66.

Hanna, D. R., & Roy, C. (2001). Roy adaptation model perspectives on family. *Nursing Science Quarterly, 14*(1), 9–13.

Pollock, S. E., Frederickson, K., Carson, M. A., Massey, V. H., & Roy, C. (1994). Contributions to nursing science: Synthesis of findings from adaptation model research. *Scholarly Inquiry for Nursing Practice, 8*(4), 361–374.

Roy, C. (1970). Adaptation: A conceptual framework in nursing. *Nursing Outlook, 18*, 42–45.

Roy, C. (1971). Adaptation: A basis for nursing practice. *Nursing Outlook, 19*, 254–257.

Roy, C. (1973). Adaptation: Implications for curriculum change. *Nursing Outlook, 21*, 163–168.

Roy, C. (1975). A diagnostic classification system for nursing. *Nursing Outlook, 23*, 90–94.

Roy, C. (1975). The impact of nursing diagnosis. *AORN Journal, 21*, 1023–1030.

Roy, C. (1976). The Roy adaptation model: Comment. *Nursing Outlook, 24*, 690–691.

Roy, C. (1979). Nursing diagnosis from the perspective of a nursing model. *Nursing Diagnosis Newsletter, 6*(3), 1–3.

Roy, C. (1979). Relating nursing theory to nursing education: A new era. *Nurse Educator, 4*(2), 16–21.

Roy, C. (1980). Exposé de Callista Roy sur theories. Exposé de Callista Roy sur l'utilisation de sa theories au nouveau de la recherche. *Acta Nursologica, 3*. [Essay by Castilla Roy on theories. Essay by Castilla Roy on utilization of her theories in new research. *Acta Nursologica, 3*]

Roy, C. (1987). Response to "Needs of spouses of surgical patients, a conceptualization within the Roy adaptation model." *Scholarly Journal for Nursing Practice, 1*(1), 45–50.

Roy, C. (1988). An explication of the philosophical assumptions of the Roy adaptation model. *Nursing Science Quarterly, 1*(1), 26–34.

Roy, C. (1988). Human information processing and nursing research. *Annual Review of Nursing Research, 6*, 237–262.

Roy, C. (1990). Case reports can provide a standard for care in nursing practice. *Journal of Professional Nursing, 6*(3), 179–180.

Roy, C. (1990). Strengthening the Roy adaptation model through conceptual clarification. *Nursing Science Quarterly, 3*(2), 64–66.

Roy, C. (1991). Theory and research for clinical knowledge development. *Journal of Japanese Nursing Research, 14*(1), 21–29.

Roy, C. (1995). Developing nursing knowledge: Practice issues raised from four philosophical perspectives. *Nursing Science Quarterly, 8*(2), 79–85.

Roy, C. (1997). Future of the Roy model: Challenge to redefine adaptation. *Nursing Science Quarterly, 10*(1), 42–48.

Roy, C. (2000). Critique: Research on cognitive consequences of treatment for childhood acute lymphoblastic leukemia. *Seminars in Oncology Nursing, 16*(4), 291.

Roy, C. (2000). A theorist envisions the future and speaks to nursing administrators. *Nursing Administration Quarterly, 24*(2), 1–12.

Roy, C. (2000). The visible and invisible fields that shape the future of the nursing care system. *Nursing Administration Quarterly, 25*(1), 119–131.

Roy, C. (2003). Reflections on nursing research and the Roy adaptation model. *Japanese Journal of Nursing Research, 36*(1), 7–11.

Roy, C. (2007). Update from the future: Thinking of theorist Sr. Callista Roy. *Nursing Science Quarterly, 20*(2), 113–116.

Roy, C. (2011). Research based on the Roy adaptation model: Last 25 years. *Nursing Science Quarterly, 24*(4), 312–320.

Roy, C. (2011). Extending the Roy adaptation model to meet changing global needs. *Nursing Science Quarterly, 24*(4), 345–351.

Whittemore, R., & Roy, C. (2002). Adapting to diabetes mellitus: A theory synthesis. *Nursing Science Quarterly, 15*(4), 311–317.

Dissertation

Roy, C. (1977). *Decision-making by the physically ill and adaptation during illness.* Unpublished doctoral dissertation, University of California, Los Angeles.

Secondary Sources

Book Chapters

Fawcett, J. (2005). Roy's adaptation model. In J. Fawcett (Ed.), *Analysis and evaluation of contemporary nursing knowledge: Nursing models and theories* (pp. 364–437). Philadelphia: F. A. Davis.

Galbreath, J. (2002). Roy adaptation model: Sister Callista Roy. In J. B. George (Ed.), *Nursing theories: The base for professional nursing practice* (pp. 295–338). Upper Saddle River, NJ: Prentice-Hall.

Phillips, K. D. (2002). Roy's adaptation model in nursing practice. In M. R. Alligood & A. M. Tomey (Eds.), *Nursing theory: Utilization & application* (pp. 289–314). St Louis: Mosby.

Tiedeman, M. E. (2005). Roy's adaptation model. In J. J. Fitzpatrick & A. L. Whall (Eds.), *Conceptual models of nursing: Analysis and application* (4th ed., pp. 146–176). Englewood Cliffs, NJ: Prentice-Hall.

Dissertations

Ahern, E. (2006). *Elaboration d'un modele theorique de l'agression en milieu psychiatrique et developpement d'instruments de mesure* (Doctoral dissertation. Universite de Montreal, 2006). *Dissertation Abstracts International, 68*, 3698.

Arcamone, A. A. (2005). *The effect of prenatal education on adaptation to motherhood after vaginal childbirth in primiparous women as assessed by Roy's four adaptive modes* (Doctoral dissertation, Widener University). *Dissertation Abstracts International, 66*, 4722.

Beck-Little, R. (2000). *Sleep enhancement interventions and the sleep of institutionalized older adults* (Doctoral dissertation, University of South Carolina). *Dissertation Abstracts International, 61*, 3503.

Black, K. D. (2004). *Physiologic responses, sense of well-being, self-efficacy for self-monitoring role, perceived availability of social support, and perceived stress in women with pregnancy-induced hypertension* (Doctoral dissertation, Widener University). *Dissertation Abstracts International, 65*, 1773.

Chayaput, P. (2004). *Development and psychometric evaluation of the Thai version of the Coping and Adaptation Processing Scale* (Doctoral dissertation, Boston College). *Dissertation Abstracts International, 65*, 2864.

Cheng, S. (2002). *A multi-method study of Taiwanese children's pain experience* (Doctoral dissertation, University of Colorado Health Sciences Center). *Dissertation Abstracts International, 63*, 1265.

Dunn, K. S. (2001). *Adaptation to chronic pain: Religious and non-religious coping in Judeo-Christian elders* (Doctoral dissertation, Wayne State University). *Dissertation Abstracts International, 62*, 5640.

Frame, K. R. (2002). *The effect of a support group on perceptions of scholastic competence, social acceptance and behavioral conduct in preadolescents diagnosed with attention deficit hyperactivity disorder* (Doctoral dissertation, Widener University). *Dissertation Abstracts International, 63*, 737.

Gipson-Jones, T. L. (2005). *The relationship between work-family conflict, job satisfaction and psychological well-being among African American nurses* (Doctoral dissertation, Hampton University). *Dissertation Abstracts International, 66*, 2512.

Harner, H. M. (2001). *Obstetrical outcomes of teenagers with adult and peer age partners* (Doctoral dissertation, University of Pennsylvania). *Dissertation Abstracts International, 62*, 2256.

Harris, R. F. (2012). *Effects of a home-based exercise program on perception of illness and adaptation in heart failure patients* (Doctoral dissertation, University of Tennessee). Retrieved from http://www.trace.tennessee.edu.

Henderson, P. D. (2002). *African-American women coping with breast cancer* (Doctoral dissertation, Hampton University). *Dissertation Abstracts International, 63*, 5764.

Huang, C. M. (2002). *Sleep and daytime sleepiness in first-time mothers during early postpartum in Taiwan* (Doctoral dissertation, University of Texas at Austin). *Dissertation Abstracts International, 64*, 3189.

Jenkins, B. E. (2006). *Emotional intelligence of faculty members, the learning environment, and empowerment of baccalaureate students* (Doctoral dissertation, Columbia University). *Dissertation Abstracts International, 67*, 3701.

Kan, E. Z. (2007). *Adaptive behaviors and perceptions of recovery following coronary artery bypass graft surgery* (Doctoral dissertation, Widener University). *Dissertation Abstracts International, 68*, 4390.

Kittiwatanapaisan, W. (2002). *Measurement of fatigue in myasthenia gravis patients* (Doctoral dissertation, University of Alabama at Birmingham). *Dissertation Abstracts International, 63*, 4595.

Klein, G. J. M. (2000). *The relationships among anxiety, self-concept, the impostor phenomenon, and generic senior baccalaureate nursing students' perceptions of clinical competency* (Doctoral dissertation, Widener University). *Dissertation Abstracts International, 61*, 5236.

Kochniuk, L. (2004). *We never buy green bananas: The oldest old. A phenomenological study* (Doctoral dissertation, University of Idaho). *Dissertation Abstracts International, 65*, 2318.

Lefaiver, C. A. (2006). *Quality of life: The dyad of caregivers and lung transplant candidates* (Doctoral dissertation, Loyola University). *Dissertation Abstracts International, 67*, 4978.

Lu, Y. (2001). *Caregiving stress effects on functional capability and self-care behavior for elderly caregivers of persons with Alzheimer's disease* (Doctoral dissertation, Case Western Reserve University, Health Sciences). *Dissertation Abstracts International, 62*, 1807.

Mahoney, E. T. (2000). *The relationships among social support, coping, self-concept, and stage of recovery in alcoholic women* (Doctoral dissertation, Catholic University of America). *Dissertation Abstracts International, 61*, 1872.

Otten, R. (2005). *History of associate degree nursing at Mount St. Mary's College: 1970–2005* (Doctoral dissertation, Pepperdine University). *Dissertation Abstracts International, 67*, 492.

Phahuwatanakorn, W. (2004). *The relationships between social support, maternal employment, postpartum anxiety, and maternal role competencies in Thai primiparous mothers* (Doctoral dissertation, Catholic University of America). *Dissertation Abstracts International, 64*, 5451.

Sabatini, M. (2003). *Exercise and adaptation to aging in older women* (Doctoral dissertation, Widener University). *Dissertation Abstracts International, 64*, 3748.

Saint-Pierre, C. (2003). *Elaboration et verification d'un modele predictif de l'adaptation aux roles associes de mere et de travailleuse a statut precaire* (Doctoral dissertation. Universite de Montreal). *Dissertation Abstracts International, 65*, 1252.

Sander, R. A. (2004). *Measurement of functional status in the spinal cord injured patient* (Doctoral dissertation, Saint Louis University). *Dissertation Abstracts International, 65*, 1783.

Senesac, P. M. (2004). *The Roy Adaptation Model: An action research approach to the implementation of a pain management organizational change project* (Doctoral dissertation, Boston College). *Dissertation Abstracts International, 65*, 2872.

Stephens, K. A. (2005). *Preoxygenation practices prior to tracheal suctioning by nurses caring for individuals with spinal cord injury* (Doctoral dissertation, Loyola University, 2005). *Dissertation Abstracts International, 66*, 2518.

Toughill, E. H. (2001). *Quality of life: The impact of age, severity of urinary incontinence and adaptation* (Doctoral dissertation, New York University). *Dissertation Abstracts International, 61*, 5240.

Wright, R. R. (2007). *Experiences of emergency nurses: What has been learned from traumatic and violent events* (Doctoral Dissertation, Columbia University). *Dissertation Abstracts International, 68*, 3698.

Wunderlich, R. J. (2003). *An exploratory study of physiological and psychological variables that predict weaning from mechanical ventilation* (Doctoral dissertation, Saint Louis University). *Dissertation Abstracts International, 64*, 3750.

Zbegner, D. K. (2003). *An exploratory retrospective study using the Roy adaptation model: The adaptive mode variables of physical energy level, self-esteem, marital satisfaction, and parenthood motivation as predictors of coping behaviors in infertile women* (Doctoral dissertation, Widener University). *Dissertation Abstracts International, 64*, 3751.

Journal Articles

Chiou, C. (2000). A meta-analysis of the interrelationships between the modes in Roy's adaptation model. *Nursing Science Quarterly, 13*(3), 252–258.

Dawson, S. (1998). Adult/elderly care nursing: Preamputation assessment using Roy's adaptation model. *British Journal of Nursing, 7*(9), 536, 538–542.

Decker, J. W. (2000). The effects of inflammatory bowel disease on adolescents. *Gastroenterology Nursing, 23*(2), 63–66.

Dixon, E. L. (1999). Community health nursing practice and the Roy adaptation model. *Public Health Nursing, 16*, 290–300.

Dunn, H. C., & Dunn D. G. (1997). The Roy adaptation model and its application to clinical nursing practice. *Journal of Ophthalmic Nursing and Technology, 6*(2), 74–78.

Harding-Okimoto, M. B. (1997). Pressure ulcers, self-concept, and body image in spinal cord injury patients. *SCI Nursing, 14*(4), 111–117.

Hennessy-Harstad, E. B. (1999). Empowering adolescents with asthma to take control through adaptation. *Journal of Pediatric Health Care, 13*(6 Part 1), 273–277.

Modrcin-McCarthy, M. A., McCue, S., & Walker, J. (1997). Preterm infants and STRESS: A tool for the neonatal nurse. *Journal of Perinatal & Neonatal Nursing, 10*(4), 62–71.

Modrcin-Talbott, M. A., Pullen, L, Ehrenberger, H., Zandstra, K., & Muenchen, B. (1998). Self-esteem in adolescents treated in an outpatient mental health setting. *Issues in Comprehensive Pediatric Nursing, 21*, 159–171.

Modrcin-Talbott, M. A., Pullen, L., Zandstra, K., Ehrenberger, H., & Muenchen, B. (1998). A study of self-esteem among well adolescents: Seeking a new direction. *Issues in Comprehensive Pediatric Nursing, 21*, 229–241.

Niska, K. J. (1999). Family nursing interventions: Mexican American early family formation: Third part of a three-part study. *Nursing Science Quarterly, 12*(4), 335–340.

Niska, K. J. (2001). Mexican American family survival, continuity, and growth: The parental perspective. *Nursing Science Quarterly, 14*(4), 322–329.

Orsi, A. J., Grandy, C., Tax, A., & McCorkle, R. (1997). Nutritional adaptation of women living with HIV: A pilot study. *Holistic Nursing Practice, 12*(1), 71–79.

Samarel, N., Fawcett, J., Krippendorf, K., Piacentino, J. C., Eliasof, B., Hughes, P., et al. (1998). Women's perception of group support and adaptation to breast cancer. *Journal of Advanced Nursing, 28*(6), 1259–1268.

Samarel, N., Fawcett, J., Tulman, L., Rothman, H., Spector, L., Spillane, P. A., et al. (1999). A resource kit for women with breast cancer: Development and evaluation. *Oncology Nursing Forum, 26*(3), 611–618.

Sheppard, V. A., & Cunnie, K. L. (1996). Incidence of diuresis following hysterectomy. *Journal of Post Anesthesia Nursing, 11*, 20–28.

Woods, S. J., & Isenberg, M. A. (2001). Adaptation as a mediator of intimate abuse and traumatic stress in battered women. *Nursing Science Quarterly, 14*(3), 215–221.

Yeh, C. H. (2001). Adaptation in children with cancer: Research with Roy's model. *Nursing Science Quarterly, 14*, 141–148.

Zhan, L. (2000). Cognitive adaptation and self-consistency in hearing-impaired older persons: Testing Roy's adaptation model. *Nursing Science Quarterly, 13*(2), 158–165.

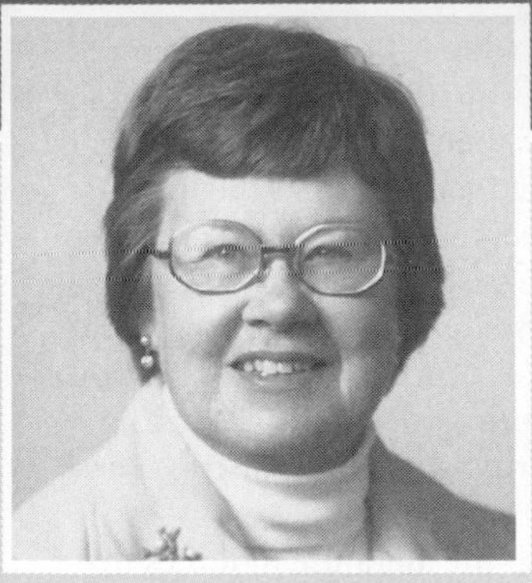

Dorothy E. Johnson
(1919–1999)

18

Behavioral System Model

*Bonnie Holaday**

"All of us, scientists and practicing professionals, must turn our attention to practice and ask questions of that practice. We must be inquisitive and inquiring, seeking the fullest and truest possible understanding of the theoretical and practical problems we encounter."

(Johnson, 1976)

CREDENTIALS AND BACKGROUND OF THE THEORIST

Dorothy E. Johnson was born on August 21, 1919, in Savannah, Georgia. She received her associate's degree from Armstrong Junior College in Savannah, Georgia (1938), her bachelor of science degree in nursing from Vanderbilt University in Nashville, Tennessee (1942), and her master's of public health degree from Harvard University in Boston (1948).

Johnson's professional experiences involved mostly teaching, although she was a staff nurse at the Chatham-Savannah Health Council from 1943 to 1944. She was an instructor and an assistant professor in pediatric nursing at Vanderbilt University School of Nursing. From 1949 until her retirement in 1978 and her subsequent move to Key Largo, Florida, Johnson was an assistant professor of pediatric nursing, an associate professor of nursing, and a professor of nursing at the University of California in Los Angeles.

In 1955 and 1956, Johnson was a pediatric nursing advisor assigned to the Christian Medical College School of Nursing in Vellore, South India. From 1965 to 1967, she served as chairperson on the committee of the California Nurses Association that developed a position statement on specifications for the clinical specialist. Johnson's publications include four books; more than 30 articles in periodicals; and many papers, reports, proceedings, and monographs (Johnson, 1980).

Of the many honors she received, Johnson (personal communication, 1984) was proudest of the 1975 Faculty Award from graduate students, the 1977 Lulu Hassenplug Distinguished Achievement Award from the California Nurses Association, and the 1981 Vanderbilt University School of Nursing Award for Excellence in Nursing. She died in February 1999 at 80 years of age. She was pleased that her behavioral system model had been found useful in furthering the development of a theoretical basis for nursing and was being used as a model for nursing practice on an institution-wide basis, but she reported that her greatest source of satisfaction came from following the productive careers of her students (D. Johnson, personal communication, 1996).

THEORETICAL SOURCES

Johnson's behavioral system model was heavily influenced by Florence Nightingale's book, *Notes on Nursing* (Johnson, 1992). Johnson began her work on the model with the premise that nursing was a profession that made a distinctive contribution to the welfare of society. Thus nursing had an explicit goal of action in patient welfare. Her task was to clarify the social mission of nursing from the "perspective of a theoretically sound view of the person we serve" (Johnson, 1977). She accepted Nightingale's belief that the first concern of nursing is with the "relationship

*Previous authors: Victoria M. Brown, Sharon S. Conner, Linda S. Harbour, Jude A. Magers, and Judith K. Watt.

between the person who is ill and their environment, not with the illness" (Johnson, 1977). Johnson (1977) noted that the "transition from this approach to the more sophisticated and theoretically sounder behavioral system orientation took only a few years and was supported by both my own, and that of many colleagues, growing knowledge about man's action systems and by the rapidly increasing knowledge about behavioral systems." Johnson (1977) came to conceive of nursing's specific contribution to patient welfare as that of fostering "efficient and effective behavioral functioning in the person, both to prevent illness and during and following illness."

Johnson used the work of behavioral scientists in psychology, sociology, and ethnology to develop her theory. The interdisciplinary literature that Johnson cited focused on observable behaviors that were of adaptive significance. This body of literature influenced the identification and the content of her seven subsystems. Talcott Parsons is acknowledged specifically in early developmental writings presenting concepts of the Johnson behavioral system model (Johnson, 1961a). Parsons' (1951, 1964) social action theory stressed a structural-functional approach. One of his major contributions was to reconcile functionalism (the idea that every observable social behavior has a function to perform) with structuralism (the idea that social behaviors, rather than being directly functional, are expressions of deep underlying structures in social systems). Thus structures (social systems) and all behaviors have a function in maintaining them. The components of the structure of a social system—goal, set, choice, and behavior—are the same in Parsons' and Johnson's theories.

Johnson also relied heavily on system theory and used concepts and definitions from Rapoport, Chin, von Bertalanffy, and Buckley (Johnson, 1980). In system theory, as in Johnson's theory, one of the basic assumptions embraces the concept of order. Another is that a system is a set of interacting units that form a whole intended to perform some function. Johnson conceptualized the person as a behavioral system in which the behavior of the individual as a whole is the focus. It is the focus on what the individual does and why. One of the strengths of the Johnson behavior system theory is the consistent integration of concepts defining behavioral systems drawn from general systems theory. Some of these concepts include holism, goal seeking, interrelationship/interdependency, stability, instability, subsystems, regularity, structure, function, energy, feedback, and adaptation.

Johnson noted that although the literature indicates that others support the idea that a person is a behavioral system and that a person's specific response patterns form an organized and integrated whole, the idea was original with her as far as she knew. Just as the development of knowledge of the whole biological system was preceded by knowledge of the parts, the development of knowledge of behavioral systems was focused on specific behavioral responses. Empirical literature supporting the notion of the behavioral system as a whole and its usefulness as a framework for nursing decisions in research, education, and nursing practice has accumulated since it was introduced (Benson, 1997; Derdiarian, 1991; Grice, 1997; Holaday, 1981, 1982; Holaday, Turner-Henson, & Swan, 1996; Lachicotte & Alexander, 1990; Martha, Bhaduri, & Jain, 2004; Oyedele, Wright, & Maja, 2013; Poster, Dee, & Randell, 1997; Turner-Henson, 1992; Wang & Palmer, 2010; Wilmoth, 2007; Wilmoth & Ross, 1997).

Developing the behavioral system model from a philosophical perspective, Johnson (1980) wrote that nursing contributes by facilitating effective behavioral functioning in the patient before, during, and after illness. She used concepts from other disciplines, such as social learning, motivation, sensory stimulation, adaptation, behavioral modification, change process, tension, and stress, to expand her theory for the practice of nursing.

MAJOR CONCEPTS & DEFINITIONS

Behavior

Johnson accepted the definition of behavior as expressed by behavioral and biological scientists—that is, the output of intraorganismic structures and processes as they are coordinated and articulated by and responsive to changes in sensory stimulation. Johnson (1980) focused on behavior affected by the actual or implied presence of other social beings that has been shown to have major adaptive significance.

System

Using Rapoport's 1968 definition of system, Johnson (1980) stated, "A system is a whole that functions as a whole by virtue of the interdependence of its parts" (p. 208). She accepted Chin's statement that there is "organization, interaction, interdependency, and integration of the parts and elements" (Johnson, 1980, p. 208). In addition, a person strives to maintain a balance in these parts through adjustments and adaptations to the impinging forces.

Behavioral System

A behavioral system encompasses the patterned, repetitive, and purposeful ways of behaving. These ways of behaving form an organized and integrated functional unit that determines and limits the interaction between the person and his or her environment and establishes the

MAJOR CONCEPTS & DEFINITIONS—cont'd

relationship of the person to the objects, events, and situations within his or her environment. Usually the behavior can be described and explained. A person as a behavioral system tries to achieve stability and balance by adjustments and adaptations that are successful to some degree for efficient and effective functioning. The system is usually flexible enough to accommodate the influences affecting it (Johnson, 1980).

Subsystems

The behavioral system has many tasks to perform; therefore parts of the system evolve into subsystems with specialized tasks. A subsystem is "a minisystem with its own particular goal and function that can be maintained as long as its relationship to the other subsystems or the environment is not disturbed" (Johnson, 1980, p. 221). The seven subsystems identified by Johnson are open, linked, and interrelated. Input and output are components of all seven subsystems (Grubbs, 1980).

Motivational drives direct the activities of these subsystems, which are continually changing through maturation, experience, and learning. The systems described appear to exist cross-culturally and are controlled by biological, psychological, and sociological factors. The seven identified subsystems are **attachment-affiliative, dependency, ingestive, eliminative, sexual, achievement,** and **aggressive-protective** (Johnson, 1980).

Attachment-Affiliative Subsystem

The attachment-affiliative subsystem is probably the most critical because it forms the basis for all social organization. On a general level, it provides survival and security. Its consequences are social inclusion, intimacy, and formation and maintenance of a strong social bond (Johnson, 1980).

Dependency Subsystem

In the broadest sense, the dependency subsystem promotes helping behavior that calls for a nurturing response. Its consequences are approval, attention or recognition, and physical assistance. Developmentally, dependency behavior evolves from almost total dependence on others to a greater degree of dependence on self. A certain amount of interdependence is essential for the survival of social groups (Johnson, 1980).

Ingestive Subsystem

The ingestive and eliminative subsystems should not be seen as the input and output mechanisms of the system. All subsystems are distinct subsystems with their own input and output mechanisms. The ingestive subsystem "has to do with when, how, what, how much, and under what conditions we eat" (Johnson, 1980, p. 213). "It serves the broad function of appetitive satisfaction" (Johnson, 1980, p. 213). This behavior is associated with social, psychological, and biological considerations (Johnson, 1980).

Eliminative Subsystem

The eliminative subsystem addresses "when, how, and under what conditions we eliminate" (Johnson, 1980, p. 213). As with the ingestive subsystem, the social and psychological factors are viewed as influencing the biological aspects of this subsystem and may be, at times, in conflict with the eliminative subsystem (Loveland-Cherry & Wilkerson, 1983).

Sexual Subsystem

The sexual subsystem has the dual functions of procreation and gratification. Including, but not limited to, courting and mating, this response system begins with the development of gender role identity and includes the broad range of sex-role behaviors (Johnson, 1980).

Achievement Subsystem

The achievement subsystem attempts to manipulate the environment. Its function is control or mastery of an aspect of self or environment to some standard of excellence. Areas of achievement behavior include intellectual, physical, creative, mechanical, and social skills (Johnson, 1980).

Aggressive-Protective Subsystem

The aggressive-protective subsystem's function is protection and preservation. This follows the line of thinking of ethologists such as Lorenz (1966) and Feshbach (1970) rather than the behavioral reinforcement school of thought, which contends that aggressive behavior is not only learned, but also has a primary intent to harm others. Society demands that limits be placed on modes of self-protection and that people and their property be respected and protected (Johnson, 1980).

Equilibrium

Johnson (1961b) stated that equilibrium is a key concept in nursing's specific goal. It is defined as "a stabilized but more or less transitory, resting state in which the individual is in harmony with himself and with his environment" (p. 65). "It implies that biological and psychological forces are in balance with each other and with impinging social forces" (Johnson, 1961a, p. 11). It is "not synonymous with a state of health, since it may be found either in health or illness" (Johnson, 1961a, p. 11).

Continued

MAJOR CONCEPTS & DEFINITIONS—cont'd

Functional Requirements and Sustenal Imperatives

For the subsystems to develop and maintain stability, each must have a constant supply of **function requirements**. The environment supplies sustenal imperatives such as protection, nurturance, and stimulation. Johnson notes that the biologic system and all other living systems have the same requirements.

Regulation/Control

The interrelated behavioral subsystems must be regulated in some fashion so that its goals can be realized. **Regulation** implies that deviations will be detected and corrected. Feedback is, therefore, a requirement of effective control. There is self-regulation by the client. The nurse can also act as a temporary external regulatory force to preserve the organization and integration of the client's behavior at an optimal level in situations of illness or under conditions where behavior constitutes a threat to health.

Tension

"The concept of **tension** is defined as a state of being stretched or strained and can be viewed as an end-product of a disturbance in equilibrium" (Johnson, 1961b, p. 10). Tension can be constructive in adaptive change or destructive in inefficient use of energy, hindering adaptation and causing potential structural damage (Johnson, 1961b). Tension is the cue to disturbance in equilibrium (Johnson, 1961a).

Stressor

Internal or external stimuli that produce tension and result in a degree of instability are called **stressors.** "Stimuli may be positive in that they are present; or negative in that something desired or required is absent. [Stimuli] . . . may be either endogenous or exogenous in origin [and] may play upon one or more of our linked open systems" (Johnson, 1961a, p. 13). The open-linked systems are in constant interchange. The open-linked systems include the physiological, personality, and meaningful small group (the family) systems and the larger social system (Johnson, 1961a).

The author acknowledges the contribution of Brown, V. M. (2006). Behavioral system model. In A. M. Tomey & M. R. Alligood (Eds.), *Nursing theorists and their work* (6th ed., pp. 386–404) Philadelphia: Mosby-Elsevier.

USE OF EMPIRICAL EVIDENCE

The empirical origins of this theory begin with Johnson's use of systems thinking (synthesis). This process concentrates on the function and behavior of the whole and is focused on understanding and explanation of the behavioral system. Johnson's work on the behavioral system model corresponded with the "systems age." Buckley's (1968) seminal text was published the same year Johnson formally presented her theory at Vanderbilt University.

System theory, as a basic science, deals on an abstract level with the general properties of systems regardless of physical form or domain of application. General system theory was founded on the assumption that all kinds of systems had characteristics in common regardless of their internal nature. Johnson used general system theory and systems thinking to bring together a body of theoretical constructs, as well as explaining their interrelationships, to identify and describe the mission of nursing. The Johnson behavioral system model provided a framework that is based on her synthesis of the component parts of this system and a description of the context of relationships with one another (subsystems) and with other systems (environment). Standing in contrast to scientific reductionism, Johnson proposed to view nursing in a holistic manner—a behavioral system. Consistent with system theory, the Johnson behavioral system model provides an understanding of a system by examining the linkages and interactions between the elements that compose the entirety of the system. The paragraphs that follow describe how Johnson incorporated empirical knowledge from other disciplines into the Johnson behavioral system model.

Concepts Johnson identified and defined in her theory are supported in the literature. She noted that Escalona and Leitch agreed that tension produces behavioral changes and that the manifestation of tension by an individual depends on both internal and external factors (Johnson, 1980). Johnson (1959a) used the work of Selye, Grinker, Simmons, and Wolff to support the idea that specific patterns of behavior are reactions to stressors from biological, psychological, and sociological sources, respectively. Johnson (1961b) suggested a difference in her model from Selye's conception of stress. Johnson's concept of stress "follows rather closely Caudill's conceptualization; that is, that stress is a process in which there is interplay between various stimuli and the defenses erected against them. Stimuli may be positive in that they are present, or negative in that something desired or required is absent" (Johnson, 1961b, pp. 7–8). Selye "conceives stress as 'a state' manifested by the specific syndrome which consists of all the nonspecifically induced changes within a biologic system" (Johnson, 1961b, p. 8).

In *Conceptual Models for Nursing Practice,* Johnson (1980) described seven subsystems that make up her behavioral system. To support the attachment-affiliative subsystem, she cited the work of Ainsworth and Robson. Heathers, Gerwitz, and Rosenthal have described and explained dependency behavior, another subsystem defined by Johnson. The response systems of ingestion and elimination, as described by Walike, Mead, and Sears, are also parts of Johnson's behavioral system. The work of Kagan and Resnik were used to support the sexual subsystem. The aggressive-protective subsystem, which functions to protect and preserve, is supported by Lorenz and Feshbach (Feshbach, 1970; Johnson, 1980; Lorenz, 1966). According to Atkinson, Feather, and Crandell, physical, creative, mechanical, and social skills are manifested by achievement behavior, another subsystem identified by Johnson (1980).

The restorative subsystem was developed by faculty and clinicians to include behaviors such as sleep, play, and relaxation (Grubbs, 1980). Although Johnson (personal communication, 1996) agreed that "there may be more or fewer subsystems" than originally identified, she did not support **restorative** as a subsystem of the behavioral system model. She believed that sleep is primarily a biological force, not a motivational behavior. She suggested that many of the behaviors identified in infants during their first years of life, such as play, are actually achievement behaviors. Johnson (personal communication, 1996) stated that there was a need to examine the possibility of an eighth subsystem that addresses explorative behaviors; further investigation may delineate it as a subsystem separate from the achievement subsystem.

MAJOR ASSUMPTIONS

Nursing

Nursing's goal is to maintain and restore the person's behavioral system balance and stability or to help the person achieve a more optimum level of balance and functioning. Thus nursing, as perceived by Johnson, is an external force acting to preserve the organization and integration of the patient's behavior to an optimal level by means of imposing temporary regulatory or control mechanisms or by providing resources while the patient is experiencing stress or behavioral system imbalance (Brown, 2006). An art and a science, nursing supplies external assistance both before and during system balance disturbance and therefore requires knowledge of order, disorder, and control (Herbert, 1989; Johnson, 1980). Nursing activities do not depend on medical authority, but they are complementary to medicine.

Person

Johnson (1980) viewed the person as a behavioral system with patterned, repetitive, and purposeful ways of behaving that link the person with the environment. The conception of the person is basically a motivational one. This view leans heavily on Johnson's acceptance of ethology theories, that innate, biological factors influence the patterning and motivation of behavior. She also acknowledged that prior experience, learning, and physical and social stimuli also influence behavior. She noted that a prerequisite to using this model is the ability to look at a person as a behavioral system, observe a collection of behavioral subsystems, and be knowledgeable about the physiological, psychological, and sociocultural factors operating outside them (class notes, 1971).

Johnson identified several assumptions that are critical to understanding the nature and operation of the person as a behavioral system. We assume that there is organization, interaction, and interdependency and integration of the parts of behavior that make up the system. An individual's specific response patterns form an organized and integrated whole. The interrelated and interdependent parts are called **subsystems.** Johnson (1977) further assumed that the behavioral system tends to achieve balance among the various forces operating within and upon it. People strive continually to maintain a behavioral system balance and steady states by more or less automatic adjustments and adaptations to the natural forces impinging upon them. Johnson also recognized that people actively seek new experiences that may temporarily disturb balance.

Johnson further (1977, 1980) assumed that a behavioral system, which both requires and results in some degree of regularity and constancy in behavior, is essential to human beings. Finally, Johnson (1977) assumed that behavioral system balance reflected adjustments and adaptations by the person that are successful in some way and to some degree. This will be true, even though the observed behavior may not always match the cultural norms for acceptable or health behavior.

Balance is essential for effective and efficient functioning of the person. Balance is developed and maintained within the subsystems(s) or the system as a whole. Changes in the structure or function of a system are related to problems with drive, lack of functional requirements or sustenal imperatives, or a change in the environment. A person's attempt to reestablish balance may require an extraordinary expenditure of energy that leaves a shortage of energy to assist biological processes and recovery.

Health

Johnson perceived health as an elusive, dynamic state influenced by biological, psychological, and social factors. Health is reflected by the organization, interaction, interdependence, and integration of the subsystems of the behavioral system (Johnson, 1980). An individual attempts to achieve a balance in this system, which will lead to functional behavior. A lack of balance in the structural or functional requirements of the subsystems leads to poor health. Thus when evaluating "health," one focuses on the behavioral system and system balance and stability, effective and efficient functioning, and behavioral system imbalance and instability. The outcomes of behavior system balance are that (1) a minimum expenditure of energy is required (implying more energy is available to maintain health, or, in the case of illness, energy is available for the biological processes needed for recovery); (2) continued biologic and social survival are ensured; and (3) some degree of personal satisfaction accrues (Grubbs, 1980; Johnson, 1980).

Environment

In Johnson's theory, the environment consists of all the factors that are not part of the individual's behavioral system, but that influence the system. The nurse may manipulate some aspects of the environment so the goal of health or behavioral system balance can be achieved for the patient (Brown, 2006).

The behavioral system "determines and limits the interaction between the person and their environment and establishes the relationship of the person to the objects, events and situations in the environment" (Johnson, 1978). Such behavior is orderly and predictable. It is maintained because it has been functionally efficient and effective most of the time in managing the person's relationship to the environment. It changes when this is no longer the case, or when the person desires a more optimum level of functioning. The behavioral system has many tasks and missions to perform in maintaining its own integrity and in managing the system's relationship to its environment.

The behavioral system attempts to maintain equilibrium in response to environmental factors by adjusting and adapting to the forces that impinge on it. Excessively strong environmental forces disturb the behavioral system balance and threaten the person's stability. An unusual amount of energy is required for the system to reestablish equilibrium in the face of continuing forces (Loveland-Cherry & Wilkerson, 1983).

The environment is also the source of the sustenal imperatives of protection, nurturance, and stimulation that are necessary prerequisites to maintain health (behavioral system balance; Grubbs, 1980). When behavioral system imbalance (disequilibrium) occurs, the nurse may need to become the temporary regulator of the environment and provide the person's supply of functional requirements so the person can adapt to stressors. The type and the amount of functional requirements needed vary by age, gender, culture, coping ability, and type and severity of illness.

THEORETICAL ASSERTIONS

The Johnson behavioral system theory addresses the metaparadigm concepts of **person, environment,** and **nursing.** The person is a behavioral system with seven interrelated subsystems (Fig. 18.1). Each subsystem is formed from a set of behavioral responses, or responsive tendencies, or action systems that share a common drive or goal. Organized around drives (some type of intraorganismic motivational structure), these responses are differentiated, developed, and modified over time through maturation, experience, and learning. They are determined developmentally and are continuously governed by a multitude of physical, biological, and psychological factors operating in a complex and interlocking fashion.

Each subsystem is described and analyzed in terms of structural and functional requirements. The four structural elements that have been identified include (1) drive or goal—the ultimate consequence of behaviors in it; (2) set—a tendency or predisposition to act in a certain way—which is subdivided into two types, **preparatory,** or what a person usually attends to, and **perseverative,** the habits one maintains in a situation; (3) choice, which represents the behavior a patient sees himself or herself as being able to use in any given situation; and (4) action or the behavior of an individual (Grubbs, 1980; Johnson, 1980). Set plays a major role both in the choices a person considers and in his or her ultimate behavior. Each of the seven subsystems has the same three functional requirements: (1) protection, (2) nurturance, and (3) stimulation. These functional requirements must be met through the person's own efforts, or with the outside assistance of the nurse. For the subsystems to develop and maintain stability, each must have a constant supply of functional requirements (sustenal imperatives) that are usually supplied by the environment. However, during illness or when the potential for illness poses a threat, the nurse may become a source of functional requirements.

The responses by the subsystems are developed through motivation, experience, and learning and are influenced by biological, psychological, and social factors (Johnson, 1980). The behavioral system attempts to achieve balance by adapting to internal and environmental stimuli. The behavioral system is made up of "all the patterned, repetitive, and purposeful ways of behaving that characterize each

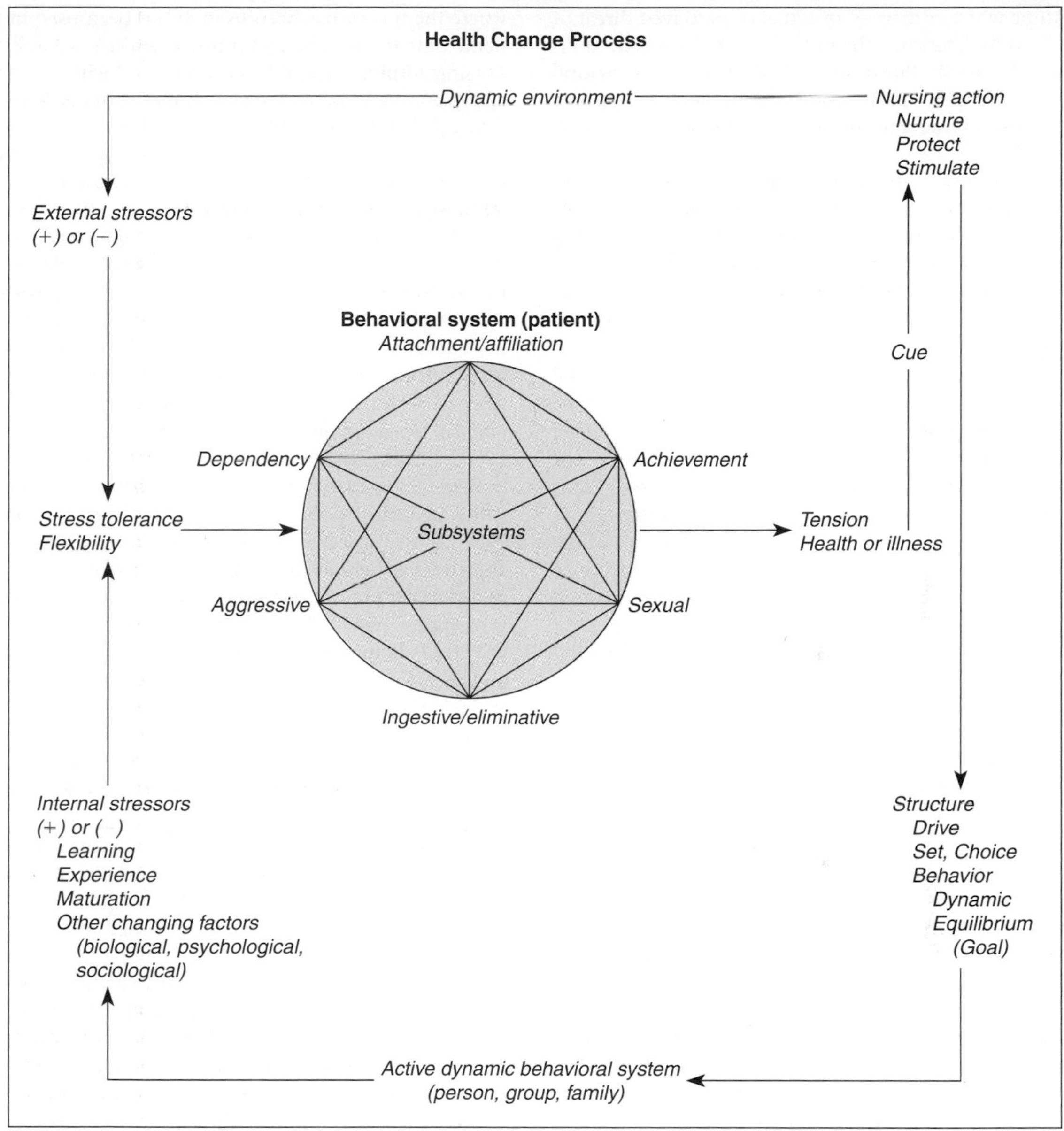

FIG. 18.1 Johnson's behavioral system model. (Conceptualized by Jude A. Magers, Indianapolis, IN.)

man's life" (Johnson, 1980, p. 209). This functional unit of behavior "determines and limits the interaction of the person and his environment and establishes the relationship of the person with the objects, events, and situations in his environment. . . . The behavioral system manages its relationship with its environment" (Johnson, 1980, p. 209). The behavioral system appears to be active and not passive. The nurse is external to and interactive with the behavioral system.

Successful use of Johnson's behavioral system theory in clinical practice requires the incorporation of the nursing process. The clinician must develop an assessment instrument that incorporates the components of the theory so they are able to assess the patient as a behavioral system to determine whether there is an actual or perceived threat of illness and to determine the person's ability to adapt to illness or threat of illness without developing behavioral system imbalance. This means developing appropriate questions and observations for each of the behavioral subsystems.

A state of instability in the behavioral system results in a need for nursing intervention. Identification of the source of the problem in the system leads to appropriate nursing action that results in the maintenance or restoration of behavioral system balance (Brown, 2006). Nursing interventions can be in such general forms as (1) repairing structural units; (2) temporarily imposing external regulatory or control measures; (3) supplying environmental conditions or resources; or (4) providing stimulation to the extent that any problem can be anticipated, and preventive nursing action is in order (Johnson, 1978). "If the source of the problem has a structural stressor, the nurse will focus on either the goal, set, choice, or action of the subsystem. If the problem is one of function, the nurse will focus on the source and sufficiency of the functional requirements since functional problems originate from an environmental excess or deficiency" (Grubbs, 1980, p. 242). The goal of nursing is to maintain or restore the person's behavioral system balance and stability or to help the person achieve a more optimum level of behavioral system functioning when this is desired and possible (Johnson, 1978).

LOGICAL FORM

Johnson approached the task of delineating nursing's mission from historical, analytical, and empirical perspectives. Deductive and inductive thinking is evident throughout the process of developing the Johnson behavioral system theory. A system, inasmuch as it is a whole, will lose its synergetic properties if it is decomposed. Understanding must therefore progress from the whole to its parts—a synthesis. Johnson first identified the behavioral system and then explained the properties and behavior of the system. Finally, she explained the properties and behavior of the subsystems as a part or function of the system. The analysis gave us description and knowledge, and the systems thinking (synthesis) gave us explanation and understanding.

ACCEPTANCE BY THE NURSING COMMUNITY

Practice

The utility of the Johnson behavioral system theory is evident from the variety of clinical settings and age groups where the theory has been used. It has been used in inpatient, outpatient, and community settings as well as in nursing administration. It has been used with a variety of client populations, and several practice tools have been developed (Fawcett, 2013).

Johnson does not use the term **nursing process. Assessment, disorders, treatment,** and **evaluation** are concepts referred to in a variety of Johnson's works. "For the practitioner, conceptual models provide a diagnostic and treatment orientation, and thus are of considerable practical import" (Johnson, 1968, p. 2). The nursing process becomes applicable in the behavioral system model when behavioral malfunction occurs "that is in part disorganized, erratic, and dysfunctional. Illness or other sudden internal or external environmental change is most frequently responsible for such malfunctions" (Johnson, 1980, p. 212). "Assistance is appropriate at those times the individual is experiencing stress of a health-illness nature which disturbs equilibrium, producing tension" (Johnson, 1961b, p. 6). However, it is important to note that systems analysis is an important component of system theory. One monitors outputs from a given subsystem to monitor performance. Signs of disequilibrium require one to identify the problem, further define the problem by gathering data, and design an intervention to restore equilibrium, or balance (Jenkins, 1969; Miller, 1965).

Johnson (1959b) implied that the initial nursing assessment begins when the cue tension is observed and signals disequilibrium. Sources for assessment data can be through history taking, testing, and structural observations (Johnson, 1980). "The behavioral system is thought to determine and limit the interaction between the person and his environment" (Johnson, 1968, p. 3). This suggests that the accuracy and quantity of the data obtained during nursing assessment are not controlled by the nurse, but by the patient (system). The only observed part of the subsystem's structure is behavior. Six internal and external regulators have been identified that "simultaneously influence and are influenced by behavior" including biophysical, psychological, developmental, sociocultural, family, and physical environmental regulators (Randell, 1991, p. 157).

The nurse must be able to access information related to goals, sets, and choices that make up the structural subsystems. "One or more of [these] subsystems is likely to be involved in any episode of illness, whether in an antecedent or a consequential way or simply in association, directly or indirectly with the disorder or its treatment" (Johnson, 1968, p. 3). Accessing the data is critical to accurate statement of the disorder.

Johnson did not define specific disorders, but she did state two general categories of disorders on the basis of the relationship to the biological system (Johnson, 1968).

"Disorders are those which are related tangentially or peripherally to disorder in the biological system; that is, they are precipitated simply by the fact of illness or the situational context of treatment; and . . . those [disorders] which are an integral part of a biological system disorder in that they are either directly associated with or a direct consequence of a particular kind of biological system disorder or its treatment."

(Johnson, 1968, p. 7)

The "means of management" or interventions do consist in part of the provision of nurturance, protection, and stimulation (Johnson, 1968, 1980). The nurse may provide "temporary imposition of external regulatory and control mechanisms, such as inhibiting ineffective behavioral responses, and assisting the patient to acquire new responses" (Johnson, 1968, p. 6). Johnson (1980) suggested that techniques include "teaching, role modeling, and counseling" (p. 211). If a problem or disorder is anticipated, preventive nursing action is appropriate with adequate methodologies (Johnson, 1980). Nurturance, protection, and stimulation are as important for preventive nursing care or health promotion as they are for managing illness (Brown, 2006).

If the problem is a structural stressor, the nurse will focus on goal, set, choice, or action of the subsystem. The nurse works to redirect the person's goals, change drive significance, broaden the range of choices, alter the set, or change the action. The nurse manipulates the structural units or imposes temporary controls. Both types of nursing actions regulate the interaction of the subsystems.

The outcome of nursing intervention is behavioral system equilibrium. "More specifically, equilibrium can be said to have been achieved at that point at which the individual demonstrates a degree of constancy in his pattern of functioning, both internally and interpersonally" (Johnson, 1961b, p. 9). The evaluation of the nursing intervention is based on whether it made "a significant difference in the lives of the persons involved" (Johnson, 1980, p. 215).

The behavioral system model has been operationalized through the development of several assessment instruments. In 1974 Grubbs (1980) used the theory to develop an assessment tool and a nursing process sheet based on Johnson's seven subsystems. Questions and observations related to each subsystem provided tools with which to collect important data, noting choices of behavior that will enable the patient to accomplish his or her goal of health.

That same year, Holaday (1980) used the theory as a model to develop an assessment tool when caring for hospitalized children. This tool allowed the nurse to describe objectively the child's behavior and to guide nursing action. In expanding the concept of "set," Holaday also identified patterns of maternal behaviors that would indicate an inadequate or poorly functioning set that was eroding to the limited choices of action in responding to the needs of chronically ill infants (Holaday, 1981, 1982).

Derdiarian (1990) investigated the effects of using two systematic assessment instruments on patient and nurse satisfaction. The Johnson behavioral system model was used to develop a self-report and observational instrument implemented with the nursing process. The Derdiarian behavioral system model instrument included assessment of the restorative subsystem and the seven subsystems advocated by Johnson. The results indicated that the instruments provided a more comprehensive and systematic approach to assessment and intervention, thereby increasing patient and nurse satisfaction with care.

Lanouette and St-Jacques (1994) used Johnson's model to compare the coping abilities and perceptions of families with premature infants with those of families with full-term infants. The results indicated that positive coping skills were relative to bonding with the infant, using resources, solving problems, and making decisions. Lanouette and St-Jacques suggested that improvement in nursing care practices in nursery, hospital, and community settings might have contributed to this outcome. This supported Johnson's statement that "the effective use of nurturance, protection, and stimulation during maternal contact at birth could significantly reduce the behavioral system problems we see today" (personal communication, 1996).

Case studies have documented the use and evaluation of the Johnson behavioral system model in clinical practice. In 1980 Rawls used the theory to systematically assess a patient who was facing the loss of function in one arm and hand. Herbert (1989) reported the outcomes of a nursing care plan developed for an elderly stroke patient. They each concluded that Johnson's theory provided a theoretical base that predicted the results of nursing interventions, formulated standards for care, and administered holistic care. Cerda and Gonzalez (2008) found it equally effective when intervening with women who were victims of domestic violence.

Some studies of practice using Johnson's model have focused on decision making and evaluation of outcomes. Grice (1997) found that the nurse, patient, and situational characteristics influenced assessment and decision making for the administration of antianxiety and antipsychotic medications for psychiatric inpatients at certain hours. Benson (1997) conducted a review of research literature on the fear of crime among older adults. The behavioral system model was used to describe the "hazards of fear of crime" that could cause disturbances in the ingestive, dependency, achievement, affiliative, and aggressive-protective subsystems (Benson, 1997, p. 26). Patient- and community-focused interventions were presented to improve quality of care and quality of life in older adults. Brinkley, Ricker, and Toumey (2007) demonstrated the use of the Johnson behavioral system theory with a morbidly obese patient with complex needs, and Tamilarasi and Kanimozhi (2009) provided theory-based interventions to improve the quality of life of breast cancer survivors.

Lachicotte and Alexander (1990) examined the use of Johnson's behavioral system model as a framework for nursing administrators to use when making decisions concerning the management of impaired nurses. They suggested that, by viewing all levels of environment, the framework encouraged nurse administrators to assess imbalance in the nursing system when nurse impairment exists and evaluate the "system's state of balance in relationship to the method chosen to deal with nurse impairment" (Lachicotte & Alexander, 1990, p. 103). Results indicated that nurse administrators preferred an assistive approach when dealing with nurse impairment. It was believed that "when the impaired nurse is confronted and assisted equilibrium begins to be restored and balance brought back to the system" (Lachicotte & Alexander, 1990, p. 103).

At the University of California, Los Angeles, the Neuropsychiatric Institute and Hospital has used Johnson's behavioral system model as the basis of their psychiatric nursing practice for many years (Auger & Dee, 1983; Dee et al., 1999; Poster, Dee, & Randell, 1997). "Patients are assessed and behavioral data are classified by subsystem. Nursing diagnoses are formulated that reflect the nature of the ineffective behavior and its relationship to the regulators in the environment" (Randell, 1991, p. 154). Johnson's theory is also incorporated into the new graduate orientation program (Puntil, 2005). A study comparing the diagnostic labels generated from the Johnson behavioral system model with those on the North American Nursing Diagnosis Association list indicated that the Johnson behavioral system model was better at distinguishing the problems and the etiology (Randell, 1991).

It has become increasingly important to document nursing care and demonstrate the effectiveness of the care on patient outcomes. Using Johnson's model, Poster and colleagues (1997) reported a positive relationship between nursing interventions and the achievement of patient outcomes at discharge. They concluded "a nursing theoretical framework made it possible to prescribe nursing care as a distinction from medical care" (Poster, Dee, & Randell, 1997, p. 73).

Dee, van Servellen, and Brecht (1998) examined the effects of managed health care on patient outcomes using Johnson's behavioral system model. Upon admission, nurses develop a behavioral profile by assessing the eight subsystems, determine the balance or imbalance of the subsystems, and rate the impact of the six regulators. This is used to determine the nursing diagnoses, plan of action, and evaluation of care for each patient. The results of this study indicated significant improvement in the level of functioning upon discharge for patients with shorter hospital stays. It is encouraging to see an undergraduate student using Johnson's theory-based research for quality improvement of care with ventricular assist device patients (Kirk, 2015) as well as dissertation research based on behavioral systems (Hernandez, 2016).

Education

Loveland-Cherry and Wilkerson (1983) analyzed Johnson's theory and concluded that it has utility in nursing education. A curriculum based on a person as a behavioral system would have definite goals and straightforward course planning. Study would center on the patient as a behavioral system and its dysfunction, which would require use of the nursing process. In addition to an understanding of systems theory, the student would need knowledge from the social and behavioral disciplines and the physical and biological sciences. The model has been used in practice and educational institutions in the United States, Canada, Australia, South Africa, and India (Derdiarian, 1981; Fleming, 1990; Grice, 1997; Hadley, 1970; Harris, 1986; Heikham & Raddi, 2015; Orb & Reilly, 1991; Puntil, 2005).

Research

Johnson (1968) stated that nursing research would need to "identify and explain the behavioral system disorders which arise in connection with illness, and develop the rationale for the means of management" (p. 7). Johnson believed the task for nurse scientists might follow one of two paths: (1) contributions to the basic understanding of the behavioral system of man, and (2) contributions to understanding behavioral system problems and treatment rationale and methodologies. She identified the important areas for research as (1) the study of the behavioral system as a whole, including such issues as stability and change, organization and interaction, and effective regulatory and control mechanisms, and (2) study of the subsystems, including the identification of additional subsystems (class notes, 1971).

Small (1980) used Johnson's theory as a conceptual framework when caring for visually impaired children. By evaluating and comparing the perceived body image and spatial awareness of normally sighted children with those of visually impaired children, Small found that the sensory deprivation of visual impairment affected the normal development of the child's body image and the awareness of his or her body in space. She concluded that when the human system is subjected to excessive stress, the goals of the system cannot be maintained.

Wilkie et al. (1988) examined cancer pain control behaviors using Johnson's behavioral system model. The results of the study demonstrated that persons used known behaviors to protect themselves from high-intensity pain. This supported the assumption that "aggressive/protective subsystem behaviors are developed and modified over time to protect the individual from pain and these behaviors represent some of the patient's pain control choices" (Wilkie et al., 1988, p. 729).

These findings were supported in a study that examined the "meanings associated with self-report and self-management decision-making" of cancer patients with metastatic bone pain (Coward & Wilkie, 2000, p. 101). Pain provided an incentive to seek treatment from health care providers; therefore it was a protective mechanism. Yet the results indicated that most of the cancer patients did not take pain medication as often as prescribed and preferred nonpharmacological methods, such as positioning or distraction, as their pain-control choices.

Believing that the model had potential in understanding cultural aspects of care, Huang (2007) used it to identify intercultural and intracultural factors that might enable or hinder Western medication adherence behavior in elderly Chinese immigrants with heart failure. Oyedele, Wright, and Maja (2013) explored South African teenagers' knowledge and perceptions regarding teenage pregnancy using the Johnson behavioral system model. They focused on four subsystems: attachment, dependency, achievement, and sexual, and assessed the drive, set, and choices of the teens in these four subsystems. Based on their findings they developed guidelines to prevent unwanted teenage pregnancies. Derdiarian (1991) examined the relationships between the aggressive and protective subsystem and the other subsystems. Her findings supported the proposition that the subsystems are interactive, interdependent, and integrated; therefore Derdiarian supported Johnson's contention that "changes in a subsystem resulting from illness cannot be well understood without understanding their relationship to changes in the other subsystems" (Johnson, 1980, p. 219).

Damus (1980) tested the validity of Johnson's theory by comparing serum alanine aminotransferase (ALT) values in patients who had various nursing diagnoses and had been exposed to hepatitis B. Damus correlated the physiological disorder of elevated ALT values with behavioral disequilibrium and found that disorder in one area reflected disorder in another area.

Nurse researchers have demonstrated the usefulness of Johnson's theory in clinical practice. Most of these studies have been conducted with individuals with long-term illnesses or chronic illnesses, such as those with urinary incontinence, chronic pain, cancer, acquired immunodeficiency syndrome, compassion fatigue, and psychiatric illnesses (Alexander, 2006; Colling et al., 2003; Coward & Wilkie, 2000; Derdiarian, 1988; Derdiarian & Schobel, 1990; Grice, 1997; Holaday & Turner-Henson, 1987; Holaday, Turner-Henson, & Swan, 1996; Martha, Bhaduri, & Jain, 2004). Studies have documented the effectiveness of using the model with children, adolescents, and the elderly population. Based on extensive practice, instrument development, and research, Holaday (1980) concluded that users of Johnson's theory are provided with a guide for planning and giving care based on scientific knowledge.

FURTHER DEVELOPMENT

Johnson (1982) acknowledged that the knowledge base for use of her model was incomplete, and she offered a challenge to researchers to complete her work. She thought that the directions provided by the model for curriculum development were clear. However, the gaps in knowledge offered challenges for educators as well as practitioners. Johnson (1989) identified a dream for nursing's growth as a scientific discipline.

> *"Since we have specified nursing's special contribution to patient—our explicit, ideal goal in patient care, nursing's growth as a scientific discipline should be rapid—even explosive. When our scientists have the general conception of the realm in which we work, i.e., the phenomena of interest to the profession and the kinds of questions to be asked, it will be possible for them to work together in a systematic fashion to build a cumulative body of knowledge."*

Primarily, the theory has been associated with individuals. However, Johnson believed that groups of individuals, such as families and communities, could be considered groups of interactive behavioral systems. With the current emphasis on quality care, health promotion, and illness and injury prevention, theory derived from the model recognizing behavioral disorders in these areas is possible.

It should be noted that preventive nursing (to prevent behavioral system disorder) is not the same as preventive medicine (to prevent biological system disorders), and disorders in both cases must be identified and explicated before approaches to prevention can be developed. At this point, not even medicine has developed many specific preventive measures (immunizations for some infectious diseases and protection against some vitamin deficiency diseases are notable exceptions). A number of general approaches to better health, including adequate nutrition, safe water, and exercise, are applicable, contributing to prevention of some disorders.

Riegel (1989) reviewed the literature to identify major factors that predict "cardiac crippled behaviors or dependency following a myocardial infarction" (p. 74). Social support, self-esteem, anxiety, depression, and perceptions of functional capacity were considered the primary factors affecting psychological adjustment to chronic coronary heart disease. This emphasized the effect of social support or nurturing on the structure and function of the dependency subsystem. Johnson stated, "If caretakers were aware of how their behaviors and family behaviors interact with patients to encourage dependency behaviors at the beginning of illness, they could easily prevent many dysfunctional problems" (D. Johnson, personal communication, 1996).

Further development is indicated to identify nursing actions that facilitate appropriate functioning of the system toward disease prevention and health maintenance. Rather than expending energy developing nursing interventions in response to the consequences of disequilibrium, nurses need to learn how to identify precursors of disequilibrium and respond with preventive interventions.

Assuming that a community is a geographical area, a subpopulation, or any aggregate of people, and assuming that a community can benefit from nursing interventions, the behavioral system framework can be applied to community health. A community can be described as a behavioral system with interacting subsystems that have structural elements and functional requirements. For example, mothers of chronically ill children have functional requirements to maintain stability within the achievement subsystem and environmental factors such as "economic, educational, and employment influence mothers' caretaking skills" (Turner-Henson, 1992, p. 97).

Communities have goals, norms, choices, and actions in addition to needing protection, nurturance, and stimulation. The community reacts to internal and external stimuli, which results in functional or dysfunctional behavior. An example of an external stimulus is health policy, and an example of dysfunctional behavior is high infant mortality rate. The behavioral system consists of yet undefined subsystems that are organized, interacting, interdependent, and integrated. Physical, biological, and psychosocial factors also affect community behavior.

System dynamics researchers have convincingly demonstrated that people's information processing capacity is limited, and that humans use bias and heuristics (e.g., anchoring and use of the available heuristic) to process information and to reduce mental effort. Groups display the same bias (Vennix et al., 1990). Research in the area of cognitive maps has illustrated the restricted character of human information processing. People seem to experience difficulty in thinking in terms of causal nets.

This body of research offers some useful insights for the study of the ingestive subsystem. How do clients process information and construct the models of reality (set) that guide their decision making (choice and action)? What potential problems or deficiencies in a client's set could be identified from a nursing assessment that incorporated tenets from system dynamics? Research could lead to development of effective assessment instruments for clinical settings.

The research in systems dynamics also provides some ideas for nursing interventions to test with our clients. System dynamicists have found that model building with clients (using flowcharts and diagrams) is helpful in improving information processing. This is based on the premise that diagramming helps with information processing (set and choice), especially with complex topics. They have also found that using simulation and training in facilitation (asking questions that foster reflection and learning, good process structuring of questions and materials) is also effective (Huz et al., 1997; Vennix et al., 1990). If a diagnosis of insufficiency or discrepancy in the ingestive subsystem were made, would these same types of interventions be helpful?

Holden (2005) noted that complexity science builds on the tradition in nursing that views clients and nursing care from a systems perspective. Complexity science seeks to understand complex adaptive systems (Miller & Page, 2007; Rickles, Hawe, & Shiell, 2007). Complex adaptive systems are a "collection of individual agents with the freedom to act in ways that are not totally predictable and whose actions are interconnected so that one agent's actions change the context for other agents" (Plsek & Greenhaligh, 2001, p. 625). The Johnson behavioral system theory emphasized the connections and interactions within a systems paradigm. The use of complexity science could expand our understanding of the environmental context and the lifestyle-related and chronic health problems we face today. Complexity science, like Johnson's system theory, indicates that a flexible range of interventions is essential to respond to health care issues. Conditions such as obesity, chronic pain, and diabetes have multiple interrelating influences such as lifestyle, social, and cultural contexts, and the way forward is not easily reduced to one uniform solution. Principles form complex adaptive systems theory, and Johnson's behavioral system theory could be used jointly to examine health care issues, allowing new and revised insights to emerge.

CRITIQUE

Clarity

Johnson's theory is comprehensive and broad enough to include all areas of nursing practice and provide guidelines for research and education. The theory is relatively simple in relation to the number of concepts. A person is described as a behavioral system composed of seven subsystems. Nursing is an external regulatory force.

Simplicity

The theory is potentially complex because there are a number of possible interrelationships among the behavioral system, its subsystems, and the environment. Potential relationships have been explored, but more empirical work is needed (Brown, 2006).

Generality

Johnson's theory has been used extensively with people who are ill or face the threat of illness. Its use with families, groups, and communities is limited. Johnson perceived a person as a behavioral system composed of seven subsystems, aggregates of interactive behavioral systems. Initially, Johnson did not clearly address nonillness situations or preventive nursing (D. Johnson, curriculum vitae, 1984). In later publications, Johnson (1992) emphasized the role of nurses in preventive health care of individuals and for society. She stated, "Nursing's special responsibility for health is derived from its unique social mission. Nursing needs to concentrate on developing preventive nursing to fulfill its social obligations" (Johnson, 1992, p. 26).

Accessibility

Accessibility is achieved by identifying empirical indicators for the abstract concepts of model. Empirical precision improves when the subconcepts and the relationships between and among them become better defined and empirical indicators are introduced to the science. The units and the relationships between the units in Johnson's theory are consistently defined. Thus an adequate degree of empirical precision has been demonstrated in research using Johnson's theory. Although some of Johnson's writings used terms such as **balance, stability, equilibrium adaptation, disturbances, disequilibrium,** and **behavior disorders** interchangeably, the programs of research of Dee, Deridarian, Holaday, Lovejoy, and Poster operationally defined terms and were consistent in their use. The clarity of these definitions and the clarity of the definitions of the subsystems add to the theory's empirical precision (Brown, 2006).

Importance

Johnson's theory guides nursing practice, education, and research; generates new ideas about nursing; and differentiates nursing from other health professions. By focusing on behavior rather than biology, the theory clearly differentiates nursing from medicine; although the concepts overlap with those of the psychosocial professions.

Johnson's behavioral system model provides a conceptual framework for nursing education, practice, and research. The theory has directed questions for nursing research. It has been analyzed and judged appropriate as a basis for the development of a nursing curriculum. Practitioners and patients have judged the resulting nursing actions to be satisfactory (Johnson, 1980). The theory has potential for continued utility in nursing to achieve valued nursing goals.

SUMMARY

Johnson's behavioral system model describes the person as a behavioral system with seven subsystems: the *achievement, attachment-affiliative, aggressive-protective, dependency, ingestive, eliminative,* and *sexual* subsystems. Each subsystem is interrelated with the others and the environment and specific structural elements and functions that help maintain the integrity of the behavioral system. Other nurse scholars added the *restorative* subsystem. The structural components of the behavioral system describe how individuals are motivated (drive) to obtain specified goals using the individual's predisposition to act in certain ways (set) using available choices to produce an action or patterned behavior. The functional requirements or sustenal imperatives protect, nurture, and stimulate the behavioral system. When the behavioral system has balance and stability, the individual's behaviors will be purposeful, organized, and predictable. Imbalance and instability in the behavioral system occur when tension and stressors affect the relationship of the subsystems or the internal and external environments.

Nursing is an external regulatory force that acts to restore balance and stability by inhibiting, stimulating, or reinforcing certain behaviors (control mechanisms), changing the structural components (patient goals, choices, actions), or fulfilling function requirements. Health is the result of the behavioral system having stability, balance, and equilibrium (Johnson, 1980).

Johnson's ultimate goals were directed toward nursing practice, a curriculum for schools of nursing, and to develop nursing science. She wanted the Johnson behavioral system model to successfully generate and disseminate nursing science; systematize nursing interventions that were ethically reflective; account for multiple perspectives; and be sensitive to society's values. It was her hope that the Johnson behavioral system model was a framework she could leave to future generations of nurses (D. Johnson, personal communication, 1991).

CASE STUDY

A 67-year-old man is admitted to the hospital for diagnostic tests after experiencing severe abdominal pain and streaks of blood in his stool. He is alert and oriented. He has a history of type 2 diabetes and hypertension. His blood glucose level is 187 mg/dL and blood pressure is 188/100 mm Hg. The patient is 5 feet 10 inches tall and weighs 145 pounds. He is currently taking antihypertensive, anticoagulant, antiinflammatory, and antidiabetic medications.

His recent history reveals that he had an acute cerebral vascular accident (CVA) 6 weeks ago that resulted in partial paralysis and numbness of the right arm and leg, expressive aphasia, and slurred speech. He completed 4 weeks of inpatient rehabilitation and is able to walk short distances with a cane and moderate assistance. The patient is weak and becomes fatigued quickly. Although he can move his right arm, he guards it because of pain with movement. He receives acetaminophen for his right arm before therapy and before sleep. He also continues to exhibit slight expressive aphasia. He is anxious about continuing his therapy and indicates concern about missing his appointment with the orthopedic physician who was to evaluate his right arm. The patient reports that food doesn't taste right anymore and he has no appetite. With encouragement from his family, he eats small portions of each meal and drinks fluids without difficulty.

The patient is a college graduate who recently retired. He has been married for 45 years and has two adult children who live in the same city. He is a leader in the church and social community. His family and friends visit him frequently in the hospital. He is cheerful and attempts to talk with them when they visit. When he doesn't have visitors, he sits quietly in a dark room or sleeps. He is tearful each time his family hugs him before leaving. He expresses appreciation for each visit and apologizes each time he "gets emotional."

Behavioral Assessment

Using Johnson's behavioral system model, the following behavioral assessment is developed:

- *Achievement:* The patient has achieved many developmental goals of adulthood. He is relearning how to do activities of daily living (ADLs), walk, talk, and perform other cognitive-motor skills such as reading, writing, and speaking.
- *Attachment-affiliative:* The patient is married with two adult children who are supportive and live in the same city. He has many friends and social contacts who visit frequently.
- *Aggressive-protective:* The patient worries about his wife traveling to the hospital at night, and he worries that she doesn't eat well while staying with him in the hospital.
- *Dependency:* His recent stroke, resulting in decreased use of his right arm and leg, has affected his mobility and independent completion of ADLs. His potential for falling, inability to feel his arm or leg if injured, and weakness are safety concerns. His wife has taken on the financial and home maintenance responsibilities.
- *Ingestive:* Since the stroke, the patient has had a decreased appetite. He has lost 20 pounds in 6 weeks. Studies reveal no swallowing difficulties. He is able to feed himself with his left hand but needs assistance with cutting foods.
- *Eliminative:* The patient is able to urinate without difficulty in a urinal but prefers walking to the bathroom. He becomes constipated easily because of decreased fluid and food intake.
- *Sexual:* There are changes in the patient's sexual relationship with his wife because of pain, limited use of his right side, and fatigue.

Environmental Assessment

The assessment of internal and external environmental factors indicates that several are creating tension and threatening the balance and stability of the behavioral system. This hospitalization and diagnostic testing adds additional stress to the already weakened biological and psychological stability of the behavioral system. The stroke produced several physical and cognitive impairments that affect independence, self-care, learning, maturation, and socialization. Hospitalization at this time can delay or decrease the prognosis of the patient's physical and speech rehabilitation. He will need assistance to move safely in the hospital environment.

The patient and his wife are active in their church and participate in many social activities. The patient taught classes in Sunday school. The recent illnesses, hospitalizations, and fatigue have decreased his ability to participate in previous activities. Although he has adapted to his right-sided weakness and decreased motor function by performing his ADLs with his left hand and walking with a cane, he still needs assistance. The patient and his wife live in a suburban neighborhood. Family members installed a ramp to facilitate access to the home. His wife states that neighbors watch the house when she is away and watch for her return to be sure she is safe.

Structural Components

- *Drive or goal:* The patient seems motivated to complete the diagnostic tests and return home. He is

CASE STUDY—cont'd

eager to get back into his outpatient rehabilitation program. It seems equally important for him to decrease stress on his wife. His wife provides positive encouragement and support for him. He looks to her for assistance with decisions.

- *Set*: It is evident that the patient is accustomed to making his own decisions and being a leader. It is also evident that he is accustomed to conferring with his wife to ensure that she is comfortable with decisions being made.
- *Choice:* Although the patient agrees to the diagnostic tests, he is no longer in pain and has had no bleeding since his hospitalization. Therefore he is more focused on achieving his rehabilitation goals. He initiates activities and seeks assistance from his family in walking to the bathroom, walking in the hall, and completing his ADLs.
- *Actions:* The patient socializes with visitors and family by actively participating in conversations. He requests assistance as needed for physical and cognitive needs. He asks for prayers from his family and friends for spiritual guidance in managing his illness.

Functional Requirements

The patient needs outside assistance for all three functional requirements including protection, nurturance, and stimulation. His inability to feel his right side and his impaired mobility increase his potential for injury. Protective devices such as hand bars and a shower chair can be used. The patient needs assistance with preparing meals but has adapted to using his left hand for eating and drinking. Socialization and performance expectations at the outpatient rehabilitation facility are important methods of providing stimulation for the patient. Stimulation is also provided by friends and family who visit the patient. Continued social stimulation is vital for this patient, because he has difficulty understanding other forms of stimulation such as radio, television, and reading.

Nursing

Nursing actions are external regulatory forces that should protect, stimulate, and nurture to preserve the organization and integration of the patient's behavioral system. Nursing actions for this patient should focus on providing explanations of diagnostic tests to be performed and the results of the tests. Identification of favorite foods and encouragement of small, frequent meals with sufficient fluids to prevent constipation will be needed. The nurse should advocate for inpatient physical and speech therapy to stimulate functional abilities and reinforce the patient's achievement behaviors and to decrease dependency requirements. It will be equally important to encourage ongoing socialization with friends and family. The patient and his wife will need support and teaching to identify methods of adapting to and managing system imbalance and instability and to identify actions that will enhance behaviors to create system balance and stability.

CRITICAL THINKING ACTIVITIES

1. Select a patient from your clinical practice and one or two of Johnson's subsystems for which there is evidence of behavioral system imbalance or the threat of loss of order. Then answer the following questions:
   a. What observation indicates there is a behavioral system imbalance or the threat of the loss of order for the subsystem(s)?
   b. Consider the patient's set. What did the patient focus on in the situation?
   c. Consider the patient's choices. Did the patient consider a range of behaviors for the situation? What role did the patient's set play in his choice of behavior?
   d. What behaviors (actions) did you see and how often? What level of intensity?
   e. What were the sources of nurturance, protection, and stimulation for the actual or desired behavior(s)? Was the source consistent and sufficient?
   f. What diagnoses did you make? Describe your intervention(s).
2. After completing activity number 1, reflect on the ways the model influenced your assessment, the description of the problem, and your diagnosis. What insights did using the theory provide for you about the patient?
3. Consider the use of Johnson's model for preventive care in a community setting. What strengths and limitations might you encounter?

POINTS FOR FURTHER STUDY

- www.stritch.edu/Library/Doing-Research/Research-by-Subject/Health-Sciences-Nursing-Theorists/Dorothy-Johnson—-Behavioral-System-Model/
- Clayton State University at http://www.clayton.edu/nursing/Nursing-Theory
- Dorothy Johnson's Theory at http://currentnursing.com/nursing_theory/
- https://nurseslabs.com/dorothy-e-johnson-behavioral-systems-model
- Johnson, D. (1988). *Portraits of excellence: The nurse theorists.* Video/DVD. Athens, OH: Fitne, Inc. https://www.fitne.net/nurse_theorists1.jsp
- Holaday, B. (2014). Johnson's behavioral system model in nursing practice. In M. R. Alligood (Ed.), *Nursing theory: Utilization & application* (5th ed., pp. 138–159). Philadelphia: Mosby Elsevier.
- Vanderbilt Medical Center at http://www.mc.vanderbilt.edu/diglib/sc-diglib/biopages/djohnson.html
- Vanderbilt University, Eskind Biomedical Library Historical Collections has a complete set of Dorothy Johnson's published and unpublished papers, personal correspondence, and photographs.

REFERENCES

Alexander, M. (2006). *Compassion fatigue experienced by emergency department nurses who provided care during and after the hurricane season of 2005*. College of Nursing Master's Thesis, Florida State University.

Auger, J. A., & Dee, V. (1983). A patient classification system based on the Johnson behavioral system model of nursing: Part 1. *Journal of Nursing Administration, 13*(4), 38–43.

Benson, S. (1997). The older adult and fear of crime. *Journal of Gerontological Nursing, 23*(10), 24–31.

Martha, L., Bhaduri, A., & Jain, A. G. (2004). Impact of oral cancer and related factors on the quality of life (QOL) of patients. *Nursing Journal of India, 95*(6), 129–131.

Brinkley, R., Ricker, K., & Toumey, K. (2007, Fall). Esthetic knowing with a hospitalized morbidly obese patient (abstract). *Journal of Undergraduate Nursing Scholarship, 9*(1).

Brown, V. M. (2006). Behavioral system model. In A. M. Tomey & M. R. Alligood (Eds.), *Nursing theorists and their work* (6th ed., pp. 386–404). Philadelphia: Mosby/Elsevier.

Buckley, W. (Ed.). (1968). *Modern systems research for the behavioral scientist: A source book*. Chicago: Aldine.

Cerda, J. A. F., & Gonzalez, M. I. (2008). Application of a theoretical model of nursing in the intervention with women, victims of domestic violence. *Enfermeria Global, 7*(13), 1–10.

Colling, J., Owen, T., McCreedy, M., & Newman, D. (2003). The effects of a continence program on frail community-dwelling elderly persons. *Urologic Nursing, 23*(2), 117–131.

Coward, D. D., & Wilkie, D. J. (2000). Metastatic bone pain: Meanings associated with self-report and self-management decision making. *Cancer Nursing, 23*(2), 101–108.

Damus, K. (1980). An application of the Johnson behavioral system model for nursing practice. In J. P. Riehl & C. Roy (Eds.), *Conceptual models for nursing practice* (2nd ed.) (pp. 274–289). New York: Appleton-Century-Crofts.

Dee, V., van Servellen, G., & Brecht, M. (1998). Managed behavioral health care patients and their nursing care problems, level of functioning, and impairment on discharge. *Journal of the American Psychiatric Nurses Association, 4*(2), 57–66.

Dee, V., Tyson, S., Capparrell, L., Rigali, J., & Gross, S. (1999). *Guide to Johnson behavioral system model patient acuity classification*. Unpublished Manual. University of California Los Angeles, Neuropsychiatric Institute & Hospital Nursing Department, Los Angeles, CA.

Derdiarian, A. K. (1981). Nursing conceptual frameworks: Implications for education, practice, and research. In D. L. Vredevae, A. K. Deridiarian, L. P. Sama, M. Eriel, & J. C. Shipaoff (Eds.), *Concepts of oncology nursing* (pp. 369–385). Englewood Cliffs, NJ: Prentice-Hall.

Derdiarian, A. K. (1988). Sensitivity of the Derdiarian behavioral system model instrument to age, site, and stage of cancer: A preliminary validation study. *Scholarly Inquiry for Nursing Practice, 2*(2), 103–124.

Derdiarian, A. K. (1990). Effects of using systematic assessment instruments on patient and nurse satisfaction with nursing care. *Oncology Nursing Forum, 17*(1), 95–100.

Derdiarian, A. K. (1991). Effects of using a nursing model–based assessment instrument on quality of nursing care. *Nursing Administration Quarterly, 15*(3), 1–16.

Derdiarian, A. K., & Schobel, D. (1990). Comprehensive assessment of AIDS patients using the behavioral systems model for nursing practice instrument. *Journal of Advanced Nursing, 15*(4), 436–446.

Fawcett, J. (2013). *Contemporary nursing knowledge: Analysis and evaluation of nursing models and theories* (3rd ed.). Philadelphia: F. A. Davis.

Feshbach, S. (1970). Aggression. In P. Mussen (Ed.), *Carmichael's manual of child psychology* (3rd ed.) (pp. 159–259). New York: Wiley.

Fleming, B. H. (1990). Use of the Johnson model in nursing education (abstract). In *Proceedings of the National Theory Conference* (pp. 109–111). Los Angeles: UCLA Nursing Department.

Grice, S. L. (1997). *Nurses' use of medication for agitation for the psychiatric inpatient*. Unpublished doctoral dissertation, Catholic University of America, Washington, DC.

Grubbs, J. (1980). An interpretation of the Johnson behavioral system model for nursing practice. In J. P. Riehl & C. Roy

(Eds.), *Conceptual models for nursing practice* (pp. 217–254). New York: Appleton-Century-Crofts.

Hadley, B. J. (1970, March). *The utility of theoretical frameworks for curriculum development in nursing; the happening at Colorado*. Paper presented at WIN (Western Interstate Council of Higher Education in Nursing), Honolulu, Hawaii.

Harris, R. B. C. (1986). Introduction of a conceptual model into a baccalaureate course. *Journal of Nursing Education, 25*(1), 66–89.

Heikham, G. C., & Raddi, S. A. (2015). Knowledge regarding complications of instrumental delivery and their management among final year B. S. nursing students of a selected nursing college, Belgaum Karnataka. *International Journal of Health Science and Research (IJHSR), 5*(5), 277–283.

Herbert, J. (1989). A model for Anna: Using the Johnson model of nursing in the care of one 75-year-old stroke patient. *Journal of Clinical Practice, Education and Management, 3*(42), 30–34.

Hernandez, R. (2016). Influencias Maternas en el sistema conductual del hijo/a relacionado con el estado nutricio (Maternal influences in their child behavioral system related to his/her nutritional status). Unpublished doctoral dissertation, Universiadad Autonoma de Tamaulipas, Mexico.

Holaday, B. (1980). Implementing the Johnson model for nursing practice. In J. P. Riehl & C. Roy (Eds.), *Conceptual models for nursing practice* (2nd ed., pp. 255–263). New York: Appleton-Century-Crofts.

Holaday, B. (1981). Maternal response to their chronically ill infant's attachment behavior of crying. *Nursing Research, 30*, 343–348.

Holaday, B. (1982). Maternal conceptual set development: Identifying patterns of maternal response to chronically ill infant crying. *Maternal-Child Nursing Journal, 11*, 47–69.

Holaday, B., & Turner-Henson, A. (1987). Chronically ill school-age children's use of time. *Pediatric Nursing, 13*(6), 410–414.

Holaday, B., Turner-Henson, A., & Swan, J. (1996). The Johnson behavioral system model: Explaining activities of chronically ill children. In P. Hinton Walker & B. Neuman (Eds.), *Blueprint for use of nursing models* (pp. 33–63). New York: NLN Press.

Holden, L. M. (2005). Complex adaptive systems: Concept analysis. *Journal of Advanced Nursing, 52*(6), 651–658.

Huang, L. (2007). Chinese culture versus western medicine: Health implications for San Francisco elder Chinese immigrants with heart failure. Unpublished doctoral dissertation, Walden University. (AAT3258410).

Huz, S., Andersen, D. F., Richardson, G. P., & Boothroyd, R. (1997). A framework for evaluating systems thinking interventions: An experimental approach to mental health system change. *Systems Dynamics Review, 13*(2), 145–169.

Jenkins, G. M. (1969). The systems approach. *Journal of Systems Engineering, 1*(1), 3–49.

Johnson, D. E. (1959a). The nature of a science of nursing. *Nursing Outlook, 7*, 291–294.

Johnson, D. E. (1959b). A philosophy of nursing. *Nursing Outlook, 7*(4), 198–200.

Johnson, D. E. (1961a). *A conceptual basis for nursing care*. Unpublished lecture, Third Conference, C. E. Program, University of California, Los Angeles.

Johnson, D. E. (1961b). *Nursing's specific goal in patient care*. Unpublished lecture, Faculty Colloquium, School of Nursing, University of California, Los Angeles.

Johnson, D. E. (1965). *Is nursing meeting the challenge of family needs?* Unpublished lecture, Wisconsin League for Nursing, Madison, WI.

Johnson, D. E. (1968). *One conceptual model of nursing*. Unpublished lecture, Vanderbilt University, Nashville, TN.

Johnson, D. E. (1976). *The search for truth*. Paper presented at the installation of officers for the new chapter (Gamma Mu) of Sigma Theta Tau at the University of California, Los Angeles.

Johnson, D. E. (1977). The behavioral system model for nursing. Paper presented at a workshop for Sigma Theta Tau.

Johnson, D. E. (1978). *Implications for research—the Johnson Behavioral System Model*. Paper presented at the Second Annual Nurse Educator Conference, New York City.

Johnson, D. E. (1980). The behavioral system model for nursing. In J. P. Riehl & C. Roy (Eds.), *Conceptual models for nursing practice* (2nd ed.) (pp. 207–216). New York: Appleton-Century-Crofts.

Johnson, D. E. (1982). *The behavioral system model for nursing*. Paper presented at Wheeling College, West Virginia.

Johnson, D. E. (1989). *Some thoughts on nursing*. Unpublished paper.

Johnson, D. E. (1992). Origins of behavioral system model. In F. Nightingale (Ed.), *Notes on nursing* (Commemorative edition, pp. 23–28). Philadelphia: Lippincott.

Kirk, N. (2015). Overall quality of life in ventricular assist device patients. Poster presented at the 14th Annual Celebration for Undergraduate Research and Creative Performance, Digital Commons. http://digitalcommons.hope.edu.

Lachicotte, J. L., & Alexander, J. W. (1990). Management attitudes and nurse impairment. *Nursing Management, 21*(9), 102–110.

Lanouette, M., & St-Jacques, A. (1994). Premature infants and their families. *Canadian Nurse, 90*(9), 36–39.

Lorenz, K. (1966). *On aggression*. New York: Harcourt.

Loveland-Cherry, C., & Wilkerson, S. (1983). Dorothy Johnson's behavioral systems model. In J. Fitzpatrick & A. Whall (Eds.), *Conceptual models of nursing: Analysis and application*. (pp. 117–135). Bowie, MD: Robert J. Brady.

Miller, J. G., & Page, S. E. (2007). *Complex adaptive systems: An introduction to computational models of social life*. Princeton, NJ: Princeton University Press.

Miller, J. G. (1965). Living systems: Basic concepts. *Behavioral Science, 10*(2), 193–237.

Orb, A., & Reilly, D. E. (1991). Changing to a conceptual base curriculum. *International Nursing Review, 38*(2), 56–60.

Oyedele, O. A., Wright, S. C. D., & Maja, T. M. M. (2013). Prevention of teenage pregnancies in Soshanguve, South Africa: Using the Johnson behavioural system model. *African Journal of Nursing & Midwifery, 15*(1), 95–108.

Parsons, T. (1951). *The social system*. Glencoe, IL: Free Press.

Parsons, T. (1964). *Societies: Comparative and evolutionary perspectives*. Englewood, NJ: Prentice-Hall.

Plsek, R., & Greenhaligh, T. T. (2001). Complexity science: The challenge of complexity in health care. *British Medical Journal, 323*(7313), 625–628.

Poster, E. C, Dee, V., & Randell, B. P. (1997). The Johnson behavioral systems model as a framework for patient outcome evaluation. *Journal of the American Psychiatric Nurses Association, 3*(3), 73–80.

Puntil, C. (2005). New graduate orientation program in geriatric psychiatric inpatient setting. *Issues in Mental Health Nursing, 56*(1), 65–80.

Randell, B. P. (1991). NANDA versus the Johnson behavioral systems model: Is there a diagnostic difference? In R. M. Carroll-Johnson (Ed.), *Classification of nursing diagnosis: Proceedings of the ninth conference.* (pp. 154–160). Philadelphia: Lippincott.

Rawls, A. C. (1980). Evaluation of the Johnson behavioral model in clinical practice: Report of a test and evaluation of the Johnson theory. *Image: The Journal of Nursing Scholarship, 12*(1), 13–16.

Rickles, D., Hawe, P., & Shiell, A. (2007). A simple guide to chaos and complexity. *Health, 61*(11), 933–937.

Riegel, B. (1989). Social support and psychological adjustment to chronic coronary heart disease: Operationalization of Johnson's behavioral system model. *Advances in Nursing Science, 11*(2), 74–84.

Small, B. (1980). Nursing visually impaired children with Johnson's model as a conceptual framework. In J. P. Riehl & C. Roy (Eds.), *Conceptual models for nursing practice* (2nd ed.). (pp. 264-273). New York: Appleton-Century-Crofts.

Tamilarasi, B., & Kanimozhi, M. (2009). Improving quality of life in breast cancer survivors: Theoretical approach. *The Nursing Journal of India, 100*(12), 276–277.

Turner-Henson, A. (1992). *Chronically ill children's mothers' perceptions of environmental variables.* Unpublished doctoral dissertation, University of Alabama at Birmingham.

Vennix, J. A. M., Gubbels, J. W., Post, D., & Poppen, H. J. (1990). A structured approach to knowledge elicitation in conceptual model-building. *Systems Dynamics Review, 6*(2), 194–208.

Wang, K., & Palmer, M. H. (2010). Women's toileting behavior related to urinary elimination: Concept analysis. *Journal of Advanced Nursing, 66*(8), 1874–1884.

Wilkie, D., Lovejoy, N., Dodd, M., & Tesler, M. (1988). Cancer pain control behaviors: Description and correlation with pain intensity. *Oncology Nursing Forum, 15*(6), 723–731.

Wilmoth, M. C. (2007). Sexuality: A critical component of quality of life in chronic disease. *Nursing Clinics of North America, 42*(4), 507–514.

Wilmoth, M. C., & Ross, J. A. (1997). Women's perception: Breast cancer and sexuality. *Cancer Practice, 5*(6), 353–359.

BIBLIOGRAPHY

Primary Sources

Book Chapters

Johnson, D. E. (1964, June). Is there an identifiable body of knowledge essential to the development of a generic professional nursing program? In M. Maker (Ed.), *Proceedings of the First Interuniversity Faculty Work Conference.* New England Board of Higher Education, Stowe, VT.

Johnson, D. E. (1973). Medical-surgical nursing: Cardiovascular care in the first person. In American Nurses Association, *ANA Clinical Sessions* (pp. 127–134). New York: Appleton-Century-Crofts.

Johnson, D. E. (1976). Foreword. In J. R. Auger (Ed.), *Behavioral systems and nursing.* Englewood Cliffs, NJ: Prentice-Hall.

Johnson, D. E. (1978). State of the art of theory development in nursing. In National League for Nursing, *Theory development: What, why, how?* (NLN Pub. No. 15–1708). New York: National League for Nursing.

Johnson, D. E. (1980). The behavioral system model for nursing. In J. P. Riehl & C. Roy (Eds.), *Conceptual models for nursing practice* (2nd ed.) (pp. 207-216). New York: Appleton-Century-Crofts.

Johnson, D. E. (1990). The behavioral system model for nursing. In M. E. Parker (Ed.), *Nursing theories in practice.* (pp. 23-32). New York: National League for Nursing.

Journal Articles

Johnson, D. E. (1943). Learning to know people. *American Journal of Nursing, 43,* 248–252.

Johnson, D. E. (1954). Collegiate nursing education. *College Public Relations Quarterly, 5,* 32–35.

Johnson, D. E. (1961). Patterns in professional nursing education. *Nursing Outlook, 9*(10), 608–611.

Johnson, D. E. (1961, Nov.). The significance of nursing care. *American Journal of Nursing, 61*(11), 63–66.

Johnson, D. E. (1962). Professional education for pediatric nursing. *Children, 9,* 153–156.

Johnson, D. E. (1964). Nursing and higher education. *International Journal of Nursing Studies, 1,* 219–225.

Johnson, D. E. (1965). Crying in the newborn infant. *Nursing Science, 3,* 339–355.

Johnson, D. E. (1965). Today's action will determine tomorrow's nursing. *Nursing Outlook, 13*(9), 38–41.

Johnson, D. E. (1966). Competence in practice: Technical and professional. *Nursing Outlook, 14*(10), 30–33.

Johnson, D. E. (1966). Year round programs set the pace in health careers promotion. *Hospitals, 40,* 57–60.

Johnson, D. E. (1967). Powerlessness: A significant determinant in patient behavior? *Journal of Nursing Educators, 6*(2), 39–44.

Johnson, D. E. (1967). Professional practice in nursing. *NLN Convention Papers, 23,* 26–33.

Johnson, D. E. (1968). Critique: Social influences on student nurses in their choice of ideal and practiced solutions to nursing problems. *Communicating Nursing Research, 1,* 150–155.

Johnson, D. E. (1968). Theory in nursing: Borrowed and unique. *Nursing Research, 17,* 206–209.

Johnson, D. E. (1968). Toward a science in nursing. *Southern Medical Bulletin, 56,* 13–23.

Johnson, D. E. (1974). Development of theory: A requisite for nursing as a primary health profession. *Nursing Research, 23,* 372–377.

Johnson, D. E. (1982). Some thoughts on nursing. *Clinical Nurse Specialist, 3*(1), 1–4.

Johnson, D. E. (1987). Evaluating conceptual models for use in critical care nursing practice. *Dimensions of Critical Care Nursing, 6,* 195–197.

Johnson, D. E., Wilcox, J. A., & Moidel, H. C. (1967). The clinical specialist as a practitioner. *American Journal of Nursing, 67,* 2298–2303.

McCaffery, M., & Johnson, D. E. (1967). Effect of parent group discussion upon epistemic responses. *Nursing Research, 16*, 352–358.

Secondary Sources

Book Chapters

Fawcett, J. (2013). Johnson's behavioral system model. In J. Fawcett (Ed.), *Contemporary nursing knowledge. Analysis and evaluation of contemporary knowledge: Nursing models and theories* (3rd ed., pp. 60–87, 104). Philadelphia: F. A. Davis.

Hoeman, S. P. (1996). Conceptual bases for rehabilitation nursing. In S. P. Hoeman (Ed.), *Rehabilitation nursing: Process and application* (2nd ed., p. 7). St Louis: Mosby.

Holaday, B. (2014). Johnson's behavioral system model in nursing practice. In M. R. Alligood (Ed.), *Nursing theory: Utilization and application* (5th ed., pp. 138–159). Philadelphia: Mosby Elsevier.

Holaday, B. (2015). Dorothy Johnson's behavioral system model and its applications (pp. 79–93). In M. E. Parker (Ed.), *Nursing theories and nursing practice* (4th ed.). Philadelphia: F. A. Davis.

Johnson, B. M., & Webber, P. B. (2005). *An introduction to theory and reasoning in nursing* (pp. 141–144). Philadelphia: Lippincott.

Lobo, M. L. (2002). Behavioral system model: Dorothy E. Johnson. In J. B. George (Ed.), *Nursing theories: The base for professional nursing practice* (5th ed., pp. 155–169). Upper Saddle River, NJ: Prentice-Hall.

McEwin, M., & Wills, E. M. (2007). *Theoretical basis for nursing* (2nd ed., pp. 148–152). Philadelphia: Lippincott.

Meleis, A. (2012). *Theoretical nursing: Development and progress* (5th ed., pp. 280–289). Philadelphia: Wolters Kluwer/Lippincott.

Wesley, R. L. (1995). *Nursing theory and models* (pp. 64–66; 152–153). Springhouse, PA: Springhouse.

Journal Articles

Botha, M. E. (1989). Theory development in perspective: The role of conceptual frameworks and models in theory development. *Journal of Advanced Nursing, 14*(1), 49–55.

Derdiarian, A. K., & Forsythe, A. B. (1983, Sept./Oct.). An instrument for theory and research development using the behavioral systems model for nursing: The cancer patient. Part II. *Nursing Research, 32*, 260–266.

Dhasaradhan, I. (2001). Application of nursing theory into practice. *Nursing Journal of India, 92*(10), 224, 236.

D'Huyvetter, D. (2000). The trauma disease. *Journal of Trauma Nursing, 7*(1), 5–12.

Dimino, E. (1988). Needed: Nursing research questions which test and expand our conceptual models of nursing. *Virginia Nurse, 56*(3), 43–46.

Hall, E. O. C. (1997). Four generations of nurse theorists in the U.S.: An overview of their questions and answers. *Nordic Journal of Nursing Research, 17*(2), 15–23.

Holaday, B. (1974). Achievement behavior in chronically ill children. *Nursing Research, 23*, 25–30.

Kaya, N. (2012). Effect of attachment styles of individuals discharged from an intensive care unit on intensive care experience. *Journal of Critical Care, 27*(1), 7–14.

Keen, J. (1982). The behavioral mode. *Nursing (Oxford), 2*(3), 71–73.

Lidell, E., Segesten, K., & Fridlund, B. (1998). Myocardial infarction patients' anxiety along the life span and interrelationship with self concept. *Nordic Journal of Nursing Research, 18*(3), 15–19.

Lovejoy, N. (1983). The leukemic child's perception of family behaviors. *Oncology Nursing Forum, 10*(4), 20–25.

Ma, T., & Gandet, D. (1997). Assessing the quality of our end-stage renal disease client population. *Journal of the Canadian Association of Nephrology Nurses and Technicians, 7*(2), 13–16.

Magnari, L. E. (1990). Hardiness, self-perceived health, and activity among independently functioning older adults. *Scholarly Inquiry for Nursing Practice, 4*(3), 177–188,

McCauley, K. C., Choromanski, J. D., Wallinger, C., & Liv, K. (1984). Current management of ventricular tachycardia: Symposium from the Hospital of the University of Pennsylvania. Learning to live with controlled ventricular tachycardia; Utilizing the Johnson mode. *Heart and Lung, 13*(6), 633–638.

Meng, M., Jiang, A., & Li, F. (2007). Research progress on Johnson's behavioral system model. *Chinese Nursing Research, 21*(35).

Moreau, D., Poster, E. C., & Niemela, K. (1993). Implementing and evaluating an attending nurse model. *Nursing Management, 24*(6), 56–58, 60, 64.

Newman, M. A. (1994). Theory for nursing practice. *Nursing Science Quarterly, 7*(4), 153–157.

Niemela, K., Poster, E. D., & Moreau, D. (1992). The attending nurse: A new role for the advanced clinician: Adolescent inpatient unit. *Journal of Child & Adolescent Psychiatric & Mental Health Nursing, 5*(3), 5–12.

Poster, E. C., & Beliz, L. (1988). Behavioral category ratings of adolescents on an inpatient psychiatric unit. *International Journal of Adolescence and Youth, 1*, 293–303.

Poster, E. C., & Beliz, L. (1992). The use of the Johnson behavioral systems model to measure changes during adolescent hospitalizations. *International Journal of Adolescence and Youth, 4*(1), 73–84.

Reynolds, W., & Cormack, D. F. S. (1991). An evaluation of the Johnson behavioral systems model for nursing. *Journal of Advanced Nursing, 16*(9), 1122–1130.

Urh, I. (1998). Dorothy Johnson's theory and nursing care of a pregnant woman. *Obzornik Zdravstvene Nege, 32*(516), 199–203.

Wilke, D. J. (1990). Cancer pain management: State-of-the-art nursing care. *Nursing Clinics of North America, 25*(2), 331–343.

Wilmoth, M. C., & Tingle, L. R. (2001). Development and psychometric testing of the Wilmoth Sexual Behaviors Questionnaire: Female. *Canadian Journal of Nursing Research, 32*(4), 135–151.

Wilmoth, M. C., & Townsend, J. (1995). A comparison of the effects of lumpectomy versus mastectomy on sexual behaviors. *Cancer Practice, 3*(5), 279–285.

Zhou, L., & Tang, L. (2010). Application of Johnson's behavioral system theory in a patient of extrahepatic bile duct stones with postoperative depression. *Nursing Journal of Chinese People's Liberation Army, 21*.

UNIT IV

Theories and Grand Theories

- Nursing theories describe, explain, or predict outcomes based on relationships among the concepts of nursing phenomena.
- Theories propose relationships by framing a nursing issue and defining relevant terms.
- Nursing theories may be developed at various levels of abstraction.
- Grand nursing theories are considered theory because although they are nearly as abstract as a conceptual model, they propose an outcome that tests the major premise of the grand theory.
- Examples of grand theories from nursing models are Roy's theory of the person as an adaptive system, Neuman's theory of optimal client stability, and King's theory of goal attainment. Other grand theory examples might be Erickson's modeling and role modeling or Meleis's theory of transitions.

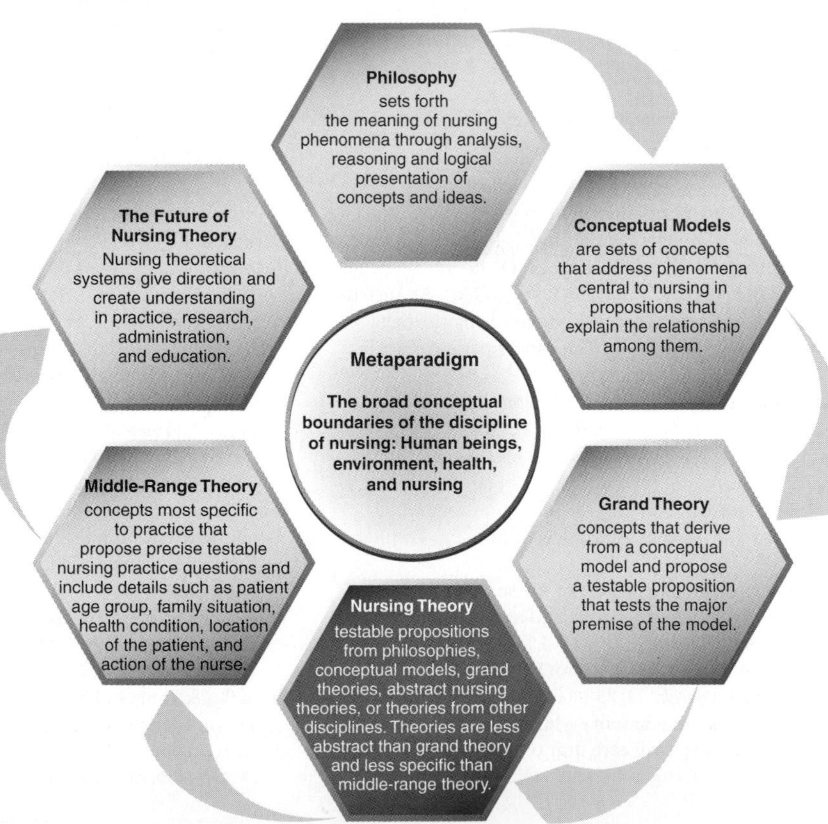

Philosophy
sets forth the meaning of nursing phenomena through analysis, reasoning and logical presentation of concepts and ideas.
Conceptual Models
are sets of concepts that address phenomena central to nursing in propositions that explain the relationship among them.
Grand Theory
concepts that derive from a conceptual model and propose a testable proposition that tests the major premise of the model.
Nursing Theory
testable propositions from philosophies, conceptual models, grand theories, abstract nursing theories, or theories from other disciplines. Theories are less abstract than grand theory and less specific than middle-range theory.
Middle-Range Theory
concepts most specific to practice that propose precise testable nursing practice questions and include details such as patient age group, family situation, health condition, location of the patient, and action of the nurse.
The Future of Nursing Theory
Nursing theoretical systems give direction and create understanding in practice, research, administration, and education.
Metaparadigm
The broad conceptual boundaries of the discipline of nursing: Human beings, environment, health, and nursing

19

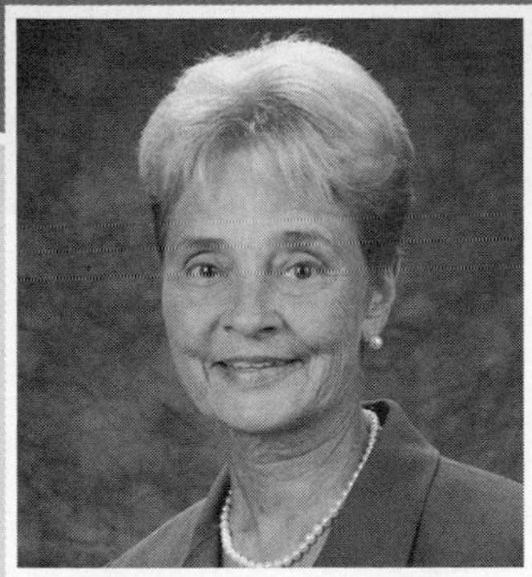

Anne Boykin

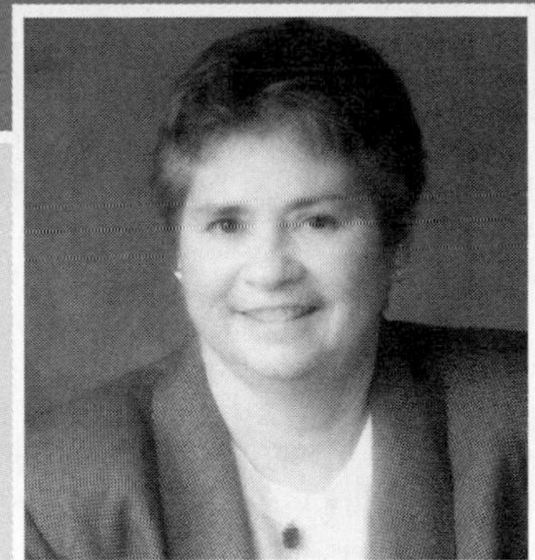

Savina O. Schoenhofer

The Theory of Nursing as Caring: A Model for Transforming Practice

Marguerite J. Purnell

"The nature of relationships is transformed through caring."
(Boykin & Schoenhofer, 2001a, p. 4)

CREDENTIALS AND BACKGROUND OF THE THEORISTS

Anne Boykin

Anne Boykin grew up in Kaukauna, Wisconsin, the eldest of six children. She began her career in nursing in 1966, graduating from Alverno College in Milwaukee, Wisconsin. She received her master's degree from Emory University in Atlanta, Georgia, and her doctorate degree from Vanderbilt University in Nashville, Tennessee. Dr. Boykin is married to Steve Staudenmeyer, and they have four children. Anne Boykin retired in the fall of 2011 and is Professor Emeritus of the Christine E. Lynn College of Nursing at Florida Atlantic University. She has relocated to Asheville, North Carolina, where she enjoys being surrounded by mountains and lakes.

Dr. Boykin is currently the Director of the college's Anne Boykin Institute for the Advancement of Caring in Nursing. Boykin has a longstanding commitment to the advancement of knowledge in the discipline, especially regarding the phenomenon of caring. Positions she has held in the International Association for Human Caring include president elect (1990–1993), president (1993–1996), and member of the nominating committee (1997–1999). As immediate past president, she served as coeditor of the journal *International Association for Human Caring* from 1996 to 1999.

Boykin's scholarly work is centered on caring as the grounding for nursing. This is evidenced in her books, *Nursing as Caring: A Model for Transforming Practice* (coauthored with Schoenhofer; 1993, 2001a) and *Living a Caring-Based Program* (1994b). The latter book illustrates how caring grounds the development of a nursing program by creating the environment for study through evaluation. In addition to these books, Dr. Boykin edited *Power, Politics and Public Policy: A Matter of Caring* (1995) and *Caring as Healing: Renewal Through Hope,* coedited with Gaut (1994). In 2014 Boykin, Schoenhofer, and Valentine coedited *Health Care System Transformation for Nursing and Health Care System Leaders: Implementing a Culture of Caring,* which provides practical strategies for living caring values for all stakeholders in the health care system. She has written numerous book chapters and articles and serves as a consultant locally, regionally, nationally, and internationally on the topic of caring.

Savina O. Schoenhofer

Savina Schoenhofer was born the second child and eldest daughter in a family of nine children and spent her formative years on the family cattle ranch in Kansas. She is named for her maternal grandfather, who was a classical musician in Kansas City, Missouri. She has a daughter, Carrie, and a granddaughter, Emma.

During the 1960s, Schoenhofer spent 3 years in the Amazon region of Brazil, working as a volunteer in community development. Her initial nursing degree was completed at Wichita State University, where she also earned graduate degrees in nursing, psychology, and counseling. She completed a PhD in educational foundations and administration at Kansas State University in 1983. In 1990 Schoenhofer cofounded *Nightingale Songs,* an early venue for communicating the beauty of nursing in poetry and prose. An early study made it apparent to Schoenhofer that caring was the service that patients overwhelmingly recognized. In addition to her work on caring, including coauthorship with Boykin of *Nursing as Caring: A Model for Transforming Practice* (1993, 2001a), Schoenhofer has written numerous articles on nursing values, primary care, nursing education, support, touch, and mentoring.

Schoenhofer's career in nursing has been influenced significantly by three colleagues: Lt. Col. Ann Ashjian (Ret.), whose community nursing practice in Brazil presented an inspiring model of nursing; Marilyn E. Parker, PhD, a faculty colleague who mentored her in the idea of nursing as a discipline, the academic role of higher education, and the world of nursing theories and theorists; and Anne Boykin, PhD, who introduced her to caring as a substantive field of study in nursing.

Dr. Schoenhofer serves on the Ethics Advisory Committee at the University of Mississippi Medical Center, where she consults and advises on questions of ethics in clinical situations that arise in practice and health care ethics education in clinical and education settings. She is Professor of Nursing at University of Mississippi Medical Center School of Nursing in Jackson and Adjunct Professor at the Florida Atlantic University College of Nursing, Boca Raton, Florida. Dr. Schoenhofer is committed to the study of nursing as caring.

THEORETICAL SOURCES

The Theory of Nursing as Caring was born out of the early curriculum development work at Florida Atlantic University College of Nursing. Anne Boykin and Savina Schoenhofer were among the faculty group revising the caring-based curriculum. When the revised curriculum was completed and instituted, each recognized the importance and human necessity of continuing to develop ideas toward a comprehensive conceptual framework that expressed the meaning and purpose of nursing as a discipline and as a profession. The Theory of Nursing as Caring is an outcome of this work. The point of departure from traditional thought was the acceptance that caring is the end rather than the means of nursing, and the intention of nursing rather than merely its instrument.

Further work to identify foundational assumptions about nursing clarified the idea of the nursing situation as a shared lived experience in which the "caring between" (Boykin & Schoenhofer, 1993, p. 26) enhances personhood. Personhood is illuminated as living grounded in caring. The clarified notions of nursing situation and focus of nursing bring to life the meaning of the assumptions underlying the theory and permit the practical understanding of nursing as both a discipline and a profession. As critique and refinement of the theory and study of nursing situations progressed, the notion of nursing being primarily concerned with health was seen as limiting. Boykin and Schoenhofer propose that nursing is concerned with the broad spectrum of human living, with the focus of nursing conceptualized as "nurturing persons living caring and growing in caring" (Boykin & Schoenhofer, 1993, p. 22).

Three bodies of work significantly influenced the initial development of the theory. Paterson and Zderad's (1988) existential phenomenological theory of humanistic nursing, viewed by Boykin and Schoenhofer as the historical antecedent of nursing as caring for such germinal ideas as "the between," "call for nursing," "nursing response," and "personhood," served as substantive and structural bases for their conceptualization of nursing as caring. Roach's (1987, 2002) thesis that caring is the human mode of being finds its natural expression and domain in the assumptions of the theory. Her "6 Cs"—*commitment, confidence, conscience, competence, compassion,* and *comportment*—contribute to a language of caring (Roach, 2002). Mayeroff's (1971) work, *On Caring,* provided rich, elemental language facilitating recognition and description of the practical meaning of living caring in the ordinariness of life. Mayeroff's (1971) major ingredients of caring—knowing, alternating rhythms, patience, honesty, trust, humility, hope, and courage—describe the wellspring of human living. In the Theory of Nursing as Caring, Mayeroff's concepts are essential for understanding living as caring and appreciating their unique expression in the reciprocal relationship of the nurse and the nursed.

Boykin and Schoenhofer's concept of nursing as a discipline was influenced by Phenix (1964), King and Brownell (1976), and Orem (1979), and as a profession by Flexner's (1910) ideas. In addition to the work of these thinkers, Boykin and Schoenhofer are longstanding members of the community of nursing scholars whose study focuses on caring. Their collegial association and mutual support undoubtedly influenced the work.

Nascent forms of the Theory of Nursing as Caring were first published in 1990 and 1991, with the first complete exposition of the theory presented at a theory conference in 1992 (Boykin & Schoenhofer, 1990, 1991; Schoenhofer & Boykin, 1993). These expositions were followed by *Nursing as Caring: A Model for Transforming Practice,* published in 1993 (Boykin & Schoenhofer, 1993) and rereleased with an epilogue in 2001 (Boykin & Schoenhofer, 2001a). Gaut notes in Boykin and Schoenhofer (2001a) that the theory is an excellent example of growth by intension, or gradual illumination, characterized by "the development of an extant bibliography, categorization of caring conceptualizations, and the further development of human care/caring theories" (p. xii).

MAJOR CONCEPTS & DEFINITIONS

Focus and Intention of Nursing

Disciplines of knowledge are communities of scholars who develop a particular perspective on the world and what it means to be in the world (King & Brownell, 1976). Disciplinary communities hold a value system in common that is expressed in its unique focus on knowledge and practice. The **focus** of nursing from the perspective of the Theory of Nursing as Caring is that the discipline of knowledge and professional practice is *nurturing persons living and growing in caring.* The general **intention** of nursing is to know persons as caring and to support and sustain them as they live caring (Boykin & Schoenhofer, 2006). This intention is expressed uniquely when the nurse enters a relationship with the nursed with the intention of knowing the other as a caring person and affirming and celebrating the person as caring (Boykin & Schoenhofer, 2001a). Caring is expressed in nursing and is "the intentional and authentic presence of the nurse with another who is recognized as living in caring and growing in caring" (Boykin & Schoenhofer, 1993, p. 24). Sensitivity and skill in creating unique and effective ways of communicating caring are developed through the nurse's intention to care.

Perspective of Persons as Caring

The fundamental assumption of the theory is that all persons are caring. Caring is lived by each person moment to moment and is an essential characteristic of being human. Caring is a process, and throughout life, each person grows in the capacity to express caring. **Person** therefore is recognized as constantly unfolding in caring. From the perspective of the theory, "fundamentally, potentially, and actually each person is caring" (Boykin & Schoenhofer, 2001a, p. 2), even though every act of the person might not be understood as caring. Knowing the person as living caring and growing in caring is foundational to the theory.

Nursing Situation

Caring is a service that nursing offers and lives in the context of the **nursing situation** (Boykin & Schoenhofer, 2006). The nursing situation is the locus of all that is known and done in nursing (Boykin & Schoenhofer, 2001a) and is conceptualized as "the shared, lived experience in which caring between nurse and nursed enhances personhood" (Boykin & Schoenhofer, 1993, p. 33). The nursing situation is what is present in the mind of the nurse whenever the intent of the nurse is "to nurse" (Boykin & Schoenhofer, 2001a). It is within the nursing situation that the nurse attends to calls for caring or reaching out to the one nursed, with the practice of nursing and the practical knowledge of nursing situated in this relational locus. The nursing situation involves an expression of values, intentions, and actions of two or more persons choosing to live a nursing relationship. In this lived relationship, all knowledge of nursing is created and understood (Boykin & Schoenhofer, 2006).

Personhood

Personhood is a process of living that is grounded in caring. Personhood implies being oneself as an authentic caring person and being open to unfolding possibilities for caring. Nurses are constantly living out the meaning of their caring from moment to moment. Within the nursing situation, the shared lived experience of caring within enhances personhood, and both the nurse and the nursed grow in caring. In the intimacy of caring, respect for self as person and respect for other are values that affirm personhood. "A profound understanding of personhood communicates the paradox of person-as-person and person-in-communion all at once" (Boykin & Schoenhofer, 2006, p. 336).

Direct Invitation

Within the nursing situation, the **direct invitation** opens the relationship to true caring between the nurse and the nursed. The direct invitation of the nurse offers the opportunity to the nursed to share what truly matters in the moment. With the intention of truly coming to know the one nursed, the nurse risks entering the other's world and comes to know what is meaningful to him or her. The

Continued

MAJOR CONCEPTS & DEFINITIONS—cont'd

focus is on what is meaningful for the one being nursed. Invitations to share what matters, such as "How might I nurse you in ways that are meaningful to you?" or "What truly matters most to you at this moment?" are communicated in the personal language of the nurse. The power of the direct invitation reaches deep into the humility of the nursing situation, uniting and guiding the intention of both the nurse and the nursed. These uniquely expressed invitations of caring call forth responses of mutual valuing in the beauty of the caring between.

Call for Nursing

Calls for nursing are calls for nurturance perceived in the mind of the nurse (Boykin & Schoenhofer, 2001a, 2001b). Intentionality (Schoenhofer, 2002a) and authentic presence open the nurse to hearing calls for nursing. The nurse responds uniquely to the one nursed with a deliberately developed knowledge of what it means to be human, acknowledging and affirming the person living caring in unique ways in the immediate situation (Boykin & Schoenhofer, 1993). Calls for nursing are uniquely situated personal expressions; they cannot be predicted, but originate within persons who are living caring in their lives and who hold hopes and aspirations for growing in caring. "Calls for nursing are individually relevant ways of saying 'Know me as caring person in the moment and be with me as I try to live fully who I truly am'" (Boykin & Schoenhofer, 2006, p. 336).

Caring Between

When the nurse enters the world of the other person with the intention of knowing the other as a caring person, the encounter gives rise to the phenomenon of **caring between**, within which personhood is nurtured (Boykin & Schoenhofer, 2001a). Through presence and intentionality, the nurse comes to know the one nursed, living and growing in caring. Constant and mutual unfolding enhances this loving relation. Without the caring between the nurse and the nursed, unidirectional activity or reciprocal exchange can occur, but nursing in its fullest sense does not occur. It is in the context of *caring between* that personhood is nurtured, each expressing self and recognizing the other as a caring person (Boykin & Schoenhofer, 2001a).

Nursing Response

Within the nursing situation, the knowing of a person clarifies the call for nursing and shapes the **nursing response**, transforming the knowledge brought by the nurse to the situation from general to particular and unique (Boykin & Schoenhofer, 2001a). The nursing response is cocreated in the immediacy of what truly matters and is a specific expression of caring nurturance to sustain and enhance the other's living and growing in caring. Nursing responses to calls for caring evolve as nurses clarify their understanding of calls through presence and dialogue. Such responses are uniquely created for the moment and cannot be predicted or applied as preplanned protocols (Boykin & Schoenhofer, 1997).

Story as Method for Knowing Nursing

Story is a method for knowing nursing and a medium for all forms of nursing inquiry. Nursing stories embody the lived experience of nursing situations involving the nurse and the nursed. As a repository of nursing knowledge, any single nursing situation has the potential to illuminate the depth and complexity of the experience as lived, that is, the caring that takes place between the nurse and the one nursed. The content of nursing knowledge is generated, developed, conserved, and known through the lived experience of nursing situations (Boykin & Schoenhofer, 2001a). The nursing situation as a unit of knowledge and practice is re-created in narrative or story (Boykin & Schoenhofer, 1991). Nursing situations are best communicated through aesthetic media such as storytelling, poetry, graphic arts, and dance to preserve the lived meaning of the situation and the openness of the situation through text. These media provide time and space for reflecting and for creativity in advancing understanding (Boykin, Parker, & Schoenhofer, 1994; Boykin & Schoenhofer, 1991, 2001a, 2006). Story as method re-creates and re-presents the essence of the experience, making the knowledge of nursing available for further study (Boykin & Schoenhofer, 2001a).

USE OF EMPIRICAL EVIDENCE

The assumptions of Nursing as Caring ground the practice of nursing in knowing, enhancing, and illuminating the caring between the nurse and the one nursed. As such, rather than providing empirical variables from which hypotheses and testable predictions are made, the Theory of Nursing as Caring *qualitatively transforms practice.* In the theory, persons are unique and unpredictable in the moment and therefore cannot and should not be manipulated or objectified as testable, researchable variables. Ellis believed that theories should reveal the knowledge that nurses must, and should, spend time pursuing (Algase & Whall,

1993). The Theory of Nursing as Caring reveals the essentiality of recognizing caring between the nurse and the one nursed as substantive knowledge that nurses must pursue. From this perspective, the outcomes of nursing care reflect the valuing of person in ways that communicate "value added" richness of the nursing experience (Boykin, Schoenhofer, Smith, et al., 2003, p. 225). Characteristics of personhood are essential to the theory, such as unity, wholeness, awareness, and intention. In nursing as caring, outcomes of nursing are articulated in terms that are subjective and descriptive, rather than objective and predictive (Boykin & Schoenhofer, 1997).

MAJOR ASSUMPTIONS

Fundamental beliefs about what it means to be human undergird the Theory of Nursing as Caring. Boykin and Schoenhofer (2001a) address six major assumptions that reflect a set of values to provide a basis for understanding and explicating the meaning of nursing.

Person

One: Persons Are Caring by Virtue of Their Humanness

The belief that persons are caring by virtue of their humanness sets forth the ontological and ethical bases on which the theory is grounded. Being a person means living caring, through which being and possibilities are known to the fullest. Each person throughout his or her life grows in the capacity to express caring. The assumption that all persons are caring does not require that each act of a person be caring, but it does require the acceptance that "fundamentally, potentially, and actually, each person is caring" (Boykin & Schoenhofer, 2001a, p. 2). Through entering, experiencing, and appreciating the life-world of other, the nature of being human is more fully understood. From the perspective of Nursing as Caring, the understanding of person as caring "centers on valuing and celebrating human wholeness, the human person as living and growing in caring, and active personal engagement with others" (Boykin & Schoenhofer, 2001a, p. 5).

Two: Persons Are Whole and Complete in the Moment

Respect for the person is communicated by the notion of a person as whole or complete in the moment. Being complete in the moment signifies that there is no insufficiency, no brokenness, and no absence of something. Wholeness, or the fullness of being, is forever present. The view of the person as caring and complete is intentional, offering a unifying lens for being present with the other that prevents segmenting into parts such as mind, body, and spirit. Through this lens, the person is at all times whole. The idea of wholeness does not preclude the idea of complexity of being. Instead, from the perspective of nursing as caring, to encounter a person as less than whole fails to truly encounter the person.

Three: Persons Live Caring, Moment to Moment

Caring is a lifetime process that is lived moment to moment and is constantly unfolding. In the rhythm of life experiences, we continually develop expressions of ourselves as caring persons. Actualization of the potential to express caring varies in the moment. As competency in caring is developed through life, we come to understand what it means to be a caring person, to live caring, and to nurture each other as caring. This awareness of self as a caring person brings to consciousness the valuing of caring and becomes the moral imperative, directing the "oughts" of actions with the persistent question, "How ought I act as caring person?" (Boykin & Schoenhofer, 2001a, p. 4).

Health

Four: Personhood Is Living Life Grounded in Caring

Personhood is a process of living caring and growing in caring: It is being authentic, demonstrating congruence between beliefs and behaviors, and living out the meaning of one's life. Personhood acknowledges the potential for unfolding caring possibilities moment to moment. From the perspective of nursing as caring, personhood is the universal human call. This implies that the fullness of being human is expressed in living caring uniquely day to day and is enhanced through participation in caring relationships (Boykin & Schoenhofer, 2001a).

Environment

Five: Personhood Is Enhanced Through Participating in Nurturing Relationships With Caring Others

As a process, personhood acknowledges the potential of persons to live caring and is enhanced through participation in nurturing relationships with caring others. The nature of relationships is transformed through caring. Caring is living in the context of relational responsibilities and possibilities, and it acknowledges the importance of knowing the person as person. "Through knowing self as caring person, I am able to be authentic to self, freeing me to truly be with others" (Boykin & Schoenhofer, 2001a, p. 4).

Nursing

Six: Nursing Is Both a Discipline and a Profession

Nursing is an "exquisitely interwoven" (Boykin & Schoenhofer, 2001a, p. 6) unity of aspects of the discipline and profession of nursing. As a discipline, nursing is a way of knowing, being, valuing, and living in the world and is envisaged as a unity of knowledge within a larger unity. The discipline of nursing attends to the discovery, creation, development, and refinement of knowledge needed for the practice of nursing. The profession of nursing attends to the application of that knowledge in response to human needs.

Nursing as caring focuses on the knowledge needed for plenary understanding of what it means to be human and the distinctive methods needed to verify this knowledge. As a human science, knowing nursing means knowing in the realms of personal, empirical, ethical, and aesthetic all at once (Carper, 1978; Phenix, 1964). These patterns of knowing provide an organizing framework for asking epistemological questions of caring in nursing.

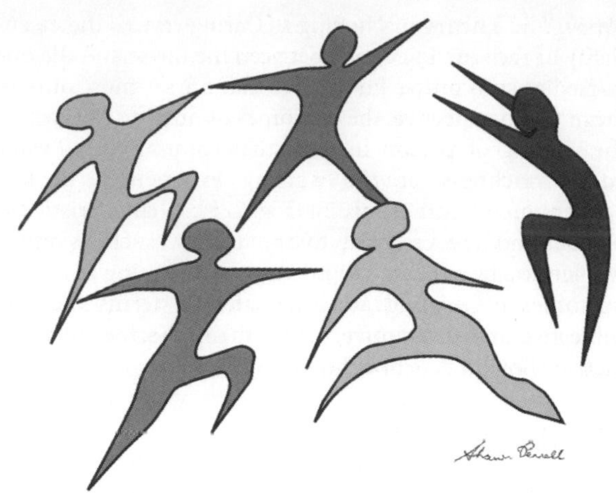

FIG. 19.1 The *Dance of Caring Persons.* (From Boykin, A., & Schoenhofer, S. O. [2001a]. *Nursing as caring: A model for transforming practice* [p. 37]. [Rerelease of original 1993 volume, with epilogue added]. Sudbury, MA: Jones & Bartlett; graphic created by Shawn Pennell, Florida Atlantic University, Boca Raton, FL.)

THEORETICAL ASSERTIONS

The broad philosophical framework of the theory ensures its congruence in a variety of nursing situations. As a general theory, Nursing as Caring is appropriate for various nursing roles, such as individual practice, group or institutional practice, and a variety of practice venues such as acute care, long-term care, nursing administration, and nursing education.

The fundamental assumptions of Nursing as Caring underpin the assertions and concepts of the theory. They are (1) to be human is to be caring, and (2) the purpose of the discipline and profession is to come to know persons and nurture them as persons living caring and growing in caring. These assumptions give rise to the concept of respect for persons as caring individuals and respect for what matters to them. The notion of respect grounds and characterizes relationships and is the starting place for all nursing caring activities.

Dance of Caring Persons

The *Dance of Caring Persons* is a visual representation of the theoretical assertion that lived caring between the nurse and the nursed expresses underlying relationships (Fig. 19.1). The egalitarian spirit of caring respect characterizes each participant in the *Dance of Caring Persons,* in which the contributions of each dancer, including the one nursed, are honored. The *Dance of Caring Persons* is also a model to guide the whole of an organization in which each person in the health care system lives caring meaningfully and has a place of value in the system—all are caregivers (Boykin, Schoenhofer, & Valentine, 2014).

Dancers enter the nursing situation, visualized as a circle of caring that provides organizing purpose and integrated functioning (Boykin, Schoenhofer, Smith, et al., 2003). Dancers move freely; some dancers touch, some dance alone, but all dance in relation to one another and to the circle. Each dancer brings special gifts as the nursing situation evolves. Some dancers may hear different notes and a different rhythm, but all harmonize in the unity of the dance and the oneness of the circle. Personal knowing of self and other is integral to the connectedness of persons in the dance, in which the nature of relating in the circle is grounded in valuing and respecting person (Boykin & Schoenhofer, 2001a). All in the nursing situation, including the nurse and the nursed, sustain the dance, being energized and resonating with the music of caring.

Outcomes of Nursing Care

Outcomes of nursing care are conceptualized from values experienced in the nursing relationship, and in normative documentation, these outcomes are unacknowledged. Boykin and Schoenhofer (1997) note that it is the responsibility of the courageous advanced practice nurse to "go beyond what is currently accepted in delimiting and languaging the value expressed by persons who participate in nursing situations" (p. 63).

LOGICAL FORM

The theory is presented in logical form grounded in nursing as a discipline of knowledge and a profession, and in general assumptions related to persons as caring in

nursing. The theory is a broad-based, general theory of nursing rendered in everyday language. Mayeroff's (1971) work, *On Caring,* and Roach's (1987) "5 Cs" provided language that illuminated the practical meaning of caring in nursing situations.

Key concepts of *caring, nursing, intention, nursing situation, direct invitation, call for nursing as caring, caring between,* and *nursing response* are described as general assumptions, and interrelated meanings are illustrated in the model of the *Dance of Caring Persons.* The direct invitation, introduced in the 2001 edition of *Nursing as Caring: A Model for Transforming Practice,* is an elaboration of the nursing situation and further clarifies the role of the nurse in initiating and sustaining caring responses. Story as a method for knowing focuses on nursing situations as the locus for nursing knowledge as a fluid and logical extension of the framework.

ACCEPTANCE BY THE NURSING COMMUNITY

Practice

Nursing is a way of living caring in the world and is revealed in personal patterns of caring. Foundations for practice of the Theory of Nursing as Caring become illumined when the nurse comes to know self as caring person "in ever deepening and broadening dimensions" (Boykin & Schoenhofer, 2001a, p. 23). Practicing nursing within this framework requires the acknowledgment that knowing self as caring matters and is integral to knowing others as caring. This is especially important in light of practice environments that depersonalize and support the notion of the nurse as an instrument and a means to an end. Rather than nursing practice focused on activities, the lens for practice becomes the intention to know and nurture the person as caring. Often, realization of the self as caring person does not occur until the nurse articulates and shares the story of the caring transpiring in the nursing situation. When reflecting upon their caring, nurses describe "Aha!" moments, signal realizations of self as always having been caring, and rediscover freedom in caring possibilities within the nursing situation: "freedom to be, freedom to choose, and freedom to unfold" (Boykin & Schoenhofer, 2001a, p. 23). Honoring caring values in explicit ways reaffirms the substance of nursing and refreshes the caring intention of the nurse. Through the sharing of story, new possibilities arise for living nursing as caring.

Nursing Service Administration

In living Nursing as Caring, the nursing administrator makes decisions through a lens in which activities are infused with a concern for shaping a transformative culture that embodies the fundamental values expressed within nursing as caring. All activities of the nursing administrator must be connected to the direct work of nursing and be "ultimately directed to the person(s) being nursed" (Boykin & Schoenhofer, 2001a, p. 33). These activities include creating, maintaining, and supporting an environment open to hearing calls for nursing and to providing nurturing responses.

Boykin and Schoenhofer (2001a) point out that contrary to the perception of nurse administrators being removed from the direct care of the nursed, they are able to directly or indirectly enter the world of the nursed, respond uniquely, and assist the nurse in securing resources to nurture persons as they live and grow in caring. The nursing administrator is also able to enter the world of the nursed indirectly, through the stories of colleagues in other roles. Other activities of the nursing administrator within the interdisciplinary environment of the organization include facilitating understanding and clarity of the focus of nursing and informing other members of the interdisciplinary health care team of the unique contributions of nurses. Sharing the depth of nursing with others through nursing situations illuminates meanings and allows for fluid reciprocity among colleagues.

The work of the nurse administrator must also reflect the uniqueness of the discipline so that nursing is being reflected, portraying respect for persons as caring and extending through mission statements, goals, objectives, standards of practice, policies, and procedures (Boykin & Schoenhofer, 2001a). The following story was related by Nancy Hilton, MSN, RN, Chief Nursing Officer at a Florida hospital. This nurse administrator, practicing from the perspective of Nursing as Caring, reflects the complexity and intentional caring expressed in living caring uniquely and courageously:

> We are intentionally refocusing our culture from a traditional bureaucratic one to a person-centered, caring-based values organization. In 2007, our Nursing Councils at St. Lucie Medical Center selected the Theory of Nursing as Caring as the theoretical model to guide our nursing practice. As a Nursing Administrator, I pondered how I could intentionally ground our hospital environment, and the practice of the nurses within its walls, in a perspective of caring. I made a deliberate commitment to deepen our knowledge and awareness by allocating time for all of us to participate in dialogues focused on knowing ourselves as caring persons.
>
> I am able to live caring uniquely as the CNO by ministering to the nurses providing direct patient care. As we transform our nursing practice, we live and grow in caring together. What I do best is utilize the art of storytelling to translate the calls for nursing into the language of the

boardroom. Through the use of strategic nursing situations, I connect the administrators directly to the one nursed. While these indirect caregivers yearn for connectedness to the patient, it takes the ingredient of courage on my part to convince the administrators why it is critical to transform an entire healthcare system by intentionally grounding it in a perspective of caring. I have been willing to conceptualize and chart the course as well as partner with key leaders in creating an environment to embody the true values of caring.

In 2014 Hilton reviewed the progress made over 6 years of enculturing and transforming the organizational practice into one based on caring. She emphatically affirmed the value of the Theory of Nursing as Caring and the ability to innovate within the model of the *Dance of Caring Persons.*

In practicing through the lens of nursing as caring, the nursing administrator assists in creating a community that appreciates, supports, and nurtures persons as they live and grow in caring. Allocation of time for dialogue allows shared meanings to emerge and demonstrates the commitment of the nursing administrator to enhance the growth of the nurse within the discipline of nursing (Boykin & Schoenhofer, 2001b). The nursing administrator interfaces with persons of many other disciplines, as well as with the one being nursed, and expresses honesty and authenticity in encouraging others to live out who they are: The nature of relating with persons whose roles range from the boardroom to the bedside is grounded in a respect for and valuing of each person.

The Theory of Nursing as Caring is gaining acceptance among large nursing organizations. In 2012 Duke University Health System adopted Nursing as Caring as their practice framework for the nursing service department. Boykin and Schoenhofer serve as consultants with the Duke University Health System on planning, implementation, evaluation, and research related to this endeavor. Boykin is also working with the Professional Practice Council of the Veteran's Administration in North Carolina as they work to articulate caring in their practice model.

Boykin, Schoenhofer, and Valentine's (2014) book is a response to the increased interest, providing a way forward for organizations desiring to transform their organizational culture to one grounded in a values-based model of caring.

Education

From the perspective of Nursing as Caring, the model for organizational design of nursing education is analogous to the *Dance of Caring Persons.* Faculty, students, and administrators dance together in the study of nursing. Each dancer is recognized, prized, and celebrated for the gifts he or she brings. The role of each person influences how the commitment to nursing education is lived out.

Nursing as caring assumptions ground the practice of nursing education and nursing education administration (Boykin & Schoenhofer, 2001a, 2001b). As expressions of the discipline, the structure and practices of the education program, including the curriculum, reflect the values and assumptions inherent in the statement of focus and the domain of the discipline, that is, nurturing persons living caring and growing in caring. Through the lens of Nursing as Caring, fundamental assumptions of the theory that honor and celebrate the uniqueness of persons as caring should be reflected. Caring, as one of the significant components of nursing knowledge, should be studied and infused throughout the curriculum (Schoenhofer, 2001). Through story—that is, the study of nursing situations—disciplinary and professional knowledge is accessed and nursing responses grounded in caring are conceptualized. All activities of the program of study should therefore be directed toward developing, organizing, and communicating nursing knowledge, the knowledge of nurturing persons living caring and growing in caring. Using the theory of Nursing as Caring, Eggenberger, Keller, and Locsin (2010) studied how students come to know persons as caring and how they express caring using a high-fidelity human simulator in emergent nursing situations. This is one exemplar of loci in which caring and technology have become a synthesis of creativity in contemporary nursing education grounded in caring.

Caring has been posited as a link between spirituality and higher education and as an ethic for being in relationship (Boykin & Parker, 1997). It is therefore a framework for knowing and the moral basis for relating. Self-discovery through an ongoing search for truth prepares learners "to receive a greater understanding of his/her reality as well as the reality of others; to develop a sense of identification, connectedness and compassion with others, and a deeper understanding of truth" (Boykin & Parker, 1997, p. 32). The challenge in higher education is to create an environment that can sustain and nurture the living of caring and spirituality (Boykin & Parker, 1997).

The role of the dean of a caring-based nursing program is "intrinsically linked" (Boykin, 1994a, p. 17) to an understanding of nursing as both a discipline and a profession and focuses actions on developing and maintaining a caring environment in which the knowledge of the discipline can be discovered. As administrator, the dean "nurtures ideas, secures resources, communicates the nature of the discipline, models living and growing in caring, cocreates a culture in which the study of nursing can be achieved freely and fully, grounds all actions in a commitment to caring as a way of being, and treats others with the same care,

concern, and understanding as those entrusted to our nursing care" (Boykin, 1994a, pp. 17–18). Such a broad scope of responsibility rests on the moral obligation inherent in the role of the dean to ensure that all actions originate in caring, and that an environment is created that fosters development of the capacity to care (Boykin, 1990).

Research

Boykin and Schoenhofer (2001a) assert that because the nature of nursing exemplified in the Nursing as Caring theory is one of reciprocal relationships, in which persons are united in oneness in caring, sciencing in nursing must be commensurate with this perspective. As a human science, nursing calls for methods of inquiry that ensure the dialogic circle in the nursing situation and fully encompass that which can be known of nursing. The ontology of nursing, with its locus in person as caring in community with others and with the universe, therefore requires an epistemology consonant with human science values and methods, with "methods and techniques that honor freedom, creativity, and interconnectedness" (Boykin & Schoenhofer, 2001a, p. 53).

Boykin and Schoenhofer (2001a) have proposed that the systematic study of nursing should include a creative methodology that recognizes the locus of study in the nursing situation. They postulate that a methodology fully adequate to capture nursing knowledge within the nursing situation might include a "phenomenological-hermeneutical process within an action research orientation" (Boykin & Schoenhofer, 2001a, p. 62). Such a method would allow the study of nursing meaning as it is being cocreated within the lived experience of the nursing situation. The idea of praxis and the theory of communicative action continue to be explored as possible underpinnings for an emergent research methodology (Schoenhofer, 2002b).

Research Studies

Research guided by the Theory of Nursing as Caring is ongoing. The practicality of Nursing as Caring is being tested and implemented in several nursing practice settings. Executive personnel, directors of nursing, and nurse administrators are calling for practice models that speak to the essentiality of caring in nursing, and these calls continue to increase.

In separate research studies within units of two major regional hospitals, JFK Medical Center and Boca Raton Community Hospital, values and outcomes of caring were reframed and rearticulated to reflect integration of the theory of Nursing as Caring. The significant courage of administrators collaborating in this caring research reflected a growing realization that caring for persons as persons is a value to which persons respond. Outcomes of care were documented within reframed institutional values of caring by nurses who contributed these values in their practice. These studies are briefly described in the following paragraphs.

A 2-year study titled "Demonstration of a Caring-Based Model for Health Care Delivery With the Theory of Nursing as Caring" was funded by the Quantum Foundation and completed at JFK Medical Center in Atlantis, Florida (Boykin et al., 2005). For this study, a practice model based on the Theory of Nursing as Caring was implemented in a telemetry unit. Persons from all stakeholder groups were invited to tell a story illustrating caring as it was lived in a nursing situation on the pilot unit. The model evolved from shared values of Nursing as Caring, including those expressed by patients, patients' families, nurses, other members and staff of the pilot unit, and members of the administrative team. Themes were uncovered in a narrative analysis and synthesis and served as explicit components of the model. Major themes of the nursing practice model were based on the theory of Nursing as Caring, and strategies and operational structures were created to reflect these themes. Support for the core of the caring-based model arising from direct invitation (Boykin & Schoenhofer, 2001a, 2001b) led to a new and renewed focus on "responding to that which matters" (Boykin et al., 2003, p. 229), which nurses now recognize as integral to caring in the nursing situation.

This project demonstrated how transformation of care occurs when nursing practice is focused intentionally on coming to know a person as caring and on nurturing and supporting the nursed as they live their caring. Within this practice model, the nursed were able to articulate the experience of being cared for, patient and nurse satisfaction increased dramatically, retention increased, and the environment for care became grounded in the values and respect for person (Boykin et al., 2003). An outcome of use of the model was that nurses sought opportunities to work in a satisfying place with caring others. When nurses transferred from the demonstration unit to other floors, they carried a new focus of nursing with them.

A similar project began in 2003 (Boykin et al., 2004; Boykin et al., 2005) in the emergency department of Boca Raton Community Hospital. The first phase of a model of care based on the Theory of Nursing as Caring was titled "Emergency Department: Transformation from Object Centered Care to Person Centered Care Through Caring." In creating the model, staff realized that changes were needed in conceptualizations of nursing practice. Initially, all emergency services staff, including physicians, nurses, and support services staff, were included, emulating the organization of the *Dance of Caring Persons.* Evaluation began early because of the success of the model in the busy venue of the emergency department. Although integration of the Theory of Nursing as Caring at JFK Medical Center and Boca Raton Community Hospital was carried out on individual units, use of the theory demonstrated flexibility and broad-based application and has been integrated systemwide at St. Lucie Medical Center, Port St. Lucie, Florida. This continuing integration was described in the Nursing Service Administration section earlier in the chapter, and is explored more thoroughly in Boykin, Schoenhofer, and Valentine (2014).

In 2007, the nursing staff and administrative personnel at St. Lucie Medical Center adopted the Theory of Nursing as Caring throughout the medical center. The first step in this process began with a study conducted to determine how best to uniquely adapt and integrate the theory of Nursing as Caring. The caring modeled in the theory was extended to all personnel throughout the hospital, from organization executives to nurses, physicians, managers, technicians, therapists, and maintenance personnel. Living caring authentically and nurturing the wholeness of others within the rigors and ordinariness of daily work were studied and exemplified in all departments and infused throughout the organization (Pross et al., 2010, 2011).

In 2009 a study was incepted at St. Mary's Medical Center, Palm Beach County, that focused on developing a dedicated education unit grounded in the Theory of Nursing as Caring (Dyess, Boykin, & Rigg, 2010). Participants included health care administrators, staff, students, and faculty. Before undertaking this project, the health care organization did not have a specific nursing theory to guide practice, and outcomes of the project proved to be rich. They included a growing appreciation for knowing one another as caring, the development of clinically seasoned and dedicated nurses who supported the advancement of theory-based caring nursing, an administrative team who were eager to mentor staff, and dedicated educators who modeled living theory-based practice to new nurses.

Caring from the heart (Touhy, 2001, 2004; Touhy & Boykin, 2008; Touhy, Strews, & Brown, 2005) is a model of practice based on the Theory of Nursing as Caring in a unit at a long-term care facility. The model of practice was designed through collaboration between project personnel and all stakeholders. All persons on the unit participated in the process to create an innovative approach that blends with the existing facility design. Major themes revolve around responding to that which matters, caring as a way of expressing spiritual commitment, devotion inspired by love for others, commitment to creating a home environment, and coming to know and respect persons as persons.

In a study titled "The Value Experienced in Relationships Involving Nurse Practitioner-Nursed Dyads," Thomas et al. (2004) sought to describe the shared experience of caring between nurse practitioners and those they nurse, and to uncover the caring experienced in the relationship. The approach used was praxis, in which dialogue that ensued among the nurse practitioner, the nursed, and the nurse researcher resulted in a portrait of caring relationships between the nurse practitioner and the nursed.

The major nursing models for acute care hospitals and the long-term care facility reflect themes that are central to Nursing as Caring, but these themes are unique to the setting and to the persons involved in each setting. The differences and similarities demonstrate the power of Nursing as Caring to transform practice in a way that reflects unity without conformity and uniqueness within oneness (Touhy, 2004; Touhy & Boykin, 2008).

FURTHER DEVELOPMENT

Theory

As a general theory of nursing, Nursing as Caring serves as a broad, conceptual framework underpinning middle-range theory development. Drawing on Nursing as Caring as the underlying theoretical framework, Locsin (1995) created a model of machine technologies and caring in nursing. Competence in machine technology and caring was presented as nursing practice when grounded in a caring perspective, without which nursing becomes the functional practice of machine proficiency. Locsin (1998) developed this critical understanding in the theory in "Technologic Competence as Caring in Critical Care Nursing." In this middle-range theory, the intention to care and to nurture the other as caring is actualized through direct knowing, technological competence, and the medium of technologically produced data. The theory is being tested in critical care settings, with development and refinement ongoing (Kongsuwan & Locsin, 2011; Locsin, 2016; Locsin & Purnell, 2015; Parcells & Locsin, 2011).

Purnell (2006) created a model for nursing education grounded in caring, with three major aspects characterizing the model: the theory of Nursing as Caring, the metaphor of the *Dance of Caring Persons* (see Fig. 19.1) as an organizing construct, and intentionality in nursing with its transformative aspect of aesthetic knowing. Caring intention that guides the creation of the course and environment is understood as a vital energy that flows through and critically interconnects every aspect of the course. The model is intended for nurses in traditional and online environments with caring intention flowing throughout. From this perspective, caring nursing intention in all its dimensions is essential in the shaping of teaching and learning. Touhy and Boykin (2008) have proposed caring as the central domain for nursing education.

Research

Research and development efforts are focused on expanding the language of caring by uncovering personal ways of living caring in everyday life (Schoenhofer, Bingham, & Hutchins, 1998) and on reconceptualizing nursing outcomes as "value experienced in nursing situations" (Boykin & Schoenhofer, 1997; Schoenhofer & Boykin, 1998a, 1998b). In consultation with graduate students, nursing faculties and health care agencies are using aspects of the theory to ground research, teaching, and practice (Dyess, Boykin, & Bulfin, 2013). Developmental efforts include the following: (1) clarification of the concept of personhood, (2) expansion of the understanding of enhancing personhood as the general outcome of nursing, (3) illuminating understanding of the concept of direct invitation, (4) innovations in nursing research, (5) use of the theory in middle-range theory work, and (6) use of the theory in the critical analysis of caring. In response to calls for transformation by health care systems to a framework grounded in caring, particular attention has focused on development and research of implementation and outcomes of caring. In a development that signifies grassroots acceptance, *Nursing as Caring* has been translated into Japanese.

CRITIQUE

Clarity

Boykin and Schoenhofer achieve semantic clarity by developing the Theory of Nursing as Caring with everyday language. The major assumptions that undergird the theory are clearly stated and interrelated. Meanings are understood intuitively and reflectively. The assumption that all persons are caring is necessary for understanding the theory, because Boykin and Schoenhofer assert that the caring between the nurse and the nursed is the source and ground of nursing. The assumption that nursing is both a discipline and a profession provides a conceptual locus for the creation of research methodologies that fluidly unite the discipline and the profession within the notion of research within praxis, or praxis as research.

Simplicity

The simplicity of the theory rests in the everyday language and in the reciprocal nature of nursing, characterized by the fundamental grounding in person as caring. The assumptions of the theory encompass a broad sweep of human understanding and lay plain conceptual groundwork for living caring. In this regard, however, the theory becomes more complex, in that assumptions and conceptual meanings are densely interconnected as the nurse comes to know self as caring person in ever greater dimensions (Boykin & Schoenhofer, 2001a). The lived meaning of Nursing as Caring is illuminated best in a nursing situation in which the notion of living caring enhances the knowing of self and other.

Generality

Boykin and colleagues (2003) describe the Theory of Nursing as Caring as a general or grand nursing theory that offers a broad philosophical framework with practical implications for transforming practice. From the perspective of Nursing as Caring, the focus of nursing knowledge and nursing action is nurturing persons who are living caring and growing in caring. The theory may be used to guide individual practice or to guide practice for the organizational level of institutions. The Theory of Nursing as Caring underpins middle-range theory development such as Locsin's (1998) theory of technological competence as caring, Dunphy and Winland-Brown's (2001) caring model for advanced practice nursing, Purnell's (2006) model of nursing education grounded in caring, and Eggenberger and Keller's (2008) approach for simulation in caring.

Accessibility

The Theory of Nursing as Caring lends itself to research methodologies with human science approaches. Because the locus of nursing inquiry is the nursing situation, the systematic study of nursing calls for a method of inquiry that can encompass the dialogic circle of understanding of persons connected in caring. Boykin and Schoenhofer (2001a) distinguish clearly between inquiry *about* nursing and inquiry *of* nursing.

Importance

When integrated into nursing practice, the Theory of Nursing as Caring illuminates and brings into consciousness and articulation the values of nursing care. These include the direct, unmediated worth of nursing care in economic terms, the value of nursing as a social and human service, the value of nursing caring as a rich, satisfying practice for nurses, and the value of regenerative nursing for the discipline. The significance of Nursing as Caring is evidenced by the adoption of the theory at multiple levels ranging from individual practice to hospital departments, to nursing administration, and now, for institution-wide and system-wide adoptions. Nursing values are being translated into values for general well-being, and caring is being infused into the domains of nonnursing personnel.

SUMMARY

The Theory of Nursing as Caring is a general or grand nursing theory that offers a broad philosophical framework with practical implications for transforming practice (Boykin et al., 2003). From the perspective of Nursing as Caring, the focus and aim of nursing as a discipline of knowledge and a professional service is "nurturing persons living caring and growing in caring" (Boykin & Schoenhofer, 2001a, p. 12). The theory is grounded in fundamental assumptions that (1) to be human is to be caring, and (2) the activities of the discipline and the profession of nursing coalesce in coming to know persons as caring and nurturing them as persons living and growing in caring.

Formed intention and authentic presence guide the nurse in selecting and organizing empirically based knowledge for practical use in each unique and unfolding nursing situation. Because caring is uniquely created in the moment in response to a uniquely experienced call for nursing caring, there can be no prescribed outcome. The caring that is experienced by the nursed and others in the nursing situation can, however, be described and valued (Boykin & Schoenhofer, 1997; Schoenhofer & Boykin, 1998a, 1998b) and in the Theory of Nursing as Caring becomes a substantive focus for study and research.

Caring in nursing is "an altruistic, active expression of love, and is the intentional and embodied recognition of value and connectedness" (Boykin & Schoenhofer, 2006, p. 336). Although caring is not unique to nursing, it is uniquely lived in nursing. The understanding of nursing as a discipline and as a profession uniquely focuses on caring as its central value, its primary interest, and the direct intention of its practice.

Models for practice are being developed in several institutional practice areas, and Nursing as Caring is being used as a conceptual basis for developing middle-range theories. As the Theory of Nursing as Caring becomes more widely known, consideration and referential inclusion in disciplinary journals have steadily increased. The theory has been used as a theoretical basis for master's and doctoral research (Drumm, 2006; Dunn, 2009; Eggenberger, 2011; Herrington, 2002; Linden, 1996, 2000; Sternberg, 2009).

From the perspective of Nursing as Caring, the nursing situation is the unit of knowledge for study for a focus on personhood as a process of living that is grounded in caring (Boykin & Schoenhofer, 1991; Touhy, 2004). The mutual relationship shared by the nurse and the nursed is one of reciprocity and subjectivity. Because nursing knowledge is found in the nursing situation, the shared, lived experience in the caring between the nurse and the nursed enhances personhood. Thus the study of story in the nursing situation is the method for knowing nursing.

Carper's (1978) fundamental patterns of *knowing, personal, empirical, ethical,* and *aesthetic* open useful pathways for organizing and understanding the rich content of nursing situations. Personal knowing centers on encountering, experiencing, and knowing self and other. Empathy, the shared knowing of other, is an expression of aesthetic knowing. Empirical knowing is factual and addresses the empirical science of nursing. Ethical knowing is concerned with moral obligations inherent in nursing situations and what ought to be. Aesthetic knowing is the subjective appreciation of phenomena as lived in the nursing situation: Nursing stories, therefore, represent both the process of creative appreciation for aesthetic knowing and illumination and integration as the product of aesthetic knowing (Boykin & Schoenhofer, 1991). The outcomes of nursing are the values experienced within the nursing situation. For this study of a nursing situation, read the following story slowly, allowing yourself to be one with the nurse and with the ones nursed, sharing in the feelings of each and dwelling in your reflections.

CASE STUDY

A Study of the Nursing Situation

I was still a student and being mentored by an experienced and loving oncology nurse. She inspired confidence in me with her quiet wisdom and gentle spirit. During one practicum, we paused briefly outside a patient's room where the door was almost closed. My mentor placed a syringe in my hand, explained its contents, and instructed me to give an IV push to her patient, Diane, inside the room. She quietly opened the door and I slipped inside. My eyes were immediately drawn to the person lying motionless in the bed, carefully draped in white sheets and blankets, and surrounded by a veil of tubes and pumps hanging over her form. She was a young woman in her 30s, with blonde, jagged hair that stuck up in all directions. On each pale

CASE STUDY—cont'd

cheek was a bright pink circle the size of a silver dollar; lying with her eyes closed, she looked like a painted doll.

Oxygen hissed in the background as I located the port and carefully administered the medication. Tears filled my eyes; in the stillness of the room, I knew Diane did not have long to live and I felt immense compassion for this young woman whose life was being cut short.

I reached over to her face and tenderly stroked her cheek with the back of my hand, the same way as I often stroked my own children's cheeks while they were sleeping. Suddenly, from the corner of the room, a man's voice barked roughly at me. "What are you doing?" he demanded.

When I turned around, a man was sitting with arms folded, rocking back and forth in a knot of misery. It was Diane's father. I answered softly that I was touching her dear heart. His shoulders started heaving and suddenly he was sobbing with deep wrenching cries. I knelt at his feet and waited, holding on to him tightly, knowing that his need was great. "My wife is bedridden—she can't even walk to come and say good-bye to our daughter. Diane is all we have." And so between gasping sobs, he told me the story of their small family, and how they had lived and loved through good times and bad. As he became calmer, I stood up and led him over to the bed, where we stood together watching over Diane. "When was the last time you held your daughter?" I asked. He looked at me wordlessly, his anguished eyes telling all. "Perhaps it is time for you to tell her the story of her life, and how much you and your wife love her. Come lie with her. She will hear you." Gently I moved the network of tubes aside, and helped him onto the bed. He turned toward Diane, his starved arms embracing her, his eyes fixed on her face, etching eternal memories. Time seemed to pause in that sacred bed.

I turned and left them with the oxygen still hissing and gave report to my mentor. She nodded wordlessly and hugged me. I remember thinking that the circle of caring that unfolded in that room had all begun with the loving nurse who was my mentor. The next day, the room was empty and devoid of life. Diane had died early that night.

CRITICAL THINKING ACTIVITIES

Find a comfortable space in which to pause, recall, and reflect. Close your eyes and dwell upon the meanings and the caring that took place within the nursing situation; then fully engage in the moment and in the meanings that emerge as you consider these questions:

1. How is the student nurse expressing caring in her responses to calls for nursing from Diane? From her father? Describe the calls for caring perceived by the student nurse.
2. How is the father expressing his caring in the nursing situation?
3. Place yourself in the shoes of the nurse, and describe the mutuality of living and growing in caring. What difference did caring nursing make in this nursing situation?
4. Describe the nurturing of the nurse mentor. What calls for nursing did she perceive from the student nurse?
5. Record your own story of caring in a journal, and reflect on your intention in that nursing situation. Review the story from time to time to see how you have grown in your caring.

POINTS FOR FURTHER STUDY

- Archives of Caring in Nursing, Christine E. Lynn Center for Caring, College of Nursing, Florida Atlantic University at http://nursing.fau.edu/outreach/archives-of-caring/
- Boykin, A., & Schoenhofer, S. O. (2001). *Nursing as caring: A model for transforming practice* [Rerelease of original 1993 volume, with epilogue added]. Sudbury, MA: Jones & Bartlett.
- Schoenhofer, S. (2016). *Nursing theorists: Portraits of excellence, vol. III: Interview,* Athens, Ohio: Fitne, Inc.
- Touhy, T., & Boykin, A. (2008). Caring as the central domain in nursing education. *International Journal for Human Caring, 12*(2), 8–15.

REFERENCES

Algase, D. L., & Whall, A. F. (1993). Rosemary Ellis' views on the substantive structure of nursing. *Image: The Journal of Nursing Scholarship, 25*(1), 69–72.

Boykin, A. (1990). Creating a caring environment: Moral obligations in the role of dean. In M. Leininger & J. Watson (Eds.), *The caring imperative in education* (pp. 247–254). New York: National League for Nursing.

Boykin, A. (1994a). Creating a caring environment for nursing education. In A. Boykin (Ed.), *Living a caring-based program* (pp. 11–25). New York: National League for Nursing.

Boykin, A. (Ed.). (1994b). *Living a caring-based program*. New York: National League for Nursing.

Boykin, A. (Ed.). (1995). *Power, politics and public policy: A matter of caring*. New York: National League for Nursing.

Boykin, A., Bulfin, S., Baldwin, J., & Southern, R. (2004). Transforming care in the emergency department. *Topics in Emergency Medicine, 26*(4), 331–336.

Boykin, A., Bulfin, S., Schoenhofer, S. O., Baldwin, J., & McCarthy, D. (2005). Living caring in practice: The transformative power of the theory of nursing as caring. *International Journal for Human Caring, 9*(3), 15–19.

Boykin, A., & Parker, M. E. (1997). Illuminating spirituality in the classroom. In M. S. Roach (Ed.), *Caring from the heart: The convergence of caring and spirituality* (pp. 21–33). Mahwah, NJ: Paulist Press.

Boykin, A., Parker, M., & Schoenhofer, S. (1994). Aesthetic knowing grounded in an explicit conception of nursing. *Nursing Science Quarterly, 7*(4), 158–161.

Boykin, A., & Schoenhofer, S. (1993). *Nursing as caring: A model for transforming practice*. New York: National League for Nursing.

Boykin, A., & Schoenhofer, S. O. (1990). Caring in nursing: Analysis of extant theory. *Nursing Science Quarterly, 3*(4), 149–155.

Boykin, A., & Schoenhofer, S. O. (1991). Story as link between nursing practice, ontology, and epistemology. *Image: The Journal of Nursing Scholarship, 23*(4), 245–248.

Boykin, A., & Schoenhofer, S. O. (1997). Reframing nursing outcomes. *Advanced Practice Nursing Quarterly, 1*(3), 60–65.

Boykin, A., & Schoenhofer, S. O. (2006). Nursing as caring: An overview of a general theory of nursing. In M. E. Parker (Ed.), *Nursing theories and nursing practice* (2nd ed., pp. 334–348). Philadelphia: F. A. Davis.

Boykin, A., & Schoenhofer, S. O. (2001a). *Nursing as caring: A model for transforming practice* [Re-release of original 1993 volume, with epilogue added]. Sudbury, MA: Jones & Bartlett.

Boykin, A., & Schoenhofer, S. O. (2001b). The role of nursing leadership in creating caring environments in health care delivery systems. *Nursing Administration Quarterly, 25*(3), 1–7.

Boykin, A., Schoenhofer, S. O., Smith, N., St. Jean, J., & Aleman, D. (2003). Transforming practice using a caring-based nursing model. *Nursing Administration Quarterly, 27*, 223–230.

Boykin, A., Schoenhofer, S., & Valentine, K. (Eds.). (2014). *Health care system transformation for nursing and health care leaders: Implementing a culture of caring*. NY: Springer Publishing.

Carper, B. A. (1978). Fundamental patterns of knowing in nursing. *Advances in Nursing Science, 1*(1), 113–124.

Drumm, J. T. (2006). *The student's experience of learning caring in a college of nursing grounded in a caring philosophy*. Florida Atlantic University. *ProQuest, UMI Dissertation Publishing*. (No. 3220671).

Dunn, D. J. (2009). *What keeps nurses in nursing: A Heideggerian hermeneutic phenomenological study*. Florida Atlantic University. *ProQuest, UMI Dissertation Publishing*. (No. 3388794).

Dunphy, L. H., & Winland-Brown, J. (2001). *Primary care: The art and science of advanced practice nursing*. Philadelphia: F. A. Davis.

Dyess, S. M., Boykin, A., & Bulfin, M. J. (2013). Hearing the voice of nurses in caring theory-based practice. *Nursing Science Quarterly, 26*(2), 167–173.

Dyess, S., Boykin, A., & Rigg, C. (2010). Integrating caring theory with nursing practice and education: Connecting with what matters. *Journal of Nursing Administration, 40*(11), 498–503.

Eggenberger, T., & Keller, K. (2008). Grounding nursing simulation in caring: An innovative approach. *International Journal for Human Caring, 12*(2), 42–49.

Eggenberger, T., Keller, K., & Locsin, R. C. (2010). Valuing caring behaviors within simulated emergent nursing situations. *International Journal for Human Caring, 14*(2), 23–29.

Eggeberger, T. L. (2011). *Holding the frontline: The experience of being a charge nurse in an acute care setting*. Florida Atlantic University. *ProQuest, UMI Dissertation Publishing*. (No. 3462565).

Flexner, A. (1910). *Medical education in the United States and Canada*. New York: The Carnegie Foundation for the Advancement of Teaching.

Gaut, D. A., & Boykin, A. (Eds.). (1994). *Caring as healing: Renewal through hope*. New York: National League for Nursing.

Herrington, C. L. (2002). The meaning of caring: From the perspective of homeless women (Master's thesis, University of Nevada, Reno, 2002). *Masters Abstracts International, 41*(01), 191.

King, A., & Brownell, J. (1976). *The curriculum and the disciplines of knowledge*. Huntington, NY: Robert E. Krieger.

Kongsuwan, W., & Locsin, R. C. (2011). Thai nurses' experiences of caring for persons with life sustaining technologies: A phenomenological study. *Intensive & Critical Care Nursing, 27*(2), 102–110.

Linden, D. (1996). Philosophical exploration in search of the ontology of authentic presence (Master's thesis, Florida Atlantic University, West Palm Beach, FL). *Masters Abstracts International, 35*(2), 519.

Linden, D. (2000). The lived experience of nursing as caring. In M. E. Parker (Ed.), *Nursing theories and nursing practice* (pp. 403–407). Philadelphia: F. A. Davis.

Locsin, R. C. (1995). Machine technologies and caring in nursing. *Image: The Journal of Nursing Scholarship, 27*(3), 201–203.

Locsin, R. C. (1998). Technologic competence as caring in critical care nursing. *Holistic Nursing Practice, 12*(4), 50–56.

Locsin, R. C. (2016). Technological competency as caring in nursing: Co-creating moments in nursing occurring within the Universal Technological Domain. *Journal of Theory Construction and Testing, 20*(1), 5–11.

Locsin, R. C., & Purnell, M. J. (2015). Advancing the theory of technological competency as caring in nursing: The universal technological domain. *International Journal for Human Caring, 19*(2), 50–54.

Mayeroff, M. (1971). *On caring*. New York: HarperCollins.

Orem, D. E. (Ed.). (1979). *Concept formalization in nursing. Process and product* (2nd ed.). Boston: Little, Brown.

Parcells, D., & Locsin, R. C. (2011). Development and psychometric testing of the Technological Competency as Caring in Nursing instrument. *International Journal for Human Caring, 15*(4), 8–13.

Paterson, J. G., & Zderad, L. T. (1988). *Humanistic nursing*. New York: National League for Nursing.

Phenix, P. (1964). *Realms of meaning*. New York: McGraw Hill.

Pross, E., Boykin, A., Hilton, N., & Gabuat, J. (2010). A study of knowing nurses as caring. *Holistic Nursing Practice, 24*(3), 142–147.

Pross, E., Hilton, N., Boykin, A., & Thomas, C. (2011). The "dance of caring persons." *Nursing Management, 42*(10), 25–30.

Purnell, M. J. (2006). Development of a model of nursing education grounded in caring and application to online nursing education. *International Journal for Human Caring, 10*(3), 8–16.

Roach, M. S. (1987). *Caring, the human mode of being*. Ottawa, Ontario, Canada: CHA.

Roach, M. S. (2002). *Caring, the human mode of being* (2nd revised ed.). Ottawa, Ontario, Canada: CHA.

Schoenhofer, S. O. (2001). Infusing the nursing curriculum with literature on caring: An idea whose time has come. *International Journal for Human Caring, 5*(2), 7–14.

Schoenhofer, S. O. (2002a). Choosing personhood: Intentionality and the theory of nursing as caring. *Holistic Nursing Practice, 16*(4), 36–40.

Schoenhofer, S. O. (2002b). Philosophical underpinnings of an emergent methodology for nursing as caring inquiry. *Nursing Science Quarterly, 15*(4), 275–280.

Schoenhofer, S. O., Bingham, V., & Hutchins, G. (1998). Giving of oneself on another's behalf: The phenomenology of everyday caring. *International Journal for Human Caring, 2*(2), 23–29.

Schoenhofer, S. O., & Boykin, A. (1998a). Discovering the value of nursing in high-technology environments: Outcomes revisited. *Holistic Nursing Practice, 12*(4), 31–39.

Schoenhofer, S. O., & Boykin, A. (1998b). The value of caring experienced in nursing. *International Journal for Human Caring, 2*(4), 9–15.

Schoenhofer, S. O., & Boykin, A. (1993). Nursing as caring: An emerging general theory of nursing. In M. E. Parker (Ed.), *Patterns of nursing theories in practice* (pp. 83–92). New York: National League for Nursing.

Sternberg, R. M. (2009). *Latinas experiencing transnational motherhood*. Florida Atlantic University. *ProQuest, UMI Dissertation Publishing*. (No. 3401817).

Thomas, J., Finch, L. P., Green, A., & Schoenhofer, S. O. (2004). The caring relationships created by nurse practitioners and the ones nursed: Implications for practice. *Topics in Advanced Nursing Practice, ejournal, 4*(4). www.medscape.com/nursingejournal.

Touhy, T. (2001). Nurturing hope and spirituality in the nursing home. *Holistic Nursing Practice, 15*(4), 45–56.

Touhy, T. A. (2004). Dementia, personhood, and nursing: Learning from a nursing situation. *Nursing Science Quarterly, 17*(1), 43–49.

Touhy, T., & Boykin, A. (2008). Caring as the central domain in nursing education. *International Journal for Human Caring, 12*(2), 8–15.

Touhy, T., Strews, W., & Brown, C. (2005). Expressions of caring as lived in nursing home staff, residents, and families. *International Journal of Human Caring, 9*(3), 31–37.

BIBLIOGRAPHY

Primary Sources

Book Chapters

Beckerman, A., Boykin A., Folden S., & Winland-Brown, J. (1994). The experience of being a student in a caring-based program. In A. Boykin (Ed.), *Living a caring-based program* (pp. 79–92). New York: National League for Nursing.

Boykin, A. (1998). Nursing as caring through the reflective lens. In C. Johns & D. Freshwater (Eds.), *Transforming nursing through reflective practice* (pp. 43–50). Oxford, England: Blackwell Science.

Boykin, A., & Schoenhofer, S. O. (2000). Nursing as caring: An overview of a general theory of nursing. In M. E. Parker (Ed.), *Nursing theories and nursing practice*. Philadelphia: F. A. Davis.

Parker, M. E., & Schoenhofer, S. O. (2007). Foundations for nursing education: Nursing as a discipline. In B. A. Moyer & R. Whittman-Price (Eds.), *Nursing education: Foundations for practice and excellence* (pp. 4–11). Philadelphia: F. A. Davis.

Schoenhofer, S. O. (2001). A framework for caring in a technologically dependent nursing practice environment. In R. C. Locsin (Ed.), *Advancing technology, caring, and nursing* (pp. 3–11). Westport, CT: Auburn House.

Schoenhofer, S. O. (2001). Outcomes of nurse caring in high technology practice environments. In R. C. Locsin (Ed.), *Advancing technology, caring, and nursing* (pp. 79–87). Westport, CT: Auburn House.

Schoenhofer, S. O., & Boykin, A. (1993). Nursing as caring: An emerging general theory of nursing. In M. E. Parker (Ed.), *Patterns of nursing theories in practice* (pp. 83–92). New York: National League for Nursing.

Schoenhofer, S. O., & Boykin, A. (2001). Caring and the advanced practice nurse. In L. Dunphy & J. Winland-Brown (Eds.), *Primary care: The art and science of advanced practice nursing*. Philadelphia: F. A. Davis.

Schoenhofer, S. O., & Coffman, S. (1993). Valuing, prizing and growing in a caring based program. In A. Boykin (Ed.), *Living a caring based program* (pp. 127–165). New York: National League for Nursing.

Touhy, T. A., Strews, W., & Brown, C. (2005). Expressions of caring as lived by nursing home staff, residents, and families. *International Journal for Human Caring, 9*(3), 31–37.

Journal Articles

Abalos, E. E., Ribera, R. Y., Locsin, R. C., & Schoenhofer, S. O. (2016). Husserlian pheonomenology and Colaizzi's method of data analysis: Exemplar in qualitative nursing inquiry using Nursing as Caring theory. *International Journal for Human Caring, 20*(1), 19–23.

Boykin, A., & Dunphy, L. (2002). Reflective essay: Justice-making: Nursing's call. Florence Nightingale. *Policy, Politics and Nursing Practice, 3*(1), 14–19.

Boykin, A., & Schoenhofer, S. O. (2000). Is there really time to care? *Nursing Forum, 35*(4), 36–38.

Boykin, A., & Winland-Brown, J. (1995). The dark side of caring: Challenges of caregiving. *Journal of Gerontological Nursing, 21*(5), 13–18.

Eggenberger, T., & Keller, K. (2008). Grounding nursing simulation in caring: An innovative approach. *International Journal for Human Caring, 12*(2), 42–49.

Finch, L. P., Thomas, J. D., Schoenhofer, S. O. (2006). Research as praxis: A mode of inquiry into caring in nursing. *International Journal for Human Caring, 10*(1), 28–31.

Schoenhofer, S. O. (1989). Love, beauty, and truth: Fundamental nursing values. *Journal of Nursing Education, 28*(8), 382–384.

Schoenhofer, S. O. (1994). Transforming visions for nursing in the timeworld of Einstein's dreams. *Advances in Nursing Science, 16*(4), 1–8.

Schoenhofer, S. O. (1995). Rethinking primary care: Connections to nursing. *Advances in Nursing Science, 17*(4), 12–21.

Schoenhofer, S. O., Dollar, C. B., & Roberson, S. (2007). Advanced practice nursing in disasters: Toward a model grounded in the theory of nursing as caring. *International Journal for Human Caring, 11*(3), 63.

Shearer, J. E. (2015). Critique of nursing as caring theory: Aesthetic knowing and caring in online nursing. *International Journal for Human Caring, 19*(2), 45–49.

Wolf, Z. R., King, B. M., & France, N. E. M. (2015). Antecedent context and structure of communication during a caring moment: Scoping review and analysis. *International Journal for Human Caring, 19*(2), 7–21.

Secondary Sources

Books

Locsin, R. C. (Ed.). (2001). *Advancing technology, caring, and nursing.* Westport, CT: Greenwood.

Locsin, R. C. (2005). *Technological competency as caring in nursing: A model for practice.* Indianapolis: Center Nursing Press, Sigma Theta Tau International.

Book Chapters

Locsin, R. C. (1995). Technology and caring in nursing. In A. Boykin (Ed.), *Power, politics, and public policy: A matter of caring* (pp. 24–36). New York: National League for Nursing.

Locsin, R., & Campling, A. (2005). Techno sapiens and post humans: Nursing, caring, and technology. In R. Locsin (Ed.), *Technological competency as caring in nursing: A model for practice* (pp. 142–155). Indianapolis: Center Nursing Press, Sigma Theta Tau International.

Journal Articles

Barry, C. D. (2001). Creating a quilt: An aesthetic expression of caring for nursing students. *International Journal for Human Caring, 6*(1), 25–29.

Blum, C. A., Hickman, C., Parcells, D. A., & Locsin, R. C. (2010). Teaching caring to RN-BSN students using simulation technology. *International Association for Human Caring, 14*(2), 41–50.

Bulfin, S., & Mitchell, G. J. (2005). Nursing as caring theory: Living theory in practice. *Nursing Science Quarterly, 18*(4), 313–319.

Carter, M. A. (1994). Book review: *Nursing as caring: A model for transforming practice. Nursing Science Quarterly, 7,* 183–184.

Eggenberger, T., & Keller, K. (2008). Grounding nursing simulation in caring: An innovative approach. *International Journal for Human Caring, 12*(2), 42–49.

Kiser-Larson, N. (2000). The concepts of caring and story viewed from three nursing paradigms. *International Journal for Human Caring, 4*(2), 26–32.

Locsin, R. C. (2002). Aesthetic expressions of the lived world of people waiting to know: Ebola at Mbarara, Uganda. *Nursing Science Quarterly, 15*(2), 123–130.

Locsin, R. C., & Purnell, M. J. (2007). Rapture and suffering with technology in nursing. *International Journal for Human Caring, 11*(1), 38–43.

McCance, T. V., McKenna, H. P., & Boore, J. R. P. (1999). Caring: Theoretical perspectives of relevance to nursing. *Journal of Advanced Nursing, 30,* 1388–1395.

Purnell, M. J., & Mead, L. J. (2007). When nurses mourn: Layered suffering. *International Journal for Human Caring, 11*(2), 47–52.

Smith, M. C. (1994). Book review: *Nursing as caring: A model for transforming practice. Nursing Science Quarterly, 7,* 184–185.

Smith, M. C. (1999). Caring and the science of unitary human beings. *Advances in Nursing Science, 21*(4), 14–28.

Touhy, T. A. (2001). Touching the spirit of elders in nursing homes: Ordinary yet extraordinary care. *International Journal for Human Caring, 6*(1), 12–17.

Touhy, T. A., Strews, W., & Brown, C. (2005). Expressions of caring as lived by nursing home staff, residents, and families. *International Journal for Human Caring, 9*(3), 31–37.

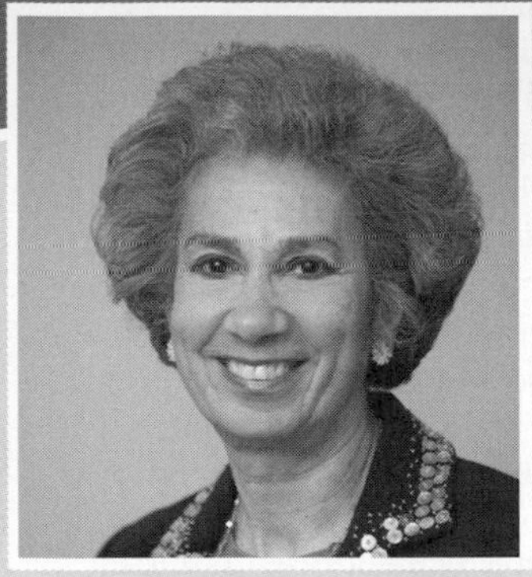

Afaf Ibrahim Meleis
(1942–Present)

Transitions Theory

Eun-Ok Im

"I believe very strongly that, while knowledge is universal, the agents for developing knowledge must reflect the nature of the questions that are framed and driven by the different disciplines about the health and well-being of individuals or populations."
(Meleis, 2007, p. ix)

CREDENTIALS AND BACKGROUND OF THE THEORIST

Afaf Ibrahim Meleis was born in Alexandria, Egypt. In personal communication with Meleis (December 29, 2007), she reckons that nursing has been part of her life since she was born. Her mother is considered the Florence Nightingale of the Middle East; she was the first person in Egypt to obtain a BSN degree from Syracuse University, and the first nurse in Egypt who obtained an MPH and a PhD from an Egyptian university. Meleis admired her mother's dedication and commitment to the profession and considered nursing to be in her blood. Under the influence of her mother, Meleis became interested in nursing and loved the potential of developing the discipline. Yet when she chose to pursue nursing, her parents objected to her choice because they knew how much nurses struggle with having a voice and affecting quality of care. However, they eventually approved of her choice and had faith that Afaf could do it.

Meleis completed her nursing degree at the University of Alexandria, Egypt. She came to the United States to pursue her graduate education as a Rockefeller Fellow to become an academic nurse (Meleis, personal communication, December 29, 2007). From the University of California, Los Angeles, she received an MS in nursing in 1964, an MA in sociology in 1966, and a PhD in medical and social psychology in 1968.

After receiving her doctoral degree, Meleis worked as administrator and acting instructor at the University of California, Los Angeles, from 1966 to 1968 and as assistant professor from 1968 to 1971. In 1971 she moved to the University of California, San Francisco (UCSF), where she spent the next 34 years and where Transitions Theory was developed. In 2002 Meleis was nominated and became the Margret Bond Simon Dean of the School of Nursing at the University of Pennsylvania. After serving 12 years as the dean at the University of Pennsylvania, she stepped "up" from her deanship in 2014, and retired from the University of Pennsylvania in June 2016. She maintains her professional title and is still active in her national and international leadership and scholarship. Her publications include an article on the undeaning transition of becoming a former dean (Meleis, 2016) and the transition toward retirement as a life cycle transition (Meleis, 2015a).

Meleis, a prominent nurse sociologist, is a sought-after theorist, researcher, and speaker on the topics of women's health and development, immigrant health care, international health care, and knowledge and theoretical development. She serves on the Counsel General of the International Council on Women's Health Issues. She received the Medal of Excellence for professional and scholarly achievements from Egyptian President Hosni Mubarak in 1990. In 2000 Meleis received the Chancellor's Medal from the University of Massachusetts, Amherst. In 2001 she received UCSF's Chancellor Award for the Advancement of Women for her role as a worldwide activist on women's issues. In 2004 she received the Pennsylvania Commission for Women Award in celebration of women's history month and the Special Recognition Award in Human Services from the Arab American Family Support Center in New York. In 2006 Meleis was presented the Robert E. Davies Award from the Penn Professional Women's Network for her advocacy on behalf of women. In 2007 she received four distinguished awards: an honorary doctorate of medicine from Linkoping University, Sweden; the Global Citizenship Award from the United Nations Association of Greater Philadelphia; the Sage Award from the University of Minnesota; and the Dr. Gloria Twine Chisum Award for Distinguished Faculty at the University of Pennsylvania for community leadership and commitment to promoting diversity. In 2008 she received the Commission on Graduates of Foreign Nursing Schools (CGFNS) International Distinguished Leadership Award based on outstanding work in the global health care community. In 2009 Meleis received the Take the Lead Award from the Girl Scouts of Southeastern Pennsylvania. In 2010 she was inducted into the UCLA School of Nursing Hall of Fame for her work in advancing and transforming nursing science.

Meleis' research focuses on global health, immigrant and international health, women's health, and the theoretical development of the nursing discipline. She authored more than 170 articles in social sciences, nursing, and medical journals; 45 chapters; and numerous monographs, proceedings, and books. Her award-winning book, *Theoretical Nursing: Development and Progress* (1985, 1991, 1997, 2007, 2011), is used widely throughout the world. In addition, her book titled *Women's Health and the World's Cities* (Meleis, Birch, & Wachter, 2011) supports her recent efforts on health issues of urban women.

The development of transitions theory began in the mid-1960s, when Meleis was working on her PhD, and it can be traced through years of research with students and colleagues. In *Theoretical Nursing: Development and Progress* (Meleis, 2007), she describes her theoretical journey from her practice and research interests. Her master's and doctoral research investigated phenomena of planning pregnancies and mastering parenting roles. She focused on spousal communication and interaction in effective or ineffective planning of the number of children in families (Meleis, 1975) and later reasoned that her ideas were incomplete because she did not consider transitions.

Subsequently her research focused on people who do not make healthy transitions and the discovery of interventions to facilitate healthy transitions. Symbolic interactionism played an important role in efforts to conceptualize the symbolic world that shapes interactions and responses. This shift in her theoretical thinking led her to role theories, as noted in her publications in the 1970s and 1980s.

Meleis' earliest work with transitions defined unhealthy transitions or ineffective transitions in relation to role insufficiency. She defined *role insufficiency* as any difficulty in the cognizance and/or performance of a role or of the sentiments and goals associated with the role behavior as perceived by the self or by significant others (Meleis, 2007). This conceptualization led Meleis to define the goal of healthy transitions as mastery of behaviors, sentiments, cues, and symbols associated with new roles and identities and nonproblematic processes. Meleis called for knowledge development in nursing to be about nursing therapeutics rather than to understand phenomena related to responses to health and illness situations. Consequently, she initiated the development of role supplementation as a nursing therapeutic as seen in her earlier research (Jones, Zhang, & Meleis, 1978; Meleis, 1975; Meleis & Swendsen, 1978).

The gist of Meleis' works published in the 1970s defined role supplementation as any deliberate process through which role insufficiency or potential role insufficiency can be identified by the incumbent role and significant others. Thus role supplementation includes both role clarification and role taking, which may be preventive and therapeutic.

With these changes in Meleis' theoretical thinking, role supplementation as a nursing therapeutic entered her research projects. Her main research questions were to further define components, processes, and strategies related to role supplementation, which she proposed would make a difference by helping patients complete a healthy transition. This led Meleis to define *health* as mastery, and she tested that definition through proxy outcome variables such as fewer symptoms, perceived well-being, and ability to assume new roles.

Meleis' theory of role supplementation was used not only in her studies on the new role of parenting (Meleis & Swendsen, 1978), but also in other studies among post–myocardial infarction patients (Dracup, Meleis, Baker, & Edlefsen, 1985), older adults (Kaas & Rousseau, 1983), parental caregivers (Brackley, 1992), caregivers of patients with Alzheimer disease (Kelley & Lakin, 1988), and women who were unsuccessful in becoming mothers and who maintained role insufficiency (Gaffney, 1992). These studies using role supplementation theory led Meleis to question the nature of transitions and the human experience of transitions. During this period, her research population interests shifted to immigrants and their health in relation to *transitions* as a concept. Norma Chick's visit to the University of California, San Francisco, from Massey University in New Zealand accelerated the development of the concept of *transitions* (Chick & Meleis, 1986) and Meleis' first transitions article as a nursing concept.

To further develop this theoretical work, Meleis initiated extensive literature searches with Karen Schumacher, a doctoral student at the University of California, San Francisco, to discover how extensively *transition* was used as a concept or framework in nursing literature. They reviewed 310 articles on transitions and developed the transition framework (Schumacher & Meleis, 1994), which was later developed as a middle-range theory. Publication of the transition framework was well received by scholars and researchers who began using it as a conceptual framework in studies that examined the following:

- Description of immigrant transitions (Meleis, Lipson, & Dallafar, 1998)
- Women's experience of rheumatoid arthritis (Shaul, 1997)
- Recovery from cardiac surgery (Shih et al., 1998)
- Family caregiving role for patients in chemotherapy (Schumacher, 1995)
- Early memory loss for patients in Sweden (Robinson et al., 1997)
- Aging transitions (Schumacher, Jones, & Meleis, 1999)
- African American women's transition to motherhood (Sawyer, 1997)

Using the transition framework, a middle-range theory for transition was developed by the researchers who had used transition as a conceptual framework. They analyzed their findings related to transition experiences and responses, identifying similarities and differences in the use of transition; findings were compared, contrasted, and integrated through extensive reading, reviewing, and dialoguing and in group meetings. The collective work was published in 2000 (Meleis et al., 2000) and has been widely used in nursing studies. Fig. 20.1 presents a diagram of the middle-range transitions theory.

Based on the early works of transitions theory, situation-specific theories that Meleis (1997) had called for were developed, including specifics in the level of abstraction, degree of specificity, scope of context, and connection to nursing research and practice (Im & Meleis, 1999a, 1999b; Schumacher, Jones, & Meleis, 1999). For example, Im and Meleis (1999b) developed a situation-specific theory of low-income Korean immigrant women's menopausal transition based on research findings, using the transition framework of Schumacher and Meleis (1994). Schumacher, Jones, and Meleis (1999) developed a situation-specific theory of elderly transition. Im (2006) also developed a situation-specific theory of Caucasian cancer patients' pain experience. These situation-specific theories were derivative of the middle-range transitions theory. In 2010 Meleis collected all the theoretical works in the literature related to transitions theory and published them in a book titled *Transitions*

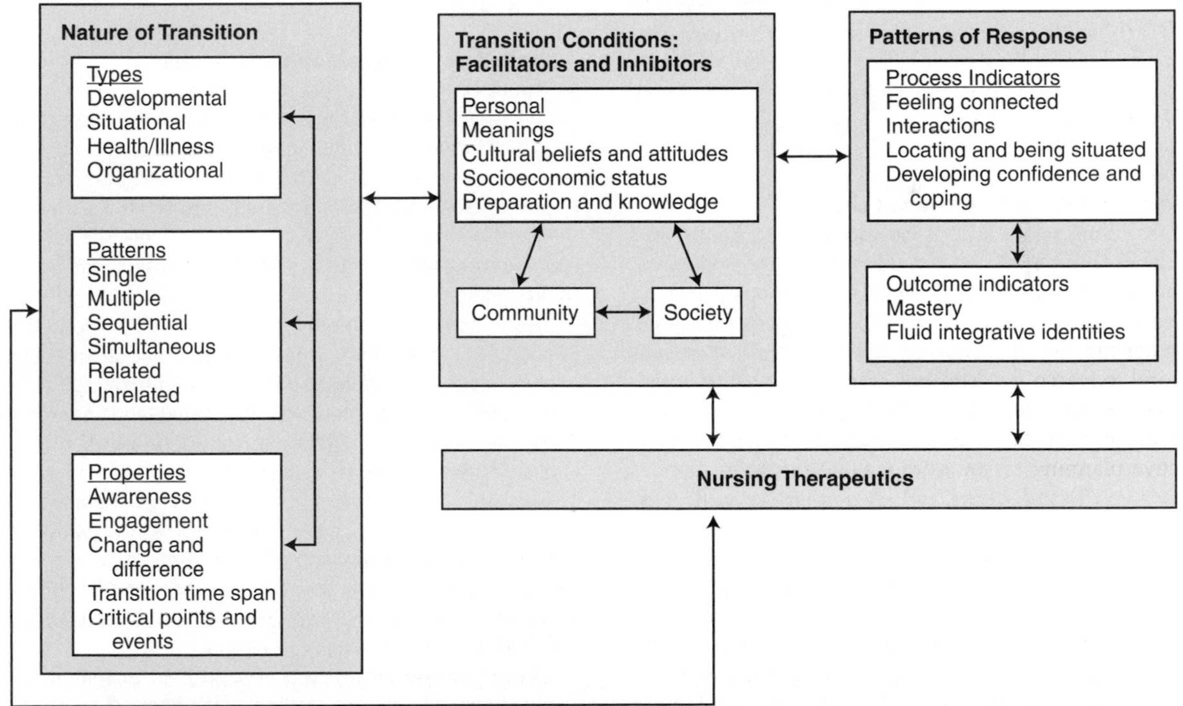

FIG. 20.1 Middle-range transitions theory. (From Meleis, A. I., Sawyer, L. M., Im, E. O., Hilfinger Messias D. K., & Schumacher, K. [2000]. Experiencing transitions: An emerging middle range theory. *Advances in Nursing Science, 23*[1], 12–28.)

Theory: Middle-Range and Situation-Specific Theories in Nursing Research and Practice. In 2011 Im analyzed the literature related to transitions theory and proposed a trajectory of theoretical development in nursing based on the theoretical works related to transitions theory in nursing. Recently Meleis (2015b) published a book chapter on transitions theory that reflects her most recent thoughts on the theory.

THEORETICAL SOURCES

Theoretical sources for transitions theory are multiple. First, Meleis' background in nursing, sociology, symbolic interactionism, and role theory and her educational background led to the development of transitions theory as described earlier in this chapter. Indeed, findings and experience from research projects, educational programs, and clinical practice in hospital and community settings have been common sources for theoretical development in nursing (Im, 2005). A systematic, extensive literature review as suggested by Walker and Avant (1995, 2005) was completed that compiled existing knowledge about nursing phenomenon. Collaborative efforts among researchers who used the transition theoretical framework and middle-range transitions theory in their studies were a source for development of transitions theory. Finally, Meleis' mentoring process could be another source for development of transitions theory. Meleis' mentoring of Schumacher led to an integrated literature review through which the first transitions theory was proposed (Schumacher & Meleis, 1994). Also, the most recent version of transitions theory by Meleis and colleagues in 2000 could also be considered a product of mentoring students in the ongoing theoretical work.

MAJOR CONCEPTS & DEFINITIONS

The major concepts and definitions from the most current transitions theory—the middle- range theory of transition proposed by Meleis and colleagues (2000)—and concepts defined earlier by Schumacher and Meleis (1994) explain major concepts of the middle-range theory of transition: (1) types and patterns of transitions; (2) properties of transition experiences; (3) transition conditions (facilitators and inhibitors); (4) patterns of response (or process indicators and outcome indicators); and (5) nursing therapeutics.

Types and Patterns of Transitions

Types of transitions include **developmental, health and illness, situational,** and **organizational**. Developmental transition includes birth, adolescence, menopause, aging (or senescence), and death. Health and illness transitions include recovery process, hospital discharge, and diagnosis of chronic illness (Meleis & Trangenstein, 1994). Organizational transitions refer to changing environmental conditions that affect the lives of clients, as well as workers within them (Schumacher & Meleis, 1994).

Patterns of transitions include multiplicity and complexity (Meleis et al., 2000). Many people experience multiple transitions simultaneously rather than experiencing a single transition, which cannot be easily distinguished from the contexts of their daily lives. Indeed, Meleis and colleagues (2000) noted that each of the studies that were the basis for the theoretical development involved people who simultaneously experienced a minimum of two types of transitions, which could not be disconnected or mutually exclusive. Thus they suggested considering whether the transitions happen sequentially or simultaneously, the degree of overlap among the transitions, and the essence of the associations among the separate events that initiate transitions for a person.

Properties of Transition Experiences

Properties of the transition experience include five subconcepts: (1) awareness; (2) engagement; (3) change and difference; (4) time span; and (5) critical points and events. Meleis et al. (2000) asserted that these properties of transition experience are interrelated as a complex process.

Awareness is defined as "perception, knowledge, and recognition of a transition experience," and level of awareness is commonly reflected in "the degree of congruency between what is known about processes and responses and what constitutes an expected set of responses and perceptions of individuals undergoing similar transitions" (Meleis et al., 2000). Although they assert that a person in transition may be somewhat aware of the changes that they are experiencing, Chick and Meleis (1986) posited that a person's unawareness of change could mean that the person may not have begun transition yet; however, Meleis and associates (2000) proposed lack of awareness doesn't necessarily mean the transition has not begun.

Engagement is another property of transition suggested by Meleis and colleagues (2000). *Engagement* refers to "the degree to which a person demonstrates involvement in the process inherent in the transition."

MAJOR CONCEPTS & DEFINITIONS—cont'd

The level of awareness is considered to influence the level of engagement; there is no engagement without awareness. Meleis and colleagues (2000) suggested that the level of engagement of a person who has this awareness of changes is different from that of a person who does not have this awareness.

Changes and differences are a property of transitions (Meleis et al., 2000). Changes that a person experiences in her or his identities, roles, relationships, abilities, and behaviors are supposed to bring a sense of movement or direction to internal as well as external processes (Schumacher & Meleis, 1994). Meleis and associates (2000) asserted that all transitions associate changes, although not all changes are associated with transitions. Rather, to comprehend a transition completely, it is essential to disclose and explain the meanings and influences of the changes and the scopes of the changes (e.g., "nature, temporality, perceived importance or severity, personal, familial, and societal norms and expectations"). Differences are also suggested as a property of transitions. Meleis and associates (2000) believed that challenging differences could be demonstrated by unsatisfied or atypical expectations, feeling dissimilar, being realized as dissimilar, or viewing the world and others in dissimilar ways, and they suggested that nurses would need to recognize the client's level of comfort and ability to deal with their changes and differences.

Time span is also a property of transitions—all transitions may be characterized as flowing and moving over time (Meleis et al., 2000). Based on Bridges (1980, 1991), **transition** is defined as "a span of time with an identifiable starting point, extending from the first signs of anticipation, perception, or demonstration of change; moving through a period of instability, confusion, and distress; to an eventual 'ending' with a new beginning or period of stability." Meleis and colleagues (2000) cautioned that it could be problematic or infeasible, and possibly even prejudicial, to frame the time span of some transition experiences.

Critical points and events are the final property of transitions suggested by Meleis and associates (2000). Critical points and events are defined as "markers such as birth, death, the cessation of menstruation, or the diagnosis of an illness." They acknowledge that specific marker events might not be evident for some transitions, although transitions usually have critical points and events. Critical points and events are usually linked to intensifying awareness of changes or dissimilarities or to a more exertive engagement in the transition process. Transitions theory conceptualizes that final critical points are differentiated by a sense of counterpoise in new schedules, competence, lifestyles, and self-care behaviors, and duration of uncertainty is characterized by variations, consecutive changes, and interruptions in existence.

Transition Conditions

Transition conditions are "those circumstances that influence the way a person moves through a transition, and that facilitate or hinder progress toward achieving a healthy transition" (Schumacher & Meleis, 1994). Transition conditions include personal, community, or societal factors that may expedite or bar the processes and outcomes of healthy transitions.

Personal conditions include meanings, cultural beliefs and attitudes, socioeconomic status, preparation, and knowledge. Meleis and colleagues (2000) considered that the meanings attached to some events accelerating a transition and to the transition process itself could expedite or bar healthy transitions. Cultural beliefs and attitudes such as stigma associated with a transition experience (e.g., Chinese stigmatization of cancer) could influence the transition experience. Socioeconomic status could influence people's transition experiences. Anticipatory preparation or lack of preparation could facilitate or inhibit people's transition experiences. **Community conditions** (e.g., community resources) or **societal conditions** (e.g., marginalization of immigrants in the host country) could be facilitators or inhibitors for transitions. Compared with personal transition conditions, the subconcepts of community conditions and societal conditions are underdeveloped.

Patterns of Response or Process and Outcome Indicators

Indicators of healthy transitions in the framework by Schumacher and Meleis (1994) were replaced by patterns of response in the middle-range theory of transitions. Patterns of response are conceptualized as **process indicators** and **outcome indicators**. These *process indicators* and *outcome indicators* characterize healthy responses. *Process indicators* that direct clients into health or toward vulnerability and risk make nurses conduct early assessment and intervention to expedite healthy outcomes. Also, *outcome indicators* may be used to check whether a transition is a healthy one, but Meleis and associates (2000) warned that outcome indicators could be associated with irrelevant events in people's lives if they are appraised early in a transition process. The process indicators suggested by Meleis and colleagues (2000) include "feeling connected, interacting, being situated, and

Continued

MAJOR CONCEPTS & DEFINITIONS—cont'd

developing confidence and coping." "The need to feel and stay connected" is a process indicator of a healthy transition; if immigrants add new contacts to their old contacts with their family members and friends, they are usually in a healthy transition. Through interactions, the meaning attached to the transition and the behaviors caused by the transition can be disclosed, analyzed, and understood, which usually results in a healthy transition. Location and being situated in terms of time, space, and relationships are usually important in most transitions; these indicate whether the person is turned in the direction of a healthy transition. The extent of increased confidence that people in transition are experiencing is another important process indicator of a healthy transition. The outcome indicators suggested by Meleis and colleagues (2000) include mastery and fluid integrative identities. "A healthy completion of a transition" can be decided by identity reformulation or the extent of mastery of the skills and behaviors that people in transition show to manage their new situations or environments.

Nursing Therapeutics

Schumacher and Meleis (1994) conceptualized nursing therapeutics as "three measures that are widely applicable to therapeutic intervention during transitions." First, they proposed assessment of readiness as a nursing therapeutic. Assessment of readiness needs to be an interdisciplinary effort and based on a full understanding of the client; it requires assessment of each of the transition conditions to generate a personal sketch of client readiness, and to allow clinicians and researchers to determine diverse patterns of the transition experience. Second, the preparation for transition is suggested as a nursing therapeutic and includes education as the main modality for generating the best condition to be ready for a transition. Third, role supplementation was proposed as a nursing therapeutic by Meleis (1975) and used by numerous researchers (Brackley, 1992; Dracup et al., 1985; Gaffney, 1992; Meleis & Swendsen, 1978). Yet in the middle-range theory of transitions, there is no further development of the concept of nursing therapeutics.

USE OF EMPIRICAL EVIDENCE

In the development of the transition framework by Schumacher and Meleis (1994), a systematic extensive literature review of more than 300 articles related to transitions provided empirical evidence of the conceptualization and theorizing. Then, as mentioned earlier in the chapter, the transition framework was tested in a number of studies to describe immigrants' transitions (Meleis, Lipson, & Dallafar, 1998), women's experiences with rheumatoid arthritis (Shaul, 1997), recovery from cardiac surgery (Shih et al., 1998), development of the family caregiving role for chemotherapy patients (Schumacher, 1995), Korean immigrant low-income women in menopausal transition (Im, 1997; Im & Meleis, 2000, 2001; Im, Meleis, & Lee, 1999), early memory loss for patients in Sweden (Robinson et al., 1997), the aging transition (Schumacher, Jones, & Meleis, 1999), African American women's transition to motherhood (Sawyer, 1997), and adult medical-surgical patients' perceptions of their readiness for hospital discharge (Weiss et al., 2007).

Development of the middle-range theory of transition builds on empirical evidence from five research studies for conceptualization and theorizing (Im, 1997; Messias, 1997; Messias et al., 1995; Sawyer, 1997; Schumacher, 1994). These studies were conducted among culturally diverse groups of people in transition, including African American mothers, Korean immigrant midlife women, parents of children diagnosed with congenital heart defects, Brazilian women immigrating to the United States, and family caregivers of persons receiving chemotherapy for cancer. Empirical findings of these five studies provided the theoretical basis for the concepts of the middle-range theory of transition, and the concepts and their relationships were developed and formulated based on a collaborative process of dialogue, constant comparison of findings across the five studies, and analysis of findings. For example, one of the personal conditions, *meanings,* was proposed based on the findings from two studies (Im, 1997; Sawyer, 1997). According to Meleis and colleagues (2000), Im (1997) found Korean immigrant midlife women had ambivalent feelings toward menopause; menopause itself did not have special meaning attached to it. She found that most participants did not connect any special health or illness concerns they were having to their menopausal transitions. Because women went through their menopause without perceiving any health or illness problems or concerns, "no special meaning" might have facilitated the women's menopausal transition. Yet Sawyer's study reported that African American women related intense enjoyment of their roles as mothers and described motherhood in terms of being responsible, protecting, supporting, and needed. Therefore meanings as a personal transition condition may or may not facilitate menopause and motherhood. The middle-range theory of transition has been used in studies to develop situation-specific theories (Im, 2006, 2010; Im & Meleis, 1999b; Schumacher, Jones, & Meleis 1999) and to test the theory in a study of relatives' experience of a move to a nursing home (Davies, 2005).

MAJOR ASSUMPTIONS

Based on Meleis' former works on role supplementation, the transition framework by Schumacher and Meleis (1994), and the middle-range theory of transitions by Meleis and colleagues (2000), the following assumptions of transitions theory may be inferred.

Nursing

- Nurses are the primary caregivers of clients and their families who are undergoing transitions.
- Transitions both result in change and are the result of change.

Person

- Transitions involve a process of movement and changes in fundamental life patterns, which are manifested in all individuals.
- Transitions cause changes in identities, roles, relationships, abilities, and patterns of behavior.
- The daily lives of clients, environments, and interactions are shaped by the nature, conditions, meanings, and processes of their transition experiences.

Health

- Transitions are complex and multidimensional. Transitions have patterns of multiplicity and complexity.
- All transitions are characterized by flow and movement over time.
- Change and difference are not interchangeable, nor are they synonymous with transition.

Environment

- Vulnerability is related to transition experiences, interactions, and environmental conditions that expose individuals to potential damage, problematic or extended recovery, or delayed or unhealthy coping.

THEORETICAL ASSERTIONS

Theoretical assertions in transitions theory were inferred in the early works of Meleis. This includes her work on role supplementation, the transition framework by Schumacher and Meleis (1994), and the middle-range theory of transitions by Meleis and colleagues (2000). Following are the theoretical assertions made in those theoretical works:

- Developmental, health and illness, and organizational transitions are central to nursing practice.
- Patterns of transition include (1) whether the client is experiencing a single transition or multiple transitions; (2) whether multiple transitions are sequential or simultaneous; (3) the extent of overlap among transitions; and (4) the nature of the relationship between the different events that are triggering transitions for a client.
- Properties of transition experience are interrelated parts of a complex process.
- The level of awareness influences the level of engagement, in which engagement may not happen without awareness.
- Humans' perceptions of and meanings attached to health and illness situations are influenced by and in turn influence the conditions under which a transition occurs.
- Healthy transition is characterized by both process and outcome indicators.
- Negotiating successful transitions depends on the development of an effective relationship between the nurse and the client (nursing therapeutic). This relationship is a highly reciprocal process that affects both the client and the nurse.

LOGICAL FORM

Transitions theory was formulated and theorized through induction using existing research literature and findings. It was initially developed as a central concept of nursing and later as a middle-range theory. Transitions theory was formulated with the goal of integrating what is known about transition experiences across different types of transitions with nursing therapeutics for people in transition. The theory provides a framework for understanding the results of previous transitions research more clearly and for proposing concepts for further study.

ACCEPTANCE BY THE NURSING COMMUNITY

Over recent decades, transitions have emerged as a central concept of nursing phenomenon, and transitions theory has been widely used throughout the world. Transitions theory was translated and used extensively in Sweden, Taiwan, South Korea, Portugal, Spain, and Singapore.

Practice

Transitions theory provides a comprehensive perspective on transition experience while considering the contexts within which people are experiencing a transition. Because of its comprehensiveness, applicability, and affinity with health, transitions theory has been applied to many human phenomena of interest and concern to nurses, such as illness, recovery, birth, death, and loss, as well as immigration.

Transitions theory is useful in explaining health and illness transitions such as the recovery process, hospital discharge, and diagnosis of chronic disease (Meleis & Trangenstein, 1994). Indeed, studies have indicated that transitions theory could be applied to nursing practice with diverse groups of people, including geriatric populations, psychiatric populations, maternal populations, family caregivers, menopausal women, patients with Alzheimer disease, immigrant women, and people with chronic illness, among others (Brackley, 1992; Im, 1997; Kaas & Rousseau, 1983; Schumacher, Dodd, & Paul, 1993; Shaul, 1997). Transitions theory could provide direction for nursing practice with people in various types of transitions by providing a comprehensive perspective on the nature and type of transitions, transition conditions, and process and outcome indicators of patterns of response to transitions. Also, transitions theory leads to development of nursing therapeutics that are congruent with the unique experience of clients and their families in transition, thus promoting healthy responses to transition.

Education

Transitions theory is used widely in graduate education and undergraduate education throughout the world (Meleis, personal communication, December 29, 2007). There is a growing international interest in integrating transitions theory into nursing curricula across countries (Meleis, personal communication, January 2008). Transitions theory was used as a curriculum framework in a number of places, including the University of Connecticut and Clayton State University in Morrow, Georgia, where transitions theory has been used in their education programs for the past 15 years. In response to increased learning needs of graduate students, Meleis taught an independent graduate elective course on transitions and health at the University of California, San Francisco. At the University of Pennsylvania, the Transitions and Health Center, directed by Mary Naylor, was established in 2007 with a $5 million endowment for support and transitions theory as its theoretical basis.

Research

Internationally a number of researchers have used transitions theory in their studies as a theoretical basis for research. Meleis' research program is naturally based on transitions theory, and other researchers have tested the empirical precision of transitions theory through their studies (Davies, 2005; Weiss et al., 2007). As mentioned earlier in the chapter, transitions theory was often used as a parent theory for situation-specific theories (Im, 2006; Im & Meleis, 1999a; Schumacher, Jones, & Meleis, 1999). A number of doctoral students, including Daphne Brewington at East Carolina University (2013), have used transitions theory in their doctoral dissertations.

FURTHER DEVELOPMENT

Transitions theory is an emerging framework that could be further developed, tested, and refined, reflecting Meleis' philosophical position on theory development as cyclic, dynamic, and evolving. Transitions theory continues to be refined and tested to explain the major concepts and relationships among diverse groups in various types of transition. Because sufficient empirical support by a number of studies using transitions theory exists, future studies should test transitions theory–based interventions, through which transitions theory gains power to direct nursing practice.

As Meleis (2007) envisioned, situation-specific theories continue to be developed based on transitions theory. In a recent analysis of the situation-specific theories that were published since 1999, transitions theory was the most commonly used middle-range theory to develop situation-specific theories (Im, 2014a). In another analysis (Im, 2014b), a total of nine situation-specific theories were found to be derived from the middle-range transitions theory during the past 10 years. The following are situation-specific theories from transitions theory:

- The situation-specific theory of migration transition for migrant farmworker women (Clingerman, 2007)
- The situation-specific theory on the transition to adult day health services (Bull & McShane, 2008)
- The situation-specific theory for guiding interventions for people with heart failure (Davidson et al., 2007)
- The situation-specific theory of care transitions (Geary & Schumacher, 2012)
- The situation-specific theory of well-being in refugee women experiencing cultural transition (Baird, 2012)
- The situation-specific theory of pain experience for Asian American cancer patients (Im, 2008)
- The situation-specific theory of Asian immigrant women's menopausal symptom experience in the United States (Im, 2010)
- The situation-specific theory of Korean immigrant women's menopausal transition (Im & Meleis, 1999)
- The situation-specific theory of Caucasian cancer patients' pain experience (Im, 2006)

CRITIQUE

Clarity

The conceptual definitions of transitions theory are clear and provide a comprehensive understanding of the complexity of transitions. The relationships among the major concepts are clearly depicted in a visually simple diagram (see Fig. 20.1). The variables are independent of one another, yet the interactive effects among the variables are clearly depicted by arrows.

Simplicity

Transitions theory is simple and clear to understand. The major concepts are logically linked, and the relationships are obvious in their theoretical assertions.

Generality

Transitions theory is a middle-range theory in scope. Middle-range theories have more limited scope and less abstraction than grand theories, and they address specific phenomena or concepts, which make them applicable in nursing practice. Transitions theory tends to be generalizable to people in transitions. When diverse types of transitions are considered, Transitions Theory is relevant for any population in transition, depending on the type of transition the population is experiencing. The research used to derive transitions theory was based on the participation of different gender and ethnic groups in various settings. This makes transitions theory more easily generalizable than theories developed for research with specific client populations.

Accessibility

Transitions theory has been tested and supported by Meleis and others as a framework for explaining the transition experiences of diverse groups of populations in different types of transitions. Transitions theory continues to evolve through planned programs of research, and continuous empirical research studies will further refine the theory. The development of situation-specific theories derived from transitions theory will further reduce its distance from the empirical world as well.

Importance

Transitions theory, with a focus on people in diverse types of transitions, provides a comprehensive and evolving guide for all health-related disciplines. Health-related disciplines always deal with a type of transition, whether single or multiple. Especially with an increasing need for culturally competent health care for diverse groups of health care clients, transitions theory provides a more appropriate theoretical fit for current health care. The inherent consideration of diversities of health care clients and its basis in research among diverse groups contribute to its importance.

SUMMARY

Current health care systems are characterized by changes, diversities, and complexities. Transitions theory, which evolved from research studies among diverse groups of people in various types of transitions, could adequately direct nursing practice and education in the current health care system. Meleis began her theoretical journey in the 1960s, and her journey continues. Transitions theory continues to be further developed through a number of studies based on the theory and the many colleagues Meleis has mentored. Recent development of situation-specific theories derived from transitions theory supports the usability and applicability of transitions theory to nursing research and practice.

CASE STUDY

Sue Kim, 49 years of age, emigrated from South Korea to the United States 6 years ago. Her family came to the United States to educate their children and moved in with family members in Los Angeles. Sue and her husband graduated from a top-ranked university in South Korea, and her husband also had a master's degree in business. However, their English skills were not adequate for them to get jobs in the United States. Instead, they opened a Korean grocery store with the money that they brought from South Korea, and they managed to settle down in Los Angeles, where a number of Koreans are living. They have two children: Mina, a 25-year-old daughter who is now the manager of a local shop, and Yujun, a 21-year-old son who is a college student. Both children were born in South Korea and moved to the United States with Sue. The children had a hard time, especially Mina, who came to the United States in her senior year of high school. However, the children finally adapted to their new environment. Now, Mina is living alone in a one-bedroom apartment near downtown, and Yujun is living in a university dormitory. The Kims are a religious family and attend their community's Protestant church regularly. They are involved in many church activities.

Sue and her husband have been too busy to have regular annual checkups for the past 6 years. About 1 year ago, Sue began to have serious indigestion, nausea, vomiting, and upper abdominal pain; she took some over-the-counter medicine and tried to tolerate the pain. Last month, her symptoms became more serious; she visited a local clinic and was referred to a larger hospital. Recently she was diagnosed with stomach cancer after a series of diagnostic tests and had surgery; she now is undergoing chemotherapy.

Continued

CASE STUDY—cont'd

You are the nurse who is taking care of Sue during this hospitalization. Sue is very polite and modest whenever you approach her. Sue is very quiet and never complains about any symptoms or pain. However, on several occasions, you think that Sue is in serious pain, when considering her facial expressions and sweating forehead. You think that Sue's English skills may not allow her to adequately communicate with health care providers. Also, you find that Sue does not have many visitors—only her husband and two children. You frequently find Sue praying while listening to some religious songs. You also find her sobbing silently. About 2 weeks are left until Sue finishes chemo therapy. You think that you should do something for Sue so she will not suffer through pain and symptoms that could be easily controlled with existing pain-management strategies. Now, you begin some preliminary planning.

1. Describe your assessment of the transition(s) Sue is experiencing. What are the types and patterns of the transition(s)? What properties of transitions can you identify from her case?
2. What personal, community, and societal transition conditions may have influenced Sue's experience? What are the cultural meanings attached to cancer, cancer pain, and symptoms accompanying chemotherapy, in this situation? What are Sue's cultural attitudes toward cancer and cancer patients? What factors may facilitate or inhibit her transition(s)?
3. Consider the patterns of response that Sue is showing. What are the indicators of healthy transition(s)? What are the indicators of unhealthy transition(s)?
4. Reflect on how transitions theory helped your assessment and nursing care for Sue.
5. If you were Sue's nurse, what would be your first action or interaction with her? Describe a plan of nursing care for Sue.

CRITICAL THINKING ACTIVITIES

1. Consider a transition you are personally engaged in now. Identify characteristics of the transition as defined in transitions theory that you have observed.
2. Analyze the changes that you are experiencing because of the specific transition. Consider how your level of awareness of these changes influences your transition experience.
3. Analyze personal, community, and societal conditions that may have influenced the transition that you are experiencing. List influences such as cultural beliefs and attitudes, socioeconomic status, and level of your preparation that have affected your approach to the transition.
4. Review your responses to the transition, and consider the outcomes of the personal transition in question 1. What would facilitate successful outcomes to the transition? What might inhibit successful outcomes?
5. How might you use this awareness in your nursing practice?

POINTS FOR FURTHER STUDY

- Meleis, A. I. (2011). *Theoretical nursing: Development and progress* (5th ed.). Philadelphia: Lippincott.
- The Transitions Theory website at the University of Pennsylvania at http://www.newcourtlandcenter@nursing.upenn.edu

REFERENCES

Baird, M. B. (2012). Well-being in refugee women experiencing cultural transition. *Advances in Nursing Science, 35*(3), 249–263.

Brackley, M. H. (1992). A role supplementation group pilot study: A nursing therapy for potential parental caregivers. *Clinical Nurse Specialist, 6*(1), 14–19.

Bridges, W. (1980). *Transitions.* Reading, MA: Addison-Wesley.

Bridges, W. (1991). *Managing transition: Making the most of change.* Menlo Park, CA: Addison Wesley.

Bull, M. J., & McShane, R. E. (2008). Seeking what's best during the transition to adult day health services. *Qualitative Health Research, 18*(5), 597–605.

Chick, N., & Meleis, A. I. (1986). Transitions: A nursing concern. In P. L. Chin (Ed.), *Nursing research methodology: Issues and implementations* (pp. 237–257). Gainsburg, MD: Aspen.

Clingerman, E. (2007). A situation-specific theory of migration transition for migrant farmworker women. *Research and Theory for Nursing Practice, 21*(4), 220–235.

Davidson, P. M., Dracup, K., Phillips, J., Padilla, G., & Daly, J. (2007). Maintaining hope in transition: A theoretical framework to guide interventions for people with heart failure. *The Journal of Cardiovascular Nursing, 22*(1), 58–64.

Davies, S. (2005). Meleis's theory of nursing transitions and relatives' experiences of nursing home entry. *Journal of Advanced Nursing, 52*(6), 658–671.

Dracup, K., Meleis, A. T., Baker, K., & Edlefsen, P. (1985). Family-focused cardiac rehabilitation: A role supplementation program for cardiac patients and spouses. *Nursing Clinics of North America, 19*(1), 113–124.

Dracup, K., Meleis, A. I., Clark, S., Clyburn, A., Shields, L., & Staley, M. (1985). Group counseling in cardiac rehabilitation: Effect on patient compliance. *Patient Education and Counseling, 6*(4), 169–177.

Gaffney, K. F. (1992). Nurse practice-model for maternal role sufficiency. *Advances in Nursing Sciences, 15*(2), 76–84.

Geary, C. R., & Schumacher, K. L. (2012). Care transitions: Integrating transition theory and complexity science concepts. *Advances in Nursing Science, 35*(3), 236–248.

Im, E. O. (1997). *Negligence and ignorance of menopause within gender multiple transition context: Low income Korean immigrant women.* Unpublished doctoral dissertation, University of California, San Francisco.

Im, E. O. (2005). Development of situation-specific theories: An integrative approach. *Advances in Nursing Science, 28*(2), 137–151.

Im, E. O. (2006). A situation-specific theory of Caucasian cancer patients' pain experience. *Advances in Nursing Science, 29*(3), 232–244.

Im, E. O. (2008). The situation-specific theory of pain experience for Asian American cancer patients. *Advances in Nursing Science, 31*(4), 319–331.

Im, E. O. (2010). A situation-specific theory of Asian immigrant women's menopausal symptom experience in the United States. *Advances in Nursing Science, 33*(2), 143–157.

Im, E. O. (2011). Transitions theory: A trajectory of theoretical development in nursing. *Nursing Outlook, 59*(5), 278–285.

Im, E. O. (2014a). The status quo of situation-specific theories. *Research and Theory for Nursing Practice, 28*(4), 278–298.

Im, E. O. (2014b). Situation-specific theories from the middle-range transitions theory. *Advances in Nursing Science, 37*(1), 19–31.

Im, E. O., & Meleis, A. I. (1999a). Situation-specific theories: Philosophical roots, properties, and approach. *Advances in Nursing Science, 22*(2), 11–24.

Im, E., & Meleis, A. I. (1999b). A situation-specific theory of Korean immigrant women's menopausal transition. *Journal of Nursing Scholarship, 31*(4), 333–338.

Im, E., & Meleis, A. I. (2000). Meanings of menopause: Low-income Korean immigrant women. *Western Journal of Nursing Research, 22*(1), 84–102.

Im, E., & Meleis, A. I. (2001). Women's work and symptoms during midlife: Korean immigrant women. *Women and Health, 33*(1/2), 83–103.

Im, E., Meleis, A. I., & Lee, K. (1999). Symptom experience of low-income Korean immigrant women during menopausal transition. *Women and Health, 29*(2), 53–67.

Jones, P. S., Zhang, X. E., & Meleis, A. I. (1978). Transforming vulnerability. *Western Journal of Nursing Research, 25*(7), 835–853.

Kaas, M. J., & Rousseau, G. K. (1983). Geriatric sexual conformity: Assessment and intervention. *Clinical Gerontologist, 2*(1), 31–44.

Kelley, L. S., & Lakin, J. A. (1988). Role supplementation as a nursing intervention for Alzheimer's disease: A case study. *Public Health Nursing, 5*(3), 146–152.

Meleis, A. I. (1975). Role insufficiency and role supplementation: A conceptual framework. *Nursing Research, 24*, 264–271.

Meleis, A. I. (1985). *Theoretical nursing: Development and progress* (1st ed.). Philadelphia: Lippincott.

Meleis, A. I. (1991). *Theoretical nursing: Development and progress* (2nd ed.). Philadelphia: Lippincott.

Meleis, A. I. (1997). *Theoretical nursing: Development and progress* (3rd ed.). Philadelphia: Lippincott.

Meleis, A. I. (2007). *Theoretical nursing: Development and progress* (4th ed.). Philadelphia: Lippincott.

Meleis, A. I. (2010). *Transitions theory: Middle-range and situation-specific theories in nursing research and practice.* New York: Springer.

Meleis, A. I. (2011). *Theoretical nursing: Development and progress* (5th ed.). Philadelphia: Lippincott.

Meleis, A. I. (2015a). Transition to retirement: A life cycle transition. In H. Loureiro (Ed.), *Transição Para a Reforma: Um Programa a Implementar Em Cuidados de Saúde Primários* (1st ed., pp. 9–15). Coimbra, Portugal: REATIVA.

Meleis, A. I. (2015b). Transitions theory. In M. Smith & M. E. Parker (Eds.), *Nursing Theories and Nursing Practice* (4th ed., pp. 361–380). Philadelphia, PA: F. A. Davis.

Meleis, A. I. (2016). The undeaning transition: Toward becoming a former dean. *Nursing Outlook, 64*(2), 186–196.

Meleis, A. I., Birch, E. L., & Wachter, S. M. (Eds.). (2011). *Women's health and the world's cities.* Philadelphia: University of Pennsylvania Press.

Meleis, A. I., Lipson, J., & Dallafar, A. (1998). The reluctant immigrant: Immigration experiences among Middle Eastern groups in Northern California. In D. Baxter & R. Krulfeld (Eds.), *Selected papers on refugees and immigrants,* vol. 5 (pp. 214–230). Arlington, VA: American Anthropological Association.

Meleis, A. I., Sawyer, L. M., Im, E. O., Hilfinger Messias, D. K., & Schumacher, K. (2000). Experiencing transitions: An emerging middle range theory. *Advances in Nursing Science, 23*(1), 12–28.

Meleis, A. I., & Swendsen, L. (1978). Role supplementation: An empirical test of a nursing intervention. *Nursing Research, 27*, 11–18.

Meleis, A. I., & Trangenstein, P. A. (1994). Facilitating transitions: Re-definition of the nursing mission. *Nursing Outlook, 42*, 255–259.

Messias, D. K. H. (1997). *Narratives of transnational migration, work, and health: The lived experiences of Brazilian women in the United States.* Unpublished doctoral dissertation, University of California, San Francisco.

Messias, D. K. H., Gilliss, C. L., Sparacino, P. S. A., Tong, E. M., & Foote, D. (1995). Stories of transition: Parents recall the diagnosis of congenital heart defects. *Family Systems Medicine, 3*(3/4), 367–377.

Robinson, P. R., Ekman, S. L., Meleis, A. I., Wahlund, L. O., & Winbald, B. (1997). Suffering in silence: The experience of early memory loss. *Health Care in Later Life, 2*(2), 107–120.

Sawyer, L. (1997). *Effects of racism on the transition to motherhood for African-American women*. Unpublished doctoral dissertation, University of California, San Francisco.

Schumacher, K. L. (1994). *Shifting patterns of self-care and caregiving during chemotherapy*. Unpublished doctoral dissertation, University of California, San Francisco.

Schumacher, K. L. (1995). Family caregiver role acquisition: Role-making through situated interaction. *Scholarly Inquiry for Nursing Practice, 9*, 211–271.

Schumacher, K. L., Dodd, M. J., & Paul, S. M. (1993). The stress process in family caregivers of persons receiving chemotherapy. *Research in Nursing & Health, 16*, 395–404.

Schumacher, K. L., Jones, P. S., & Meleis, A. I. (1999). Helping elderly persons in transition: A framework for research and practice. In L. Swanson & T. Tripp Reimer (Eds.), *Advances in gerontological nursing: Life transitions in the older adult,* vol. 3 (pp. 1–26). New York: Springer.

Schumacher, K. L., & Meleis, A. I. (1994). Transitions: A central concept in nursing. *Image: Journal of Nursing Scholarship, 26*(2), 119–127.

Shaul, M. P. (1997). Transition in chronic illness: Rheumatoid arthritis in women. *Rehabilitation Nursing, 22*, 199–205.

Shih, F. J., Meleis, A. I., Yu, P. J., Hu, W. Y., Lou, M. F., & Huang, G. S. (1998). Taiwanese patients' concerns and coping strategies: Transitions to cardiac surgery. *Heart and Lung, 27*(2), 82–98.

Walker, L. O., & Avant, K. C. (1995). *Strategies for theory construction in nursing* (3rd ed.). Norwalk, CT: Appleton & Lange.

Walker, L. O., & Avant, K. C. (2005). *Strategies for theory construction in nursing* (4th ed.). Norwalk, CT: Appleton & Lange.

Weiss, M. E., Piacentine, L. B., Lokken, L., Ancona, J., Archer, J., Gresser, S., et al. (2007). Perceived readiness for hospital discharge in adult medical-surgical patients. *Clinical Nurse Specialist, 21*(1), 31–42.

BIBLIOGRAPHY

Primary Sources

Books

Meleis, A. I. (2007). *Theoretical nursing: Development and progress* (4th ed.). Philadelphia: Lippincott.

Book Chapters

Brooten, D., & Naylor, M. D. (1999). Transitional environments. In A. S. Hinshaw, S. L. Feetham & J. Shaver (Eds.), *Handbook of clinical nursing research* (pp. 641–654). Thousand Oaks, CA: Sage.

Lipson, J. G., & Meleis, A. I. (1999). Research with immigrants and refugees. In A. S. Hinshaw, S. L. Feetham, & J. Shaver (Eds.), *Handbook of clinical nursing research* (pp. 87–106). Thousand Oaks, CA: Sage.

Meleis, A. I. (1997). *On transitions and knowledge development. Nursing beyond art and science* (annotated ed.). Japan: Japan Academy of Nursing Science.

Meleis, A. I. (1998). Research on role supplementation. In J. J. Fitzpatrick (Ed.), *Encyclopedia of nursing research*. New York: Springer.

Meleis, A. I., Lipson, J., & Dallafar, A. (1998). The reluctant immigrant: Immigration experiences among Middle Eastern groups in Northern California. In D. Baxter & R. Krulfeld (Eds.), *Selected papers on refugees and immigrants,* vol. 5 (pp. 214–230). Arlington, VA: American Anthropological Association.

Meleis, A. I., Lipson, J. G., Muecke, M., & Smith, G. (1998). *Immigrant women and their health: An olive paper*. Indianapolis: Sigma Theta Tau International.

Meleis, A. I., & Schumacher, K. L. (1998). Transitions and health. In J. J. Fitzpatrick (Ed.), *Encyclopedia of nursing research* (pp. 570–571). New York: Springer.

Meleis, A. I., & Swendsen, L. (1977). *Does nursing intervention make a difference? A test of the ROSP. Communicating nursing research: Nursing research priorities: Choice or chance,* vol. 8 (pp. 308–324). Boulder, CO: Western Interstate Commission for Higher Education.

Meleis, A. I., Swendsen, L., & Jones, D. (1980). Preventive role supplementation: A grounded conceptual framework. In M. H. Miller & B. Flynn (Eds.), *Current perspectives in nursing: Social issues and trends,* vol. 2 (pp. 3–14). St Louis: Mosby.

Dissertations

Almendarez, B. L. (2007). *Mexican American elders and nursing home transition*. Unpublished doctoral dissertation, University of Texas Health Science Center at San Antonio, TX.

Lenz, B. K. (2002). *Correlates of tobacco use and non-use among college students at a large university: Application of a transition framework*. Unpublished doctoral dissertation, University of Minnesota.

McMillan, E. S. (2002). *Education to practice questionnaire: A content analysis*. Unpublished doctoral dissertation, Wilmington College Division of Nursing, Delaware.

Missal, B. E. (2003). *The Gulf Arab woman's transition to motherhood*. Unpublished doctoral dissertation, University of Minnesota.

O'Brien-Barry, P. (2003). *The contribution of sex-role orientation and role commitment to interrole conflict in working first-time mothers at 6 to 9 months postpartum*. Unpublished doctoral dissertation, New York University.

Vardaman, S. (2011). *Lived experiences of transitions in international nursing students*. Unpublished doctoral dissertation, University of Texas, Tyler.

Journal Articles

Brown, M. A., & Olshansky, E. F. (1997). From limbo to legitimacy: A theoretical model of the transition to the primary care nurse practitioner role. *Nursing Research, 46*(1), 46–51.

Duchscher, J. B. (2008). A process of becoming: The stages of new nursing graduate professional role transition. *Journal of Continuing Education in Nursing, 39*(10), 441–450.

Elmberger, E., Bolund, C., & Lutzen, K. (2000). Transforming the exhausting to energizing process of being a good parent in the face of cancer. *Health Care for Women International, 21*(6), 485–499.

McCain, G. C., & Deatrick, J. A. (1994). The experience of high-risk pregnancy. *Journal of Obstetric, Gynecologic, and Neonatal Nursing, 23*(5), 421–427.

Meleis, A. I. (1975). Role/insufficiency and role supplementation: A conceptual framework. *Nursing Research, 24*, 264–271.

Meleis, A. I. (1987). Role transition and health. *Kango Kenkyo: The Japanese Journal of Nursing Research, 20*(1), 81, 69–89.

Meleis, A. I. (1991). Between two cultures: Identity, roles, and health. *Health Care for Women International, 12*, 365–378.

Meleis, A. I. (1997). Immigrant transitions and health care: An action plan. *Nursing Outlook, 45*(1), 42.

Meleis, A. I., & Rogers, S. (1987). Women in transition: Being vs. becoming or being and becoming. *Health Care for Women International, 8*, 199–217.

Meleis, A. I., & Swendsen, L. (1978). Role supplementation: An empirical test of a nursing intervention. *Nursing Research, 27*, 11–18.

Meleis, A. I., & Trangenstein, P. A. (1994). Facilitating transitions: Redefinition of a nursing mission. *Nursing Outlook, 42*(6), 255–259.

Messias, D. K. H. (2002). Transnational health resources, practices, and perspectives: Brazilian immigrant women's narratives. *Journal of Immigrant Health, 4*(4), 183–200.

Messias, D. K. H., Gilliss, C. L., Sparacino, P. S. A., Tong, E. M., & Foote, D. (1995). Stories of transition: Parents recall the diagnosis of congenital heart defect. *Family Systems Medicine, 13*(3/4), 367–277.

Schumacher, K. L. (1995). Family caregiver role acquisition: Role-making through situated interaction. *Scholarly Inquiry for Nursing Practice, 9*, 211–271.

Schumacher, K. L. (1996). Reconceptualizing family caregiving: Family-based illness care during chemotherapy. *Research in Nursing & Health, 19*, 261–272.

Schumacher, K. L., Dodd, M. J., & Paul, S. M. (1993). The stress process in family caregivers of persons receiving chemotherapy. *Research in Nursing & Health, 16*, 395–404.

Schumacher, K. L., Stewart, B. J., & Archbold, P. G. (1998). Conceptualizing and measurement of doing family caregiving well. *Image: Journal of Nursing Scholarship, 30*(1), 63–69.

Shih, F., & Huang, L. H. (1996). Patients' needs and their coping strategies transition to cardiac surgery. *Kaohsiung Journal of Medical Sciences, 12*(2), 114–127.

Shih, F. J., Meleis, A. I., Yu, P. J., Hu, W. Y., Lou, M. F., & Huang, G. S. (1998). Taiwanese patients' concerns and coping strategies: Transitions to cardiac surgery. *Heart and Lung, 27*(2), 82–98.

Swendsen, L., Meleis, A. I., & Jones, D. (1978). Role supplementation for new parents: A role mastery plan. *American Journal of Maternal Child Nursing, 3*, 84–91.

Watson, N., & Pulliam, L. (2000). Transgenerational health promotion. *Holistic Nursing Practice, 14*(4), 1–11.

Weiss, M. E., & Lokken, L. (2009). Predictors and outcomes of postpartum mothers' perceptions of readiness for discharge after birth. *Journal of Obstetric, Gynecologic, and Neonatal Nursing, 38*(4), 406–417.

Weiss, M. E., Piacentine, L. B., Lokken, L., Ancona, J., Archer, J., Gresser, S., et al. (2007). Perceived readiness for hospital discharge in adult medical-surgical patients. *Clinical Nurse Specialist, 21*(1), 31–42.

Wilkins, K. L., & Woodgate, R. L. (2006). Transition: A conceptual analysis in the context of siblings of children with cancer. *Journal of Pediatric Nursing, 21*(4), 256–265.

Wilson, S. A. (1997). The transition to nursing home life: A comparison of planned and unplanned admissions. *Journal of Advanced Nursing, 26*, 864–871.

Secondary Sources

Books

Meleis, A. I., Isenberg, M., Koerner, J. E., Lacey, B., & Stern, P. (1995). *Diversity, marginalization, and culturally competent health care: Issues in knowledge development*. Washington: American Academy of Nursing.

Meleis, A. I., Lipson, J. G., Muecke, M., & Smith, G. (1998). *Immigrant women and their health: An olive paper*. Indianapolis, IN: Sigma Theta Tau International.

Meleis, A. I., Birch, E. L., & Wachter, S. M. (Eds.). (2011). *Women's health and the world's cities*. Philadelphia: University of Pennsylvania Press.

St. Hill, P., Lipson, J., & Meleis, A. I. (Eds.). (2002). *Caring for women cross-culturally: A portable guide*. Philadelphia: F. A. Davis.

Journal Articles

Dracup, K., Cronenwett, L., Meleis, A. I., & Benner, P. E. (2005). Reflections on the doctorate of nursing practice. *Nursing Outlook, 53*(4), 177–182.

Dracup, K., Cronenwett, L., Meleis, A. I., & Benner, P. E. (2005). Reply to letter to the editor on reflections on the doctorate of nursing practice. *Nursing Outlook, 53*(6), 269.

Hall, J. M., Stevens, P. E., & Meleis, A. I. (1992). Developing the construct of role integration: A narrative analysis of women clerical workers' daily lives. *Research in Nursing & Health, 15*(6), 447–457.

Hall, J. M., Stevens, P. E., & Meleis, A. I. (1992). Experiences of women clerical workers in patient care areas. *Journal of Nursing Administration, 22*(5), 11–17.

Hall, J. M., Stevens, P. E., & Meleis, A. I. (1994). Marginalization: A guiding concept for valuing diversity in nursing knowledge development. *Advances in Nursing Science, 16*(4), 23–41.

Hattar-Pollara, M., & Meleis, A. I. (1995). Parenting adolescents: The experiences of Jordanian immigrant women in California. *Health Care for Women International, 16*(3), 195–211.

Hattar-Pollara, M., & Meleis, A. I. (1995). Stress of immigration and the daily lived experience of Jordanian immigrant women. *Western Journal of Nursing Research, 17*(5), 521–539.

Hattar-Pollara, M., Meleis, A. I., & Nagib, H. (2000). A study of the spousal role of Egyptian women in clerical jobs. *Health Care for Women International, 21*(4), 305–317.

Hattar-Pollara, M., Meleis, A. I., & Nagib, H. (2003). Multiple role stress and patterns of coping of Egyptian women in clerical jobs. *Transcultural Nursing, 14*(2), 125–133.

Im, E., Meleis, A. I., & Park, Y. S. (1999). A feminist critique of the research on menopausal experience of Korean women. *Research In Nursing and Health, 22*, 410–420.

Jones, P., & Meleis, A. I. (2002). Caregiving between two cultures: An integrative experience. *Journal of Transcultural Nursing, 13*(3), 202–209.

Jones, P. S., Jaceldo, K. B., Lee, J. R., Zhang, X. E., & Meleis, A. I. (2001). Role integration and perceived health in Asian American women caregivers. *Research in Nursing and Health, 24*, 133–144.

Jones, P. S., & Meleis, A. I. (1993). Health is empowerment. *Advances in Nursing Science, 15*(3), 1–14.

Jones, P. S., Zhang, X. E., & Meleis, A. I. (1978). Transforming vulnerability. *Western Journal of Nursing Research, 25*(7), 835–853.

Laffrey, S. C., Meleis, A. I., Lipson, J. G., Solomon, M., & Omidian, P. A. (1989). Assessing Arab-American health care needs. *Social Science and Medicine, 29*(7), 877–883.

Meleis, A. I. (1992). Community participation and involvement: Theoretical and empirical issues. *Health Services Management Research, 5*(10), 5–16.

Meleis, A. I. (1992). Directions for nursing theory development in the 21st century. *Nursing Science Quarterly, 5*(3), 112–117.

Meleis, A. I. (1992). Nursing: A caring science with a distinct domain. *Sairaanhoitaja*, (6), 8–12.

Meleis, A. I. (1992). On the way to scholarship: From master's to doctorate. *Journal of Professional Nursing, 8*(6), 328–334.

Meleis, A. I. (1996). Culturally competent scholarship: Substance and rigor. *Advances in Nursing Science, 19*(2), 1–16.

Meleis, A. I. (2001). Small steps and giant hopes: Violence on women is more than wife battering. (Editorial). *Health Care for Women International, 23*, 313–315.

Meleis, A. I. (2001). Women's work, health and quality of life: It is time we redefine women's work. *Women and Health, 33*(1/2), xv–xviii.

Meleis, A. I. (2002). Whither international research? (Editorial). *Journal of Nursing Scholarship, 34*(1), 4–5.

Meleis, A. I. (2003). Brain drain or empowerment. (Guest Editorial). *Journal of Nursing Scholarship, 35*(2), 105.

Meleis, A. I. (2005). Arabs. In J. Lipson & S. Dibble (Eds.), *Culture and clinical care: A practical guide* (pp. 42–57). San Francisco: University of California San Francisco Nursing Press.

Meleis, A. I. (2005). Safe womanhood is not safe motherhood: Policy implications. *Health Care for Women International, 26*(2), 464–471.

Meleis, A. I. (2005). Shortage of nurses means a shortage of nurse scientists. (Editorial). *Journal of Advanced Nursing, 49*(2), 111.

Meleis, A. I. (2006). Human capital in health care: A resource crisis of a caring crisis? *Global Health Link, 139*, 6–7, 21–22.

Meleis, A. I., Arruda, E. N., Lane, S., & Bernal, P. (1994). Veiled, voluminous and devalued: Narrative stories about low-income women from Brazil, Egypt & Colombia. *Advances in Nursing Science, 17*(2), 1–15.

Meleis, A. I., & Bernal, P. (1994). Domestic workers in Colombia as spouses: Security and servitude. *Holistic Nursing, 8*(4), 33–43.

Meleis, A. I., & Bernal, P. (1995). The paradoxical world of muchacha de por dia ín Colombia. *Human Organization, 54*, 393–400.

Meleis, A. I., Douglas, M., Eribes, C., Shih, F., & Messias, D. (1996). Employed Mexican women as mothers and partners: Valued, empowered and overloaded. *Journal of Advanced Nursing, 23*, 82–90.

Meleis, A. I., & Fishman, J. (2001). Rethinking the work in health: Gendered and cultural expectations. (Editorial). *Health Care for Women International, 22*, 195–197.

Meleis, A. I., Hall, J. M., & Stevens, P. E. (1994). Scholarly caring in doctoral nursing education: Promoting diversity and collaborative mentorship. *Image: Journal of Nursing Scholarship, 26*(3), 177–180.

Meleis, A. I., & Im, E. (1999). Transcending marginalization in knowledge development. *Nursing Inquiry, 6*(2), [illegible]–102.

Meleis, A. I., & Im, E. O. (2002). Grandmothers and women's health: From fragmentation to coherence. *Health Care for Women International, 23*(2), 207–224.

Meleis, A. I., Kulig, J., Arruda, E. N., & Beckman, A. (19[illegible]). Maternal role of women in clerical jobs in southern Brazil: Stress and satisfaction. *Health Care for Women International, 11*(4), 369–382.

Meleis, A. I., & Lindgren, T. (2001). Show me a woman who does not work! *Journal of Nursing*, 209–210.

Meleis, A. I., & Lipson, J. (2003). Cross-cultural health and strategies to lead development of nursing practice. In J. Daly, S. Speedy & D. Jackson (Eds.), *Nursing Leadership* (pp. 69–88). Philadelphia: Churchill Livingstone.

Meleis, A. I., Lipson J. G., & Paul, S. M. (1992). Ethnicity and health among five Middle Eastern immigrant groups. *Nursing Research, 41*(2), 98–103.

Meleis, A. I., Messias, D. K. H., & Arruda, E. N. (1995). Women's work environment and health: Clerical workers in Brazil. *Research in Nursing and Health, 19*, 53–62.

Meleis, A. I., & Stevens, P. E. (1992). Women in clerical jobs: Spousal role satisfaction stress and coping. *Women & Health, 18*(1), 23–40.

Messias, D. K. H., Hall, J. M., & Meleis, A. I. (1996). Voices of impoverished Brazilian women: Health implications of roles and resources. *Women and Health, 24*(1), 1–20.

Messias, D. K. H., Im, E., Page, A., Regev, H., Spiers, J., & Meleis, A. I. (1997). Defining and redefining work: Implications for women's health. *Gender and Society, 11*(3), 296–323.

Messias, D. H., Regev, H., Im, E., Spiers, J., Van, P., & Meleis, A. I. (1997). Expanding the visibility of women's work: Policy implications. *Nursing Outlook, 45*, 258–264.

Siantz, M. L., & Meleis, A. I. (2007). Integrating cultural competence into nursing education and practice: 21st century action steps. *Journal of Transcultural Nursing, 18*(1), 86–90.

Van, P., & Meleis, A. I. (2003). Coping with grief after involuntary pregnancy loss: Perspectives of African-American women. *Journal of Obstetric, Gynecologic, & Neonatal Nursing, 32*(1), 28–39.

21

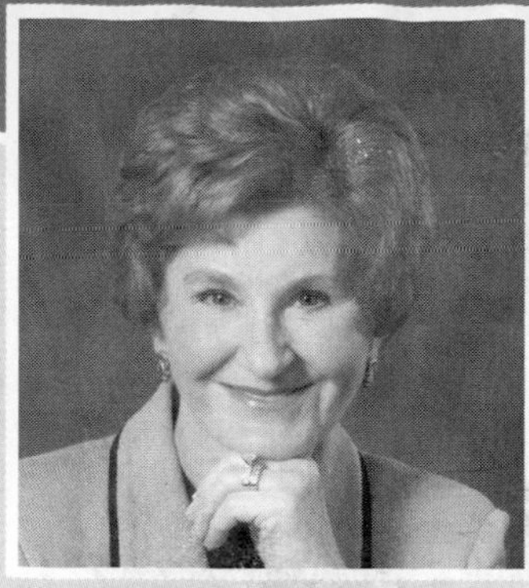

Nola J. Pender
(1941–Present)

Health Promotion Model

*Teresa J. Sakraida and Jane Wilson**

"Middle range theories that have been tested in research provide evidence for evidence-based practice, thus facilitating translation of research into practice."
(Nola J. Pender, personal communication, April 2008)

CREDENTIALS AND BACKGROUND OF THE THEORIST

Nola J. Pender's first encounter with professional nursing occurred at 7 years of age, when she observed the nursing care given to her hospitalized aunt. "The experience of watching the nurses caring for my aunt in her illness created in me a fascination with the work of nursing," noted Pender (Pender, personal communication, May 6, 2004). This experience and her subsequent education instilled in her a desire to care for others and influenced her belief that the goal of nursing was to help people care for themselves. Pender contributes to nursing knowledge of health promotion through her research, teaching, presentations, and writings.

Pender was born August 16, 1941, in Lansing, Michigan. She was the only child of parents who advocated education for women. Family encouragement to become a registered nurse led her to the School of Nursing at West Suburban Hospital in Oak Park, Illinois. This school was chosen for its ties with Wheaton College and its strong Christian foundation. She received her nursing diploma in 1962 and began working on a medical-surgical unit and subsequently in a pediatric unit in a Michigan hospital (Pender, personal communication, May 6, 2004).

In 1964, Pender completed her baccalaureate in nursing at Michigan State University. She credits Helen Penhale, assistant to the dean, who streamlined her program for fostering her options for further education. As was common in the 1960s, Pender changed her major from nursing as she pursued her graduate degrees. She earned a master's degree in human growth and development at Michigan State University in 1965. "The M.A. in growth and development influenced my interest in health over the human life span. This background contributed to the formation of a research program for children and adolescents," stated Pender. She completed her doctorate in psychology and education in 1969 at Northwestern University. Pender's (1970) dissertation research investigated developmental changes in encoding processes of short-term memory in children. She credits Dr. James Hall, doctoral program advisor, with "introducing me to considerations of how people think and how a person's thoughts motivate behavior." Several years later, she completed master's-level work in community health nursing at Rush University (Pender, personal communication, May 6, 2004).

After earning her doctorate, Pender notes a shift in her thinking toward defining the goal of nursing care as the optimal health of the individual. A series of conversations with Dr. Beverly McElmurry at Northern Illinois University and reading *High-Level Wellness* by Halpert Dunn (1961) inspired expanded notions of health and nursing. Her marriage to Albert Pender, an associate professor of business and economics who has collaborated with his wife

*Previous author: Lucy Anne Tillett. The author wishes to express appreciation to Nola J. Pender for reviewing the chapter.

in writing about the economics of health care, and the birth of a son and a daughter provided increased personal motivation to learn more about optimizing human health.

In 1975, Pender published "A Conceptual Model for Preventive Health Behavior" as a basis for studying how individuals made decisions about their own health care in a nursing context. This article identified factors that were found in earlier research to influence decision making and actions of individuals in preventing disease. Pender's original health promotion model was presented in the first edition of her text, *Health Promotion in Nursing Practice,* which was published in 1982. Based on subsequent research, the health promotion model was revised and presented in a second edition in 1987 and in a third edition in 1996. The fourth edition of *Health Promotion in Nursing Practice* was coauthored by Pender, Carolyn L. Murdaugh (PhD), and Mary Ann Parsons (PhD) and published in 2002, and a fifth edition was published in 2006.

In 1988, Pender and colleagues conducted a study at Northern Illinois University, DeKalb, which was funded by the National Institutes of Health. Susan Walker, Karen Sechrist, and Marilyn Frank-Stromborg tested the validity of the health promotion model (Pender et al., 1988). The research team developed the Health Promoting Lifestyle Profile, an instrument used to study the health-promoting behavior of working adults, older adults, patients undergoing cardiac rehabilitation, and ambulatory patients with cancer (Pender, Murdaugh, & Parsons, 2002). Results from these studies supported the health promotion model (Pender, personal communication, July 19, 2000). Subsequently, more than 40 studies tested the predictive capability of the model for health-promoting lifestyle, exercise, nutrition practices, use of hearing protection, and avoidance of exposure to environmental tobacco smoke (Pender, 1996; Pender, Murdaugh, & Parsons, 2002).

Pender provided leadership in the development of nursing research in the United States. Her support of the National Center for Nursing Research in the National Institutes of Health was instrumental to its formation. She has promoted scholarly activity in nursing through involvement with Sigma Theta Tau International, as president of the Midwest Nursing Research Society from 1985 to 1987, and as chairperson of the Cabinet on Nursing Research of the American Nurses Association. She has served as a Trustee of the Midwest Nursing Research Society since 2009 (Pender, n.d.). Inducted as a fellow of the American Academy of Nursing in 1981, she served as President of the Academy from 1991 until 1993. In 1998 she was appointed to a 4-year term on the U.S. Preventive Services Task Force, an independent panel charged to evaluate scientific evidence and to make age-specific and risk-specific recommendations for clinical preventive services (Pender, n.d.).

As a leader in nursing education, Dr. Pender guided many students and mentored others. Over her 40 years as an educator, she facilitated the learning of baccalaureate, master's, and doctorate students. She has mentored a number of postdoctoral fellows. In 1998 the University of Michigan School of Nursing honored Pender with the Mae Edna Doyle Award for excellence in teaching. She is a Distinguished Professor at Loyola University of Chicago School of Nursing.

A recipient of many awards and honors, Dr. Pender has served as a distinguished scholar at a number of universities. She received an honorary doctorate from Widener University in 1992. In 1988 she received the Distinguished Research Award from the Midwest Nursing Research Society for her contributions to research and research leadership, and in 1997 she received the American Psychological Association Award for outstanding contributions to nursing and health psychology. Her widely used text, *Health Promotion in Nursing Practice* (Pender, Murdaugh, & Parsons, 2002), was the American Nurses Association Book of the Year for contributions to community health nursing (Pender, n.d.).

Pender was Associate Dean for Research at the University of Michigan School of Nursing from 1990 to 2001. In this position, she facilitated external funding of faculty research, supported emerging centers of research excellence in the School of Nursing, promoted interdisciplinary research, supported translating research into science-based practice, and linked nursing research to formulation of health policy (Pender, n.d.). A child and adolescent health behavior research center initiated at the University of Michigan in 1991 represents Pender's efforts to build a large interdisciplinary research team to study and influence the health-promoting behaviors of individuals by understanding how these behaviors are established in youth (Pender, personal communication, May 24, 2000). Her program of research includes two major foci: (1) understanding how self-efficacy effects the exertion and affective (activity-related affect) responses of adolescent girls to the physical activity challenge and (2) developing an interactive computer program as an intervention to increase physical activity among adolescent girls. The Design of a Computer Based Physical Activity Counseling Intervention for Adolescent Girls was a research program led by Dr. Lorraine Robbins (Robbins et al., 2006).

Pender has published numerous articles on exercise, behavior change, and relaxation training as aspects of health promotion and has served on editorial boards and as an editor for journals and books. Pender is recognized as a scholar, presenter, and consultant on health promotion. She has consulted with nurse scientists in Japan, Korea, Mexico, Thailand, the Dominican Republic, Jamaica, England, New Zealand, and Chile (Pender, Murdaugh, & Parsons, 2006). Her book has been translated into Japanese and Korean (Pender, 1997a, 1997b). Pender continues influencing the nursing profession by providing leadership as a consultant to research centers and providing early scholar consultation (Pender, n.d.). As a nationally and internationally known leader, Pender speaks at conferences and seminars. She collaborates with the editor of the *American Journal of Health Promotion,* advocating for legislation to fund health promotion research (Pender, personal communication, May 6, 2004).

Pender's plans include travel to offer consultation and speaking opportunities. She engages in some graduate teaching, including courses on theories of nursing and scientific writing as a Distinguished Professor at Loyola University in Chicago (Pender, personal communication, February 27, 2008). She mentors through e-mail exchanges about scholarly research programs.

THEORETICAL SOURCES

Pender's background in nursing, human development, experimental psychology, and education led her to use a holistic nursing perspective, social psychology, and learning theory as foundations for the health promotion model. The health promotion model (Fig. 21.1) integrates several constructs. Central to the health promotion model is the social learning theory of Albert Bandura (1977), which postulates the importance of cognitive processes in the changing of behavior. Social learning theory, now titled *social cognitive theory,* includes the following self-beliefs: self-attribution, self-evaluation, and self-efficacy. Self-efficacy is a central construct of the health promotion model (HPM) (Pender, 1996; Pender, Murdaugh, & Parsons,

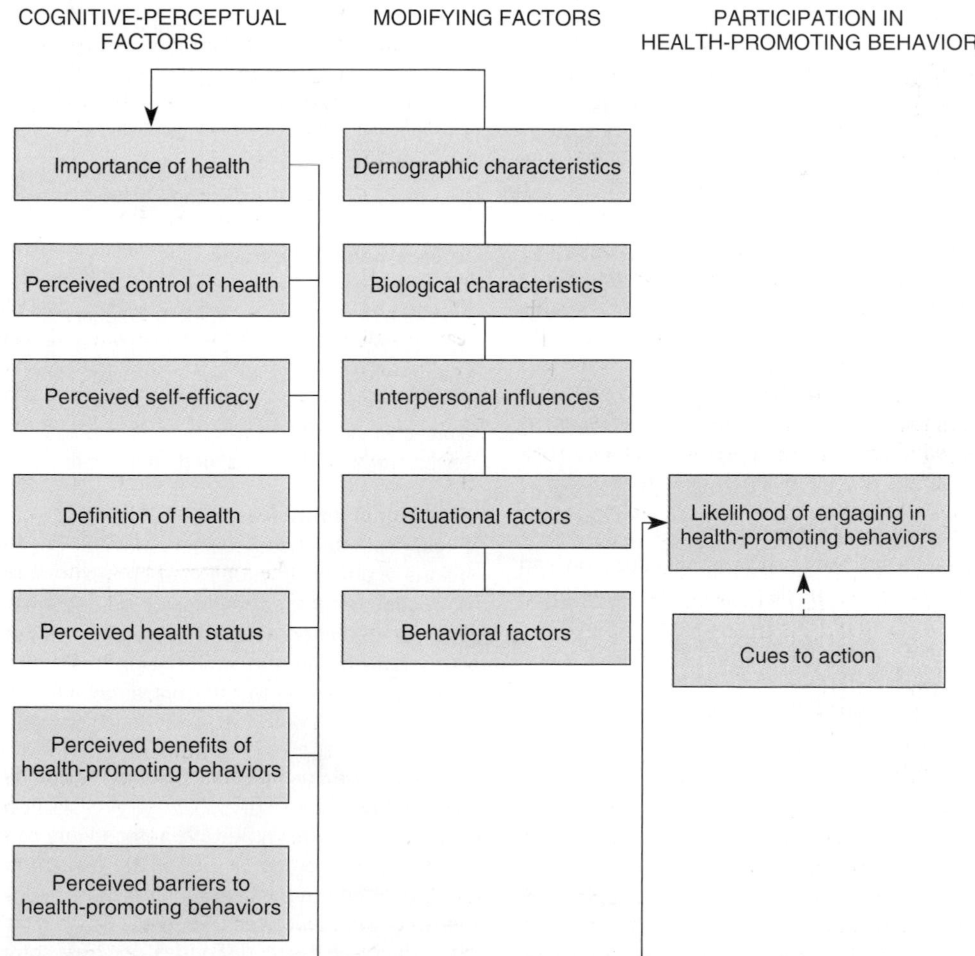

FIG. 21.1 Health promotion model. (From Pender, N. J. [1987]. *Health promotion in nursing practice* [2nd ed., p. 58]. New York: Appleton & Lange. Copyright Pearson Education, Upper Saddle River, NJ.)

2002). The expectancy value model of human motivation described by Feather (1982) proposes that behavior is rational and economical and was important to the model's development.

The Health Promotion Model is similar in construction to the health belief model (Becker, 1974), which explains disease prevention behavior; but the HPM differs from the health belief model in that it does not include fear or threat as a source of motivation for health behavior. The HPM expands to encompass behaviors for enhancing health and applies across the life span (Pender, 1996; Pender, Murdaugh, & Parsons, 2002).

MAJOR CONCEPTS & DEFINITIONS

The major concepts and definitions presented here are found in the revised health promotion model (Pender et al., 2006).

Prior Related Behavior

Prior related behavior refers to the frequency of the same or similar behavior in the past. This has direct and indirect effects on the likelihood of engaging in health-promoting behaviors.

Personal Factors

Personal factors are categorized as biological, psychological, and sociocultural. These factors are predictive of a given behavior and are shaped by the nature of the target behavior being considered.

Personal Biological Factors

Included in personal biological factors are variables such as age, gender, body mass index, pubertal status, menopausal status, aerobic capacity, strength, agility, and balance.

Personal Psychological Factors

Personal psychological factors include variables such as self-esteem, self-motivation, personal competence, perceived health status, and definition of health.

Personal Sociocultural Factors

Factors such as race, ethnicity, acculturation, education, and socioeconomic status are included in sociocultural factors.

Behavioral-Specific Cognitions and Affects

The following are behavioral-specific cognitions and affects that are considered of major motivational significance; these variables are modifiable through nursing actions (Pender, 1996).

Perceived Benefits of Action

Perceived benefits of action are anticipated positive outcomes that will result from health behavior.

Perceived Barriers to Action

Perceived barriers to action are anticipated, imagined, or real blocks and personal costs of undertaking a given behavior.

Perceived Self-Efficacy

Perceived self-efficacy is judgment of personal capability to organize and execute a health-promoting behavior. Perceived self-efficacy influences perceived barriers to action, so higher efficacy results in lowered perceptions of barriers to the performance of the behavior.

Activity-Related Affect

An activity-related affect describes subjective positive or negative feelings that occur before, during, and after behavior based on the stimulus properties of the behavior itself. Activity-related affect influences perceived self-efficacy, which means the more positive the subjective feeling, the greater is the feeling of efficacy. In turn, increased feelings of efficacy can generate further positive affect.

Interpersonal Influences

These influences are cognitions concerning behaviors, beliefs, or attitudes of others. Interpersonal influences include norms (expectations of significant others), social support (instrumental and emotional encouragement), and modeling (vicarious learning through observing others engaged in a particular behavior). Primary sources of interpersonal influences are families, peers, and health care providers.

Situational Influences

Situational influences are personal perceptions and cognitions of any given situation or context that can facilitate or impede behavior. They include perceptions of available options, demand characteristics, and aesthetic features of the environment in which given health-promoting behavior is proposed to take place. Situational influences may have direct or indirect influences on health behavior.

Immediate Antecedents of Behavior and Behavior Outcomes

The following are immediate antecedents of behavior or behavioral outcomes. A behavioral event is initiated by a commitment to action unless there is a competing demand that cannot be avoided or a competing preference that cannot be resisted (Pender, personal communication, July 19, 2000).

MAJOR CONCEPTS & DEFINITIONS—cont'd

Commitment to a Plan of Action
This commitment describes the concept of intention and identification of a planned strategy that leads to implementation of health behavior.

Immediate Competing Demands and Preferences
Competing demands are alternative behaviors over which individuals have low control, because there are environmental contingencies such as work or family care responsibilities. Competing preferences are alternative behaviors over which individuals exert relatively high control, such as the choice of ice cream or an apple for a snack.

Health-Promoting Behavior
A health-promoting behavior is an end point or action outcome that is directed toward attaining positive health outcomes such as optimal well-being, personal fulfillment, and productive living. Examples of health-promoting behavior are eating a healthy diet, exercising regularly, managing stress, gaining adequate rest and spiritual growth, and building positive relationships.

USE OF EMPIRICAL EVIDENCE

The health promotion model, as depicted in Fig. 21.1, served as a framework for research aimed at predicting overall health-promoting lifestyles and specific behaviors such as exercise and use of hearing protection (Pender, 1987). Pender and colleagues conducted a program of research funded by the National Institute of Nursing Research to evaluate the health promotion model in the following populations: (1) working adults, (2) older community-dwelling adults, (3) ambulatory patients with cancer, and (4) patients undergoing cardiac rehabilitation. These studies tested the validity of the health promotion model (Pender, personal communication, May 24, 2000). A summary of findings from earlier studies is included in the 1996 edition of *Health Promotion in Nursing Practice* (Pender, 1996). Studies further testing the model are discussed in the fifth edition of *Health Promotion in Nursing Practice* (Pender, Murdaugh, & Parsons, 2006). The fifth edition includes an emphasis on the health promotion model as applied to diverse and vulnerable populations and addresses evidence-based practice.

The rationale for revision of the health promotion model stemmed from research. The process of refining the health promotion model, as published in 1987, led to several changes in the model (Pender, 1996) (see Fig. 21.1).

First, importance of health, perceived control of health, and cues for action were deleted. Second, the definition of health, perceived health status, and demographic and biological characteristics were repositioned as personal factors in the 1996 revision of the health promotion model (Pender, 1996) and the fourth edition of *Health Promotion in Nursing Practice* (Pender, Murdaugh, & Parsons, 2002) (Fig. 21.2). Third, the revised health promotion model (see Fig. 21.2) added three new variables that influenced the individual to engage in health-promoting behaviors (Pender, 1996):

- Activity-related affect
- Commitment to a plan of action
- Immediate competing demand and preferences

The revised health promotion model focuses on 10 categories of determinants of health-promoting behavior. The revised model identifies concepts relevant to health-promoting behaviors and facilitates the generation of testable hypotheses (Pender, Murdaugh, & Parsons, 2002).

The health promotion model provides a paradigm for the development of instruments. The Health Promoting Lifestyle Profile and the Exercise Benefits-Barriers Scale (EBBS) are two examples.* These instruments serve to test the model and support further model development.

The purpose of the Health Promotion Lifestyle Profile instrument is to measure health-promoting lifestyle (Pender, 1996). The Health Promotion Lifestyle Profile II (HPLP-II), is a revision of the original instrument for research.† The 52-item, four-point, Likert-style instrument has six subscales: (1) health responsibility, (2) physical activity, (3) nutrition, (4) interpersonal relations, (5) spiritual growth, and (6) stress management. The mean can be derived for each subscale, or a total mean can be calculated to signify overall health-promoting lifestyle (Walker, Sechrist, & Pender, 1987). The instrument provides assessment of a health-promoting lifestyle of individuals and is used clinically by nurses for patient support and education.

*The EBBS can be obtained from the Health Promotion Research Program, Social Science Research Institute, Northern Illinois University, DeKalb, IL 60115.

†The HPLP-II can be obtained through the faculty-staff profile for Dr. Susan Noble Walker, EdD, RN, at the College of Nursing, University of Nebraska Medical Center. The link to download is available at swalker@unmc.edu

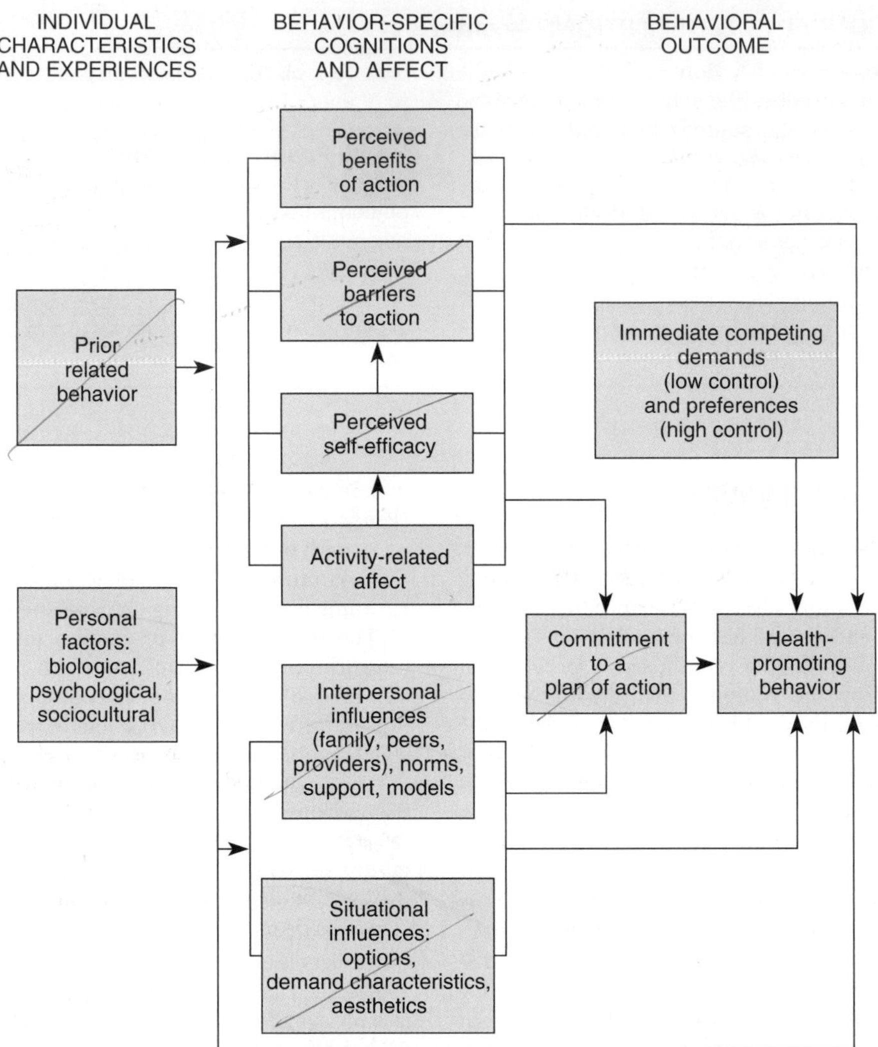

FIG. 21.2 Revised health promotion model. (From Pender, N. J., Murdaugh, C. L., & Parsons, M. A. [2002]. *Health promotion in nursing practice* 4th Ed., ©2002. Reprinted by permission of Pearson Education, Inc., New York, New York.)

The health promotion model identifies cognitive and perceptual factors as major determinants of health-promoting behavior. The EBBS measures the cognitive and perceptual factors of perceived benefits and perceived barriers to exercise (Sechrist, Walker, & Pender, 1987). The 43-item, four-point, Likert-styled instrument consists of a 29-item benefits scale and a 14-item barriers scale that may be scored separately or as a whole. The higher the overall score on the 43-item instrument, the more positively the individual perceives the benefits to exercise in relation to barriers to exercise (Sechrist, Walker, & Pender, 1987). The EBBS is useful clinically for evaluating exercise perceptions.

MAJOR ASSUMPTIONS

The assumptions reflect the behavioral science perspective and emphasize the active role of the patient in managing health behaviors by modifying the environmental context. In the third edition of *Health Promotion in Nursing Practice,* Pender (1996) stated the major assumptions of the health promotion model that address person, environment, and health are as follows:

1. Persons seek to create conditions of living through which they can express their unique human health potential.

2. Persons have the capacity for reflective self-awareness, including assessment of their own competencies.
3. Persons value growth in directions viewed as positive and attempt to achieve a personally acceptable balance between change and stability.
4. Individuals seek to actively regulate their own behavior.
5. Individuals in all their biopsychosocial complexity interact with the environment, progressively transforming the environment and being transformed over time.
6. Health professionals constitute a part of the interpersonal environment, which exerts influence on persons throughout their life spans.
7. Self-initiated reconfiguration of person-environment interactive patterns is essential to behavioral change (pp. 54–55).

THEORETICAL ASSERTIONS

The model depicts the multifaceted natures of persons interacting with the environment as they pursue health. The HPM has a competence- or approach-oriented focus (Pender, 1996). Health promotion is motivated by the desire to enhance well-being and to actualize human potential (Pender, 1996). In her first book, *Health Promotion in Nursing Practice,* Pender (1982) asserts that complex biopsychosocial processes motivate individuals to engage in behaviors directed toward the enhancement of health. Fourteen theoretical assertions derived from the model appear in the fourth edition of the book (Pender, Murdaugh, & Parsons, 2002):

1. Prior behavior and inherited and acquired characteristics influence beliefs, affect, and enactment of health-promoting behavior.
2. Persons commit to engaging in behaviors from which they anticipate deriving personally valued benefits.
3. Perceived barriers can constrain the commitment to action, the mediator of behavior, and the actual behavior.
4. Perceived competence or self-efficacy to execute a given behavior increases the likelihood of commitment to action and actual performance of behavior.
5. Greater perceived self-efficacy results in fewer perceived barriers to specific health behavior.
6. Positive affect toward a behavior results in greater perceived self-efficacy, which, in turn, can result in increased positive affect.
7. When positive emotions or affect is associated with a behavior, the probability of commitment and action is increased.
8. Persons are more likely to commit to and engage in health-promoting behaviors when significant others model the behavior, expect the behavior to occur, and provide assistance and support to enable the behavior.
9. Families, peers, and health care providers are important sources of interpersonal influences that can increase or decrease commitment to and engagement in health-promoting behavior.
10. Situational influences in the external environment can increase or decrease commitment to or participation in health-promoting behavior.
11. The greater the commitment to a specific plan of action, the more likely health-promoting behaviors are to be maintained over time.
12. Commitment to a plan of action is less likely to result in the desired behavior when competing demands over which persons have little control require immediate attention.
13. Commitment to a plan of action is less likely to result in the desired behavior when other actions are more attractive and thus preferred over the target behavior.
14. Persons can modify cognitions, affect, and the interpersonal and physical environments to create incentives for health actions (pp. 63–64).

LOGICAL FORM

The health promotion model was formulated through induction by use of existing research to form a pattern of knowledge about health behavior. The health promotion model is a conceptual model from which middle-range theories may be developed. It was formulated with the goal of integrating what is known about health-promoting behavior to generate questions for further testing. This model illustrates how a framework of previous research fits together and how concepts can be manipulated for further study.

ACCEPTANCE BY THE NURSING COMMUNITY

Practice

Wellness as a nursing specialty has grown in prominence, and current state-of-the-art clinical practice includes health promotion education. Nursing professionals find the health promotion model relevant, as it applies across the life span and is useful in a variety of settings (Pender, 1996; Pender, Murdaugh, & Parsons, 2002). The model applies the formation of community partnerships with its consideration of the environmental context and extends to global health promotion (Pender, Murdaugh, & Parsons, 2010).

Clinical interest in health behaviors represents a philosophical shift that emphasizes quality of lives alongside the saving of lives. In addition, there are financial, human, and environmental burdens upon society when individuals do not engage in prevention and health promotion. The health promotion model contributes a nursing solution to health policy and health care reform by providing a means for understanding how consumers can be motivated to attain personal health. The utility of the model in nursing practice is illustrated by Valek, Greenwald, and Lewis (2016), who applied the health promotion model to develop an intervention for practitioners to monitor psychological factors associated with the maintenance of weight loss in patients.

Education

The health promotion model is used widely in graduate education and increasingly in undergraduate nursing education in the United States (Pender, personal communication, May 24, 2000). In the past, health promotion was placed behind illness care, because clinical education was conducted primarily in acute care settings (Pender et al., 1992). Increasingly, the health promotion model is incorporated in nursing curricula as an aspect of health assessment, community health nursing, and wellness-focused courses (N. Pender, personal communication, May 24, 2000). Growing international efforts across a number of countries are working to integrate the health promotion model into nursing curricula (Pender, personal communication, May 6, 2004; Pender, Murdaugh, & Parsons, 2002).

Research

The health promotion model is a tool for research. Pender's research agenda and that of other researchers have tested and report the empirical precision of the model. The Health Promoting Lifestyle Profile, derived from the model, serves as the operational definition for health-promoting behaviors. Drawing upon the Health Promoting Lifestyle Profile, the Adolescent Lifestyle Profile demonstrates the adaptability of the health promotion model to the life span (Hendricks, Murdaugh, & Pender, 2006). The health promotion model has applications emphasizing the importance of the assessment of factors believed to influence health behavior changes Wilk and colleagues (2013) studied the sweat patterns among pubertal girls during exercise and Bryer, Cherkis, and Raman (2013) conducted a survey of health behaviors of undergraduate nursing students. Further research is indicated to examine the environmental context and expand its application to include global health-promotion strategies.

FURTHER DEVELOPMENT

The model continues to be refined (Pender, Murdaugh, & Parsons, 2010) and tested for its power to explain the relationships among factors believed to influence changes in a wide array of health behaviors. Sufficient empirical support for model variables now exists for some behaviors to warrant design and conduct of intervention studies to test model-based nursing interventions.

Lusk and colleagues (Lusk, Hong, et al., 1999; Lusk, Kwee, et al., 1999) used important predictors of construction workers' use of hearing protection from the health promotion model (self-efficacy, barriers, interpersonal influences, and situational influences) to develop an interactive, video-based program to increase use. This large, multiple-site study found that the intervention increased the use of worker hearing protection by 20% compared with the group without intervention—a statistically significant improvement from baseline (Lusk, Hong, et al., 1999). Intervention studies such as those by Wilk and colleagues (2013) and Padden and colleagues (2013) and practice applications like that of Valik and colleagues (2016) represent the use of the model to build and use nursing science. Finally, there have been many dissertations in recent years (see the dissertation list in the bibliography) based on Pender's work.

CRITIQUE

Clarity

The conceptual definitions provide clarity and lead to greater understanding of the complexity of health behavior phenomena. Visual diagrams illustrate the relationships clearly (see Fig. 21.2).

Simplicity

The health promotion model is easy to understand. The factors in each set are linked logically, and the relationships are clarified in the theoretical assertions. The sets of factors, which are direct or indirect influences, are clear in visual diagrams that display their associations. Factors are seen as independent, but the sets have an interactive effect that results in action.

Generality

The model is middle range in scope. It is highly generalizable to adult populations. The research used to derive the model was based on male, female, young, old, well, and ill samples. The research agenda includes application in a variety of settings. A research program tested the applicability of the model to children 10 to 16 years of age (Robbins et al., 2006). Cultural and diversity considerations support model testing in diverse populations.

Accessibility

Pender and others have supported the model through empirical testing as a framework for explaining health promotion. The Health Promoting Lifestyle Profile is an instrument used to assess health-promoting behaviors (Pender, Murdaugh, & Parsons, 2006). The model continues to evolve through planned programs of research. Continued empirical research, especially intervention studies, further refine the model. Research foci continue upon evidence-based and effective health promotion strategies that serve the individual within the context of the community (Pender, Murdaugh, & Parsons, 2010).

Importance

Pender identified health promotion as a goal for the 21st century, just as disease prevention was a task of the 20th century. The model describes the interaction between the nurse and the consumer while considering the role of environment in health promotion (Pender, Murdaugh, & Parsons, 2010). Pender responded to the political, social, and personal environment of her time to clarify nursing's role in delivering health promotion services to persons of all ages. The model fosters thinking about future opportunities and influences the use of technological advances such as the electronic health record as a means to achieve prevention and health promotion (Pender, Murdaugh, & Parsons, 2010).

SUMMARY

The movement to greater responsibility and accountability for successful personal health practices requires the support of the nursing profession through development of evidence-based practice. The health promotion model evolved from a substantive research program and continues to provide direction for better health practices. The model guides further research in various populations. Pender's visionary leadership continues to influence health promotion–related education, research, and policy.

CASE STUDY

Thomas, a 26-year-old graduate student of Cuban descent, comes to the college health clinic to discuss his perceived weight problem. He tells you that he wants a more business-like look and wants to have more energy. He says that he is tired of having his belly fall over his belt. In your physical assessment, you find that Thomas is 5 feet 11 inches, weighs 260 pounds, and has mild hypertension (132/90 mm Hg). His mother has a history of diabetes mellitus, and he tells you that high blood pressure runs in the family. His 64-year-old father had a heart attack 1 year ago. His electrocardiogram demonstrates normal sinus rhythm. He does not smoke. He says that his stress level is high, because he is working on his master's thesis. Thomas leaves to have some screening blood work and makes an appointment to see you next week. You begin some preliminary planning.

Analysis of this case study follows to illustrate the critical thinking process with the health promotion model for care of Thomas:

1. What online state-of-the-science resources might you use to help you in planning disease prevention and health promotion?
   - The Agency for Healthcare Research and Quality provides a "Guide to Clinical Preventive Services," which lists the latest available recommendations on preventive interventions: screening tests, counseling, immunizations, and medication regimens for more than 80 conditions. Age-specific periodic screenings based on gender and individual risk factors are available from the website (http://www.ahrq.gov/clinic/uspstfix.htm). The consumer section offers downloadable files.
   - *Healthy People 2020* includes a comprehensive set of disease prevention and health promotion objectives developed to improve the health of all people in the United States during the first decade of the 21st century (http://www.healthypeople.gov).
   - The U.S. Department of Health and Human Services website contains information about safety and wellness and more (http://www.hhs.gov). Pertinent information can be found under the category of Prevention.
2. What were some of the emotional and behavioral cues provided that suggest Thomas is ready for a weight loss management plan?
   - Thomas demonstrated self-direction, because he came to the clinic on his own.
   - He told you that he wants a more business-like look and wants to have more energy.
   - He stated that he is tired of having his belly fall over his belt.
   - He stated that his stress level is high.
3. In establishing a behavior change plan with Thomas, what are some interpersonal facilitators and potential barriers to change?
   - *Facilitators* include self-direction, motivation by family medical history, and desire for change.
   - *Potential barriers* include the fact that graduate students may have limited financial resources; stress level is high; and Thomas may believe he

Continued

CASE STUDY—cont'd

has limited time for physical activity, possibly using eating as a coping mechanism. (Additional assessment is indicated to validate barriers.)

4. List some alternatives in the behavior change plan that you will discuss with Thomas at your next meeting. In general, discuss diet, physical activity, and stress management.
   - Complete a behavioral contract as a commitment to a plan of action. In the plan, establish a long-term weight loss goal and short-term progress goals.
   - Review kinds of foods he enjoys, and assess dietary concerns, if any.
   - Discuss ways to increase physical activity and which of the activities he intends to carry out, and establish a calendar.
   - Provide a referral to the campus physical activity trainer.
   - Discuss stress management.
   - Establish follow-up.
   - Schedule weight checks every week.
   - Begin reward-reinforcement planning.

CRITICAL THINKING ACTIVITIES

1. Choose one health-promoting behavior in which you personally could but don't engage. Identify factors, as defined in the health promotion model, which contribute to your decision not to participate. Include immediate competing alternatives.
2. Analyze factors that contribute to your participation in a health-promoting activity and place each factor under the appropriate label from the health promotion model.
3. Consider your own philosophy of health and prepare your description of wellness. Is absence of disease more prominent than positive, active statements of health?
4. Anticipate the health-promoting behaviors important at various stages of development across the life span. What health promotion topics do you include in your practice?

POINTS FOR FURTHER STUDY

- Pender, N. J. (1986, Oct.). *Enhancing wellness through nursing research* (Videotape). Recorded at the Nursing Conference, October 16–17, Memphis, TN. Available through University of Tennessee, Memphis, School of Nursing.
- Pender, N. J. (1989, May). *Expressing health through beliefs and actions* (Videotape). Recorded live at Discovery International, Inc., Nurse Theorist Conference, May 11–12, Pittsburgh. Available through Meetings International, Louisville, KY.
- Pender, N. J. (2008). *Portraits of excellence: The nurse theorists*, vol. 2. Athens, Ohio: Fitne, Inc.

REFERENCES

Bandura, A. (1977). Self-efficacy: Toward a unifying theory of behavioral change. *Psychology Review, 84*(2), 191–215.

Becker, M. H. (1974). *The health belief model and personal behavior*. Thorofare, NJ: Charles B. Slack.

Bryer, J., Cherkis, F., & Raman, J. (2013). Health-promotion behaviors of undergraduate nursing students: A survey analysis. *Nursing Education Perspectives, 34*(6), 410–415.

Dunn, H. L. (1961). *High-level wellness*. Arlington, VA: Beatty.

Feather, N. T. (1982). *Expectations and actions: Expectancy-value models in psychology*. Hillsdale, NJ: Lawrence Erlbaum Associates.

Hendricks, C., Murdaugh, C., & Pender, N. (2006). The adolescent lifestyle profile: Development and psychometric characteristics. *Journal of National Black Nurses Association, 17*(1), 1–5.

Lusk, S. L., Hong, O. S., Ronis, S. L., Eakin, B. L., Kerr, M. J., & Early, M. R. (1999). Effectiveness of an intervention to increase construction worker's use of hearing protection. *Human Factors, 41*(3), 487–494.

Lusk, S. L., Kwee, M. J., Ronis, D. L., & Eakin, B. L. (1999). Applying the health promotion model to development of a worksite intervention. *American Journal of Health Promotion, 13*(4), 219–226.

Padden, D. L., Connors, R. A., Posey, S. M., Ricciardi, R., & Agazio, J. G. (2013). Factors influencing a health promoting lifestyle in spouses of active duty military. *Health Care for Women International, 34*(8), 674–693.

Pender, N. J. (1970). A developmental study of conceptual, semantic differential, and acoustical dimensions as encoding categories in short-term memory (Doctoral dissertation, Northwestern University). *Dissertation Abstracts International, A, 30*(10), 4283.

Pender, N. J. (1975). A conceptual model for preventive health behavior. *Nursing Outlook, 23*(6), 385–390.

Pender, N. J. (1982). *Health promotion in nursing practice.* New York: Appleton-Century-Crofts.
Pender, N. J. (1987). *Health promotion in nursing practice* (2nd ed.). New York: Appleton & Lange.
Pender, N. J. (1996). *Health promotion in nursing practice* (3rd ed.). Stamford, CT: Appleton & Lange.
Pender, N. J. (1997a). *Health promotion in nursing practice* (3rd ed.). Stamford, CT: Appleton & Lange. [Japanese translation].
Pender, N. J. (1997b). *Health promotion in nursing practice* (3rd ed.). Stamford, CT: Appleton & Lange. [Korean translation].
Pender, N. J. (n.d.). *Faculty-Staff profile, University of Michigan School of Nursing.* Retrieved from http://nursing.umich.edu/faculty-staff/nola-j-pender.
Pender, N. J., Baraukas, V. H., Hayman, L., Rice, V. H., & Anderson, E. T. (1992). Health promotion and disease prevention: Toward excellence in nursing practice and education. *Nursing Outlook, 40*(3), 106–120.
Pender, N. J., Murdaugh, C. L., & Parsons, M. A. (2002). *Health promotion in nursing practice* (4th ed.). Upper Saddle River, NJ: Prentice-Hall.
Pender, N. J., Murdaugh, C. L., & Parsons, M. A. (2006). *Health promotion in nursing practice* (5th ed.). Upper Saddle River, NJ: Pearson/Prentice-Hall.
Pender, N. J., Murdaugh, C. L., & Parsons, M. A. (2010). *Health promotion in nursing practice* (6th ed.). Upper Saddle River, NJ: Pearson.
Pender, N. J., Walker, S. N., Sechrist, K. R., & Stromborg, M. F. (1988). Development and testing of the health promotion model. *Cardiovascular Nursing, 24*(6), 41–43.
Robbins, L. B., Gretebeck, K. A., Kazanis, A. S., & Pender, N. J. (2006). Girls on the Move program to increase physical activity participation. *Nursing Research, 55*(3), 206–216.
Sechrist, K. R., Walker, S. N., & Pender, N. J. (1987). Development and psychometric evaluation of the exercise/barriers scale. *Research in Nursing and Health, 10,* 357–365.
Valek, R. M., Greenwald, B. J., & Lewis, C. C. (2016). Psychological factors associated with weight loss maintenance. *Nursing Science Quarterly, 28*(2), 129–135.
Walker, S. N., Sechrist, K. R., & Pender, N. J. (1987). The health-promoting lifestyle profile: Development and psychometric characteristics. *Nursing Research, 36*(2), 76–80.
Wilk, B., Pender, N., Volterman, K., Bar-Or, O., & Timmons, B. W. (2013). Influence of pubertal stage on local sweating patterns of girls exercising in the heat. *Pediatric Exercise Science, 25*(2), 212–220.

BIBLIOGRAPHY

Primary Sources

Books

Pender, N. J. (1982). *Health promotion in nursing practice.* New York: Appleton-Century-Crofts.
Pender, N. J. (1987). *Health promotion in nursing practice* (2nd ed.). New York: Appleton & Lange.
Pender, N. J. (1996). *Health promotion in nursing practice* (3rd ed.). Stamford, CT: Appleton & Lange.
Pender, N. J., Murdaugh, C. L., & Parsons, M. A. (2002). *Health promotion in nursing practice* (4th ed.). Upper Saddle River, NJ: Prentice Hall.
Pender, N. J., Murdaugh, C. L., & Parsons, M. A. (2006). *Health promotion in nursing practice* (5th ed.). Upper Saddle River, NJ: Pearson/Prentice Hall.
Pender, N. J., Murdaugh, C. L., & Parsons, M. A. (2010). *Health promotion in nursing practice* (6th ed.). Upper Saddle River, NJ: Pearson.

Book Chapters

Pender, N. J. (1984). Health promotion and illness prevention. In H. Werley & J. Fitzpatrick (Eds.), *Annual review of nursing research* (pp. 83–105). New York: Springer.
Pender, N. J. (1985). Self modification. In G. Bulechek & J. McCloskey (Eds.), *Interventions: Treatments for nursing diagnosis* (pp. 80–91). Philadelphia: Saunders.
Pender, N. J. (1986). Health promotion: Implementing strategies. In B. Logan & C. Dawkins (Eds.), *Family-centered nursing in the community* (pp. 295–334). Menlo Park, CA: Addison-Wesley.
Pender, N. J. (1987). Health and health promotion: The conceptual dilemmas. In M. E. Duffy & N. J. Pender (Eds.), *Conceptual issues in health promotion: Report of proceedings of a wingspread conference* (pp. 7–23). Indianapolis: Sigma Theta Tau International.
Pender, N. J. (1989). Languaging a health perspective for NANDA taxonomy on research and theory. In R. M. Carroll-Johnson (Ed.), *Classification of nursing diagnoses* (pp. 31–36). Philadelphia: Lippincott.
Pender, N. J. (1989). The pursuit of happiness, stress, and health. In S. Wald (Ed.), *Community health nursing: Issues and topics* (pp. 145–175). Englewood Cliffs, NJ: Prentice-Hall.
Pender, N. J. (1998). Motivation for physical activity among children and adolescents. In J. Fitzpatrick & J. S. Stevenson (Eds.), *Annual review of nursing research,* vol. 16 (pp. 139–172). New York: Springer.
Pender, N. J. (2004). Health promotion interventions for culturally diverse populations: Can we meet the challenge? In W. Kunaviktikul (Ed.), *Improving life through health promotion: Nurses making a difference* (pp. 11–26). Chaing Mai, Thailand: Chotana Press.
Pender, N. J. (2005). A global agenda for health promotion. In W. Kunaviktikul (Ed.), *Toward success in health promotion* (pp. 11–23). Chaing Mai, Thailand: Chotana Press.
Pender, N. J., & Pender, A. R. (1989). Attitudes, subjective norms, and intentions to engage in health behaviors. In C. A. Tanner (Ed.), *Using nursing research* (NLN Pub. No. 15–2232, pp. 466–472). New York: National League for Nursing.
Pender, N. J., & Sallis, J. (1995). Exercise counseling by health professionals. In R. Dishman (Ed.), *Exercise adherence* (2nd ed.) (pp. 213–235). Champaign, IL: Human Kinetics.
Pender, N. J., Sallis, J., Long, B. J., Calfas, K. J. (1994). Health care provider counseling to promote physical activity. In R. K. Dishman (Ed.), *Advances in exercise adherence* (pp. 213–235). Champaign, IL: Human Kinetics.
Pender, N. J., & Stein, K. F. (2002). Social support, the self system and adolescent health and health behaviors. In L. L. Hayman,

M. M. Mahon, & J. R. Turner (Eds.), *Health behavior in childhood and adolescence* (pp. 37–66). New York: Springer.

Journal Articles

Berg, A. O., Allan, J. D., Frame, P. S., Homer, C. J., Johnson, M. S., Klein, J. D., et al. (2002). Newborn hearing screening: Recommendations and rationale. *American Journal of Nursing, 102*(11), 83–89.

Berg, A. O., Allan, J. D., Frame, P. S., Homer, C. J., Lieu, T. A., Mulrow, C. D., et al; U S Preventive Services Task Force. (2002). Screening for chlamydia infection: Recommendations and rationale. U.S. Preventive Services Task Force. *American Journal of Nursing, 102*(10), 87–92; discussion 93.

Eden, K. B., Orleans, C. T., Mulrow, C. D., Pender, N. J., & Teutsch, S. M. (2002). Does counseling by clinicians improve physical activity? A summary of the evidence for the U. S. Preventive Services Task Force. *Annals of Internal Medicine, 137*(3), E208–E215.

Frank-Stromborg, M., Pender, N. J., Walker, S. N., & Sechrist, K. R. (1990). Determinants of health-promoting lifestyle in ambulatory cancer patients. *Social Science and Medicine, 31*(10), 1159–1168.

Garcia, A. W., Broda, M. A. N., Frenn, M., Coviak, C., Pender, N. J., & Ronis, D. L. (1995). Gender and developmental differences in exercise beliefs among youth and prediction of their exercise behavior. *Journal of School Health, 65*(6), 213–219.

Garcia, A. W., Broda, M. A. N., Frenn, M., Coviak, C., Pender, N. J., & Ronis, D. L. (1997). Gender differences: Exercise beliefs among youth. *Reflections, 23*(1), 21–22.

Garcia, A. W., Pender, N. J., Antonakos, C. L., & Ronis, D. L. (1998). Changes in physical activity beliefs and behaviors of boys and girls across the transition to junior high school. *Journal of Adolescent Health, 5*, 394–402.

Hendricks, C., Murdaugh, C., & Pender, N. (2006). The adolescent lifestyle profile: Development and psychometric characteristics. *Journal of National Black Nurses Association, 17*(2), 1–5.

Pender, N. J. (1975). A conceptual model for preventive health behavior. *Nursing Outlook, 23*(6), 385–390.

Pender, N. J. (1984). Physiologic responses of clients with essential hypertension to progressive muscle relaxation training. *Research in Nursing and Health, 7*, 197–203.

Pender, N. J. (1985). Effects of progressive muscle relaxation training on anxiety and health locus of control among hypertensive adults. *Research in Nursing and Health, 8*, 67–72.

Pender, N. J. (1988). Research agenda: Identifying research ideas and priorities. *American Journal of Health Promotion, 2*(4), 42–51.

Pender, N. J. (1988). Research agenda: The influences of health policy on an evolving research agenda. *American Journal of Health Promotion, 2*(3), 51–54.

Pender, N. J. (1989). Health promotion in the workplace: Suggested directions for research. *American Journal of Health Promotion, 3*(3), 38–43.

Pender, N. J. (1990). Expressing health through lifestyle patterns. *Nursing Science Quarterly, 3*(3), 115–122.

Pender, N. J. (1990). Research agenda: A revised research agenda model. *American Journal of Health Promotion, 4*(3), 220–222.

Pender, N. J. (1992). Making a difference in health policy. *Nursing Outlook, 40*(3), 104–105.

Pender, N. J. (1992). The NIH strategic plan: How will it affect the future of nursing science and practice? *Nursing Outlook, 40*(2), 55–56.

Pender, N. J. (1992). Reforming health care: Future direction. *Nursing Outlook, 40*(1), 8–9.

Pender, N. J. (1993). Creating change through partnerships. *Nursing Outlook, 41*(1), 8–9.

Pender, N. J. (1993). Health care reform: One view of the future. *Nursing Outlook, 41*(2), 56–57.

Pender, N. J. (1993). Reaching out. *Nursing Outlook, 41*(3), 103–104.

Pender, N. J., Barkaukas, V. H., Hayman, L., Rice, V. H., & Anderson, E. T. (1992). Health promotion and disease prevention: Toward excellence in nursing practice and education. *Nursing Outlook, 40*(3), 106–112, 120.

Pender, N. J., Bar-Or, O., Wilk, B., & Mitchell, S. (2002). Self-efficacy and perceived exertion of girls during exercise. *Nursing Research, 51*(2), 86–91.

Pender, N. J., & Pender, A. R. (1980). Illness prevention and health promotion services provided by nurse practitioners: Predicting potential consumers. *American Journal of Public Health, 70*(8), 798–803.

Pender, N. J., & Pender, A. R. (1986). Attitudes, subjective norms, and intentions to engage in health behaviors. *Nursing Research, 35*(1), 15–18.

Pender, N. J., Sechrist, K. R., Stromborg, M., & Walker, S. N. (1987). Collaboration in developing a research program grant. *Image: The Journal of Nursing Scholarship, 19*(2), 75–77.

Pignone, M. P., Ammerman, A., Fernandez, L., Orleans, C. T., Pender, N., Woolf, S., et al. (2003). Counseling to promote a healthy diet in adults: A summary of the evidence for the U.S. Preventive Services Task Force. *American Journal of Preventive Medicine, 24*(1), 75–92.

Robbins, L. B., Gretebeck, K. A., Kazanis, A. S., & Pender, N. J. (2006). Girls on the Move program to increase physical activity participation. *Nursing Research, 55*(3), 206–216.

Robbins, L. B., Pender, N. J., Conn, V. S., Frenn, M. D., Neuberger, G. B., Nies, M. A., et al. (2001). Physical activity research in nursing. *Journal of Nursing Scholarship, 33*(4), 315–321.

Robbins, L. B., Pender, N. J., & Kazanis, A. S. (2003). Barriers to physical activity perceived by adolescent girls. *Journal of Midwifery & Women's Health, 48*(3), 206–212.

Robbins, L. B., Pender, N. J., Ronis, D. L., Kazanis, A. S., & Pis, M. B. (2004). Physical activity, self-efficacy, and perceived exertion among adolescents. *Research in Nursing & Health, 27*(6), 435–446.

Robbins, L. B., Pis, M. B., Pender, N. J., & Kazanis, A. S. (2004). Exercise self-efficacy, enjoyment, and feeling states among adolescents. *Western Journal of Nursing Research, 26*(7), 699–715; discussion 716–621.

Robbins, L. B., Pis, M. B., Pender, N. J., & Kazanis, A. S. (2004). Physical activity self-definition among adolescents. *Research & Theory for Nursing Practice, 18*(4), 317–330.

Walker, S. N., Kerr, M. J., Pender, N. J., & Sechrist, K. R. (1990). A Spanish language version of the health promoting lifestyle profile. *Nursing Research, 39*(5), 268–273.

Whitlock, E. P., Orleans, C. T., Pender, N., & Allan, J. (2002). Evaluating primary care behavioral counseling interventions: An evidence-based approach. *American Journal of Preventive Medicine, 22*(4), 267–284.

Wu, T. Y., & Pender, N. (2002). Determinants of physical activity among Taiwanese adolescents: An application of the health promotional model. *Research in Nursing & Health, 25*(1), 25–36.

Wu, T. Y., Pender, N., & Yang, K. P. (2002). Promoting physical activity among Taiwanese and American adolescents. *Journal of Nursing Research, 10*(1), 57–64.

Wu, T. Y., Ronis, D. L., Pender, N., & Jwo, J. (2002). Development of questionnaires to measure physical activity cognitions among Taiwanese adolescents. *Preventive Medicine, 35*(1), 54–64.

Secondary Sources

Dissertations

Alatrash, M. H. (2015). *Behaviors and views of three Arab American women subgroups regarding breast cancer screening: A comparative study. ProQuest Dissertations & Theses Global.* (UMI No. 3727060).

Anderson, J. K. (2008). *Predictors of health promoting behaviors and health-related quality of life in post myocardial infarction adults.* Doctoral dissertation. Retrieved from *ProQuest Dissertations & Theses A&I* database. (UMI No. 304324280).

Baker, O. G. (2003). *Relationship of parental tobacco use, peer influence, self-esteem, and tobacco use among Yemeni American adolescents: Mid-range theory testing. Dissertation Abstracts International, 64–03B,* 1175. (University Microfilms No. AAT3086416.)

Browning, G. A. (2011). *Health promotion and the older rural adult.* Retrieved from *ProQuest Dissertations & Theses Global.* (No. 3498672).

Costanzo, C. (2005). *Physical activity counseling intervention for women age 50–75 within the community.* University of Nebraska Medical Center. Retrieved from *ProQuest Digital Dissertations* database. (Publication No. AAT: 3165167).

Cyphers, N. A. (2015). *The relationship between religiosity and health-promoting behaviors of pregnant women at pregnancy resource centers.* Retrieved from *ProQuest Dissertations & Theses Global.* (UMI No. 3724837.)

Davis, L. (2013). *The effects of cardiovascular education on knowledge and perceptions of self-efficacy to implement behavior change among African Americans in a church setting.* Retrieved from *ProQuest Dissertations & Theses Global.* (UMI No. 3568213.)

DouchandBrown, S. E. (2009). *Health promotion behaviors among African American women.* Doctoral dissertation. Retrieved from *ProQuest Dissertations & Theses A&I* . (UMI No. 304929507.)

Easom, L. R. (2003). *Determinants of participation in health promotion activities in rural elderly caregivers. Dissertation Abstracts International, 64–02B,* 636. (University Microfilms No. AAT3081342.)

Edmonds, J. C. (2006). *The relationship of weight, body image, self-efficacy, and stress to health-promoting behaviors: A study of college educated African American women.* The Catholic University of America, Washington, D.C. Retrieved from *ProQuest Digital Dissertations* database. (Publication No. AAT 3214670.)

Espelin, J. M. (2010). *Substance abuse education for undergraduate nursing students: A target approach to program evaluations.* Doctoral Nursing Practice Thesis. Retrieved from *ProQuest Dissertations & Theses A&I.* (UMI No. 759116956.)

Gabry, H. (2005). *Understanding the relationship between health behavior during pregnancy and health locus of control among Arab and non-Arab women to reduce high risk pregnancy.* George Mason University, Washington, D.C. Retrieved from *ProQuest Digital Dissertations.* (Publication No. AAT 3167540.)

Gautam, B. (2011). *Factors predicting exercise behavior of graduate students.* Doctoral dissertation. *ProQuest Dissertations & Theses A&I* database. (UMI No. 3497803.)

Grund, F. J. (2013). *Predictors of health promoting lifestyles in baccalaureate nursing students. ProQuest Dissertations & Theses Global.* (UMI No. 3588289).

Hagerstrom, G. (2010). *Personal factors, perceptions, influences and their relationship with adherence behaviors in patients with diabetes.* Doctoral dissertation. Retrieved from *ProQuest Dissertations & Theses A&I* database. (UMI No. 3442416).

Haus, C. S. (2003). *Medication management strategies used by community-dwelling older adults living alone. Dissertation Abstracts International, 64–07B,* 3188. (University Microfilms No. AAT3097641.)

Hubbard, A. B. (2002). *The impact of curriculum design on health promoting behaviors at a community college in south Florida. Dissertation Abstracts International, 63–06,* 2112.

Hung, S. L. (2009). *The relationship of lifestyle behavior and occupational characteristics to selected health problems among truck drivers in Taiwan.* Doctoral dissertation. Retrieved from *ProQuest Dissertations & Theses A&I* database. (UMI No. 3383206.)

Jadalla, A. A. (2007). *Acculturation, health, and health behaviors of adult Arab Americans.* Loma Linda University, California. Retrieved from *ProQuest Digital Dissertations.* (Publication No. AAT 3282707.)

Kalampakorn, S. (2000). *Stages of construction workers' use of hearing protection. Dissertation Abstracts International, 61–07B,* 3508.

Keegan, J. P. (2011). *Predictive ability of Pender's Health Promotion Model for physical activity and exercise participation for people with spinal cord injury: A hierarchical regression analysis.* Doctoral dissertation. Retrieved from *ProQuest Dissertations & Theses A&I* database. (UMI No. 3488940.)

Khalil, K. (2014). *Factors affecting health promotion lifestyle behaviors among Arab American women.* Retrieved from *ProQuest Dissertations & Theses Global.* (UMI No. 3580965.)

Luther, C. H. (2003). *Living the coming of osteoporosis: Health promotion behaviors of women at risk for osteoporosis in Mississippi. Dissertation Abstracts International, 64–08B,* 3746. (University Microfilms No. AAT3101544.)

Nodine, P. M. (2011). *The contribution of physical activity to sleep parameters in pregnancy within the context of prepregnant body mass index.* Doctoral dissertation. Retrieved from *ProQuest Dissertations & Theses A&I* database. (UMI No. 3467224.)

Pichayapinyo, P. (2005). *The relationship of perceived benefits, perceived barriers, social support, and sense of mastery on adequacy of prenatal care for first-time Thai mothers.* The Catholic University of America, Washington, D.C. Retrieved from *ProQuest Digital Dissertations.* (Publication No. AAT 3169867.)

Politsky, S. (2013). *Relationships among self-care behaviors and professional quality of life in oncology nurses.* Retrieved from *ProQuest Dissertations & Theses.* (UMI No. 3579580.)

Polsingchan, S. (2010). *Health-promoting behaviors in Thai persons with chronic renal failure.* Doctoral dissertation. Retrieved from *ProQuest Dissertations & Theses A&I* database. (UMI No. 3446004.)

Putnam, K. F. (2008). *The relationship of inner strength and health promoting behaviors and their effect on quality of life in midlife women.* Retrieved from *ProQuest Dissertations & Theses Global.* (UMI No. 3345133.)

Sakraida, T. J. (2002). *Divorce transition, coping responses, and health promoting behavior of midlife women. Dissertation Abstracts International, 62–12B*, 5646. (University Microfilms No. AAT3037817.)

Sapp, C. J. (2003). *Adolescents with asthma: Effects of personal characteristics and health-promoting lifestyle behaviors on health-related quality of life. Dissertation Abstracts International, 64–05B*, 2131. (University Microfilms No. AAT3092071.)

Vitztum, C. M. (2015). *Physical activity in adolescents with orthopedic limitations: The use of human-animal interaction in the form of dog-walking.* Retrieved from *ProQuest Dissertations & Theses Global.* (UMI No. 3741545)

Warner, K. D. (2000). *Health-related lifestyle behaviors of twins: Interpersonal and situational influences. Dissertation Abstracts International, 61–03B*, 1331.

Zamora, R. I. (2015). *Fall risks in an inpatient gero-psychiatric unit: Can they be predicted?* Retrieved from *ProQuest Dissertations & Theses Global.* (UMI No. 3663265.)

Journal Articles

Agazio, J. G., Ephraim, P. M., Flaherty, N. B., & Gurney, C. A. (2002). Health promotion in active-duty military women with children. *Women Health, 35*(1), 65–82.

Alaviani, M., Khosravan, S., Alami, A., & Moshki, M. (2015). The effect of a multi-strategy program on developing social behaviors based on Pender's Health Promotion Model to prevent loneliness of old women referred to Gonabad urban health centers. *International Journal of Community Based Nursing & Midwifery, 3*(2), 132–140.

Alkhalaileh, M. A., Khaled, M. H. B., Baker, O. G., & Bond, E. A. (2011). Pender's health promotion model: An integrative literature review. *Middle East Journal of Nursing, 5*(5), 12–22.

Callaghan, D. (2005). Healthy behaviors, self-efficacy, self-care, and basic conditioning factors in older adults. *Journal of Community Health Nursing, 22*(3), 169–178.

Callaghan, D. (2006). Basic conditioning factors' influences on adolescents' healthy behaviors, self-efficacy, and self-care. *Issues in Comprehensive Pediatric Nursing, 29*(4), 191–204.

Callaghan, D. (2006). The influence of basic conditioning factors on healthy behaviors, self-efficacy, and self-care in adults. *Journal of Holistic Nursing, 24*(3), 178–185.

Callaghan, D. M. (2005). The influence of spiritual growth on adolescents' initiative and responsibility for self-care. *Pediatric Nursing, 31*(2), 91–95.

Calvert, W. J., & Bucholz, K. K. (2008). Adolescent risky behaviors and alcohol use. *Western Journal of Nursing Research, 30*(1), 147–148.

Campbell, M., & Torrance, C. (2005). Coronary angioplasty: Impact on risk factors and patients' understanding of the severity of their condition. *Australian Journal of Advanced Nursing, 22*(4), 26–31.

Canaval, G. E., & Sãnchez, M. A. N. (2011). Lifestyle and cancer prevention in female employees at a health institution. *Colombia Medica, 42*(2), 177–183.

Chen, C., Kuo, S., Chou, Y., & Chen, H. (2007). Postpartum Taiwanese women: Their postpartum depression, social support and health-promoting lifestyle profiles. *Journal of Clinical Nursing, 16*(8), 1550–1560.

Chen, M., James, K., Hsu, L., Chang, S., Huang, L., & Wang, E. K. (2005). Health-related behavior and adolescent mothers. *Public Health Nursing, 22*(4), 280–288.

Conway, A. E., McClune, A. J., & Nosel, P. (2007). Down on the farm: Preventing farm accidents in children. *Pediatric Nursing, 33*(1), 45–48.

Costanzo, C., Walker, S. N., Yates, B. C., McCabe, B., & Berg, K. (2006). Physical activity counseling for older women. *Western Journal of Nursing Research, 28*(7), 786–810.

Daggett, L. M., & Rigdon, K. L. (2006). A computer-assisted instructional program for teaching portion size versus serving size. *Journal of Community Health Nursing, 23*(1), 29–35.

Dehdari, T., Rahimi, T., Aryaeian, N., & Gohari, M. R. (2014). Effect of nutrition education intervention based on Pender's Health Promotion Model in improving the frequency and nutrient intake of breakfast consumption among female Iranian students. *Public Health Nutrition, 17*(3), 657–666.

Esperat, C., Feng, D., Zhang, Y., & Owen, D. (2007). Health behaviors of low-income pregnant minority women. *Western Journal of Nursing Research, 29*(3), 284–300.

Esposito, E. M., & Fitzpatrick, J. J. (2011). Registered nurses' beliefs of the benefits of exercise, their exercise behaviour and their patient teaching regarding exercise. *International Journal of Nursing Practice, 17*(4), 351–356.

Evio, B. D. (2005). The relationship between selected determinants of health behavior and lifestyle profile of older adults. *Philippine Journal of Nursing, 75*(1), 23–31.

Guarnero, P. A. (2006). Health promotion behaviors among a group of 18–29 year old gay and bisexual men. *Communicating Nursing Research, 39*, 298.

Guarnero, P. A. (2007). Staying healthy: How are young gay and bisexual men doing? *Communicating Nursing Research, 40*, 429.

Gusain, S. (2008). Nursing and self-motivation for elderly. *Nursing Journal of India, 99*(1), 5–7.

Hacihasanoğlu, R., & Gözüm, S. (2011). The effect of patient education and home monitoring on medication compliance, hypertension management, healthy lifestyle behaviours and bmi in a primary health care setting. *Journal of Clinical Nursing, 20*(5/6), 692–705.

Hageman, P. A., Walker, S. N., & Pullen, C. H. (2005). Tailored versus standard internet-delivered interventions to promote physical activity in older women. *Journal of Geriatric Physical Therapy, 28*(1), 28–33.

Hensley, R. D., Jones, A. K., Williams, A. G., Willsher, L. B., & Cain, P. P. (2005). One-year clinical outcomes for Louisiana residents diagnosed with type 2 diabetes and hypertension. *Journal of the American Academy of Nurse Practitioners, 17*(9), 363–369.

Ho, A. Y. K., Berggren, I., & Dahlborg-Lyckhage, E. (2010). Diabetes empowerment related to Pender's health promotion model: A meta-synthesis. *Nursing & Health Sciences, 12*(2), 259–267.

Holstein, P., & Berg, J. A. (2007). Premenstrual symptoms and academic stress in rural college women. *Communicating Nursing Research, 40*, 540.

Huang, T., & Dai, F. (2007). Weight retention predictors for Taiwanese women at six-month postpartum. *Journal of Nursing Research, 15*(1), 11–20.

Hui, W. H. (2002). The health-promoting lifestyles of undergraduate nurses in Hong Kong. *Journal of Professional Nursing, 18*(2), 101–111.

Johnson, R. L. (2005). Gender differences in health-promoting lifestyles of African Americans. *Public Health Nursing, 22*(2), 130–137.

Johnson, R. L., & Nies, M. A. (2005). A qualitative perspective of barriers to health-promoting behaviors of African Americans. *ABNF Journal, 16*(2), 39–41.

Kaewthummanukul, T., Brown, K. C., Weaver, M. T., & Thomas, R. R. (2006). Predictors of exercise participation in female hospital nurses. *Journal of Advanced Nursing, 54*(6), 663–675.

Lohse, J. L. (2003). A bicycle safety education program for parents of young children. *Journal of School Nursing, 19*(2), 100–110.

Lucas, J. A., Orshan, S. A., & Cook, F. (2000). Determinants of health-promoting behavior among women ages 65 and above living in the community. *Scholarly Inquiry for Nursing Practice, 14*(1), 77–100.

Maes, C., & Louis, M. (2007). Advanced nurse practitioners and sexual history taking practices among older adults. *Communicating Nursing Research, 40*, 464.

McCullagh, M., Lusk, S. L., & Ronis, D. L. (2002). Factors influencing use of hearing protection among farmers: A test of the Pender health promotion model. *Nursing Research, 51*(1), 33–39.

McDonald, P. E., Brennan, P. F., & Wykle, M. L. (2005). Perceived health status and health-promoting behaviors of African-American and white informal caregivers of impaired elders. *Journal of National Black Nurses' Association, 16*(1), 8–17.

McGrath, J. A., O'Malley, M., & Hendrix, T. J. (2011). Group exercise mode and health-related quality of life among healthy adults. *Journal of Advanced Nursing, 67*(3), 491–500.

McMurry, T. B. (2006). A comparison of pharmacological tobacco cessation relapse rates. *Journal of Community Health Nursing, 23*(1), 15–28.

Mendias, E. P., & Paar, D. P. (2007). Perceptions of health and self-care learning needs of outpatients with HIV/AIDS. *Journal of Community Health Nursing, 24*(1), 49–64.

Milne, J. L., & Moore, K. N. (2006). Factors impacting self-care for urinary incontinence. *Urologic Nursing, 26*(1), 41–51.

Montgomery, K. S. (2002). Health promotion with adolescents: Examining theoretical perspectives to guide research. *Research & Theory for Nursing Practice, 16*(2), 119–134.

Nies, M. A., & Motyka, C. L. (2006). Factors contributing to women's ability to maintain a walking program. *Journal of Holistic Nursing, 24*(1), 7–14.

Olson, A. F., & Berg, J. A. (2006). Theoretical foundations of promoting perimenopausal bone health. *Communicating Nursing Research, 39*, 279.

Piazza, J., Conrad, K., & Wilbur, J. (2001). Exercise behavior among female occupational health nurses. Influence of self-efficacy, perceived health control, and age. *AAOHN Journal, 49*(2), 79–86.

Ronis, D. L., Hong, O., & Lusk, S. L. (2006). Comparison of the original and revised structures of the health promotion model in predicting construction workers' use of hearing protection. *Research in Nursing & Health, 29*(1), 3–17.

Rothman, N. L., Lourie, R. J., Brian, D., & Foley, M. (2005). Temple Health Connection: A successful collaborative model of community-based primary health care. *Journal of Cultural Diversity, 12*(4), 145–151.

Sisk, R. J. (2000). Caregiver burden and health promotion. *International Journal of Nursing Studies, 37*(1), 37–43.

Smith, A. B., & Bashore, L. (2006). The effect of clinic-based health promotion education on perceived health status and health promotion behaviors of adolescent and young adult cancer survivors. *Journal of Pediatric Oncology Nursing, 23*(6), 326–334.

Smith, S. A., & Michel, Y. (2006). A pilot study on the effects of aquatic exercises on discomforts of pregnancy. *Journal of Obstetric, Gynecologic, and Neonatal Nursing, 35*(3), 315–323.

Srof, B. J., & Velsor-Friedrich, B. (2006). Health promotion in adolescents: A review of Pender's Health Promotion Model. *Nursing Science Quarterly, 19*(4), 366–373.

Stark, M. A., Chase, C., & DeYoung, A. (2010). Barriers to health promotion in community dwelling elders. *Journal of Community Health Nursing, 27*(4), 175–186 112p.

Walker, S. N., Pullen, C. H., Hertzog, M., Boeckner, L., & Hageman, P. A. (2006). Determinants of older rural women's activity and eating. *Western Journal of Nursing Research, 28*(4), 449–474.

Wilson, M. (2005). Health-promoting behaviors of sheltered homeless women. *Family & Community Health, 28*(1), 51–63.

International Journal Articles

Adeyemi, A. A., Jarad, F., Pender, N., & Higham, S. M. (2007). Assessing the efficacy of denture cleaners with quantitative light-induced fluorescence (QLF). *European Journal of Prosthodontics & Restorative Dentistry, 15*(4), 165–170.

Garcia, A. W., Broda, M. A., Frenn, M., Coviak, C., Pender, N. J., & Ronis, D. L. (1997). Gender and developmental differences in exercise beliefs among youth and prediction of their exercise behavior [Japanese translation]. *The Japanese Journal of Nursing Research, 30*(3), 51–61.

Kahawong, W., Phancharoenworakul, K., Khampalikit, S., Taboonpong, S., & Chittchang, U. (2005). Nutritional health-promoting behavior among women with hyperlipidemia. *Thai Journal of Nursing Research, 9*(2), 91–102.

Kemppainen, J., Bomar, P. J., Kikuchi, K., Kanematsu, Y., Ambo, H., & Noguchi, K. (2011). Health promotion behaviors of residents with hypertension in Iwate, Japan and North Carolina, USA. *Japan Journal of Nursing Science, 8*(1), 20–32.

Kerr, M. J., Lusk, S. L., & Ronis, D. L. (2002). Explaining Mexican American worker's hearing protection use with the health promotion model. *Nursing Research, 51*(2), 100–109.

Kerr, M. J., Savik, K., Monsen, K. A., & Lusk, S. L. (2007). Effectiveness of computer-based tailoring versus targeting to promote use of hearing protection. *Canadian Journal of Nursing Research, 39*(1), 80–97.

Mafutha, G. N., & Wright, S. C. D. (2013). Compliance or noncompliance of hypertensive adults to hypertension management at three primary healthcare day clinics in Tshwane. *Curationis, 36*(1), 1–6.

Meethien, N., Pothiban, L., Ostwald, S. K., Sucamvang, K., & Panuthai, S. (2011). Effectiveness of nutritional education in promoting healthy eating among elders in northeastern Thailand. *Pacific Rim International Journal of Nursing Research, 15*(3), 188–201.

Mete, S., Yenal, K., Tokat, M. A., & Serçekus, P. (2012). Effects of vaginal douching education on Turkish women's vaginal douching practice. *Research & Theory for Nursing Practice, 26*(1), 41–53.

Mohamadian, H., Eftekhar, H., Rahimi, A., Mohamad, H. T., Shojaiezade, D., & Montazeri, A. (2011). Predicting health-related quality of life by using a health promotion model among Iranian adolescent girls: A structural equation modeling approach. *Nursing & Health Sciences, 13*(2), 141–148.

Morowatisharifabad, M. A., & Shirazi, K. K. (2007). Determinants of oral health behaviors among preuniversity (12th-grade) students in Yazd (Iran): An application of the health promotion model. *Family & Community Health, 30*(4), 342–350.

Phuphaibul, R., Leucha, Y., Putwattana, P., Nuntawan, C., Tapsart, C., Tachudhong, A., et al. (2005). Health promoting behaviors of Thai adolescents, family health related lifestyles and parent modeling. *Thai Journal of Nursing Research, 9*(1), 28–37.

Pichayapinyo, P., O'Brien, M. E., Duffy, J. R., & Agazio, J. (2007). The relationship of perceived benefits, perceived barriers, social support, and sense of mastery on adequacy of prenatal care for first-time Thai mothers. *Thai Journal of Nursing Research, 11*(2), 106–117.

Rezaei-Adaryani, M., & Rezaei-Adaryani, M. (2012). Health-promoting lifestyle of a group of Iranian medical, nursing and allied health students. *Journal of Clinical Nursing, 21*(23/24), 3587–3589.

Schlickau, J. M., & Wilson, M. E. (2005). Breastfeeding as health-promoting behaviour for Hispanic women: Literature review. *Journal of Advanced Nursing, 52*(2), 200–210.

Shin, K. R., Kang, Y., Park, H. J., Cho, M. O., & Heitkemper, M. (2008). Testing and developing the health promotion model in low-income, Korean elderly women. *Nursing Science Quarterly, 21*(2), 173–178.

Shin, Y., Jang, H., & Pender, N. J. (2001). Psychometric evaluation of the Exercise Self-Efficacy Scale among Korean adults with chronic diseases. *Research in Nursing & Health, 24*(1), 68–76.

Shin, Y., Pender, N. J., & Yun, S. (2003). Using methodological triangulation for cultural verification of commitment to a plan for exercise scale among Korean adults with chronic diseases. *Research in Nursing & Health, 26*(4), 312–321.

Shin, Y., Yun, S., Pender, N. J., & Jang, H. (2005). Test of the health promotion model as a causal model of commitment to a plan for exercise among Korean adults with chronic disease. *Research in Nursing & Health, 28*(2), 117–125.

Shin, Y. H., Hur, H. K., Pender, N. J., Jang, H. J., & Kim, M. (2006). Exercise self-efficacy, exercise benefits and barriers, and commitment to a plan for exercise among Korean women with osteoporosis and osteoarthritis. *International Journal of Nursing Studies, 43*(1), 3–10.

Vakili, M., Rahaei, Z., Nadrian, H., & YarMohammadi, P. (2011). Determinants of oral health behaviors among high school students in Shahrekord, Iran based on Health Promotion Model. *Journal of Dental Hygiene, 85*(1), 39–48.

Victor, J. F., de Oliveira Lopes, M. V., & Ximenes, L. B. (2005). Analysis of diagram the health promotion model of Nola J. Pender [Portuguese]. *ACTA Paulista de Enfermagem, 18*(3), 235–240.

Wang, H. H. (2001). A comparison of two models of health-promoting lifestyle in rural elderly Taiwanese women. *Public Health Nursing, 18*(3), 204–211.

Wang, W., Wang, C., Tung, Y., & Peng, J. (2007). Factors influencing adolescent second-hand smoke avoidance behavior from the perspective of Pender's health promotion model [Chinese]. *Journal of Evidence-Based Nursing, 3*(4), 280–288.

Waring, D. T., Pender, N., & Counihan, D. (2005). Mandibular arch changes following nonextraction treatment. *Australian Orthodontic Journal, 21*(2), 111–116.

Wu, T. Y., & Pender, N. (2005). A panel study of physical activity in Taiwanese youth: Testing the revised health-promotion model. *Family & Community Health, 28*(2), 113–124.

Wu, T. Y., Pender, N., & Noureddine, S. (2003). Gender differences in the psychosocial and cognitive correlates of physical activity among Taiwanese adolescents: A structural equation modeling approach. *International Journal of Behavioral Medicine, 10*(2), 93–105.

Yang, K., Laffrey, S. C., Stuifbergen, A., Im, E., May, K., & Kouzekanani, K. (2007). Leisure-time physical activity among midlife Korean immigrant women in the US. *Journal of Immigrant and Minority Health, 9*(4), 291–298.

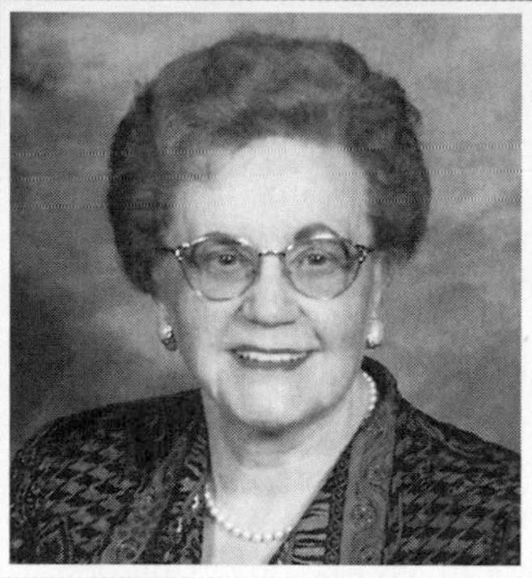

Madeleine M. Leininger (1927–2012)

22

Theory of Culture Care Diversity and Universality

Marilyn R. McFarland

"Care is the essence of nursing and a distinct, dominant, central and unifying focus."
Madeleine Leininger (Leininger & McFarland, 2002, p. 192)

CREDENTIALS AND BACKGROUND OF THE THEORIST

Madeleine M. Leininger, founder of transcultural nursing and leader in transcultural nursing and human care theory, was the first professional nurse with graduate preparation in nursing to hold a doctorate in cultural and social anthropology. Born in Sutton, Nebraska, she began her nursing career after graduating from the diploma program at St. Anthony's School of Nursing in Denver, Colorado. In 1950 she obtained a bachelor's degree in biological science from Benedictine College in Atchison, Kansas, with a minor in philosophy and humanistic studies. After graduation she served as an instructor, staff nurse, and head nurse on a medical-surgical unit and opened a psychiatric unit while director of nursing service at St. Joseph's Hospital in Omaha, Nebraska. During this time, she pursued advanced study in nursing, nursing administration, teaching and curriculum in nursing, and tests and measurements at Mount St. Scholastica College in Atchison, Kansas, and Creighton University in Omaha, Nebraska.

In 1954 Leininger obtained a master's degree in psychiatric nursing from Catholic University of America in Washington, D.C. She was then employed at the College of Health at the University of Cincinnati, where she developed the first master's level clinical specialist program in child psychiatric nursing. She initiated and directed the first graduate nursing program in psychiatric nursing at the University of Cincinnati and Therapeutic Psychiatric Nursing Center at University Hospital (Cincinnati). In 1960 she cowrote one of the first basic psychiatric nursing texts with Hofling, titled *Basic Psychiatric Concepts in Nursing,* which was published in 11 languages and used worldwide (Hofling & Leininger, 1960).

While working at a child guidance home in the mid-1950s in Cincinnati, Leininger discovered that the staff lacked understanding of cultural factors influencing the behavior of children. Among these children of diverse cultural backgrounds, she observed differences in response to care and psychiatric treatments that deeply concerned her. Psychoanalytical theories and therapy strategies did not seem to reach children from diverse cultural backgrounds. She became increasingly concerned that her nursing decisions and actions, and those of other staff, did not appear to help these children adequately. Leininger posed many questions to herself and the staff about cultural differences among children and therapy outcomes. However, few staff members were interested or knowledgeable about cultural factors in the diagnosis and treatment of clients. Margaret Mead became a visiting professor in the Department of Psychiatry at the University of Cincinnati, and Leininger discussed the interrelationships between nursing and anthropology with Mead. Leininger recalled a stimulating discussion wherein she asked Dr. Mead whether *she* saw

Photo credit: Dr. Madeleine Leininger, Madonna University, Livonia, MI, *circa* 1999. *Source:* The Madeleine M. Leininger Collection on Human Caring and Transcultural Nursing, ARC-008, Photo 03, Archives of Caring in Nursing, Florida Atlantic University, Boca Raton, FL.

This chapter is dedicated in memory of Dr. Madeleine Leininger.

any relationship between nursing and anthropology and "theoretical notions," to which Mead replied, "Well, that is something for you to discover" (Leininger, 1991). Thereafter, Leininger decided to pursue her interests with focused doctoral study on cultural, social, and psychological anthropology at the University of Washington, Seattle.

During the 1950s and 1960s, Leininger (1970, 1978) identified common areas of theory interests and research foci between the disciplines of nursing and anthropology, which aided her in formulating transcultural nursing concepts, theory, principles, and practices. As a doctoral student, Leininger studied many cultures. She found anthropology fascinating and believed it should be of interest to all nurses. She focused on the Gadsup people of the Eastern Highlands of New Guinea; she lived alone with these indigenous people for nearly 2 years and undertook an ethnographic and ethnonursing study in their villages (Leininger, 1995, 1996). She was not only able to observe unique features of the culture, but also observed a number of marked differences between Western and non-Western cultures in caring health and well-being practices. From her experiences with the Gadsup, she continued to develop her theory of culture care diversity and universality (culture care theory) and the ethnonursing research method (Leininger, 1978, 1991, 1995). Her research and theory helped nursing students understand cultural differences in human care and caring, health, and illness. She encouraged many students and faculty to pursue graduate nursing education and practice. Her enthusiasm and interest in developing the field of transcultural nursing with a human care focus sustained her for more than 6 decades.

The first course in transcultural nursing was offered in 1966 at the University of Colorado, where Leininger was professor of nursing and anthropology—one of the first joint appointments for a professor of nursing in another discipline. She initiated the Committee on Nursing and Anthropology with the American Anthropological Association in 1968 and served as its chair for several years (Leininger, 1991, 1995).

Leininger served as director of the Nurse Scientist PhD Program in the United States in 1969, when she was appointed Dean and Professor of Nursing and Lecturer in Anthropology at the University of Washington, Seattle, where she remained until 1974. There she established the first academic nursing department on comparative nursing care systems to support master's and doctoral programs. She initiated several transcultural nursing courses and mentored the nurses in a doctoral program with a focus on transcultural nursing.

In 1974 Leininger was appointed Dean and Professor of Nursing at the College of Nursing and Adjunct Professor of Anthropology at the University of Utah in Salt Lake City. At this institution, she initiated the first master's and doctoral programs in transcultural nursing and established the first doctoral program offerings at this institution (Leininger, 1978). These programs were the first to offer substantive courses focused specifically on transcultural nursing. She initiated and was director of a new research facilitation office at the University of Utah. In 1974 Leininger founded the International Transcultural Nursing Society and remained an active leader in the organization throughout her lifetime. She established the National Research Care Conferences in 1978 (later renamed the International Society for Human Caring) to help nurses focus on the study of human care phenomena (Leininger, 1988a, 1988b, 1991). She served as an early president of the American Association of Colleges of Nursing and was one of the first members of the American Academy of Nursing in 1975.

Leininger's book, *Nursing and Anthropology: Two Worlds to Blend* (1970), laid the foundation for developing the field of transcultural nursing, the culture care theory, and culturally based health care. Her next book, *Transcultural Nursing: Concepts, Theories, and Practice* (1978), identified major concepts, theoretical ideas, and practices in transcultural nursing and was the first definitive publication on transcultural nursing. During the next 60 years Leininger established, explicated, and used the culture care theory to study many cultures within the United States and worldwide. She developed an ethnonursing research method to be used with the theory to qualitatively discover the insider or emic view of cultures (Leininger, 1991; Leininger & McFarland, 2002, 2006) for nurse researchers to study and discover culture care phenomena from the perspective of human science philosophy and through the lens of qualitative analysis (Leininger, 1978, 1985a, 1991, 1995; Leininger & McFarland, 2002, 2006; McFarland & Wehbe-Alamah, 2015).

In 1981 Leininger was recruited to Wayne State University in Detroit, where she was Professor of Nursing and Adjunct Professor of Anthropology and Director of Transcultural Nursing Offerings until her semiretirement in 1995. She served as Director of the Center for Health Research at Wayne State for 5 years. In 1989 Leininger launched the *Journal of Transcultural Nursing,* serving as its editor until her retirement. While at Wayne State, she again developed courses and seminars in transcultural nursing, caring, and qualitative research methods for baccalaureate, master's, doctoral, and postdoctoral nursing and nonnursing students. In addition, Dr. Leininger taught and mentored students and nurses in field research in transcultural nursing and continued to teach these methods at various universities within the United States and worldwide.

Leininger wrote or edited more than 30 books. Some of her most significant books after 1978 included *Caring: An Essential Human Need* (Leininger, 1981); *Care: The Essence of Nursing and Health* (1984); *Qualitative Research Methods in Nursing* (1985a); *Ethical and Moral Dimensions of Care: Chapters from Conference on the Ethics and Morality of Caring* (1990a); *The Caring Imperative in Education* (Leininger & Watson, 1990); *Culture Care Diversity and Universality: A Theory of Nursing* (1991); *Transcultural Nursing: Concepts, Theories, Research, and Practice* (Leininger & McFarland, 2002a); and *Culture Care Diversity and Universality: A Worldwide Theory of Nursing* (Leininger and McFarland, 2006), which contain full accounts of her theory and method. She published more than 200 articles and 45 book chapters plus films, videos, DVDs, and research reports focused on transcultural nursing; human care and health phenomena; the future of nursing; and related topics relevant to nursing and anthropology. Dr. Leininger served on eight editorial boards and refereed several publications in addition to her active involvement with the Transcultural Nursing Scholars Group and the development of and contributions to her website (www.madeleine-leininger.com). She is known as one of the most creative, productive, innovative, and futuristic authors in nursing who provided new and substantive research-based transcultural nursing content and ideas to advance nursing as a discipline and a profession.

Leininger had many lifelong areas of expertise and interest. In addition to transcultural nursing with care as a central focus, comparative education and administration, nursing theories, politics, ethical dilemmas of nursing and health care, qualitative research methods, the future of nursing and health care, and nursing leadership were all areas of interest to her. As a certified transcultural nurse and transcultural nurse researcher, Leininger studied 15 individual and unique cultures; mentored or supervised approximately 200 master's and doctoral students focused on transcultural nursing, human caring and care, and related areas worldwide; and consulted with researchers and institutions, especially those using culture care theory. Culture care theory is used worldwide and continues to grow important culture care phenomena about diverse cultures.

She found time to give lectures to anthropologists, physicians, social workers, pharmacists, and educators and conduct research with colleagues. She was one of the few nurses who was active in both nursing and anthropology, making contributions at national and international transcultural conferences and association meetings. She worked enthusiastically to encourage nursing educators and practitioners to integrate transcultural nursing and culture-specific care concepts into nursing curricula and clinical practices of nursing (Leininger, 1991, 1995; McFarland & Leininger, 2002, 2006; McFarland & Wehbe-Alamah, 2015). Across seven decades, numerous nurses with advanced degrees and baccalaureate students have been certified in transcultural nursing and used Leininger's culture care theory (Leininger, 1991, 1995; Leininger & McFarland, 2002, 2006; McFarland & Wehbe-Alamah, 2015).

Dr. Leininger gained international recognition in nursing and related fields through her transcultural nursing and care writings, theory, research, consultation, courses, and dynamic addresses. She received many awards and honors for her lifetime professional and academic accomplishments. She was listed in *Who's Who of American Women; Who's Who in Health Care; Who's Who in Community Leaders; Who's Who of Women in Education; International Who's Who in Community Service;* and *Who's Who in International Women*, to name a few. Her name appears on the National Register of Prominent Americans and International Notables, International Women, and the National Register of Prominent Community Leaders. She received several honorary degrees from Benedictine College in Atchison, Kansas; a doctorate from the University of Kuopio, Finland; and a Doctor of Science from the University of Indiana, Indianapolis. In 1976 and 1995 she was recognized for her unique and significant contribution to the American Association of Colleges of Nursing as its first full-time president. Leininger received the Russell Sage Outstanding Leadership Award in 1995. Leininger was a fellow in the American Academy of Nursing, a fellow of the American Anthropology Society, a fellow of the Society for Applied Anthropology, and a Fellow of the Royal College of Nursing in Australia. She was a member of Sigma Theta Tau International, Delta Kappa Gamma, and the Scandinavian College of Caring Science in Stockholm, Sweden. She served as a distinguished visiting scholar and lecturer at 85 universities in the United States and worldwide and was a visiting professor at universities in Sweden, Wales, Japan, China, Australia, Finland, New Zealand, and the Philippines. While at Wayne State University she received the Board of Regents' Distinguished Faculty Award, the Distinguished Research Award, the President's Excellence in Teaching, and the Outstanding Graduate Faculty Mentor Award. In 1996 Madonna University in Livonia, Michigan, honored her with its dedication of the Leininger Book Collection and a special Leininger Reading Room for her outstanding contributions to nursing and the social sciences and humanities. Leininger was honored as a Living Legend of the American Academy of Nursing in 1998.

Dr. Leininger's last works on the culture care theory were publications in peer-reviewed professional journals. She coauthored an interview for *Nursing Science Quarterly* (Clarke et al., 2009) where she discussed the history and future of transcultural care, the nursing profession, and global health care. In 2011 she authored a reflective article about father protective care in the *Online Journal of Cultural Competence in Nursing and Healthcare*. She conducted this retrospective comparative study of three Western and one non-Western culture (Old Order Amish Americans, Anglo Americans, Mexican Americans, and the Gadsup of the Eastern Highlands of New Guinea) about father protective care beliefs and practices with the goal of using that knowledge to provide culturally congruent care. She reported on culture care decision and action modes of similar and diverse care findings discussed with the informant fathers as ways they might integrate their cultural values and care practices to help their sons. Fathers from the Old Order Amish and the Gadsup wished to preserve (culture care preservation) their traditional protective care practices to maintain healthy and active cultural lifeways. Anglo American and Mexican American fathers wanted to negotiate (culture care negotiation) ways to transmit spiritual and religious traditions knowledge to their sons. Leininger then began work on a new culture care construct, **collaborative care**, which she presented with Marilyn McFarland via a keynote videocast at the 37th Annual Conference of Transcultural Nursing Society in October 2011, and her article based on this construct was accepted for publication in the *Online Journal of Cultural Competence in Health Care.*

Dr. Madeleine Leininger died peacefully on August 10, 2012, in Omaha, Nebraska. She continued to work until shortly before her passing, collaborating with colleagues on contributions to several projects and other publications in progress as well as revisions to her website. Among these works was a chapter contribution, "Leininger's Father Protective Care," to the 2015 third edition of her theory book, *Leininger's Culture Care Diversity and Universality: A Worldwide Nursing Theory* by McFarland and Wehbe-Alamah.

THEORETICAL SOURCES

Leininger's theory derives from the disciplines of anthropology and nursing (Leininger, 1991, 1995; Leininger & McFarland, 2002, 2006; McFarland & Wehbe-Alamah, 2015). She described *transcultural nursing* as a major area of nursing focused on comparative study and analysis of diverse cultures and subcultures in the world with respect to their caring values, expressions, and health-illness beliefs and patterns of behavior.

The purpose of the theory is to discover human care diversities and universalities in relation to worldview, cultural and social structure dimensions, and ways to provide culturally congruent care with people of various cultures to maintain or regain their well-being or health, or face death in a culturally appropriate way (Leininger, 1991, 1995; Leininger & McFarland, 2002, 2006; McFarland & Wehbe-Alamah, 2015). The goal of the theory is to provide culturally congruent care to people that is beneficial and fits with the client, family, or culture group healthy lifeways (Leininger, 1991, 1995; Leininger & McFarland, 2002, 2006; McFarland & Wehbe-Alamah, 2015). Transcultural nursing goes from an awareness state to use of culture care nursing knowledge to practice culturally congruent and responsible care (Leininger, 1991, 1995; Leininger & McFarland, 2002, 2006; McFarland & Wehbe-Alamah, 2015).

Leininger predicted that in time there would be a new kind of nursing practice reflecting nursing practices that are culturally defined, grounded, and specific guiding nursing care for individuals, families, groups, and institutions. She contended that because culture and care knowledge are the broadest and most holistic means to conceptualize and understand people, they are central to and imperative to nursing education and practice (Leininger, 1991, 1995; Leininger & McFarland, 2002, 2006; McFarland & Wehbe-Alamah, 2015).

In addition, she stated that transcultural nursing had become one of the most important, relevant, and highly promising areas of formal study, research, and practice in the multicultural world (Leininger, 1988a, 1995; Leininger & McFarland, 2002, 2006; McFarland & Wehbe-Alamah, 2015). Leininger predicted that for nursing to be meaningful and relevant to clients and other nurses in the world, transcultural nursing knowledge and competencies would be imperative to guide all nursing care decisions and actions for effective and successful health outcomes (Leininger, 1991, 1995, 1996; Leininger & McFarland, 2002, 2006; McFarland & Eipperle, 2008; McFarland & Wehbe-Alamah, 2015). Leininger (2002a) distinguished between **transcultural nursing** and **cross-cultural nursing**. The former refers to nurses prepared in transcultural nursing who are committed to developing knowledge and practice in transcultural nursing, whereas cross-cultural nursing refers to nurses who use applied or medical anthropological concepts (Leininger, 1995; Leininger & McFarland, 2002, 2006; McFarland & Wehbe-Alamah, 2015). She said international nursing occurs when nurses travel to or have nursing practice or service-learning experiences in other nations or countries, and transcultural nursing involves multiple *cultures* and has comparative theoretical and practice-based foci (Leininger, 1995; Leininger & McFarland, 2002, 2006; McFarland & Wehbe-Alamah, 2015). Leininger described the certified transcultural nurse **generalist** (CTN-B) as a nurse prepared at the baccalaureate level who is able to apply transcultural nursing concepts, principles, and practices that are generated by transcultural nurse specialists (Leininger, 1991, 1995; Leininger & McFarland, 2002, 2006; McFarland & Wehbe-Alamah, 2015). The transcultural nurse **specialist** (CTN-A) is prepared in graduate programs and receives in-depth preparation and mentorship in transcultural nursing knowledge and practice. The CTN-A has acquired competency through post-baccalaureate educational knowledge about selected cultures in sufficient depth (values, beliefs, and lifeways) to provide high-quality, safe, and effective transcultural nursing care (Leininger, 1991,

1995; Leininger & McFarland, 2002, 2006; McFarland & Wehbe-Alamah, 2015). The transcultural CTN-A serves as an expert field practitioner, teacher, researcher, and consultant with respect to select cultures. This individual values and uses nursing theory to develop and advance knowledge within transcultural nursing (Leininger, 1991, 1995; Leininger & McFarland, 2002, 2006; McFarland & Wehbe-Alamah, 2015).

Leininger defined theory as the systematic and creative discovery of knowledge about a domain of interest that appears important to understand or to account for some unknown phenomenon. She believed that nursing theory must take into account creative discovery about individuals, families, and groups and their caring, values, expressions, beliefs, and actions or practices based on their cultural lifeways to provide effective, satisfying, and culturally congruent care. If nurses recognize the cultural aspects of human needs, there are signs of beneficial or efficacious nursing care practices and evidence of satisfaction with nursing services, with healing and well-being (Leininger, 1991, 1995; Leininger & McFarland, 2002, 2006; McFarland & Wehbe-Alamah, 2015).

Leininger (1991) developed her theory of culture care diversity and universality based on the belief that people of different cultures are capable of guiding professionals to receive the kind of care they desire or need from others. Culture is the patterned and valued lifeways of people that influence their decisions and actions; therefore the theory is directed toward nurses to discover and document the world of the client and to use their emic (insider) viewpoints, knowledge, and practices with appropriate etic (outsider) as the bases for making culturally congruent professional care actions and decisions (Leininger, 1991, 1995).

The culture care theory is inductive and deductive and derived from emic and etic knowledge (Leininger, 1991). Leininger (1991) encouraged nurses and others to obtain grounded insider knowledge from people or the culture, because it is more credible. The theory is viewed holistically with specific domains of interest (Leininger, 1991, 1995; Leininger & McFarland, 2002, 2006; McFarland & Wehbe-Alamah, 2015). The culture care theory is a broad holistic nursing theory, because it takes into account the totality and holistic perspective of human life and existence, including social structure factors, worldview, cultural history and values, environmental context (Leininger, 1988b), language expressions, and folk (generic) and professional care patterns. These are some of the critical and essential bases for the discovery of care knowledge that leads to the health and well-being of clients and guides therapeutic nursing practices.

Leininger's (2002c) theory of culture care diversity and universality has distinct features that differ from other nursing theories. This theory is focused explicitly on discovering holistic and comprehensive culture care, and it can be used *across* Western and non-Western cultures because it includes multiple holistic factors universally found in cultures. It is focused on discovering comprehensive factors influencing human care such as worldview, social structure factors, language, generic and professional care, ethnohistory, and the environmental context. The theory has abstract and practice dimensions that can be examined systematically to achieve culturally congruent, meaningful, and acceptable care outcomes (McFarland & Wehbe-Alamah, 2015). It is the only nursing theory explicitly focused on culture and care of diverse cultures, using three theory-based culture care modes of decisions and actions in practice to reach outcomes for well-being, health, and satisfactory lifeways for people. The theory is designed to discover care—what is diverse and what is universally related to care and health—and has an integrated comparative focus to discover different or contrasting transcultural nursing care practices with specific care constructs. The theory with the ethnonursing method has enablers designed to tease out in-depth informant emic data and health-related information. Thus the enablers are used for cultural health care assessments. The theory guides the generation of new knowledge in nursing and health care, arriving at culturally congruent, meaningful, and beneficial care.

MAJOR CONCEPTS & DEFINITIONS

Leininger developed constructs relevant to her culture care theory. The major constructs are listed here. The reader is referred to her definitive works to study the full theory (Leininger, 1991, 1995; Leininger & McFarland, 2002, 2006; McFarland & Wehbe-Alamah, 2015).

Care and Caring

Care refers to abstract and manifest phenomena with expressions of assistive, supportive, enabling, and facilitating ways toward or about self or others. **Caring** refers to actions, attitudes, or practices to assist others toward healing and well-being (Leininger, 1991, 1995; Leininger & McFarland, 2002, 2006; McFarland et al., 2012; McFarland & Wehbe-Alamah, 2015). "*Care* . . . includes generic/folk care and professional care which are major parts of the theory that have been predicted to influence and explain the health and wellbeing of diverse cultures" (McFarland & Wehbe-Alamah, 2015, pp. 9–10).

Continued

MAJOR CONCEPTS & DEFINITIONS—cont'd

Generic Care

"**Generic care** refers to the learned and transmitted lay, indigenous, traditional or local folk (emic) knowledge and practices to provide assistance, supportive, enabling, and facilitative acts for or toward others with evident or anticipated health needs in order to improve wellbeing or to help with dying or other human conditions" (McFarland & Wehbe-Alamah, 2015, p. 14).

Professional Care

"**Professional nursing care** refers to formal and explicit cognitively learned professional care knowledge and practices obtained generally through educational institutions [usually nongeneric] [that] are taught to nurses and others to provide assistive, supportive, enabling, or facilitative acts for or to another individual or group in order to improve their health, prevent illnesses, or to help with dying or other human conditions" (McFarland & Wehbe-Alamah, 2015, p. 14).

Culture

"**Culture** refers to learned, shared, and transmitted values, beliefs, norms, and lifeways of a particular culture that guide thinking, decisions, and actions in patterned ways. Culture is equally as important as care; is not an adverb or adjective to care. Leininger conceptualized culture care as synthesized and closely linked phenomena with interrelated ideas" (Leininger & McFarland, 2006, p. 18; McFarland & Wehbe-Alamah, 2015, p. 10).

Culture Care

Culture care refers to the synthesis of the two major constructs (*care* and *culture*) that guide the researcher to discover, explain, and account for health, well-being, care expressions, and other human conditions (Leininger & McFarland, 2006).

Culturally Congruent Care

Culturally congruent care is culturally based care knowledge, acts, and decisions used in sensitive, creative, and meaningful ways to appropriately fit the cultural values, beliefs, and lifeways of clients for their health and well-being, or to prevent or face illness, disabilities, or death. "The provision of culturally congruent and safe care has been the major goal of the culture care theory" (McFarland & Wehbe-Alamah, 2015, p. 14).

Culture Care Diversity

"**Culture care diversity** refers to the variabilities or differences in culture care beliefs, meanings, patterns, values, symbols, lifeways, symbols, and other features among human beings related to providing beneficial care for clients from a designated culture" (McFarland & Wehbe-Alamah, 2015, p. 14).

Culture Care Universality

"**Culture care universality** refers to commonly shared or similar cultural care phenomena features of human beings or groups with recurrent meanings, patterns, values, symbols, or lifeways that serve as a guide for caregivers to provide assistive, supportive facilitative, or enabling people care for healthy outcomes" (McFarland & Wehbe-Alamah, 2015, p. 15).

Worldview

"**Worldview** refers to the way people look out on their world or universe to form a picture or value stance about life or the world around them. Worldview provides a broad perspective about one's orientation to life, people, or groups that influence care or caring responses and guides one's decisions or actions, especially related to matters of health or well-being" (McFarland & Wehbe-Alamah, 2015, p. 15).

Cultural and Social Structure Dimensions

The "**cultural and social structure dimensions** refer to the dynamic, holistic, and interrelated patterns of structured features of a culture (or subculture) that include but are not limited to technology factors; religious and philosophical factors; kinship and social factors; cultural values, beliefs, and lifeways; political and legal factors; economic factors; and educational factors as well as environmental context, language, and ethnohistory" (McFarland & Wehbe-Alamah, 2015, p. 75).

Environmental Context

"**Environmental context** refers to the totality of an event, situation, or particular experience that gives meaning to people's expressions, interpretations, and social interactions within particular geophysical, ecological, spiritual, sociopolitical, and technological factors in specific cultural settings" (McFarland & Wehbe-Alamah, 2015, p. 15).

Ethnohistory

"**Ethnohistory** refers to the sequence of past facts, events, instances, or experiences of human beings, groups, cultures, or institutions over time in particular contexts that help explain past and current lifeways about culture care influencers affecting the health and well-being, disability, or death of people" (McFarland & Wehbe-Alamah, 2015, p. 15).

MAJOR CONCEPTS & DEFINITIONS—cont'd

Emic

"**Emic** refers to local, indigenous, or the insider cultural knowledge and views about specific phenomena" (McFarland & Wehbe-Alamah, 2015, p. 14).

Etic

"**Etic** refers to the outsider or stranger (often health professionals) views or institutional or system knowledge and interpreted values about cultural phenomena" (McFarland & Wehbe-Alamah, 2015, p. 14).

Health

Health refers to a state of well-being that is culturally defined, valued, and practiced that reflects the ability of individuals or groups to perform their daily role activities in culturally expressed, beneficial, and patterned lifeways (Leininger, 1991; McFarland & Wehbe-Alamah, 2015); a state of restorative well-being that is culturally constituted, defined, valued, and practiced by individuals or groups and enables them to perform their daily lives (Leininger & McFarland, 2002; McFarland & Wehbe-Alamah, 2015).

Culture Care Preservation or Maintenance

Culture care preservation or maintenance refers to assistive, supportive, facilitative, or enabling professional actions and decisions that help people of a particular culture to retain, preserve, or maintain meaningful care beliefs and values for their well-being, to recover from illness, or to deal with handicaps or dying (Leininger 1991, 1995; Leininger & McFarland, 2002, 2006; McFarland & Wehbe-Alamah, 2015).

Culture Care Accommodation or Negotiation

Culture care accommodation or negotiation refers to those assistive, accommodating, facilitative, or enabling creative professional care actions and decisions that help people of a designated culture (or subculture) to adapt to or negotiate with others for culturally congruent, safe, effective care for meaningful and beneficial health outcomes (Leininger 1991, 1995; Leininger & McFarland, 2002, 2006; McFarland & Wehbe-Alamah, 2015).

Culture Care Repatterning or Restructuring

Culture care repatterning or restructuring refers to the assistive, supportive facilitative, or enabling professional actions and decisions that help clients reorder, change, or modify their lifeways for beneficial health care patterns, practices, or outcomes (Leininger 1991, 1995; Leininger & McFarland, 2002, 2006; McFarland & Wehbe-Alamah, 2015).

USE OF EMPIRICAL EVIDENCE

For more than 6 decades, Leininger held that care was the essence of nursing and the dominant, distinctive, and unifying feature of nursing (Leininger, 1970, 1988b, 1991; Leininger & McFarland, 2002, 2006; McFarland & Wehbe-Alamah, 2015). She believed care to be complex, elusive, and often embedded in social structure and other aspects of culture (Leininger, 1991; Leininger & McFarland, 2006). She held that different forms, expressions, and patterns of care were diverse, and some were universal (Leininger, 1991; Leininger & McFarland, 2002, 2006). Leininger (1985b, 1990b; Leininger & McFarland, 2002, 2006) used qualitative ethnomethods, especially ethnonursing, to study care. These methods are directed toward discovering the people-truths, views, beliefs, and patterned lifeways of cultural groups, families, and individuals. During the 1960s, Leininger blended nursing and anthropology and developed the ethnonursing method to study transcultural nursing phenomena specifically and systematically. This method focuses on discovery of care beliefs, values, and practices as cognitively or subjectively known by the people of a culture through their local people-centered language, experiences, beliefs, and values about actual or potential nursing phenomena such as care, health, and environmental factors (Leininger, 1991, 1995; Leininger & McFarland, 2002, 2006; McFarland et al., 2012; McFarland & Wehbe-Alamah, 2015). Although nursing used the words *care* and *caring* for more than a century, the definitions and usage were without specific meanings to the culture of the client or nurse (Leininger, 1988a, 1988b). "Indeed, the concepts about caring have been some of the least understood and studied of all human knowledge and research areas within and outside of nursing" (Leininger, 1978, p. 33). With transcultural culture care theory and ethnonursing method it is possible to get close to the discovery of people-based care, because data come directly from people and not from outsider views. An important purpose of the theory is to document, know, predict, and explain systematically through field data what is diverse and universal about the generic and professional care of cultures being studied (Leininger, 1991).

Leininger (1988a) held that detailed and culturally based caring knowledge and practices should distinguish nursing's contributions from those of other disciplines. The first reason for studying culture care theory is that the construct of *care* has been critical to human growth, development, and survival for human beings from the beginning of the human species (Leininger, 1988a, 1988b). The second reason is to explicate and fully understand cultural knowledge and the roles of caregivers and care recipients in different cultures to provide culturally congruent care (Leininger, 1991, 1995; Leininger & McFarland, 2002, 2006; McFarland & Wehbe-Alamah, 2015). Third, care knowledge is discovered and can be used as essential to promote the healing and well-being of clients, to face death or disability, or to ensure the survival of human cultures over time (Leininger, 1991, 1995). Fourth, the nursing profession needs to systematically study care from a broad and holistic cultural perspective to discover the expressions and meanings of care, health, illness, and well-being (Leininger, 1991, 1995; Leininger & McFarland, 2002, 2006; McFarland & Wehbe-Alamah, 2015). Leininger (1991, 1995) found that care was largely an elusive phenomenon often embedded in cultural lifeways and values. This knowledge serves as a sound basis for nurses to guide their practice for culturally congruent care and specific therapeutic ways to maintain health, prevent illness, heal, or help people face death (Leininger, 1991, 1995; Leininger & McFarland, 2002, 2006; McFarland & Wehbe-Alamah, 2015).

A central thesis of the theory is that if the meaning of care can be fully grasped, the well-being or health care of individuals, families, and groups can be predicted, and culturally congruent care can be provided (Leininger, 1991, 1994, 1995). Leininger (1991) viewed care as one of the most powerful constructs and the central phenomenon of nursing. However, such care constructs and patterns must be fully documented, understood, and used to ensure that culturally based knowledge is the major guide to transcultural nursing decisions and actions and is used to guide culturally congruent nursing practices (Leininger 1991, 1995; Leininger & McFarland, 2002, 2006; McFarland & Wehbe-Alamah, 2015). Leininger studied several cultures in depth, including with undergraduate and graduate students and faculty using qualitative research methods. She extensively explicated care constructs through many cultures that had different cultural meanings, cultural experiences, and uses of diverse and similar care values, beliefs, patterns, and expressions by their people (Leininger 1991, 1995; Leininger & McFarland, 2002, 2006; McFarland & Wehbe-Alamah, 2015). Culture care knowledge continues to be discovered by transcultural nurses in the development of culture-specific care practices with diverse and similar cultures. Leininger (1991) believed, in time, both diverse and universal features of care and health would be documented as the essence of nursing knowledge and practice.

Leininger stated that the goal of the culture care theory is to provide culturally congruent care (Leininger, 1991, 1995; Leininger & McFarland, 2002, 2006; McFarland & Wehbe-Alamah, 2015). She maintained that nurses could not separate worldviews, social structure factors, and cultural beliefs (lay/folk/generic and professional) from health, wellness, illness, or care when working with cultures because these factors are closely linked and interrelated (Leininger, 1994; McFarland & Wehbe-Alamah, 2015). Social structure factors such as religion, politics, culture, economics, and kinship are significant forces affecting care and influencing illness patterns and well-being. She emphasized the importance of discovering generic (folk or lay, local, and indigenous) care beliefs, values, and expressions held by cultures and comparing them with professional care practices (Leininger, 1991, 1995; Leininger & McFarland, 2002, 2006; McFarland & Wehbe-Alamah, 2015).

Leininger found that cultural blindness, cultural shock, cultural imposition, and ethnocentrism by nurses continued to greatly reduce the quality of care offered to clients from diverse cultures (Leininger, 1991, 1995; Leininger & McFarland, 2002, 2006; McFarland & Wehbe-Alamah, 2015). Moreover, nursing diagnoses and medical diagnoses that are not culturally based and known may create serious problems for those of some cultures that lead to unfavorable and sometimes serious outcomes (Leininger, 1995, 1996; Leininger & McFarland, 2002, 2006). Providing culturally congruent care enhances client satisfaction about the care they have received; it is a powerful healing force in the provision of quality health care. *Quality* care is what clients want most when they seek care from nurses, and it can be provided only when culturally derived and congruent care is known and used.

MAJOR ASSUMPTIONS

The universality of care reflects the common nature of human beings and humanity, whereas the diversity of care reflects the discovered variability and unique features of human beings. Major assumptions of the theory of culture care diversity and universality presented here were derived from Leininger's definitive works on the theory and subsequent evolutionary changes (Leininger 1991; Leininger & McFarland, 2002, 2006; McFarland & Wehbe-Alamah, 2015):

- Care is the essence and the central dominant, distinct, and unifying focus of nursing.
- Humanistic and scientific care is essential for human growth, well-being, health, survival, and to face death and disabilities.
- Care (caring) is essential to curing or healing, because there can be no curing without caring (this assumption was held to have profound relevance worldwide).
- Culture care is the synthesis of two major constructs (culture and care) that guide the researcher to discover, explain, and account for health, well-being, care expressions, and other human conditions.
- Culture care expressions, meanings, patterns, processes, and structural forms are diverse, but some commonalities (universalities) exist among and between cultures.
- Culture care values, beliefs, and practices are influenced by and embedded in the worldview, social structure factors (e.g., religion, philosophy of life, kinship, politics, economics, education, technology, and cultural values) and the ethnohistorical and environmental contexts.
- Every culture has generic (lay, folk, naturalistic; mainly emic) and usually some professional (etic) care to be discovered and used for culturally congruent care practices.
- Culturally congruent and therapeutic care occurs when culture care values, beliefs, expressions, and patterns are explicitly known and used appropriately, sensitively, and meaningfully with people of diverse or similar cultures.
- Leininger's three theoretical modes of care offer new, creative, and different therapeutic ways to help people of diverse cultures.
- The ethnonursing research method and other qualitative research paradigmatic methods offer important means to discover largely embedded, covert, epistemic, and ontological culture care knowledge and practices.
- Transcultural nursing is a discipline with a body of knowledge and practices to attain and maintain the goal of culturally congruent care for health and well-being.

THEORETICAL ASSERTIONS OR TENETS

In developing culture care theory, four major theoretical tenets were conceptualized and formulated by the theorist (Leininger & McFarland, 2002, 2006; McFarland & Wehbe-Alamah, 2015):

1. Culture care expressions, meaning, patterns, and practices are diverse, and yet there are shared commonalities and some universal attributes.
2. The worldview, multiple social structure factors, ethnohistory, environmental context, language, and generic and professional care are critical influencers of culture care patterns to predict health, well-being, illness, healing, and ways people face disabilities and death.
3. Generic emic (folk) and etic (professional) health factors in different environmental contexts greatly influence health and illness outcomes.
4. From an analysis of these influencers, three major decision and action modes (culture care preservation or maintenance; culture care accommodation or negotiation; and culture care repatterning or restructuring) were predicted to provide ways to give culturally congruent, safe, and meaningful health care to cultures (Leininger & McFarland, 2002, 2006; McFarland & Wehbe-Alamah, 2015; Wehbe-Alamah, 2008).

These decision and action modes were predicted to be key factors in the provision of culturally congruent, meaningful, and acceptable care for beneficial outcomes. When using these modes, individual, family, group, or community factors are assessed and responded to in dynamic and participatory nurse–client relationships.

In conceptualizing the theory, the first major and central theoretical tenet was "care diversities (differences) and universalities (commonalities) existed among and between cultures in the world" (Leininger & McFarland, 2002, p. 78). However, Leininger asserted that culture care meanings and uses first had to be discovered to establish a body of transcultural knowledge. A second major theoretical tenet was that the "worldview, social structure factors such as religion, economics, education, technology, politics, kinship (social), ethnohistory, environment, language, and generic care and professional care factors would greatly influence culture care meanings, expressions, and patterns in different cultures" (Leininger & McFarland, 2002, p. 78).

Leininger maintained that knowing the cultural and social structure factors was necessary to provide meaningful and satisfying care to people and predicted they would be powerful influencers on culturally based care. These factors also needed to be discovered directly from cultural informants to confirm them as being influencing factors related to health, well-being, illness, and death. The third major theoretical tenet was "both generic (emic) and professional (etic) care needs to be taught, researched, and brought together into care practices for satisfying care for clients which leads to their health and wellbeing" (Leininger, 2002, p. 78).

The fourth major theoretical tenet was the conceptualization of the three major care modes of decisions and actions (stated previously) to arrive at culturally congruent care for the general health and well-being of clients, or to help them face death or disabilities (Leininger & McFarland, 2002, 2006; McFarland & Wehbe-Alamah, 2015).

The researcher or clinician draws upon findings from the social structure, generic care and professional practices, and other influencing factors to study or provide culturally based care for individuals, families, and groups. These factors need to be studied, assessed, and responded to in a dynamic and coparticipatory nurse–client relationship (Leininger 1991; Leininger & McFarland, 2002, 2006; McFarland & Wehbe-Alamah, 2015).

LOGICAL FORM

Leininger derived concepts for her theory of culture care diversity and universality from anthropology and nursing and reconceptualized them into a set of constructs for a transcultural nursing theory with a human care perspective (1991, 1995). She developed the ethnonursing research method emphasizing the importance of studying people from their local knowledge and experiences and later compares this knowledge with their outsider beliefs and practices. Her book, *Qualitative Research Methods in Nursing* (Leininger, 1985a), and subsequent publications (Leininger, 1990b, 1995; Leininger 1991; Leininger & McFarland, 2002, 2006; McFarland & Wehbe-Alamah, 2015) provide substantive knowledge about qualitative methods in nursing.

Leininger was skilled in ethnonursing, ethnography, life histories, life stories, photography, and phenomenological methods for a holistic study approach of cultural behavior in diverse environmental contexts (Leininger, 1991, 2015; Leininger & McFarland, 2002, 2006; McFarland & Wehbe-Alamah, 2015). With these qualitative methods, the researcher moves with people in their daily living activities toward understanding their world.

With the ethnonursing research method, the nurse researcher inductively obtains data of documented descriptive and interpretative narratives from informants through observation and participation explicating culture care values (Leininger, 1991, 2015; Leininger & McFarland, 2002, 2006; McFarland & Wehbe-Alamah, 2015). The qualitative approach is important for developing basic and substantive data-based culture care knowledge to guide nurses in care practices. From the beginning, ethnonursing has been based primarily on the direct discovery of data from the cultural groups under study.

Although other methods of research, such as **hypothesis testing** and **experimental quantitative methods**, can be used to study transcultural care, the method depends on the researcher's purposes, research question, and goals of the study. Creativity and the willingness of the nurse researcher to use various research methods to discover nursing knowledge is encouraged. However, Leininger believed qualitative methods were important to establish meanings and discover accurate cultural knowledge, and quantitative methods were of limited value for studying cultures and care. Leininger also believed the use of both qualitative and quantitative methods in the same study obscured the findings (Leininger, 1991, 1995; Leininger & McFarland, 2002, 2006; McFarland & Wehbe-Alamah, 2015).

The Sunrise Enabler and the theory of cultural care diversity and universality are not fully addressed here. Rather, selected ideas are presented to introduce the reader to Leininger's pioneering and creative work of the evolving holistic and comprehensive theory. Leininger developed the Sunrise Enabler (Fig. 22.1) in the 1970s to depict the essential components of the theory. The Sunrise Enabler was refined by Leininger in 2006 and subsequently updated by McFarland & Wehbe-Alamah (2015). It has evolved to be a definitive enabler to comprehensively guide and focus studies and with which to make culturally congruent care decisions and actions. The upper half of the Sunrise Enabler depicts key theoretical constructs related to worldview and cultural and social structure dimensions. These dimensions include technology factors; religious and philosophical factors; kinship and social factors; cultural values, beliefs, and lifeways; political and legal factors; economic factors; and educational factors as well as environmental context, language, and ethnohistory.

These factors influence culture care expressions and patterns and the folk, professional, and nursing care systems depicted in the middle section of the Sunrise Enabler. The upper and lower halves together form a full sun, representing the universal care constructs that nurses would consider to appreciate human care and health (Leininger, 1991, 1995; Leininger & McFarland, 2002, 2006; McFarland & Wehbe-Alamah, 2015).

According to Leininger, *nursing* acts as a bridge between generic (folk) and professional care (Leininger & McFarland, 2002, 2006; McFarland & Wehbe-Alamah, 2015). Nurses use the three culture care modes of nursing decisions and actions in practice as predicted in the theory: *Culture care preservation or maintenance, culture care accommodation or negotiation,* and *culture care repatterning or restructuring* (Leininger 1991, 1995; Leininger & McFarland, 2002, 2006; McFarland & Wehbe-Alamah, 2015).

The Sunrise Enabler depicts human beings as inseparable from their cultural backgrounds and social structure factors, worldview, history, and environmental context (Leininger 1991, 1995; Leininger & McFarland, 2002, 2006; McFarland & Wehbe-Alamah, 2015). Gender, race, age, and

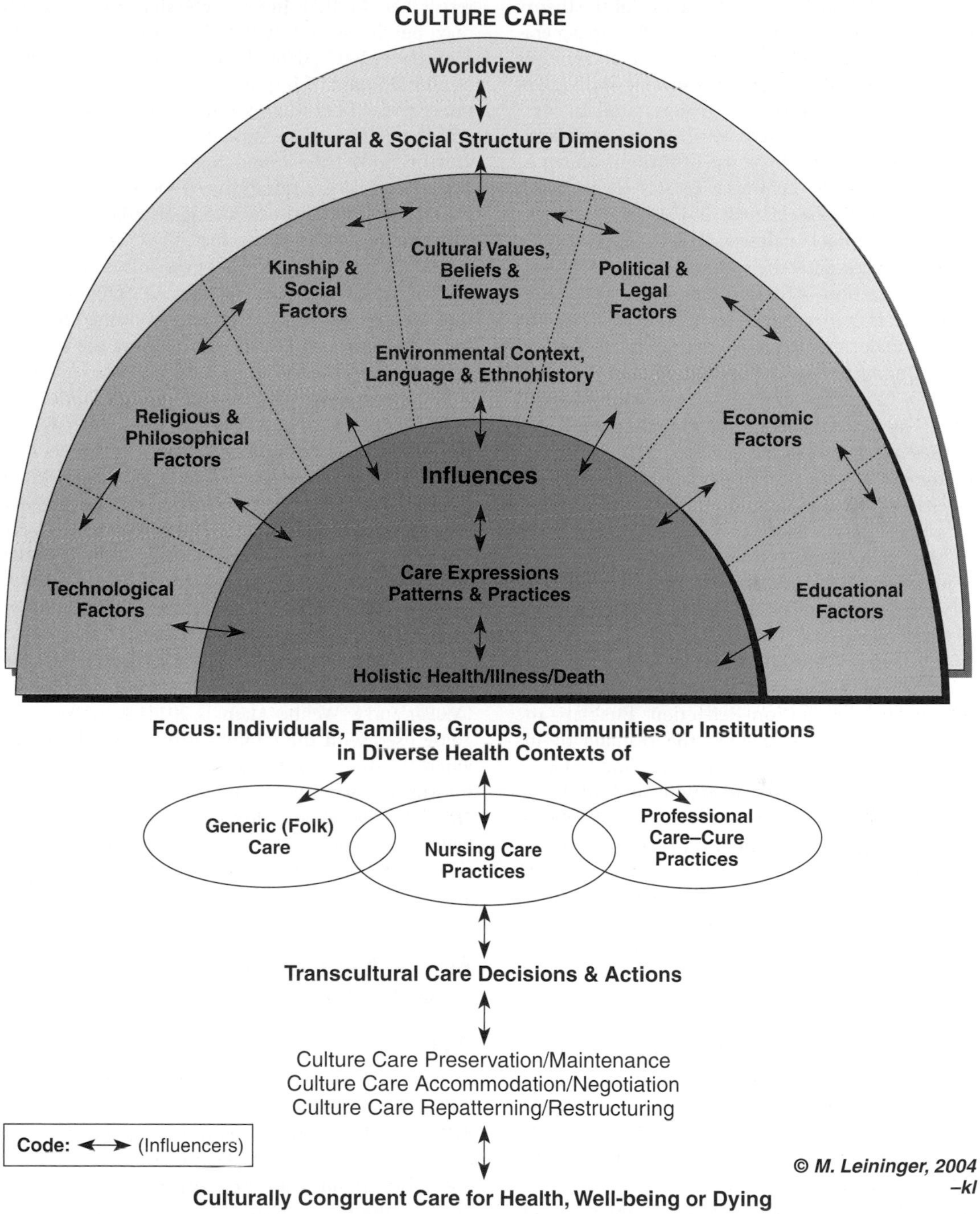

FIG. 22.1 Leininger's Sunrise Enabler. *(Copyright Madeleine Leininger, 2004. Used by permission.)*

class are embedded in social structure factors of the theory and are studied from a holistic perspective. Theory generation from ethnonursing studies may occur at multiple levels, from small-scale studies with specific individuals (micro level) to larger studies with groups, families, communities, or institutions (macro level). Leininger developed several enablers to facilitate use of the four phases of qualitative data analysis (Leininger & McFarland, 2002, 2006; McFarland & Wehbe-Alamah, 2015).

The first phase of data analysis is collecting, describing, and documenting raw data; the second phase is identification and categorization of descriptors and components; the third phase is pattern and contextual analysis; the fourth phase is major themes, research findings, theoretical formulations, and recommendations (McFarland & Wehbe-Alamah, 2015). Criteria to evaluate ethnonursing research findings are "used to challenge discovered universalities and diversities in relation to the Culture Care Theory and the qualitative paradigm . . . and to systematically examine and discover in-depth care and culture meanings and interpretive findings" (McFarland & Wehbe-Alamah, 2015, p. 56). These criteria are **credibility**; **confirmability**; **meaning-in-context**; **saturation**; **recurrent patterning**; and **transferability** (Leininger, 1995; Leininger & McFarland, 2002, 2006; McFarland & Wehbe-Alamah, 2015).

Leininger developed several additional enablers to assist nurse researchers in their use of the ethnonursing method: the Observation-Participation-Reflection Enabler; the Stranger-to-Trusted Friend Enabler; the Domain of Inquiry Enabler; Leininger's Semi-Structured Inquiry Guide Enabler to Assess Culture Care and Health; and the Acculturation Health Assessment Enabler for Cultural Patterns in Traditional or Nontraditional Lifeways. "Enablers sharply contrast with mechanistic devices such as tools, scales, measurement instruments, and other tools generally used in quantitative studies" (Leininger, 2002c, p. 89).

The Observation-Participation-Reflection Enabler is used to facilitate the researcher to enter and remain with informants in their familiar or natural context during the study. The researcher gradually moves slowly and politely with permission from the role of observer and listener to participant and reflector with the informants. The researcher does not disrupt and is therefore able to observe what is occurring naturally in the environment or with the people (Leininger & McFarland, 2002, 2006; McFarland & Wehbe-Alamah, 2015).

With the Stranger-to-Trusted Friend Enabler, the researcher learns much about oneself and the people and culture being studied. The goal with this guide is to move from distrusted stranger to become a trusted friend, and thereby more accurately observe cultural attitudes, behaviors, and expressions. This process is essential for the researcher so that honest, credible, and in-depth data may be discovered with the informants (Leininger & McFarland, 2002, 2006; McFarland & Wehbe-Alamah, 2015).

The Domain of Inquiry Enabler is a statement made by nurse researchers when guided by the culture care theory and the ethnonursing method to clearly focus his or her area of study (McFarland & Wehbe-Alamah, 2015). The domain comprises questions or ideas related to the focus of the study, its purpose, and goals related to culture and care and as such is a "succinct, tailor-made statement focused directly and specifically on culture care and health phenomena" (Leininger, 2002c, p. 92). This domain is carefully worded and then rigorously examined for adherence to theory tenets and assumptions using the six qualitative or evaluation criteria (McFarland & Wehbe-Alamah, 2015).

Leininger's Semi-Structured Inquiry Guide Enabler to Assess Culture Care and Health was developed by Leininger with open-ended questions "to assist researchers [during interviews and observations] to enter the world of informants, hear their stories, and make holistic and culture specific discoveries" (McFarland & Wehbe-Alamah, 2015, p. 84). This enabler correlates closely with the social structure factors of the culture care theory as depicted in the Sunrise Enabler (Leininger & McFarland, 2002, 2006; McFarland & Wehbe-Alamah, 2015).

The Acculturation Health Assessment Enabler for Cultural Patterns in Traditional or Nontraditional Lifeways (McFarland & Wehbe-Alamah, 2015) is another important guide used with the ethnonursing method. It is essential when studying cultures to assess the extent of the informants' **acculturation**, whether they are more or less "traditionally or nontraditionally oriented in their values, beliefs, and general lifeways" (Leininger & McFarland, 2002, p. 92). This enabler is used for both cultural assessments and ethnonursing research studies.

ACCEPTANCE BY THE NURSING COMMUNITY

Practice

Leininger identified several factors associated with the reluctance by nursing to recognize and value transcultural nursing and cultural factors in nursing practices and education (Leininger, 1991; Leininger & McFarland, 2002, 2006; McFarland & Wehbe-Alamah, 2015).

First, the theory was conceptualized during the 1950s when very few nurses were prepared in anthropology or had cultural knowledge to help them understand transcultural concepts, models, or theories. In those early days, most nurses did not have knowledge about the nature of anthropology and how anthropological knowledge might contribute to human care and health behaviors, or serve as background knowledge for understanding nursing phenomena or problems. Second, although people had longstanding and inherent cultural needs, clients were reluctant to press health care providers to meet their cultural needs and therefore their cultural and social needs were not recognized or met (Leininger, 1970, 1978, 1995; Leininger & McFarland, 2002, 2006; McFarland & Wehbe-Alamah, 2015). Third, until the 1990s, transcultural nursing articles submitted for publication were often rejected because journal editors did not know, value, or understand the relevance of cultural knowledge or transcultural nursing as essential to nursing. Fourth, the concept of culture *care* was of limited interest to nurses until the late 1970s, when Leininger began promoting the importance of nurses studying human care, obtaining background knowledge in anthropology, and obtaining graduate preparation in transcultural nursing, research, and practice. Fifth, Leininger contended that nursing remained too ethnocentric and far too adherent to following interest and directions of organized Western medicine. Sixth, nursing progress in the development of a distinct body of knowledge was limited, because many nurse researchers were dependent on using quantitative research methods. The contemporary acceptance and use of qualitative research methods in nursing continues to provide new insights and knowledge related to nursing and transcultural nursing. The interest in using transcultural nursing knowledge, research, education, and practices by nurses worldwide has continued to grow and evolve as the discipline of nursing has developed (Leininger, 1991, 1995; Leininger & McFarland, 2002, 2006; McFarland & Wehbe-Alamah, 2015).

As the world becomes more culturally diverse, nurses will find a more urgent need to be prepared to provide culturally congruent care. Some nurses experience culture shock, conflict, and clashes as they move from one location to another or from rural settings to urban communities without having first had some transcultural nursing preparation. As cultural conflicts arise, individuals and families experience less satisfaction with nursing and medical professional care practices (Leininger, 1988a, 1991; Leininger & McFarland, 2002, 2006; McFarland & Wehbe-Alamah, 2015). Nurses who travel and seek employment globally experience cultural stresses. Transcultural nursing education has thus become imperative for all nurses worldwide. Transcultural Nurse Certification by the Transcultural Nursing Society has provided a major step toward ensuring safe and culturally competent nursing practices (Leininger, 1991, 1995; Leininger & McFarland, 2002, 2006; McFarland & Wehbe-Alamah, 2015). Accordingly, more nurses are seeking transcultural certification to be able to provide culturally congruent care for their clients. The *Journal of Transcultural Nursing,* the *Online Journal of Cultural Competence in Nursing and Healthcare,* and other transculturally focused professional journals provide published research and theorctical perspectives about numerous diverse cultures worldwide to guide nursing practices.

Application of the culture care theory to advanced practice nursing has been explicated by several contemporary transcultural authors (Eipperle, 2015; Embler, Mixer, & Gunther, 2015; McFarland & Eipperle, 2008; Raymond & Omeri, 2015; Strang & Mixer, 2016; Wehbe-Alamah, 2008, 2011) as a "foundational basis for the educational preparation, primary care contextual practice, and outcomes-focused research endeavors of advanced practice nursing" (McFarland & Eipperle, 2008, p. 48) using the three culture care modes, the enablers, and the ethnonursing method. These authors emphasized integration of culturally congruent or sensitive care through direct and explicit approaches to be used by the nurse practitioner, who "needs to be able to sensitively and competently integrate culture care into contextual routines, clinical ways, and approaches to primary care practice through role modeling, policy making, procedural performance and performance evaluation, and the use of the advance practice nursing process" (McFarland & Eipperle, 2008, p. 49). Concepts and methods for integrating emic and etic care approaches into primary care practice and use of the education-research-practice continuum form the basis for clinical care decisions and actions.

Education

The inclusion of culture and comparative care in nursing curricula began in 1966 at the University of Colorado, where Leininger was professor of nursing and anthropology. Nurses' awareness of the importance of culture care began during the late 1960s, but very few nurse educators were adequately prepared to teach courses about transcultural nursing. After the world's first master's and doctoral programs in transcultural nursing were approved and implemented in 1977 at the University of Utah, many nurses became specifically prepared in transcultural nursing. With the heightened public awareness of health care costs, diverse cultures, and human rights extant in contemporary society worldwide, there is a much greater demand for comprehensive, holistic, and transcultural health care professionals to provide high-quality, comprehensive, and holistic care. Leininger's advocacy for culture-specific care based on theoretical constructs has been critical for the discovery of diverse and universal aspects of care (Leininger, 1991, 1995, 1996; Leininger & McFarland, 2002, 2006; McFarland & Wehbe-Alamah, 2015). A critical need remains for nurses to be educated in transcultural nursing in undergraduate, master's, and doctoral programs. There is a need for well-qualified faculty prepared in transcultural nursing to teach and guide research in nursing schools within the United States and in other countries (Leininger, 1991, 1995; Leininger & McFarland, 2002, 2006; McFarland & Wehbe-Alamah, 2015; Mixer, 2008).

Leininger received numerous requests to teach courses, give lectures, and conduct workshops on human care and transcultural nursing in the United States and other countries until her death in 2012. Leininger had called for schools of nursing to offer transcultural programs to meet the worldwide demand for transculturally prepared nurses in many cultures (Leininger, 1991, 1995). These nursing programs remain urgently needed for practice, education, research, administration, consultation, and in the preparation of transcultural nurses for certification. The demand for transcultural nurses far exceeds available transculturally prepared nursing faculty, educational funding, or resources (Leininger, 1991, 1995; Leininger & McFarland, 2002, 2006; McFarland & Wehbe-Alamah, 2015).

Research

Nurses worldwide use Leininger's culture care theory in practice, research, education, and administration. This theory is the only one in nursing focused specifically on culture care with a specific research method (ethnonursing) to study cultures and care practices (Leininger, 1991, 1995; Leininger & McFarland, 2002, 2006; McFarland et al., 2012; McFarland & Wehbe-Alamah, 2015). Transcultural nurses, like many nurses, conduct their studies despite limited funds. Nurses conducting transcultural studies are leaders in sharing their research with students and colleagues at conferences and instructional programs related to transcultural nursing worldwide and have been instrumental in opening doors to transcultural nursing in many organizations. Despite societal demands for culturally competent, sensitive, and responsible care, national and international organizations began to support transcultural nursing only in the 1990s. Through the persistent efforts and exacting competencies of transcultural nurse specialists, progress has been made. Transcultural nurses have inspired other nurses to pursue research and discover new culture care knowledge in nursing. This knowledge will greatly reshape and transform current and future nursing care practices (McFarland & Wehbe-Alamah, 2015).

McFarland (1997) conducted a 2-year ethnonursing study comparing Anglo American and African American groups living in a residence home for the elderly in a large Midwestern United States city. The research was an in-depth emic and etic culture care investigation that revealed several significant findings, including the importance of using the three theory-based culture care modes of decision and action when caring for the elderly. The culturally congruent care findings were as follows:

- Anglo American and African American elderly expect culture care preservation or maintenance for their lifelong generic or folk care patterns.
- Doing for other residents rather than having a self-care focus was a major care maintenance value for both cultures and was a dominant finding.
- Protective care was more important to African American than to Anglo American elders, but nursing staff provided protective care and practiced culture care or negotiation for both groups of elders, such as accompanying them when they desired to go for walks in the surrounding inner-city neighborhood.
- African American nurses practiced culture care accommodation or negotiation when they linked their emic care with generic care values and practices.

Culture care maintenance or preservation; **culture care accommodation or negotiation**; and **culture care repatterning or restructuring** were new ways for nurses to provide culturally congruent and safe lifeways care practices for the elderly of both cultures. Based on the findings of this study, several institutional culture care policies were developed to guide professional elderly care.

FURTHER DEVELOPMENT

Leininger believed that all professional nurses in the world should be prepared in transcultural nursing and demonstrate competencies in transcultural nursing (Leininger, 1988b, 1995; Leininger & McFarland, 2002, 2006; McFarland & Wehbe-Alamah, 2015; Mixer, 2008). Transcultural nursing must become an integral part of education and practice for nurses to be relevant in the 21st century. Currently, the demand for prepared transcultural nurses far exceeds the numbers of nurses, faculty, and clinical specialists in the world. Significantly transcultural nurse theorists, researchers, and scholars are urgently needed to continue developing a body of transcultural knowledge and transform nursing education and practice. All nurses need basic knowledge about diverse cultures in the world and in-depth knowledge of two or three cultures (Leininger, 1995, 1996; Leininger & McFarland, 2002, 2006; McFarland & Wehbe-Alamah, 2015). Leininger believed that transcultural nursing research was already leading to some highly promising and different ways to advance nursing education and practice (Leininger, 1991, 1995; Leininger & McFarland, 2002, 2006; McFarland & Wehbe-Alamah, 2015). Health disciplines including medicine, pharmacy, and social work have begun to integrate transcultural health knowledge and practices into their programs of study (Leininger, 1995). This trend has increased the demand for culturally competent faculty to teach transcultural health care.

Present and future theories and studies in transcultural nursing are essential to meet the needs of culturally diverse people. The culture care theory continues to grow in importance worldwide. Both universal and diverse care knowledge are important to establish a substantive body of transcultural nursing knowledge and to support nursing as a transcultural profession and discipline. Leininger's theory has gained global interest and use because it is holistic, relevant, and futuristic and deals with specific, yet abstract, care knowledge (Leininger, 1991, 1995; Leininger & McFarland, 2002, 2006; McFarland & Wehbe-Alamah, 2015).

CRITIQUE

Simplicity

The culture care theory enables a broad, holistic, comprehensive perspective of individuals, families, cultures, communities, and populations. The theory is truly transcultural and global in scope; it is both intricate, elegant in its simplicity, and applicable to nursing practice. It is used by researchers to guide the discovery of transcultural nursing knowledge and qualitative research methods to explicate culture care phenomena. Nurse researchers develop domains of inquiry using the theory to pursue scientific and humanistic culture care knowledge. Nurses seek both universal and diverse culturally based care phenomena held by diverse cultures. Leininger's culture care theory is relevant worldwide to help guide nurse researchers to conceptualize theoretically based research questions, producing findings to guide practice (McFarland & Wehbe-Alamah, 2015). It is holistic and comprehensive, with key constructs related to worldview and key cultural and social structure dimensions as depicted in the Sunrise Enabler (McFarland et al., 2012; McFarland & Wehbe-Alamah, 2015). The theory allows for the explication of multiple conceptual interrelationships and diverse social structure factors that influence care and health (McFarland et al., 2012; McFarland & Wehbe-Alamah, 2015). Leininger found that undergraduate and graduate nursing students alike were able to use the theory and discover how practical, relevant, and useful it was to their work. The cognitive map of the theory, the Sunrise Enabler, helps nurses visualize the theory and understand its application to nursing practice and research.

Generality

The culture care theory demonstrates the criterion of generality because it is a qualitatively oriented theory that is broad, comprehensive, and worldwide in scope. The theory enables the nurse to address the provision of care from the perspective of a multicultural worldview. It is useful and applicable to groups and individuals with the goal of providing culture-specific nursing care (McFarland & Wehbe-Alamah, 2015). The broad constructs are well organized and described for study with specific cultures. The body of culture care research has led to a vast amount of expert knowledge. Many aspects of culture, care, and health have been identified as influencers of the practice of culturally congruent nursing care. More research is needed for comparative study of culture-specific and universal care knowledge (McFarland & Wehbe-Alamah, 2015). More cultural groups need to be studied to confirm their care constructs for transferability of discoveries to diverse groups and settings (McFarland & Wehbe-Alamah, 2015). Findings from the use of the culture care theory and the ethnonursing research method provide culturally congruent client care in a variety of health and community settings worldwide and transform nursing education and practice (McFarland & Wehbe-Alamah, 2015).

Accessibility

The ethnonursing research method, the qualitative method developed by Leininger for use with the theory of culture care diversity and universality, uses the criteria of **credibility**; **confirmability**; **meaning-in-context**; **recurrent patterning**; **saturation**; and **transferability** to evaluate ethnonursing research findings (McFarland & Wehbe-Alamah, 2015). Using these criteria within the ethnonursing research method, 164 care constructs have been confirmed, with more continually being discovered. The data discovered with the ethnonursing method and discovered from the people's worldview lead to credibility and confirmability of the research findings (McFarland & Wehbe-Alamah, 2015). Ongoing and future research is predicted to reveal additional culture care and health findings with implications for culturally congruent transcultural care practices and nursing education. The body of transcultural nursing knowledge that has been discovered and met the evaluative criteria over the past 6 decades has had an influence on professional nursing care practices and on the structure and function of many health care systems (Leininger, 1991, 1995; Leininger & McFarland 2002, 2006; McFarland & Wehbe-Alamah, 2015).

Importance

The theory of culture care diversity and universality has guided the provision of nursing care for meaningful and beneficial client outcomes. Providing culture-specific, culturally congruent care is an essential established goal in contemporary nursing (Eipperle, 2015; McFarland & Eipperle, 2008). The theory is central to the domain of nursing for culture care knowledge acquisition and application (McFarland & Wehbe-Alamah, 2015; Wehbe-Alamah, 2008).

The theory is highly useful, applicable, and essential to nursing practice, consultation, education, leadership, research, and administration. The concept of *care* as the central focus of nursing and the basis for building nursing knowledge and its application to practice is essential to advance culturally congruent nursing knowledge and care practices (Eipperle, 2015; McFarland & Eipperle, 2008; McFarland & Wehbe-Alamah, 2015; Wehbe-Alamah, 2008). The social structure factors of the Sunrise Enabler and the three culture care modes of decisions and actions guide the provision of culturally congruent care. The theory of culture care diversity and universality supports a sound, culturally and socially responsible discipline and profession to meet the care and health needs of a multicultural world (Wehbe-Alamah, 2008, 2011).

SUMMARY

As a holistic human care theory in nursing, the Culture Care Theory of Diversity and Universality is valued worldwide. Practicing nurses now have holistic, culturally based research findings for use in caring for clients of diverse and similar cultures or subcultures. Disciplines other than nursing have found the theory and method helpful and valuable. Newcomers to the theory and the method benefit from experienced expert mentors, in addition to studying previous transcultural research that used the theory and the method. Most important, nurses often express that the theory is natural to nursing and helps one gain fresh insights about care, health, and well-being. Unquestionably, the theory will continue to guide the building of nursing knowledge and the discovery of new applications of practice using the three culture care modes of decisions and actions in an increasingly multicultural and global society (Wehbe-Alamah, 2008, 2011). Research guided by the theory provides a credible pathway to advance the profession of nursing and the body of transcultural knowledge for application in nursing practice, consultation, education, leadership, and research worldwide.

CASE STUDY

An elderly Arab American Muslim man who spoke little English was admitted to the hospital for increasing pain at rest in his left foot. His foot was cool and pale, and he had a history of vascular surgical procedures. He had many chronic health problems, including type 2 diabetes, hypertension, and chronic obstructive pulmonary disease. He also had had a myocardial infarction and several cerebral vascular accidents. While in the hospital, he developed abdominal pain and underwent a cholecystectomy. This elderly grandfather had a large family, including a wife, nine children, and many grandchildren. His wife insisted that all family members visit him daily while he was in the hospital. The family wanted the man's face turned toward Mecca (toward the east) while they prayed with him. They brought audiotaped passages from the Koran, which they played at his bedside. Other families who were visiting their sick relatives complained to the nurses that the Arab family was taking up the entire waiting room, and there was no place for anyone else to sit.

As a transcultural nurse, how might you use the three modes of culture care decisions and actions from the theory of culture care diversity and universality to provide culturally congruent care for this elderly man and his family and for the other clients and their families in the critical care unit?

CRITICAL THINKING ACTIVITIES

1. Form a group of four students for this exercise. Each member of the group should select an ethnonursing research study reported in the *Journal of Transcultural Nursing* that used Leininger's theory of culture care diversity and universality. Each student should select a study unique to his or her own culture and different from the other students in the group. Review each study and identify its theoretical domain of inquiry, purpose, assumptions, definitions, methods, research design, data analysis, culture care modes of decisions and actions, and nursing implications.
2. Discuss the applicability of the theory of culture care diversity and universality to discover nursing knowledge and provide culturally congruent care. Take into consideration the current trends of consumers of health care, cultural diversity factors, and changes in medical and nursing school curricula. The following are examples of trends you may use as a thread to start your discussion:
   a. The importance of transcultural nursing knowledge in an increasingly diverse world
   b. The growth of lay support groups to provide information and sharing of experiences and support for

clients, families, and groups experiencing chronic, terminal, or life-threatening illnesses or treatment modalities from diverse or similar cultures

c. Cultural values, beliefs, health practices, and research knowledge in undergraduate and graduate nursing curricula across the life span
d. Inclusion of alternative or generic care in nursing curricula, such as medicine men, Native American healers, curers, and herbalists in the Southwest and selected substantiated Chinese and Ayurvedic medicine methods shown to be effective for the treatment of both acute and chronic diseases
e. The increased access to health care information from the Internet and the growing number of books, audio recordings, and video recordings published on health maintenance, alternative medicine, herbs, vitamins, minerals, and over-the-counter medications and preparations
f. Spiraling health care costs; use of health maintenance organizations, preferred provider organizations (PPO), or internal plan provider lists; lack of health insurance; increased reliance on self-diagnosis, treatment, and care; and increased availability of diagnostic kits for home-based self-diagnostic testing
g. Problems related to cultural conflicts, stress, pain, and cultural imposition practices
h. Increased suspiciousness and mistrust or distrust of cultural, religious, and political groups because of increased terrorist activities worldwide

3. Consider the patients on a unit, health department, or community-based clinic where you have clinical experience in relation to the following:
   a. Identify the cultures represented by the clients using Leininger's theory with the Sunrise Enabler and the Acculturation Health Assessment Enabler for Cultural Patterns in Traditional or Nontraditional Lifeways.
   b. Compare the cultural mix of the staff (physicians, nurses, social workers, medical and technical assistant staff, and clerks) in the area where you are considering the culture of the patients. How do they differ from their clients?
   c. Review the printed materials, such as educational and visual aids, and observe artifacts and paintings in the waiting room, examination rooms, and classrooms of the department or center to identify the cultures depicted and languages used.
   d. On the basis of data obtained from these exercises, use the theory of culture care diversity and universality to develop a plan for the provision of culturally sensitive and congruent care for clients.
4. Discuss the relevance of the theory of culture care diversity and universality for nurses in various roles working in diverse practice settings.

REFERENCES

Clarke, P. N., McFarland, M. R., Andrews, M. M., & Leininger, M. M. (2009). Caring: Some reflections on the impact of the culture care theory by McFarland & Andrews and a conversation with Leininger. *Nursing Science Quarterly*, *22*(3), 233–239.

Eipperle, M. K. (2015). Application of the three modes of culture care decisions and actions in advanced practice primary care. In M. R. McFarland & H. B. Wehbe-Alamah (Eds.). *Leininger's culture care diversity and universality: A worldwide nursing theory* (3rd ed., pp. 317–344). Burlington, MA: Jones and Bartlett Learning.

Embler, P., Mixer, S. J., & Gunther, M. (2015). End-of-life culture care practices among Yup'ik Eskimo. *Online Journal of Cultural Competence in Nursing and Healthcare*, *5*(1), 36–49.

Hofling, C. K., & Leininger, M. M. (1960). *Basic psychiatric concepts in nursing*. Philadelphia, PA: J. B. Lippincott.

Leininger, M. M. (1970). *Nursing and anthropology: Two worlds to blend*. New York: John Wiley & Sons.

Leininger, M. M. (Ed.). (1978). *Transcultural nursing: Concepts, theories, and practice*. New York: John Wiley & Sons.

Leininger, M. M. (Ed.). (1981). *Caring: An essential human need*. Thorofare, NJ: Charles B. Slack.

Leininger, M. M. (Ed.). (1984). *Care: The essence of nursing and health*. Thorofare, NJ: Charles B. Slack.

Leininger, M. M. (Ed.). (1985a). *Qualitative research methods in nursing*. New York: Grune & Stratton.

Leininger, M. M. (1985b). Transcultural care diversity and universality: A theory of nursing. *Nursing and Health Care*, *6*(4), 202–212.

Leininger, M. M. (Ed.). (1988a). *Care: The essence of nursing and health*. Detroit: Wayne State University Press.

Leininger, M. M. (Ed.). (1988b). *Caring: An essential human need*. Detroit: Wayne State University Press.

Leininger, M. M. (1990a). *Ethical and moral dimensions of care: Chapters from conference on the ethics and morality of caring*. Detroit, MI: Wayne State University Press.

Leininger, M. M. (1990b). Ethnomethods: The philosophic and epistemic bases to explicate transcultural nursing knowledge. *Journal of Transcultural Nursing*, *1*(2), 40–51.

Leininger, M. M. (Ed.). (1991). *Culture care diversity and universality: A theory of nursing*. New York, NY: National League for Nursing Press.

Leininger, M. M. (1994). Quality of life from a transcultural nursing perspective. *Nursing Science Quarterly*, *7*(1), 22–28.

Leininger, M. M. (1995). *Transcultural nursing: Concepts, theories, and practice* (2nd ed.). Columbus, OH: McGraw-Hill College Custom Series.

Leininger, M. M. (1996). Culture care theory, research and practice. *Nursing Science Quarterly*, *9*(2), 71–78.

Leininger, M. M. (2011). Leininger's reflection on the ongoing father protective care research. *The Online Journal of Cultural Competence in Nursing and Healthcare*, *1*(2), 1–13.

Leininger, M. M. (2015). Leininger's father protective care. In M. R. McFarland & H. B. Wehbe-Alamah (Eds.). *Leininger's culture care diversity and universality: A worldwide nursing theory* (3rd ed., pp. 119–136). Burlington, MA: Jones and Bartlett Learning.

Leininger, M. M., & McFarland, M. R. (2002). *Transcultural nursing: Concepts, theories, research, & practice* (3rd ed.). New York: McGraw-Hill Medical.

Leininger, M. M., & McFarland, M. R. (Eds.). (2006). *Culture care diversity and universality: A worldwide theory of nursing* (2nd ed.). Sudbury, MA: Jones & Bartlett.

Leininger, M. M., & Watson, J. (Eds.). (1990). *The caring imperative in education*. New York: National League for Nursing Press.

McFarland, M. R. (1997). Use of the culture care theory with Anglo and African Americans in a long-term care setting. *Nursing Science Quarterly*, *10*(4), 186–192.

McFarland, M. R., & Eipperle, M. K. (2008). Culture care theory: A proposed theory guide for nurse practitioner practice in primary care settings. *Contemporary Nurse*, *28*(2), 48–63.

McFarland, M. R., Mixer, S. J., Wehbe-Alamah, H. B., & Burk, R. (2012). Ethnonursing: A qualitative research method for studying culturally competent care across disciplines. *International Journal of Qualitative Methods*, *11*(3), 259–279.

McFarland, M. R., & Wehb-he-Alamah, H. B. (Eds.). (2015). *Leininger's culture care diversity and universality: A worldwide theory of nursing* (3rd ed.). Burlington, MA: Jones and Bartlett Learning.

Mixer, S. J. (2008). Use of the culture care theory and ethnonursing method to discover how nursing faculty teach culture care. *Contemporary Nurse*, *28*(2), 23–36.

Raymond, L. M., & Omeri, A. (2015). Transcultural midwifery: Culture care for Mauritian immigrant childbearing families living in New South Wales, Australia. In M. R. McFarland & H. B. Wehbe-Alamah (Eds.). *Culture care diversity and universality: A worldwide nursing theory* (3rd ed., pp. 183–254). Burlington, MA: Jones and Bartlett Learning.

Strang, C. W., & Mixer, S. J. (2016). Discovery of the meanings, expressions, and practices related to malaria care among the Maasai. *Journal of Transcultural Nursing*, *27*(4), 333–341.

Webhe-Alamah, H. B. (2008). Bridging generic and professional care practices for Muslim patients through the use of Leininger's culture care modes. *Contemporary Nurse*, *2*(28), 83–97.

Wehbe-Alamah, H. B. (2011). The use of culture care theory with Syrian Muslims in the Midwestern United States. *Online Journal of Cultural Competence in Nursing and Healthcare*, *1*(3), 1–12.

BIBLIOGRAPHY

Selected Primary Sources

Websites

International Association for Human Caring at https://iafhc.wildapricot.org/page-18059

Madeleine M. Leininger at http://www.madeleine-leininger.com/resources.shtml

Transcultural Nursing Society at www.tcns.org

Book Chapters

Leininger, M. M. (1993). Evaluation criteria and critique of qualitative research studies. In J. Morse (Ed.), *Qualitative nursing research: A contemporary dialogue* (pp. 393–414). Newbury Park, CA: Sage Publications.

Leininger, M. M. (2002). Culture care assessments for congruent competency practices. In M. M. Leininger & M. R. McFarland (Eds.), *Transcultural nursing: Concepts, theories, research, & practice* (3rd ed., pp. 117–143). New York: McGraw-Hill Medical.

Leininger, M. M. (2002). Essential transcultural nursing concepts, principles, examples, and policy statements. In M. M. Leininger & M. R. McFarland (Eds.). *Transcultural nursing: Concepts, theories, research, & practice* (3rd ed., pp. 45–69). New York: McGraw-Hill Medical.

Leininger, M. M. (2002). Lifecycle culturally-based care and health patterns of the Gadsup of New Guinea: A non-Western culture. In M. M. Leininger & M. R. McFarland (Eds.), *Transcultural nursing: Concepts, theories, research, & practice* (3rd ed., pp. 217–237). New York: McGraw-Hill Medical.

Leininger, M. M. (2002). Part I. The theory of culture care and the ethnonursing research method. In M. M. Leininger & M. R. McFarland (Eds.), *Transcultural nursing: Concepts, theories, research, & practice* (3rd ed., pp. 71–98). New York: McGraw-Hill Medical.

Leininger, M. M. (2002). Part I. Toward integrative generic and professional health care. In M. M. Leininger & M. R. McFarland (Eds.), *Transcultural nursing: Concepts, theories, research, & practice* (3rd ed., pp. 145–154). New York: McGraw-Hill Medical.

Leininger, M. M. (2002). The future of transcultural nursing: A global perspective. In M. M. Leininger & M. R. McFarland (Eds.), *Transcultural nursing: Concepts, theories, research, & practice* (3rd ed., pp. 577–595). New York: McGraw-Hill Medical.

Leininger, M. M., & McFarland, M. R. (2002). Transcultural nursing: Curricular concepts, principles, and teaching and learning activities for the 21st century. In M. M. Leininger & M. R. McFarland (Eds.), *Transcultural nursing: Concepts, theories, research, & practice* (3rd ed., pp. 527–561). New York: McGraw-Hill Medical.

Leininger, M. M. (2002). Transcultural mental health nursing. In M. M. Leininger & M. R. McFarland (Eds.), *Transcultural nursing: Concepts, theories, research, & practice* (3rd ed., pp. 239–262). New York, NY: McGraw-Hill Medical.

Leininger, M. M. (2002). Transcultural nursing and globalization of health care: Importance, focus, and historical aspects. In M. M. Leininger & M. R. McFarland (Eds.), *Transcultural nursing: Concepts, theories, research, & practice* (3rd ed., pp. 3–43). New York, NY: McGraw-Hill Medical.

Leininger, M. M. (2006). Culture care diversity and universality theory and evolution of the ethnonursing method. In M. M. Leininger & M. R. McFarland (Eds.), *Culture care diversity and universality: A worldwide theory of nursing* (2nd ed., pp. 1–41). Sudbury, MA: Jones & Bartlett.

Leininger, M. M. (2006). The ethnonursing research method and enablers. In M. M. Leininger & M. R. McFarland (Eds.), *Culture care diversity and universality: A worldwide theory of nursing* (2nd ed., pp. 43–81). Sudbury, MA: Jones & Bartlett.

Leininger, M. M. (2006). Culture care of the Gadsup Akuna of the Eastern Highlands of New Guinea: The first transcultural nursing study [revised reprint]. In M. M. Leininger & M. R. McFarland (Eds.), *Culture care diversity and universality: A worldwide theory of nursing* (2nd ed., pp. 115–157). Sudbury, MA: Jones & Bartlett.

Leininger, M. M. (2006). Culture care of the Southern Sudanese of Africa. In M. M. Leininger & M. R. McFarland (Eds.), *Culture care diversity and universality: A worldwide theory of nursing* (2nd ed., pp. 255–279). Sudbury, MA: Jones & Bartlett.

Leininger, M. M. (2015). The benefits of the theory of culture care diversity and a look to the future for transcultural nursing. In M. R. McFarland & H. B. Wehbe-Alamah (Eds.), *Culture care diversity and universality: A worldwide nursing theory* (3rd ed., pp. 101–118). Burlington, MA: Jones and Bartlett Learning.

Journal Articles

Leininger, M. M. (1997). [Classic] Overview of the theory of culture care with the ethnonursing research method. *Journal of Transcultural Nursing, 8*(2), 32–52.

Leininger, M. M. (2002). Culture care theory: A major contribution to advance transcultural nursing and practices. *Journal of Transcultural Nursing, 13*(3), 189–192.

Leininger, M. M. (2007). Theoretical questions and concerns: Response from the theory of culture care diversity and universality perspective. *Nursing Science Quarterly, 20*(1), 9–13.

Media Sources

Leininger, M. M., & McFarland, M. R. (Co-producers). (2006). *Transcultural nursing: The theory of culture care. Second of a Three-DVD Set, Transcultural Nursing*. Livonia, MI: Leininger.

Leininger, M. M., Andrews, M. M., & McFarland, M. R. (1994). *Transcultural nursing: Transforming the profession*. [Videotape]. Livonia, MI: Transcultural Nursing Society.

Secondary Sources

Media Sources

McFarland, M. R. (2011). Dr. Madeleine Leininger reflects on her father protective care research with Dr. Marilyn McFarland [Video]. *Online Journal of Cultural Competence in Nursing and Healthcare, 2*(1). doi: http://dx.doi.org/10.9730/ojccnh.org/v1n2d1.

Wehbe-Alamah, H. B., McFarland, M. R., & Vanderlaan, J. S. (2012). Leininger's early experiences in nursing and anthropology: A conversation with Dr. Madeleine Leininger [Video]. *Online Journal of Cultural Competence in Nursing and Healthcare, 4*(2). doi: http://dx.doi.org/10.9730/ojccnh.org/v2n4d1.

Books

McFarland, M. R., & Wehbe-Alamah, H. B. (Eds.). (2016). *Transcultural nursing: Concepts, theories, research, & practice* (4th ed.). New York: McGraw-Hill.

Book Chapters

Andrews, M. M. (2006). Globalization of the transcultural nursing theory and research. In M. M. Leininger & M. R. McFarland (Eds.), *Culture care diversity and universality: A worldwide theory of nursing* (2nd ed., pp. 83–114). Sudbury, MA: Jones & Bartlett.

Andrews, M. M., & Collins, J. (2015). Using the culture care theory as an organizing framework for a federal project on cultural competence. In M. R. McFarland & H. B. Wehbe-Alamah (Eds.), *Culture care diversity and universality: A worldwide nursing theory* (3rd ed., pp. 537–552). Burlington, MA: Jones and Bartlett Learning.

Courtney, R., & Wolgamott, S. (2015). Using Leininger's theory as the building block for cultural competence and cultural assessment for a collaborative care team in a primary care setting. In M. R. McFarland & H. B. Wehbe-Alamah (Eds.), *Leininger's culture care diversity and universality: A worldwide nursing theory* (3rd ed., pp. 345–368). Burlington, MA: Jones and Bartlett Learning.

Curren, D. (2006). Clinical nursing aspects discovered with the culture care theory. In M. M. Leininger & M. R. McFarland (Eds.), *Culture care diversity and universality: A worldwide theory of nursing* (2nd ed., pp. 159–180). Sudbury, MA: Jones & Bartlett.

Farrell, L. S. (2006). Culture care of the Potawatomi Native Americans who experienced family violence. In M. M. Leininger & M. R. McFarland (Eds.), *Culture care diversity and universality: A worldwide theory of nursing* (2nd ed., pp. 207–238). Sudbury, MA: Jones & Bartlett.

Knecht, L., & Sabatine, C. (2015). Application of the culture care theory to international service-learning experiences in Kenya. In M. R. McFarland & H. B. Wehbe-Alamah (Eds.), *Culture care diversity and universality: A worldwide nursing theory* (3rd ed., pp. 475–501). Burlington, MA: Jones and Bartlett Learning.

McFarland, M. R. (2014). Leininger's theory of culture care diversity and universality in nursing practice. In M. R. Alligood (Ed.), *Nursing theory: Utilization and application* (5th ed., pp. 350–367). St Louis, MO: Elsevier.

McFarland, M. R., Mixer, S. J., Lewis, A. E., & Easley, C. E. (2006). Use of the culture care theory and as a framework for the recruitment, engagement, and retention of culturally diverse students in a traditionally European American baccalaureate nursing program. In M. M. Leininger & M. R. McFarland (Eds.), *Culture care diversity and universality: A worldwide theory of nursing* (2nd ed., pp. 239–254). Sudbury, MA: Jones & Bartlett.

McFarland, M. R., Wehbe-Alamah, H. B., Vossos, H. B., & Wilson, M. (2015). Synopsis of findings discovered within a descriptive metasynthesis of doctoral dissertations guided by the culture care theory with use of the ethnonursing research method. In M. R. McFarland & H. B. Wehbe-Alamah (Eds.), *Culture care diversity and universality: A worldwide nursing theory* (3rd ed., pp. 287–315). Burlington, MA: Jones and Bartlett Learning.

McFarland, M. R., & Zehnder, N. (2006). Culture care of German American elders in a nursing home context. In M. M. Leininger & M. R. McFarland (Eds.), *Culture care diversity and universality: A worldwide nursing theory* (2nd ed., pp. 181–205). Sudbury, MA: Jones & Bartlett.

Mixer, S. J. (2015). Application of the culture care theory in teaching cultural competence and culturally congruent care. In M. R. McFarland & H. B. Wehbe-Alamah (Eds.), *Culture care diversity and universality: A worldwide nursing theory* (3rd ed., pp. 369–387). Burlington, MA: Jones and Bartlett Learning.

Morris, E. J. (2015). An examination of subculture as a theoretical construct through an ethnonursing study of urban African American adolescent gang members. In M. R. McFarland & H. B. Wehbe-Alamah (Eds.), *Culture care diversity and universality: A worldwide nursing theory* (3rd ed., pp. 255–285). Burlington, MA: Jones and Bartlett Learning.

Wehbe-Alamah, H. B. (2006). Culture care of Lebanese Muslim women in the Midwestern USA. In M. M. Leininger & M. R. McFarland (Eds.), *Culture care diversity and universality: A worldwide theory of nursing* (2nd ed., pp. 307–325). Sudbury, MA: Jones & Bartlett.

Wehbe-Alamah, H. B. (2015). Folk care beliefs and practices of traditional Lebanese and Syrian Muslims in the Midwestern United States. In M. R. McFarland & H. B. Wehbe-Alamah (Eds.), *Culture care diversity and universality: A worldwide nursing theory* (3rd ed., pp. 137–182). Burlington, MA: Jones and Bartlett Learning.

Wehbe-Alamah, H. B. (2015). Madeleine Leininger's theory of culture care diversity and universality. In M. C. Smith & M. E. Parker (Eds.), *Nursing theories and nursing practice* (4th ed., pp. 303–319). Philadelphia: F. A. Davis.

Wehbe-Alamah, H. B., & McFarland, M. R. (2015). Leininger's enablers for use with the ethnonursing research method. In M. R. McFarland & H. B. Wehbe-Alamah (Eds.), *Culture care diversity and universality: A worldwide nursing theory* (3rd ed., pp. 73–100). Burlington, MA: Jones and Bartlett Learning.

Wehbe-Alamah, H. B., & McFarland, M. R. (2015). The ethnonursing research method. In M. R. McFarland & H. B. Wehbe-Alamah (Eds.), *Culture care diversity and universality: A worldwide nursing theory* (3rd ed., pp. 35–71). Burlington, MA: Jones and Bartlett Learning.

Wehbe-Alamah, H. B., & McFarland, M. R. (2015). Transcultural nursing course outline, educational activities, and syllabi using the culture care theory. In M. R. McFarland & H. B. Wehbe-Alamah (Eds.), *Culture care diversity and universality: A worldwide nursing theory* (3rd ed., pp. 553–577). Burlington, MA: Jones and Bartlett Learning.

Wenger, A. F. Z. (2006). Culture care and health of Russian and Vietnamese refugee communities in the United States. In M. M. Leininger & M. R. McFarland (Eds.), *Culture care diversity and universality: A worldwide theory of nursing* (2nd ed., pp. 327–348). Sudbury, MA: Jones & Bartlett.

Journal Articles

Andrews, M. M. (2008). Global leadership in transcultural practice, education, and research. *Contemporary Nurse, 28*(2), 13–16.

Andrews, M. M., Thompson, T., Wehbe-Alamah, H. B., et al. (2011). Developing a culturally competent workforce through collaborative partnerships. *Journal of Transcultural Nursing, 22*(3), 300–306.

Bhat, A., Wehbe-Alamah, H. B., McFarland, M. R., Filter, M. S., & Keiser, M. (2015). Advancing cultural assessments in palliative care using web-based education. *Journal of Hospice and Palliative Nursing, 17*(4), 348–355.

Coleman, S., Garretson, B., Wehbe-Alamah, H. B., McFarland, M. R., & Wood, M. (2016). RESPECT: Reducing 30-day emergency department visits and readmissions of bariatric surgical patients effectively through cultural competency training of nurses. *Online Journal of Cultural Competence in Nursing and Healthcare, 6*(1).

Hubbert, A. O. (2005). An ethnonursing research study: Adults residing in a Midwestern Christian philosophy urban homeless shelter. *Journal of Transcultural Nursing, 16*(3), 236–244.

Hubbert, A. O. (2008). A partnership of a Catholic-based health system, nursing, and American Indian traditional medicine practitioners. *Contemporary Nurse, 28*(2), 64–72.

McFarland, M. R. (2010, October). Theoretical basis for transcultural care: Theory of culture care diversity and universality (Madeleine Leininger). In M. K. Douglas & D. F. Pacquiao (Eds.), *Core curriculum for transcultural nursing and health care*. Thousand Oaks, CA: Dual printing as supplement to *Journal of Transcultural Nursing, 21*(1), 92S–101S.

Mixer, S. J., & McFarland, M. R. (2010, October). Cross cultural communication: Use of Leininger's action modes in conflict resolution. In M. K. Douglas & D. F. Pacquiao (Eds.), *Core curriculum for transcultural nursing and health care*. Thousand Oaks, CA: Dual printing as supplement to *Journal of Transcultural Nursing, 21*(1), 147S–150S.

Mixer, S. J., McFarland, M. R., Andrews M. M., & Strang, C. W. (2013). Exploring faculty health and well-being: Creating a caring scholarly community. *Nurse Education Today, 33*(2013), 1471–1476.

Mixer, S. J., Fornehed, M. L., Varney, J., & Lindley, L. C. (2014). Culturally congruent end-of-life care for rural Appalachian people and their families. *Journal of Hospice and Palliative Nursing, 16*(8), 526–534.

Wehbe-Alamah, H. B., Farmer, M. E., McFarland, M. R., Tower, A., Jones, M., Shah, V., & El Hayek, J. (2015). Development of an extensible game architecture for teaching transcultural nursing. *Online Journal of Cultural Competence in Nursing and Healthcare, 5*(1), 64–74.

Wehbe-Alamah, H. B., McFarland, M. R., Macklin, J., & Riggs, N. (2011). The lived experiences of African American women receiving care from nurse practitioners in a nurse-managed clinic in an urban context. *Online Journal of Cultural Competence in Nursing and Health Care, 1*(1), 15–26.

Wolf, K. M., Zoucha, R., McFarland, M. R., Salman, K., Dagane, A., & Hashi, N. (2014, September 16). Somali immigrant perceptions of mental health and illness: An ethnonursing study. *Journal of Transcultural Nursing, 25* e1–e10.

23

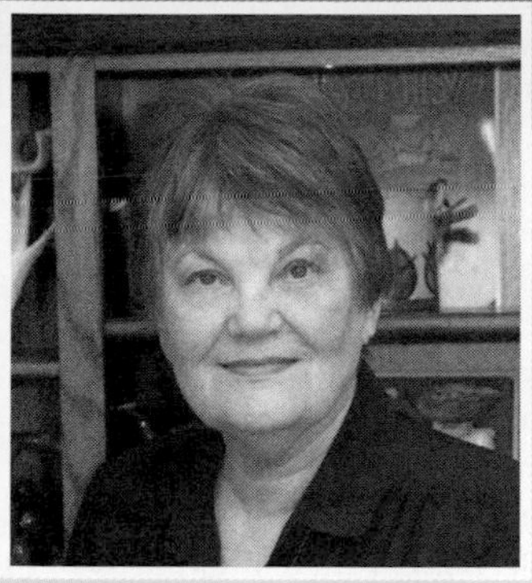
Margaret A. Newman
(1933–Present)

Health as Expanding Consciousness

Dorothy Jones and Mary Antonelli

"We have to embrace a new vision of health. Our caring must be linked with a concept of health that encompasses and goes beyond disease. The theory of health as expanding consciousness provides that perspective."
(Newman, 2008, p. 2)

CREDENTIALS AND BACKGROUND OF THE THEORIST

Margaret A. Newman was born on October 10, 1933, in Memphis, Tennessee. She earned a bachelor's degree in home economics and English from Baylor University in Waco, Texas, and a second bachelor's degree in nursing from the University of Tennessee in Memphis (M. Newman, curriculum vitae, 1996). Her master's degree in medical-surgical nursing and teaching is from the University of California, San Francisco. She earned her doctorate in nursing science and rehabilitation nursing in 1971 from New York University.

Newman held academic positions at the University of Tennessee, New York University, Pennsylvania State University, and the University of Minnesota in Minneapolis (where she is Professor Emeritus) until her retirement in 1996. During her nursing education career, she was Director of Nursing for the Clinical Research Center at the University of Tennessee, Acting Director of the PhD Program in the Division of Nursing at New York University, Professor-in-Charge of the Graduate Program and Research in Nursing at Pennsylvania State University, and Professor and nurse theorist at the University of Minnesota.

Newman achieved numerous honors and awards, including the American Academy of Nursing, 1976; Outstanding Alumnus Award, University of Tennessee College of Nursing in Memphis, 1975 and 2002; Distinguished Alumnus Award, Division of Nursing, New York University, 1984; Hall of Fame, University of Mississippi School of Nursing, 1988; Latin American teaching fellow, 1976 and 1977; *American Journal of Nursing* scholar in 1979; Distinguished Faculty, Seventh International Conference on Human Functioning, Wichita, Kansas, 1983; E. Louise Grant Award for Nursing Excellence, University of Minnesota, 1996; mention in *Who's Who in American Women, Who's Who in America,* and *Who's Who in American Nursing;* Distinguished Resident at Westminster College, Salt Lake City, Utah, 1991; Distinguished Scholar in Nursing, New York University Division of Nursing, 1992; Sigma Theta Tau Founders Elizabeth McWilliams Miller Award for Excellence in Research, 1993; and Nurse Scholar Award, Saint Xavier University School of Nursing, 1994, and she became an American Academy of Nursing Living Legend in 2008.

Newman presented her ideas on a theory of health in 1978 at a conference on nursing theory in New York. At that time, she was researching the relationship of movement, time, and consciousness and development of her theory of health as expanding consciousness. In 1985 Newman conducted workshops in New Zealand and the University of Tampere in Finland, at a weeklong conference

Previous authors: Janet Witucki Brown, Martha Raile Alligood, Snehlata Desai, M. Jan Keffer, DeAnn M. Hensley, Kimberly A. Kilgore-Keever, Jill Vass Langfitt, and LaPhyllis Peterson.
Photo courtesy of New York University, 2009

on the theory of consciousness as it relates to nursing (M. Newman, personal communication, 1988).

Newman published numerous papers, articles, book chapters, and books on theory and her theory of health as expanding consciousness. She published several books, including *Theory Development in Nursing* (1979), *Health as Expanding Consciousness* (1986, 1994), *A Developing Discipline: Selected Works of Margaret Newman* (1995a), and *Transforming Presence: The Difference That Nursing Makes* (2008). In 2011 *Nursing Science Quarterly* published an issue (volume 24, issue 3) devoted to Newman's accomplishments and honoring her work.

Many publications reflect her passion for integration of nursing theory, practice, and research; evolving viewpoints on trends in philosophy of nursing; and analysis of theoretical models of nursing practice and nursing research (Newman, 1992, 1997b, 1999, 2003). During 1989 and 1990, Newman was principal investigator of a project exploring the theory and structure of a professional model of nursing practice at Carondelet St. Mary's Community Hospitals and Health Centers in Tucson, Arizona (Newman, 1990b; Newman, Lamb, & Michaels, 1991).

Over the years, Newman provided consultation regarding the expansion of her theory of health in more than 40 states and numerous countries and served on editorial review panels, including *Nursing Research, Western Journal of Nursing Research, Nursing and Health Care, Advances in Nursing Science, Nursing Science Quarterly,* and the advisory board of *Advances in Nursing Science* (M. Newman, personal communication, 2004).

THEORETICAL SOURCES

The theory of health as expanding consciousness emanated from Newman's early personal family experiences. While caring for her mother who was experiencing restricted body movement because of amyotrophic lateral sclerosis, Newman became interested in nursing. From undergraduate years through her doctoral studies, Newman's thinking about nursing knowledge was shaped by scholars from nursing and other disciplines. These influences, life experiences, and scholarly pursuits contributed to development of Newman's theory of health as expanding consciousness.

Rogers' (1970) science of unitary human beings and her assumptions regarding wholeness, pattern, and unidirectionality are foundational to Newman's theory (M. Newman, personal communication, 2004). Hegel's fusion of opposites (Acton, 1967) helped Newman conceptualize health and illness into a new concept of health. Bentov's (1977) explication of life as the process of expanding consciousness prompted Newman to assert her concept of health as the process of expanding consciousness (M. Newman, personal communication, 2004). Newman's postulate of disease as a manifestation of the pattern of health is supported by Bohm's (1980) theory of implicate order. Newman (1994) stated that she began to comprehend "the underlying, unseen pattern that manifests itself in varying forms, including disease, and the interconnectedness and omnipresence of all that there is" (p. xxvi). Young's (1976) theory of human evolution pinpointed the role of pattern recognition for Newman. She explained that Young's ideas provided the impetus for integration of the basic concepts of her new theory—movement, space, time, and consciousness—into a dynamic portrayal of life and health (Newman, 1994). Moss's (1981) experience of love as the highest level of consciousness was important to Newman, providing affirmation and elaboration of her intuition regarding the nature of health. Newman (1997a) acknowledges contributions of multiple theories to her theory; she clarifies that her theory "was enriched by them, but was not based on them" (p. 23).

MAJOR CONCEPTS & DEFINITIONS

Health

Health is the "pattern of the whole" of a person and includes disease as a manifestation of the pattern of the whole, based on the premise that life is an ongoing process of expanding consciousness (Newman, 1986). It is regarded as the evolving pattern of the person and environment and is viewed as an increasing ability to perceive alternatives and respond in a variety of ways (Newman, 1986). Health is "a transformative process to more inclusive consciousness" (Newman, 2008, p. 16).

Using Hegel's dialectical fusion of opposites, Newman explained conceptually how disease fuses with its opposite, nondisease or absence of disease, to create a new concept of health that is relational and is "patterned, emergent, unpredictable, unitary, intuitive, and innovative," rather than a traditional linear view that is "causal, predictive, dichotomous, rational, and controlling" (Newman, 1994, p. 13). Health and the evolving pattern of consciousness are the same. The essence of the emerging paradigm of health is recognition of pattern. Newman (1994) sees the life process as progression toward higher levels of consciousness.

MAJOR CONCEPTS & DEFINITIONS—cont'd

Pattern

Pattern is information that depicts the whole and understanding of the meaning of all of the relationships at once (M. Newman, personal communication, 2004). It is conceptualized as a fundamental attribute of all there is, and it gives unity in diversity (Newman, 1986). Pattern is what identifies an individual as a particular person. Examples of explicit manifestations of the pattern of a person are the genetic pattern that contains information that directs becoming, the voice pattern, and the movement pattern (Newman, 1986). Characteristics of pattern include movement, diversity, and rhythm. Pattern is conceptualized as being somehow intimately involved in energy exchange and transformation (Newman, 1994). According to Newman (1987b), "Whatever manifests itself in a person's life is the explication of the underlying implicate pattern . . . the phenomenon we call health is the manifestation of that evolving pattern" (p. 37).

In *Health as Expanding Consciousness,* Newman (1986, 1994) developed pattern as a major concept that is used to understand the individual as a whole being. Newman described a paradigm shift in the field of health care: the shift from treatment of disease symptoms to a search for patterns and the meaning of those patterns. Newman (1994) stated that the patterns of interaction of person and environment constitute health. Individual life patterns according to Newman (2008) move "through peaks and troughs, variations in order-disorder that are meaningful for the person" (p. 6). An event such as a disease occurrence is part of a larger process. By interacting with the event, no matter how destructive the force might be, its energy augments the person's energy and enhances his or her power. One must grasp the pattern of the whole to see this (Newman, 1986). Newman notes she now views the process of unfolding pattern as evolving and unidirectional rather than fixed (i.e., stages), suggesting choice can be a moment of conscious awareness and recognition of new opportunities. As individuals select new actions and behaviors, their responses can be transforming, leading to new choices and experiences (M. Newman, personal communication, April 2016).

Consciousness

Consciousness is both the informational capacity of the system and the ability of the system to interact with its environment (Newman, 1994). Newman asserts that understanding of her definition of consciousness is essential to understanding the theory. Consciousness includes not only cognitive and affective awareness, but also the "interconnectedness of the entire living system which includes physicochemical maintenance and growth processes as well as the immune system" (Newman, 1990a, p. 38).

In 1978 Newman identified three correlates of consciousness (time, movement, and space) as manifestations of the pattern of the whole. The life process is seen as a progression toward higher levels of consciousness. Newman (1979) views the expansion of consciousness as what life and health is all about, and the sense of time is an indicator in the changing level of consciousness.

Newman (1986) integrates Bentov's (1977) definition of absolute consciousness as "a state in which contrasting concepts become reconciled and fused. Movement and rest fuse into one" (p. 67). Absolute consciousness is equated with love, where all opposites are reconciled and all experiences are accepted equally and unconditionally, such as love and hate, pain and pleasure, and disease and nondisease. Reed (1996) concurred with Newman's theory that the phase of evolutionary development is when the person moves beyond a focus on self that is limited by time, space, and physical concerns, suggesting transcendence as a process through which the person moves to a high level of consciousness.

Movement-Space-Time

Newman emphasizes the importance of examining **movement-space-time** together as dimensions of emerging patterns of consciousness rather than as separate concepts of the theory (M. Newman, personal communication, 2004).

USE OF EMPIRICAL EVIDENCE

The basic idea for the theory of health as expanding consciousness emanated from Newman's personal family experiences. Her mother's struggle with amyotrophic lateral sclerosis sparked her interest in nursing. From that experience, the idea that "illness reflected the life patterns of the person and that what was needed was the recognition of that pattern and acceptance of it for what it meant to that person" (Newman, 1986, p. 3).

Throughout Newman's writings, terms such as *call to nursing, growing conscience-like feeling, fear, power, meaning of life and health, belief of life after death, rituals of health,* and *love* suggest Newman endeavored to make a disturbing life experience logical. Her life experience triggered beginning maturation toward theory development in nursing. Within her philosophical framework, Newman began to develop a synthesis of disease–nondisease–health as recognition of the total patterning of a person.

Research has been conducted on the theoretical sources (Newman, 1987b). In 1979 Newman wrote that for nursing research to have meaning in terms of theory development, it must have three components: (1) having as its purpose the testing of theory, (2) making explicit the theoretical framework upon which the testing relies, and (3) reexamining the theoretical underpinnings in light of the findings (Newman, 1979). She believed that if health is considered an individual personal process, then research should focus on studies that explore changes and similarities in personal meaning and patterns.

MAJOR ASSUMPTIONS

The foundation for Newman's assumptions (M. Newman, personal communication, 2000) is her definition of health, which is grounded in Rogers' 1970 model for nursing, specifically, the focus on wholeness, pattern, and unidirectionality. From this, Newman developed the following assumptions that continue to support her theory (Newman, 2008).

1. Health encompasses conditions heretofore described as illness or, in medical terms, pathology.
2. These "pathological" conditions can be considered a manifestation of the total pattern of the individual.
3. The pattern of the individual that eventually manifests itself as pathology is primary and exists before structural or functional changes.
4. Removal of the pathology in itself will not change the pattern of the individual.
5. If becoming "ill" is the only way an individual's pattern can manifest itself, then that is health for that person.

From these assumptions, Newman set forth her thesis: *Health is the expansion of consciousness* (M. Newman, personal communication, 2008).

Newman's implicit assumptions about human nature include being unitary, an open system, in continuous interconnectedness with the open system of the universe, and continuously engaged in an evolving pattern of the whole (M. Newman, personal communication, 2000). She views unfolding consciousness as a process that occurs regardless of what actions nurses perform. However, nurses assist clients who are getting in touch with what is going on and in that way facilitate the process (Newman, 1994).

Newman designated "caring in the human health experience" (M. Newman, personal communication, 2004; Newman, Sime, & Corcoran-Perry, 1991, p. 3) as the focus of nursing and specified this focus as the metaparadigm of the discipline. She asserts the interrelated concepts of nursing, person, health, and environment as inherent in this focus (M. Newman, personal communication, 2004). Coming from a unitary, transformative disciplinary paradigm, Newman does not see these concepts in isolation and therefore does not discuss them separately, but has elaborated on nursing and health. In the following paragraphs, implicit definitions from Newman's work are used to discuss the four components.

Nursing

Newman emphasizes the primacy of relationships as a focus of nursing, both nurse–client relationships and relationships within clients' lives (Newman, 2008). During dialectic nurse–client relationships, clients get in touch with the meaning of their lives through identification of meanings in the process of their evolving patterns of relating (Newman, 2008). "The emphasis of this process is on knowing/caring through pattern recognition" (Newman, 2008, p. 10). Insight into these patterns provides clients with illumination of action possibilities, which then opens the way for transformation (Newman, 1990a).

Nurses facilitate pattern recognition in clients by forming relationships with them at critical points in their lives and connecting with them in authentic ways. The nurse–client relationship is characterized by "a rhythmic coming together and moving apart as clients encounter disruption of their organized, predictable state" (Newman, 1999, p. 228). She states that nurses continue to connect with clients as they move through periods of disorganization and unpredictability to arrive at a higher, organized state (Newman, 1999). The nurse comes together with clients at critical choice points in their lives and participates with them in the process of expanding consciousness. The relationship is one of rhythmicity and timing, with the nurse letting go of the need to direct the relationship or fix things. As the nurse relinquishes the need to manipulate or control, there is greater ability to enter into this fluctuating, rhythmic partnership with the client (Newman, 1999). Newman has diagrammed this nurse–client interaction of coming together and moving apart through the processes of recognition, insight, and transformation (Fig. 23.1). Nurses are partners in the process of expanding consciousness and are also transformed and have their lives enhanced in the dialogical process (Newman, 2008). As facilitator, the nurse helps an individual, family, or community focus on patterns of relating (M. Newman, personal communication, 2004; Pharris, 2005). Thus the nursing process is one of pattern recognition.

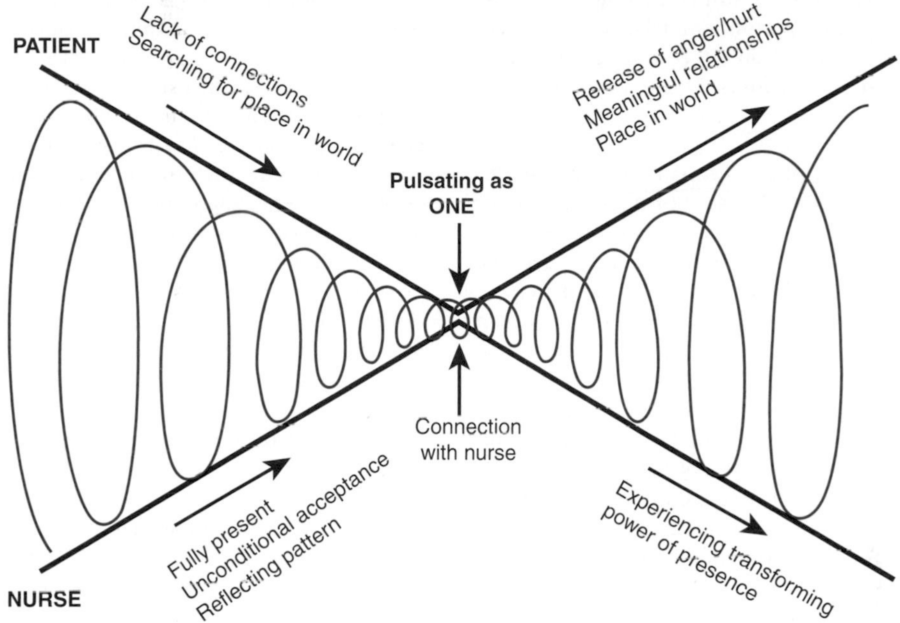

FIG. 23.1 Nurse and patient coming together and moving apart in process recognition, insight, and transformation. (From Newman, M. A. [2008]. *Transforming presence: The difference that nursing makes*. Philadelphia: F. A. Davis.)

Newman's early suggestion (Newman, 1995b) was that unitary person–environment patterns of interaction could be used to facilitate clients' pattern recognition. At that time patterns were intended to guide nurses to make holistic observations of "person-environment behaviors that together depict a very specific pattern of the whole for each person" (Newman, 1995b, p. 261). Newman (2008) subsequently has emphasized concentrating on what is most meaningful to clients in their own stories and patterns of relating.

Within the theory, the role of the nurse in nurse–client interactions is seen as a "caring, pattern-recognizing presence" (Newman, 2008, p. 16). The nurse perceives patterns in client's stories or sequences of events that change with new information. According to Newman (2008), it is important for nurses to view clients' stories comprehensively. Through active listening, nurses enter the whole through the parts and intuit the whole from the pattern. Differences are viewed as part of a unified whole. The nurse facilitates client insight through sharing in the process of pattern recognition, opening action possibilities (Newman, 1987b).

Person

Throughout Newman's work, the terms *client, patient, person, individual,* and *human being* are used interchangeably. Clients are viewed as participants in the transformative process.

Persons as individuals are identified by their individual patterns of consciousness (Newman, 1986) and defined as "centers of consciousness within an overall pattern of expanding consciousness" (Newman, 1986, p. 31). The definition of *persons* includes family and community (Newman, 1994).

Environment

Although environment is not explicitly defined, it is described as being the larger whole, which contains the consciousness of the individual. The pattern of person consciousness interacts within the pattern of family consciousness and within the pattern of community interactions (Newman, 1986). A major assumption is that "consciousness is coextensive in the universe and resides in all matter" (Newman, 1986, p. 33). Client and environment are viewed as a unitary evolving pattern (Newman, 2008).

Newman identifies interaction between person and environment as a key process that creates unique configurations for each individual. Patterns of person–environment evolve to higher levels of consciousness. The assumption is that all matter in the universe-environment possesses consciousness, but at different levels. Interpretation of

Newman's view clarifies that health is the interaction pattern of a person with the environment. Disease in a human energy field is a manifestation of a unique pattern of person–environment interaction.

Health

Health is the major concept of Newman's theory of health as expanding consciousness. A fusion of disease and nondisease creates a synthesis regarded as health (Newman, 1979, 1991, 1992). Disease and nondisease each reflect the larger whole; therefore a new concept of health, "pattern of the whole," was formed (Newman, 1986, p. 12). Newman (1999) further elaborated her view of health by stating that "health is the pattern of the whole, and wholeness *is*" (p. 228). Wholeness cannot be gained or lost. Becoming ill does not diminish wholeness within this perspective, but wholeness takes on a different form. Newman (2008) states that pattern recognition is the essence of emerging health. "Manifest health, encompassing disease and nondisease, can be regarded as the explication of the underlying pattern of person-environment" (Newman, 1994, p. 11). Therefore health and evolving pattern of consciousness are the same; specifically, health is viewed "as a transformative process to more inclusive consciousness" (Newman, 2008, p. 16).

THEORETICAL ASSERTIONS

Early Designation of Concepts and Propositions

Early writings focused on the concepts of *movement, space, time,* and *consciousness.* In *Theory Development in Nursing,* Newman (1979) delineated the relationships among movement, space, time, and consciousness. One proposition proposed a complementary relationship between time and space (Newman, 1979, 1983). Examples of this relationship were given at the macrocosmic, microcosmic, and humanistic (everyday) levels. At the humanistic level, highly mobile individuals live in a world of expanded space and compartmentalized time. There is an inverse relationship between space and time, so when a person's life space is decreased, by physical or social immobility, that person's time is increased (Newman, 1979).

Movement is a "means whereby space and time become a reality" (Newman, 1983, p. 165). Humankind is in a constant state of motion and is constantly changing internally (at the cellular level) and externally (through body movement and interaction with the environment). This movement through time and space is what gives humankind a unique perception of reality. Movement brings change and enables the individual to experience the world (Newman, 1979).

Movement was also referred to as a "reflection of consciousness" (Newman, 1983, p. 165). It is the means of experiencing reality and the means by which an individual expresses thoughts and feelings about the reality of experiences. An individual conveys awareness of self through the movement involved in language, posture, and body movement (Newman, 1979). An indication of the internal organization of a person and of that person's perception of the world can be found in the rhythm and pattern of the person's movement. Movement patterns provide additional communication beyond that which language can convey (Newman, 1979).

The concept of **time** is seen as a function of movement (Newman, 1979). This assertion was supported by Newman's (1972) studies of the experience of time as related to movement and gait tempo. Newman's research demonstrated that the slower an individual walks the less subjective time is experienced. However, compared with clock time, time seems to "fly." Although individuals who are moving quickly subjectively feel that they are "beating the clock," they report that time seems to be dragging when checking a clock (Newman, 1972, 1979).

Time is also conceptualized as a measure of consciousness (Newman, 1979). Bentov (1977) measured consciousness with a ratio of subjective to objective time and proposed this assertion. Newman applied this measure of consciousness to subjective and objective data from her research and found "increasing consciousness with age" (Newman, 1982, p. 293). Newman cited this evidence as support for her position that the life process evolves toward consciousness expansion. However, she asserted that certain moods, such as depression, might be accompanied by a diminished sense of time (Newman & Gaudiano, 1984).

Synthesis of Patterns of Movement, Space-Time, and Consciousness

As the theory evolved, Newman developed a synthesis of the pattern of movement, space, time, and consciousness (M. Newman, personal communication, 2004, 2008). Time was not merely conceptualized as subjective or objective, but was viewed in a holographic sense (M. Newman, personal communication, 2000). According to Newman (1994), "Each moment has an explicate order and also enfolds all others, meaning that each moment of our lives contains all others of all time" (p. 62). Newman (1986) illustrated the centrality of space-time in the following example:

> *"Mrs. V. made repeated attempts to move away from her husband and to move into an educational program to become more independent. She felt she had no space for herself, and she tried to distance herself (space) from her husband. She felt she had no time for leisure (self), was overworked, and was constantly meeting other people's needs. She was submissive to the demands and criticism of her husband."*
>
> ***(p. 56)***

Space, time, and movement later became linked with Newman's (1986) assertion that the intersection of movement-space-time represented the person as a center of consciousness. Furthermore, this varied from person to person, place to place, and time to time. Newman (1986) emphasized that the crucial task of nursing is to be able to see the concepts of movement-space-time in relation to one another and consider them all at once, recognizing patterns of evolving consciousness.

In *Health as Expanding Consciousness* (Newman, 1986, 1994), Newman's theory encompassed the work of Young's spectrum of consciousness (Young, 1976). She saw Young's central theme as one in which self and universe were of the same nature. This essential nature could not be defined but was characterized by complete freedom and unrestricted choice at both the beginning and the end of life's trajectory (Newman, 1986).

Newman established a corollary between her model of health as expanding consciousness and Young's conception of the evolution of human beings (Fig. 23.2). She explained that individuals came into being from a state of consciousness, and that they were bound in time, found their identity in space, and, through movement, learned the "law" of the way that things worked; they then made choices that ultimately took them beyond space and time to a state of absolute consciousness (Newman, 1994).

Newman (1994) also stated that restrictions in movement-space-time have the effect of forcing an awareness that extends beyond the physical self. When natural movement is altered, space and time are also altered. When movement is restricted (physical or social), it is necessary for an individual to move beyond self, thereby making movement an important choice point in the process of evolving human consciousness (Newman, 1994). She assumed that the awareness corresponded to the "inward, self-generated reformation that Young [spoke] of as the turning point of the process" (Newman, 1994, p. 46). When a person progresses to the state of timelessness, there is increasing freedom from time. Finally, the last stage is absolute consciousness, which Newman (1994) asserted is equated with love.

Emphasis on the Experiential Process of Nurse–Client

With the realization that the early research testing of propositional statements stemmed from a mechanistic view of movement-space-time consciousness and failed to honor the basic assumptions of her theory, Newman shifted focus to authentic involvement of the nurse researcher as a participant with the client in the unfolding pattern of expanding consciousness (Newman, 2008). The unitary, transformative paradigm demanded that the

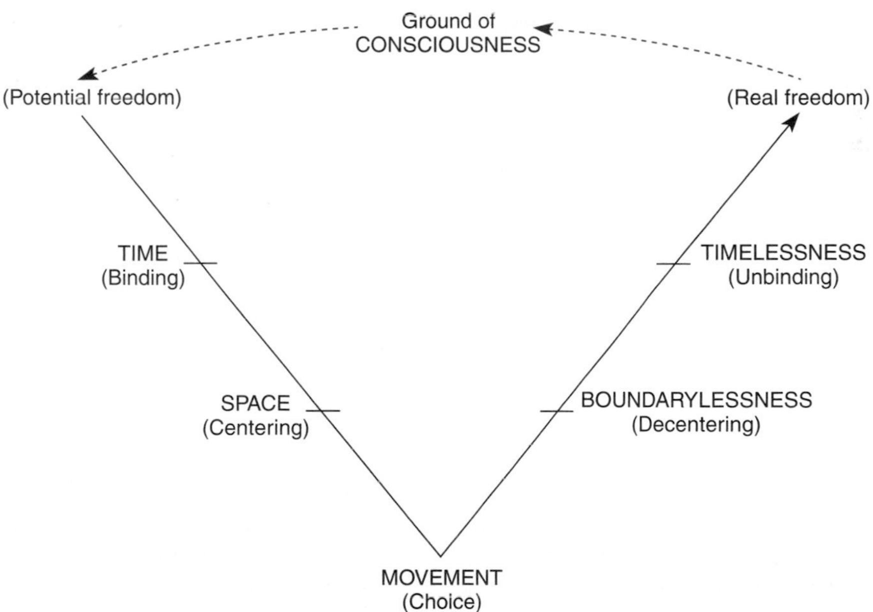

FIG. 23.2 Parallel between Newman's theory of expanding consciousness and Young's stages of human evolution. (From Newman, M. A. [1990]. Newman's theory of health as praxis. *Nursing Science Quarterly, 3*[1], 37–41.)

research honor and reveal the mutuality of interaction between nurse and client, the uniqueness and wholeness of pattern in each client situation, and movement of the life process toward higher consciousness.

"With the unitary, transformative paradigm the researcher honors and reveals the mutuality of interaction between nurse and client with the intent to help" (Newman, 2008, p. 21). Further, this process focuses "on transformation from one point to another and incorporates the uniqueness and wholeness of pattern in each client situation, and movement of the life process toward higher consciousness" (Newman, 2008, p. 21). Newman (2008) states, "The nature of nursing practice is the caring, pattern-recognizing relationship between nurse and client—a relationship that is a transforming presence" (p. 52).

The protocol for this research was first started in 1994, and variations of this guide continue to be implemented in current praxis research. Litchfield (1999) explicated this process as "practice wisdom" in her work with families of hospitalized children, and Endo (1998) analyzed the phases of the process in her work with women with ovarian cancer. The data of this praxis research reveal evidence of expanding consciousness in the quality and connectedness of the client's relationships and support the importance of the nurse's creative presence in participants' insight (M. Newman, personal communication, 2004, 2008). Variations of the praxis research have been used in numerous populations and settings (Newman, 2008; Picard & Jones, 2007).

This method of inquiry is called **cooperative inquiry** or **interactive, integrative participation**. Newman (1989, 1990a) developed a method to describe patterns as unfolding and evolving over time. Newman (1990a) stated that during the development of a methodology to test the theory of health, "sharing our (researcher's) perception of the person's pattern with the person was meaningful to the participants and stimulated new insights regarding their lives" (p. 37).

In 1994, she described the research protocol as **hermeneutic dialectic**, a method that allows the pattern of person–environment to reveal itself without disturbing the unity of the pattern (M. Newman, personal communication, 2000).

LOGICAL FORM

Newman used both inductive and deductive logic in early theory development. Inductive logic is based on observing particular instances and then relating those instances to form a whole. Newman's theory development was derived from her earlier research on time perception and gait tempo. Time and movement, with space and consciousness, were subsequently used as central components in her early conceptual framework. These concepts helped explain "the phenomena of the life process and therefore of health" (Newman, 1979, p. 59). Newman (1997a) describes the evolution of the theory as it moved from linear explication and testing of concepts of time, space, and movement to an elaboration of interacting patterns as manifestations of expanding consciousness. Evolution of the theory of health as expanding consciousness as a process of evolving in conjunction with research progressed through several stages (Newman, 1997a, 1997b). These stages included testing the relationships of the concepts of movement, space, and time; identifying sequential person–environmental patterns; and recognizing the centrality of nurse–client relationships or dialogue in the clients' evolving insight and accompanying potential for action. The process actually became cyclical as the original concepts of movement-space-time emerged as dimensions in the unitary evolving process of consciousness (Newman, 1997a).

ACCEPTANCE BY THE NURSING COMMUNITY

Practice

Newman believes that research within the theory of health as expanding conscious is praxis, which she defines as a "mutual process between nurse and client with the intent to help" (Newman, 2008, p. 21). Furthermore, this mutual process focuses "on transformation from one point to another and incorporates the guidance of an a priori theory" (Newman, 2008, p. 21). Research and practice are interwoven with the theory.

In Newman's view, the responsibility of nurses is to establish a primary relationship with the individual-participant for the purpose of identifying meaningful patterns and facilitating the individual-participant's action potential and decision-making ability (Newman, 2008). Communication and collaboration with other nurses, associates, and health care professionals are essential (Newman, 1989). Nurses as primary care providers who are focused completely on relationships with the individual(s) can relate well to her view of the professional nurse role. From the Newman perspective, nursing is the study of "caring in the human health experience" (Newman, Lamb, & Michaels, 1991, p. 3). The role of the nurse in this experience is to help individuals recognize their patterns, which results in the illumination of action possibilities that open the way for transformation.

The theory has been used in practice with various client populations. Kalb (1990) applied Newman's theory of health in the clinical management of pregnant women hospitalized for complications of maternal–fetal health.

Smith's (1995) work focused on the health of rural African American women. Yamashita (1999) studied Japanese and Canadian family caregivers, Rosa (2006, 2016) worked with persons living with chronic skin wounds. Benzein, Olin, and Persson (2014) found Swedish family conversations that reflected Newman's well-being also managed their health better. Kamau, Rotich, and Mwembe (2015) applied Newman's theory to design nursing care of patients infected with human immunodeficiency virus (HIV) in Kenya, Africa. Pierre-Louis and colleagues (2011) studied patterns in the lives of African American women with diabetes, MacLeod (2011) studied experiences of spousal caregivers, and Ness (2009) applied the theory to study pain expression in perioperative Somali women.

Studies have focused on patterns of persons with rheumatoid arthritis (Brauer, 2001; Neill, 2002; Schmidt, Brauer, & Peden-McAlpine, 2003), patterns of patients with cancer (Barron, 2005; Endo, 1998; Endo et al., 2000; Karian, Jankowski, & Beal, 1998; Kiser-Larson, 2002; Moch, 1990; Newman, 1995c; Roux, Bush, & Dingley, 2001; Utley, 1999), coronary heart disease (Newman & Moch, 1991), chronic obstructive pulmonary disease (Jonsdottir, 1998), hepatitis C (Thomas, 2002), and HIV and acquired immune deficiency syndrome (AIDS) (Kamau, Rotaich, & Mwembe, 2015; Lamendola & Newman, 1994).

Hayes (2015) used Newman's theory to study the patterns of incarcerated women. Hatzfeld and colleagues (2015) studied factors influencing health behavior in military personnel and reported that the descriptions aligned with Newman's theory. Tiffany and Hoglund (2016) applied Newman's theory in nursing education with a simulated case study.

Litchfield (1999) described the patterning of nurse–client relationships in families with frequent illness and hospitalization of toddlers and its use in family health. Weingourt (1998) reported on the use of Newman's theory of health with elderly nursing home residents, and Capasso (2005) reported increased emotional and physical client healing as a result of use of the theory in nurse–client interactions.

Additional research includes studies that involved recognizing health patterns in persons with multiple sclerosis (Neill, 2005), spousal caregivers of partners with dementia (Brown & Alligood, 2004; Brown et al., 2007), adolescent males incarcerated for murder (Pharris, 2002), and life experiences of black Caribbean women (Peters-Lewis, 2006). Additional studies have included life patterns of women who successfully lost weight and maintained weight loss (Berry, 2002), a focus on victimizing sexuality and healing patterns (Smith, 1997), the meaning of death of an adult child to an elder (Weed, 2004), the experience of family members living through the sudden death of a child (Picard, 2002), nurse facilitation of health as expanding consciousness in families of children with special health care needs (Falkenstern, 2003), and health as expanding consciousness to conceptualize adaptation in burn patients (Casper, 1999).

Newman's research as praxis has also been used to describe the lived experience of life passing in middle-adolescent females (Shanahan, 1993), patterns of expanding consciousness in women in midlife (Picard, 2000) and women transitioning through menopause (Musker, 2005), and patterns in families of medically fragile children (Tommet, 2003). Endo and colleagues (2005) conducted action research involving practicing nurses and found that nurses experienced deeper meaning in their lives as a result of the transformative power of pattern recognition in their work with clients. Flanagan (2005) found that preoperative nurses working within the theory saw the effect of their presence in changing patient experiences. Ruka (2005) developed a model of nursing home practice for use in pattern recognition with persons with dementia. Bateman and Merryfeather (2014) describe the personal positive benefit in the lives of nurses whose practice is based on Newman's theory of health as expanding consciousness. Dyess (2011) focused on the concept of faith in the context of health as expanding consciousness. Haney and Tufts (2012) used health as expanding consciousness to frame a home health care study of electronic communication for parental well-being and satisfaction in relation to medically fragile children.

Education

Newman (1986) stated that ideally, "Nurses need to be free to relate to patients in an ongoing partnership that is not limited to a particular place or time" (Newman, 1986, p. 89). She suggested that nursing education revolve around pattern as a concept, substance, process, and method. Education by this method enables nurses to be recognized as an important resource for the continued development of health care. Newman (2008) proposes that, "attention to the nature of transformative learning will help to establish the priorities of the discipline" (p. 73). As students and teachers engage in intuitive awareness, they resonate with each other in a transforming way (Endo et al., 2007).

Newman's theory in relation to nursing education reveals that teaching the praxis research method also teaches students a practice method that is congruent with the theory, and it is a means for students to experience transformation through pattern recognition (Newman, 2008). Newman sees theory, practice, and research as process rather than separate domains. Teaching the theory of health as expanding consciousness moves from a dichotomous view of health to a view that accepts disease as a manifestation of health. Learning to let go of the professional's control and respecting the individual patient's choices are integral parts of practice within this framework. Students and practicing nurses who use Newman's theory face personal transformation by learning to recognize patterns through nurse–client interactions. An individual's personal experience is the core not just of teaching and practice, but of research as well. Newman (1994) explains that nurses need to sense their own pattern of relating as an indication of the nurse–client interacting pattern. She emphasizes that there needs to be a sense of the process of the relationship with clients from within, giving attention to the "we" in the nurse–client relationship (Newman, 1997b).

Newman's theory has been used in nursing education to provide content into a model called the **healing web.** This model was designed to integrate nursing education and nursing service with private and public education programs for baccalaureate and associate nursing degree programs in South Dakota (Bunkers et al., 1992). A number of scholars describe the application of the health as expanding consciousness theory in various aspects of nursing education (Clarke & Jones, 2011; Endo et al., 2007; Picard & Mariolis, 2002, 2005; Tiffany & Hoglund, 2016). Sethares and Gramling (2014) demonstrated how using the theory within a clinical curriculum allowed the students to know their patients from a more holistic perspective. This experience was transformative for students and their patients. These experiences allow for the "possibility of bringing this knowledge forward into the understanding of professional nursing" (Sethares & Gramling, 2014, p. 307).

Research

From the beginning Newman's theory of health was useful in the practice of nursing because it contained the concepts of movement and time that are used by the nursing profession and intrinsic to nursing interventions such as range of motion and ambulation (Newman, 1987a). Early research with the theory manipulated concepts of space, time, and movement. Besides Newman, several researchers conducted research about time, space, or movement. Newman and Gaudiano (1984) focused on depression in older adults and decreased subjective time. Mentzer and Schorr (1986) used Newman's model of duration of time as a consciousness index in a study of institutionalized older adults. Engle (1986) addressed the relationship between movement, time, and assessment of health. Schorr and Schroeder (1989) studied differences in consciousness with regard to time and movement, and in another study examined relationships among type A behavior, temporal orientation, and death anxiety as manifestations of consciousness with mixed results (Schorr & Schroeder, 1991). During the 1980s, using health as expanding consciousness, Marchione investigated the meaning of disabling events in families in which an additional person became part of the nuclear family. The addition was a disruptive event for the family and created disturbances in time, space, movement, and consciousness, suggesting that Newman's work with patterns could be used to understand family interactions (Marchione, 1986). This awareness ushered in decades of research and progress with the hermeneutic pattern process of nursing research and practice. Newman sees health as expanding consciousness as emerging from a Rogerian perspective, incorporating theories of caring and projecting a transformative process (Newman, 2005). Future researchers will be greatly assisted by Smith's (2011) comprehensive review of the theory of health as expanding consciousness research literature.

FURTHER DEVELOPMENT

Previously discussed research studies and application in nursing practice in this chapter support the theory of health as expanding consciousness, illuminating the importance of pattern recognition in the process of expanding consciousness. The theory has been used extensively to explore and understand the experience of health within illness, supporting the premise of the theory, that disruptive situations provide a catalytic effect and facilitate movement to higher levels of consciousness.

CRITIQUE

Clarity

There is semantic clarity in the definitions, descriptions, and dimensions of the concepts of the theory. The language used, the logical order, and the explanatory process contribute to the clarity of this theory.

Simplicity

The deeper meaning of the theory of health as expanding consciousness is complex. The theory must be understood as a whole rather than isolating the concepts. Newman advocated in the 1994 edition of her book, *Health as Expanding Consciousness,* that the holistic approach of the hermeneutic dialectic method is consistent with the theory and requires a high level of understanding of the theory on the part of the researcher to extend the theory in praxis research (M. Newman, personal communication, 1996).

Generality

The concepts in Newman's theory are broad in scope, and they all relate to health. The theory has been applied in many cultures and across the spectrum of nursing care situations (M. Newman, personal communication, 2004). Application of the theory is universal in nature. The broad scope has provided a focus for middle-range theory development. Consideration of findings from the research continues to expand the generalizability of the theory.

Accessibility

The early stages of development of the theory were tested with the traditional quantitative scientific mode. The hermeneutic dialectic approach developed subsequently has been used extensively for full explication of its meaning and application, demonstrating areas of application as well as its modality for clinical practice. Health as expanding consciousness is used in different cultures nationally and internationally. The theory is used with individuals as well as with groups and is used to influence health policy development, practice, and research. Its application changes the way care is delivered and affects the lives of the nurse and the patient. Nurses have said that once they come to know the person and pattern using the framework, it is difficult to practice any other way (Newman, 2008).

Importance

The focus of Newman's theory of health as expanding consciousness provides an evolving guide for all health-related disciplines. In the quest for understanding the phenomenon of health, this unique view of health challenges nurses to make a difference in nursing practice by the application of this theory. Newman's health as expanding consciousness provides a perspective of nursing that recognizes and honors clients' histories, unique attributes and experiences, desires and goals, and life journeys (Bateman & Merryfeather, 2014; Newman, 1994). The volume of literature cited in this chapter illustrates the global importance of Newman's nursing theory.

SUMMARY

Although Newman started with a rational, empirical approach that was both inductive and deductive, she found it restrictive and "not consistent with the paradigm from which the theory was drawn" (1997a, p. 23). With time her work evolved to a more interactive, integrative approach but continued to be objective and controlled. When she shifted from the scientific paradigm with its objectivity and control and allowed the principles of her theoretical paradigm to guide her research, she began to see the core of pattern and process as nursing practice. She saw that the evolving pattern in process required an approach of mutual process, rather than objective observation. Patterns showed that expanding consciousness was related to quality and connectedness of relationships. The nurse researcher's creative presence was vital to the participant's insight. Newman (1986) concluded that individuals experience a theory in living it. She labeled her research as hermeneutic dialectic. The Theory of Health as Expanding Consciousness, along with the research as praxis method, has been used extensively in nursing practice with a variety of individuals, family and community situations, nursing education, and practice models and nursing research in the United States and other countries of the world. Newman continues to write, consult, and lecture, advancing her work.

CASE STUDY

Alice is an 81-year-old widow who has lived alone in a low-income apartment complex in a small rural Appalachian town since her husband's death 8 years ago. She has one surviving family member, a granddaughter, who lives 30 miles away. Alice never learned to drive and depends on her granddaughter for all transportation to physician appointments and for shopping and getting medications. Her income is $824 monthly, and she requires several expensive prescriptions for arthritis, hypertension, and cardiac problems. She has osteoarthritis in her knees and requires a quad cane for support and safety when getting around her apartment. A visiting nurse stops by weekly to check her blood pressure and to give her an injection for her arthritis. The visiting nurse notes that Alice's blood pressure is elevated, and Alice states that she has been unable to get her medication because her granddaughter's car is broken. Alice mentions that she is low on food in the apartment because she can't get out to shop.

Alice admits that she hardly knows or speaks to her neighbors despite having lived there for 8 years, and she still feels like a stranger and doesn't want to "push myself in." She says that she hates to bother people and "won't

Continued

CASE STUDY—cont'd

hardly unless I just have to." She says she sometimes gets lonely for "her people," who are all deceased.

The visiting nurse, working with Alice, recognizes the current situation as a choice point, with potential for increased interaction with others and increased consciousness. The old ways no longer work for Alice, and new ways of relating are necessary. The nurse incorporates the elements of Newman's method to assist Alice in pattern recognition for the purpose of discovering new potentials for action. As the nurse has Alice relate her story, through dialogue and interaction Alice recognizes past patterns of relating and how present circumstances changed those patterns. Alice talks about how she and her husband lived for 56 years in a rural mountain cabin with few neighbors except for two sisters and their daughter. They were very self-sufficient, grew large gardens, had their own livestock, and rarely went into town. All the family members are deceased now except the granddaughter, who insisted that Alice leave the cabin and move into town after the death of her husband. It seems apparent that Alice's past patterns have been those of independence and limiting social contact to mainly family members.

The nurse shares her perceptions with Alice, who confirms and verifies the pattern. Alice states, "I just don't know how long I am going to manage by myself anymore." The nurse helps her explore sources of aid, in addition to the granddaughter, that may help Alice remain in her apartment as independently as possible. Alice relates that there is one man, a few doors away, who has stopped several times to ask if she needed anything from the grocery store, but she hasn't asked him because she hates to bother him and doesn't want "to be beholden." After further discussion, she decides that she will ask him to pick up staples and medications for her and will pay him back by baking him bread, saying, "I just love to bake anyway and haven't had anyone much to bake for."

In subsequent weekly visits, Alice and the nurse explore the possibility of getting medications at a reduced price through the local nurse-managed clinic. Alice states that she might try getting to know some of her neighbors. The nurse helps Alice make arrangements to be picked up by the Senior Van for physician appointments. As Alice begins to build her own support system, she finds that she relies on the nurse less for help with maintaining her independence, and they resume their pattern of the nurse checking her blood pressure and giving her injections weekly. However, Alice and the nurse have now developed a relationship that has transformed them both, and the nurse is often met at the door with the smell of fresh-baked bread and an invitation to "have a bite." They both enjoy this new relationship.

CRITICAL THINKING ACTIVITIES

1. Describe your own view of health, health care practice, and nursing practice, and compare your views with those of Newman.
2. What is the view of nursing with health as expanding consciousness?
3. How does this view guide the nurse–patient relationship?
4. How does this view direct nursing knowledge development?
5. What changed Newman's view of health, nursing practice, and research?
6. Consider a patient you have cared for in the past, and describe how health as expanding consciousness (pattern of the whole) might have changed your practice with that patient.

POINTS FOR FURTHER STUDY

- Brown, J. W., & Alligood, M. R. (2014). Newman's theory of health and nursing practice. In M. R. Alligood (Ed.), *Nursing theory: Utilization & application* (5th ed., pp. 394–411). St Louis, MO: Mosby-Elsevier.
- Newman, M. A. (1997). *Margaret Newman: Health as expanding consciousness* (video). Available from Fitne, Inc, 5 Depot Street, Athens, OH 45701, (800) 691–8480.
- Newman, M. A. (2008). *Transforming presence: The difference that nursing makes.* Philadelphia: F. A. Davis.
- Smith, M. C. (2011). Integrative review of research related to Margaret Newman's theory of health as expanding consciousness. *Nursing Science Quarterly, 24*(3), 256–263.

REFERENCES

Acton, H. B. (1967). George Wilhelm Freidrich Hegel 1770–1831. In P. Edwards (Ed.), *The encyclopedia of philosophy* (Vols. 3 & 4). New York: Macmillan & Free Press.

Barron, A. (2005). Suffering, growth, and possibility: Health as expanding consciousness in end-of-life care. In C. Picard & D. Jones (Eds.), *Giving voice to what we know: Margaret Newman's theory of health as expanding consciousness in nursing practice, research, and education* (pp. 43–50). Sudbury, MA: Jones & Bartlett.

Bateman, G. C., & Merryfeather, L. (2014). Newman's theory of health as expanding consciousness: A person evolution. *Nursing Science Quarterly, 27*(1), 57–61.

Bentov, I. (1977). *Stalking the wild pendulum*. New York: Dutton.

Benzein, E., Olin, C., & Persson, C. (2015). "You get it all together"—families' evaluation of participating in family health conversations. *Scandinavian Journal of Caring Sciences, 29*(1), 136–144.

Berry, D. C. (2002). *Newman's theory of health as expanding consciousness in women maintaining weight loss.* Doctoral dissertation, Boston College. *Dissertation Abstracts International, 63*, 2300.

Bohm, D. (1980). *Wholeness and the implicate order*. London: Routledge and Kegan Paul.

Brauer, D. J. (2001). Common patterns of person-environment interaction in persons with rheumatoid arthritis. *Western Journal of Nursing Research, 23*, 414–430.

Brown, J. W., & Alligood, M. R. (2004). Realizing wrongness: Stories of older wife caregivers. *Journal of Applied Gerontology, 23*(2), 104–119.

Brown, J. W., Chen, S. L., Mitchell, C., & Province, A. (2007). Help-seeking by older husbands caring for wives with dementia. *Journal of Advanced Nursing, 59*(4), 352–360.

Bunkers, S. S., Bendtro, M., Holmes, P. K., et al. (1992). The healing web: A transformative model for nursing. *Nursing and Health Care, 13*, 68–73.

Capasso, V. A. (2005). The theory is the practice: An exemplar. In C. Picard & D. Jones (Eds.), *Giving voice to what we know: Margaret Newman's theory of health as expanding consciousness in nursing practice, research, and education* (pp. 65–71). Sudbury, MA: Jones & Bartlett.

Casper, S. A. (1999). *Psychological adaptation as a dimension of health as expanding consciousness: Effectiveness of burn survivors support groups.* Master's thesis, D'Youville College Buffalo, New York. *Masters Abstracts International, 37*, 1433.

Clarke, P. N., & Jones, D. A. (2011). Expanding consciousness in nursing education and practice. *Nursing Science Quarterly, 24*(3), 223–226.

Dyess, S. M. (2011). Faith: A concept analysis. *Journal of Advanced Nursing, 12*, 2723–2731.

Endo, E. (1998). Pattern recognition as a nursing intervention with Japanese women with ovarian cancer. *Advances in Nursing Science, 20*(4), 49–61.

Endo, E., Miyahara, T., Sizuli, S., & Ohmasa, T. (2005). Partnering of researcher and practicing nurses for transformative nursing. *Nursing Science Quarterly, 18*(2), 138–145.

Endo, E., Nitta, N., Inayoshi, M., et al. (2000). Pattern recognition as a caring partnership in families with cancer. *Journal of Advanced Nursing, 32*, 603–610.

Endo, E., Takaki, M., Abe, K., Terashima, K., & Nitta, N. (2007). *Creating a helping model with nursing students who want to quit smoking: Patterning in a nursing student-teacher partnership based on M. Newman's theory of health.* Paper presented at The Power of Caring: The Gateway to Healing, 29th Annual International Association for Human Caring Conference, St Louis, MO, May 16–19.

Engle, V. (1986). The relationship of movement and time to older adults' functional health. *Research in Nursing and Health, 9*, 123–129.

Falkenstern, S. K. (2003). *Nursing facilitation of health as expanding consciousness in families who have a child with special health care needs.* Unpublished doctoral dissertation, Pennsylvania State University, University Park, PA.

Flanagan, J. M. (2005). Creating a healing environment for staff and patients in a pre-surgery clinic. In C. Picard & D. Jones (Eds.), *Giving voice to what we know: Margaret Newman's theory of health as expanding consciousness in nursing practice, research, and education*. Sudbury, MA: Jones & Bartlett.

Haney, T., & Tufts, K. A. (2012). A pilot study using electronic communication in home healthcare: Implications on parental well-being and satisfaction caring for medically fragile children. *Home Healthcare Nurse, 30*(4), 216–224.

Hatzfeld, J., Nelson, M., Waters, C., & Jennings, B. (2016). Factors influencing health behaviors among active duty Air Force personnel. *Nursing Outlook, 64*(5), 440–449.

Hayes, M. (2015). The life patter of incarcerated women: The complex and interwoven lives of trauma, mental illness, and substance abuse. *Journal of Forensic Nursing, 11*(4), 214–222.

Jonsdottir, H. (1998). Life patterns of people with chronic obstructive pulmonary disease: Isolation and being closed in. *Nursing Science Quarterly, 11*(4), 160–166.

Kalb, K. A. (1990). The gift: Applying Newman's theory of health in nursing practice. In M. Parker (Ed.), *Nursing theories in practice* (pp. 163–186). New York: National League for Nursing.

Kamau, S. M., Rotich, R. J., & Mwembe, D. J. (2015). Applying Margaret Newman's theory of health as expanding consciousness to psychosocial nursing care of HIV infected patients in Kenya. *American Journal of Nursing Science, 4*(1), 6–11.

Karian, V. E., Jankowski, S. M., & Beal, J. A. (1998). Exploring the lived experience of childhood cancer survivors. *Journal of Pediatric Oncology, 15*, 153–162.

Kiser-Larson, N. (2002). Life pattern of native women experiencing breast cancer. *International Journal for Human Caring, 6*(2), 61–68.

Lamendola, F. P., & Newman, M. A. (1994). The paradox of HIV/AIDS as expanding consciousness. *Advances in Nursing Science, 16*(3), 13–21.

Litchfield, M. (1999). Practice wisdom. *Advances in Nursing Science, 22*(2), 62–73.

MacLeod, C. E. (2011). Understanding experiences of spousal caregivers with health as expanding consciousness. *Nursing Science Quarterly, 24*(3), 245–255.

Marchione, J. M. (1986). Pattern as methodology for assessing family health: Newman's theory of health. In P. Winstead-Fry (Ed.), *Case studies in nursing theory*. (214–240). New York: National League for Nursing.

Mentzer, C., & Schorr, J. A. (1986). Perceived situational control and perceived duration of time: Expressions of life patterns. *Advances in Nursing Science, 9*(1), 13–20.

Moch, S. D. (1990). Health within the experience of breast cancer. *Journal of Advanced Nursing, 15*, 1426–1435.

Moss, R. (1981). *The I that is we*. Millbrae, CA: Celestial Arts.

Musker, K. M. (2005). *Life patterns of women transitioning through menopause*. Doctoral dissertation, Loyola University, Chicago.

Neill, J. (2002). Transcendence and transformation in the life patterns of women living with rheumatoid arthritis. *Advances in Nursing Science, 24*(4), 27–47.

Neill, J. (2005). Recognizing pattern in the lives of women with multiple sclerosis. In C. Picard & D. Jones (Eds.), *Giving voice to what we know* (pp. 153–165). Sudbury, MA: Jones & Bartlett.

Ness, S. M. (2009). Pain expression in the perioperative period: Insights from a focus group of Somali women. *Pain Management Nursing, 10*(2), 65–75.

Newman, M. A. (1972). Time estimation in relation to gait tempo. *Perceptual and Motor Skills, 34*, 359–366.

Newman, M. A. (1979). *Theory development in nursing*. Philadelphia: F. A. Davis.

Newman, M. A. (1982). Time as an index of expanding consciousness with age. *Nursing Research, 31*, 290–293.

Newman, M. A. (1983). Newman's health theory. In I. W. Clements & F. B. Roberts (Eds.), *Family health: A theoretical approach to nursing care*. (pp. 161–175). New York: Wiley.

Newman, M. A. (1986). *Health as expanding consciousness*. St Louis: Mosby.

Newman, M. A. (1987a). Aging as increasing complexity. *Journal of Gerontological Nursing, 13*(9), 16–18.

Newman, M. A. (1987b). Patterning. In M. Duffy & N. J. Pender (Eds.), *Conceptual issues in health promotion. A* report of proceedings *of a Wingspread Conference, Racine, WI, April 13–15, 1987*. (pp. 36–50). Indianapolis: Sigma Theta Tau.

Newman, M. A. (1989). The spirit of nursing. *Holistic Nursing Practice, 3*(3), 1–6.

Newman, M. A. (1990a). Newman's theory of health as praxis. *Nursing Science Quarterly, 3*(1), 37–41.

Newman, M. A. (1990b). Shifting to higher consciousness. In M. Parker (Ed.), *Nursing theories in practice* (pp. 129–139). New York: National League for Nursing.

Newman, M. A. (1991). Health conceptualizations. In J. J. Fitzpatrick, R. L. Taunton, & A. K. Jacox (Eds.), *Annual review of nursing research* (vol. 9). (pp. 221–242). New York: Springer.

Newman, M. A. (1992). Nightingale's vision of nursing theory and health. In F. Nightingale (Ed.), *Notes on nursing: What it is, and what it is not* (commemorative edition, pp. 44–47). Philadelphia: Lippincott.

Newman, M. A. (1994). *Health as expanding consciousness* (2nd ed.). Sudbury MA: Jones & Bartlett (NLN Press).

Newman, M. A. (1995a). *A developing discipline: Selected works of Margaret Newman*. New York: National League for Nursing Press.

Newman, M. A. (1995b). Dialogue: Margaret Newman and the rhetoric of nursing theory. *Image: The Journal of Nursing Scholarship, 27*, 261.

Newman, M. A. (1995c). Recognizing a pattern of expanding consciousness in persons with cancer. In M. A. Newman (Ed.), *A developing discipline: Selected works of Margaret Newman* (pp. 159–171). New York: National League for Nursing Press.

Newman, M. A. (1997a). Evolution of the theory of health as expanding consciousness. *Nursing Science Quarterly, 10*(1), 22–25.

Newman, M. A. (1997b). Experiencing the whole. *Advances in Nursing Science, 20*, 34–39.

Newman, M. A. (1999). The rhythm of relating in a paradigm of wholeness. *Image: The Journal of Nursing Scholarship, 31*, 227–230.

Newman, M. A. (2003). A world of no boundaries. *Advances in Nursing Science, 26*(4), 240–245.

Newman, M. A. (2005). Foreword. In C. Picard & D. Jones (Eds.), *Giving voice to what we know: Margaret Newman's theory of health as expanding consciousness* (pp. xii–xv). Sudbury, MA: Jones & Bartlett.

Newman, M. A. (2008). *Transforming presence: The difference that nursing makes*. Philadelphia: F. A. Davis.

Newman, M. A., & Autio, S. (1986). *Nursing in a prospective payment system health care environment*. Minneapolis: University of Minnesota.

Newman, M. A., & Gaudiano, J. K. (1984). Depression as an explanation for decreased subjective time in the elderly. *Nursing Research, 33*, 137–139.

Newman, M. A., Lamb, G. S., & Michaels, C. (1991). Nurse case management: The coming together of theory and practice. *Nursing and Health Care, 12*, 404–408.

Newman, M. A., & Moch, S. D. (1991). Life patterns of persons with coronary heart disease. *Nursing Science Quarterly, 4*(4), 161–167.

Newman, M. A., Sime, M. A., & Corcoran-Perry, S. A. (1991). The focus of the discipline of nursing. *Advances in Nursing Science, 14*, 1–6.

Peters-Lewis, A. (2006). *How the strong survive: Health as expanding consciousness and the life experiences of Black Caribbean women*. Doctoral dissertation, Boston College.

Pharris, M. D. (2002). Coming to know ourselves as community through a nursing partnership with adolescents convicted of murder. *Advances in Nursing Science, 24*(3), 21–42.

Pharris, M. D. (2005). Engaging with communities in a pattern recognition process. In C. Picard & D. Jones (Eds.), *Giving voice to what we know: Margaret Newman's theory of health as expanding consciousness in nursing practice, research, and education* (pp. 83–93). Sudbury, MA: Jones & Bartlett.

Picard, C. A. (2000). Pattern of expanding consciousness in midlife women: Creative movement and the narrative as modes of expression. *Nursing Science Quarterly, 13*(2), 150–157.

Picard, C. (2002). Family reflections on living through sudden death of a child. *Nursing Science Quarterly, 15*(3), 242–250.

Picard, C., & Jones, D. (Eds.). (2007). *Giving voice to what we know: Margaret Newman's theory of health as expanding*

consciousness in nursing practice, research, and education. Sudbury, MA: Jones & Bartlett.
Picard, C., & Mariolis, T. (2002). Teaching-learning process. Praxis as a mirroring process: Teaching psychiatric nursing grounded in Newman's health as expanding consciousness. *Nursing Science Quarterly, 15*(2), 118–122.
Picard, C., & Mariolis, T. (2005). Praxis as a mirroring process: Teaching psychiatric nursing grounded in Newman's health as expanding consciousness. In C. Picard & D. Jones (Eds.), *Giving voice to what we know: Margaret Newman's theory of health as expanding consciousness in nursing practice, research, and education* (pp. 169–177). Sudbury, MA: Jones & Bartlett.
Pierre-Louis, B., Akoh, V., White, P., & Pharris, M. D. (2011). Patterns in the lives of African-American women with diabetes. *Nursing Science Quarterly, 24*(3), 227–236.
Reed, P. G. (1996). Transcendence: Formulating nursing perspectives. *Nursing Science Quarterly, 9*(1), 2–4.
Rogers, M. E. (1970). Nursing, a science of unitary man. In J. P. Riehl & C. Roy (Eds.), *Conceptual models for nursing practice.* New York: Appleton-Century-Crofts.
Rosa, K. C. (2006). A process model of healing and personal transformation in persons with chronic skin wounds. *Nursing Science Quarterly, 19*(4), 359–358.
Rosa, K. C. (2016). Integrative review on the use of Newman praxis relationship in chronic illness. *Nursing Science Quarterly, 29*(3), 211–218.
Roux, G., Bush, H. A., & Dingley, C. E. (2001). Inner strength in women with breast cancer. *Journal of Theory Construction and Testing, 5*(1), 19–27.
Ruka, S. (2005). Creating balance: Rhythms and patterns in people with dementia living in a nursing home. In C. Picard & D. Jones (Eds.), *Giving voice to what we know: Margaret Newman's theory of health as expanding consciousness in nursing practice, research, and education.* (pp. 95–104). Sudbury, MA: Jones & Bartlett.
Schmidt, B. J., Brauer, D. J., & Peden-McAlpine, C. (2003). Experiencing health in the context of rheumatoid arthritis. *Nursing Science Quarterly, 16*(2), 155–162.
Schorr, J. A., & Schroeder, C. A. (1989). Consciousness as a dissipative structure: An extension of the Newman model. *Nursing Science Quarterly, 2*(4), 183–193.
Schorr, J. A., & Schroeder, C. A. (1991). Movement and time: Exertion and perceived duration. *Nursing Science Quarterly, 4*(3), 104–112.
Sethares, K. A., & Gramling, K. L. (2014). Newman's health as expanding consciousness in baccalaureate education. *Nursing Science Quarterly, 27*(4), 302–307.
Shanahan, S. M. (1993). The lived experience of life-passing in middle adolescent females. *Masters Abstracts International, 32,* 1376.
Smith, C. A. (1995). The lived experience of staying healthy in rural African American families. *Nursing Science Quarterly, 8*(1), 17–21.
Smith, M. C. (2011). Integrative review of research related to Margaret Newman's theory of health as expanding consciousness. *Nursing Science Quarterly, 24*(3), 256–263.
Smith, S. K. (1997). Women's experiences of victimizing socialization. Part I: Responses related to abuse and home and family environment. *Issues in Mental Health Nursing, 18,* 395–416.
Thomas, J. A. (2002). What are the life patterns of people with hepatitis C? Doctoral dissertation, University of Nevada, Reno. *Dissertation Abstracts International, 41,* 194.
Tiffany, J. M., & Hoglund, B. A. (2016). Using virtual simulation to teach inclusivity: A case study. *Clinical Simulation in Nursing, 12*(4), 115–122.
Tommet, P. A. (2003). Nurse-parent dialogue: Illuminating the evolving pattern of families of children who are medically fragile. *Nursing Science Quarterly, 16*(3), 239–246.
Utley, R. (1999). The evolving meaning of cancer for long-term survivors of breast cancer. *Oncology Nursing Forum, 26,* 1519–1523.
Weed, L. D. (2004). *The meaning of the death of an adult child to an elder: A phenomenological investigation.* Unpublished doctoral dissertation, University of Tennessee, Knoxville, TN.
Weingourt, R. (1998). Using Margaret A. Newman's theory of health with elderly nursing home residents. *Perspectives in Psychiatric Care, 34*(3), 25–30.
Yamashita, M. (1999). Newman's theory of health applied to family caregiving in Canada. *Nursing Science Quarterly, 12*(1), 73–79.
Young, A. M. (1976). *The reflexive universe: Evolution of consciousness.* San Francisco: Robert Briggs.

BIBLIOGRAPHY

Primary Sources

Newman, M. A. (1971). *An investigation of the relationship between gait tempo and time perception.* Unpublished doctoral dissertation, New York University.
Newman, M. A. (1990). Shifting to higher consciousness. In M. Parker (Ed.), *Nursing theories in practice* (pp. 129–139). New York: National League for Nursing.
Newman, M. A. (1994). Theory for nursing practice. *Nursing Science Quarterly, 7*(4), 153–157.
Newman, M. A. (1999). Letters to the editor: A commentary on Newman's theory of health as expanding consciousness. *Advances in Nursing Science, 21*(3), viii–ix.
Newman, M. A. (2002). Caring in the human health experience. *International Journal for Human Caring, 6*(2), 8–12.
Newman, M. A. (1981). The meaning of health. In G. E. Laskar (Ed.), *Applied systems research and cybernetics: Vol. 4. Systems research in health care, biocybernetics and ecology* (pp. 1739–1743). New York: Pergamon.
Newman, M. A. (1987). Nursing's emerging paradigm: The diagnosis of pattern. In A. M. McLane (Ed.), *Classification of nursing diagnoses. Proceedings of the seventh conference, North American Nursing Diagnosis Association* (pp. 53–60). St Louis: Mosby.
Newman, M. A. (1993). Prevailing paradigms in nursing. *Nursing Outlook, 40*(1), 10–14.
Newman, M. A. (1996). Prevailing paradigms in nursing. In J. W. Kenney (Ed.), *Philosophical and theoretical perspectives for*

advanced nursing practice (pp. 302–307). Sudbury, MA: Jones & Bartlett.

Newman, M. A. (1996). Theory of the nurse-client partnership. In E. Cohen (Ed.), *Nurse case management in the 21st century* (pp. 119–123). St Louis: Mosby.

Newman, M. A. (1997). A dialogue with Martha Rogers and David Bohm about the science of unitary human beings. In M. Madrid (Ed.), *Patterns of Rogerian knowing* (pp. 3–10). New York: National League for Nursing.

Newman, M. A. (2003). The immediate applicability of nursing praxis. *Quality Nursing: The Japanese Journal of Nursing Education and Nursing Research, 9*(5), 4–6.

Secondary Sources

Batty, M. L. E. (1999). *Pattern identification and expanding consciousness during the transition of "low risk" pregnancy. A study embodying Newman's health as expanding consciousness (Margaret Newman).* Master's thesis, University of New Brunswick, Canada. *Masters Abstracts International, 39,* 826.

Brown, J. W. (2011). Health as expanding consciousness: A nursing perspective for Grounded Theory research. *Nursing Science Quarterly, 24*(3), 197–201.

Cowling, W. R. III, Newman, M., Watson, J., & Smith, M. (2007). The power of wholeness, consciousness, and caring: a dialogue on nursing science, art, and healing. (Abstract). *International Journal for Human Caring, 11*(3), 52.

Dean, P. J. (2002). Aesthetic expression. A poem dedicated to the nursing theories of Martha Rogers and Margaret Newman. *International Journal for Human Caring, 6,* 70.

Ford-Gilboe, M. V. (1994). A comparison of two nursing models: Allen's developmental health model and Newman's theory of health as expanding consciousness. *Nursing Science Quarterly, 7*(3), 113–118.

Jacono, B. J., & Jacono, J. J. (1996). The benefits of Newman and Parse in helping nurse teachers determine methods to enhance student creativity. *Nurse Education Today, 16,* 356–362.

Jonsdottir, H., Litchfield, M., & Pharris, M. D. (2003). Partnership in practice. *Research and Theory for Nursing Practice, 17,* 51–63.

Lamb, G. S., & Stempel, J. E. (1994). Nurse case management from the client's view: Growing as insider-expert. *Nursing Outlook, 42,* 7–13.

Lamendola, F. P., & Newman, M. A. (1994). The paradox of HIV/AIDS as expanding consciousness. *Advances in Nursing Science, 16*(3), 13–21.

Litchfield, M. (1999). Practice wisdom. *Advances in Nursing Science, 22*(2), 62–73.

Moch, S. D. (1998). Health-within-illness: Concept development through research and practice. *Journal of Advanced Nursing, 28,* 305–310.

Neill, J. (2002). From practice to caring praxis through Newman's theory of health as expanding consciousness: A personal journey. *International Journal for Human Caring, 6*(2), 48–54.

Nelson, M. L., Howell, J. K., Larson, J. C., & Karpiuk, K. L. (2001). Student outcomes of the healing web: Evaluation of a transformative model for nursing education. *Journal of Nursing Education, 40,* 404–413.

Pharris, M. D. (2001). Margaret A. Newman, health as expanding consciousness. In M. Parker (Ed.), *Nursing theories and nursing practice.* Philadelphia: F. A. Davis.

Picard, C. (2002). Family reflections on living through sudden death of a child. *Nursing Science Quarterly, 15*(3), 242–250.

Quinn, J. F. (1992). Holding sacred space: The nurse as healing environment. *Holistic Nursing Practice, 6*(4), 26–36.

Schorr, J. A., Farnham, R. C., & Ervin, S. M. (1991). Health patterns in aging women as expanding consciousness. *Advances in Nursing Science, 13*(4), 52–63.

Schorr, J. A., & Schroeder, C. A. (1989). Consciousness as a dissipative structure: An extension of the Newman model. *Nursing Science Quarterly, 2*(4), 183–193.

Schorr, J. A., & Schroeder, C. A. (1991). Movement and time: Exertion and perceived duration. *Nursing Science Quarterly, 4*(3), 104–112.

Smith, C. A. (1995). The lived experience of staying healthy in rural African American families. *Nursing Science Quarterly, 8*(1), 17–21.

Yamashita, M. (1997). Family caregiving: Application of Newman's and Peplau's theories. *Journal of Psychiatric and Mental Health Nursing, 4,* 401–405.

Yamashita, M. (1998). Family coping with mental illness: A comparative study. *Journal of Psychiatric and Mental Health Nursing, 5,* 515–523.

Yamashita, M. (1998). Newman's theory of health as expanding consciousness: Research on family caregiving in mental illness in Japan. *Nursing Science Quarterly, 11*(3), 110–115.

24

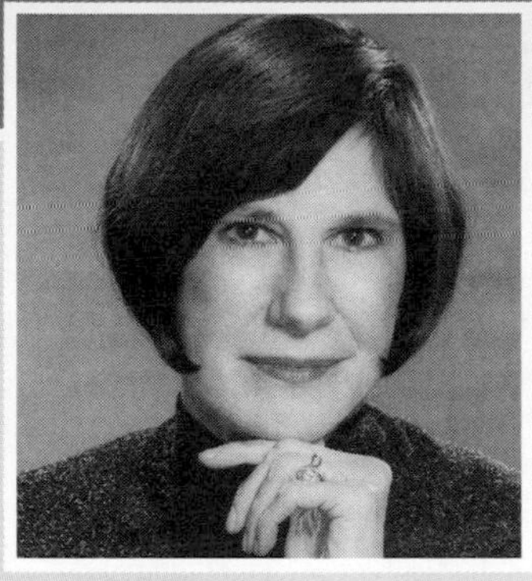
Rosemarie Rizzo Parse

Humanbecoming

Debra A. Bournes, Sandra Schmidt Bunkers, and Gail J. Mitchell

"The assumptions and principles of humanbecoming incarnate a deep concern for the delicate sentiments of being human and show a profound recognition of human freedom and dignity."
(Parse, 2007b, p. 310)

CREDENTIALS AND BACKGROUND OF THE THEORIST

Rosemarie Rizzo Parse is a graduate of Duquesne University in Pittsburgh and received her master's and doctorate degrees from the University of Pittsburgh. She was a faculty member of the University of Pittsburgh, Dean of the Nursing School at Duquesne University (1977–1982), Professor and Coordinator of the Center for Nursing Research at Hunter College of the City University of New York (1983–1993), Professor and Niehoff Chair at Loyola University Chicago (1993–2006), and Distinguished Professor Emeritus at Loyola University Chicago (2006 to present). In January 2007, she became a Consultant and Visiting Scholar at New York University College of Nursing, where she was also an adjunct professor until 2012. Dr. Parse is founder and current editor of *Nursing Science Quarterly* and President of Discovery International. She founded the Institute of Humanbecoming, where she teaches the humanbecoming paradigm in nursing (Parse, 1981, 1998, 2005, 2007b, 2010, 2011b, 2012b, 2014).

Dr. Parse is a Fellow in the American Academy of Nursing, where she initiated and chaired the nursing theory–guided practice expert panel. As editor of *Nursing Science Quarterly,* she has spearheaded a well-known, highly cited venue for nurse scholars to share and debate matters important to nursing research and theory development for over 30 years. For this and other works, Dr. Parse has received several honors. She has received two Lifetime Achievement Awards (one from the Midwest Nursing Research Society and one from the Asian American Pacific Islander Nurses Association), the Rosemarie Rizzo Parse Scholarship was endowed in her name at the Henderson State University School of Nursing, her books were twice named "best picks" by Sigma Theta Tau International, and the Society of Rogerian Scholars honored her with the Martha E. Rogers Golden Slinky Award. In 2008 she received the *New York Times* Nurse Educator of the Year Award, and in 2012 she received the Medal of Honor at the University of Lisbon in Portugal.

Throughout her career, Dr. Parse has made outstanding contributions to the discipline and profession of nursing through progressive leadership in nursing knowledge development, research, education, and practice. She has explored the ethics of human dignity, set forth humanbecoming tenets of human dignity (Parse, 2010), and developed teaching-learning (Parse, 2004), mentoring (Parse, 2008b), leading-following (Parse, 2008a, 2011a), community (Parse, 2003, 2012b), and family (Parse, 2009a) models that are used worldwide. She has published 10 books (Morrow, 2012b; Parse, 1974, 1981, 1987, 1995, 1998, 1999a, 2001b, 2003, 2014) and more than 150 articles and editorials about matters pertinent to nursing and other health-related disciplines. Dr. Parse has shared her knowledge in more than 300 local, national, and international presentations and workshops in more than 35 countries on five continents. Her works have been translated into many languages, and she consults throughout the world with nursing education programs and health care settings that are using her work to guide research, practice, leadership, education, and regulation of quality standards. She has planned and implemented many international conferences on nursing theory, the humanbecoming paradigm, qualitative research, and quality of life.

Parse has chaired more than 40 doctoral dissertations, guided more than 300 students with creative research conceptualizations, and mentored faculty and students on qualitative and quantitative research proposals, grant applications, and manuscripts for publications. She developed basic and applied science research methods (Parse, 2001b, 2005, 2011b, 2014, 2016a, 2016b); conducted multiple qualitative research studies about living experiences of health and quality of life (such as hope, laughing, joy-sorrow, feeling respected, contentment, feeling very tired, and quality of life for persons with Alzheimer disease); and taught theory and research courses in institutions of higher learning, including Loyola University Chicago, University of Cincinnati, University of Dayton, University of South Carolina, and others.

Parse is an articulate, courageous, and vibrant leader with a strong vision and deliberate determination to advance the discipline of nursing. She is well known internationally for the humanbecoming paradigm—a nursing perspective focused on living quality and human dignity from the perspective of patients, families, and communities. She is an inspirational mentor whose diligent loving presence, consistent and willing availability, and respectful and gentle urgings have helped many seasoned and budding nurse scholars to pursue their dreams. Those who have had the honor of working with her as students and colleagues have been mentored by this truly outstanding nurse leader (Bournes, 2007; Cody, 2012).

THEORETICAL SOURCES

The humanbecoming theory has evolved over time. First, it was the humanbecoming nursing theory, then it became the humanbecoming school of thought; by 2016 it had evolved to the humanbecoming paradigm (Parse, 2016). The humanbecoming paradigm makes explicit that "cocreating reality as a seamless symphony of becoming is the central thought foundational to the ontology of humanbecoming" (p. 26). Several new concepts have emerged with the new paradigm and they include the following: humanuniverse as indivisible, unpredictable, and everchanging cocreation; the ethos of humanbecoming is dignity—presence, existence, trust, and worth; and living quality as the becoming visible–invisible becoming of the emerging now (Parse, 2014). The epistemology of the humanbecoming paradigm is universal humanuniverse living experiences (Parse, 2016a, 2016b) and the basic sciencing methodologies, include Parsesciencing and humanbecoming hermeneutic sciencing (Parse, 2016a, 2016b). (See referenced articles for further descriptions of the methods.) Parse no longer uses the term *research,* but rather uses *sciencing,* which is more in line with the thinking of the new paradigm. *Nursing practice* is no longer the language used for this paradigm, but rather *living the art of nursing in true presence* is the way a nurse is with others in illuminating meaning, shifting rhythms, and inspiring transcending (the person does this in the true presence of the nurse) (Parse, 2014, 2016b). This is the language of the humanbecoming paradigm.

The humanbecoming paradigm is grounded in human science proposed by Dilthey and others (Cody & Mitchell, 2002; Mitchell & Cody, 1992; Parse, 1981, 1987, 1996, 1998, 2007b, 2010, 2012b, 2014). The humanbecoming paradigm is "consistent with Martha E. Rogers' principles and postulates about unitary human beings, and it is consistent with major tenets and concepts from existential-phenomenological thought, but it is a new product, a different conceptual system" (Parse, 1998, p. 4). Parse developed her theory while working at Duquesne University in Pittsburgh (during the 1960s and 1970s) when Duquesne was regarded as the center of the existential-phenomenological movement in the United States. Dialogue with scholars such as van Kaam and Giorgi stimulated her thinking on the living experiences of humans and their situated freedom and participation in life.

Parse synthesized the science of unitary human beings, developed by Martha E. Rogers (1970, 1992) with the fundamental tenets from existential-phenomenological thought, articulated by Heidegger, Sartre, and Merleau-Ponty, and secured nursing as a human science. She contends that humans cannot be reduced to component parts and be understood. Rather, persons are living beings who are different from schemata that divide them. Parse challenges the traditional medical view of nursing and distinguishes the discipline of nursing as a unique, basic science focused on universal humanuniverse living experiences. She supports the notion that nurses require a unique knowledge base that informs their living the art and sciencing that is essential to fulfill their commitment to humankind (Parse, 1981, 1987, 1993, 2007b, 2010, 2012b, 2014, 2016a, 2016b).

In creating humanbecoming, Parse (1981) drew on Rogers' principles of helicy, integrality, and resonancy and her postulates (energy field, openness, pattern, and pandimensionality) (Parse, 1981; Rogers, 1970, 1992). These ideas underpin Parse's notions about persons as open beings who relate with the universe illimitably, that is, "with indivisible, unbounded knowing extended to infinity" (Parse, 2007b, p. 308), and who are indivisible, unpredictable, everchanging, and recognizable by pattern (Parse, 1981, 1998, 2007b, 2012b).

From existential-phenomenological thought, Parse drew on the tenets of intentionality and human subjectivity and the corresponding concepts of coconstitution, coexistence, and situated freedom (Parse, 1981, 1998, 2007b, 2012b). She uses the prefix *co-* on many of her words to denote the participative nature of persons. *Co-* means "together with," and, for Parse, humans can never be separated from their relationships with the universe—thus her 2007(b) conceptualizations of *humanbecoming* and humanuniverse as one word. Relationships with the universe include all the linkages humans have with other people and with ideas, projects, predecessors, history, and culture (Parse, 1981, 1998, 2007b, 2012b).

From Parse's perspective, humans are intentional. That is, humans have an open and meaningful stance with the universe and people, projects, and ideas that constitute living experiences. Being intentional means that humans' involvements are not random. They are chosen for reasons known and not known. Intentionality is also about purpose and how persons choose direction, ways of thinking, and acting with projects and people. People choose attitudes and actions with illimitable options (Parse, 1981, 1998, 2007b, 2012b, 2014).

The basic tenet, human subjectivity, means viewing humans not as things or objects, but as indivisible, unpredictable, everchanging beings (Parse, 1998, 2007b) and as a mystery of being with nonbeing. Humans live all-at-onceness as the becoming visible–invisible becoming of the emerging now (Parse, 2012b). Parse posits that humans' presence with the world is personal and that humans live meaning as their becoming who they are. As people choose meanings and projects according to their value priorities, they coparticipate with the world in indivisible, unbounded ways (Parse, 1981, 1998, 2007b, 2012b, 2014). Persons are inseparable from the world and craft unique relationships. A person's becoming is complex and full of explicit-implicit meaning (Parse, 1981, 1998, 2007b, 2012b, 2014).

Coconstitution means any moment is cocreated with the constituents of the situation (Parse, 1981, 1998, 2007b, 2012b, 2014). Humans choose meaning with the particular constituents of day-to-day life. Life happens, events unfold in expected and unexpected ways, and the human being coconstitutes personal meaning and significance. Coconstitution surfaces with opportunities and limitations for humans as they live their presence with the world, and as they make choices about what things mean and how to proceed. The term *coconstitution* refers to creating different meanings from the same situations. People change and are changed through their personal interpretations of life situations. Various ways of thinking and acting unite familiar patterns with newly emerging ones as people craft their unique realities.

Coexistence means "the human is not alone in any dimension of becoming" (Parse, 1998, p. 17). Humans are always with the world of things, ideas, language, unfolding events, and cherished traditions, and they also are always with others—not only contemporaries, but also predecessors and successors. Humans are community (Parse, 2003). Indeed, Parse posits that "without others, one would not know that one is a being" (1998, p. 17). Persons think about themselves in relation to others and how they might be with their plans and dreams. Connected with freedom, Parse describes an abiding respect for human change and possibility.

Finally, situated freedom means that human beings emerge in the context of a time and history, a culture and language, physicality, and potentiality. Parse suggests that human freedom means "reflectively and prereflectively one participates in choosing the situations in which one finds oneself as well as one's attitude toward the situations" (Parse, 1998, p. 17). Humans are always choosing what is important in their lives. They decide the attention to give to situations, projects, and people. In day-to-day living, people choose and act on their value priorities, and value priorities shift as life unfolds. Sometimes acting on beliefs is as important as achieving a desired outcome. Personal integrity is intimately connected to situated freedom.

In 2007, 2012, and 2014, Parse published important conceptual refinements for the humanbecoming paradigm. First, in 2007, she changed human becoming and human-universe to *humanbecoming* and *humanuniverse*. These changes, according to Parse (2007b), further specify her commitment to the indivisibility of cocreation. Parse's new concepts of humanbecoming and humanuniverse demonstrate through language that there is no space for thinking that humans can be separated from becoming or the universe—these notions are irreducible.

In addition, Parse (2007b) specified four postulates that permeate all principles of humanbecoming. The four postulates are *illimitability, paradox, freedom,* and *mystery*. The four postulates further specify ideas embedded within Parse's school of thought. Illimitability represents Parse's thinking about the indivisible, unpredictable, everchanging nature of humanbecoming. Parse (2007b) stated, "Illimitability is the 'unbounded knowing extended to infinity, the all-at-once remembering and prospecting with the moment'" (p. 308). Indivisible, unbounded knowing "is a privileged knowing accessible only to the individual living the life" (Parse, 2008e, p. 46). Paradox has always been affiliated with humanbecoming, and Parse's bringing it forth as a postulate that permeates all theoretical principles emphasizes the importance of paradox with humanuniverse cocreation. She stated, "paradoxes are not opposites to be reconciled or dilemmas to be overcome but, rather, are lived rhythms . . . expressed as a pattern preference" (Parse, 2007b, p. 309), "incarnating an individual's choices in day-to-day living" (Parse, 2008e, p. 46). Humans make choices about how they will be with paradoxical experiences and continuously make choices about where to focus their attention. For example, all humans live paradoxical rhythms of certainty–uncertainty, joy–sorrow, and others, and they move with the rhythm of their paradoxical experiences—at times focusing on certainty or joy, for instance, yet always having an awareness of living the uncertainty or sorrow inherent in situations. Likewise, freedom, although a cornerstone of Parse's early thinking, is seen in a new light in her most recent thinking. Parse (2007b) stated that freedom is "contextually construed liberation" (p. 309). People have freedom within their situations to choose ways of being. Finally, mystery, the fourth postulate, is presented in a more specific way as something special that transcends the conceivable and as the unfathomable and unknowable that always accompanies the "indivisible, unpredictable, everchanging humanuniverse" (p. 309).

In 2012 Parse introduced new conceptualizations that further specify the meaning of the all-at-onceness of human experience from a humanbecoming perspective. Her belief system (ontology) underpinning humanbecoming "specifies that with humanuniverse the human is an august presence, a seamless symphony of becoming, living the emerging now. **Becoming visible–invisible becoming of the emerging now** is the living moment that brings to the fore the idea that meaning changes with each unfolding living experience incarnating the remembered with the prospected all-at-once" (Parse, 2012b, p. 44). The becoming visible–invisible becoming of the emerging now is the universe of histories and experiences and hopes and dreams that cocreate each moment, as humans live and shape their lives with their illimitable, unbounded knowing. Human living experiences surface moment to moment like waves surfacing from an ocean. What is becoming visible in human experience is what is happening in the moment that is explicitly known and described by the person living it. It is like waves that are swelling to the top of the ocean—visible for a moment, yet always shifting and changing and being cocreated with what is happening in the entirety of the ocean, invisible beneath the surface yet cocreating the waves that are becoming visible with their invisible becoming. Then in 2013 Parse identified **living quality** as "the individual's core whatness, the stuff of a life" (p. 112). Living quality is the becoming visible–invisible becoming of the emerging now (Parse, 2013, 2014).

Based on her latest thinking, Parse (2007b, 2012b, 2014) refined the wording of the three principles of her theory (see the Major Concepts & Definitions box).

MAJOR CONCEPTS & DEFINITIONS

Three principles constitute the humanbecoming theory flowing from these themes—meaning, rhythmicity, and transcendence (Parse, 1981, 1998, 2007b, 2012b, 2014). Each principle contains three concepts that require thoughtful exploration to understand the depth of the humanbecoming theory. The principles (Parse, 2014) are as follows:

1. Structuring meaning is the imaging and valuing of languaging.
2. Configuring rhythmical patterns is the revealing–concealing and enabling–limiting of connecting–separating.
3. Cotranscending with possibles is the powering and originating of transforming (p. 36).

Principle I: Structuring Meaning

"**Structuring meaning** is the imaging and valuing of languaging" (Parse, 2014, p. 36). This principle specifies that persons structure, or choose, the meaning of their realities, and this choosing happens with explicit-tacit knowing. Sometimes questions are not answerable, because people may not know why they think or feel one way or another. This first principle posits that people create their reality illimitably with others, and they show or language their reality in the ways they speak and remain silent and in the ways they move and stay still. As people language their realities, they language their value priorities and meanings according to this principle. This principle has three concepts: (1) imaging, (2) valuing, and (3) languaging.

Imaging

Paradoxes: Explicit–Tacit and Reflective–Prereflective

Imaging is the first concept of the first principle. The paradoxes of imaging are explicit–tacit and reflective–prereflective (Parse, 1998, 2007b, 2012b, 2014). Imaging is an individual's view of reality. It is the shaping of personal knowledge in explicit and tacit ways (Parse, 1981, 1998, 2007b, 2012b, 2014). Some knowing is a reflective, deliberate process, whereas other knowing is prereflective. For Parse, people are inherently curious and seek answers. The answers to questions emerge as persons explore meaning in light of reality and their view of things. Imaging is a personal interpretation of meaning, possibility, and consequence. Nurses cannot completely know another's imaging, but they explore, respect, and bear witness as people struggle with shaping, exploring, integrating, rejecting, and interpreting.

MAJOR CONCEPTS & DEFINITIONS—cont'd

Valuing

Paradox: Confirming–Not Confirming

Valuing is the second concept of the first principle. The paradox of valuing is confirming–not confirming (Parse, 1998, 2007b, 2012b, 2014). This concept is about how persons confirm and do not confirm beliefs in light of a personal perspective or worldview (Parse, 1981, 1998, 2007b, 2012b, 2014). Persons are continuously confirming–not confirming beliefs as they are making choices about how to think, act, and feel. These choices may be consistent with prior choices, or they may be radically different and require a shifting of value priorities. Sometimes people may think about anticipated choices, and once the choice arrives they change their thinking and direction in life. Values reflect what is important in life to a person or a family. For Parse, living one's value priorities is how an individual expresses humanbecoming. Nurses learn about persons' values by asking them what is most important.

Languaging

Paradoxes: Speaking–Being Silent and Moving–Being Still

Languaging is the third concept of the first principle. The paradoxes of languaging are speaking–being silent and moving–being still (Parse, 1998, 2007b, 2012b, 2014). Languaging is a concept that is visible and relates to how humans symbolize and express their imaged realities and their value priorities. When languaging is visible to others, it is expressed in patterns that are shared with those who are close. Family members or close friends often share similar patterns, such as speaking, moving, and being quiet (Parse, 1981, 1998, 2007b, 2012b, 2014). People disclose things about themselves when they language and when they are silent and remain still. Nurses witness the languaging that people show, but cannot know the meaning of the languaging. To understand the languaging, nurses ask people what their words, actions, and gestures mean. It is possible that persons still may not know the meaning of their languaging, and in that case the nurse respects the process of coming to understand the meaning of a situation. Explicating meaning takes time, and people know when it is right to illuminate the meaning and significance of an event or happening.

Principle 2: Configuring Rhythmical Patterns

The second principle of humanbecoming is "**configuring rhythmical patterns** is the revealing-concealing and enabling-limiting of connecting-separating" (Parse, 2014, p. 36). This principle means that human beings create patterns in day-to-day life, and these patterns tell about personal meanings and values. In the patterns of relating that people create, many freedoms and restrictions surface with choices; all patterns involve complex engagements and disengagements with people, ideas, and preferences. The second principle has three concepts: (1) revealing–concealing, (2) enabling–limiting, and (3) connecting–separating.

Revealing–Concealing

Paradox: Disclosing–Not Disclosing

Revealing–concealing is the first concept of the second principle. The paradox of revealing–concealing is disclosing–not disclosing (Parse, 2007b, 2012b, 2014). Revealing–concealing is the way persons disclose and keep hidden the persons they are becoming with the becoming visible–invisible becoming of the emerging now (Parse, 1981, 1998, 2007b, 2012b, 2014). There is always more to tell and more to know about self as well as others. Sometimes people know what they want to say, and they deliver messages about what is becoming visible to them with great clarity; at other times, people may surprise themselves with the messages they give as what is becoming visible shifts and changes with the invisible becoming of their emerging now. Some aspects of reality and experience remain concealed. People also disclose–not disclose differently in different situations and with different people. Patterns of revealing–concealing are cocreated and intimately connected with the intentions of those persons cocreating the moment. In choosing how to be with others, nurses cocreate what happens when they are with persons.

Enabling–Limiting

Paradox: Potentiating–Restricting

Enabling–limiting is the second concept of the second principle. It is connected with the paradox potentiating–restricting (Parse, 2007b, 2012b, 2014). Enabling–limiting is related to the potentials and opportunities that surface with the restrictions and obstacles of everyday living. Every choice, even those made prereflectively, has potentials and restrictions. It is not possible to know all the consequences of any given choice; therefore people make choices amid the reality of ambiguity. Every choice is pregnant with possibility in both opportunity and restriction. This is verified in practice daily when patients and families say things like, "This is the worst thing that could have happened to our family, but it has helped us in many ways." Enabling–limiting is about choosing from the possibilities and living with the consequences of those choices. Nurses bear witness to others as they contemplate the options and anticipated consequences of difficult choices.

Continued

MAJOR CONCEPTS & DEFINITIONS—cont'd

Connecting–Separating

Paradox: Attending–Distancing

Connecting–separating is the third concept of the second principle. The paradox connected with connecting–separating is attending–distancing (Parse, 2007b, 2012b, 2014). This concept relates to the ways persons create patterns of connecting and separating with people and projects. Patterns created reveal value priorities. Connecting–separating is about communion–aloneness and the ways people separate from some to join with others. Connecting–separating is also about the paradox attending–distancing and explains the way two people can be very close and yet separate. Sometimes there is connecting when people are separating because persons can dwell with an absent presence with great intimacy, especially when grieving for another (Bournes, 2000a; Cody, 1995b; Pilkington, 1993). Nurses learn about persons' patterns of connecting–separating by asking about their important relationships and projects.

Principle 3: Cotranscending With Possibles

The third principle of humanbecoming is, "**cotranscending with possibles** is the powering and originating of transforming" (Parse, 2014, p. 36). The meaning of this principle is that persons continuously change and unfold in life as they engage with and choose from infinite possibilities about how to be, what attitude or approach to have, whom to relate with, and what interests or concerns to explore. Choices reflect the person's ways of moving and changing with the becoming visible–invisible becoming of the emerging now. The three concepts of this principle are as follows: (1) powering, (2) originating, and (3) transforming.

Powering

Paradoxes: Pushing–Resisting, Affirming–Not Affirming, Being–Nonbeing

Powering, the first concept of the third principle, is connected with the paradoxes pushing–resisting, affirming–not affirming, and being–nonbeing (Parse, 1998, 2007b, 2012b, 2014). Powering is a concept that conveys meaning about struggle and life and the will to go on despite hardship and threat. Parse (1981, 1998, 2012b, 2014) describes powering as pushing–resisting that is always happening and that affirms being in light of the possibility of nonbeing. People constantly engage being and nonbeing. Nonbeing is about loss and the risk of death and rejection. Powering is the force exerted, the pushing to act and live with purpose amid possibilities for affirming and holding what is cherished while simultaneously living with loss and the threat of nonbeing. There is resistance with the pushing force of powering, because persons live with others who are powering with different possibilities in the visible–invisible becoming of the emerging now. Conflict, according to Parse (1981, 1998, 2007b, 2012b, 2014), presents opportunities to clarify meanings and values, and nurses enhance this process by being present with persons who are exploring issues, conflicts, and options.

Originating

Paradoxes: Certainty–Uncertainty, Conforming–Not Conforming

Originating, the second concept of the third principle, is about human uniqueness and holds the following two paradoxes: (1) certainty–uncertainty and (2) conforming–not conforming (Parse, 1998, 2007b, 2012b, 2014). People strive to be like others, yet they also strive to be unique. Choices about originating occur with the reality of certainty–uncertainty. It is not possible to know all that may come from choosing to be different or from choosing to be like others. For some, there is danger in being too much like others; for others, the danger is in being different. Each person defines and lives originating in light of their worldview and values. Originating and creating anew is a pattern that coexists with constancy and conformity (Parse, 1981, 1998, 2007b, 2012b, 2014). Humans craft their unique patterning of originating as they engage the possibilities of everyday life. Nurses witness originating with persons choosing how they are going to be with their changing health patterns.

Transforming

Paradox: Familiar–Unfamiliar

Transforming, the third concept of the third principle, is explicated with the paradox familiar–unfamiliar (Parse, 1998, 2007b, 2012b, 2014). Transforming is about the continuously changing and shifting views that people have about their lives as they live what is becoming visible to them with the invisible becoming of their emerging now. People are always struggling to integrate the unfamiliar with the familiar in living everydayness. When new discoveries are made, people change their understanding and life patterns, and worldviews shift with insights that illuminate a familiar situation in a new light. Transforming is the ongoing change cocreated as new information and insights become visible in the emerging now, as people find ways to change in the direction of their cherished hopes and dreams (Parse, 1981, 1998, 2007b, 2012b, 2014). Nurses, in the way they are present with others, help or hinder a person's efforts to clarify their hopes, dreams, and desired directions.

USE OF EMPIRICAL EVIDENCE

In 2016 Parse presented two basic science methods that are consistent with the new humanbecoming paradigm: humanbecoming hermeneutic sciencing (Parse, 2016a) and Parsesciencing (Parse, 2016b). As mentioned previously, Parse no longer uses the term *research,* but rather uses the term *sciencing.* "From a humanbecoming perspective, sciencing is ongoing, indivisible, unpredictable, everchanging coming to know" (Parse, 2016b). These methods can be further explored in the identified references. The dated language that follows has not been changed for historical purposes, but new language and meanings are also added.

Research (sciencing) guided by the humanbecoming theory is meant to enhance understanding of the theoretical foundation, or the knowledge contained in the assumptions, postulates, principles, and concepts of humanbecoming (Doucet & Bournes, 2007; Parse, 1998, 2007b, 2012b, 2014). Research (sciencing) is not used to test Parse's theory. Nurses assume persons, who are free to choose, have unique meanings of life situations. They are indivisible, unpredictable, ever changing beings who relate with others in paradoxical patterns. To test these beliefs would be comparable to testing the assumption that humans are spiritual beings or that people are composed of complex systems. These statements are abstract beliefs based on experience, observation, and beliefs about the nature of reality. The foundational or ontological statements are value laden, and, as noted earlier, a nurse either has an attraction and commitment to these foundational beliefs or not. The idea of a human being who is indivisible, unpredictable, everchanging, and free to choose meaning is an assumption that is either believable or not. Assumptions about humans are theoretical, not factual. A student or a nurse relates to one notion of human being or another. According to Parse (1991, 1999b, 2008c, 2008d, 2009b) this is why there is a need for multiple views; the discipline of nursing can and does accommodate different views and different theories about phenomena of concern to nursing. In agreement with Hall, Parse stated the following when discussing the issue of testing the humanbecoming theory:

> *"The [humanbecoming] theory does not lend itself to testing, since it is not a predictive theory and is not based on a cause-effect view of [humanuniverse]. The purpose of the research [sciencing] is not to verify the theory or test it but, rather, the focus is on uncovering the essences of lived phenomena to gain further understanding of universal [humanuniverse living experiences]. This understanding evolves from connecting the descriptions given by people to the theory, thus making more explicit the essences of being human."*
>
> ***(1993, p. 12)***

Therefore sciencing with Parse's theory expands understanding about universal humanuniverse living experiences and builds new knowledge about humanbecoming (Doucet & Bournes, 2007; Parse, 2012b, 2014, 2016a, 2016b). Knowledge of humanbecoming contributes to the substantive knowledge of the nursing discipline. Disciplinary knowledge is different from the practical or technical knowledge that nurses use in health care settings. Disciplinary knowledge is theoretical knowledge that identifies the phenomena of concern for nurses—which for Parse (1998, 2007b, 2012b, 2014, 2016a, 2016b) is humanuniverse living experiences. According to Parse (1998), "scholarly research is formal inquiry leading to the discovery of new knowledge with the enhancement of theory" (p. 59). The idea of new knowledge with enhancement of theory requires attention to clarify distinctions among different ways of thinking.

Research (sciencing) guided by humanbecoming explores universal humanuniverse living experiences with people as they live them with the becoming visible–invisible becoming of their day-to-day lives. Parse contends there are universal humanuniverse living experiences, such as hope, joy, sorrow, grief, fear, and confidence. Research participants' (now referred to as **historians**) accounts of their **living experiences** in humanbecoming-guided sciencing are descriptions of their "remembering-prospecting of the phenomenon [being studied] as it is appearing with the emerging now. It is *living* the experience being described" (Parse, 2012b, p. 49) in light of what is becoming visible to them about the experience in the moment. This means that sciencing guided by humanbecoming explores universal humanuniverse living experiences as people live them. People live in the moment, and what is remembered and what is hoped for are always viewed within the context of what is becoming visible in the emerging now. Universal humanuniverse living experiences are not reduced to linear time frames, because living experiences are cocreated with "indivisible, unbounded knowing" (Parse, 2007b, p. 308). A nurse researcher (now referred to as a **nurse scholar**) conducting a Parsesciencing investigation invites persons to speak about a particular universal humanuniverse living experience. For instance, a historian might talk about his or her experience of grieving (Cody, 1995a, 2000; Pilkington, 1993). The scholar guided by humanbecoming knows that the person's reality encompasses what is remembered and what is imagined or hoped for as it is appearing in the moment (Parse, 2007b). The scholar assumes that the person knows his or her experience and can offer an account of the experience as he or she lives and knows it. What is shared about the experience under investigation is what Parse (2008e) calls "truth for the moment" (p. 46). Truth for the moment is the person's description of his or her reality, an expression of "personal wisdom" (Parse, 2008e,

p. 46) about the phenomenon under study in light of what is happening and known in that instant. Truth, from this perspective, is "unfolding evidence, testimony to everchanging knowing, as new insights shift meaning and truth for the moment" (Parse, 2008e, p. 46). Thus sciencing evidence is "truth for the moment" (p. 46).

In 1987 Parse first developed a specific research method (now called **sciencing**) consistent with the humanbecoming theory (this method was originally called the *Parse research method* and has evolved to the **Parsesciencing method**); since then, a humanbecoming hermeneutic method has been articulated and now has evolved to humanbecoming hermeneutic sciencing (Cody, 1995c; Parse, 1998, 2001b, 2005, 2007a, 2011b, 2014, 2016a). For more information about these methods, see *The Human Becoming School of Thought: A Perspective for Nurses and Other Health Professionals* (Parse, 1998); *Qualitative Inquiry: The Path of Sciencing* (Parse, 2001b); and *The Humanbecoming Paradigm: A Transformational Worldview* (Parse, 2014). Additional detail and updates about humanbecoming sciencing can be found in Parse's and others' articles (Doucet & Bournes, 2007; Parse, 2005, 2011b, 2014, 2016a, 2016b). Parsesciencing records accounts of personal experiences and systematically examines these accounts to identify the aspects of living experiences shared across participants. Core ideas shared across all participants form a structure of the phenomenon under study. The structure (this is now referred to as the **discerning extant moment**) (Parse, 2016b) is defined by Parse (2011b) as "a description of the emerging now. . . . The emerging now incarnates remembering-prospecting about the [living] experience" (p. 13). The discerning extant moment of the universal humanuniverse living experience is created by "the fusion of horizons of the historians and the scholars" (Parse, 2016b). New knowledge is embedded in the core concepts and, once discovered, enhances theory and understanding in ways beyond the particular study. The weaving of new knowledge with the theoretical concepts expands understanding of the content of the humanbecoming theory (this weaving is now referred to as **transubstantiating**) (Parse, 2016b), and new knowledge develops disciplinary and interdisciplinary thinking and dialogue.

A metaphor of panning for gold describes Parsesciencing. The scholar gathers descriptions from historians like a person panning for gold gathers up the earth. The extraction-synthesis processes (this process is now referred to as **distilling-fusing**) (Parse, 2016b) of Parsesciencing is likened to the gathering, sifting, swirling, seeking, and separating, as when panning. Scholars following Parsesciencing work to separate particular context from core ideas. The gathering and discovering happen over and over as context and earth are separated from the core ideas or nuggets that eventually stand out from the surrounding context or earth. Panning for gold is backbreaking work. Parsesciencing is also arduous. Both processes include excitement and anticipation of what is to be discovered. The distilling-fusing process of Parsesciencing separates out core ideas that are present in all participants' descriptions of the living experience under investigation. Core ideas, like gold nuggets, are isolated but not yet refined to a form that makes them meaningful in the world at large. Gold nuggets are refined into coins or jewelry. Core ideas are refined to the language of humanbecoming and nursing science, so other nurses see not only the gold nuggets but also the meaningfulness of the newly refined ideas in light of a language of nursing science. Because all sciencing is theory driven, sciencing findings are interpreted in light of the guiding frame of reference to advance disciplinary knowledge.

MAJOR ASSUMPTIONS

In her original work, Parse (1981, 1998) synthesized "principles, tenets, and concepts from Rogers, Heidegger, Merleau-Ponty, and Sartre . . . in the creation of the assumptions about the human and becoming, underpinning a view of nursing grounded in the human sciences. Each assumption is unique and represents a synthesis of three of the postulates and concepts drawn from Rogers' work and from existential phenomenology" (Parse, 1998, p. 19). Parse drew upon the work of other theorists to build a solid foundation for a new nursing science. Accordingly, the original assumptions underpinning humanbecoming focused on beliefs about humans and about their becoming visible–invisible becoming, which is health (Parse, 2012a). Parse does not specify separate assumptions about the universe because the universe is illimitable and cocreated with humans—rather than separate from humans. In fact, in her more recent work, Parse (2014) has updated her assumptions to make clear that humans and universe are inseparable. Her assumptions now describe her beliefs about humanuniverse, living quality, and the ethos of humanbecoming (Parse, 2014). Three themes arise from the assumptions of the humanbecoming paradigm: (1) **meaning**, (2) **rhythmicity**, and (3) **transcendence** (Parse, 1998, 2014). The postulates **illimitability**, **paradox**, **freedom**, and **mystery** (Parse, 2007b) permeate the three themes.

Meaning is borne in the messages that persons give and take with others in speaking, moving, silence, and stillness (Parse, 1998, 2012b, 2014). Meaning indicates the significance of something and is chosen by people. Outsiders cannot decide the meaning or significance of something for another person. Nurses cannot know what it will mean for a family to hear news of an unexpected illness or change in health until they learn the meaning it holds from the family's perspective. Sometimes the significance of something is not known until meaning is explored and possibilities examined. Personal meanings are shared with others when people express their views, concerns, hopes, and dreams. According to Parse (1998, 2014) meaning is connected with moments of day-to-day living, as well as with the meaning or purpose of life.

Rhythmicity is about patterns and possibility. Parse (1981, 1998, 2014) suggests that people live unrepeatable patterns of relating with others, ideas, objects, and situations. Their patterns of relating incarnate their priorities, and these patterns are changing constantly as they integrate new experiences and ideas with what is becoming visible–invisible in the emerging now. For Parse, people are recognized by their unique patterns. People change their patterns when they integrate new priorities, ideas, and dreams and show consistent patterns that continue like threads of familiarity and sameness throughout life.

Transcendence is the third major theme of the humanbecoming paradigm. Transcendence is about change and possibility, the infinite possibility that is humanbecoming. "The possibilities arise with . . . [humanuniverse] . . . as options from which to choose personal ways of becoming" (Parse, 1998, p. 30). To believe one thing or another, to go in one direction or another, to be persistent or let go, to struggle or acquiesce, to be certain or uncertain, to hope or despair—all these options surface in day-to-day living. Considering and choosing from these options is cotranscending with the possibles.

Nursing

Consistent with her beliefs, Parse writes about nursing as a basic science. Parse (2000) wrote, "It is the hope of many nurses that nursing as a discipline will enjoy the recognition of having a unique knowledge base and the profession will be sufficiently distinct from medicine that people will actually seek nurses for nursing care, not medical diagnoses" (p. 3). For more than 35 years, Parse has advanced the belief that nursing is a basic science, and that nurses require theories that are different from other disciplines. Parse believes that nursing is a unique service to humankind. This does not mean that nurses do not benefit from and employ knowledge from other disciplines and fields of study. It means that nurses primarily rely on and value the knowledge of nursing theory in their practice and sciencing activities. Parse (1992) has articulated clearly that she believes "nursing is a science, the practice of which is a performing art" (p. 35). From this view, nursing is a learned discipline, and nursing theories guide sciencing (research) and living the art (practice).

Nursing practice for those choosing Parse's theory is guided by a methodology that emerges directly from humanbecoming ontology. Parse (2014) posited that with the ontological base of humanbecoming, "the term *living*, not *practice*, is the proper way to describe the humanbecoming professionals' way of *being with* persons" (p. 91). Living the art of humanbecoming involves true presence. Parse suggested the following concerning true presence: "True presence is a powerful humanuniverse whole-in-motion connection, a special way of *being with* others, attentive to moment-to-moment changes in meaning with the becoming visible-invisible becoming of the emerging now" (p. 93). When the humanbecoming professional is living true presence with another, the person develops new insights in illuminating meaning, shifting rhythms, and inspiring transcending (Parse, 2014). For examples of living the art of nursing guided by humanbecoming, see the following: Bournes and Naef (2006); Bunkers (2011, 2012b); Hayden (2010); Hegge (2012); Jasovsky and colleagues (2010); Jonas-Simpson (2010); Oaks and Drummond (2009); Peterson-Lund (2011); Smith (2010); and Tanaka, Katsuno, and Takahashi (2012). Parse describes nursing practice as living the art of humanbecoming in the following way:

> *"The nurse is in true presence with the individual (or family) as the individual (or family) uncovers the personal meaning of the situation and makes choices to move forward in the now moment with cherished hopes and dreams. The focus is on the meaning of the liv[ing] experience for the person (or family) unfolding 'there with' the presence of the nurse. . . . The living of the theory in practice is indeed what makes a difference to the people touched by it."*
>
> ***(1993, p. 12)***

Nursing, for Parse, is a science, and the performing art of nursing is practiced in relationships with persons (individuals, groups, and communities). Parse (1989) set forth the following set of fundamentals for practicing the art of nursing:

- Know and use nursing frameworks and theories.
- Be available to others.
- Value the other as a human presence.
- Respect differences in view.
- Own what you believe and be accountable for your actions.
- Move on to the new and untested.
- Connect with others.
- Take pride in self.
- Like what you do.
- Recognize the moments of joy in the struggles of living.
- Appreciate mystery and be open to new discoveries.
- Be competent in your chosen area.
- Rest and begin anew. (p. 111)

Person, Environment, Health Viewed as Humanuniverse, Humanbecoming, and Living Quality

As mentioned previously, Parse (1998, 2007b, 2012b) views the concepts *human and universe* as inseparable and irreducible. To emphasize this inseparability, she specified *humanuniverse* and *humanbecoming* as one word (Parse, 2007b). Parse no longer refers to *health* in the new humanbecoming paradigm. What is important is the concept of living quality (Parse, 2014). Living quality is the becoming visible–invisible becoming of the emerging now as humans live their lives structuring meaning, configuring rhythmical patterns, and cotranscending with possibles (Parse, 2012a). Living quality conveys the idea that people are constantly changing. "*Living quality* refers to a person's core whatness, the stuff of a life. What is the whatness? It is the living community that each individual's august presence is—the humanuniverse cocreation with predecessors, contemporaries, and successors" (Parse, 2013, p. 112). Living quality has three core knowings: "fortifying wisdom, discerning witness, and penetrating silence" (Parse, 2013, p. 112). In living fortifying wisdom persons choose ways of being according to their value priorities. "Fortifying wisdom dwells with the individual's explicit-tacit knowings, as the individual is moving and at once initiating ways to strengthen personal value priorities" (p. 114). In living discerning witness, a person chooses certain pattern preferences that create both opportunities and restrictions all-at-once. "Discerning witness moves individuals at every unfolding moment in anchoring with persisting amid shifting with diversifying in cautiously attending with the everchanging" (p. 114). In living penetrating silence an individual ponders in silence the illimitable opportunities available to him or her for creating anew. "*Penetrating silence* is piercing quiet in solemn stillness. It is the perfect intimacy of the unutterable that permeates the whatness of being" (p. 114). These core knowings of living quality cocreate humanuniverse becoming.

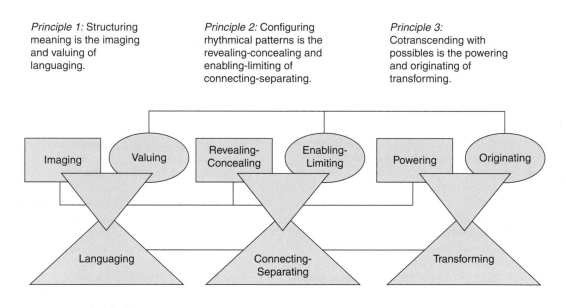

THEORETICAL ASSERTIONS

Parse's (1981, 1998, 2012b, 2014) principles are the assertions of the humanbecoming theory. Each principle interrelates the nine concepts of humanbecoming: (1) imaging, (2) valuing, (3) languaging, (4) revealing–concealing, (5) enabling–limiting, (6) connecting–separating, (7) powering, (8) originating, and (9) transforming (Fig. 24.1). Sciencing projects generate discerning extant moments (previously known as *structures*) of the universal

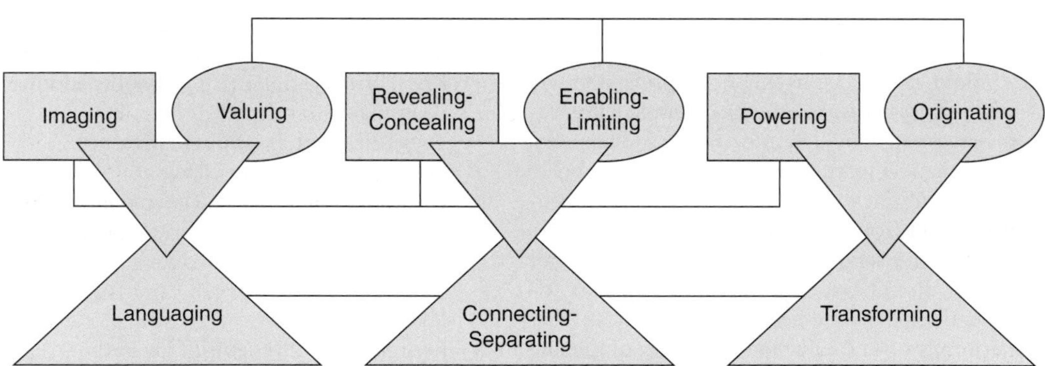

Concepts in the *squares*: *Powering* emerges with the *revealing-concealing* of *imaging*.
Concepts in the *ovals*: *Originating* emerges with the *enabling-limiting* of *valuing*.

FIG. 24.1 Relationship of principles, concepts, and theoretical structures of the humanbecoming theory. (From Parse, R. R. [1998]. *The human becoming school of thought: A perspective for nurses and other health professionals* [p. 56]. Thousand Oaks, CA: Sage. Principles updated from Parse, R. R. [2012]. New humanbecoming conceptualizations and the humanbecoming community model: Expansions with sciencing and living the art. *Nursing Science Quarterly, 25,* 44–52.)

humanuniverse living experiences that further specify relationships among theoretical concepts. For example, Naef and Bournes (2009) studied the living experience of waiting for persons on a list to receive a lung transplant and presented the following discerning extant moment: "The lived experience of waiting is enabling-limiting the imaging-valuing of powering connecting-separating" (p. 145). Discerning extant moments are used to enhance understanding of phenomena as readers consider historian descriptions that connect to the concepts of humanbecoming. For more examples of humanbecoming sciencing, the reader is referred to an overview of studies (Doucet & Bournes, 2007, and other recent publications; Baumann, 2008, 2012b, 2016; Bournes & Milton, 2009; Bunkers, 2010b, 2012a; Condon, 2010a, 2010c; Doucet, 2012a, 2012b; Florczak, 2010, 2012; Maillard-Struby, 2012; Morrow, 2010; Parse, 2005, 2008e, 2009c, 2011b, 2012b, 2014, 2016a; Peterson-Lund, 2012; Smith, 2012).

LOGICAL FORM

The inductive–deductive process was central to the creation of the humanbecoming theory. The theory originated from Parse's personal experiences with her readings and in living the art of nursing. She deductively–inductively crafted major components of humanbecoming from the science of unitary human beings and existential-phenomenological thought. She intuitively and methodically derived the assumptions, postulates, principles, concepts, practice (living the art), and sciencing methodologies of the humanbecoming paradigm. Fig. 24.1 illustrates how the principles, concepts, and theoretical structures connect in simplicity and complexity. Abstraction and complexity create possibility for growth, scholarship, and sustainability.

ACCEPTANCE BY THE NURSING COMMUNITY

Practice

The range of publications about humanbecoming demonstrates the broad scope of acceptance by the nursing community (Bournes, 2013; Bournes & Ferguson-Paré, 2007; Bournes & Flint, 2003; Bournes & Naef, 2006; Bunkers, 2010a, 2010c, 2011, 2012b; Hayden, 2010; Hegge, 2012; Jasovsky et al., 2010; Mitchell, Bournes, & Hollett, 2006; Oaks & Drummond, 2009; Peterson-Lund, 2011; Smith, 2010; Tanaka, Katsuno, & Takahashi, 2012). A community of nurse scholars is advancing humanbecoming in living the art, sciencing, and education. The theory has made a difference to nurses and to persons (patients) experiencing humanbecoming professionals living true presence. This includes nurses who work with older adults and with children. The theory guides living the art of nursing for nurses who work with families (Parse, 2009a) and with persons in hospital settings, clinics, and community settings (Parse, 2003, 2012b). A community-based health action model, for instance, has been developed and has received support from the local community and other funding agencies (Crane, Josephson, & Letcher, 1999). The theory was used as an overarching theoretical guide to develop a decisioning model for nurse regulators at a state board of nursing (Benedict et al., 2000; Damgaard & Bunkers, 1998, 2012). The theory has generated controversy and scholarly dialogue about nursing as an evolving discipline and a distinct human science. It is not a question of whether the theory works in a particular area of nursing; it has been lived by nurses in the operating theater, in parishes, in shelters, in boards of nursing, in acute care hospitals, in long-term and community settings, and in any setting where nurses have relationships with persons and families.

Education

The humanbecoming paradigm and the philosophical assumptions and theoretical beliefs specified by Parse (1981, 1998, 2012b, 2013, 2014) have fueled many scholarly dialogues about outcomes in living the art of nursing, in sciencing, and in education when different theories guide nursing endeavors. In *Nursing Science Quarterly* and other journals, nurses have advanced dialogue and debate about the role of theory in nursing, the limitations and contributions of the medical model, the ethics of nursing diagnoses and the nurse–person relationship, paternalism and health care, the knowledge of advanced nursing practice, paradigmatic issues in nursing, the limitations of evidence-based nursing, the possibilities and politics of human science, freedom and choice, the focus of community-based nursing, the nature of truth, leadership and nursing theory, and the scope of mistakes in nursing.

Parse (2004, 2014) created a humanbecoming teaching–learning model that has been used in a variety of ways with students in academic settings (Baumann, 2012a; Bunkers, 2009; Condon, 2009, 2012a, 2012b; Condon & Hegge, 2011; Delis, 2012; Letcher & Yancey, 2004; Milton, 2012b; Ursel & Aquino-Russell, 2010) and practice settings (Bournes & Naef, 2006). Teachers in academic and practice settings have contributed new understanding and new processes of teaching–learning, and Parse's theory was used as a model for explicating pros and cons of tele-apprenticeship (Norris, 2002). The humanbecoming paradigm is included in nursing courses at the undergraduate and graduate levels in many schools of nursing.

In *Man-Living-Health: A Theory of Nursing,* Parse (1981) presented a sample master's in nursing curriculum. She outlined this process-based curriculum in detail, including course descriptions and course sequencing. The curriculum plan was updated in 1998 in *The Human Becoming School of Thought: A Perspective for Nurses and Other Health Professionals.* Parse outlined philosophy, goals, conceptual framework, themes, program indicators, culture content, and evaluation in a sample curriculum plan consistent with humanbecoming. In *The Humanbecoming Paradigm: A Transformational Worldview,* Parse (2014) presented an educational plan for humanbecoming professionals. The disciplinary knowledge in this plan has the base of the humanbecoming paradigm. Outlined in the plan are a program philosophy, aims, conceptual framework, and indicators.

A master's curriculum consistent with humanbecoming was developed at Olivet Nazarene University in Kankakee, Illinois (Milton, 2003). To date, most students who study the humanbecoming paradigm are guided by the theory in their living the art of nursing and in sciencing. Parse's ideas and theory are increasingly integrated into undergraduate programs to expand options for students being taught that nursing is an art and a science. For example, an undergraduate curriculum was designed, implemented, and accredited at California Baptist University in Riverside, California (C. Milton, personal communication, July 6, 2012). Also, students at the master's and doctorate (PhD and DNP) levels at South Dakota State University, Brookings and Sioux Falls, South Dakota, study the humanbecoming paradigm, and several PhD students have used it as a guide in their dissertation sciencing projects.

Research

Humanbecoming theory has guided sciencing studies in many different countries about numerous living experiences, including feeling loved, feeling very tired, having courage, waiting, feeling cared for, grieving, caring for a loved one, persisting while wanting to change, feeling understood, and being listened to, as well as time passing, quality of life, health, lingering presence, hope, and contentment (Doucet & Bournes, 2007). Parsesciencing and humanbecoming hermeneutic sciencing (Parse, 2016a, 2016b) generate new knowledge about humanuniverse universal living experiences (Cody, 1995b, 1995c; Parse, 2001a, 2001b, 2005, 2007a, 2011b, 2012b). Sciencing findings have enhanced understanding of how people experience hope while imaging new possibilities and how people create moments of respite amid the anguish of grieving a loss. Sciencing findings are woven with the theory, so findings also inform thinking beyond any particular study.

In the grieving and loss studies, researchers described a rhythm of engaging and disengaging with the one lost and with others who remind the one grieving about the one who was lost (Cody, 1995a; Florczak, 2008; Pilkington, 1993, 2008). Women who had a miscarriage already had a relationship with their babies, and the anguish of losing the child was so intense that women invented ways to distance themselves from the reality of the lost child. When they were alone, the pain was unbearable, and when they were with others, the anguish was both eased and intensified as consoling expressions mingled with words acknowledging the reality of the lost child (MacDonald & Jonas-Simpson, 2009; Pilkington, 1993). Women described rhythms of engaging–disengaging with the lost child and close others, pain, and respite. Connecting the rhythm to the theoretical concept of *connecting–separating* and to the idea of *lingering presence* means nurses can think about and be present with those experiencing grieving and loss. How do families in palliative care express their engaging and distancing from the one who is moving toward death? How do parents losing adult children engage and disengage with the absent children? Sciencing studies about loss and grieving may further enhance understanding about connecting–separating with knowledge for nursing practice.

In 2004 Mitchell developed a framework for critiquing humanbecoming sciencing that expanded options for critics engaging humanbecoming-guided nursing science. Parse (2011b) continues to refine the sciencing methods. In the first changes, Parse changed the name of the participant proposition to **language-art**, and she added a process requiring the researcher to select or create an artistic expression showing how the researcher was transfigured through the research process (Parse, 2005). The artistic expression enhances understanding of what the scholar learned about the phenomenon under study. For instance, in a study on the experience of feeling respected, Parse (2006) reported that 10 adult historians in her study described feeling respected as "an acknowledgement of personal worth" (p. 54). They described, for example, feeling confident, being trusted, feeling appreciated, and experiencing joy when feeling respected (Parse, 2006). Parse showed that in each case, the historian spoke about feeling respected as a "fortifying assuredness amid potential disregard emerging with the fulfilling delight of prized alliances" (p. 54). Parse's (2006) artistic expression for this study—that is, her depiction of her own learning about the phenomenon of feeling respected that surfaced through the sciencing process—was the following poem:

The oak tree stands
noble on the hill
even in
cherry blossom time.

Basho (1644–1694/1962)

Parse (2006) interpreted the artistic expression saying, "The oak tree stands noble, acknowledged as such with the potential of being disregarded amid the beauty of cherry blossoms, yet there is delight in the fortification of being known as oak tree. Oak tree and cherry blossoms live a mutuality of being prized as individually unique and uniquely together" (p. 55). Subsequently, Parse introduced **metaphorical emergings** to the Parse research method. She did this after examining reports of many Parse research method studies and noting:

> *"Linguistic descriptions of universal [living] experiences by participants were rife with metaphors that creatively expressed the meaning of universal [living] experiences. Metaphors are phrases, attributions to objects or ideas that offer surprise twists on meanings. . . . To extract metaphors expressed by participants from dialogues about universal [living] experiences and to creatively conceptualize them in light of the ontology of humanbecoming expands knowledge of the experiences."*
>
> ***(2011b, p. 13)***

Parse (2011b) used the 2006 study on feeling respected to illustrate the use of metaphorical emergings with the Parse research method. The metaphorical emergings that arose from the participants' descriptions of feeling respected in that study (Parse, 2006) included: "Feeling respected feels like everything is firing on all cylinders; I'm just euphoric for half an hour after class" (p. 53). Describing what can be learned from this metaphor in light of the study, Parse wrote the following:

> *"This metaphor further illuminates the meaning of feeling respected when connected to the core concepts (fortifying assuredness amid potential disregard, fulfilling delight, and prized alliances) and when elaborated with the ontology of humanbecoming. Firing on all cylinders is the driving force of pushing-resisting in powering onward with the buoyant momentum of fortifying assuredness. The fortifying assuredness with feeling respected arises with illimitable imaginings that cocreate anew the familiar-unfamiliar preferred preferences lived with opportunities amid limitations. The euphoric feeling in the metaphor is the fulfilling delight of being elevated with regard, yet with the remembered and ever-present potential for disregard. The living paradox of regard-disregard reveals and at once conceals the diversity in connecting-separating with prized alliances that surface with feeling respected. The metaphor 'firing on all cylinders . . . [with euphoria]' brings feeling respected to light as a powerful force of unwavering buoyancy in confirming human engagements. It shows the lived experience of feeling respected as a cocreation languaged in the emerging now that all-at-once incarnates the mystery of being human."*
>
> ***(2011b, p. 14)***

Further changes in Parsesciencing and humanbecoming hermeneutic sciencing can be explored by reading cited references at the end of this chapter.

CRITIQUE

Clarity

Humanbecoming is an abstract and complex paradigm in nursing that includes the humanbecoming theory (the principles). It is a theory, rather than a model, because its concepts and interrelationships are in principles written at an abstract level of discourse—the language of science. The theory penetrates the foundations of traditional nursing and health care in general. This penetration may be limited to cracklike fissures or streams of activity to expand opportunities and advance thinking. This requires nurses to explore ways that are helpful to foster the betterment of humankind.

Simplicity

In keeping with the theoretical discourse, the major concepts of humanbecoming are defined in abstract philosophical terms. The language has been a source of comfort and discomfort for nurses (Mitchell & Bournes, 2000; Mitchell, Bournes, & Hollett, 2006). Discomfort with the language is sometimes related more with unfamiliar beliefs and assumptions about humanuniverse than with the actual concepts. The nondirectional statements that do not specify causal or predictive relationships about humanuniverse are discomforting for some.

The concepts of humanbecoming often resonate with people when considered at the level of human experience. For instance, the concept of valuing at the level of human experiences focuses on the ways persons choose and act on what is important in their lives. This idea should be inherently familiar, as should the idea that people sometimes disclose intimate details about their lives and sometimes keep secrets from others (revealing–concealing). Pickrell and colleagues (1998) noted that a first-time reader might be tempted to dismiss the concepts as too simple to convey the complexity inherent in the theory, but they caution that to do so would be a mistake. Parse's principles describe a complex and realistic picture of humanbecoming that provides a meaningful framework for understanding the illimitability, mystery, freedom, and paradox of humanuniverse.

Generality

The humanbecoming paradigm has been selected as a theoretical guide by nurses and other health professionals in different settings, including acute care, long-term care, community, and nursing regulation. The theory has helped nurses be with individuals, families, and groups and has been evaluated in nursing settings where patients commented on the positive difference it made (Bournes & Ferguson-Paré, 2007; Jonas, 1995; Mitchell, Bernardo, & Bournes, 1997; Northrup & Cody, 1998; Williamson, 2000). Humanbecoming has helped leaders create beneficial change in organizational culture and informed development of standards of care (Mitchell & Bournes, 1998), best-practice guidelines (Nelligan et al., 2002; Registered Nurses Association of Ontario, 2002), decision-making tools for nurse regulators (Benedict et al., 2000; Bunkers, 2016; Damgaard & Bunkers, 1998, 2012), mentoring programs for novice nurses (Bournes & Plummer, 2011; Bournes et al., 2011), and leadership and sciencing programs for nurses who work at the point of care (Bournes, 2013). The theory of humanbecoming changes what professionals see when they engage with persons in living the art of nursing and in sciencing. The theory changes the thinking, acting, attitudes, and approaches that professionals rely on to fulfill their intentions with others. Indeed, the humanbecoming theory changes the intentions and purposes of professionals, and there is no limit to how this learning may contribute to meaningful practices and approaches for all professional activities linked with research, education, and leadership.

Accessibility

Accessibility of the theory is evaluated with evidence addressed in the following questions:

- Does evidence (taken here to mean "does reality") support the theory?
- Do the principles and concepts of the humanbecoming theory make sense to nurses when they are with people in living the art of nursing (practice)?
- Does the humanbecoming theory help nurses be with people in ways that are helpful and that make a difference from the person's perspective?
- Is the theory useful for administrators and scholars (researchers)?
- Do sciencing (research) findings expand knowledge and enhance the theoretical base?

The answer to these questions is, clearly, an enthusiastic "yes." The theory is useful because it provides a meaningful foundation that is helpful for nurses who want to live certain values in practice and research (Bournes & Ferguson-Paré, 2007; Mitchell, Jonas-Simpson, & Ivonoffski, 2006).

A nurse who is learning the theory might ask the following questions:

- What does humanbecoming theory say about people, and do I believe in these ideas as they are presented?
- Am I comfortable with the basic beliefs espoused in the humanbecoming theory?

The answers to the initial questions about evidence or congruence with reality often lead to a decision to pursue the more difficult task of studying the theory. A commitment to learn more requires some attraction to the basic underlying values and assumptions about humanuniverse, living quality, and the ethos of humanbecoming (Parse, 2014). These values recognize that people have their own unique views about life and their living quality. They speak about what things mean on a personal level; value their priorities and pursue what is important to them; want to make their own choices; and speak about paradoxical thoughts and feelings, saying "on the one hand this and on the other hand that." Finally nurses ask, "How do I believe people change? Do people make choices that help them move in the direction of their own hopes and dreams?" Humanbecoming theory explores these questions.

Importance

Parse calls nursing a *human science,* and, as such, it represents particular beliefs that have been around for longer than 100 years. The humanbecoming theory has taken human science beliefs into service and knowledge development in new and important ways. The humanbecoming living the art of nursing and sciencing methodologies are generating transformations in care and a renewed sense of professional purpose. Consider these examples:

1. Nurses in two Canadian provinces spent 24 months evaluating humanbecoming-guided care, and these acute care nurses reported enhanced satisfaction and purpose in their work as professional nurses (Bournes & Ferguson-Paré, 2007; Mitchell, Bournes, & Hollett 2006).
2. Teams of humanbecoming scholars, practitioners, artistic writers, actors, and consumers produced a research-based drama called *I'm Still Here* about living with Alzheimer disease. The Murray Alzheimer Research and Education Program at the University of Waterloo funded the production of a DVD version of the drama, as well as an educational guide informed by humanbecoming theory, research, and self-reflective practice (Mitchell, Jonas-Simpson, & Ivonoffski, 2006). Hundreds of health professionals and families in countries around the globe have purchased the DVD and educational guide. Researchers Mitchell, Dupuis, and Jonas-Simpson toured a live performance of *I'm Still Here* to complete a longitudinal study funded by the Social Sciences and Humanities Research Council of Canada (SSHRC); this study evaluated knowledge translation through artistic performance.

3. Jonas-Simpson's work on loss for mothers who experience the loss of their baby has been informed by humanbecoming and findings presented in New York in an interactive exhibit of stories, poetry, photographs, and research-inspired paintings by artist Ann Bayly for professionals and mothers invited to share their own stories in a journal. Most recently, it has informed the cocreation of two videos: *Enduring Love: Transforming Loss* is about how mothers and their families live with the loss of a child, and *Why Did Baby Die? Mothering Children Living With the Loss, Love and Continuing Presence of a Baby Sibling* focuses on the surviving children. Both videos are available from http://bookstore.yorku.ca.
4. The humanbecoming mentoring model (Parse, 2008b) was used in a study (Bournes & Plummer, 2011) that examined the impact of a mentoring program with experienced critical care nurses and new graduate nurses interested in a career in critical care. It was designed to address important issues relating to recruitment and retention of critical care nurses, to enhance nurse mentoring capacity at a university-affiliated teaching hospital, to evaluate a mentoring program for staff nurses, and to extend knowledge about the effectiveness and generalizability the humanbecoming 80/20 model (Bournes & Ferguson-Paré, 2007). A total of 11 experienced critical care nurse participants and 13 new graduate nurse participants engaged in the program together. They spent 80% of their time in direct patient care and 20% on professional development, with a focus on learning about humanbecoming-guided nursing practice and mentoring and working together in mentoring dyads. The experienced critical care nurses also participated in separate humanbecoming mentor development workshops throughout the study. Findings demonstrated an overall increase in satisfaction of critical care nurses shown in the results of serial employee opinion surveys. Sick time, overtime, and turnover trended downward among the participant group compared with nonparticipants. Mentor group participants shifted in the ways in which they described the importance of the mentorship experience. Mentor participants, though frustrated at times with having to learn theory, appreciated the refreshing and satisfying opportunity to engage with their protégés. They described feeling respected, feeling supported, and being challenged in their learning to view the importance of nursing in a new way. They also described deeper, more connected relationships than they had anticipated before the study. They spoke about respect and concern for one another and the importance of listening and being nonjudgmental. They also described being more satisfied in their roles, understanding how humanbecoming can guide their relationships with their colleagues and with patients and families, feeling renewed in their commitment to nursing, and learning from younger nurses. Protégé participants also shifted in the way they described the importance of the mentoring experience. They appreciated the guidance and advice about work and skills that they had anticipated would come with the mentoring experience, but they also shared that the mentorship was inspiring to them and helped them to imagine many career possibilities for their future in nursing. They also described respecting others' views, being less judgmental and more understanding, listening more attentively to others' stories, and gaining new friends. They described acquiring new insights about people and about nursing, feeling more rounded, and understanding themselves and their career goals more clearly. They also appreciated seeing the bigger picture in relation to having a better understanding of the variety of nursing roles and of the various practice settings represented by participants in the study.
5. The humanbecoming leading–following and teaching–learning models are used in Geneva, Switzerland, in health care settings and community centers for families of persons living with cancer.
6. The humanbecoming paradigm, including the theory and the humanbecoming human dignity model (Parse, 2014), are used by the South Dakota Board of Nursing, Sioux Falls, South Dakota, to guide the regulatory-decisioning model for the protection of the public.

There are convincing indications that the humanbecoming theory is a fitting guide for practitioners who want to create respectful partnerships with people seeking assistance with living quality. Three decades ago, Phillips (1987) suggested that Parse's work would transform the knowledge base and the practice of nursing to a unitary perspective. Indeed, the humanbecoming theory is transforming practitioners who live the art of nursing in numerous settings, and evaluations are positive (Bournes, 2002b; Bournes & Ferguson-Paré, 2007; Bournes et al., 2011; Jonas, 1995; Legault & Ferguson-Paré, 1999). The humanbecoming theory directs attention to persons' meanings of living quality and to their wishes, needs, concerns, and preferences for information and care. The future of health care is based on the development of theories and practices that honor and respect people as experts in their own lives. At least five of the largest teaching hospitals in Canada have supported nurses piloting and implementing standards of practice that are explicitly informed by humanbecoming. University Health Network, the largest teaching hospital affiliated with the University of Toronto, supported nurses to use 20% of their time to participate in teaching–learning sessions informed by humanbecoming. A 2-year pilot study evaluated changes when a surgical unit used humanbecoming patient-centered care (Bournes & Ferguson-Paré, 2007). This pilot was replicated on a cardiosciences unit at Regina General Hospital in Saskatchewan, Canada (Bournes et al., 2009) and on two additional units at University Health Network in Toronto, Canada, with similar results (Bournes & Ferguson-Paré, 2007).

SUMMARY

Work with the humanbecoming paradigm continues to evolve, as does the theory itself. An important development happened in 1998, when Parse extended the humanbecoming school of thought and introduced the text *Community: A Humanbecoming Perspective* (2003), which offers new concepts about change in community. Further explication of the community model is found in Parse's (2012b) article, "New Humanbecoming Conceptualizations and the Humanbecoming Community Model: Expansions With Sciencing and Living the Art." Parse has created humanbecoming teaching–learning (Parse, 2004), mentoring (Parse, 2008b), leading–following (Parse, 2008a, 2011a), and family models (Parse, 2009a) that are being used in research, leadership, practice, and education settings (Bournes, 2013; Condon, 2010b, 2011; Florczak, Falkenstern, & Baumann, 2010; Kim, Lee, & Baumann, 2011; Maillard-Struby, 2012; Milton, 2010a, 2010b, 2011, 2012a; Morrow, 2012a). Most recently, the publication *The Humanbecomng Paradigm: A Transformational Worldview* (2014) presents many of Parse's current changes in the paradigm, theory, and related models. Ongoing sciencing expands understanding and illuminates new relationships among theoretical concepts. As schools of nursing introduce and teach the humanbecoming paradigm, more nurses explore the theory in practice. Learning the theory requires formal study, quiet contemplation, and creative synthesis. As more nurses use the theory in living the art and in sciencing and leadership, their scholarly dialogue advances the nursing discipline.

The theory of humanbecoming continues as a theory for the future. As nurses question how they are relating with others and question the knowledge base of the discipline, the humanbecoming theory provides a perspective and field of possibilities for change and growth. Administrators who engage nurses are continuing to clarify not only what they want from professionals, but also how they want professionals to perform. The mechanistic approach continues to lose appeal for health care professionals whose mandate is to relate to people as human beings living with hope and no hope, joy and sorrow, and life and death. This theory is a humanbecoming approach for nurses and even more as humankind evolves.

CASE STUDY

Mrs. Brown, a 48-year-old woman, is living with a diagnosis of breast cancer. She has just come into the oncology clinic for her third round of chemotherapy. When asked how she is doing, Mrs. Brown starts speaking about how tired she is and how she is feeling burdened with keeping secrets from her daughter. Mrs. Brown has not told her daughter about her cancer diagnosis because she is afraid of how her daughter might react. Mrs. Brown says she is just barely holding on to things at this time, and she cannot take much more. She is also concerned about the chemotherapy and what she can expect, because the side effects are getting more intense. Consider Mrs. Brown in the critical thinking activities that follow.

CRITICAL THINKING ACTIVITIES

1. Think about Parse's (2014) living the art of nursing—illuminating meaning (explicating), shifting rhythms (dwelling with), and inspiring transcending (moving with). Nurses live true presence with persons, and this means centering and preparing to bear witness to Mrs. Brown's reality. To invite Mrs. Brown to speak, the nurse may initially ask her to say more about her situation. In the cadence of speech, Mrs. Brown may pause, giving the nurse an opening to pose questions that assist Mrs. Brown's exploration of how she is feeling. The nurse may ask: "What is the burden about? What does it mean? What does she think will happen if her daughter gets upset?" Thinking about and picturing an anticipated event is, according to Parse (1990, 1998), an opportunity to rehearse and to clarify how best to be in light of anticipated consequences. In this way, the person is helped with decisions about how best to go forward or how to change the situation.

2. Articulate the judgments that are called for in the humanbecoming theory. The nurse refrains from summarizing, comparing, judging, or labeling Mrs. Brown as she struggles with the possibilities and choices in her situation. The unconditional regard called for by the humanbecoming theory is extremely challenging. It can be much easier to give advice or to try to teach, but what is called for is for the nurse to bear witness to the person's own value priorities. What might you say to Mrs. Brown to encourage her to explore her possibilities?
3. Where does experience lie for nurses guided by the humanbecoming theory? The nurse guided by humanbecoming theory believes that Mrs. Brown knows the best way to proceed—the nurse cannot possibly know the way for another person. Mrs. Brown said she cannot take much more in her life, and yet she is burdened with her secret. This struggle is hers to wrestle with and choose a way to move on. The mother knows her daughter, and she also knows how much upset she can take in her life. The nurse's true presence and theory-guided questions can help Mrs. Brown to figure out how to be in light of her value priorities in the moment. The nurse also knows that Mrs. Brown's value priorities may change at any time, leading to a different course of action. The nurse may have expertise in other areas, based on her knowledge and experience, and trusts that persons will seek information when ready.
4. Mrs. Brown spoke about being tired. The nurse might explore this further. How does the tiredness show itself? What does Mrs. Brown find helpful? What would she like to do about it? Until these things are known, the nurse cannot know how to proceed. The nurse may discover helpful suggestions to offer. The nurse guided by humanbecoming offers information as people indicate their readiness to hear it. The nurse believes that providing information or suggestions as persons seek it in the flow of dialogue and listening are the most respectful and meaningful ways of teaching.
5. Specify three benefits for humanity when nurses follow the humanbecoming theory. Humanbecoming living the art of true presence is consistent with what people say they want from health professionals. Persons have indicated in numerous reports and publications that they want to be listened to, respected, involved in their care, and provided with meaningful information—when they want and need it. People do not want to be judged or labeled when it comes to their choices or ways of living. Persons want to be believed, understood, and respected. Humanbecoming theory provides a guide for nurses who want to live the art of nursing in ways that clients want. It has been shown that nurses guided by the humanbecoming perspective are more vigilant, more inclined to act on client concerns, and more likely to involve clients and families in their care (Mitchell & Bournes, 1998; Parse, 2011c).

POINTS FOR FURTHER STUDY

- Discovery International at www.discoveryinternational online.com.
- International Consortium of Parse Scholars. *Humanbecoming* at www.humanbecoming.org.
- Parse, R. R. (2004). A human becoming teaching-learning model. *Nursing Science Quarterly, 17,* 33–35.
- Parse, R. R. (2007). Hope in "Rita Hayworth and Shawshank Redemption": A human becoming hermeneutic study. *Nursing Science Quarterly, 20,* 148–154.
- Parse, R. R. (2007). The humanbecoming school of thought in 2050. *Nursing Science Quarterly, 20,* 308–311.
- Parse, R. R. (2008). The humanbecoming leading-following model. *Nursing Science Quarterly, 21,* 369–375.
- Parse, R. R. (2008). The humanbecoming mentoring model. *Nursing Science Quarterly, 21,* 195–198.
- Parse, R. R. (2008). Truth for the moment: Personal testimony as evidence. *Nursing Science Quarterly, 21,* 45–48.
- Parse, R. R. (2009). The humanbecoming family model. *Nursing Science Quarterly, 22,* 305–309.
- Parse, R. R. (2010). Human dignity: A humanbecoming ethical phenomenon. *Nursing Science Quarterly, 23,* 257–262.
- Parse, R. R. (2011). Humanbecoming leading-following: The meaning of holding up the mirror. *Nursing Science Quarterly,* 24, 169–171.
- Parse, R. R. (2011). What people want from professional nurses. *Nursing Science Quarterly, 24,* 93.
- Parse, R. R. (2012). New humanbecoming conceptualizations and the humanbecoming community model: Expansions with sciencing and living the art. *Nursing Science Quarterly, 25,* 44–52.
- Parse, R. R. (2014). *The humanbecoming paradigm: A transformational worldview.* Discovery International Publication: Pittsburgh, PA.
- Parse, R. R. (2016). Humanbecoming hermeneutic sciencing: Reverence, awe, betrayal, and shame in the lives of others. *Nursing Science Quarterly, 29,* 128–135.
- *Rosemarie Parse, Theory of Humanbecoming. (1990). Nurse Theorists: Portraits of Excellence,* Volume 1. Available at https://www.fitne.net/nurse_theorists1.jsp.

REFERENCES

Basho. (1962). *Haiku harvest.* White Plains, NY: Peter Pauper Press. (Original work published 1644–1694).

Baumann, S. L. (2008). Wisdom, compassion, and courage in the Wizard of Oz: A humanbecoming hermeneutic study. *Nursing Science Quarterly, 21,* 322–329.

Baumann, S. L. (2012a). Educating international students. *Nursing Science Quarterly, 25,* 97–98.

Baumann, S. L. (2012b). A humanbecoming program of research. *Nursing Science Quarterly, 25,* 17–19.

Baumann, S. L. (2016). The living experience of difficulty telling the truth: A Parse method study. *Nursing Science Quarterly, 28,* 49–56.

Benedict, L. L., Bunkers, S. S., Damgaard, G. A., Duffy, C. E., Hohman, M. L., & Vander Woude, D. L. (2000). The South Dakota board of nursing theory–based regulatory decisioning model. *Nursing Science Quarterly, 13,* 167–171.

Bournes, D. (2000a). A commitment to honoring people's choices. *Nursing Science Quarterly, 13,* 18–23.

Bournes, D. A. (2002b). Research evaluating human becoming in practice. *Nursing Science Quarterly, 15,* 190–195.

Bournes, D. A. (2007). Rosemarie Rizzo Parse over the years. *Nursing Science Quarterly, 20,* 305.

Bournes, D. A. (2013). Cultivating a spirit of inquiry using the humanbecoming leading-following model: The nursing research challenge. *Nursing Science Quarterly, 26,* 182–188.

Bournes, D. A., & Ferguson-Paré, M. (2007). Human becoming and 80/20: An innovative professional development model for nurses. *Nursing Science Quarterly, 20,* 237–253.

Bournes, D. A., Ferguson-Paré, M., Plummer, C., & Kyle, C. (2009, February). *Innovations in nurse retention and professional development: The 80/20 humanbecoming patient-centered care model in Regina, Saskatchewan.* Paper presented at the 2009 National Nursing Leadership Conference, Toronto, Ontario.

Bournes, D. A., & Flint, F. (2003). Mis-takes: Mistakes in the nurse-person process. *Nursing Science Quarterly, 16,* 127–130.

Bournes, D. A., & Milton, C. L. (2009). Nurses' experiences of feeling respected–not respected. *Nursing Science Quarterly, 22,* 47–56.

Bournes, D. A., & Naef, R. (2006). Human becoming practice around the globe: Exploring the art of living true presence. *Nursing Science Quarterly, 19,* 109–115.

Bournes, D. A., & Plummer, C. (2011). *Critical care mentoring study: Testing a program to enhance recruitment and retention of nurses.* Final report submitted to the Ontario Ministry of Health and Long-Term Care (Grant no. 06505). Toronto, Ontario.

Bournes, D. A., Plummer, C., Hollett, J., & Sherman, D. (2011, March). *Critical care mentoring study: Testing a program to enhance recruitment and retention of nurses.* Abstract submitted for paper presentation at the Nursing Leadership Network of Ontario Conference, "Setting the Bar for a High Performing Healthcare System." Toronto, Ontario.

Bunkers, S. S. (2009). Fostering the creative spirit in teaching-learning. *Nursing Science Quarterly, 21,* 323–325.

Bunkers, S. S. (2010a). A focus on human flourishing. *Nursing Science Quarterly, 23,* 290–295.

Bunkers, S. S. (2010b). The lived experience of feeling sad. *Nursing Science Quarterly, 23,* 231–239.

Bunkers, S. S. (2010c). The power and possibility in listening. *Nursing Science Quarterly, 23,* 22–27.

Bunkers, S. S. (2011). What is not yet: Cultivating the imagination. *Nursing Science Quarterly, 24,* 324–328.

Bunkers, S. S. (2012a). The lived experience of feeling disappointed: A Parse research method study. *Nursing Science Quarterly, 25,* 53–61.

Bunkers, S. S. (2012b). Presence: The eye of the needle. *Nursing Science Quarterly, 25,* 10–14.

Bunkers, S. S. (2016). I am community. *Nursing Science Quarterly, 29*(2), 103–107.

Cody, W. K. (1995a). The lived experience of grieving for families living with AIDS: Family-centered research using Parse's method. In R. R. Parse (Ed.), *Illuminations: The humanbecoming theory in practice and research* (pp. 197–242). New York: National League for Nursing.

Cody, W. K. (1995b). The meaning of grieving for families living with AIDS. *Nursing Science Quarterly, 8,* 104–114.

Cody, W. K. (1995c). Of life immense in passion, pulse, and power: Dialoguing with Whitman and Parse. A hermeneutic study. In R. R. Parse (Ed.), *Illuminations: The humanbecoming theory in practice and research* (pp. 269–308). New York: National League for Nursing.

Cody, W. K. (2000). The lived experience of grieving for persons living with HIV who have used injection drugs. *Journal of the Association of Nurses in AIDS Care, 11,* 82–92.

Cody, W. K. (2012). A brave and startling truth: Parse's humanbecoming school of thought in the context of the contemporary nursing discipline. *Nursing Science Quarterly, 25,* 7–9.

Cody, W. K., & Mitchell, G. J. (2002). Nursing knowledge and human science revisited: Practical and political considerations. *Nursing Science Quarterly, 15,* 4–13.

Condon, B. B. (2009). Artistic expression in teaching-learning. *Nursing Science Quarterly, 21,* 326–331.

Condon, B. B. (2010a). The lived experience of feeling misunderstood. *Nursing Science Quarterly, 23,* 138–147.

Condon, B. B. (2010b). A story of family. *Nursing Science Quarterly, 23,* 210–214.

Condon, B. B. (2010c). Understanding-misunderstanding: A philosophical and theoretical exploration. *Nursing Science Quarterly, 23,* 306–314.

Condon, B. B. (2011). Hidden treasures in co-shaping community environment. *Nursing Science Quarterly, 24,* 112–117.

Condon, B. B. (2012a). Celebrating now in teaching-learning. *Nursing Science Quarterly, 25,* 28–33.

Condon, B. B. (2012b). Thinking unleashed. *Nursing Science Quarterly, 25,* 225–230.

Condon, B. B., & Hegge, M. (2011). Human dignity: A cornerstone of doctoral education in nursing. *Nursing Science Quarterly, 24,* 209–214.

Crane, J., Josephson, D., & Letcher, D. (1999, Nov.). *The human becoming health action model in community.* Paper presented at The Seventh Annual International Colloquium on Human Becoming, Loyola University, Chicago.

Damgaard, G., & Bunkers, S. S. (1998). Nursing science-guided practice and education: A state board of nursing perspective. *Nursing Science Quarterly, 11*, 142–144.

Damgaard, G., & Bunkers, S. S. (2012). Revisited: The South Dakota Board of Nursing theory-based regulatory decision-ing model. *Nursing Science Quarterly, 25*, 211–216.

Delis, P. C. (2012). Illumination of Parse's theory of humanbecoming: Modern literature as situation study. *Nursing Science Quarterly, 25*, 144–146.

Doucet, T. J. (2012a). Feeling strong: A Parse research method study. *Nursing Science Quarterly, 25*, 62–71.

Doucet, T. J. (2012b). A humanbecoming program of research: Having faith. *Nursing Science Quarterly, 25*, 20–24.

Doucet, T., & Bournes, D. A. (2007). Review of research related to Parse's theory of human becoming. *Nursing Science Quarterly, 20*, 16–32.

Florczak, K. L. (2008). The persistent yet everchanging nature of grieving a loss. *Nursing Science Quarterly, 21*, 7–11.

Florczak, K. L. (2010). Gathering information on spirituality: From whose perspective? *Nursing Science Quarterly, 23*, 201–205.

Florczak, K. L. (2012). Stories and programs of research: Revelations about humanbecoming. *Nursing Science Quarterly, 25*, 15–16.

Florczak, K., Falkenstern, S. K., & Baumann, S. L. (2010). A glimmer into the understanding of family. *Nursing Science Quarterly, 23*, 105–112.

Hayden, S. J. (2010). Disaster care through a human becoming lens. *Nursing Science Quarterly, 23*, 125–128.

Hegge, M. J. (2012). Humanbecoming and practice: Fairness-unfairness. *Nursing Science Quarterly, 25*, 141–143.

Jasovsky, D. A., Morrow, M. R., Clementi, P. S., & Hindle, P. A. (2010). Theories in action and how nursing practice changed. *Nursing Science Quarterly, 23*, 29–38.

Jonas, C. M. (1995). Evaluation of the human becoming theory in family practice. In R. R. Parse (Ed.), *Illuminations: The human becoming theory in practice and research* (pp. 347–366). New York: National League for Nursing.

Jonas-Simpson, C. (2010). Awakening to space consciousness and timeless transcendent presence. *Nursing Science Quarterly, 23*, 195–200.

Kim, H. K., Lee, O. J., & Baumann, S. L. (2011). Nursing practice with families without a country. *Nursing Science Quarterly, 24*, 273–278.

Legault, F., & Ferguson-Paré, M. (1999). Advancing nursing practice: An evaluation study of Parse's theory of human becoming. *Canadian Journal of Nursing Leadership, 12*(1), 30–35.

Letcher, D. C., & Yancey, N. R. (2004). Witnessing change with aspiring nurses: A human becoming teaching-learning process in nursing education. *Nursing Science Quarterly, 17*, 36–41.

MacDonald, C. A., & Jonas-Simpson, C. M. (2009). Living with changing expectations for women with high risk pregnancies. *Nursing Science Quarterly, 21*, 74–82.

Maillard-Struby, F. (2012). Feeling unsure: A lived experience of humanbecoming. *Nursing Science Quarterly, 25*, 72–81.

Milton, C. L. (2003). A graduate curriculum guided by human becoming: Journeying with the possible. *Nursing Science Quarterly, 16*, 214–218.

Milton, C. L. (2010a). Doing the right thing with families during critical life events. *Nursing Science Quarterly, 23*, 113–116.

Milton, C. L. (2010b). Failing to do the right thing: Nurse practice and the family experience. *Nursing Science Quarterly, 23*, 206–208.

Milton, C. L. (2011). Reading between the lines: A leading-following phenomenon. *Nursing Science Quarterly, 24*, 321–323.

Milton, C. L. (2012a). Acting faithfully in community. *Nursing Science Quarterly, 25*, 25–27.

Milton, C. L. (2012b). Teaching-learning in community: The metaphor of nurse as guest. *Nursing Science Quarterly, 25*, 137–139.

Mitchell, G. J. (2004). An emerging framework for human becoming criticism. *Nursing Science Quarterly, 17*, 103–109.

Mitchell, G. J., Bernardo, A., & Bournes, D. (1997). Nursing guided by Parse's theory: Patient views at Sunnybrook. *Nursing Science Quarterly, 10*, 55–56.

Mitchell, G. J., & Bournes, D. A. (1998). *Finding the way: A video guide to patient focused care* (Videotape). Toronto, Ontario, Canada: Sunnybrook & Women's Health Science Centre.

Mitchell, G. J., & Bournes, D. A. (2000). Nurse as patient advocate? In search of straight thinking. *Nursing Science Quarterly, 13*, 204–209.

Mitchell, G. J., Bournes, D. A., & Hollett, J. (2006). Human becoming-guided patient centered care: New perspectives transform nursing practice. *Nursing Science Quarterly, 19*, 218–224.

Mitchell, G. J., & Cody, W. K. (1992). Nursing knowledge and human science: Ontological and epistemological considerations. *Nursing Science Quarterly, 5*, 54–61.

Mitchell, G. J., Jonas-Simpson, C., & Ivonoffski, V. (2006). Research-based theatre: The making of *I'm Still Here*. *Nursing Science Quarterly, 19*, 198–206.

Morrow, M. R. (2010). Feeling unsure: A universal lived experience. *Nursing Science Quarterly, 23*, 315–325.

Morrow, M. R. (2012a). Fairness and justice in leading-following: Opportunities to foster integrity in the first 100 days. *Nursing Science Quarterly, 25*, 188–193.

Morrow, M. R. (2012b). Reviews of books written by Rosemarie Rizzo Parse. *Nursing Science Quarterly, 25*, 114–118.

Naef, R., & Bournes, D. A. (2009). The lived experience of waiting: A Parse method study. *Nursing Science Quarterly, 22*, 141–153.

Nelligan, P., Grinspun, D., Jonas-Simpson, C., McConnell, H., Peter, E., & Pilkington, B. (2002). Client centered care: Making the ideal real. *Hospital Quarterly, 5*(4), 70–76.

Norris, J. R. (2002). One-to-one teleapprenticeship as a means for nurses teaching and learning Parse's theory of human becoming. *Nursing Science Quarterly, 15*, 143–149.

Northrup, D. T., & Cody, W. K. (1998). Evaluation of the human becoming theory in practice in an acute care psychiatric setting. *Nursing Science Quarterly, 11*, 23–30.

Oaks, G., & Drummond, S. (2009). Envisioning human dignity to enhance practice while journeying with Rwandan women: Student nurses teaching-learning Parse's theory of humanbecoming. *Nursing Science Quarterly, 22*, 229–232.

Parse, R. R. (1974). *Nursing fundamentals*. Flushing, NY: Medical Examination.

Parse, R. R. (1981). *Man-living-health: A theory of nursing*. New York: Wiley.

Parse, R. R. (1987). *Nursing science: Major paradigms, theories, and critiques*. Philadelphia: Saunders.
Parse, R. R. (1989). Essentials for practicing the art of nursing. *Nursing Science Quarterly, 2*, 111.
Parse, R. R. (1990). Health: A personal commitment. *Nursing Science Quarterly, 3*, 136–140.
Parse, R. R. (1991). Growing the discipline of nursing. *Nursing Science Quarterly, 4*, 139.
Parse, R. R. (1992). Human becoming: Parse's theory of nursing. *Nursing Science Quarterly, 5*, 35–42.
Parse, R. R. (1993). Scholarly dialogue: Theory guides research and practice. *Nursing Science Quarterly, 6*, 12.
Parse, R. R. (Ed.). (1995). *Illuminations: The human becoming theory in practice and research*. New York: National League for Nursing.
Parse, R. R. (1996). The human becoming theory: Challenges in practice and research. *Nursing Science Quarterly, 9*, 55–60.
Parse, R. R. (1998). *The human becoming school of thought: A perspective for nurses and other health professionals*. Thousand Oaks, CA: Sage.
Parse, R. R. (1999a). *Hope: An international human becoming perspective*. Sudbury, MA: Jones & Bartlett.
Parse, R. R. (1999b). Nursing: The discipline and the profession. *Nursing Science Quarterly, 12*, 275.
Parse, R. R. (2000). Into the new millennium. *Nursing Science Quarterly, 13*, 3.
Parse, R. R. (2001a). The lived experience of contentment: A study using the Parse research method. *Nursing Science Quarterly, 14*, 330–338.
Parse, R. R. (2001b). *Qualitative inquiry: The path of sciencing*. Boston: Jones & Bartlett.
Parse, R. R. (2003). *Community: A human becoming perspective*. Sudbury, MA: Jones & Bartlett.
Parse, R. R. (2004). A human becoming teaching-learning model. *Nursing Science Quarterly, 17*, 33–35.
Parse, R. R. (2005). The human becoming modes of inquiry: Emerging sciencing. *Nursing Science Quarterly, 18*, 297–300.
Parse, R. R. (2006). Feeling respected: A Parse method study. *Nursing Science Quarterly, 19*, 51–56.
Parse, R. R. (2007a). Hope in "Rita Hayworth and Shawshank Redemption": A human becoming hermeneutic study. *Nursing Science Quarterly, 20*, 148–154.
Parse, R. R. (2007b). The humanbecoming school of thought in 2050. *Nursing Science Quarterly, 20*, 308–311.
Parse, R. R. (2008a). The humanbecoming leading-following model. *Nursing Science Quarterly, 21*, 369–375.
Parse, R. R. (2008b). The humanbecoming mentoring model. *Nursing Science Quarterly, 21*, 5.
Parse, R. R. (2008c). Is there a tipping point for congruence in nursing knowledge? *Nursing Science Quarterly, 21*, 193.
Parse, R. R. (2008d). Nursing knowledge development: Who's to say how? *Nursing Science Quarterly, 21*, 101.
Parse, R. R. (2008e). Truth for the moment: Personal testimony as evidence. *Nursing Science Quarterly, 21*, 45–48.
Parse, R. R. (2009a). The humanbecoming family model. *Nursing Science Quarterly, 22*, 305–309.
Parse, R. R. (2009b). Knowledge development and programs of research. *Nursing Science Quarterly, 22*, 5–6.
Parse, R. R. (2009c). Mixed methods or mixed meanings in research? *Nursing Science Quarterly, 22*, 101.
Parse, R. R. (2010). Human dignity: A humanbecoming ethical phenomenon. *Nursing Science Quarterly, 23*, 257–262.
Parse, R. R. (2011a). Humanbecoming leading-following: The meaning of holding up the mirror. *Nursing Science Quarterly, 24*, 169–171.
Parse, R. R. (2011b). The humanbecoming modes of inquiry: Refinements. *Nursing Science Quarterly, 24*, 11–15.
Parse, R. R. (2011c). What people want from professional nurses. *Nursing Science Quarterly, 24*, 93.
Parse, R. R. (2012a, June). *The humanbecoming school of thought*. Paper presented at the Institute of Humanbecoming, Pittsburgh, PA.
Parse, R. R. (2012b). New humanbecoming conceptualizations and the humanbecoming community model: Expansions with sciencing and living the art. *Nursing Science Quarterly, 25*, 44–52.
Parse, R. R. (2013). Living quality: A humanbecoming phenomenon. *Nursing Science Quarterly, 26*, 111–115.
Parse, R. R. (2014). *The humanbecoming paradigm: A transformational worldview*. Pittsburgh: Discovery International.
Parse, R. R. (2016a). Humanbecoming hermeneutic sciencing: Reverence, awe, betrayal, and shame in *The Lives of Others*. *Nursing Science Quarterly, 29*, 128–135.
Parse, R. R. (2016b). Parsesciencing. *Nursing Science Quarterly, 29*(4), 271–274.
Peterson-Lund, R. (2011). The beauty of the moment: Lakota and humanbecoming perspective of time. *Nursing Science Quarterly, 24*, 386–390.
Peterson-Lund, R. (2012). Living on the edge: Frontier voices. *Nursing Science Quarterly, 25*, 90–96.
Phillips, J. R. (1987). A critique of Parse's man-living-health theory. In R. R. Parse (Ed.), *Nursing science: Major paradigms, theories, and critiques* (pp. 181–204). Philadelphia: Saunders.
Pickrell, K. D., Lee, R. E., Schumacher, L. P., & Twigg, P. (1998). Rosemarie Rizzo Parse: Human becoming. In A. M. Tomey & M. R. Alligood (Eds.), *Nursing theorists and their work* (4th ed., pp. 463–481). St Louis: Mosby.
Pilkington, F. B. (1993). The lived experience of grieving the loss of an important other. *Nursing Science Quarterly, 6*, 130–139.
Pilkington, F. B. (2008). Expanding nursing perspectives on loss and grieving. *Nursing Science Quarterly, 21*, 6–7.
Registered Nurses Association of Ontario. (2002). *Client centered care: Nursing best practice guideline*. Toronto, Ontario, Canada: Registered Nurses Association of Ontario.
Rogers, M. E. (1970). *An introduction to the theoretical basis of nursing*. Philadelphia: F. A. Davis.
Rogers, M. E. (1992). Nursing science and the space age. *Nursing Science Quarterly, 5*, 27–34.
Smith, S. M. (2010). Humanbecoming: Not just a way of being. *Nursing Science Quarterly, 23*, 216–219.
Smith, S. M. (2012). The lived experience of doing the right thing: A Parse method study. *Nursing Science Quarterly, 25*, 82–89.
Tanaka, J., Katsuno, T., & Takahashi, T. (2012). Using Parse's humanbecoming theory in Japan. *Nursing Science Quarterly, 25*, 99–102.
Ursel, K. L., & Aquino-Russell, C. E. (2010). Illuminating person-centered care with Parse's teaching-learning model. *Nursing Science Quarterly, 23*, 118–123.
Williamson, G. J. (2000). The test of a nursing theory: A personal view. *Nursing Science Quarterly, 13*, 124–128.

BIBLIOGRAPHY

Primary Sources

Books

Parse, R. R. (1974). *Nursing fundamentals*. Flushing, NY: Medical Examination.

Parse, R. R. (1981). *Man-living-health: A theory of nursing*. New York: Wiley.

Parse, R. R. (1987). *Nursing science: Major paradigms, theories, and critiques*. Philadelphia: Saunders.

Parse, R. R. (Ed.). (1995). *Illuminations: The human becoming theory in practice and research*. New York: National League for Nursing.

Parse, R. R. (1998). *The human becoming school of thought: A perspective for nurses and other health professionals*. Thousand Oaks, CA: Sage.

Parse, R. R. (1999). *Hope: An international human becoming perspective*. Sudbury, MA: Jones & Bartlett.

Parse, R. R. (2001). *Qualitative inquiry: The path of sciencing*. Boston: Jones & Bartlett.

Parse, R. R. (2003). *Community: A human becoming perspective*. Sudbury, MA: Jones & Bartlett.

Parse, R. R. (2014). *The humanbecoming paradigm: A transformational worldview*. Pittsburgh, PA: Discovery International.

Parse, R. R., Coyne, A. B., & Smith, M. J. (1985). *Nursing research: Qualitative methods*. Bowie, MD: Brady.

Journal Articles

Parse, R. R. (1967). Advantages and disadvantages of associate degree nursing programs. *Journal of Nursing Education, 6*(15), 5–8.

Parse, R. R. (1988). Beginnings. *Nursing Science Quarterly, 1*(1), 1–2.

Parse, R. R. (1988). Creating traditions: The art of putting it together. *Nursing Science Quarterly, 1*(2), 45.

Parse, R. R. (1988). Scholarly dialogue: The fire of refinement. *Nursing Science Quarterly, 1*(4), 141.

Parse, R. R. (1988). The mainstream of science: Framing the issue. *Nursing Science Quarterly, 1*(3), 93.

Parse, R. R. (1989). Essentials for practicing the art of nursing. *Nursing Science Quarterly, 2*(3), 111.

Parse, R. R. (1989). Making more out of less. *Nursing Science Quarterly, 2*(4), 155.

Parse, R. R. (1989). Martha E. Rogers: A birthday celebration. *Nursing Science Quarterly, 2*(2), 55.

Parse, R. R. (1989). Qualitative research: Publishing and funding. *Nursing Science Quarterly, 2*(1), 1–2.

Parse, R. R. (1990). A time for reflection and projection. *Nursing Science Quarterly, 3*(4), 143.

Parse, R. R. (1990). Health: A personal commitment. *Nursing Science Quarterly, 3*(3), 136–140.

Parse, R. R. (1990). Nursing theory–based practice: A challenge for the 90s. *Nursing Science Quarterly, 3*(2), 53.

Parse, R. R. (1990). Parse's research methodology with an illustration of the lived experience of hope. *Nursing Science Quarterly, 3*(1), 9–17.

Parse, R. R. (1990). Promotion and prevention: Two distinct cosmologies. *Nursing Science Quarterly, 3*(3), 101.

Parse, R. R. (1991). Electronic publishing: Beyond browsing. *Nursing Science Quarterly, 4*(1), 1.

Parse, R. R. (1991). Growing the discipline of nursing. *Nursing Science Quarterly, 4*(4), 139.

Parse, R. R. (1991). Mysteries of health and healing: Two perspectives. *Nursing Science Quarterly, 4*(3), 93.

Parse, R. R. (1991). Phenomenology and nursing. *Japanese Journal of Nursing, 17*(2), 261–269.

Parse, R. R. (1991). The right soil, the right stuff. *Nursing Science Quarterly, 4*(2), 47.

Parse, R. R. (1992). Human becoming: Parse's theory of nursing. *Nursing Science Quarterly, 5*(1), 35–42.

Parse, R. R. (1992). Moving beyond the barrier reef. *Nursing Science Quarterly, 5*(3), 97.

Parse, R. R. (1992). Nursing knowledge for the 21st century: An international commitment. *Nursing Science Quarterly, 5*(1), 8–12.

Parse, R. R. (1992). The performing art of nursing. *Nursing Science Quarterly, 5*(4), 147.

Parse, R. R. (1992). The unsung shapers of nursing science. *Nursing Science Quarterly, 5*(2), 47.

Parse, R. R. (1993). Cartoons: Glimpsing paradoxical moments. *Nursing Science Quarterly, 6*(1), 1.

Parse, R. R. (1993). Critical appraisal: Risking to challenge. *Nursing Science Quarterly, 6*(4), 163.

Parse, R. R. (1993). Nursing and medicine: Two different disciplines. *Nursing Science Quarterly, 6*(3), 109.

Parse, R. R. (1993). Plant now; reap later. *Nursing Science Quarterly, 6*(2), 55.

Parse, R. R. (1993). Scholarly dialogue: Theory guides research and practice. *Nursing Science Quarterly, 6*(1), 12.

Parse, R. R. (1993). The experience of laughter: A phenomenological study. *Nursing Science Quarterly, 6*(1), 39–43.

Parse, R. R. (1994). Charley Potatoes or mashed potatoes? *Nursing Science Quarterly, 7*(3), 97.

Parse, R. R. (1994). Laughing and health: A study using Parse's research method. *Nursing Science Quarterly, 7*(2), 55–64.

Parse, R. R. (1994). Martha E. Rogers: Her voice will not be silenced. *Nursing Science Quarterly, 7*(2), 47.

Parse, R. R. (1994). Quality of life: Sciencing and living the art of human becoming. *Nursing Science Quarterly, 7*(1), 16–21.

Parse, R. R. (1994). Scholarship: Three essential processes. *Nursing Science Quarterly, 7*(4), 143.

Parse, R. R. (1995). Again: What is nursing? *Nursing Science Quarterly, 8*(4), 143.

Parse, R. R. (1995). Building the realm of nursing knowledge. *Nursing Science Quarterly, 8*(2), 51.

Parse, R. R. (1995). Commentary: Parse's theory of human becoming: An alternative to nursing practice for pediatric oncology nurses. *Journal of Pediatric Oncology Nursing, 12*(3), 128.

Parse, R. R. (1995). Nursing theories and frameworks: The essence of advanced practice nursing. *Nursing Science Quarterly, 8*(1), 1.

Parse, R. R. (1996). Building knowledge through qualitative research: The road less traveled. *Nursing Science Quarterly, 9*(1), 10–16.

Parse, R. R. (1996). Critical thinking: What is it? *Nursing Science Quarterly, 9*(3), 138.

Parse, R. R. (1996). Hear ye, hear ye: Novice and seasoned authors! *Nursing Science Quarterly, 9*(1), 1.

Parse, R. R. (1996). Nursing theories: An original path. *Nursing Science Quarterly, 9*(2), 85.

Parse, R. R. (1996). Quality of life for persons living with Alzheimer's disease: A human becoming perspective. *Nursing Science Quarterly, 9*(3), 126–133.

Parse, R. R. (1996). Reality: A seamless symphony of becoming. *Nursing Science Quarterly*, *9*(4), 181–183.

Parse, R. R. (1996). The human becoming theory: Challenges in practice and research. *Nursing Science Quarterly*, *9*(1), 55–60.

Parse, R. R. (1997). Concept inventing: Unitary creations. *Nursing Science Quarterly*, *10*(2), 63–64.

Parse, R. R. (1997). The human becoming theory: The was, is, and will be. *Nursing Science Quarterly*, *10*(1), 32–38.

Parse, R. R. (1997). Investing the legacy: Martha E. Rogers' voice will not be silenced. *Visions: The Journal of Rogerian Science*, *5*(1), 7–11.

Parse, R. R. (1997). Joy-sorrow: A study using the Parse research method. *Nursing Science Quarterly*, *10*(2), 80–87.

Parse, R. R. (1997). Leadership: The essentials. *Nursing Science Quarterly*, *10*(3), 109.

Parse, R. R. (1997). New beginnings in a quiet revolution. *Nursing Science Quarterly*, *10*(1), 1.

Parse, R. R. (1997). Transforming research and practice with the human becoming theory. *Nursing Science Quarterly*, *10*(4), 171–174.

Parse, R. R. (1998). The art of criticism. *Nursing Science Quarterly*, *11*(2), 43.

Parse, R. R. (1998). Moving on. *Nursing Science Quarterly*, *11*(4), 135.

Parse, R. R. (1998). Will nursing exist tomorrow? A reprise. *Nursing Science Quarterly*, *11*(1), 1.

Parse, R. R. (1999). Authorship: Whose responsibility? *Nursing Science Quarterly*, *12*(2), 99.

Parse, R. R. (1999). Community: An alternative view. *Nursing Science Quarterly*, *12*(2), 119–124.

Parse, R. R. (1999). Expanding the vision: Tilling the field of nursing knowledge. *Nursing Science Quarterly*, *12*, 3.

Parse, R. R. (1999). Integrity and the advancement of nursing knowledge. *Nursing Science Quarterly*, *12*(3), 187.

Parse, R. R. (1999). Nursing science: The transformation of practice. *Journal of Advanced Nursing*, *30*(6), 1383–1387.

Parse, R. R. (1999). Nursing: The discipline and the profession. *Nursing Science Quarterly*, *12*(4), 275.

Parse, R. R. (1999). Witnessing as true presence. *Illuminations: Newsletter for the International Consortium of Parse Scholars*, *8*(3), 1.

Parse, R. R. (2000). Into the new millennium. *Nursing Science Quarterly*, *13*(1), 3.

Parse, R. R. (2000). Language: Words reflect and co-create meaning. *Nursing Science Quarterly*, *13*(3), 187.

Parse, R. R. (2000). Obfuscating: The persistent practice of misnaming. *Nursing Science Quarterly*, *13*(2), 91–92.

Parse, R. R. (2000). Paradigms: A reprise. *Nursing Science Quarterly*, *13*(4), 275–276.

Parse, R. R. (2001). Contributions to the discipline. *Nursing Science Quarterly*, *14*(1), 5.

Parse, R. R. (2001). The lived experience of contentment: A study using the Parse research method. *Nursing Science Quarterly*, *14*, 330–338.

Parse, R. R. (2001). Nursing: Still in the shadow of medicine. *Nursing Science Quarterly*, *14*(3), 181.

Parse, R. R. (2001). The universe is flat. *Nursing Science Quarterly*, *14*(2), 93.

Parse, R. R. (2002). 15th anniversary celebration. *Nursing Science Quarterly*, *15*, 3.

Parse, R. R. (2002). Aha! Ah! Haha! Discovery, wonder, laughter. *Nursing Science Quarterly*, *15*, 273.

Parse, R. R. (2002). Mentoring moments. *Nursing Science Quarterly*, *15*, 97.

Parse, R. R. (2002). Transforming healthcare with a unitary view of human. *Nursing Science Quarterly*, *15*, 46–50.

Parse, R. R. (2002). Words, words, words: Meanings, meanings, meanings! *Nursing Science Quarterly*, *15*, 183.

Parse, R. R. (2003). A call for dignity in nursing. *Nursing Science Quarterly*, *16*, 193.

Parse, R. R. (2003). Research approaches: Likenesses and differences. *Nursing Science Quarterly*, *16*, 5.

Parse, R. R. (2003). Silos and schools of thought. *Nursing Science Quarterly*, *16*, 101.

Parse, R. R. (2003). The lived experience of feeling very tired: A study using the Parse research method. *Nursing Science Quarterly*, *16*, 319–325.

Parse, R. R. (2003). What constitutes nursing research? *Nursing Science Quarterly*, *16*, 287.

Parse, R. R. (2004). Another look at vigilance. *Illuminations: Newsletter for the International Consortium of Parse Scholars*, *13*(2), 1.

Parse, R. R. (2004). A human becoming teaching-learning model. *Nursing Science Quarterly*, *17*, 33–35.

Parse, R. R. (2004). The many meanings of unitary: A plea for clarity. *Nursing Science Quarterly*, *17*, 293.

Parse, R. R. (2004). New directions. *Nursing Science Quarterly*, *17*, 5.

Parse, R. R. (2004). Person-centered care. *Nursing Science Quarterly*, *17*, 193.

Parse, R. R. (2004). Power in position. *Nursing Science Quarterly*, *17*, 101.

Parse, R. R. (2004). Quality of life: A human becoming perspective. *Japanese Journal of Nursing Research*, *37*(5), 21–26.

Parse, R. R. (2004). The ubiquitous nature of unitary: Major change in human becoming language. *Illuminations: Newsletter for the International Consortium of Parse Scholars*, *13*(1), 1.

Parse, R. R. (2005). Attentive reverence. *Illuminations: Newsletter for the International Consortium of Parse Scholars*, *14*(2), 1.

Parse, R. R. (2005). Challenges for global nursing. *Nursing Science Quarterly*, *18*, 285.

Parse, R. R. (2005). Choosing a doctoral program in nursing: What to consider. *Nursing Science Quarterly*, *18*, 5.

Parse, R. R. (2005). A community of scholars. *Nursing Science Quarterly*, *18*, 119.

Parse, R. R. (2005). The human becoming modes of inquiry: Emerging sciencing. *Nursing Science Quarterly*, *18*, 297–300.

Parse, R. R. (2005). The meaning of freely choosing. *Illuminations: Newsletter for the International Consortium of Parse Scholars*, *14*(1), 1–2.

Parse, R. R. (2005). Nursing and medicine: Continuing challenges. *Nursing Science Quarterly*, *18*, 5.

Parse, R. R. (2005). Parse's criteria for evaluation of theory with a comparison of Parse and Fawcett. *Nursing Science Quarterly*, *18*, 135–137.

Parse, R. R. (2005). Scientific standards: A renewed alert. *Nursing Science Quarterly*, *18*, 97.

Parse, R. R. (2005). Symbols and meanings in academia. *Nursing Science Quarterly*, *18*, 197.

Parse, R. R. (2006). Concept inventing: Continuing clarification. *Nursing Science Quarterly, 19,* 289.
Parse, R. R. (2006). Feeling respected: A Parse method study. *Nursing Science Quarterly, 19,* 51–57.
Parse, R. R. (2006). Nursing and medicine: Continuing challenges. *Nursing Science Quarterly, 19,* 5.
Parse, R. R. (2006). Outcomes: Saying what you mean. *Nursing Science Quarterly, 19,* 189.
Parse, R. R. (2006). Research findings evince benefits of nursing theory-guided practice. *Nursing Science Quarterly, 19,* 87.
Parse, R. R. (2007). Building a research culture. *Nursing Science Quarterly, 20,* 197.
Parse, R. R. (2007). Data-based articles and duplicate publication. *Nursing Science Quarterly, 20,* 301.
Parse, R. R. (2007). Hope in "Rita Hayworth and Shawshank Redemption": A human becoming hermeneutic study. *Nursing Science Quarterly, 20,* 148–154.
Parse, R. R. (2007). A human becoming perspective on quality of life. *Nursing Science Quarterly, 20,* 217.
Parse, R. R. (2007). The humanbecoming school of thought in 2050. *Nursing Science Quarterly, 20,* 308.
Parse, R. R. (2007). Nursing knowledge and health policy. *Nursing Science Quarterly, 20,* 105.
Parse, R. R. (2007). Twenty years of commitment to nursing's uniqueness as a discipline. *Nursing Science Quarterly, 20,* 5.
Parse, R. R. (2008). The humanbecoming leading-following model. *Nursing Science Quarterly, 21,* 369–375.
Parse, R. R. (2008). The humanbecoming mentoring model. *Nursing Science Quarterly, 21,* 195–198.
Parse, R. R. (2008). Is there a tipping point for congruence in nursing knowledge? *Nursing Science Quarterly, 21,* 193.
Parse, R. R. (2008). Nursing knowledge development: Who's to say how? *Nursing Science Quarterly, 21,* 101.
Parse, R. R. (2008). Proliferation of degrees in nursing: A call for clarity. *Nursing Science Quarterly, 21,* 5.
Parse, R. R. (2008). Truth for the moment: Personal testimony as evidence. *Nursing Science Quarterly, 21,* 45–48.
Parse, R. R. (2008). Time: The inevitable presence. *Nursing Science Quarterly, 21,* 281–282.
Parse, R. R. (2009). Knowledge development and programs of research. *Nursing Science Quarterly, 22,* 5–6.
Parse, R. R. (2009). Mixed methods or mixed meanings in research? *Nursing Science Quarterly, 22,* 101.
Parse, R. R. (2009). Visionary leadership: Making a difference in healthcare through research. *Nursing Science Quarterly, 22,* 197–198.
Parse, R. R. (2009). What a difference a word makes. *Nursing Science Quarterly, 22,* 301.
Parse, R. R. (2009). The humanbecoming family model. *Nursing Science Quarterly, 22,* 305–309.
Parse, R. R. (2010). Human dignity: A humanbecoming ethical phenomenon. *Nursing Science Quarterly, 23,* 257–262.
Parse, R. R. (2010). Imagine! *Nursing Science Quarterly, 23,* 97.
Parse, R. R. (2010). Nursing education: Issues reminiscent of the last century. *Nursing Science Quarterly, 23,* 273.
Parse, R. R. (2010). Respect! *Nursing Science Quarterly, 23,* 193.
Parse, R. R. (2011). Humanbecoming leading-following: The meaning of holding up the mirror. *Nursing Science Quarterly, 24,* 169–171.
Parse, R. R. (2011). The humanbecoming modes of inquiry: Refinements. *Nursing Science Quarterly, 24,* 11–15.
Parse, R. R. (2011). What people want from professional nurses. *Nursing Science Quarterly, 24,* 93.
Parse, R. R. (2012). Impact factor—one-size-fits-all: What's wrong with this picture? *Nursing Science Quarterly, 25,* 209–210.
Parse, R. R. (2012). New humanbecoming conceptualizations and the humanbecoming community model: Expansions with sciencing and living the art. *Nursing Science Quarterly, 25,* 44–52.
Parse, R. R. (2012). The things we make, make us. *Nursing Science Quarterly, 25,* 125.
Parse, R. R. (2012). The 25-year evolution of *Nursing Science Quarterly*: Keeping the dream alive. *Nursing Science Quarterly, 25,* 5–6.
Parse, R. R. (2013). Living quality: A humanbecoming phenomenon. *Nursing Science Quarterly, 26,* 111–115.
Parse, R. R. (2013). Move over nurses: There's a new professional on the block. *Nursing Science Quarterly, 26,* 301.
Parse, R. R. (2013). Research as evidence: The many meanings. *Nursing Science Quarterly, 26,* 109.
Parse, R. R. (2013). "What we've got here is failure to communicate": The meaning of the term *nursing* perspective. *Nursing Science Quarterly, 26,* 5–6.
Parse, R. R. (2013). Words: What do they really mean? *Nursing Science Quarterly, 26,* 209.
Parse, R. R. (2014). Evidence-based practice in nursing: Here or gone with the wind of disenchantment? *Nursing Science Quarterly, 27,* 189.
Parse, R. R. (2014). Integrity in publication. *Nursing Science Quarterly, 27,* 95.
Parse R. R. (2014). More on leadership: Ambiguity, integrity, wisdom. *Nursing Science Quarterly, 27,* 5.
Parse, R. R. (2014). Research language: A call for consistency. *Nursing Science Quarterly, 27,* 273.
Parse, R. R. (2015). Does one size fit all? *Nursing Science Quarterly, 28,* 261.
Parse, R. R. (2015). Interdisciplinary and interprofessional: What are the differences? *Nursing Science Quarterly, 28,* 5–6.
Parse, R. R. (2015). Nursing: A basic or applied science. *Nursing Science Quarterly, 28,* 181–182.
Parse, R. R. (2015). Nursing science or is it the science of nursing? *Nursing Science Quarterly, 28,* 101–102.
Parse, R. R. (2016). Humanbecoming hermeneutic sciencing: Reverence, awe, betrayal, and shame in *The Lives of Others*. *Nursing Science Quarterly, 29,* 128–135.
Parse, R. R. (2016). Parsesciencing: A basic science mode of inquiry. *Nursing Science Quarterly, 29.*
Parse, R. R. (2016). Quality of life: A ubiquitous term. *Nursing Science Quarterly, 29,* 185.
Parse, R. R. (2016). Scientific merit: Integrity in research. *Nursing Science Quarterly, 29,* 5.
Parse, R. R. (2016). Where have all the *nursing* theories gone? *Nursing Science Quarterly, 29,* 101–102.
Parse, R. R., Bournes, D. A., Barrett, E. A. M., Malinski, V. M., & Phillips, J. R. (1999). A better way: 10 things health professionals can do to move toward a more personal and meaningful system. *On Call: A Magazine for Nurses and Healthcare Professionals, 2*(8), 14–17.

25

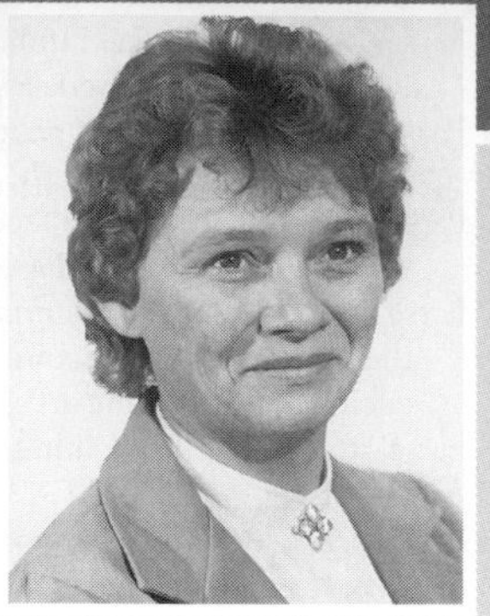

Helen C. Erickson
(1937–Present)

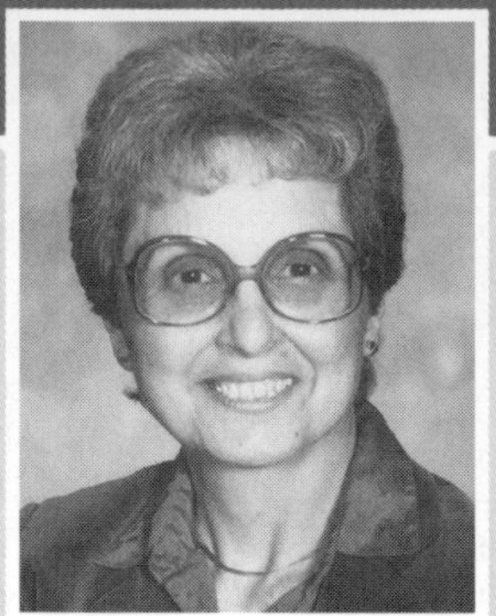

Evelyn M. Tomlin
(1929–Present)

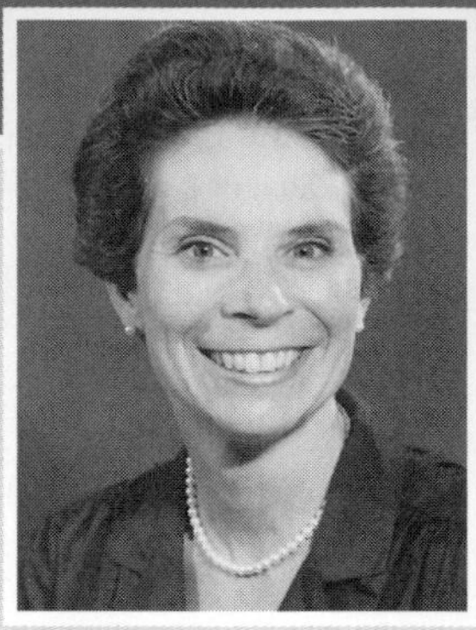

Mary Ann P. Swain
(1941–Present)

Modeling and Role-Modeling

Margaret E. Erickson

"Unconditional acceptance of the person as a human in the process of Being and Becoming is basic to the Modeling and Role-Modeling paradigm. It is a prerequisite to facilitating holistic growth. . . . Unconditional acceptance of the person as a human being who has an inherent need for dignity and respect from others, and for connectedness—that kind of Unconditional Acceptance is based on Unconditional Love."

(Erickson, 2006, p. 343)

CREDENTIALS AND BACKGROUND OF THE THEORISTS

Helen C. Erickson

Helen C. Erickson received a diploma in 1957 from Saginaw General Hospital in Saginaw, Michigan. Her degrees include a baccalaureate in nursing in 1974, dual master's degrees in psychiatric nursing and medical-surgical nursing in 1976, and a doctorate of educational psychology in 1984, all from the University of Michigan. Erickson began her professional experience as Head Nurse of the Midland Community Hospital Emergency Room in Midland, Texas; she then worked as Night Supervisor at the Michigan State Home for the Mentally Impaired and Handicapped in Mount Pleasant. In 1960 she moved to Puerto Rico with her husband and was Director of Health Services at Inter-American University in San German, Puerto Rico, until 1964. On return to the United States, she worked as a staff nurse at St. Joseph's and University of Michigan Hospitals in Ann Arbor, Michigan. Later she was a Mental Health nurse consultant to the Pediatric Nurse Practitioner Program at the University of Michigan and Adult Care units at the University of Michigan Hospitals.

Erickson's academic career began at the University of Michigan School of Nursing as Assistant Instructor in the RN Studies Program; later she was named Chairperson of the Undergraduate Program and Dean for Undergraduate Studies. She served as Assistant Professor at the University

Previous authors: Margaret E. Erickson, Jane A. Caldwell-Gwin, Lisa A. Carr, Brenda Kay Harmon, Karen Hartman, Connie Rae Jarlsberg, Judy McCormick, and Kathryn W. Noone.
The authors express appreciation to Helen C. Erickson, Evelyn M. Tomlin, and Mary Ann P. Swain for critiquing earlier editions of this chapter.

of Michigan from 1978 to 1986. In 1986 she moved to the University of South Carolina College of Nursing, where she served as Associate Professor, Assistant Dean for Academic Programs, and Associate Dean for Academic Affairs. In 1988 she became Professor of Nursing, Chair of Adult Health, and Special Assistant to the Dean, Graduate Programs, at the University of Texas School of Nursing in Austin, Texas. In 1997 she was honored with Emeritus Professor status at the University of Texas at Austin. She has maintained an independent nursing practice since 1976.

Erickson is a member of the American Nurses Association, American Nurses Foundation, the Charter Club, American Holistic Nurses Association, Texas Nurses Association, Sigma Theta Tau, and the Institute for the Advancement of Health. She served as President of the Society for the Advancement of Modeling and Role-Modeling from 1986 to 1990; as chairperson of the First National Symposium on Modeling and Role-Modeling in 1986; and on the planning boards for many national biannual conferences.

Erickson was in *Who's Who Among University Students* and is a member of Phi Kappa Phi. She received the Sigma Theta Tau Rho Chapter Award of Excellence in Nursing in 1980 and the Amoco Foundation Good Teaching Award in 1982. She was accepted into Adara (a University of Michigan honor society for women in leadership from 1980 to 1986) in 1982. In 1990 she received the Faculty Teaching Award from the University of Texas School of Nursing, a Founders award from the Sigma Theta Tau International Honor Society in Nursing. She also received the Excellence in Education Award from the Epsilon Theta chapter in 1993 and the Graduate Faculty Teaching Award from the University of Texas School of Nursing in 1995. Erickson was inducted as a Fellow into the American Academy of Nursing in 1996. She received the Distinguished Faculty citation from Humboldt State University in California in 2001. The Helen Erickson Endowed Lectureship in Holistic Health Nursing was established in her honor in 1997 at the University of Texas at Austin. The biennial lectureship highlights international holistic nursing leaders. She was honored with the American Holistic Nurses Association, Holistic Nurse of the Year Award in 2014 for her outstanding and ongoing work in furthering holistic nursing.

Erickson consults on research using the modeling and role-modeling theory and presents seminars, conferences, keynotes, and papers on the theory nationally and internationally. She has consulted on implementation of the theory in practice at the University of Michigan Medical Center; Brigham and Women's Hospital in Boston; Oregon Health Science University Hospital in Portland; the University Health Systems in San Antonio, Texas; and the University of Pittsburgh hospitals as well as other institutions. In academic settings and service practice–based institutions and agencies, she mentors and facilitates faculty members, staff nurses, and administrators on use of the theory in their curricula and practice. Humboldt University School of Nursing in Arcata, California, was first to use the modeling and role-modeling theory as a conceptual curriculum base. Metropolitan State University at St. Paul adopted the modeling and role-modeling theory for their nursing programs. Similarly, St. Catherine's College in St. Paul, Minnesota, and the Joanne Gay Dishman Department of Nursing at Lamar University in Beaumont, Texas adopted it for many of their programs.

Erickson has been invited to speak at many national and international conferences. She has been involved in activities of the American Holistic Nurses' Association, served as a content expert for certification curricula, and was included in a book featuring nurse healers (H. Erickson, personal communication, July 1992). Although retired from the University of Texas at Austin, she is still actively involved in the promotion of holistic nursing, serving as Chair for the Board of Directors of the American Holistic Nurses' Certification Corporation (AHNCC) from 2002 to 2012, she remains involved and committed to the work of the AHNCC. She provides consultation and educational programs nationally and internationally and is actively involved in the Society for the Advancement of Modeling and Role-Modeling (H. Erickson, personal communication, June 2000); she also serves on the Milton H. Erickson Foundation Board of Directors.

Evelyn M. Tomlin

Evelyn M. Tomlin's nursing education began in Southern California. She attended Pasadena City College, Los Angeles County General Hospital School of Nursing, and the University of Southern California, where she received her bachelor of science degree in nursing. In 1976 she received a master's of science degree in psychiatric nursing from the University of Michigan.

Tomlin's professional experiences are varied. She began as a clinical instructor at Los Angeles County General Hospital School of Nursing and later lived in Kabul, Afghanistan, where she taught English at the Afghan Institute of Technology. She served as a school nurse and practiced family nursing in the overseas American and European communities where she lived and participated in more than 46 home deliveries with a certified nurse-midwife. After she established medical services at the United States Embassy Hospital, she practiced as a staff nurse. Upon returning to the United States, she was employed by the Visiting Nurse Association (VNA) in Ann Arbor, Michigan. At the VNA, she was coordinator and clinical instructor for student practical nurses. In addition, she was a staff nurse in a coronary care unit, worked in the respiratory intensive care unit, and was head nurse in the emergency department at St. Joseph's Mercy Hospital in Ann Arbor. She later taught fundamentals of nursing as Assistant Professor in the RN Studies Program at the University of Michigan. During this time, she served as mental health consultant to the pediatric nurse practitioner program at the University of Michigan.

Tomlin was among the first 16 nurses in the United States to be certified by the American Association of Critical Care Nurses. With several colleagues, she opened one of the first offices for independent nursing practice in Michigan and continued independent practice until 1993. She is a member of Sigma Theta Tau Rho Chapter, California Scholarship Federation, and the Philomathian Society. Tomlin presented programs based on the Modeling and Role-Modeling Theory, with emphasis on clinical applications. She was the first editor for the newsletter of the Society for the Advancement of Modeling and Role-Modeling (E. Tomlin, curriculum vitae, 1992).

In 1985 Tomlin moved to Big Rock, Illinois, where she enjoyed teaching small community and nursing groups and working in a community shelter serving the women and children of Fox Valley. She later moved to Geneva, Illinois, where she resides with her husband. Tomlin identifies herself as a Christian in retirement from nursing for pay, but not from nursing practice. She is pursuing interests in the practice of healing prayer, stating that she has always been interested in the interface of the modeling and role-modeling theory and Judeo-Christian principles. She is now retired after many years on the Board of Directors and as a volunteer at Wayside Cross Ministries in Aurora, Illinois, where she taught and counseled homeless women, many of whom were single mothers.

Mary Ann P. Swain

Mary Ann P. Swain's educational background is in psychology. She received her bachelor's degree in psychology from DePauw University and her master's and doctoral degrees in psychology from the University of Michigan. Swain taught psychology, research methods, and statistics as a teaching assistant at DePauw University and later as a lecturer and professor of psychology and nursing research at the University of Michigan. At the University of Michigan, she was Director of the Doctoral Program in Nursing in 1975 for 1 year, was Chairperson of Nursing Research from 1977 to 1982, and became Associate Vice President for Academic Affairs in 1983.

Swain is a member of the American Psychological Association and an associate member of the Michigan Nurses Association. She developed and taught classes in psychology, research, and nursing research methods and collaborated with nurse researchers on projects, including health promotion among diabetic patients and ways to influence compliance among patients with hypertension. She helped Erickson publish a model that assessed an individual's potential to mobilize resources and adapt to stress, which is significant to the modeling and role-modeling theory.

Swain received the Alpha Lambda Delta, Psi Chi, Mortar Board, and Phi Beta Kappa awards while at DePauw University. In 1981 she was recognized by the Rho Chapter of Sigma Theta Tau for Contributions to Nursing, and in 1983 she became an honorary member of Sigma Theta Tau. In 1994 she moved to Appalachia, New York, with her husband, where she served as Provost and Vice President for Academic Affairs for Binghamton University for nearly 20 years. Currently she is director of the doctoral (PhD in nursing) program at Decker School of Nursing and Chair of the Department of Student Affairs at Binghamton University in Binghamton, New York. Her research interests are modeling and role-modeling theory; health development across the life span; self-care; leadership and management; and interrelationships among life stressors, healthy development, and illness.

THEORETICAL SOURCES

The theory and paradigm of modeling and role-modeling was developed with a retroductive process. The original model was derived inductively from Erickson's clinical and personal life experiences. The works of Maslow, Erikson, Piaget, Engel, Selye, and Milton H. Erickson were then integrated and synthesized into the original model to name, articulate, and refine a holistic theory and paradigm for nursing. H. Erickson (1976) argued that people have mind-spirit-body relations and an identifiable resource potential that predicts their ability to contend with stressors and resulting stress. She articulated a relationship between needs status and developmental processes, satisfaction with needs and attachment objects, loss and illness, and health and need satisfaction. Tomlin and Swain validated and affirmed Erickson's practice model and helped her expand and articulate phenomena, concepts, and theoretical relationships.

Maslow's theory of human needs was used to label and articulate Erickson and her colleagues' personal observations that "all people want to be the best that they can possibly be; unmet basic needs interfere with holistic growth whereas satisfied needs promote growth" (M. Erickson, 1996a, 1996b, 2006; Erickson, Tomlin, & Swain, 2002, p. 56; Jensen, 1995). Erickson further developed the model to state that unmet basic needs create need deficits that lead to initiation or aggravation of physical or mental distress or illness, whereas needs satisfaction creates assets that provide resources needed to contend with stress and promote health, growth, and development.

Piaget's theory of cognitive development provided a framework for understanding development of thinking, and Erik Erikson's work on psychosocial development through the life span provided a theoretical basis for understanding the psychosocial evolution of the individual. His eight stages represent developmental tasks. As an individual resolves each task, he or she gains strengths that contribute to character development and health. As an outcome of each stage, people develop a sense of their own worth and projection of themselves into the future. "The utility of Erikson's theory is the freedom we may take to view aspects of people's problems as uncompleted tasks. This perspective provides a hopeful expectation for the individual's future since it connotes something still in progress" (Erickson, Tomlin, & Swain, 2002, pp. 62–63).

The works of Winnicott, Klein, Mahler, and Bowlby on object attachment were integrated to develop and articulate the concept of affiliated individuation (AI). Object relations theory proposes that an infant initially forms an attachment to his or her caregiver after having repeated positive contacts. As the child grows and begins to move toward a more separate and individuated state, a sense of autonomy develops, and he or she usually transfers some attachment to an inanimate object such as a cuddly blanket or a teddy bear. Later, the child may attach to a favorite baseball glove, doll, or pet, and finally onto more abstract things in adulthood, such as an educational degree, professional role, or relationship. Erickson drew on these works and proposed a theoretical relationship between object attachment and needs satisfaction, theorizing that when an object repeatedly meets an individual's basic needs, attachment or connectedness to that object occurs. From synthesis of these theoretical linkages and research findings, a new concept of AI was identified and defined as the "need to be dependent on support systems while simultaneously maintaining independence from these support systems" (Erickson et al., 1983, p. 252)—that all people have an inherent need to be connected with significant others at the same time that there is a sense of separateness and individuation from them (H. Erickson, 2006, 2010; M. Erickson, 1996b; Erickson, Erickson, & Jensen, 2006; Erickson, Tomlin, & Swain, 1983). From the time of birth until a person takes their last breath, AI and object attachment are essential to needs satisfaction, adaptive coping, and healthy growth and development. Furthermore, "object loss results in basic need deficits" (Erickson, Tomlin, & Swain, 2002, p. 88). Loss is real, threatened, or perceived; it may be a normal part of the developmental process, or it may be situational. Loss always results in grief; normal grief is resolved in approximately 1 year. When loss occurs and only inadequate or inappropriate objects are available to meet needs, morbid grief results. Morbid grief interferes with the individual's ability to grow and develop to his or her maximal potential (M. Erickson, 2006; Erickson, Tomlin, & Swain, 2002). The work of Selye and Engel, cited by Erickson, Tomlin, and Swain (1983), provided additional conceptual support for the propositions regarding loss and an individual's stress responses to loss or losses. Selye's theory pertains to an individual's biophysical responses to stress, and Engel explores psychosocial responses to stressors.

The integration and synthesis of these theories, with Erickson's clinical observations and lived experiences, resulted in the conception of the adaptive potential assessment model (APAM). The APAM focuses on an individual's ability to mobilize resources when confronted with stressors rather than adapt to them. This model was first developed by Erickson (1976) and later described in publication by Erickson and Swain (1982).

Erickson credits Milton H. Erickson with influencing her clinical practice and providing inspiration and direction in the development of this theory. Initially, he articulated the formulation of the modeling and role-modeling theory when he urged H. Erickson to "model the client's world, understand it as they do, then role-model the picture the client has drawn, building a healthy world for them" (H. Erickson, personal communication, November 1984).

MAJOR CONCEPTS & DEFINITIONS

Modeling

The act of **modeling** is the process the nurse uses as she or he develops an image and an understanding of the client's world—an image and understanding developed within the client's framework and from the client's perspective. The art of modeling is the development of a mirror image of the situation from the client's perspective. "The science of modeling is the scientific aggregation and analysis of data collected about the client's model" (Erickson, Tomlin, & Swain, 2002, p. 95). "Modeling occurs as the nurse accepts and understands her client" (Erickson, Tomlin, & Swain, 2002, p. 96).

Role-Modeling

The art of **role-modeling** occurs when the nurse plans and implements interventions that are unique for the client. The science of role-modeling occurs as the nurse plans interventions with respect to her theoretical base

Continued

MAJOR CONCEPTS & DEFINITIONS—cont'd

for the practice of nursing. "Role-modeling is the essence of nurturance. It requires an unconditional acceptance of the person as the person is, while gently encouraging and facilitating growth and development at the person's own pace and within the person's own model" (Erickson, Tomlin, & Swain, 2002, p. 95). "Role-modeling starts the second the nurse moves from the analysis phase of the nursing process to the planning of nursing interventions" (Erickson, Tomlin, & Swain, 2002, p. 95).

Nursing

"**Nursing** is the holistic helping of persons with their self-care activities in relation to their health. This is an interactive, interpersonal process that nurtures clients' strengths to enable the development, release, and channeling of resources for coping with their circumstances and environment. The goal is to achieve a state of perceived optimum health and contentment" (Erickson, Tomlin, & Swain, 2002, p. 49).

Nurturance

"**Nurturance** fuses and integrates cognitive, physiological, and affective processes, with the aim of assisting a client to move toward holistic health. Nurturance implies that the nurse seeks to know and understand the client's personal model of his or her world and to appreciate its value and significance for that client from the client's perspective" (Erickson, Tomlin, & Swain, 2002, pp. 48–49).

Unconditional Acceptance

"Being accepted as a unique, worthwhile, important individual—with no strings attached—is imperative if the individual is to be facilitated in developing his or her own potential. The nurse's use of empathy helps the individual learn that the nurse accepts and respects him or her as is. The acceptance will facilitate the mobilization of resources needed as this individual strives for adaptive equilibrium" (Erickson, Tomlin, & Swain, 2002, p. 49).

Person

People are alike because they have holism, lifetime growth and development, and a need for affiliated individuation (AI). They are different because they have inherent endowment, adaptation, and self-care knowledge (Erickson, Tomlin, & Swain, 1983).

How People Are Alike

Holism

"Human beings are holistic persons who have multiple interacting subsystems. Permeating all subsystems are the inherent bases. These include genetic makeup and spiritual drive. Body, mind, emotion, and spirit are a total unit, and they act together. They affect and control one another interactively. The interaction of the multiple subsystems and the inherent bases creates **holism:** Holism implies that the whole is greater than the sum of the parts" (Erickson, Tomlin, & Swain, 2002, pp. 44–45).

Basic Needs

"All human beings have basic needs that can be satisfied, but only from within the framework of the individual" (Erickson, Tomlin, & Swain, 2002, p. 58). "Basic needs are met only when the individual perceives that they are met" (Erickson, Tomlin, & Swain, 2002, p. 57).

Lifetime Development

Lifetime development evolves through psychological and cognitive stages.

Psychological Stages

"Each stage represents a developmental task or a decisive encounter resulting in a turning point, a moment of decision between alternative basic attitudes (e.g., trust versus mistrust or autonomy versus shame and doubt). As a maturing individual negotiates or resolves each age-specific crisis or task, the individual gains enduring strengths and attitudes that contribute to the character and health of the individual's personality in his or her culture" (Erickson, Tomlin, & Swain, 2002, p. 61).

Cognitive Stages

"Consider how thinking develops rather than what happens in psychosocial or affective development. Piaget believed that cognitive learning develops in a sequential manner and in stages. He identified four distinct stages in this process: sensorimotor, preoperational, concrete operations, and formal operations" (Erickson, Tomlin, & Swain, 2002, pp. 63–64).

Affiliated Individuation

"Individuals have an instinctual need for AI. They need to be able to depend on support systems while simultaneously maintaining independence from these support systems. They need to feel a deep sense of both the "I" and the "we" states of being and to perceive freedom and acceptance in both states" (Erickson, Tomlin, & Swain, 2002, p. 47).

MAJOR CONCEPTS & DEFINITIONS—cont'd

How People Are Different

Inherent Endowment

"Each individual is born with a set of genes that will to some extent predetermine appearance, growth, development, and responses to life events. Clearly, both genetic makeup and inherited characteristics influence growth and development. They might influence how one perceives oneself and one's world. They make individuals different from one another, each unique in his or her own way" (Erickson, Tomlin, & Swain, 2002, pp. 74–75).

Adaptation

Adaptation occurs as the individual responds to external and internal stressors in a health-directed and growth-directed manner. Adaptation involves mobilizing internal and external coping resources. No subsystem is left in jeopardy when adaptation occurs (Erickson, Tomlin, & Swain, 2002).

The individual's ability to mobilize resources is depicted by the adaptive potential assessment model (APAM). "The APAM identifies three different coping potential states: (1) arousal, (2) equilibrium (adaptive and maladaptive), and (3) impoverishment. Each of these states represents a different potential for the individual to mobilize self-care resources. . . . Movement among the states is influenced by one's ability to cope [with ongoing stressors] and the presence of new stressors" (Erickson, Tomlin, & Swain, 2002, pp. 80–81).

Nurses can use this model to predict an individual's potential to mobilize self-care resources in response to stress.

Mind-Body-Emotion-Spirit Relationships

"We are all biophysical, psychosocial beings who want to develop our potential—that is, to be the best we can be" (Erickson, Tomlin, & Swain, 2002, p. 70). Permeating all the subsystems is humans' spiritual drive.

Self-Care

Self-care involves the use of knowledge, resources, and actions.

Self-Care Knowledge

"At some level, a person knows what has made him or her sick, lessened his or her effectiveness, or interfered with his or her growth. The person also knows what will make him or her well, optimize his or her effectiveness or fulfillment (given circumstances), or promote his or her growth" (Erickson, Tomlin, & Swain, 2002, p. 48).

Self-Care Resources

Self-care resources are "the internal resources, as well as additional resources, mobilized through self-care action that help gain, maintain, and promote an optimum level of holistic health" (Erickson, Tomlin, & Swain, 2002, pp. 254–255).

Self-Care Action

Self-care action is "the development and utilization of self-care knowledge and self-care resources" (Erickson, Tomlin, & Swain, 2002, p. 254).

USE OF EMPIRICAL EVIDENCE

Several studies provided initial evidence for philosophical premises and theoretical linkages implied in the original book by Erickson, Tomlin, and Swain (1983) and later specified by Erickson (1990b). The APAM (Figs. 25.1 and 25.2) has been tested as a classification model (Barnfather,

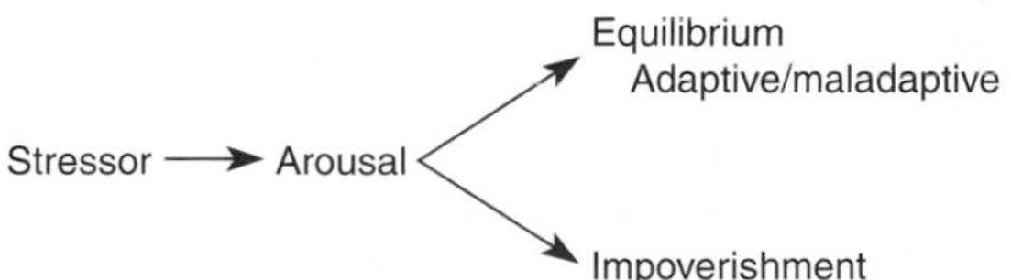

FIG. 25.1 Adaptive potential assessment model. (From Erickson, H. C., Tomlin, E. M., & Swain, M. A. P. [1983]. *Modeling and role-modeling: A theory and paradigm for nursing.* Englewood Cliffs, NJ: Prentice Hall.)

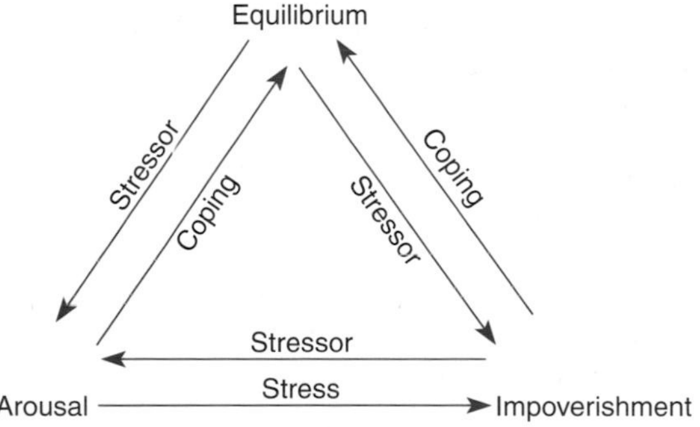

FIG. 25.2 Dynamic relationship among the states of the adaptive potential assessment model. (From Erickson, H. C., Tomlin, E. M., & Swain, M. A. P. [1983]. *Modeling and role-modeling: A theory and paradigm for nursing.* Englewood Cliffs, NJ: Prentice Hall.)

1987; Erickson, 1976) (1) as a predictor for health status (Barnfather, 1990b) (2) for length of hospital stay (Erickson & Swain, 1982), and (3) for assessing basic needs status (Barnfather, 1993). Findings from these studies provided beginning evidence for the proposed three states across populations, a relationship between health and ability to mobilize resources, and an ability to mobilize resources and needs status. Benson (2003, 2006, 2011) studied the APAM as applied to small groups.

Relationships among self-care knowledge, resources, and activities were demonstrated in several studies (Acton, 1993; Baas, 1992; Goldstein, 2013; Irvin, 1993; Jensen, 1995; Miller, 1994). The self-care knowledge construct first studied by Erickson (1990c) was replicated and found to be significantly associated with perceived control; perceived autonomy (Hertz & Anschutz, 2002; Matsui & Capezuti, 2008); and quality of life (Baas, Fontana, & Bhat, 1997; Goldstein, 2013). Self-directedness, need for harmony (affiliation), and need for autonomy (individuation) were found when multidimensional scaling was used to explore relationships among self-care knowledge, resources, and actions. The author concluded that a positive attitude was a major factor when health-directed self-care actions were assessed (Rosenow, 1991). Physical activity in patients after myocardial infarction was affected by life satisfaction (not physical condition); life satisfaction was predicted by availability of self-care resources and resources needed; and resources needed served as a suppressor for resources available (Baas, 1992). Bray (2005) found in an adolescent population that needs satisfaction was associated with development of internal resources and the ability to cope adaptively with stressors related to cognitive and psychological health challenges. In a sample of caregivers, social support predicted stress level and self-worth had an indirect effect on hope through self-worth (Irvin, 1993; Irvin & Acton, 1997), whereas persons with diabetes and spiritual well-being were better able to cope (Landis, 1991).

Using modeling and role-modeling theory as a guideline, interviews were conducted to determine the client's model of the world, and seven themes emerged (Erickson, 1990a):

1. Cause of the problem, which was unique to the individual
2. Related factors, also unique to the individual
3. Expectations for the future
4. Types of perceived control
5. Affiliation
6. Lack of affiliation
7. Trust in the caregiver

Each was unique and warranted individualized interventions. Other qualitative research studies on self-care knowledge revealed that acutely ill patients perceived monitoring, caring, presence, touch, and voice tones as comforting (Kennedy, 1991); healthy adults sought needs satisfaction from the nurse practitioner in primary care (Boodley, 1986, 1990); and hospice patients benefited from nurse empathy (Raudonis, 1991). Additional studies addressed the experience of persons 85 years of age and older as they managed their health (Beltz, 1999), the perceptions of hope in elementary school children (Baldwin, 1996), the experiences and perceptions of mothers using child health services in South Africa (Jonker, 2012), the experiential meaning of well-being and the lived experience of employed mothers (Weber, 1995, 1999), the meaning and effects of suffering in people with rheumatoid arthritis (Dildy, 1992), the relationship between experiences of prolonged family suffering and evolving spiritual identity (Clayton, 2001), the quality of life of older adults with urinary incontinence (Liang, 2008), practice challenges when caring for morbidly obese patients (Pokorny et al., 2009), unmet needs of patients with schizophrenia (Perese & Wu, 2010), promotion of optimum health outcomes among children of incarcerated parents (Falk, 2013, 2014), and human–environment relationships when healing from an episodic illness (Bowman, 1998).

Case study methods have shown relationships among needs, attachment, and developmental residual needs (Kinney, 1990; Kinney & Erickson, 1990) and coping (Jensen, 1995) and challenges in the treatment of factitious disorder (Hagglund, 2009).

Studies revealed relationships among mistrust and length of stay in hospitalized subjects; perceived enactment of autonomy, self-care, and holistic health in older adults (Anschutz, 2000; Hertz & Anschutz, 2002; Hertz, Rossetti, & Nelson, 2005); perceived enactment of autonomy and self-care resources among senior center users (Matsui & Capezuti, 2008); perceived enactment of autonomy, self-care, support, control, and well-being in older adults (Chen, 1996); perceived enactment of autonomy and related sociodemographic factors among older adults (Hwang & Lin, 2004); loss, morbid grief, and onset of symptoms of Alzheimer disease (Erickson et al., 1994; Irvin & Acton, 1996); AI and self-care knowledge in adults undergoing chronic warfarin therapy (Goldstein, 2013); and basic needs satisfaction and health-promoting self-care behaviors in adults (Acton & Malathum, 2000).

Other studies addressed linkages between role-modeled interventions and outcomes (Erickson et al., 1994; Hertz, 1991; Irvin, 1993; Jensen, 1995; Kennedy, 1991; Lamb, 2005; Sung & Yu, 2006). University students who perceived satisfaction of needs were more successful in school (Smith, 1980), older adults who felt supported reported higher needs satisfaction and were better able to cope (Keck, 1989), adolescent mothers who felt supported and perceived needs satisfaction had a more positive maternal–infant attachment (M. Erickson, 2006; Erickson, 1996a, 1996b), and persons convicted of sexual offenses who were provided with support to remodel their worlds were able to develop new behaviors and move on with their lives (Scheela, 1991). Families and post–myocardial infarction patients who were able to participate in planning their own care through contracting had less anxiety and better perceived control and support (Holl, 1992). Caregivers of adults with dementia who experienced theory-based nursing using the modeling and role-modeling theory perceived that their needs were met and were healthier, and they were encouraged, which helped them accept the situation and transcend the experience of caregiving (Hopkins, 1995). Self-care resources, measured as needs, are related to perceived support and coping in women with breast cancer (Keck, 1989), physical well-being in persons with chronic obstructive pulmonary disease (Kline, 1988; Leidy, 1990), and anxiety in hospitalized patients who had cardiac surgery and their families (Holl, 1992). Finally, when AI was tested as a buffer between stress and well-being, a mediation effect was found (Acton, 1993, 1997; Acton et al., 1997).

Chen (1996) found that feelings of control over one's health (health control orientation) status in older adults with hypertension correlated highly with self-efficacy and self-care. In addition, her work supported that health control orientation, self-efficacy, and self-care were associated with well-being. Other researchers found that trust predicts adolescent clients' involvement in a prescribed medical regimen (Finch, 1987); perceived support and adaptation are related to developmental residual in families with newborn infants (Darling-Fisher, 1987; Darling-Fisher & Leidy 1988); and mistrust predicts length of hospital stay, and positive residual serves as a buffer (Finch, 1987). Positive residual in the intimacy stage of healthy adults predicts health behaviors (MacLean, 1990, 1992). Developmental residual predicts hope, trust-mistrust residual predicts generalized hope and autonomy-shame, and doubt residual predicts particularized hope in the elderly (Curl, 1992).

Studies have also been used to explore perceived enactment of autonomy and life satisfaction in older adults (Anschutz, 2000), self-care knowledge in informants in the hospital (Erickson, 1985), developmental growth in adults with heart failure (Baas et al., 1999), the ability to mobilize coping resources and basic needs (Barnfather, 1990a), the relationship between basic needs satisfaction and emotionally motivated eating (Cleary, & Crafti, 2007; Timmerman & Acton, 2001); relations among hostility, self-esteem, self-concept, and psychosocial residual in persons with coronary heart disease (Sofhauser, 1996, 2003); and hostility among nurses in the workplace setting (Sofhauser, 2015). Researchers have explored the relationship between spiritual well-being and heart failure (Beery et al., 2002); spirituality in caregivers of family members with dementia (Acton & Miller, 1996); the implementation of a mind, body, spirit self-empowerment program for adolescents (Nash, 2007a, 2007b); and spirituality in women with breast cancer (Kinney et al., 2003). Baas (2004) studied self-care resources and quality of life in patients after myocardial infarction and self-care resources and well-being in clients with cardiac disorders (Baas, 2011). She and colleagues examined the psychosocial aspects of heart failure management (Baas & Conway, 2004), explored body awareness in heart failure or transplant patients (Baas et al., 2004), and reported patient adjustments to cardiac devices (Beery, Baas, & Henthorn, 2007).

Tools that have been developed to test the modeling and role-modeling theory include the Basic Needs Satisfaction Inventory (Kline, 1988), the Erikson Psychosocial Stage Inventory (Darling-Fisher & Leidy, 1988), the Perceived Enactment of Autonomy tool designed to measure prerequisites to self-care actions in the elderly (Hertz, 1991, 1999; Hertz & Anschutz, 2002), the Self-Care Resource Inventory (Baas, 1992, 2011), an adjustment scale designed to measure self-report with implanted devices in cardiac patients (Beery et al., 2005), the Robinson Self-Appraisal Inventory to measure denial (the first stage in the grief process) in patients after myocardial infarction (Robinson, 1994), the Erickson Maternal Bonding-Attachment Tool designed to measure self-care knowledge as motivational style (deficit or being motivated) and self-care resource (maternal needs satisfaction) (Erickson, 1996b), the Family Experience With Eating Disorders Scale (FEEDS) to measure self-care knowledge regarding parental perceptions of the family environment and family dynamics specific to eating disorders (Folse, 2007), and the Hopkins Clinical Assessment of the APAM (Hopkins, 1995).

MAJOR ASSUMPTIONS

Nursing

"The nurse is a facilitator, not an effector. Our nurse-client relationship is an interactive, interpersonal process that aids the individual to identify, mobilize, and develop his or her own strengths to achieve a perceived optimal state of health and well-being" (H. Erickson, personal communication, 2004). Rogers (1996) defined this relationship as facilitative-affiliation. The five aims of nursing interventions are to build trust, affirm and promote client strengths, promote positive orientation, facilitate perceived control, and set health-directed mutual goals (Erickson, Tomlin, & Swain, 2002).

Person

Differentiation is made between patients and clients in this theory. A patient is given treatment and instruction; a client participates in his or her own care. "Our goal is for nurses to work with clients" (Erickson, Tomlin, & Swain, 2002, p. 21). "A client is one who is considered to be a legitimate member of the decision-making team, who always has some control over the planned regimen, and who is incorporated into the planning and implementation of his or her own care as much as possible" (Erickson et al., 1990, p. 20; Erickson, Tomlin, & Swain, 2002, p. 253). In alignment with this premise is the belief that the client is always the primary source of data.

Health

"Health is a state of physical, mental, and social wellbeing, not merely the absence of disease or infirmity. It connotes a state of dynamic equilibrium among the various subsystems [of a holistic person]" (Erickson, Tomlin, & Swain, 2002, p. 46) and "is affected by the individual's spiritual drive, which has greater influence on the person's total state of well-being than any of the subsystems" (Erickson, 2006, p. 480).

Environment

"Environment is not identified in the theory as an entity of its own. The theorists see environment in the social subsystems as the interaction between self and others both cultural and individual. Biophysical stressors are seen as part of the environment" (H. Erickson, personal communication, March 1988).

THEORETICAL ASSERTIONS

The theoretical assertions of the modeling and role-modeling theory are based on the linkages between completion of developmental tasks and basic needs satisfaction; among basic needs satisfaction, object attachment and loss, and developmental tasks; and between the ability to mobilize coping resources and needs satisfaction. Three generic theoretical assertions constitute the following theoretical linkages implied in the theory:

1. "The degree to which developmental tasks are resolved is dependent on the degree to which human needs are satisfied" (Erickson, Tomlin, & Swain, 2002, p. 87).
2. "The degree to which needs are satisfied by object attachment depends on the availability of those objects and the degree to which they provide comfort and security as opposed to threat and anxiety" (Erickson, Tomlin, & Swain, 1983, p. 90).
3. "An individual's potential for mobilizing resources, the person's state of coping according to the APAM, is directly associated with the person's need satisfaction level" (Erickson, Tomlin, & Swain, 2002, p. 91).

LOGICAL FORM

The modeling and role-modeling theory was formulated using retroductive thinking. The theorists went through four levels of theory development and then cycled from inductive to deductive reasoning (H. Erickson, personal communication, March 1988). Erickson identified theoretical concepts and relationships to label and define her practice-based observations. These observations were then tested within the context of the theoretical bases identified. Integration and synthesis of the theoretical concepts and linkages with the clinical observations resulted in the development of a "new multidimensional theory and paradigm for nursing—modeling and role-modeling" (H. Erickson, personal communication, November 1984). Modeling and role-modeling may be viewed as a theory and a paradigm according to Merton (1968), who said that paradigms "provide a compact arrangement of central concepts and their interrelations that are utilized for description and analysis" (p. 70).

ACCEPTANCE BY THE NURSING COMMUNITY

Practice

Their book *Modeling and Role-Modeling: A Theory and Paradigm for Nursing* (Erickson, Tomlin, & Swain, 2002), chapters in nursing theory texts, and published research studies have exposed nurses in practice to this theory. Based on the applicability and interest in using this theory to guide holistic nursing practice, the modeling and role-modeling theory has been implemented in many hospitals throughout the country. For example, nurses on surgical units at the University of Michigan Medical Center use an assessment tool based on the modeling and role-modeling theory. The tool is used to gather information to identify the client's need assets, deficits, developmental residual, attachment-loss and grief status, and potential therapeutic interventions (see Appendix at the end of this chapter) (Bowman, 1998; H. Erickson, personal communication, March 1988).

Helen Erickson has lectured extensively, nationally and internationally and held one-on-one consultations with nurses from various practice and educational backgrounds. Nurses who practice in adult health; case management; community health; critical and intensive care; infant, adolescent, and family health; gerontology; mental health; emergency rooms; and hospices use this theory. The beauty of the theory is that it can be applied within any setting and with any population. Erickson noted that what seemed to be a revolutionary idea as recently as 1972 (calling for the client to be the head of the health care team) has gained acceptance, as has the notion that nurses can practice independently (H. Erickson, personal communication, November 1984). According to Erickson, negative responses to the theory came from individuals who cannot accept the idea of listening to the client first, or who do not take the concept of holism seriously (H. Erickson, personal communication, November 1984).

Brigham and Women's Hospital in Boston has used the modeling and role-modeling theory as a theoretical basis for the professional practice model for years. The nurses use the theory as a framework to structure care planning and case conferences. Jenny James, former vice president for nursing, stated that "consistency of language, the way care is talked about and planned" is one of the major advantages of using this theoretical basis (J. James, personal communication, July 1992). Nurses at Brigham and Women's Hospital use an adaptation of the assessment tool developed at the University of Michigan Medical Center. At the Fourth National Conference on Modeling and Role-Modeling (Boston, October 1992), implementation of the professional practice model at Brigham and Women's Hospital and case studies were first presented by the staff nurses (J. James, personal communication, July 1992). Nurses at the University of Pittsburgh Medical Center; Children's Hospital of the University of Wisconsin at Madison; University of Tennessee Medical Center in Knoxville; Oregon Health Sciences University Hospital; University Health System in San Antonio, Texas; Salina Regional Health Center; and other hospitals and state agencies across the United States have also adopted the modeling and role-modeling theory as the foundation for their professional practice as well as for staff development (Alligood, 2011; Arruda, 2010; Bales, 2010; Haylock, 2008, 2010; Hodge et al., 2014; Knapp, 2013; Knox-Woodward, 2014; Koren & Papmiditriou 2013; Raudonis & Acton, 1997; Shams, 2014; Sofhauser, 2015; Veo, 2010).

Education

The modeling and role-modeling theory has been introduced into the curriculum in nursing programs throughout the country. Faculty members have contacted and continue to contact Erickson regarding the use of the theory in their curricula and for specific courses. Metropolitan State University in St. Paul, Minnesota, selected modeling and role-modeling as the conceptual framework for their curriculum, and students are taught theory-based practice throughout the program. Other programs that use modeling and role-modeling theory as a basis for curriculum include but are not limited to St. Catherine's University in St. Paul, Minnesota; the Alternate Entry master's nursing program at the University of Texas at Austin; the University of Texas at Brownsville; Lamar University, Joanne Gay Dishman Department of Nursing in Beaumont, Texas; State University of New York at Buffalo; University of Tennessee at Knoxville; Capital University in Columbus, Ohio; and Foo Yin College of Nursing and Medical Technology in Taiwan. The theory has been used in academic settings to facilitate student learning (Ackerman-Barger, 2010; Aghebati et al., 2015; Faye, 2011; Gregg & Twibell, 2016; Levine & Perpetua, 2006; McElligott, 2010; Merryfeather, 2015; Perese, 2002; Schultz, 1998).

Research

Nurses throughout the world use modeling and role-modeling as the theoretical framework for their research. Findings from research studies continue to support and validate the self-care knowledge construct and the importance of support and control as well as other theoretical linkages. Erickson's (1976) initial study provided evidence that psychosocial factors are significantly related to physical health. A follow-up study in 1988 conducted by Erickson, Lock, and Swain supported those findings, and subsequent research has provided expansion and enrichment of major theoretical concepts. As described earlier in the chapter, perceived support, perceived control, hope for the future, satisfaction with daily life, needs satisfaction, perceived autonomy, AI, self-care knowledge, self-care actions, and self-care resources are some key concepts that have been supported and validated through research. Several master's and doctoral students at the University of Michigan School of Nursing, the University of Texas at Austin, and other universities have pursed research based on the theory. Campbell and colleagues (1985) conducted research at the University of Michigan Medical Center hypothesizing that the length of hospital stay was correlated with the stages of development. They used a nursing assessment tool adapted from the assessment model to measure a patient's psychosocial development and to relate developmental status to the length of hospitalization and the number of health problems identified during hospitalization. Findings indicated that trust–mistrust balance accounts for a large percentage of the variance in the length of hospitalization.

Erickson, principal investigator of research on Modeling and Role-Modeling with Alzheimer's Patients, was funded by the National Institutes of Health, National Center for Nursing Research. This project included 10 other investigators. Findings supported the constructs of self-care knowledge, adaptive potential, and AI (H. Erickson, personal communication, July 1992).

Numerous graduate students have based their theses and dissertations on modeling and role-modeling theory. In addition, extensive published work substantiates the major constructs and theoretical linkages of the theory (Erickson, 1990a). Research continues to expand the modeling and role-modeling theory.

FURTHER DEVELOPMENT

As this theory is practiced, explored, examined, and researched, much potential exists for further development. The theory has gained national and international attention. The founding of the Society for the Advancement of Modeling and Role-Modeling has enhanced involvement. The society was formed to develop and maintain a network of colleagues to advance the development and application of the modeling and role-modeling theory. One of the society's goals is to promote continued research related to the theory. The first national symposium of the society was in 1986, and it meets biennially. At the 1988 conference in Hilton Head, South Carolina, society members came from 12 states (H. Erickson, personal communication, November 1988). By the 1990 conference in Austin, Texas, members represented more than 33 states (H. Erickson, personal communication, July 1992). These biennial conferences continue to provide a forum for researchers, educators, and practitioners to disseminate knowledge pertaining to the modeling and role-modeling theory and paradigm (H. Erickson, personal communication, May 2016).

Presentations included studies based in critical care units and community-based practice, in multiple types of educational settings, and across the life span. In 2010 nurses from all over the United States as well as Egypt, Canada, South Africa, China, and Great Britain attended the conference in San Antonio, Texas. The international biennial conferences provide an opportunity for nurses to discuss interrelationships among holistic nursing practice, theory, research, and education.

CRITIQUE

Clarity

Erickson, Tomlin, and Swain present their theory clearly. Definitions in the theory are denotative, with the concepts explicitly defined. They use everyday language and offer examples to illustrate their meaning. Their definitions and assumptions are consistent, and there is a logical progression from assumptions to assertions.

Simplicity

The theory appears simple; however, closer inspection reveals its depth and complexity. It is based on biological and psychological theories and on several theorists' philosophical assumptions. The interactions among the major concepts, assumptions, and assertions add to the theory and increase its complexity.

Generality

The modeling and role-modeling theory is generalizable to all aspects and most settings of professional nursing practice. Major assumptions that deal with developmental tasks, basic needs satisfaction, object attachment and loss, and adaptive potential are broad enough to be applicable in diverse nursing situations. Numerous examples of the applicability of the theory in educational settings, clinical practice, and research were cited earlier in this chapter.

Accessibility

Accessibility refers to the testability, application of a *theory*, and the extent that defined concepts are grounded in observable reality. The theory has operationally defined concepts, identifiable subconcepts, and clearly defined and denotative definitions. The major concepts, modeling and role-modeling, are reality-based, making them empirical. Definitions are clearly articulated, making concept testing possible. The theorists have provided an outline for collecting, analyzing, and synthesizing data and guidelines for implementing the theory. These explicit guidelines increase empirical precision, allowing any practitioner to test the theory using those tools.

Midrange theories are identified, supported, and substantiated. Data obtained through critical analyses and testing provides evidence for and validation of the theory. Modeling and role-modeling theory gains even greater empirical precision with new and ongoing studies. The need for practicing nurses to continue research with the theory is recognized and welcomed.

Importance

One of the challenges facing the profession of nursing is the development of its unique, scientific knowledge base and the use of nursing theory as a basis for professional practice. The modeling and role-modeling theory contributes steady progress toward this goal. Although relatively young, the theory has gained recognition in the nursing community. Interest has grown, and research has supported its theoretical statements. Numerous nurses cited earlier in this chapter have engaged in research based on this theory, lending more and more credence to the theoretical propositions.

Chinn and Kramer (2015) propose that the importance of a theory is relative to how it addresses nursing practice, education, and administration goals. Modeling and role-modeling theory guides research, directs practice, and generates new ideas; thus this theory possesses inherent value and importance for the discipline of nursing (Alligood, 2011). Finally, the theory is aligned with current and future holistic health care needs and trends that include foci on "client satisfaction and experience, self-care knowledge, engagement, experience," and other important issues in health care (*ANA Nursing Scope and Standards of Practice,* 3rd ed. American Nurses Association, 2015, pp. 11, 20, 227).

SUMMARY

Nurses have the opportunity to share in important, intimate life experiences with clients. They have the ability and responsibility to facilitate healing and achievement of clients' perceived maximal state of health and well-being. The modeling and role-modeling theory provides nurses with a practice-based theoretical framework to attain these goals, in any setting and with any population. Numerous research studies and ongoing scientific work provide empirical support for this nursing theory. As the theory matures, the extent of its merit and worth continues to become more evident.

CASE STUDY

Robert, a 75-year-old rancher with a history of chronic obstructive pulmonary disease (COPD), is admitted with shortness of breath, angina, and nausea (unmet physiological needs). It is his fourth admission in 6 months (he is having difficulty adapting to stressors in his life). The nurse introduces herself in a quiet, calm voice and tells him she will be his primary nurse during his stay (interventions designed to establish trust and a sense of safety and security and to facilitate a sense of connectedness). She asks him why he came in (he is the primary data source). He states, "I can't breathe, and my chest hurts." After he is stabilized (physiological needs are met, so the nurse can focus on his other needs), she says, "I notice that you have had multiple admissions in the last few months. Why do you think you are here today?" (The nurse seeks information from the client who is the primary data source and facilitates a sense of client control.) He replies, "My wife of 49 years died a few months ago; she took care of me, and my heart is broken. My life no longer has meaning." (He is experiencing unmet needs, is having problems with the developmental stage of generativity, and is grieving the loss of his wife.)

During her assessment, the nurse discovers that Robert lives on a ranch by himself. His nearest neighbor is 4 miles away, his son lives out of state, he has no help with his daily living activities, he is housebound because he can no longer drive, he has no support system, and he feels unable to get on with his life without his wife. The nurse asks him what he needs to feel better and to help him get through the next few weeks (promoting positive future orientation). He replies, "I need to be closer to my friends and the hospital. I am so lonely and afraid out there by myself" (unmet love and belonging and safety and security needs).

After a lengthy discussion, they decide together to implement a plan of care. (The nurse is facilitating client control, affirming his strengths and his self-care knowledge that he knows what will make him heal; together they are setting mutual goals.) Robert calls and speaks to his son, who plans to visit (this action facilitates his sense of perceived support and AI). His minister is called, and grief counseling is arranged (support is perceived, facilitation of grief resolution is initiated, and the client is facilitated in being future-focused).

Robert decides that he will move to town into a senior citizen apartment that provides meals and other services, and arrangements are made for him to have help with the moving process. He will be closer to the hospital and other people if he needs them (this will help him feel safer and more secure). He can then choose when to visit with friends or participate in social activities that are offered at the complex (his love and belonging needs can be met, and this facilitates his sense of control). He can also receive assistance with basic physiological needs when needed (meals, housekeeping services). After he is settled into his new home, the nurse provides him with her telephone number, so he can call if he needs anything or if he just wants to check in (support and love and belonging needs are met). This action facilitates the client's trust and AI. His control is maintained, and his strengths and self-care knowledge are affirmed (he will know how to and be able to call when he needs assistance, or will be connected to the nurse). Finally, the nurse schedules regular telephone calls (based on the client's schedule) to check in and see how he is doing and to address any concerns or questions he has. This action facilitates trust, his safety and security and love and belonging, and AI needs are met.

CRITICAL THINKING ACTIVITIES

1. Interview a client, and use the theory to interpret the data. Identify nursing diagnoses based on the interpretations.
2. Propose a nursing plan of care based on the interview and interpretation in question 1.
3. Assuming the goal is to promote the client's health and development, predict the client outcome based on the proposed nursing plan of care. Predict the client outcome if the care is not given.
4. Assess the client from primary, secondary, and tertiary sources. Compare for congruency among the three types of sources.

POINTS FOR FURTHER STUDY

- Erickson, H. (Ed.). (2006). *Modeling and role-modeling: A view from the client's world.* Cedar Park, TX: Unicorns Unlimited.
- Erickson, H. C., Tomlin, E. M., & Swain, M. A. (2002). *Modeling and role-modeling: A theory and paradigm for nursing.* Cedar Park, TX: EST Co. (Original work published 1983, Englewood Cliffs, NJ: Prentice-Hall.)
- The Society for the Advancement of Modeling and Role-Modeling at http://www.mrmnursingtheory.org/

  [Research and conceptual references are available on the website on midrange theories, major constructs, and philosophical assumptions of the modeling and role-modeling theory.]

REFERENCES

Ackerman-Barger, P. (2010). Embracing multiculturalism in nursing learning environments. *Journal of Nursing Education, 49*(12), 677–682.

Acton, G. (1993). *The relationships among stressors, stress, affiliated-individuation, burden, and well-being in caregivers of adults with dementia: A test of the theory and paradigm for nursing, modeling and role-modeling.* Unpublished doctoral dissertation, University of Texas, Austin.

Acton, G. (1997). The mediating effect of affiliated-individuation in caregivers of adults with dementia. *Journal of Holistic Nursing, 15*(4), 336–357.

Acton, G., & Malathum, P. (2000). Basic need satisfaction and health-promoting self-care behaviors in adults. *Western Journal of Nursing Research, 22*(7), 796–811.

Acton, G. J., Irvin, B. L., Jensen, B. A., Hopkins, B. A., & Miller, E. W. (1997). Explicating midrange theory through methodological diversity. *Advances in Nursing Science, 19*(3), 78–85.

Acton, G. J., & Miller, E. W. (1996). Affiliated individuation in caregivers of adults with dementia. *Issues in Mental Health Nursing, 17*, 245–260.

Aghebati, N., Mohammadi, E., Ahmadi, F., & Noaparast, K. (2015). Principle-based concept analysis: Intentionality in holistic nursing theory. *Journal of Holistic Nursing, 33*(1), 68–83.

Alligood, M. R. (2011). Theory-based practice in a major medical centre. *Journal of Nursing Management, 19*, 981–988.

American Nurses Association. (2015). *ANA Nursing: Scope and standards of practice* (3rd ed.). Silver Spring, MD: American Nurses Association.

Anschutz, C. A. (2000). *Perceived enactment of autonomy and life satisfaction: An elderly perspective.* Unpublished master's thesis, Fort Hays State University, Fort Hays, KS.

Arruda, E. (2010). Better retention through nursing theory. *Journal for Nurses in Staff Development, 26*(1), 17–22.

Baas, L. S. (1992). *The relationships among self-care knowledge, self-care resources, activity level and life satisfaction in persons three to six months after a myocardial infarction. Dissertation Abstracts International, 53*, 1780B.

Baas, L. S. (2004). Self-care resources and activity as predictors of quality of life in persons after myocardial infarction. *Dimensions of Critical Care Nursing, 23*(3), 131–138.

Baas, L. S. (2011). Construct validity of the revised Self-Care Resources Inventory. Retrieved from http://hdl.handle.net/10755/178037.

Baas, L. S., Beery, T. A., Allen, G. A., Wizer, M., & Wagoner, L. E. (2004). An exploratory study of body awareness in persons with heart failure or transplant. *Journal of Cardiovascular Nursing, 19*(1), 32–40.

Baas, L. S., Beery, T. A., Fontana, J. A., & Wagoner, L. E. (1999). An exploratory study of developmental growth in adults with heart failure. *Journal of Holistic Nursing, 17*(2), 117–138.

Baas, L. S., & Conway, G. A. (2004). Psychosocial aspects of heart failure management. In S. Stewart, D. D. Moser, & D. Thompson (Eds.), *Caring for the heart failure patient: A textbook for the healthcare professional* (pp. 197–209). London: Martin Bunitz.

Baas, L. S., Fontana, J. A., & Bhat, G. (1997). Relationships between self-care resources and the quality of life of persons with heart failure: A comparison of treatment groups. *Progress in Cardiovascular Nursing, 12*(1), 25–38.

Baldwin, C. M. (1996). Perceptions of hope: Lived experiences of elementary school children in an urban setting. *Journal of Multicultural Nursing & Health, 2*(3), 41–45.

Bales, I. (2010). Testing a computer-based ostomy care training resource for staff nurses. *Ostomy Wound Management, 56*(5), 60–69.

Barnfather, J. (1993). Testing a theoretical proposition for modeling and role-modeling: A basic need and adaptive potential status. *Issues in Mental Health Nursing, 13*, 1–18.

Barnfather, J. S. (1987). *Mobilizing coping resources related to basic need status in healthy, young adults. Dissertation Abstracts International*, 49/02-B, 0360.

Barnfather, J. S. (1990a). An overview of the ability to mobilize coping resources related to basic needs. In H. Erickson & C. Kinney (Eds.), *Modeling and role-modeling: Theory, practice and research* (vol. 1). (pp. 156–169). Austin, TX: Society for the Advancement of Modeling and Role-Modeling.

Barnfather, J. S. (1990b). Mobilizing coping resources related to basic need status. In H. Erickson & C. Kinney (Eds.), *Modeling and role-modeling: Theory, practice and research* (vol. 1). Austin, TX: Society for the Advancement of Modeling and Role-Modeling.

Beery, T., Baas, L. S., & Henthorn R. (2007). Self-reported adjustment to implanted cardiac devices. *Journal of Cardiovascular Nursing, 22*(6), 516–524.

Beery, T. A., Baas, L. S., Fowler, C., & Allen, G. (2002). Spirituality in persons with heart failure. *Journal of Holistic Nursing, 20*(10), 5–30.

Beery, T. A., Baas, L. S., Mathews, H., Burroughs, J., & Henthorn R. (2005). Development of the Implanted Devices Adjustment Scale. *Dimensions of Critical Care Nursing, 24*(5), 242–248.

Beltz, S. (1999). *How persons 85 years and older, living in congregate housing, experience managing their health: Preservation of self.* Unpublished doctoral dissertation, University of Texas, Austin.

Benson, D. (2003). *Adaptive potential assessment model as applied to small groups.* Unpublished doctoral dissertation, University of LaVerne, LaVerne, CA.

Benson, D. (2006). Coping with stress. In H. Erickson (Ed.), *Modeling and role-modeling: A view from the client's world* (pp. 240–274). Cedar Park, TX: Unicorns Unlimited.

Benson, D. (2011). *A theoretical model for group adaptive expansion.* Retrieved from http://hdl.handle.net/10755/153865.

Boodley, C. A. (1986). *A nursing study of the experience of having a health examination.* Unpublished doctoral dissertation, University of Michigan, Ann Arbor, MI.

Boodley, C. A. (1990). The experience of having a healthy examination. In H. Erickson & C. Kinney (Eds.), *Modeling and role-modeling: Theory, practice and research* (vol. 1). Austin, TX: Society for the Advancement of Modeling and Role-Modeling.

Bowman, S. S. (1998). *The human-environment relationship in self-care when healing from episodic illness.* Unpublished doctoral dissertation, University of Texas, Austin, TX.

Bray, C. O. (2005). *The relationship between psychosocial attributes, self-care resources, basic need satisfaction and measures of cognitive and psychological health of adolescents: A test of the modeling and role-modeling theory.* Unpublished doctoral dissertation, University of Texas, Austin, TX.

Campbell, J., Finch, D., Allport, C., Erickson, H. C., & Swain, M. A. (1985). A theoretical approach to nursing assessment. *Journal of Advanced Nursing, 10*, 111–115.

Chen, Y. (1996). *Relationships among health control orientation, self-efficacy, self-care, and subjective well-being in the elderly with hypertension.* Unpublished doctoral dissertation, University of Texas, Austin, TX.

Chinn, P. L., & Kramer, M. K. (2015). *Integrated knowledge development in nursing* (9th ed.). St Louis: Mosby.

Clayton, D. (2001). *Journeys through chaos: Experiences of prolonged family suffering and evolving spiritual identity.* Unpublished doctoral dissertation, University of Texas, Austin, TX.

Cleary, J., & Crafti, N. (2007). Basic need satisfaction, emotional eating, and dietary restraint as risk factors for recurrent overeating in a community sample. *E-Journal of Applied Psychology. Clinical and Social Issues, 3*(2).

Curl, E. D. (1992). *Hope in the elderly: Exploring the relationship between psychosocial developmental residual and hope. Dissertation Abstracts International, 47*, 992B.

Darling-Fisher, C. S. (1987). *The relationship between mothers' and fathers' Eriksonian psychosocial attributes, perceptions of family support, and adaptation to parenthood.* Unpublished doctoral dissertation, University of Michigan, Ann Arbor, MI.

Darling-Fisher, C., & Leidy, N. (1988). Measuring Eriksonian development of the adult: The modified Erikson psychosocial stage inventory. *Psychological Reports, 62*, 747–754.

Dildy, S. M. P. (1992). *A naturalistic study of the meaning and impact of suffering in people with rheumatoid arthritis.* Unpublished doctoral dissertation, University of Texas, Austin, TX.

Erickson, H. (1990a). Modeling and role-modeling with psychophysiological problems. In J. K. Zeig & S. Gilligan (Eds.), *Brief therapy: Myths, methods, and metaphors.* (pp. 473–490). New York: Brunner/Mazel.

Erickson, H. (1990b). Theory based nursing. In H. Erickson & C. Kinney (Eds.), *Modeling and role-modeling: Theory, practice and research* (vol. 1). (pp. 1–27). Austin, TX: Society for the Advancement of Modeling and Role-Modeling.

Erickson, H. (1990c). Self-care knowledge: An exploratory study. In C. Kinney & H. Erickson (Eds.), *Modeling and role-modeling: Theory, practice and research* (vol. 1, pp. 178–202). Austin, TX: Society for the Advancement of Modeling and Role-Modeling.

Erickson, H. (2006). *Modeling and role-modeling: A view from the client's world.* Cedar Park, TX: Unicorns Unlimited.

Erickson, H. (2010). *Exploring the interface between the philosophy and discipline of holistic nursing. Modeling and role-modeling at work.* Cedar Park, TX: Unicorns Unlimited.

Erickson, H., Tomlin, E., & Swain, M. (2002). *Modeling and role-modeling: A theory and paradigm for nursing.* Cedar Park, TX: EST Co.

Erickson, H. C. (1976). *Identification of states of coping utilization physiological and psychological data.* Unpublished master's thesis, University of Michigan, Ann Arbor, MI.

Erickson, H. C., Kinney, C., Becker, H., Acton, G., Irvin, B., Hopkins, R., et al. (1994). *Modeling and role-modeling with*

Alzheimer's patients (National Institutes of Health funded grant). Unpublished manuscript, University of Texas, Austin, TX.

Erickson, H. C., & Swain, M. A. (1982). A model for assessing potential adaptation to stress. *Research in Nursing and Health, 5*, 93–101.

Erickson, H. C., Tomlin, E. M., & Swain, M. A. P. (1983). *Modeling and role-modeling: A theory and paradigm for nursing.* Englewood Cliffs, NJ: Prentice-Hall.

Erickson, M. (1996a). Factors that influence the mother-infant dyad relationships and infant well-being. *Issues in Mental Health Nursing, 17*, 185–200.

Erickson, M. (1996b). *Relationships among support, needs satisfaction, and maternal attachment in the adolescent mother.* Unpublished doctoral dissertation, University of Texas, Austin, TX.

Erickson, M. (2006). Attachment, loss, and reattachment. In H. Erickson (Ed.), *Modeling and role-modeling: A view from the client's world.* (pp. 208–239). Cedar Park, TX: Unicorns Unlimited.

Erickson, M., Erickson, H., & Jensen, B. (2006). Affiliated individuation and self-actualization: Need satisfaction as a prerequisite. In H. Erickson (Ed.), *Modeling and role-modeling: A view from the client's world.* (pp. 182–207). Cedar Park, TX: Unicorns Unlimited.

Falk, K. (2013). *Appreciative inquiry to transform nursing practice for mentoring children of promise.* Unpublished doctoral dissertation, City University of New York, New York.

Falk, K. (2014). Appreciative inquiry with nurses who work with children of incarcerated parents. *Nursing Science Quarterly, 27*(4), 315–323.

Faye, F. (2011). Integrating nursing science in the education process. *Creative Nursing, 17*(3), 113–117.

Finch, D. (1987). *Testing a theoretically based nursing assessment.* Unpublished doctoral dissertation, University of Michigan, Ann Arbor, MI.

Folse, V. (2007). The family experience with eating disorders scale: Psychometric analysis. *Archives of Psychiatric Nursing, 21*(4), 210–221.

Goldstein, L. (2013). *Relationships among quality of life, self-care, and affiliated individuation in persons on chronic warfarin therapy. UT Electronic Theses & Dissertations,* University of Texas, Austin, Texas. Retrieved from https://repositories.lib.utexas.edu/handle/2152/21865.

Gregg, S. R., & Twibell, K. R. (2016). Try-it-on. Experiential learning of holistic stress management in a graduate nursing curriculum. *Journal of Holistic Nursing, 34*(3), 300–308.

Hagglund, L. A. (2009). Challenges in the treatment of factitious disorder: A case study. *Archives of Psychiatric Nursing, 23*(1), 58–64.

Haylock, P. (2008). *Giving voice to the vulnerable: Advocacy and oncology nursing. Electronic Theses & Dissertations,* University of Texas Medical Branch, Galveston, TX.

Haylock, P. J. (2010). Advanced cancer: A mind-body-spirit approach in life and living. *Seminars in Oncology Nursing, 26*(3), 183–194.

Hertz, J. E. (1999). Testing two self-care measures in elderly home care clients. In S. H. Gueldner & L. W. Poon (Eds.), *Gerontological nursing issues for the 21st century* (pp. 195–205). Indianapolis: Center Nursing Press.

Hertz, J. E. G. (1991). *The perceived enactment of autonomy scale: Measuring the potential for self-care action in the elderly. Dissertation Abstracts International, 52*, 1953B.

Hertz, J. E., & Anschutz, C. A. (2002). Relationships among perceived enactment of autonomy, self-care, and holistic health in community-dwelling older adults. *Journal of Holistic Nursing, 20*(2), 166–186.

Hertz, J. E., Rossetti J., & Nelson, C. M. (2005). Perceived autonomy and self-care resources in older residents of senior apartments. *Virginia Henderson Global e-Repository.* Retrieved from http://hdl.handle.net/10755/161167.

Hodge, D., Bonifas, R., Sun, F., & Wolosin, R. (2014). Developing a model to address African Americans' spiritual needs during hospitalization. *Clinical Gerontologists, 37*(4), 386–405.

Holl, R. M. (1992). *The effect of role-modeled visiting in comparison to restricted visiting on the well-being of clients who had open heart surgery and their significant family members in the critical care unit. Dissertation Abstracts International, 53*, 4030B.

Hwang, H., & Lin, H. (2004). Perceived enactment of autonomy and related sociodemographic factors among non-institutionalized elders. *The Kaohsiung Journal of Medical Sciences, 20*(4), 166–173.

Irvin, B. L. (1993). *Social support, self-worth and hope as self-care resources for coping with caregiver stress. Dissertation Abstracts International, 54*(06), B2995.

Irvin, B. L., & Acton, G. (1996). Stress mediation in caregivers of cognitively impaired adults: Theoretical model testing. *Nursing Research, 45*(3), 160–166.

Irvin, B. L., & Acton, G. J. (1997). Stress, hope and well-being of women caring for family members with Alzheimer's disease. *Holistic Nursing Practices, 11*(2), 69–79.

Jensen, B. (1995). *Caregiver responses to a theoretically based intervention program: Case study analysis.* Unpublished doctoral dissertation, University of Texas, Austin, TX.

Jonker, L. (2012). *The experiences and perceptions of mothers utilizing child health services.* Thesis, Stellenbosch University. Stellenbosch, South Africa. Retrieved from http://scholar.sun.ac.za.

Keck, V. E. (1989). *Perceived social support, basic needs satisfaction, and coping strategies of the chronically ill. Dissertation Abstracts International, 50*, 3921B.

Kennedy, G. T. (1991). *A nursing investigation of comfort and comforting care of the acutely ill patient. Dissertation Abstracts International, 52*, 6318B.

Kinney, C. K. (1990). Facilitating growth and development: A paradigm case for modeling and role-modeling. *Issues in Mental Health Nursing, 11*, 375–395.

Kinney, C., & Erickson, H. (1990). Modeling the client's world: A way to holistic care. *Issues in Mental Health Nursing, 11*, 93–108.

Kinney, C. K., Rodgers, D. R., Nash, K., & Bray, C. (2003). Holistic healing for women with breast cancer through a mind, body, and spirit self-empowerment program. *Journal of Holistic Nursing, 21*, 260–279.

Kline, N. W. (1988). *Psychophysiological processes of stress in people with a chronic physical illness. Dissertation Abstracts International, 49*, 2129B.

Knapp, S. (2013). The effects of a violence assessment checklist on the incidence of violence for emergency department nurses. *Evidence-Based Practice Project Reports*. Retrieved from http://scholar.valpo.edu/ebpr/23.

Knox-Woodward, J. (2014). Employing provider mentoring/coaching to improve preventative quality ordering. Retrieved from http://scholarworks.waldenu.edu/dissertations/119/.

Koren, M. E., & Papmiditriou, C. (2013). Spirituality of staff nurses: Application of modeling and role-modeling theory. *Holistic Nursing Practice, 27*(1), 37–44.

Lamb, P. B. (2005). *Application of the modeling role-modeling theory to mentoring in nursing*. Unpublished master's thesis, Montana State University, Bozeman, MT.

Landis, B. J. (1991). *Uncertainty, spiritual well-being, and psychosocial adjustment to chronic illness. Dissertation Abstracts International, 52*, 4124B.

Leidy, N. K. (1990). A structural model of stress, psychosocial resources, and symptomatic experience in chronic physical illness. *Nursing Research, 39*(4), 230–236.

Levine, M. A., & Perpetua, E. (2006). International immersion programs in baccalaureate nursing education: Professor and student perspectives. *Journal of Cultural Diversity, 13*(1), 20–26.

Liang, C. V. (2008). *Urinary incontinence among rural elders residing in long-term care*. Unpublished doctoral dissertation, Assessment of Bladder Health Initiative Program, State University of New York at Binghamton, NY.

MacLean, T. T. (1990). *Erikson's development and stressors as factors in healthy lifestyle. Dissertation Abstracts International, 48*, 1710A.

MacLean, T. T. (1992). Influence of psychosocial development and life events on the health practices of adults. *Issues in Mental Health, 13*, 403–414.

Matsui, M., & Capezuti, E. (2008). Perceived autonomy and self-care resources among senior center users. *Geriatric Nursing, 29*(2), 141–147.

McElligott, D. (2010). Healing: The journey from concept to nursing practice. *Journal of Holistic Nursing, 28*(4), 251–259.

Merryfeather, L. (2015). Passionate scholarship or academic safety: An ethical issue. *Journal of Holistic Nursing, 33*(1), 60–67.

Merton, R. K. (1968). *Social theory and social structure*. New York: The Free Press.

Miller, E. W. (1994). *The meaning of encouragement and its connection to the inner-spirit as perceived by caregivers of the cognitively impaired*. Unpublished doctoral dissertation, University of Texas, Austin, TX.

Nash, K. (2007a). Implementation and evaluation of the Empower Youth program. *Journal of Holistic Nursing, 25*(1), 26–36.

Nash, K. (2007b). Evaluation of the empower peer support and education program for middle school–aged adolescents. *Journal of Holistic Health, 25*, 26–36.

Perese, E. (2002). Integrating psychiatric nursing into a baccalaureate nursing curriculum. *Journal of the American Psychiatric Nurses Association, 8*(5), 152–158.

Perese, E. F., & Wu, Y. B. (2010). Shortfalls of treatment for patients with schizophrenia: Unmet need, obstacles to recovery. *International Journal of Psychosocial Rehabilitation, 14*(2), 43–56.

Pokorny, M., Scott, E., Rose, M. A., et al. (2009). Challenges in caring for the morbidly obese patients. *Home Healthcare Nurse, 27*(1), 43–52.

Raudonis, B. (1991). *A nursing study of empathy from the hospice patient's perspective*. Unpublished doctoral dissertation, University of Texas, Austin, TX.

Raudonis, B., & Acton, G. (1997). Theory based nursing practice. *Journal of Advanced Nursing, 26*(1), 138–145.

Robinson, K. R. (1994). Developing a scale to measure denial levels of clients with actual or potential myocardial infarctions. *Heart and Lung, 23*, 36–44.

Rogers, S. (1996). Facilitative affiliation: Nurse-client interactions that enhance healing. *Issues in Mental Health Nursing, 17*, 171–184.

Rosenow, D. J. (1991). *Multidimensional scaling analysis of self-care actions for reintegrating holistic health after a myocardial infarction: Implications for nursing. Dissertation Abstracts International, 53*, 1789B.

Scheela, R. (1991). *The remodeling process: A grounded study of adult male incest offenders' perceptions of the treatment process*. Unpublished doctoral dissertation, University of Texas, Austin, TX.

Schultz, E. (1998). Academic advising from a nursing theory perspective. *Nurse Educator, 23*(1), 22–25.

Shams, M., Favara, I., Meneghello, E., & Barzon, F. (2014). Nursing and psychological issues in obese patients. *The Globesity Challenge to General Surgery*. Milan, Italy: Springer-Verlag Italia.

Smith, K. (1980). *Relationship between social support and goal attainment*. Unpublished master's thesis, University of Michigan, Ann Arbor, MI.

Sofhauser, C. (1996). *The relations among hostility, self-esteem, self-concept, psychosocial residual in persons with coronary heart disease. Dissertations Abstracts International*, 5B/01-B.

Sofhauser, C. (2015). Hostility patterns: Implications for nursing practice. *Nursing Science Quarterly, 28*(3), 202–208.

Sofhauser, C. D. (2003). Psychosocial antecedents of hostility in persons with coronary heart disease. *Journal of Holistic Nursing, 21*(3), 280–300.

Sung, P. H., & Yu, S. K. (2006). The nursing experience of applying MRM model to personality disorder. *Hu Li Za Zhi, 53*(4), 89–95.

Timmerman, G., & Acton, G. (2001). The relationship between basic need satisfaction and emotional eating. *Issues in Mental Health Nursing, 22*(7), 691–701.

Veo, P. (2010). Concept mapping for applying theory to nursing practice. *Journal for Nurses in Professional Development, 26*(1), 17–22.

Weber, G. J. (1999). The experiential meaning of well-being for employed mothers. *Western Journal of Nursing Research, 21*(6), 785–795.

Weber, G. J. T. (1995). *Employed mothers with pre-school-aged children: An exploration of their lived experiences and the nature of their well-being. Dissertation Abstracts International, 56–06*(B), 3131.

BIBLIOGRAPHY

Primary Sources

Books

Erickson, H. (1986). *Synthesizing clinical experiences: A step in theory development*. Ann Arbor, MI: Biomedical Communications.

Erickson, H., & Kinney, C. (Eds.). (1990). *Modeling and role-modeling: Theory, practice and research* (vol. 1). Austin, TX: Society for the Advancement of Modeling and Role-Modeling.

Book Chapters

Erickson, H. (1977). Communication in nursing. In H. Erickson (Ed.), *Professional nursing matrix: A workbook* (pp. 1–150). Ann Arbor, MI: Media Library, University of Michigan.

Erickson, H. (1985). Modeling and role-modeling: Ericksonian approaches with physiological problems. In J. Zeig & S. Langton (Eds.), *Ericksonian psychotherapy: The state of the art*. New York: Brunner/Mazel.

Erickson, H. (1990). Modeling and role-modeling with psychophysiological problems. In J. K. Zeig & S. Gilligan (Eds.), *Brief therapy: Myths, methods, and metaphors* (pp. 473–491). New York: Brunner/Mazel.

Erickson, H. (1990). Theory based nursing. In C. Kinney & H. Erickson (Eds.), *Modeling and role-modeling: Theory, practice and research* (vol. 1, pp. 1–27). Austin, TX: Society for the Advancement of Modeling and Role-Modeling.

Journal Articles

Barnfather, J., Swain, M. A., & Erickson, H. (1989). Construct validity of an aspect of the coping process: Potential adaptation to stress. *Issues in Mental Health Nursing, 10*, 23–40.

Barnfather, J., Swain, M. A., & Erickson, H. (1989). Evaluation of two assessment techniques. *Nursing Science Quarterly, 4*, 172–182.

Erickson, H. (1983). Coping with new systems. *Journal of Nursing Education, 22*(3), 132–135.

Erickson, H. (1991). Modeling y role-modeling con psychophysiological problemas. *Rapport: Hipnosis de Milton H. Erickson—Revista del Instituto Milton H. Erickson de Buenos Aires* (Argentina), *1*(1), 41–53.

Erickson, H., & Swain, M. A. (1982). A model for assessing potential adaptation to stress. *Research in Nursing and Health, 5*, 93–101.

Erickson, H., & Swain, M. A. (1990). Mobilizing self-care resources: A nursing intervention for hypertension. *Issues in Mental Health Nursing, 11*, 217–236.

Secondary Sources

Books

Bowlby, J. (1969). *Attachment*. New York: Basic Books.

Bowlby, J. (1973). *Separation*. New York: Basic Books.

Bowlby, J. (1980). *Loss*. New York: Basic Books.

Engel, G. S. (1962). *Psychological development in health and disease*. Philadelphia: Saunders.

Erikson, E. (1963). *Childhood and society*. New York: W. W. Norton.

Haley, J. (1973). *Uncommon therapy: The psychiatric techniques of Milton H. Erickson, M.D.* New York: W. W. Norton.

Maslow, A. H. (1968). *Toward a psychology of being* (2nd ed.). New York: D. Von Nostrand.

Maslow, A. H. (1970). *Motivation and personality* (2nd ed.). New York: Harper & Row.

Piaget, J. (1952). *The origins of intelligence in children*. New York: International Universities Press.

Piaget, J., & Inhelder, B. (1969). *The psychology of the child*. New York: Basic Books.

Journal Articles

Bartholomew, K. (1990). Avoidance of intimacy: An attachment perspective. *Journal of Social and Personal Relationships, 7*, 147–178.

Beery, T., & Baas, L. (1996). Medical devices and attachment: Holistic healing in the age of invasive technology. *Issues in Mental Health Nursing, 17*, 233–243.

Hertz, J. (1996). Conceptualization of perceived enactment of autonomy in the elderly. *Issues in Mental Health Nursing, 17*, 261–273.

Kinney, C. (1996). Transcending breast cancer: Reconstructing one's self. *Issues in Mental Health Nursing, 17*, 201–216.

Leidy, N. (1994). Operationalizing Maslow's theory: Development and testing of the Basic Needs Satisfaction Inventory. *Issues in Mental Health Nursing, 15*, 277–295.

Leidy, N. K., & Traver, G. A. (1995). Psychophysiological factors contributing to functional performance in people with COPD: Are there gender differences? *Research in Nursing and Health, 18*(6), 535–546.

Mahler, M. S. (1967). On human symbiosis and the vicissitudes of individuation. *Journal of the American Psychoanalytic Association, 15*, 740–763.

Miller, E. W. (1995). Encouraging Alzheimer's caregivers. *Journal of Christian Nursing, 12*(4), 7–12.

Sappington, J., & Kelley, J. H. (1996). Modeling and role-modeling theory: A case study of holistic care. *Journal of Holistic Nursing, 14*(2), 130–141.

Walsh, K. K., Vanden Bosch, T. M., & Boehm, S. (1989). Modeling and role-modeling: Integrating nursing theory into practice. *Journal of Advanced Nursing, 14*, 755–761.

APPENDIX

Assessment Tool Based on Modeling and Role-Modeling*

- I. Description of the situation
  - A. Overview of the situation
  - B. Etiology
    1. Eustressors
    2. Stressors
    3. Distressors
  - C. Therapeutic needs
- II. Expectations
  - A. Immediate
  - B. Long-term
- III. Resource potential
  - A. External
    1. Social network
    2. Support system
    3. Health care system
  - B. Internal
    1. Strengths
    2. Adaptive potential
       - a. Feeling states
       - b. Physiological parameters
- IV. Goals and life tasks
  - A. Current
  - B. Future

Data Interpretation Tool Based on Modeling and Role-Modeling†

- I. Interpret data for ability to mobilize resources (APAM)
- II. Interpret data for needs status (assets and deficits related to type of need), attachment objects, loss, grief (normal or morbid), life tasks (developmental: actual and chronological)

Data Analysis Tool Based on Modeling and Role-Modeling‡

- I. Step one
  - A. Articulate relationships between stressors and needs status.
  - B. Articulate relationships between needs status and ability to mobilize resources.
  - C. Articulate relationships between needs status and loss of attachment.
  - D. Articulate relationships between loss and type of grief response.
  - E. Articulate relationships between the type of need assets and deficits and the developmental residual.
  - F. Articulate relationships between chronological developmental task and developmental residual.
- II. Step two
  - A. Articulate relationships among stressors, resource potential, needs status, loss, grief status, developmental residual, chronological task, and attachment potential.
  - B. Articulate relationships among needs status, potential resources, developmental residual, and personal goals.

AI, Affiliated individuation; *APAM,* adaptive potential assessment model.

*Interview questions and thoughts that guide critical thinking are suggested in Erickson, H. C., Tomlin, E. M., & Swain, M. A. (1983). *Modeling and role-modeling: A theory and paradigm for nursing* (pp. 116–168). Englewood Cliffs, NJ: Prentice-Hall. Suggestions for interviewing techniques are found in Erickson, H. C. (1990). Self-care knowledge. In H. C. Erickson & C. Kinney (Eds.), *Modeling and role-modeling: Theory, practice and research* (vol. 1). Austin, TX: Society for the Advancement of Modeling and Role-Modeling.

†Critical thinking guidelines for data interpretation are suggested in Erickson, H. C., Tomlin, E. M., & Swain, M. A. (1983). *Modeling and role-modeling: A theory and paradigm for nursing* (pp. 148–166). Englewood Cliffs, NJ: Prentice-Hall; and Erickson, H. C. (1990). Theory based nursing. In H. C. Erickson & C. Kinney (Eds.), *Modeling and role-modeling: Theory, practice and research* (vol. 1). Austin, TX: Society for the Advancement of Modeling and Role-Modeling.

‡Critical thinking guidelines for data analysis are suggested in Erickson, H. C., Tomlin, E. M., & Swain, M. A. (1983). *Modeling and role-modeling: A theory and paradigm for nursing* (pp. 148–166). Englewood Cliffs, NJ: Prentice-Hall; and Erickson, H. C. (1990). Theory-based nursing. In H. C. Erickson & C. Kinney (Eds.), *Modeling and role-modeling: Theory, practice and research* (vol. 1). Austin, TX: Society for the Advancement of Modeling and Role-Modeling.

APPENDIX—cont'd

Planning Tool Based on Modeling and Role-Modeling[§]

I. Aims of interventions
   A. Build trust
   B. Promote positive orientation
   C. Promote client control
   D. Promote strengths
   E. Set health-directed goals

II. Intervention goals
   A. Develop a trusting and functional relationship between yourself and your client.
   B. Facilitate a self-projection that is futuristic and positive.
   C. Promote AI with the minimal degree of ambivalence possible.
   D. Promote a dynamic, adaptive, and holistic state of health.
   E. Promote and nurture a coping mechanism that satisfies basic needs and permits growth-need satisfaction.
   F. Facilitate congruent actual and chronological developmental stages.

[§]Critical thinking guidelines for planning are suggested in Erickson, H. C., Tomlin, E. M., & Swain, M. A. (1983). *Modeling and role-modeling: A theory and paradigm for nursing* (pp. 169–220). Englewood Cliffs, NJ: Prentice-Hall; and Erickson, H. C. (1990). Theory-based nursing. In H. C. Erickson & C. Kinney (Eds.), *Modeling and role-modeling: Theory, practice and research* (vol. 1). Austin, TX: Society for the Advancement of Modeling and Role-Modeling.

26

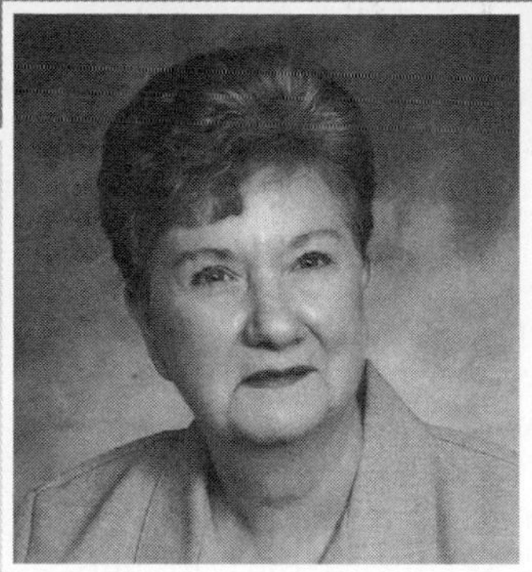
Gladys L. Husted
(1941–Present)

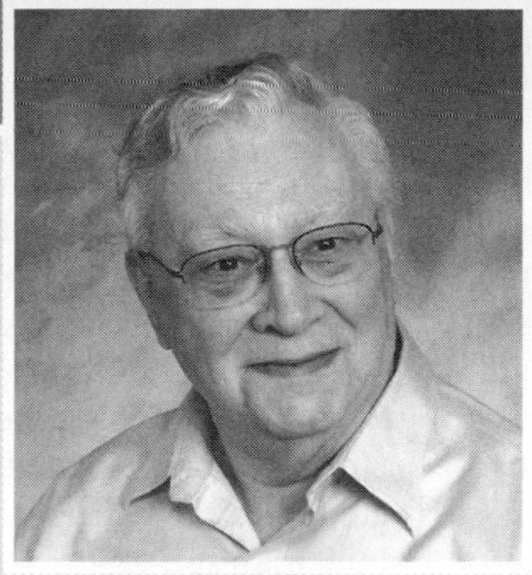
James H. Husted
(1931–Present)

Symphonological Bioethical Theory

Carrie Scotto

"Symphonology (from 'symphonia,' a Greek word meaning agreement) is a system of ethics based on the terms and preconditions of an agreement."
(Husted & Husted, 2001, p. 34)

CREDENTIALS AND BACKGROUND OF THE THEORISTS

Gladys Husted was born in Pittsburgh, where her life, practice, education, and teaching continue to influence the nursing profession. Husted received a Bachelor of Science in Nursing degree from the University of Pittsburgh in 1962 and began practice in public health and acute inpatient medical-surgical care. Observations of interactions between nurses and patients initiated her interest in ethical issues. In 1968 she earned a master's degree in nursing education while teaching at the Louise Suyden School of Nursing at St. Margaret's Memorial Hospital in Pittsburgh. Her love of teaching prompted doctoral study that resulted in a terminal degree from the University of Pittsburgh Department of Curriculum and Supervision.

G. Husted is professor emeritus at Duquesne University School of Nursing, where in 1998 she was awarded the title of School of Nursing Distinguished Professor. She was also recognized for teaching excellence at all levels of the curriculum with the Duquesne University School of Nursing Recognition Award for Excellence, 1990/1991, and the Faculty Award for Excellence in Teaching, 1994/1995. The Medical College of Ohio chose Husted as Distinguished Lecturer in 2000. She is a member of Sigma Theta Tau International, Phi Kappa Phi, and the National League for Nursing.

G. Husted consulted with the Western Pennsylvania Hospital Nursing Division developing an ethics committee, educating staff and management, and providing guidance for the newly formed committee. She also consulted with Allegheny General Medical Center for staff development and the National Nursing Ethics Advisory Group for the Department of Veterans Affairs. G. Husted served as curriculum consultant for several schools of nursing and has presented at many national-level conferences.

James Husted was born in Kingston, Pennsylvania, and has had a lifelong interest in philosophy. While in the army in Germany, he became interested in ethics through conversations with a former ethics professor, particularly the work of Benedict Spinoza. His post-army career focused on sales and on hiring and training agents for health insurance companies. However, he continued to read and develop his philosophical and ethical ideas. During the 1980s he joined the high-IQ societies Mensa and Intertel, serving as a philosophy expert for Mensa and a regional director for Intertel.

The theorists met and were married in 1974, establishing and cultivating a dialogue that brought about the theory of symphonology. They are coauthors of several editions of

Ethical Decision Making in Nursing. Their book was selected as one of Nursing and Health Care's Notable Books of 1991, 1995, and 2001. It also won the Nursing Society Award in 2001. Their regular column, "A Practice Based Bioethic," appeared in *Advanced Practice Nursing Quarterly* from 1997 to 1998. In addition to publishing books, book chapters, and journal articles, they have presented their ethical theory at conferences and workshops.

The Husteds reside in Pittsburgh and for many years continued to develop and disseminate their work through teaching, writing, presenting at conferences and workshops, and serving as consultants for ethics committees. Both are now retired.

THEORETICAL SOURCES

The authors define **symphonology** as "the study of agreements and the elements necessary to forming agreements," (Husted et al, 2015, p. x). In health care, it is the study of agreements between health care professionals and patients. An agreement is based on the nature of the relationship between the parties involved. In its ethical dimensions, it outlines the commitments and obligations of each. Although the theory developed from the observation of nurses and nursing practice, it later expanded to include all health care professionals. The development of this theory has led to the construction of a practice-based decision-making model that assists in determining when and what actions are appropriate for health care professionals and patients. The name of the theory is derived from the Greek word *symphonia,* which means "agreement."

Ethics is "a system of standards to motivate, determine, and justify actions directed to the pursuit of vital and fundamental goals" (Husted et al, 2015, p. 1). Ethics examines what ought to be done, within the realm of what can be done, to preserve and enhance human life. The Husteds, therefore, describe ethics as the science of living well.

Bioethics is concerned with the ethics of interactions between a patient and a health care professional, what ought to be done to preserve and enhance human life within the health care arena. Within the past century, the expanding knowledge base and growth of technology altered existing health care practice and created threatening and confusing circumstances not previously encountered. Increasing numbers and types of treatment options allowed patients to survive conditions they would not have in the past. However, the morbidity of the survivors brought new questions: Who should receive treatment? What is the appropriateness of treatments under particular circumstances? Who should decide what treatments are appropriate? In this way, bioethics became a central issue in what previously had been a prescriptive environment. It became essential to consider ethical concerns, as well as scientific solutions, to questions of health (Jecker, Jonsen, & Pearlman, 1997). Through personal experience and observation of nurses, the Husteds recognized the increasingly complex nature of bioethical dilemmas and the failure of the health care system to adequately address them.

To clarify the reasons for the deficiency of the health care system in addressing the issue of delivering ethical care, the Husteds examined traditional ideas and concepts used to guide ethical behavior. These ideas include deontology, utilitarianism, emotivism, and social relativism. Deontology is a duty-based ethic in which the consequences of one's actions are irrelevant. One acts in accordance with preset standards regardless of the outcome. The inappropriateness of this type of guideline is obvious in relation to health care professionals, because they are responsible for foreseeing the effects of their actions and acting only in ways that benefit a patient. Utilitarian thought would have health care professionals acting to bring about the greatest good for the greatest number of people. This is inconsistent with the practice of health care professionals who act as agents for individual patients. Emotivism promotes ethical actions in accordance with the emotions of those involved. Rational thought has no place in emotive choices, making this type of decision-making process inappropriate in the health care arena. Social relativism imposes the beliefs of a society onto the individual. This approach is incongruous with the increasing diversity of our emerging global society. The Husteds recognized that the inappropriateness of traditional methods of ethical reasoning brought about the failure of the health care system to successfully address bioethical issues.

Because traditional models proved inadequate to guide ethical behavior for health care professionals, the Husteds began to conceive and develop a method by which health care professionals might determine appropriate ethical actions. The theory was based on logical thinking, emphasizing the provision of holistic, individualized care. They drew from the work of Aristotle, Benedict Spinoza, and Michael Polanyi. These philosophers adhere to rational thought and value persons as individuals. Aristotle, a student of Plato, advanced his teacher's work by recognizing that there is more to understanding phenomena than simple rationality. He believed that one must develop insight and perception to recognize how principles can be applied to each situation (McKeon, 1941).

The Dutch philosopher Spinoza examined the nature of humans and human knowledge. He recognized that although the process and outcomes of reasoning may be comparable for each person, intuitive and discerning thought is unique to each. Spinoza believed that reason must be coupled with intuitive thought for true understanding (Lloyd, 1996). Spinoza was noted for taking well-worn philosophical concepts and transforming them into new and engaging ideas. This is true of the Husteds' development of symphonology, particularly in the evolution of the meaning of bioethical standards.

Polanyi (1964) proposed that understanding is derived from awareness of the entirety of a phenomenon, that the lived experience is greater than separate, observable parts. Tacit knowledge, that which is implied, is necessary to understand and interpret that which is explicit (Polanyi, 1964). These concepts, the uniqueness of the individual and the extension of reason and rationality with insight and discernment to create true understanding, are the foundations of the symphonological method.

MAJOR CONCEPTS & DEFINITIONS

Agency

Agency is the capacity of an agent to initiate action toward a chosen goal. The shared goal of a nurse and patient is to restore the patient's agency (Husted et al., 2015).

Context

The "**context** is the interweaving of the relevant facts of a situation" (Husted et al, 2015, p. 77). There are three interrelated elements of context: the context of the situation, the context of knowledge, and the context of an agent's awareness. The context of the situation includes all aspects of the situation that provide understanding of the situation and promote the ability to act effectively within it. The context of knowledge is an agent's preexisting knowledge, which includes factors usually found within the situation. In the context of an agent's awareness, the first two contexts are interwoven. It is an agent's present awareness of all the relevant aspects of the situation (knowledge and circumstances) that are necessary to understand and act effectively within it (Husted et al., 2015).

Environment Agreement

The **environment** established by symphonology is formed by agreement within a context. **Agreement** is a shared state of awareness on the basis of which interaction occurs (Husted & Husted, 2015). Agreement creates the realm in which nursing and all other human interactions occur. Every agreement is aimed toward a final value to be attained through interactions made possible by understanding.

The health care professional–patient agreement is formed by a meeting of the professional's and the patient's needs. Their agreement is one in which the needs and desires of the patient are central. The professional's commitment is defined in terms of the patient's needs. Without this agreement, there would be no context for interaction between the two; the relationship would be unintelligible to both (Husted & Husted, 1999).

Health

Health is a concept applicable to every potential of a person's life. Health involves not only thriving of the physical body, but also happiness. Happiness is realized as individuals pursue and progress toward the goals of their chosen life plan (Husted & Husted, 2001). Health is evident when individuals experience, express, and engage in the fundamental bioethical standards.

Nursing

A nurse acts as the agent of the patient, doing for her patient what he would do for himself if he were able (Husted et al, 2015). The nurse's ethical responsibility is to encourage and strengthen those qualities in the patient that serve life, health, and well-being through their interaction (Fedorka & Husted, 2004).

Person-Patient

A person is an individual with a unique character structure, possessing the right to pursue vital goals as he chooses (Husted et al, 2015). These characteristics are unique to an individual and also may be shared by others (Husted & Husted, 2008). Vital goals are related to survival and the enhancement of life. A **person** takes on the role of **patient** when he has a loss or a decrease in agency resulting in an inability to take the actions required for survival or happiness (Husted & Husted, 1998).

Rights

Rights is the product of an implicit agreement among rational beings, by virtue of their rationality, not to obtain actions or the product of actions from others except through voluntary consent, objectively gained (Husted et al, 2015). **Rights** is a singular term that represents the critical agreement of nonaggression among rational people (Husted & Husted, 1997b).

USE OF EMPIRICAL EVIDENCE

Study and dialogue between the two theorists, coupled with experience of the overall evolution of health care and observation of individual nurse–patient relationships, provided the impetus to develop symphonology theory. G. Husted's dissertation focused on the effect of teaching ethical principles on a student's ability to use these in practical ways through case studies. J. Husted was very instrumental in the selection of the dissertation topic and was used as a consultant during the process. Development of G. Husted's doctoral work led to numerous publications and presentations before the first edition of the book *Ethical Decision Making in Nursing* was published in 1991. This first edition presented their work as a conceptual model only. As they continued to develop their ideas, incorporating feedback from graduate students, the symphonological theory emerged. Before publication of the second edition, the Husteds (1995a) continued to clarify the theoretical concepts and developed the model for practice.

Beginning in 1990, Duquesne University offered a course devoted to this bioethical theory. The authors continued to seek critique and examples about their work from students, practitioners, and other experts. The third edition of the book, *Ethical Decision Making in Nursing and Healthcare: The Symphonological Approach* (Husted & Husted, 2001), offered a clarified description of the theory, with advanced concepts separated from the basic concepts. In addition, the model was redrawn to better represent the nonlinear nature of the theory in practice. The fourth edition offers further clarification of concepts and the integration of concepts in the theory as a whole. In addition, the text is rearranged to present the concepts from simple to more complex. The fifth edition, published in 2015, includes two former doctoral students as coauthors who use the model in practice and have added to the continued development and clarification of the model. In the fifth edition the concepts of freedom and self-assertion were merged. The authors agreed that these concepts were the same and distinguished from each other only by time. They chose to keep the term *freedom* because most people can relate to that term.

As the theory emerged, the need for an emphasis on the individual became apparent and essential. In recent years, it has become accepted practice in the literature to designate patients and nurses as "he/she," or simply use the plural form, referring to nurses and their patients. The authors recognized that these awkward and anonymous terms distract readers from thinking in terms of real people within the context of a particular situation. Therefore they chose to refer to individuals as *he,* in the case of patients, and *she,* in the case of health care professionals in particular situations and examples. This chapter continues with that practice.

MAJOR ASSUMPTIONS

The assumptions from this theory arise from the practical reasoning. The model is meant to provide nurses and other health care professionals with a logical method of determining appropriate ethical actions. Although many of the terms are familiar to nurses and health care professionals, some have been redefined to support the reality of human interaction and ethical delivery of health care.

Nursing

Symphonology holds that a nurse or any other health care professional acts as the agent of the patient. Using her education and experience, a nurse does for her patient what he would do for himself if he were able. Nursing cannot occur without both nurse and patient. "A nurse takes no actions that are not interactions" (Husted & Husted, 2001, p. 37). The nurse's ethical responsibility is to encourage and strengthen those qualities in the patient that serve life, health, and well-being through their interaction (Fedorka & Husted, 2004).

Agency is the capacity of an agent to take action toward a chosen goal. A nurse as agent takes action for a patient, one who cannot act on his own behalf. The shared goal of a nurse and a patient is to restore the patient's agency. The nurse acts with and for the patient toward this end.

Person or Patient

The Husteds define a *person* as an individual with a unique character structure possessing the right to pursue vital goals as he chooses (Husted et al, 2015). Vital goals are concerned with survival and the enhancement of life. A person takes on the role of patient when he has lost or experienced a decrease in agency, resulting in his inability to take the actions required for survival or happiness. The inability to take action may result from physical or mental problems or from a lack of knowledge or experience (Husted & Husted, 1998).

Health

Health is not defined directly by the Husteds. The entire theory is driven by the concept of health in the broadest, most holistic sense. Health is a concept applicable to every potential of a person's life. Health involves not only thriving of the physical body, but also happiness. Happiness is realized as individuals pursue and progress toward the goals of their chosen life plan (Husted et al, 2015). Health is evident when individuals experience, express, and engage in the fundamental bioethical standards.

Environment or Agreement

The environment established by symphonology is formed by agreement. "Agreement is a shared state of awareness on the basis of which interaction occurs" (Husted et al, 2015, p. 32). Agreement creates the realm in which nursing and all other human interactions occur. Every agreement is aimed toward a final value to be attained through interactions made possible by understanding.

The health care professional–patient agreement is formed by a meeting of the professional's and the patient's needs. Their agreement is one in which the needs and desires of the patient are central. The professional's commitment is defined in terms of the patient's needs. Without this agreement, there would be no context for interaction between the two. The relationship would be unintelligible to both (Husted & Husted, 1999).

Symphonology theory is not a compilation of traditional cultural platitudes. It is a method of determining what is practical and justifiable in the ethical dimensions of professional practice. Symphonology recognizes that what is possible and desirable in the agreement is dependent on the context.

The context is the interweaving of the relevant facts of a situation—the facts that are necessary to act upon to bring about a desired result (Husted & Husted, 2001). There are three interrelated elements of context: the context of the situation, the context of knowledge, and the context of awareness. The context of the situation includes all facts relevant to the situation that provide understanding of the situation and promote the ability to act effectively within it. The context of knowledge is an agent's preexisting knowledge of the relevant facts of the situation. The context of awareness represents an integration of the agent's awareness of the facts of the situation and her preexisting knowledge about how to most effectively deal with these facts (Husted & Husted, 2008).

THEORETICAL ASSERTIONS

Symphonology is classified as a grand theory because of its broad scope. Grand theories structure goals related to a specific view of the discipline (Walker & Avant, 2011). Grand theories are broader than conceptual models and may be used as a model to guide practice and research (Fawcett & Garity, 2009). The authors developed symphonology theory from the recognition of a need for theoretical guidelines related to the ethical delivery of health care. The understanding and use of this theory are based on a fundamental ethical element that describes the rational relationship between human beings: human rights.

Rights

The Husteds describe *rights* as the fundamental ethical element. Traditionally, rights are viewed as a list of options to which one is entitled, a list of items or actions to which one has a just claim. Symphonology holds rights as a singular concept. It is the implicit, species-wide agreement that one will not force another to act, or take by force the products of another's actions. Rights are viewed as the critical agreement among rational people, the agreement of nonaggression (Husted & Husted, 1997a). This agreement emerged as humans became rational and developed a civilized social structure. A nonaggression agreement is preconditional to all civilized human interaction. It serves as a foundation on which all other agreements rest. The formal definition is as follows: "the product of an implicit agreement among rational beings, held by virtue of their rationality, not to obtain actions or the products of actions from others except through voluntary consent, objectively gained" (Husted et al, 2015, p. 20). The operation of this is evident in human interaction.

Symphonology theory can ensure ethical action in the provision of health care. Agreement is the foundation of symphonology. Agreements occur based on the implicit understanding of human rights. The understanding of nonaggression that exists among rational persons constitutes human rights. This understanding makes negotiation and cooperation among individuals possible.

Ethical Standards

Ethical standards have been the benchmarks of ethical behavior. The standards include terms familiar to health care professionals such as beneficence, veracity, and confidentiality. However, the Husted et al, (2015) have conceived new meanings for ethical standards that correspond to the foundational concepts of symphonology: the person as a unique individual and the use of insight and discernment in addition to reason and rationality to achieve a deeper understanding.

Traditionally, bioethical concepts have been used to guide ethical action by mandating concrete directives for action. For instance, the concept of beneficence conventionally maintains that one must see that no harm comes to a patient. However, it is not always possible to predict how and when harm will occur, making adherence to this directive an unrealistic goal. The concept of beneficence, viewed as a mandate, could also imply that defending oneself against a physical attack is unethical. Similarly, veracity, or truth telling, holds that one must always speak the truth regardless of the consequences. Therefore it is unethical to withhold potentially harmful information, regardless of the consequences. Adhering to veracity may interfere with one's commitment to beneficence. Clearly, ethical standards taken as concrete directives do not allow for the consideration of context.

Ethical standards have been redefined, not as concrete rules, but as human qualities or character structures that can and must be recognized and respected in the individual (Husted & Husted, 1995b). For example, in symphonological terms, beneficence includes the idea of acting in the patient's best interest, but it begins with the patient's evaluation of what is beneficial. In this way, ethical standards are presuppositions in the health care professional–patient agreement and ethical guides to decision making. The participants work together with the implicit understanding that each is possessed of human characteristics. The description and names of the bioethical standards have changed over time based on feedback from practitioners. Symphonological theory holds that patients have a right to receive the benefits specified in the bioethical standards. Box 26.1 provides definitions and examples of bioethical standards.

BOX 26.1 Bioethical Standards

Autonomy

Autonomy is the uniqueness of the individual, the singular character structure of the individual. Every person has the right to act on his or her unique and independent purposes.

Beneficence

Beneficence is the capability to act to acquire desired benefits and necessary life requirements. Each person may act to obtain the things he or she needs and prefers.

Fidelity

Fidelity is an individual's faithfulness to his or her own uniqueness. Each person manages, maintains, and sustains his or her unique life. For the health care professional, fidelity in agreement means commitment to the obligations accepted in the professional role.

Freedom

Freedom is the capability and right to take action based on the agent's own evaluation of the situation. Every person may choose his or her course of action without interference.

Objectivity

Objectivity is the right to achieve and sustain the exercise of objective awareness. Every person has an awareness and understanding of the universe outside himself or herself. Every person has the right to manage, maintain, and sustain this understanding as he or she chooses.

Just as the bioethical standards are not to be considered as concrete directives, so too, they are not distinct entities. Each standard blends with the others as representative of the unique character structure of the individual (J. Husted, personal communication, March 2004). As stated earlier, recognition of these standards is preconditional to the implicit patient–health care professional agreement. When recognized and respected in each individual, these human qualities and capabilities form the basis for ethical interaction. When they are disregarded, the context of the situation is lost. Interaction is then based on whatever is served by concrete directives or on the whim of the participants.

Certainty

There are circumstances in health care when a patient is unable to communicate his unique character structure, as in the case of an infant or a comatose patient. Health care professionals also interact with individuals from different cultures for whom a common language is lacking. In these cases, the bioethical standards can provide a measure of certainty when knowledge of an individual's unique character is unobtainable.

> *"If you know nothing whatever about an individual's uniqueness, then you are justified in acting on the basis that, as a member of the human species, he shares much in common with every other individual"*
> ***(Fedorka & Husted, 2004, p. 58).***

These commonalities are the bioethical standards. Each person needs the power to sustain his unique nature; the power to be objectively aware of his surroundings; and the power to control his time and effort, to pursue benefit, and to avoid harm. Lacking other information, nurses and health care professionals are justified to do all they can to restore these powers to the individual.

Decision-Making Model

Fig. 26.1 demonstrates the way the concepts of the theory interact with direct decision making. The elements of ethical decision making interact in the following way:

- A person is a rational being with a unique character structure. Each person has the right to choose and pursue, without interference, a course of action in accordance with his needs and desires.
- Agreements between individuals are demonstrated by a shared state of awareness directed toward a goal.
- The health care professional–patient agreement is directed toward preserving and enhancing the life of the patient.
- Context is the basis for determining what actions are ethical within the health care professional–patient agreement. "Context is the interweaving of the relevant

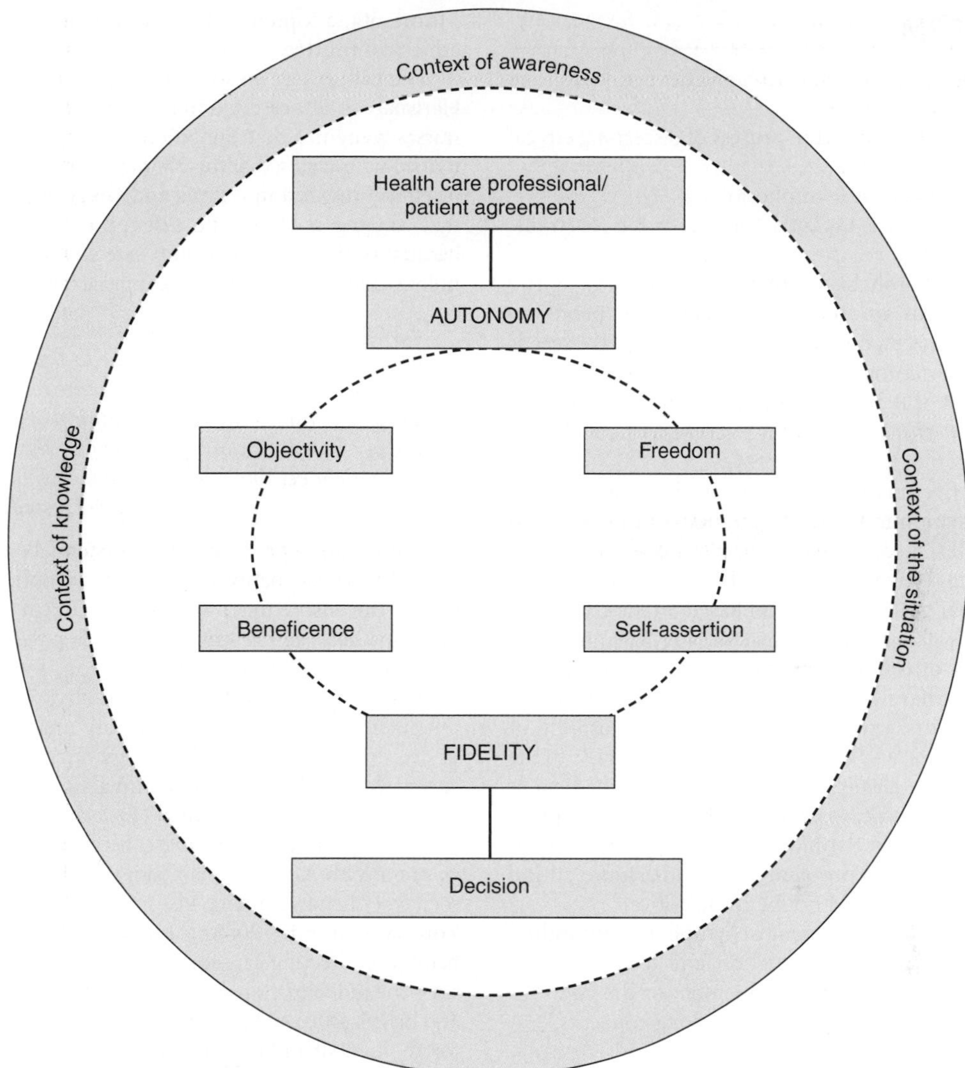

FIG. 26.1 Bioethical decision-making model. (Husted, G.L., Husted, J. H., Scotto, C., & Wolf, K. [2015]. *Ethical decision making in nursing and healthcare* [5th ed.]. New York: Springer.)

facts of the situation—the facts that are necessary to act upon to bring about a desired result, an agent's awareness of these facts, and the knowledge an agent has of how to deal most effectively with these facts" (Husted & Husted, 2008, p. 84). In this way, there are no universal ethical principles.

- Ethical decisions are the result of reasoning from the context to a decision rather than applying a decision or principle to a situation without regard for the context.

The Husteds described the ultimate application and practice of these assumptions by health care professionals in the following way. The professional will come to understand and work from the philosophy that:

> *"My patient's virtues (autonomy) are such that he is moving toward his goal (freedom) in these circumstances (objectivity) for this reason (beneficence). My virtues (autonomy) are such that I must act with him (interactive freedom) to assist him (his freedom) within the possibilities (of beneficence) in his circumstances to achieve every possible benefit that can be discovered (by objective awareness)."*
>
> ***(Husted & Husted, 2001, p. 154)***

LOGICAL FORM

Abductive reasoning, like induction and deduction, follows a pattern:

- A is a collection of data (the process of discerning ethical action).
- B (if true) explains A (symphonology).
- No other hypothesis explains A as well as B does (traditional methods).
- Therefore B is probably correct.

The strength of an abductive conclusion depends on how solidly B can stand by itself, how clearly B exceeds alternatives, how comprehensive was the search for alternatives, the cost of B being wrong and the benefits of being right, and how strong the need is to come to a conclusion at all (Josephson & Josephson, 1994).

The abductive method is evident in the inception and evolution of symphonology. The strength of this theory is evident as well. The concepts of symphonology clearly can be observed not only in health care but also in other walks of life. It is clear that ethical action based on the context of an individual's particular circumstances is far superior to the imposition of concrete directives that often contradict one another or have little relationship to the situation at hand. The authors' extensive study of the philosophy of knowledge, science, and the human condition attests to the comprehensive search for alternative answers. The benefit to patients and health care professionals of receiving practice-based ethical care would be immeasurable. Finally, the need to address the problem of how to achieve ethical action in health care could not be more critical.

Since the initial development of symphonology, inductive reasoning based on observation and feedback from practitioners has provided for refinement of the concepts and clarification of the relationships among concepts.

ACCEPTANCE BY THE NURSING COMMUNITY

Practice

The Husted symphonological model for ethical decision making (Husted & Husted, 2001) was developed as a practice model for applying the concepts of symphonology. This model, stressing the centrality of the individual and the necessity of reason directed by context, is vital in existing and emerging health care systems. The model provides a philosophical framework to ensure ethical care delivery by nurses and all other disciplines of health care. Unlike traditional models, the symphonological model provides for logically justifiable ethical decision making. The North Memorial Medical Center in Robbinsdale, Minnesota, adopted the model for use by their nursing ethics committee.

The call to care in nursing is central to the profession. Hartman (1998) asserted that caring is demonstrated when nurses recognize that the bioethical standards are so intertwined with caring that together they provide a perfect circle of ethical justification. Enns and Gregory (2006) proposed that nursing is losing the essence and practice of caring because of the changing health care environment. Symphonology offers a practice-based approach to care, as follows:

> *"A practice-based approach is derived from, and therefore is intended to be appropriate to the situation of a patient, the purpose of the health care setting, and the role of the nurse. The more an ethical system restricts practice based on abstract principles the more nurse and patient become alienated from each other."*
>
> ***(Husted & Husted, 1997b, p. 14)***

Many nurses practice within systems bound by protocols and critical pathways. Using a symphonological approach can ensure that nursing practice remains ethical and does not become prescriptive. This is particularly important when considering making decisions for those who can no longer make decision for themselves (Gropelli, 2005). Often clinical emergency patients are unable to participate in decision making. Symphonology offers a method of ensuring that ethical conclusion and actions are based on the best interests of the individual (Fedorka & Husted, 2004).

Offering culturally sensitive care is increasingly important as our health care systems change in response to a global society (Chenowethm et al., 2006; Wehbe-Alamah, 2008; Zoucha & Broome, 2008). Although cultural factors can be helpful in directing care for a patient, nurses must also consider the individual's personal commitment to the traditions and beliefs of his culture. In this way, the nurse provides care for the patient rather than the culture (Zoucha & Husted, 2000). Using the Husted model, care is directed within the context of the individual's circumstances. Imposition of a false context, cultural or otherwise, is prevented. Brown (2001b) advocated the use of symphonology theory to direct discussion and education of patients regarding advance directives. Bioethical standards are used to guide discussion about what type of treatment an individual would or would not want, given particular circumstances. Hardt (2004) proposed an intervention for nurses in ethical dilemmas. The emergence of health care teams as a method of delivering comprehensive care brings many disciplines together to serve patients' needs. Overlapping roles and disparate goals can cause confusion among team members. Symphonological theory, with its patient-centered focus, can serve as common ground to initiate and promote collaboration among health care professionals of all disciplines. Symphonology can be applied to all caring disciplines. Khechane (2008) developed a model for pastoral care practice based on symphonology. Using the decision-making model, pastoral care practitioners provide for the relief of suffering using the bioethical standards.

Education

As symphonology is disseminated, it is easy to integrate it into nursing education. Ethics is increasingly being addressed throughout nursing curricula rather than as a separate topic, particularly for advanced nursing students. The broad applicability for symphonology makes it an excellent framework for nursing curricula. Beginning students can easily grasp and apply the theoretical concepts. Using this theory as a basis for nursing interactions directs the student in ethical practice from the beginning of learning nursing practice. The concept of context can be used as the basis for assessment. The bioethical standards direct the student in choosing appropriate approaches, timing, and type of interventions for each patient. Because of the holistic approach and central concern for the patient, symphonology can be incorporated easily into existing nursing curricula.

Brown (2001a) addressed the importance of ethical interaction between nurse educator and student. The agreement in this case is more explicit, because both parties are more aware of the commitments and responsibilities. Recognizing the bioethical standards in both the educator and the student serves to direct ethical actions between them. Above all, the educator and student recall that the educator–student–patient agreement is central to the learning process.

The Husted model not only identifies and organizes professional values and ethical principles for learners, but it also helps the educator to develop a consistent professional ethical orientation. Cutilli (2009) used case study applications with the symphonological theory approach to patient and family education. Burger et al. (2014) used the Husted model to examine incivility among faculty in education. The model provides a mechanism to explore interactions based on the bioethical standards and facilitates ethical decision making within interactions. This led to the conclusion that the integration of ethics into academia is essential for nursing education.

Administration

Health care administrators make decisions at several levels. They have a responsibility to the community at large and the financial viability of the institution within the community, the employees, and those receiving care. Hardt (2004) described how administrators use the principles of symphonology to guide their decision making to produce ethically justifiable outcomes. At the community and institutional levels, one considers the needed services provided by the institution. In cases in which the services needed would not be feasible for the institution, resources within the community can be shared and supported by the institution so that needed services are available with the least amount of loss to the institution. At the employee level, the administrators are concerned with care delivery as well as interpersonal relations. Symphonology guides decision making into equitable rather than equal solutions. For example, an employer may choose to forgo the use of a harsh sanction for absenteeism when the employee is able to show extenuating circumstances that prevented her attendance. This is also true for the development of policy regarding employees' behavior. Ethical policy provides guidelines for examining situations rather than prescribed rules with concrete directives for action. With regard to individual patients, administrators act as role models and consultants when addressing ethical issues.

Hardt and Hopey (2001) described the problematic situations that occur within managed care systems. Difficulties that have been identified include the refusal of the organization to provide care deemed appropriate by health care professionals and the inappropriate demands of patients and families. Using the principles of symphonology, health care professionals can examine the context and determine appropriate ethical actions within the implicit and explicit agreements.

Nurse administrators and managers can also use symphonology to mediate inappropriate situations between patients and nurses (Bavier, 2007)—for example, cases in which patients wish to give an inappropriate gift as a sign of appreciation to a particular nurse.

Research

Symphonology in research is useful in relation to the researcher-subject agreement. The health care professional–patient relationship is to some extent implicit, but the relationship between a researcher and a subject must be thoroughly explicit. Brown (2001c) suggested using the bioethical standards to develop an ethical informed consent protocol. Particularly when the research involves vulnerable populations, the consent of surrogates is made more acceptable and is obtained more easily if the good of the individual is made central by using the bioethical standards.

FURTHER DEVELOPMENT

Initial testing of symphonological theory included two phases. First, a qualitative study examined the perceptions and satisfaction of nurses and patients and their significant others as they engaged in ethical decision making for health care issues (Husted, 2001). The themes that emerged from this study were used to develop visual analog tools to measure feelings in nurses and patients. In the second phase, a pilot study to test the tool was completed. The

Cronbach alpha was reported as 0.74 for the nurse's tool and 0.82 for the patient's tool (Husted, 2004).

Irwin (2004) used a sample of 30 participants involved in a variety of decisions about health care and treatment during hospitalization in an acute care setting. The study included a decision support intervention for patients to determine the following: (1) whether key concepts of symphonological theory describe the experience of individuals making health care decisions, and (2) whether application of the decision-making framework enables nurses and patients to make ethically justifiable decisions. Results confirmed that patients expressed all the concepts of symphonology when discussing their experiences with health care decision making. Statistical analysis of pretest and posttest scores on the Bioethical Decision Making Preference Scale for Patients demonstrated that subjects had a more positive experience of being involved in decision making ($p = 0.02$) and felt more sufficiency of knowledge ($p = 0.013$), less frustration ($p = 0.014$), and more sense of power ($p = 0.009$) after the intervention. These findings support the validity of symphonology theory. The theory can be used to describe the experience of being involved in decision making, and symphonology has utility as a model for assisting patients through the decision-making process.

A graduate student used the nursing visual analog tool to discover how nurses felt when dealing with disclosure issues with patients and reported a Cronbach alpha of 0.82 (Bavier, 2003). Testing of the theory continues; a doctoral graduate analyzed data from a study designed to determine the effect of a symphonology-based educational intervention on the ethical decision-making performance of advanced-level nursing students and compared student understanding of the application of symphonology with other theories (Mraz, 2012).

CRITIQUE

Clarity

In *Ethical Decision Making in Nursing* (Husted & Husted, 1995a), the authors presented the emerging concepts of symphonology and the relationships among the concepts. The book may be difficult for beginning nurses to follow, because deeper concepts meant for advanced practitioners are included along with basic ideas. The third edition, *Ethical Decision Making in Nursing and Healthcare: The Symphonological Approach,* begins with the basic concepts for understanding and using the theory and then moves to more advanced concepts in later sections (Husted & Husted, 2001). Along with this improved organization, the third edition shows the emergence of increasing clarity for all concepts, the bioethical standards in particular. The fourth edition provides yet further clarity using tables and figures and includes a user-friendly teacher manual.

This work challenges traditional methods of thought and requires the reader to develop a new understanding of familiar concepts. Storytelling and examples provide the opportunity to recognize and understand the importance of alternative and extended meanings for familiar terms. The conversational tone of the writing is appealing and creates a comfortable atmosphere for a complex subject.

Simplicity

The authors first challenge the truth and efficacy of traditional ideas about ethical behavior and decision making. This is a simple matter if the reader is open-minded to a different view of nursing events. As the reader accepts the challenge, the simplicity of the theory is evident. There are few concepts, and the relational statements flow logically from the definitions. The model clearly demonstrates the elements of the process of ethical reasoning and the manner in which these elements interact.

Generality

Symphonology is applicable at all levels of nursing practice and in all areas of health care. The principles can be applied between nurse and patient, researcher and subject, manager and employee, and educator and student. Health care professionals of all types can use this method to determine appropriate ethical behaviors in practice. This theory can also be applied to the process of establishing health care policy that is ethical in nature. Indeed, these principles can be applied in all walks of life, depending on the nature of the agreement between the parties involved.

Accessibility

Symphonology is a theory grounded in ethical principles and based in reality. Evidence has demonstrated support of the theory in nursing practice decision research, and the reality of the usefulness of the theory in practice is evident. Nurses and other health care professionals can easily understand the concepts and apply them in all situations. The result of using the symphonological model is a patient-centered, ethically justifiable decision.

Importance

Being able to identify ethical actions in health care is of vital importance to patients, health care professionals, and the health care industry itself. Understanding ethical dilemmas of nursing practice is important for nursing education, research, and practice. Before a nurse or any health care professional takes action (regardless of how effective the action has been in the past), the action must be justified as ethical with regard to the particular patient. Reliance on concrete directives to guide action serves the directives, but only by chance serves the patient. Therefore the pursuit of a practice-based ethical theory is essential for nursing practice and health care.

SUMMARY

The Husteds recognized that the traditional methods of decision making were insufficient to address the bioethical problems emerging in the evolving health care system. They developed a theory of ethics and a decision-making model based on rational thought combined with ethical principles, insight, and understanding. Their theory is founded on the singular concept of human rights, the essential agreement of nonaggression among rational people that forms the foundation of all human interaction. Upon this foundation, health care professionals and patients enter into an agreement to act to achieve the patient's goals. Preconditional to this agreement are recognition and respect for each person's unique character structure and the attendant properties of that structure: freedom, objectivity, beneficence, and fidelity. Ethical decisions are established within the context of a particular situation, using knowledge pertaining to the situation. Symphonological theory and the model for practice ensure ethically justifiable, individualized decisions.

CASE STUDY

Alvin, 66 years of age, has been in the hospital for 12 weeks with multiple trauma after a motor vehicle accident. His condition worsens each day, and his prognosis is very grave. He is not alert, but he grimaces and withdraws from stimulation. Before his injury, Alvin signed a living will and discussed with his family his desire not to be kept alive in the event he was ill or injured and recovery was not possible. The health care team tells his family that, despite aggressive treatment, many of Alvin's body systems are failing. Even if Alvin survives, there is no hope that he will be able to live without a ventilator because of extensive lung damage. The team suggests supportive care for Alvin and a do-not-resuscitate order. Most of the family members express the desire to ensure Alvin's comfort. Two family members believe Alvin will survive and recover. They refuse the team's suggestion and demand that Alvin receive every available treatment to keep him alive.

Analysis

- Autonomy: Alvin's desires should be given priority over his family members' desires.
- Freedom: Not to honor Alvin's wishes is a violation of his freedom.
- Objectivity: The subjective feelings of two family members are in conflict with objective reality. Only the patient's feelings are considered in ethical decisions.
- Beneficence: The patient's goals cannot be obtained by aggressive treatment; however, aggressive treatment may well cause the patient further harm.
- Fidelity: The health care professional's agreement with Alvin was to act as his agent in pursuing goals that are possible to attain.

CRITICAL THINKING ACTIVITIES

Using the Husted model, analyze the following ethical situations:

1. Christina, 46 years of age, has been in the hospital for 2 weeks after a traumatic injury. Her condition was very grave, but she is beginning to show signs of recovery. The health care team suggests that a blood transfusion will provide the necessary support to continue her improvement. Christina and her family practice a religious faith that does not permit blood transfusions. Christina's husband and religious leader insist that she not be given the transfusion regardless of the consequences. When the visitors leave, Christina tells the nurse that she would like to receive the transfusion, but only if it could be kept secret from her family. What should the nurse do?
2. Angela, 34 years of age, is dying of lung cancer. Despite counseling and support, she is very frightened. When her death is imminent, she screams over and over, "Don't let me die! Don't let me die!" Despite all efforts, Angela succumbs before her husband arrives. He asks, "How was she? Was she afraid?" What should the nurse say?
3. Johnny, 7 years of age, is a psychiatric inpatient with a diagnosis of trichomania (hair pulling). His parents are very concerned about stopping his destructive behavior and have developed a series of punishments for incidents of hair pulling. Johnny has been seen pulling his hair out several times during the day. His parents arrive and ask how many times Johnny pulled his hair. What should the nurse say?

4. Eugene, 47 years of age, has several chronic illnesses. Despite education and support, he declines to adhere to prescribed health care practices. Mark, a home health care nurse, has been seeing Eugene for several months and has made little progress in helping Eugene improve his health. While discussing the situation, Eugene tells Mark that he has no intention of changing his behaviors. Is Mark justified in asking the physician to discontinue home health visits?
5. Agnes is a nurse on a busy medical nursing unit. Mr. Brown frequently asks Agnes to interrupt her work to answer questions and perform nonemergent tasks for him. Agnes's other patients complain of neglect. What should Agnes do, and how can she justify her actions?
6. Burt, a 34-year-old manic depressive patient, lives in a group home with others. Sometimes, Burt stops taking his medication and disappears for weeks at a time. He has been arrested for vagrancy, but has never been violent. He states he enjoys his "vacations," because his medicine makes his life seem boring, dull, and difficult. Burt's family calls the director of the group home and insists that Burt be required to take his medicine each morning under supervision. What should the director say, and how could he justify various courses of action?

POINTS FOR FURTHER STUDY

- Burger, K., Kramlich, D., Malitas, M., Page-Cutrara, K., & Whitfield-Harris, L. (2014). Application of the symphonological approach to faculty-to-faculty incivility in nursing education. *Journal of Nursing Education, 53*(10), 563–568.
- Husted, J., Husted, G., Scotto, C., & Wolf, K. (2015). *Ethical decision making in nursing and healthcare* (5th ed.). New York: Springer.

REFERENCES

Bavier, A. (2003). *Types of disclosure discussion between oncology nurses and their patients/families: An exploratory study*. Unpublished manuscript, Duquesne University, Pittsburgh, PA.

Bavier, A. (2007). Practice matters. Beyond a box of chocolates. *American Nurse Today, 11*(2), 14–15.

Brown, B. (2001a). The educator student/patient agreement. In G. L. Husted & J. H. Husted (Eds.), *Ethical decision making in nursing and healthcare: The symphonological approach* (3rd ed., pp. 215–217). New York: Springer.

Brown, B. (2001b). The professional/patient agreement and advanced directives. In G. L. Husted & J. H. Husted (Eds.), *Ethical decision making in nursing and healthcare: The symphonological approach* (3rd ed., pp. 233–237). New York: Springer.

Brown, B. (2001c). The researcher/subject agreement. In G. L. Husted & J. H. Husted (Eds.), *Ethical decision making in nursing and healthcare: The symphonological approach* (3rd ed., pp. 229–231). New York: Springer.

Chenowethm, L., Jeon, Y., Goff, M., & Burke, C. (2006). Cultural competency and nursing care: An Australian perspective. *International Nursing Reviews, 53*, 34–40.

Cutilli, C. C. (2009). Ethical considerations in patient and family education: Using the symphonological approach. *Orthopaedic Nursing, 28*(4), 187–192.

Enns, C., & Gregory, D. (2007). Lamentation and loss: Expressions of caring by contemporary surgical nurses. *Journal of Advanced Nursing, 58*(4), 339–347.

Fawcett, J., & Garity, J. (2009). *Evaluating research for evidence-based nursing practice*. Philadelphia: F. A. Davis.

Fedorka, P., & Husted, G. L. (2004). Ethical decision making in clinical emergencies. *Topics in Emergency Medicine, 26*, 52–60.

Gropelli, T. (2005). A decision for Sam. *Journal of Gerontological Nursing, 31*(1), 45–48.

Hardt, M. (2001). Core then care: The nursing leader's role in caring. *Nursing Administration Quarterly, 25*(3), 37–45.

Hardt, M. (2004). *Efficacy of a symphonological intervention in promoting a positive experience for nurses and patients experiencing bioethical dilemmas*. Unpublished manuscript, Duquesne University, Pittsburgh, PA.

Hartman, R. (1998). Revisiting the call to care: An ethical perspective. *Advanced Practice Nursing Quarterly, 4*(2), 14–18.

Husted, G. L. (2001). The feelings nurses and patients/families experience when faced with the need to make bioethical decisions. *Nursing Administration Quarterly, 25*(3), 1–9.

Husted, G. L. (2004). *The feelings of nurses and patients/families involved in the bioethical decision making process: The psychometric testing of two instruments*. Unpublished manuscript, Duquesne University, Pittsburgh, PA.

Husted, G. L., & Husted, J. H. (1991). *Ethical decision making in nursing*. St Louis: Mosby.

Husted, G. L., & Husted, J. H. (1995a). *Ethical decision making in nursing* (2nd ed.). St Louis: Mosby.

Husted, G. L., & Husted, J. H. (1995b). The bioethical standards: The analysis of dilemmas through the analysis of persons. *Advanced Practice Nursing Quarterly, 1*(2), 69–76.

Husted, G. L., & Husted, J. H. (1997a). An ethical defense against the plague of cloning. *Advanced Practice Nursing Quarterly, 3*(2), 82–84.

Husted, G. L., & Husted, J. H. (1997b). Is a return to a caring perspective desirable? *Advanced Practice Nursing Quarterly, 3*(1), 14–17.

Husted, G. L., & Husted, J. H. (2001). *Ethical decision making in nursing and healthcare: The symphonological approach* (3rd ed.). New York: Springer.

Husted, G. L., & Husted, J. H. (2008). *Ethical decision making in nursing and healthcare: The symphonological approach* (4th ed.). New York: Springer.

Husted, G. L., Husted, J. H, Scotto, C., & Wolf, K. (2015). *Ethical decision making in nursing and healthcare* (5th ed.). New York: Springer.

Husted, J. H., & Husted, G. L. (1998). The role of the nurse in ethical decision making. In G. DeLoughery (Ed.), *Issues and trends in nursing* (pp. 216–242). St Louis: Mosby.

Husted, J. H., & Husted, G. L. (1999). Agreement: The origin of ethical action. *Critical Care Nursing, 22*(3), 12–18.

Irwin, M. (2004). *Effect of symphonology on patients' experience of involvement in health care decision making: A qualitative and quantitative study*. Unpublished dissertation, Duquesne University, Pittsburgh, PA.

Jecker, N., Jonsen, A., & Pearlman, R. (1997). *Bioethics: An introduction to the history, methods and practice*. Sudbury, MA: Jones & Bartlett.

Josephson, J., & Josephson, S. (1994). *Abductive inference: Computation, philosophy, technology*. New York: Cambridge University Press.

Khechane, M. (2008). Application and adaptation of the symphonology bioethical theory (SBT) in pastoral care practice. *Hervormde Teologiese Studies, 64*(2), 959–976.

Lloyd, G. (1996). *Spinoza and the ethics*. New York: Routledge.

McKeon, R. (Ed.). (1941). *The basic works of Aristotle*. New York: Random House.

Mraz, M. (2012). *The impact of the symphonological approach to ethical decision making on advanced level nursing students.* Unpublished dissertation. Duquesne University, Pittsburgh, PA.

Polanyi, M. (1964). *Personal knowledge*. New York: Harper & Row.

Walker, L., & Avant, K. (2011). *Strategies of theory construction in nursing* (5th ed.). Boston: Prentice Hall.

Wehbe-Alamah, H. (2008). Bridging generic and professional care practices for Muslim patients through use of Leininger's culture care modes. *Contemporary Nurse, 28*(1), 83–97.

Zoucha, R., & Broome, B. (2008). The significance of culture in nursing: Examples from the Mexican-American culture and knowing the unknown. *Urologic Nursing, 28*(2), 140–142.

Zoucha, R., & Husted, G. (2000). The ethical dimensions of delivering cultural congruent nursing and health care. *Issues in Mental Health Nursing, 21*(3), 325–340.

BIBLIOGRAPHY

Primary Sources

Book Chapters

Husted, G. L., & Husted, J. H. (1999). Strength of character through the ethics of nursing. In S. Osgood (Ed.), *Essential readings in nursing managed care* (pp. 102–106). Gaithersburg, MD: Aspen.

Husted, G. L., & Husted, J. H. (2005). The ethical experience of caring for vulnerable populations: The symphonological approach. In M. DeChesnay (Ed.), *Caring for vulnerable populations* (pp. 71–79). St Louis: Mosby.

Husted, J., Husted, G., & Scotto, C. (2012). Ethics and the advanced practice nurse. In A. Joel (Ed.), *Advanced Practice Nursing* (3rd ed.) (pp. 522–543). Philadelphia: F. A. Davis.

Journal Articles

Husted, G. L., & Husted, J. H. (1995). The bioethical standards: The analysis of dilemmas through the analysis of persons. *Advanced Practice Nursing Quarterly, 1*(2), 69–76.

Husted, G. L., & Husted, J. H. (1996). Ethical dilemmas: Time and fidelity. *American Journal of Nursing, 96*(11), 74.

Husted, G. L., & Husted, J. H. (1997). A modest proposal concerning policies. *Advanced Practice Nursing Quarterly, 3*(3), 17–19.

Husted, G. L., & Husted, J. H. (1997). An ethical defense against the plague of cloning. *Advanced Practice Nursing Quarterly, 3*(2), 82–84.

Husted, G. L., & Husted, J. H. (1997). An ethical examination of in-vitro fertilization and cloning. *AORN Journal, 65*(6), 1–2.

Husted, G. L., & Husted, J. H. (1997). Is a return to a caring perspective desirable? *Advanced Practice Nursing Quarterly, 3*(1), 14–17.

Husted, G. L., & Husted, J. H. (1997). Is cloning moral? *Nursing and Health Care: Perspectives on Community, 18*, 168–169.

Husted, G. L., & Husted, J. H. (1998). Ethical balance versus ethical anomaly. *Advanced Practice Nursing Quarterly, 4*(1), 51–53.

Husted, G. L., & Husted, J. H. (1998). Strength of character through the ethics of nursing. *Advanced Practice Nursing Quarterly, 3*(4), 23–25.

Husted, G. L., & Husted, J. H. (1998). With the ethical agreement: Where are you now? *Advanced Practice Nursing Quarterly, 4*(2), 34–35.

Husted, J. H., & Husted, G. L. (2000). When is a health care system not an ethical health care system? Suspending the do-not-resuscitate order in the operating room. *Critical Care Nursing Clinics of North America, 12*, 157–163.

Husted, G. L., Miller, M. C., & Brown, B. (1999). Test of an educational brochure on advance directives designed for the well-elderly. *Journal of Gerontological Nursing, 25*(1), 34–40.

Husted, G. L., Miller, M. C., Zaremba, J. A., Clutter, S. L., Jennings, K. R., & Stainbrook, D. (1997). Advance directives and what attracts elderly people to particular brochures. *Journal of Gerontological Nursing, 23*(2), 41–45.

Zoucha, R., & Husted, G. L. (2000). Is delivering culturally congruent psychosocial healthcare ethical? *Issues in Mental Health Nursing, 21*(3), 325–340.

Zoucha, R. D., & Husted, G. L. (2002). The ethical dimensions of delivering culturally congruent nursing and health care. *Review Series Psychiatry, Sweden, 3*, 10–11.

Secondary Sources

Books

Burkhardt, M. A., & Nathaniel, A. K. (2002). *Ethics and issues in contemporary nursing* (2nd ed.). Clifton Park, NJ: Delmar.

Daly, J., Speedy, S., & Jackson, D. (2005). *Professional nursing: Concepts, issues, and challenges*. New York: Springer.

de Chesnay, M., & Anderson, B. (2008). *Caring for the vulnerable: Perspectives in nursing theory, practice, and research*. Sudbury, MA: Jones & Bartlett.

Fry, S., & Johnstone, M. (2002). *Ethics in nursing practice: A guide to ethical decision making*. Malden, MD: Blackwell Science.

Journal Articles

Anderson, J., Biba, S., & Hartman, R. L. (1996). Ethical case comment. To tell or not to tell . . . the case for ethical analysis. *Dimensions of Critical Care Nursing, 15*(6), 318–323.

Baldonado, A. (1996). Ethnicity and morality in a multicultural world. *Journal of Cultural Diversity, 3*(4), 105–108.

Best, J. T. (2001). Effective teaching for the elderly: Back to basics. *Orthopedic Nursing, 20*(3), 46–52.

Bridger, J. C. (1997). A study of nurses' views about the prevention of nosocomial urinary tract infections. *Journal of Clinical Nursing, 6*(5), 379–387.

Brown, B. (2003). Historical perspectives. The history of advance directives: A literature review. *Journal of Gerontological Nursing, 29*(9), 4–14.

Burcham, J. L. R. (2002). Cultural competence: An evolutionary perspective. *Nursing Forum, 37*(4), 5–15.

Caitlin, A. (1997). Pediatric ethics, issues, & commentary. Creating a beginning ethics library. *Pediatric Nursing, 23*(5), 495–496.

Cioffi, R. (2003). Communicating with culturally and linguistically diverse patients in an acute care setting: Nurses' experiences. *International Journal of Nursing Studies, 40*(3), 299–306.

Claassen, M. (2000). A handful of questions: Supporting parental decision making. *Clinical Nurse Specialist, 14*(4), 189–195.

DeLikkis, A., & Sauer, R. (2004). Respect as ethical foundation for communication in employee relations. *Laboratory Medicine, 35*(5), 262–266.

Dennis, B. (1999). The origin and nature of informed consent: Experiences among vulnerable groups. *Journal of Professional Nursing, 15*(5), 281–287.

Goldblatt, D. (2001). A messy necessary end—Health care proxies need our support. *Neurology, 56*(2), 148–152.

Groupp, E. (2005). Recruiting seniors with chronic low back pain for a randomized controlled trial of a self-management program. *Journal of Manipulative & Physiological Therapeutics, 28*(2), 97–102.

Hardt, M. (2001). Core then care: The nurse leader's role in "caring." *Nursing Administration Quarterly, 25*(3), 37–45.

Hunt, S. (1996). Ethics of resource distribution: Implications for palliative care services. *International Journal of Palliative Nursing, 2*(4), 222–226.

Jeffery, D. (2005). Adapting de-escalation techniques with deaf service users. *Nursing Standard, 19*(49), 41–47.

Jirwe, M. (2006). The theoretical framework of cultural competence. *Journal of Multicultural Nursing & Health, 12*(3), 6–16.

Johnson, J. E. (2002). Six steps to ethical leadership in health care. *Patient Care Management, 18*(2), 5–9.

Mariano, C. (2001). Holistic ethics. *American Journal of Nursing, 101*(1 part 1), Hospital Extra: 24A-C.

Martindale, A., & Collins, D. (2005). Professional judgment and decision making: The role of intention for impact. *The Sport Psychologist, 19*(3), 303–313.

McFadden, E. A. (1996). Moral development and reproductive health decisions. *Journal of Obstetric, Gynecologic, & Neonatal Nursing, 25*(6), 507–512.

Oberle, K., & Tenove, S. (2000). Ethical issues in public health nursing. *Nursing Ethics: An International Journal for Health Care Professionals, 7*(5), 425–438.

Oddi, L. F., Cassidy, V. R., & Fisher, C. (1995). Nurses' sensitivity to the ethical aspects of clinical practice. *Nursing Ethics: An International Journal for Health Care Professionals, 2*(3), 197–209.

Perry, J. (2006). Resisting vulnerability: The experiences of families who have kin in hospital—a feminist ethnography. *International Journal of Nursing Studies, 43*(2), 173–184.

Reveillere, C., Pham, T., Masclet, G., Nandrino, J. L., & Beaune, D. (2000). The relationship between burn-out and personality in care-givers in a palliative care unit. *Annals Medico Psychologiques, 158*(9), 716–721.

Rice, V. H., Beck, C., & Stevenson, J. S. (1997). Ethical issues relative to autonomy and personal control in independent and cognitive impaired elders. *Nursing Outlook, 45*(1), 27–34.

Roberson, D. (2007). Inequities in screening for sexually transmitted infections in African American adolescents: Can health policy help? *Journal of Transcultural Nursing, 18*(3), 286–291.

Saulo, M. (1996). How good case managers make tough choices: Ethics and mediation. Part I. *Journal of Care Management, 2*(1), 8, 10, 12.

Scotto, C. (2003). A new view of caring. *Journal of Nursing Education, 42*(7), 289–291.

Scotto, C. (2005). Symphonological bioethical theory. In A. M. Tomey & M. R. Alligood (Eds.), *Nursing theorists and their work* (6th ed., pp. 584–601). St Louis: Mosby.

Sellar, B. (2006). Subjective leisure experiences of older Australians. *Australian Occupational Therapy Journal, 53*(3), 211–219.

Simko, L. (1999). Adults with congenital heart disease: Utilizing quality of life and Husted's nursing theory as a conceptual framework. *Critical Care Nursing Quarterly, 22*(3), 1–11.

Steckler, J. (1998). Examination of ethical practices in nursing continuing education using the Husted model. *Advanced Practice Nursing Quarterly, 4*(2), 59–64.

Szirony, T., Price, J., Wolfe, E., Telljohann, S., & Dake, J. (2004). Perceptions of nursing faculty regarding ethical issues in nursing research. *Journal of Nursing Education, 43*(6), 270–279.

Thomas, A. (1997). Patient autonomy and cancer treatment decisions. *International Journal of Palliative Nursing, 3*(6), 317–323.

Viney, C. (1996). A phenomenological study of ethical decision-making experiences among senior intensive care nurses and doctors concerning withdrawal of treatment. *Nursing in Critical Care, 4*, 182–187.

Von Post, I. (1996). Exploring ethical dilemmas in perioperative nursing practice through critical incidents. *Nursing Ethics: An International Journal for Health Care Professionals, 3*(3), 236–249.

Weiner, C., Tabak, N., & Bergman, R. (2001). The use of physical restraints for patients suffering from dementia. *Nursing Ethics, 56*(2), 148–152.

Wilmot, S. (2000). Nurses and whistleblowing: The ethical issues. *Journal of Advanced Nursing, 32*(5), 1051–1057.

Wilson, D. M. (1998). Administrative decision making in response to sudden health care agency funding reductions: Is there a role for ethics? *Nursing Ethics, 5*(4), 319–329.

Wurzbach, M. E. (1999). Acute care nurses' experiences of moral certainty. *Journal of Advanced Nursing, 30*(2), 287–293.

Zoucha, R. (2006). Considering culture in understanding interpersonal violence. *Journal of Forensic Nursing, 2*(4), 195–196.

UNIT V

Middle-Range Theories

- Middle-range theories are the least abstract theory level for concrete practice applications.
- Middle-range theories include the characteristics of nursing practice or situations.
- Middle-range theories are theoretical evidence of applicability and outcome.
- Middle-range theories develop evidence for nursing practice outcomes.
- Middle-range theories are recognizable as such because they contain characteristics of nursing practice. Characteristics of middle-range theories include the following:
  - The situation or health condition of the client or patient
  - Client or patient population or age group
  - Location or area of practice (e.g., community)
  - Action of the nurse or intervention
  - The client or patient outcome anticipated

Philosophy sets forth the meaning of nursing phenomena through analysis, reasoning and logical presentation of concepts and ideas.
Conceptual Models are sets of concepts that address phenomena central to nursing in propositions that explain the relationship among them.
Grand Theory concepts that derive from a conceptual model and propose a testable proposition that tests the major premise of the model.
Nursing Theory testable propositions from philosophies, conceptual models, grand theories, abstract nursing theories, or theories from other disciplines. Theories are less abstract than grand theory and less specific than middle-range theory.
Middle-Range Theory concepts most specific to practice that propose precise testable nursing practice questions and include details such as patient age group, family situation, health condition, location of the patient, and action of the nurse.
The Future of Nursing Theory Nursing theoretical systems give direction and create understanding in practice, research, administration, and education.
Metaparadigm
The broad conceptual boundaries of the discipline of nursing: Human beings, environment, health, and nursing

27

Maternal Role Attainment—Becoming a Mother

*Molly Meighan**

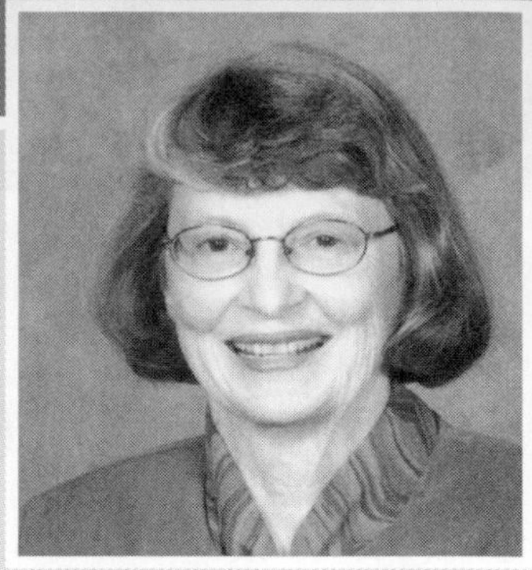

Ramona T. Mercer (1929–Present)

"The process of becoming a mother requires extensive psychological, social, and physical work. A woman experiences heightened vulnerability and faces tremendous challenges as she makes this transition. Nurses have an extraordinary opportunity to help women learn, gain confidence, and experience growth as they assume the mother identity."

(Mercer, 2006, p. 649)

CREDENTIALS AND BACKGROUND OF THE THEORIST

Ramona T. Mercer began her nursing career in 1950, when she received her diploma from St. Margaret's School of Nursing in Montgomery, Alabama. She graduated with the L. L. Hill Award for Highest Scholastic Standing. She returned to school in 1960 after working as a staff nurse, head nurse, and instructor in the areas of pediatrics, obstetrics, and contagious diseases. She completed a bachelor's degree in nursing in 1962, graduating with distinction from the University of New Mexico, Albuquerque. She went on to earn a master's degree in maternal-child nursing from Emory University in 1964 and completed a doctorate in maternity nursing at the University of Pittsburgh in 1973.

After receiving her doctorate degree, Mercer moved to California and accepted the position of Assistant Professor in the Department of Family Health Care Nursing at the University of California, San Francisco. She was promoted to associate professor in 1977 and to full professor in 1983. She remained in that role until her retirement in 1987. Currently, Dr. Mercer is Professor Emeritus in Family Health Nursing at the University of California, San Francisco (http://www.nurses.info/nursing_theory_midrange_theories_ramona_mercer.htmMercer).

Mercer received awards throughout her career. In 1963, while working and pursuing studies in nursing, she received the Department of Health, Education, and Welfare Public Health Service Nurse Trainee Award at Emory University and was inducted into Sigma Theta Tau. She received this award again during her years at the University of Pittsburgh. She also received the Bixler Scholarship for Nursing Education and Research, Southern Regional Board, for doctoral study. In 1982 she received the Maternal Child Health Nurse of the Year Award from the National Foundation of the March of Dimes and American Nurses Association, Division of Maternal Child Health Practice. She was presented with the Fourth Annual Helen Nahm Lecturer Award at the University of California, San Francisco School of Nursing in 1984. Mercer's research awards include the American Society for Psychoprophylaxis in Obstetrics (ASPO)/Lamaze National Research Award in 1987; the Distinguished Research Lectureship Award, Western Institute of Nursing, Western Society for Research in Nursing in 1988; and the American Nurses Foundation's Distinguished Contribution to Nursing Science Award in 1990 (Mercer, curriculum vitae, 2002). Mercer has authored numerous articles, editorials, and

*Previous authors: Mary M. (Molly) Meighan, Alberta M. Bee, Denise Legge, and Stephanie Oetting.
Photo credit: Marie Cox, M&M Studios, San Francisco, CA.

commentaries. In addition, she has published six books and six book chapters.

In early research efforts, Mercer focused on the behaviors and needs of breastfeeding mothers, mothers with postpartum illness, mothers of infants born with defects, and teenage mothers. Her first book, *Nursing Care for Parents at Risk* (1977), received an *American Journal of Nursing* Book of the Year Award in 1978. Her study of teenage mothers over the first year of motherhood resulted in the 1979 book *Perspectives on Adolescent Health Care,* which also received an *American Journal of Nursing* Book of the Year Award in 1980. Preceding research led Mercer to study family relationships, antepartal stress as related to familial relationships and the maternal role, and mothers of various ages. In 1986 Mercer's research on three age groups of mothers was drawn together in her third book, *First-Time Motherhood: Experiences from Teens to Forties* (1986a). Mercer's fifth book, *Parents at Risk,* published in 1990, also received an *American Journal of Nursing* Book of the Year Award. *Parents at Risk* (1990) focused on strategies for facilitating early parent-infant interactions and promoting parental competence in relation to specific risk situations. Mercer's sixth book, *Becoming a Mother: Research on Maternal Identity from Rubin to the Present,* was published in 1995. This book contains a more complete description of Mercer's theory of maternal role attainment and her framework for studying variables that affect the maternal role.

Since her first publication in 1968, Mercer has written numerous articles for both nursing and nonnursing journals. She published several online courses for *Nurseweek* during the 1990s and through early 2000, including "Adolescent Sexuality and Child-bearing," "Transitions to Parenthood," and "Helping Parents When the Unexpected Occurs."

Mercer maintained membership in several professional organizations, including the American Nurses Association and the American Academy of Nursing, and was an active member on many national committees. From 1983 to 1990, she was Associate Editor of *Health Care for Women International.* Mercer served on the review panel for *Nursing Research and Western Journal of Nursing Research* and on the editorial board of the *Journal of Adolescent Health Care,* and she was on the executive advisory board of *Nurseweek.* She also served as a reviewer for numerous grant proposals. In addition, she was actively involved with regional, national, and international scientific and professional meetings and workshops (Mercer, curriculum vitae, 2002). She was honored as a Living Legend by the American Academy of Nursing during the Annual Meeting and Conference in Carlsbad, California, in November 2003. Mercer was honored by the University of New Mexico in 2004, receiving the first College of Nursing Distinguished Alumni Award. In 2005 she was recognized as among the most outstanding alumni and faculty, and her name appears on the Wall of Fame at the University of California, San Francisco.

THEORETICAL SOURCES

Mercer's theory of maternal role attainment was based on her extensive research on the topic beginning in the late 1960s. Mercer's professor and mentor, Reva Rubin at the University of Pittsburgh, was a major stimulus for both research and theory development. Rubin (1977, 1984) was well known for her work in defining and describing maternal role attainment as a process of binding-in, or being attached to, the child and achieving a maternal role identity or seeing oneself in the role and having a sense of comfort about it. Mercer's framework and study variables reflect many of Rubin's concepts.

In addition to Rubin's work, Mercer based her research on both role and developmental theories. She relied heavily on an interactionist approach to role theory, using Mead's (1934) theory on role enactment and Turner's (1978) theory on the core self. In addition, Thornton and Nardi's (1975) role acquisition process helped shape Mercer's theory, as did the work of Burr et al. (1979). Werner's (1957) developmental process theories also contributed. In addition, Mercer's work was influenced by von Bertalanffy's (1968) general system theory. Her model of maternal role attainment, depicted in Fig. 27.1, uses Bronfenbrenner's (1979) concepts of nested circles as a means of portraying interactional environmental influences on the maternal role. The complexity of her research interest led Mercer to rely on several theoretical sources to identify and study variables that affect maternal role attainment. Although much of her work involved testing and extending Rubin's theories, she has consistently looked to the research of others in the development and expansion of her theory.

USE OF EMPIRICAL EVIDENCE

Mercer selected both maternal and infant variables for her studies on the basis of her review of the literature and findings of researchers in several disciplines. She found that many factors may have a direct or indirect influence on the maternal role, adding to the complexity of her studies. Maternal factors in Mercer's research included age at first birth, birth experience, early separation from the infant, social stress, social support, personality traits, self-concept, child-rearing attitudes, and health. She included the infant variables of temperament, appearance, responsiveness, health status, and ability to give cues. Mercer (1995) and Ferketich and Mercer (1995a, 1995b, 1995c) also noted the importance of the father's role and applied many of Mercer's previous findings in studying the paternal response to parenthood. Her research required numerous instruments to measure the variables of interest.

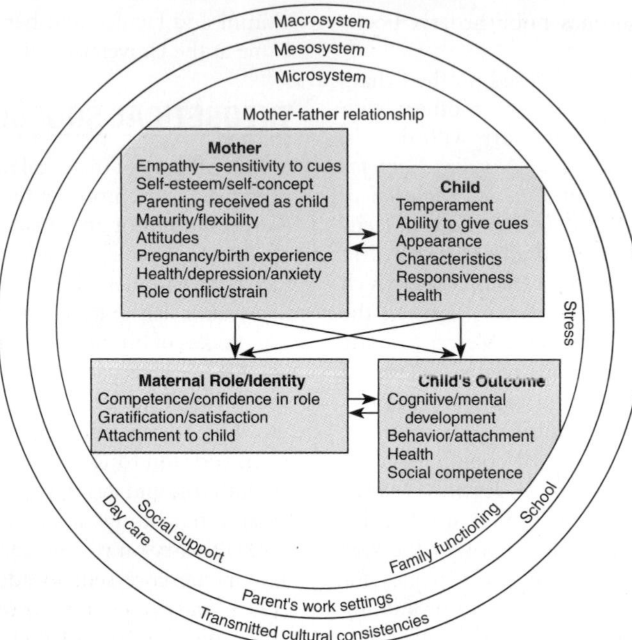

FIG. 27.1 Model of maternal role attainment. (Modified from Mercer, R. T. [1991]. *Maternal role: Models and consequences.* Paper presented at the International Research Conference sponsored by the Council of Nurse Researchers and the American Nurses Association, Los Angeles, CA. Copyright Ramona T. Mercer, 1991. NOTE: This figure has been modified based on personal communication with R. T. Mercer [January 4, 2003]. The word exosystem was replaced with mesosystem to be more consistent with Bronfenbrenner's [1979] model, on which it is based.)

MAJOR CONCEPTS & DEFINITIONS

Maternal Role Attainment

Maternal role attainment is an interactional and developmental process occurring over time in which the mother becomes attached to her infant, acquires competence in the caretaking tasks involved in the role, and expresses pleasure and gratification in the role (Mercer, 1986a). "The movement to the personal state in which the mother experiences a sense of harmony, confidence, and competence in how she performs the role is the end point of maternal role attainment—maternal identity" (Mercer, 1981, p. 74).

Maternal Identity

Maternal identity is defined as having an internalized view of the self as a mother (Mercer, 1995).

Perception of Birth Experience

A woman's perception of her performance during labor and birth is her perception of the birth experience (Mercer, 1990).

Self-Esteem

Mercer et al. (1986) describe **self-esteem** as "an individual's perception of how others view oneself and self-acceptance of the perceptions" (p. 341).

Self-Concept (Self-Regard)

Mercer (1986a) outlines **self-concept**, or **self-regard**, as "The overall perception of self that includes self-satisfaction, self-acceptance, self-esteem, and congruence or discrepancy between self and ideal self" (p. 18).

Flexibility

Roles are not rigidly fixed; therefore who fills the roles is not important (Mercer, 1990). "**Flexibility** of childrearing attitudes increases with increased development. Older mothers have the potential to respond less rigidly to their infants and to view each situation in respect to the unique nuances" (Mercer, 1990, p. 12).

MAJOR CONCEPTS & DEFINITIONS—cont'd

Child-Rearing Attitudes

Child-rearing attitudes are maternal attitudes or beliefs about child rearing (Mercer, 1986a).

Health Status

Health status is defined as "The mother's and father's perception of their prior health, current health, health outlook, resistance-susceptibility to illness, health worry concern, sickness orientation, and rejection of the sick role" (Mercer et al., 1986, p. 342).

Anxiety

Mercer and colleagues (1986) describe **anxiety** as "a trait in which there is specific proneness to perceive stressful situations as dangerous or threatening, and as a situation-specific state" (p. 342).

Depression

According to Mercer and colleagues (1986), **depression** is "having a group of depressive symptoms and in particular the affective component of the depressed mood" (p. 342).

Role Strain–Role Conflict

Role strain is the conflict and difficulty felt by the woman in fulfilling the maternal role obligation (Mercer, 1985a).

Gratification-Satisfaction

Mercer (1985b) describes **gratification** as "the satisfaction, enjoyment, reward, or pleasure that a woman experiences in interacting with her infant, and in fulfilling the usual tasks inherent in mothering."

Attachment

Attachment is a component of the parental role and identity. It is viewed as a process in which an enduring affectional and emotional commitment to an individual is formed (Mercer, 1990).

Infant Temperament

An easy versus a difficult **temperament** is related to whether the infant sends hard-to-read cues, leading to feelings of incompetence and frustration in the mother (Mercer, 1986a).

Infant Health Status

Infant health status relates to illness causing maternal-infant separation, interfering with the attachment process (Mercer, 1986a).

Infant Characteristics

Characteristics include infant temperament, appearance, and health status (Mercer, 1981).

Infant Cues

Infant cues are infant behaviors that elicit a response from the mother (R. T. Mercer, personal communication, September 2003).

Family

Mercer and colleagues (1986) define **family** as "a dynamic system that includes subsystems—individuals (mother, father, fetus/infant) and dyads (mother-father, mother-fetus/infant, and father-fetus/infant) within the overall family system" (p. 339).

Family Functioning

Family functioning is the individual's view of the activities and relationships between the family and its subsystems and broader social units (Mercer & Ferketich, 1995).

Father or Intimate Partner

The **father** or **intimate partner** contributes to the process of maternal role attainment in a way that cannot be duplicated by any other person (R. T. Mercer, personal communication, January 2003). The father's interactions help diffuse tension and facilitate maternal role attainment (Donley, 1993; Mercer, 1995).

Stress

Stress is made up of positively and negatively perceived life events and environmental variables (Mercer, 1990).

Social Support

According to Mercer and colleagues (1986), **social support** is "the amount of help actually received, satisfaction with that help, and the persons (network) providing that help" (p. 341). Four areas of social support are as follows:

1. **Emotional support**: "Feeling loved, cared for, trusted, and understood" (Mercer, 1986a, p. 14)
2. **Informational support**: "Helping the individual help herself by providing information that is useful in dealing with the problem and/or situation" (Mercer, 1986a, p. 14)
3. **Physical support**: A direct kind of help (Mercer, Hackley, & Bostrom, 1984)
4. **Appraisal support**: "A support that tells the role taker how she is performing in the role; it enables the individual to evaluate herself in relationship to others' performance in the role" (Mercer, 1986a, p. 14)

Mother-Father Relationship

The **mother-father relationship** is the perception of the mate relationship that includes intended and actual values, goals, and agreements between the two (Mercer, 1986b). The maternal attachment to the infant develops within the emotional field of the parents' relationship (Donley, 1993; Mercer, 1995).

Mercer has studied the influence of these variables on parental attachment and competence over several intervals, including the immediate postpartum period and 1 month, 4 months, 8 months, and 1 year after birth (Mercer & Ferketich, 1990a, 1990b). In addition, she has included adolescents, older mothers, ill mothers, mothers dealing with congenital defects, families experiencing antepartal stress, parents at high risk, mothers who had cesarean deliveries, and fathers in her research (Mercer, 1989; Mercer & Ferketich, 1994, 1995; Mercer, Ferketich, & DeJoseph, 1993). As a recent step, she compared her findings and the basis for her original theory with current research. As a result, Mercer (2004) has proposed that the term *maternal role attainment* be replaced with *becoming a mother,* because this more accurately describes the continued evolvement of the role across the woman's life span. In addition, she proposed using more recent nursing research findings to describe the stages and process of becoming a mother.

MAJOR ASSUMPTIONS

For maternal role attainment, Mercer (1981, 1986a, 1995) stated the following assumptions:

- A relatively stable core self, acquired through lifelong socialization, determines how a mother defines and perceives events; her perceptions of her infant's and others' responses to her mothering, with her life situation, are the real world to which she responds (Mercer, 1986a).
- In addition to the mother's socialization, her developmental level and innate personality characteristics also influence her behavioral responses (Mercer, 1986a).
- The mother's role partner, her infant, will reflect the mother's competence in the mothering role through growth and development (Mercer, 1986a).
- The infant is considered an active partner in the maternal role-taking process, affecting and being affected by the role enactment (Mercer, 1981).
- The father's or mother's intimate partner contributes to role attainment in a way that cannot be duplicated by any other supportive person (Mercer, 1995).
- Maternal identity develops concurrently with maternal attachment, and each depends on the other (Mercer, 1995; Rubin, 1977).

Nursing

Mercer (1995) stated that "Nurses are the health professionals having the most sustained and intense interaction with women in the maternity cycle" (p. xii). Nurses are responsible for promoting the health of families and children; nurses are pioneers in developing and sharing assessment strategies for these patients. Her definition of nursing provided in a personal communication is as follows:

> *"Nursing is a dynamic profession with three major foci: health promotion and prevention of illness, providing care for those who need professional assistance to achieve their optimal level of health and functioning, and research to enhance the knowledge base for providing excellent nursing care. Nurses provide health care for individuals, families, and communities. Following assessment of the client's situation and environment, the nurse identifies goals with the client, provides assistance to the client through teaching, supporting, providing care the client is unable to provide for self, and interfacing with the environment and the client."*
>
> ***(R. Mercer, personal communication, March 2004)***

In her writing, Mercer (1995) refers to the importance of nursing care. In *Becoming a Mother: Research on Maternal Identity from Rubin to the Present,* Mercer does not specifically mention nursing care; however, she emphasizes that the kind of help or care a woman receives during pregnancy and the first year after giving birth can have long-term effects for her and her child. Nurses in maternal-child settings play a sizable role in providing both care and information during this period.

Person

Mercer (1985a) does not specifically define *person* but refers to the *self* or *core self.* She views the self as separate from the roles that are played. Through maternal individuation, a woman may regain her own personhood as she extrapolates herself from the mother-infant dyad (Mercer, 1985b). The core self evolves from a cultural context and determines how situations are defined and shaped (Mercer, 1985a). The concepts of self-esteem and self-confidence are important in attainment of the maternal role. The mother as a separate person interacts with her infant and with the father or her significant other. She is both influential and is influenced by both of them (Mercer, 1995).

Health

In her theory, Mercer defines *health status* as the mother's and father's perception of their prior health, current health, health outlook, resistance-susceptibility to illness, health worry or concern, sickness orientation, and rejection of the sick role. Health status of the newborn is the extent of disease present and infant health status by parental rating of overall health (Mercer, 1986b). The health status of a family is affected negatively by antepartum stress (Mercer, Ferketich, et al., 1988; Mercer, May, et al., 1986). Health status is an important indirect influence on satisfaction with relationships in childbearing families. Health is also viewed as a desired outcome for the child. It is influenced by both maternal and infant variables. Mercer (1995) stresses the importance of health care during the childbearing and childrearing processes.

Environment

Mercer conceptualized the environment from Bronfenbrenner's definition of the ecological environment and based her earliest model (see Fig. 27.1) on it (Mercer, 1995; R. Mercer, personal communication, June 2000). This model illustrates the ecological interacting environments in which maternal role attainment develops. During a personal communication on January 4, 2003, Mercer explained, "Development of a role/person cannot be considered apart from the environment; there is a mutual accommodation between the developing person and the changing properties of the immediate settings, relationships between the settings, and the larger contexts in which the settings are embedded." Stresses and social support within the environment influence both maternal and paternal role attainment and the developing child.

THEORETICAL ASSERTIONS

Mercer's original theory and model of maternal role attainment were introduced in 1991 during a symposium at the International Research Conference sponsored by the Council of Nursing Research and American Nurses Association in Los Angeles, California (Mercer, 1995). It was refined and presented more clearly in her 1995 book, *Becoming a Mother: Research on Maternal Identity from Rubin to the Present* (see Fig. 27.1).

Mercer's (2004) more recent revision of her theory has focused on the woman's transition in becoming a mother. Motherhood involves an extensive change in a woman's life that requires her ongoing development. According to Mercer, becoming a mother is more extensive than just assuming a role. It is unending and continuously evolving. Therefore she proposed that the term *maternal role attainment* be retired. She based that recommendation on the published research of Walker, Crain, and Thompson (1986a, 1986b), Koniak-Griffin (1993), and McBride and Shore (2001), who had examined the process of mothering and raised questions about the appropriateness of maternal role attainment as an end point in the process.

Maternal Role Attainment: Mercer's Original Model and Theory

Mercer's model of maternal role attainment was placed within Bronfenbrenner's (1979) nested circles of the *microsystem, mesosystem,* and *macrosystem* (see Fig. 27.1). The original model proposed by Mercer was altered in 2000, changing the term *exosystem,* originally found in the second circle, and replacing it with the term *mesosystem.* Mercer (personal communication, January 2003) explained that this change made the model more consistent with Bronfenbrenner's terminology, as follows:

1. The microsystem is the immediate environment in which maternal role attainment occurs. It includes factors such as family functioning, mother-father relationships, social support, economic status, family values, and stressors. The variables contained within this immediate environment interact with one or more of the other variables in affecting the transition to motherhood. The infant as an individual is embedded within the family system. The family is viewed as a semiclosed system maintaining boundaries and control over interchange between the family system and other social systems (Mercer, 1990).

The microsystem is the most influential on maternal role attainment (Mercer, 1995; R. Mercer, personal communication, January 2003). In 1995 Mercer expanded her earlier concepts and model to emphasize the importance of the father in role attainment, stating that he helps "diffuse tension developing within the mother-infant dyad" (p. 15). Maternal role attainment is achieved through the interactions of father, mother, and infant. The microsystem in Fig. 27.2, first introduced in Mercer's (1995) sixth book, *Becoming a Mother: Research on Maternal Identity from Rubin to the Present,* depicts this interaction. The layers *a* through *d* represent the stages of maternal role attainment from anticipatory to personal (role identity) and the infant's growth and developmental stages (Mercer, 1995).

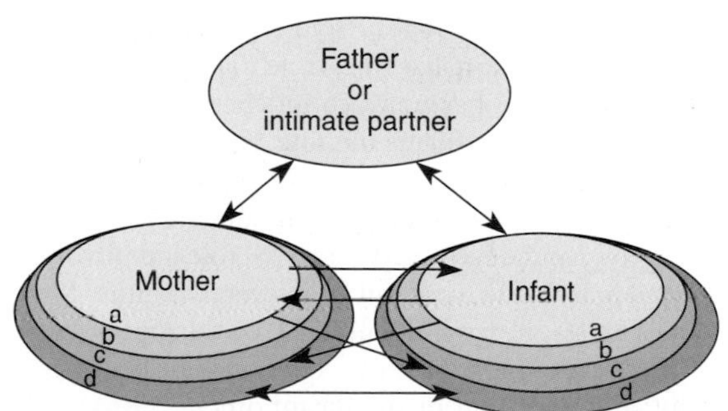

FIG. 27.2 A microsystem within the evolving model of maternal role attainment. (From Mercer, R. T. [1995]. *Becoming a mother: Research on maternal identity from Rubin to the present.* New York: Springer; used by permission.)

2. The mesosystem encompasses, influences, and interacts with persons in the microsystem. Mesosystem interactions may influence what happens to the developing maternal role and the child. The mesosystem includes day care, school, work setting, places of worship, and other entities within the immediate community.
3. The macrosystem refers to the general prototypes existing in a particular culture or transmitted cultural consistencies. The macrosystem includes the social, political, and cultural influences on the other two systems. The health care environment and the current health care system policies that affect maternal role attainment originate in this system (Mercer, 1995). National laws regarding women and children and health priorities that influence maternal role attainment are within the macrosystem.

Maternal role attainment is a process that follows four stages of role acquisition; these stages have been adapted from Thornton and Nardi's 1975 research. The following stages are indicated in Fig. 27.2 as the layers *a* through *d:*

a. **Anticipatory**: The anticipatory stage begins during pregnancy and includes the initial social and psychological adjustments to pregnancy. The mother learns the expectations of the role, fantasizes about the role, relates to the fetus *in utero,* and begins to role-play.
b. **Formal**: The formal stage begins with the birth of the infant and includes learning and taking on the role of mother. Role behaviors are guided by formal, consensual expectations of others in the mother's social system.
c. **Informal**: The informal stage begins as the mother develops unique ways of dealing with the role not conveyed by the social system. The woman makes her new role fit within her existing lifestyle based on past experiences and future goals.
d. **Personal**: The personal or role-identity stage occurs as the woman internalizes her role. The mother experiences a sense of harmony, confidence, and competence in the way she performs the role, and the maternal role is achieved.

Stages of role attainment overlap and are altered as the infant grows and develops. A maternal role identity may be achieved in a month, or it can take several months (Mercer, 1995). The stages are influenced by social support, stress, family functioning, and the relationship between the mother and the father or significant other.

Traits and behaviors of both the mother and the infant may influence maternal role identity and child outcome. Maternal traits and behaviors included in Mercer's model are empathy, sensitivity to infant cues, self-esteem and self-concept, parenting received as a child, maturity and flexibility, attitudes, pregnancy and birth experience, health, depression, and role conflict. Infant traits that affect maternal role identity include temperament, ability to send cues, appearance, general characteristics, responsiveness, and health. Examples of the infant's developmental responses that interact with the mother's developing maternal identity, depicted as *a* through *d* in Fig. 27.2, include the following:

a. Eye contact with the mother as she talks to her or him; grasp reflex
b. Smile reflex and quieting behavior in response to the mother's care
c. Consistent interactive behaviors with the mother
d. Eliciting responses from the mother; increasing mobility

According to Mercer:

> *"The personal role identity stage is reached when the mother has integrated the role into her self system with a congruence of self and other roles; she is secure in her identity as mother, is emotionally committed to her infant, and feels a sense of harmony, satisfaction, and competence in the role."*
>
> ***(1995, p. 14)***

Using Burke and Tully's (1977) work, Mercer (1995) stated that a role identity has internal and external components; the identity is the internalized view of self (recognized maternal identity), and role is the external, behavioral component.

Becoming a Mother: A Revised Model and Theory

Mercer has continued to use both her own research and the research of others as building blocks for her theory. In 2003 she began reexamining the theory of maternal role attainment, proposing that the term *becoming a mother* more accurately reflects the process based on recent research. According to Mercer (2004), the concept of role attainment suggests an end point rather than an ongoing process and may not address the continued expansion of the self as a mother. Mercer's conclusions are based largely on current nursing research about the cognitive and behavioral dimensions of women becoming mothers. Walker, Crain, and Thompson's (1986a, 1986b) questions about maternal role attainment as a continuing process contributed to Mercer's reexamination of her theory. Koniak-Griffin (1993) also questioned the behavioral and cognitive dimensions of maternal role attainment. Hartrick (1997) reported in her study that mothers of children from 3 to 16 years of age undergo a continual process of self-definition. McBride and Shore (2001), in their research on mothers and grandmothers, suggested that there may be a need to retire the term *maternal role attainment,* because "it implies a static situation rather than fluctuating process"

(p. 79). Finally, in a synthesis of nine qualitative studies, Nelson (2003) described continued growth and transformation in women as they become mothers. Mercer (2004) acknowledged that new challenges in motherhood require making new connections to regain confidence in the self and proposed replacing the term *maternal role attainment* with *becoming a mother.*

Qualitative studies have identified stages of maternal role attainment using the descriptive terms of participants. A compilation of the results of several of these studies has led Mercer (2004, 2006) to the following proposed changes in the names of stages leading to maternal role identity:

- Commitment and preparation (pregnancy)
- Acquaintance, practice, and physical restoration (first 2 weeks)
- Approaching normalization (second week to 4 months)
- Integration of maternal identity (approximately 4 months)

These stages parallel the original stages in Mercer's theory, but they embrace the maternal experience more completely and use terminology derived from new mothers' descriptions of their experiences.

Theory building, according to Mercer (personal communication, September 2003), is a continual process as research provides evidence for clarifying concepts, additions, and deletions. Although many of the more recent studies support the findings of both Rubin and Mercer, Mercer (2004) recognized the evidence for needed changes in her original theory for greater clarity and consistency. It is with this insight that she proposed retiring the term *maternal role attainment.* Mercer (2004) acknowledges that becoming a mother, which connotes continued growth in mothering, is more descriptive of the process, which is much larger than a role. Although some roles may be terminated, motherhood is a lifelong commitment.

Mercer has continued to use Bronfenbrenner's concept of interacting nested ecological environments. However, she renamed them to reflect the living environments: family and friends, community, and society at large (Fig. 27.3).

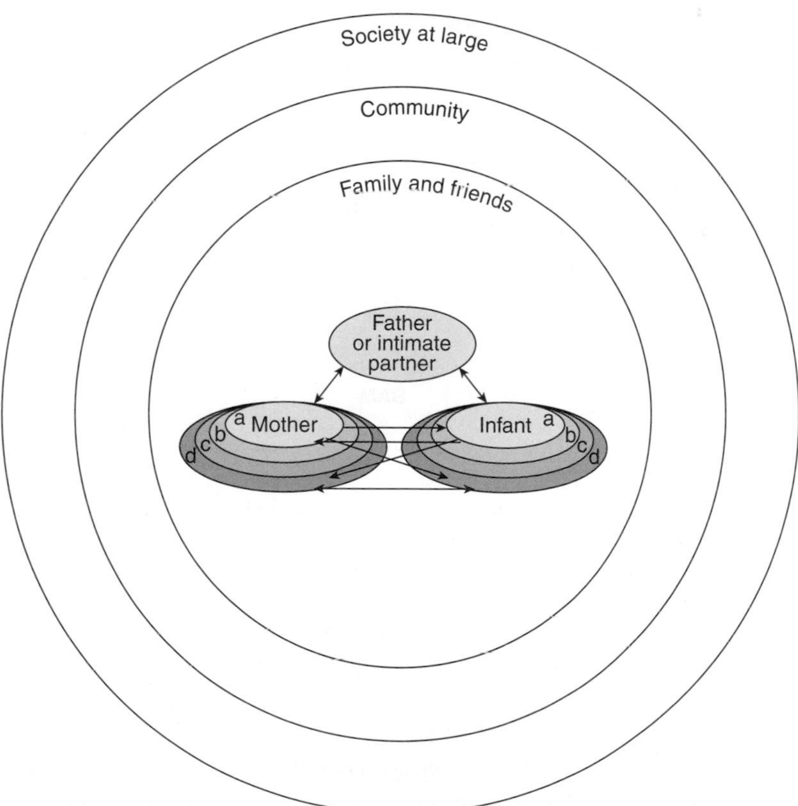

FIG. 27.3 Becoming a mother: a revised model. (From R. T. Mercer, personal communication, September 2003.)

This model places the interactions between mother, infant, and father at the center of the interacting, living environments (R. Mercer, personal communication, September 2003; Mercer & Walker, 2006). Variables within the family and friends environment include physical and social support, family values, cultural guidelines for parenting, knowledge and skills, family functioning, and affirmation as a mother. The community environment includes day care, places of worship, schools, work settings, health care facilities, recreational facilities, and support groups. Within the society at large, influences come from laws affecting woman and children, evolving reproductive and neonatal science, national health care programs, various social programs, and funding for research promoting becoming a mother.

The newest model (Fig. 27.4) shows interacting environments that affect the process of becoming a mother. The model was developed in 2006 based on a review of the nursing research about the effectiveness or interventions aimed at fostering the process of becoming a mother. This model depicts the complex issues that have the potential to either facilitate or inhibit the process of becoming a mother (Mercer & Walker, 2006). According to Mercer and Walker (2006), the model presents both environmental variables and maternal-infant characteristics that are important considerations for both nursing practice and future research.

LOGICAL FORM

Mercer used both deductive and inductive logic in developing the theoretical framework for studying factors that influence maternal role attainment during the first year of motherhood and in her theory. Deductive logic is

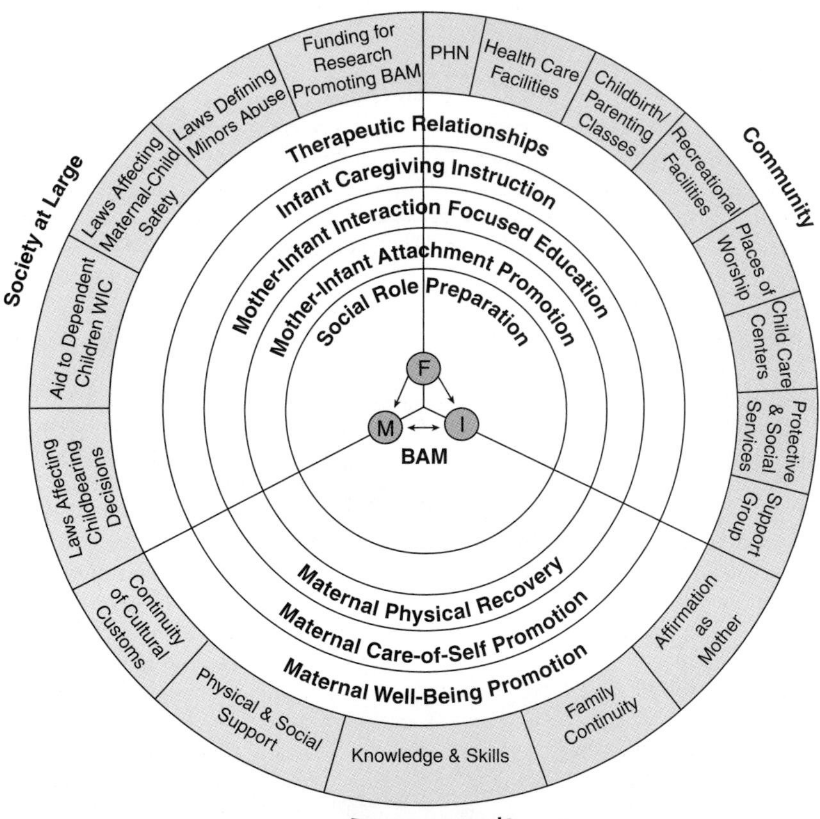

FIG. 27.4 Interacting environments that affect the process of becoming a mother. (From Mercer, R. T., & Walker, L. O. [2006]. A review of nursing interventions to foster becoming a mother. *Journal of Obstetric, Gynecologic, and Neonatal Nursing, 35*[5], 570–581.)

demonstrated in Mercer's use of works from other researchers and disciplines. Role and developmental theories and the work of Rubin on maternal role attainment provided a base for the original framework. Mercer also used inductive logic in the development of her theory of maternal role attainment. Through practice and research, she observed adaptation to motherhood from a variety of circumstances. She noted that differences existed in adaptation to motherhood when maternal illness complicated the postpartum period, when a child with a defect was born, and when a teenager became a mother. These observations directed the research about those situations and the subsequent development of her theory. Changes to her original theory have been based on more recent research and deductive reasoning coupled with her belief in continually improving the clarity and usefulness of her theory.

ACCEPTANCE BY THE NURSING COMMUNITY

Practice

Mercer's theory is highly practice oriented. The concepts in her theory have been cited in many obstetrical textbooks and have been used in practice by nurses and those in other disciplines. Both the theory and the model are capable of serving as a framework for assessment and planning, implementing, and evaluating nursing care of new mothers and their infants. The utility of Mercer's theory in nursing practice is described and illustrated by Meighan (2014) in Chapter 17 of the fifth edition of *Nursing Theory: Utilization & Application* by Alligood. Mercer's theory is useful to practicing nurses across many maternal-child settings. Mercer (1986a, 1986b) linked her research findings with nursing practice at each interval from birth through the first year, making her theory applicable in a variety of pediatric settings.

In addition, Mercer's theory has been used in organizing patient care. Concepts in the research conducted by Neeson et al. (1983), "Pregnancy Outcome for Adolescents Receiving Prenatal Care by Nurse Practitioners in Extended Roles," were used in setting up a clinical practice. Clark and colleagues (2001) used Mercer's theory to establish and test a parent education curriculum for substance-abusing women in a residential treatment facility. Meighan and Wood (2005) used the theory of maternal role attainment to explore the effect of hyperemesis gravidarum on maternal role assumption.

Education

Mercer's work has appeared extensively in both maternity and pediatric nursing texts. Many of the current concepts in maternal-child nursing are based on Mercer's research. Her theory and models help simplify the very complex process of becoming a parent. The theory of maternal role attainment is credited with enhancing understanding and making Mercer's contribution extremely valuable to nursing education. The theory of maternal role attainment provides a framework for students as they learn to plan and provide care for parents in a wide variety of settings. Mercer's recognition of the need to examine research evidence supporting her original work and her effort to continually update and improve her theory have served as examples for nursing students. Renaming the theory *becoming a mother* represented the ongoing growth process of motherhood more accurately and has gained acceptance since introduced in 2004. However, the *theory of maternal role attainment* is still used by some. Mercer's theory and research have also been used in other disciplines as they relate to parenting and maternal role attainment. It has been shown to be helpful to students in psychology, sociology, and education.

Research

Mercer advocated the involvement of students in faculty research. During her tenure at the University of California, San Francisco, she chaired committees and was a committee member for numerous graduate theses and dissertations. Collaborative research with a graduate student and junior faculty member in 1977 and 1978 led to the development of a highly reliable, valid instrument to measure mothers' attitudes about the labor and delivery experience. Numerous researchers have requested and received permission to use the instrument.

Mercer's work has served as a springboard for other researchers. The theoretical framework for her correlational study exploring the differences between three age groups of first-time mothers (15–19, 20–29, and 30–42 years of age) was tested by others, including Walker and colleagues (1986a, 1986b). Sank (1991) used Mercer's theory in her doctoral dissertation research titled *Factors in the Prenatal Period That Affect Parental Role Attainment During the Postpartum Period in Black American Mothers and Fathers.* Mercer's theory of maternal role attainment served as the framework for Washington's (1997) dissertation, *Learning Needs of Adolescent Mothers When Identifying Fever and Illnesses in Infants Less Than Twelve Months of Age.* Bacon (2001) used Mercer's theory in her dissertation, *Maternal Role Attainment and Maternal Identity in Mothers of Premature Infants.* Dilmore (2003) based her study, *A Comparison of Confidence Levels of Postpartum Depressed and Non-Depressed First Time Mothers,* on Mercer's research.

McBride wrote the following:

> *"Maternal role attainment has been a fundamental concern of nursing since the pioneering work of Mercer's mentor, Rubin, almost two decades ago. It is now becoming the research-based, theoretically sound construct that nurse researchers have been searching for in their analysis of the experience of new mothers."*
>
> ***(1984, p. 72)***

Recent studies include those by Rode and Kiel (2015), who studied maternal depression and infant temperament on maternal role, and Mackintosh and Callister (2015), who studied identity in childbearing adolescents.

FURTHER DEVELOPMENT

Mercer used her initial research as a building block for other studies. In later research, she aimed at identifying predictors of maternal-infant attachment on the basis of maternal experience with childbirth and maternal risk status. Mercer also examined paternal competence on the basis of experience with childbirth and pregnancy risk status. She developed and tested a causal model to predict partner relationships in high-risk and low-risk pregnancy. More work and refinement of the original model and theory have taken place over the years. She included the importance of the father in maternal role attainment, adding this to her model and theory in her 1995 book, *Becoming a Mother: Research on Maternal Identity from Rubin to the Present.*

In *First-Time Motherhood: Experiences from Teens to Forties,* Mercer (1986a) presented a model of the following four phases that occur in the process of maternal role attainment during the first year of motherhood:

1. The physical recovery phase (from birth to 1 month)
2. The achievement phase (from 2 to 4 or 5 months)
3. The disruptions phase (from 6 to 8 months)
4. The reorganization phase (from after the eighth month and still in process at 1 year)

In addition, adaptation to the maternal role was proposed to occur at three levels (biological, psychological, and social), which interact and are interdependent throughout the phases. These phases and levels of adaptation were described briefly and applied to her research. In 2003 Mercer proposed additional changes to the theory (2004), which included abandoning the term *maternal role attainment* for the term *becoming a mother.* Changes to the model and adoption of the following four descriptive phases to the process of becoming a mother were also proposed:

1. Commitment and preparation (pregnancy)
2. Acquaintance, practice, and physical restoration (first 2 weeks)
3. Approaching normalization (second week to 4 months)
4. Integration of maternal identity (approximately 4 months)

These changes were based on research studies by other nurses and are evidence of Mercer's continued scrutiny and critique of her theory to improve its utility in practice and research.

According to Mercer and Walker (2006), research into specific nursing interventions that foster becoming a mother is needed. They encourage the involvement of nursing staff, students, and faculty in the development and testing of assessment guidelines and instruments to measure outcomes of nursing interventions that support maternal role identity and the process of becoming a mother. Mercer and Walker also encourage further research with mothers who face special challenges, including mothers who face childbirth complications, mothers with low social and economic resources, adolescent mothers, and mothers with high-risk infants. According to Mercer and Walker, development and testing of nursing interventions that support and empower parents are warranted. They encourage research to determine how best to foster becoming a mother in culturally diverse groups, explaining that each culture has customs and values attached to childbearing that affect the transition to motherhood.

Mercer's concern for the utility and applicability of her theory is evident in her continued work toward clarity and usefulness. Revisions of her theory in 2003, although based on nursing research, are still being tested in other studies. Although qualitative research to describe the phases of becoming a mother uses the exact words of women experiencing this transition, these phases have not been confirmed among women in other cultures or in different circumstances.

CRITIQUE

Clarity

The concepts, variables, and relationships have not always been defined explicitly, but they were described and implied in Mercer's earlier work. However, the concepts were defined theoretically and operationalized consistently. Work toward improving clarity is evident. Concepts, assumptions, and goals have been organized into a logical and coherent whole, so understanding the interrelationships among the concepts is relatively easy. Some interchanging of terms and labels used to identify concepts, such as *adaptation and attainment, social support,* and *support network,* is potentially confusing for the reader, and *maternal role attainment* has not been defined consistently, which can obstruct clarity. *Maternal identity,* a term that Mercer defines as the final stage of role attainment (personal or role identity stage), is sometimes substituted for *maternal role attainment.* According to Mercer (1995), when the maternal role has been attained, the mother has achieved a maternal identity, the internalized role of mother. However, the terms *attainment* and *role identity* are sometimes confusing.

Mercer continued to work toward greater clarity and proposed using terms derived from nursing researchers that would be understood more clearly by users of her theory. She questioned the use of the term *maternal role attainment,* because it connotes a static state rather than the continuously evolving role as a mother. Mercer examined qualitative research containing the exact words of women experiencing motherhood, and she favored using those words to describe the stages of becoming a mother.

Simplicity

Despite numerous concepts and relationships, the theoretical framework for maternal role attainment or becoming a mother organizes a rather complex phenomenon into an easily understood and useful form. The theory is predictive in nature and readily lends itself as a guide for practice. Concepts are not specific to time and place, and, although abstract, they are described and operationalized to the extent that meanings are not easily misinterpreted. The process of becoming a mother is multifaceted and varies considerably according to the individual and to environmental influences. Mercer's theory provides a framework for understanding this complex, multidimensional process.

Generality

Mercer's theory is derived from and is specific to parent-child nursing and also has been used by other disciplines concerned with mothering and parenting. The theory can be generalized to all women during pregnancy through the first year after birth, regardless of age, parity, or environment. It is among the few theories applicable to high-risk perinatal patients and their families. Mercer (1995) specified her theory for the study and prediction of parental attachment, including that of the pregnant woman's partner. Therefore it is useful for studying and working with family members after birth. Mercer's work has broadened the range of application of previously existing theories on maternal role attainment, because her studies have spanned various developmental levels and situational contexts.

Accessibility

Mercer's work has evolved from extensive research efforts. The concepts, assumptions, and relationships are grounded predominantly in empirical observations and are congruent. The degree of concreteness and the completeness of operational definitions increase the empirical precision. The theoretical framework for exploring differences among age groups of first-time mothers lends itself well to further testing and is being used by others for this purpose. The continued scrutiny by Mercer herself has continually improved her theory and solidified her concepts.

Importance

The theoretical framework for maternal role attainment during the first year has proved to be useful, practical, and valuable to nursing. Mercer's work is used repeatedly in nursing research, practice, and education. The framework is also applicable to any discipline that works with mothers and children during the first year of motherhood. McBride (1984) wrote, "Dr. Mercer is the one who developed the most complete theoretical framework for studying one aspect of parental experience, namely, the factors that influence the attainment of the maternal role in the first year of motherhood" (p. 72).

Throughout her career, Mercer consistently has linked research and practice. Applications for nursing care or nursing interventions are addressed and provide the bond between research and practice. As she has said, nursing research is the "bridge to excellence" in nursing practice (Mercer, 1984, p. 47).

SUMMARY

The theory of maternal role attainment has been shown to be useful in both research and practice for nurses and other disciplines concerned with parenting. Mercer's continued devotion to improving the usefulness and clarity of her theory and model is evident and has served well those who use her theory. Mercer's use of both her own research and the research of others strengthens her work. Her proposal to adopt the theory of becoming a mother is based solidly on the research process. Motherhood and attainment of the parenting role is a very complex, multilevel process. Mercer's theory and her work make this process logical and understandable and provide a solid foundation for practice, education, and research.

CASE STUDY

Susan, a 19-year-old woman, delivered her first infant prematurely 5 days ago. Although her postpartum course has been relatively uneventful, the infant has had difficulty and must remain hospitalized. Susan and her young husband visit the nursery every afternoon to be with the baby, but they ask very few questions. In talking with the couple, the nurse learns that the only living grandparents of the baby live a great distance away. Susan will not have any family or friends to turn to when she takes the baby home.

In this high-risk perinatal case, Mercer's framework should be useful for nursing assessment and intervention to facilitate maternal role attainment. How would you use it as a guide in planning care for Susan?

CRITICAL THINKING ACTIVITIES

1. Consider Mercer's theory and model of maternal role attainment as a guide for practice. List the ways it is useful to plan care of a new mother.
2. High-risk families often continue to experience problems for years after the birth of a child with a congenital problem. What areas of Mercer's theory might be adapted for assessment and intervention for these mothers and their families?
3. Does the model proposed by Mercer adequately address current changes in health care delivery and the impact on the family? What changes in Mercer's model, if any, need to be addressed?
4. Mercer advanced her theory from *maternal role attainment* to include *becoming a mother* to address the evolving role of motherhood. Consider the difference between attaining the maternal role and becoming a mother. What different processes do attaining the maternal role and becoming a mother involve?

POINTS FOR FURTHER STUDY

Publications

- Meighan, M. (2014). Mercer's becoming a mother theory in nursing practice. In M. R. Alligood (Ed.), *Nursing theory: Utilization & application* (5th ed., pp. 332–349) St Louis: Mosby-Elsevier.
- Mercer, R. T. (2004). Becoming a mother versus maternal role attainment. *Journal of Nursing Scholarship, 36*(3), 226–232.
- Mercer, R. T. (2006). Nursing support of the process of becoming a mother. *Journal of Obstetric, Gynecologic, and Neonatal Nursing, 35*(5), 649–651.
- Mercer, R. T., & Walker, L. O. (2006). A review of nursing interventions to foster becoming a mother. *Journal of Obstetric, Gynecologic, and Neonatal Nursing, 35*(5), 568–582.

Websites

- Ahid, A. (2013). Life and work of Ramona Mercer slide presentation at http://www.slideshare.net/azizahid1/maternal-role-attainment-theory
- Cardinal Stritch University Library: Mercer's maternal role attainment at http://www.stritch.edu/Library/Doing-Research/Research-by-Subject/Health-Sciences-Nursing-Theorists/Ramona-T—Mercer—-Maternal-Role-Attainment/
- Necor, J. A. (2014). Ramona Mercer's maternal role attainment theory at http://www.slideshare .net/JosephineAnnNecor/ramona-mercers-maternal-role-attainment-theory
- Prezi Presentation (2013): Mercer's maternal role attainment theory at https://prezi.com/pieoko6bgbku/ramona-mercers-maternal-role-attainment-theory/
- University of New Mexico Past Distinguished Alumni Award: Ramona Mercer at http://nursing.unm.edu/alumni-and-friends/daa-profiles/ramona-mercer.html

REFERENCES

Bacon, A. C. (2001). *Maternal role attainment and maternal identity in mothers of premature infants.* Doctoral dissertation, Chicago School of Professional Psychology. *Dissertation Abstracts International,* 61, 8-B (University Microfilms No. 2001–95004–447.)

Bronfenbrenner, U. (1979). *The ecology of human development: Experiment by nature and design.* Cambridge, MA: Harvard University Press.

Burke, P. J., & Tully, J. C. (1977). The measurement of role identity. *Social Forces, 55,* 881–897.

Burr, W. R., Leigh, G. K., Day, R. D., & Constantine, J. (1979). Symbolic interaction and the family. In W. R. Burr, R. Hill, F. I. Nye, & I. L. Reiss (Eds.), *Contemporary theories about the family* (vol. 2, pp. 42–111). New York: Free Press.

Clark, B. S., Rapkin, D., Busen, N. H., & Vasquez, E. (2001). Nurse practitioners and parent education: A partnership for health. *Journal of the American Academy of Nurse Practitioners, 13*(7), 310–316.

Dilmore, D. L. (2003). *A comparison of confidence levels of postpartum depressed and non-depressed first time mothers.* Unpublished thesis, Gainesville, FL: University of Florida.

Donley, M. G. (1993). Attachment and the emotional unit. *Family Process, 32,* 3–20.

Ferketich, S. L., & Mercer, R. T. (1995a). Paternal-infant attachment of experienced and inexperienced fathers during infancy. *Nursing Research, 44,* 31–37.

Ferketich, S. L., & Mercer, R. T. (1995b). Predictors of paternal role competence by risk status. *Nursing Research, 43,* 80–85.

Ferketich, S. L., & Mercer, R. T. (1995c). Predictors of role competence for experienced and inexperienced fathers. *Nursing Research, 44,* 89–95.

Hartrick, G. A. (1997). Women who are mothers: The experience of defining self. *Health Care for Women International, 18,* 263–277.

Koniak-Griffin, D. (1993). Maternal role attainment. *Image: The Journal of Nursing Scholarship, 25,* 257–262.

Mackintosh, J., & Callister, L. (2015). Discovering self: Childbearing adolescents' maternal identity. *Journal of Maternal Child Nursing, 40*(4), 243–248.

McBride, A. B. (1984). The experience of being a parent. *Annual Review of Nursing Research, 2,* 63–81.

McBride, A. B., & Shore, C. P. (2001). Women as mothers and grandmothers. *Annual Review of Nursing Research, 19,* 63–85.

Mead, G. H. (1934). *Mind, self and society.* Chicago: University of Chicago Press.

Meighan, M. (2014). Mercer's becoming a mother theory in nursing practice. In M. R. Alligood (Ed.), *Nursing theory: Utilization & application* (5th ed., pp. 332–349). St Louis: Mosby.

Meighan, M., & Wood, A. F. (2005). The impact of hyperemesis gravidarum on maternal role assumption. *Journal of Obstetric, Gynecologic, and Neonatal Nursing, 34*(2), 172–179.

Mercer, R. T. (1977). *Nursing care for parents at risk.* Thorofare, NJ: Charles B. Slack.

Mercer, R. T. (1979). *Perspectives on adolescent health care.* Philadelphia: Lippincott.

Mercer, R. T. (1981). A theoretical framework for studying factors that impact on the maternal role. *Nursing Research, 30,* 73–77.

Mercer, R. T. (1984). Nursing research: The bridge to excellence in practice. *Image: The Journal of Nursing Scholarship, 16*(2), 47–51.

Mercer, R. T. (1985a). The process of maternal role attainment over the first years. *Nursing Research, 34,* 198–204.

Mercer, R. T. (1985b). The relationship of age and other variables to gratification in mothering. *Health Care for Women International, 6,* 295–308.

Mercer, R. T. (1986a). *First-time motherhood: Experiences from teens to forties.* New York: Springer.

Mercer, R. T. (1986b). The relationship of developmental variables to maternal behavior. *Research in Nursing Health, 9,* 25–33.

Mercer, R. T. (1989). Responses to life-span development: A review of theory and practice for families with chronically ill members. *Scholarly Inquiry for Nursing Practice: An International Journal, 3,* 23–26.

Mercer, R. T. (1990). *Parents at risk.* New York: Springer.

Mercer, R. T. (1995). *Becoming a mother: Research on maternal identity from Rubin to the present.* New York: Springer.

Mercer, R. T. (2004). Becoming a mother versus maternal role attainment. *Journal of Nursing Scholarship, 36*(3), 226–232.

Mercer, R. T. (2006). Nursing support of the process of becoming a mother. *Journal of Obstetric, Gynecologic, and Neonatal Nursing, 35*(5), 649–651.

Mercer, R. T., & Ferketich, S. L. (1990a). Predictors of family functioning eight months following birth. *Nursing Research, 39,* 76–82.

Mercer, R. T., & Ferketich, S. L. (1990b). Predictors of parental attachment during early parenthood. *Journal of Advanced Nursing, 15,* 268–280.

Mercer, R. T., & Ferketich, S. L. (1994). Maternal-infant attachment of experienced and inexperienced mothers during infancy. *Nursing Research, 43,* 344–350.

Mercer, R. T., & Ferketich, S. L. (1995). Experienced and inexperienced mothers' maternal competence during infancy. *Research in Nursing Health, 18,* 333–343.

Mercer, R. T., Ferketich, S. L., & DeJoseph, J. F. (1993). Predictors of partner relationships during pregnancy and infancy. *Research in Nursing Health, 16,* 45–56.

Mercer, R. T., Ferketich, S. L., DeJoseph, J., May, K. A., & Sollid, D. (1988). Effects of stress on family functioning during pregnancy. *Nursing Research, 37,* 268–275.

Mercer, R. T., Hackley, K. C., & Bostrom, A. (1984). Social support of teenage mothers. *Birth Defects: Original Article Series, 20*(5), 245–290.

Mercer, R. T., May, K. A., Ferketich, S., & DeJoseph, J. (1986). Theoretical models for studying the effect of antepartum stress on the family. *Nursing Research, 35,* 339–346.

Mercer, R. T., & Walker, L. O. (2006). A review of nursing interventions to foster becoming a mother. *Journal of Obstetric, Gynecologic, and Neonatal Nursing, 35*(5), 568–582.

Neeson, J. D., Patterson, K. A., Mercer, R. T., & May, K. A. (1983). Pregnancy outcome for adolescents receiving prenatal care by nurse practitioners in extended roles. *Journal of Adolescent Health Care, 4*, 94–99.

Nelson, A. M. (2003). Transition to motherhood. *Journal of Obstetric, Gynecologic, & Neonatal Nursing, 32*, 465–477.

Rode, J., & Kiel, E. (2015). The mediated effects of maternal depression and infant temperament on maternal role. *Archives of Women's Mental Health*, 1–8. Online at Springer Link: http://link.springer.com/article/10.1007/s00737-015-0540-1.

Rubin, R. (1977). Binding-in in the postpartum period. *Maternal Child Nursing Journal, 6*, 67–75.

Rubin, R. (1984). *Maternal identity and the maternal experience.* New York: Springer.

Sank, J. C. (1991). *Factors in the prenatal period that affect parental role attainment during the postpartum period in black American mothers and fathers.* Doctoral dissertation, University of Texas, Austin, Texas, 1991. (University Microfilms No. 1993–155453.)

Thornton, R., & Nardi, P. M. (1975). The dynamics of role acquisition. *American Journal of Sociology, 80*, 870–885.

Turner, J. H. (1978). *The structure of sociological theory* (revised ed.). Homewood, IL: Dorsey Press.

von Bertalanffy, L. (1968). *General system theory.* New York: George Braziller.

Walker, L. O., Crain, H., & Thompson, E. (1986a). Maternal role attainment and identity in the postpartum period: Stability and change. *Nursing Research, 35*(2), 68–71.

Walker, L. O., Crain, H., & Thompson, E. (1986b). Mothering behavior and maternal role attainment during the postpartum period. *Nursing Research, 35*(6), 322–325.

Washington, L. J. (1997). *Learning needs of adolescent mothers when identifying fever and illnesses in infants less than twelve months of age.* Doctoral dissertation, University of Miami. *Dissertation Abstracts International, 57*, (12-B). (University Microfilms No. 1997–95012–208.)

Werner, H. (1957). The concept of development from a comparative and organismic point of view. In D. H. Harris (Ed.), *The concept of development* (pp. 125–148). Minneapolis: University of Minnesota.

BIBLIOGRAPHY

Primary Sources

Books

Mercer, R. T. (1977). *Nursing care for parents at risk.* Thorofare, NJ: Charles B. Slack.

Mercer, R. T. (1979). *Perspectives on adolescent health care.* Philadelphia: Lippincott.

Mercer, R. T. (1986). *First-time motherhood: Experiences from teens to forties.* New York: Springer.

Mercer, R. T. (1990). *Parents at risk.* New York: Springer.

Mercer, R. T. (1995). *Becoming a mother: Research on maternal identity from Rubin to the present.* New York: Springer.

Journal Articles

Ferketich, S. L., & Mercer, R. T. (1995). Paternal-infant attachment of experienced and inexperienced fathers during infancy. *Nursing Research, 44*, 31–37.

Ferketich, S. L., & Mercer, R. T. (1995). Predictors of role competence for experienced and inexperienced fathers. *Nursing Research, 44*, 89–95.

Mercer, R. T. (1995). A tribute to Reva Rubin. *Maternal Child Nursing, 20*, 184.

Mercer, R. T. (1997). Chronically ill children: How families adjust. *Nurseweek, 10*(9), 14–15, 17.

Mercer, R. T. (1997). The employed mother's challenges. *Nurseweek, 10*(17), 10–11, 15.

Mercer, R. T. (2000). Response to "Life-span development: A review of theory and practice for families with chronically ill members." *Scholarly Inquiry for Nursing Practice, 14*(4), 375–378.

Mercer, R. T., & Ferketich, S. L. (1995). Experienced and inexperienced mothers' maternal competence during infancy. *Research in Nursing Health, 18*, 333–343.

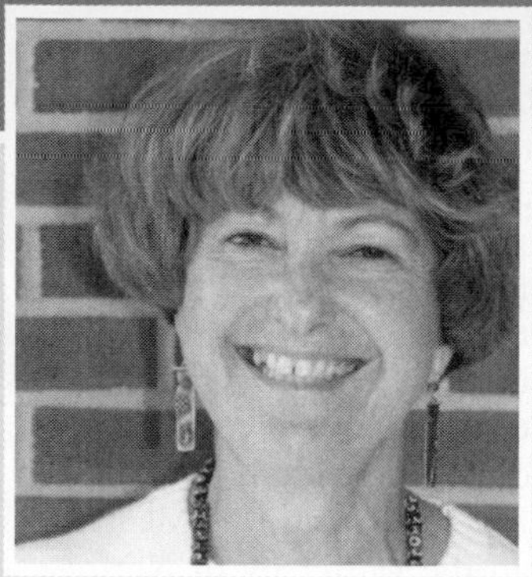

Merle H. Mishel
(1939–Present)

28

Uncertainty in Illness Theory

Donald E. Bailey, Jr. and Janet L. Stewart*

"My theory can be applied to both practice and research. It has been used to explain clinical situations and design interventions that lead to evidence-based practice. Current and future nurse scientists have and will continue to extend the theory to different patient populations. This work has the potential to transform health care."
(Mishel, personal communication, May 2008)

CREDENTIALS AND BACKGROUND OF THE THEORIST

Merle H. Mishel was born in Boston, Massachusetts. She graduated from Boston University with a bachelor of arts degree in 1961 and received her master's of science in psychiatric nursing from the University of California in 1966. Mishel completed her master's of arts and doctorate in social psychology at the Claremont Graduate School in Claremont, California, in 1976 and 1980, respectively. Her dissertation research was supported by a National Research Service Award to develop and test the Perceived Ambiguity in Illness Scale, later named the Mishel Uncertainty in Illness Scale (MUIS-A). The original scale has been used as the basis for the following three additional scales:

1. A community version (MUIS-C) for chronically ill individuals who are not hospitalized or receiving active medical care
2. A measure of parents' perceptions of uncertainty (PPUS) with regard to their child's illness experience
3. A measure of uncertainty in spouses or other family members when another member of the family is acutely ill (PPUS-FM)

Early in her professional career, Mishel practiced as a psychiatric nurse in acute care and community settings. While pursuing her doctorate, she was on the nursing faculty at California State University at Los Angeles, rising from assistant professor to full professor. She practiced as a nurse therapist in community and private practice settings from 1973 to 1979. After completing her doctorate in social psychology, Mishel became associate professor at the University of Arizona College of Nursing in 1981 and full professor in 1988. She was Division Head of Mental Health Nursing from 1984 to 1991. While at Arizona, Mishel received numerous intramural and extramural research grants that supported the continued development of the theoretical framework of uncertainty in illness. During this period, she continued practicing as a nurse therapist with the heart transplant program at the University Medical Center. She was inducted as a fellow in the American Academy of Nursing in 1990.

Mishel moved back east in 1991 and joined the faculty at the University of North Carolina at Chapel Hill School of Nursing as professor, and was awarded the endowed Kenan Professor of Nursing Chair in 1994. Friends of the National Institute of Nursing Research presented her with a Research Merit Award in 1997 and invited her to present her research as an exemplar of federally funded nursing

*The authors wish to think Dr. Merle Mishel for her review and input for this chapter.
Photo Credit: Dr. Michael Belyea, University of North Carolina, Chapel Hill, NC.

intervention studies at a Congressional Breakfast in 1999. She was Director of the T-32 Institutional National Research Service Award Training Grant, Interventions for Preventing and Managing Chronic Illness, which awards predoctoral and postdoctoral fellowships to nurses who are interested in developing interventions for underserved chronically ill patients. Mishel's research program is noteworthy for being funded continually by the National Institutes of Health from 1984 through 2011. Each grant was built on findings from prior studies moving systematically toward theoretically derived and scientifically tested nursing interventions. Mishel coled the Hillman Scholars Program designed to produce a new generation of nurse innovators with knowledge and research skills to solve complex health problems and improve patient care.

Among her many awards, Mishel received a Sigma Theta Tau Sigma Xi Chapter Nurse Research Predoctoral Fellowship from 1977 to 1979 and received the Mary Opal Wolanin Research Award in 1986. She has been a visiting scholar at many institutions throughout North America, including the University of Nebraska, University of Texas at Houston, University of Tennessee at Knoxville, University of South Carolina, University of Rochester, Yale University, and McGill University. Mishel was doctoral program consultant for the University of Cincinnati College of Nursing from 1991 to 1992 and Rutgers University School of Nursing in 1993. In 2004 she received the Linnea Henderson Research Fellowship Program Award from the Kent State University School of Nursing. Over the past 20 years, she presented more than 80 invited addresses at schools of nursing throughout the United States and Canada. With growing international interest in her theory and measurement tools, Mishel conducted an International Symposium on Uncertainty at Kyungpook National University in Daegu, South Korea; was a visiting scholar at Mahidol University in Bangkok, Thailand; and delivered the keynote address for the Japanese Society of Nursing Research annual convention in Sapporo, Japan.

Mishel was a member of many professional organizations, including the American Academy of Nursing, Sigma Theta Tau International, American Psychological Association, American Nurses Association, Society of Behavioral Medicine, Oncology Nursing Society, Southern Nursing Research Society, and Society for Education and Research in Psychiatric Nursing. She served as a grant reviewer for the National Cancer Institute, National Center for Nursing Research, and National Institute on Aging, and was a charter member of the study section on human immunodeficiency virus (HIV) at the National Institute of Mental Health. Dr. Mishel retired from the University of North Carolina at Chapel Hill in 2014.

THEORETICAL SOURCES

When Mishel began her research into uncertainty, the concept had not been applied in the health and illness context. Her original uncertainty in illness theory (Mishel, 1988) drew from existing information-processing models (Warburton, 1979) and personality research (Budner, 1962) from psychology that characterized uncertainty as a cognitive state resulting from insufficient cues with which to form a cognitive schema or internal representation of a situation or event. Mishel attributes the underlying stress-appraisal-coping-adaptation framework in the original theory to the work of Lazarus and Folkman (1984). The unique aspect of this framework was its application to uncertainty as a stressor in the context of illness, a particularly meaningful proposal for nursing.

With the reconceptualization of the theory, Mishel (1990) recognized that the Western approach to science supported a mechanistic view with emphasis on control and predictability. She used critical social theory to recognize bias inherent in the original theory, an orientation toward certainty and adaptation. Mishel incorporated tenets from chaos theory and open systems for a more accurate representation of how chronic illness creates disequilibrium and how people incorporate continual uncertainty to find new meaning in illness.

MAJOR CONCEPTS & DEFINITIONS

Uncertainty

Uncertainty is the inability to determine the meaning of illness-related events, occurring when the decision maker is unable to assign definite value to objects or events, or is unable to predict outcomes accurately (Mishel, 1988).

Cognitive Schema

Cognitive schema is a person's subjective interpretation of illness, treatment, and hospitalization (Mishel, 1988).

Stimuli Frame

Stimuli frame is the form, composition, and structure of the stimuli that a person perceives, which are then structured into a cognitive schema (Mishel, 1988).

Symptom Pattern

Symptom pattern is the degree to which symptoms occur with sufficient consistency to be perceived as having a pattern or configuration (Mishel, 1988).

MAJOR CONCEPTS AND DEFINITIONS—cont'd

Event Familiarity

Event familiarity is the degree to which a situation is habitual or repetitive or contains recognized cues (Mishel, 1988).

Event Congruence

Event congruence refers to the consistency between the expected and the experienced in illness-related events (Mishel, 1988).

Structure Providers

Structure providers are the resources available to assist the person in the interpretation of the stimuli frame (Mishel, 1988).

Credible Authority

Credible authority is the degree of trust and confidence a person has in his or her health care providers (Mishel, 1988).

Social Supports

Social supports influence uncertainty by assisting the individual to interpret the meaning of events (Mishel, 1988).

Cognitive Capacities

Cognitive capacities are the information-processing abilities of a person, reflecting both innate capabilities and situational constraints (Mishel, 1988).

Inference

Inference refers to the evaluation of uncertainty using related, recalled experiences (Mishel, 1988).

Illusion

Illusion refers to beliefs constructed out of uncertainty (Mishel, 1988).

Adaptation

Adaptation reflects biopsychosocial behavior occurring within persons' individually defined range of usual behavior (Mishel, 1988).

New View of Life

New view of life refers to the formulation of a new sense of order, resulting from the integration of continual uncertainty into one's self-structure, in which uncertainty is accepted as the natural rhythm of life (Mishel, 1988).

Probabilistic Thinking

Probabilistic thinking refers to a belief in a conditional world in which the expectation of continual certainty and predictability is abandoned (Mishel, 1988).

USE OF EMPIRICAL EVIDENCE

The uncertainty in illness theory grew out of Mishel's dissertation research with hospitalized patients, using both qualitative and quantitative findings to generate the first conceptualization of uncertainty in the context of illness. With the publication of Mishel's Uncertainty in Illness Scale (Mishel, 1981), extensive research began into adults' experiences with uncertainty related to chronic and life-threatening illnesses. Considerable empirical evidence has accumulated to support Mishel's theoretical model in adults. Several integrative reviews of uncertainty research have comprehensively summarized and critiqued the state of the science (Cahill et al., 2012; Hansen et al., 2012; Mishel, 1997a, 1999; Stewart & Mishel, 2000). The authors included studies that directly support the elements of Mishel's uncertainty model.

Most empirical studies have been focused on two antecedents of uncertainty, stimuli frame and structure providers, and the relationship between uncertainty and psychological outcomes. Mishel tested other elements of the model in her early research, such as the mediating roles of appraisal and coping (Mishel et al., 1991; Mishel & Braden, 1987; Mishel & Sorenson, 1991), and these elements have recently been incorporated into several uncertainty management intervention studies (Cohen et al., 2016; Rains & Tukachinsky, 2015).

Studies have shown that objective or subjective indicators of the severity of life-threat or illness symptoms associate positively with uncertainty (Baird & Eliasziw, 2011; Cohen et al., 2016; Somjaivong et al., 2011). Across a sustained illness trajectory, unpredictability in symptom onset, duration, and intensity has been related to perceived uncertainty (Arroll et al., 2012; Kim, Lee, & Lee, 2012). Similarly, the ambiguous nature of illness symptoms and the consequent difficulty in determining the significance of physical sensations have been identified as sources of uncertainty (Hilton, 1988; Lin et al., 2015).

Social support has been shown to have a direct effect on uncertainty by reducing perceived complexity and an indirect effect through its effect on the predictability of symptom pattern (Donovan et al., 2014; Lin, 2012; Mishel &

Braden, 1988; Scott et al., 2011; Somjaivong et al., 2011). The perception of stigma associated with some conditions, particularly HIV infection (Regan-Kubinski & Sharts-Hopko, 1995) and Down syndrome (Van Riper & Selder, 1989), served to create uncertainty when families were unsure about how others would respond to the diagnosis. Family members have been shown to experience high levels of uncertainty as well, which may further reduce the amount of support experienced by the patient (Baird & Eliasziw, 2011; Brown & Powell-Cope, 1991; Fedele et al., 2013; Hilton, 1996). Uncertainty was heightened by interactions with health care providers when patients and family members received unclear information, received simplistic explanations that did not fit their experience, or perceived that care providers were not expert or responsive enough to help them manage the intricacies of the illness (Checton & Greene, 2012; Step & Ray, 2011).

Numerous studies have reported the negative effects of uncertainty on psychological outcomes, characterized variously as anxiety, depression, hopelessness, psychological distress (Arroll et al., 2012; Kim & So, 2012; Miles, Funk, & Kasper, 1992; Mishel & Sorenson, 1991; Page et al., 2012), posttraumatic stress disorder (Tackett et al., 2016), quality of life (Lasker et al., 2011; Somjaivong et al., 2011; Song et al., 2011), satisfaction with family relationships (Wineman et al., 1993), satisfaction with health care services (Tai-Seale et al., 2012), and family caregivers' maintenance of their own self-care activities (O'Brien, Wineman, & Nealon, 1995). Uncertainty has also been shown to have an effect on the negative symptom experience of survivors of breast cancer treatment (Hall, Mishel, & Germino, 2014).

In 1990 the original theory was expanded to include the idea that uncertainty may not be resolved but may become part of an individual's reality. In this context, uncertainty is appraised as an opportunity that prompts the formation of a new, probabilistic view of life. To adopt this new view of life, the patient must be able to rely on social resources and health care providers who themselves accept the idea of probabilistic thinking (Mishel, 1990). When uncertainty is framed as a normal part of life, it becomes a positive force for multiple opportunities and resulting positive mood states (Mishel, 1990).

Support for the reconceptualized uncertainty in illness theory has been found in predominantly qualitative studies of people with chronic and life-threatening illnesses. The process of formulating a new view of life is described as a revised life perspective (Hilton, 1988), new life goals (Carter, 1993), new ways of being in the world (Mast, 1998), growth through uncertainty (He et al., 2016), and new levels of self-organization (Fleury, Kimbrell, & Kruszewski, 1995). In studies of men with chronic illness or their caregivers, the process is described as transformed self-identity and new goals for living (Brown & Powell-Cope, 1991), a more positive perspective on life (Katz, 1996), reevaluating what is worthwhile (Nyhlin, 1990), contemplation and self-appraisal (Charmaz, 1995), uncertainty viewed as opportunity (Baier, 1995), and redefining normal and building new dreams (Mishel & Murdaugh, 1987).

MAJOR ASSUMPTIONS

Person

Mishel's uncertainty in illness theory is middle range and focused on persons. Mishel's original uncertainty in illness theory, published in 1988, included several major assumptions (Fig. 28.1). The first two reflect how uncertainty was conceptualized within psychology's information-processing models, as follows:

1. Uncertainty is a cognitive state, representing the inadequacy of an existing cognitive schema to support the interpretation of illness-related events.
2. Uncertainty is an inherently neutral experience, neither desirable nor aversive until it is appraised as such.

Two more assumptions reflect the uncertainty theory's roots in traditional stress and coping models that posit a linear stress to coping to adaptation relationship as follows:

3. Adaptation represents the continuity of an individual's usual biopsychosocial behavior and is the desired outcome of coping efforts to either reduce uncertainty appraised as danger or maintain uncertainty appraised as opportunity.
4. The relationships among illness events, uncertainty, appraisal, coping, and adaptation are linear and unidirectional, moving from situations promoting uncertainty toward adaptation.

Mishel challenged assumptions 3 and 4 in her 1990 reconceptualization of the theory. The reconceptualization came about as a result of contradictory findings when the theory was applied to people with chronic illnesses. The original formulation of the theory held that uncertainty typically is appraised as an opportunity only in conditions that represent a known downward trajectory; in other words, uncertainty is appraised as opportunity when it is the alternative to negative certainty. However, Mishel and others found that people appraised uncertainty as an opportunity in situations without a certain downward trajectory, particularly in long-term chronic illnesses, and that in this context people often developed a new view of life.

It was at that time that Mishel turned to chaos theory to explain how prolonged uncertainty could function as a catalyst to change a person's perspective on life and illness. Chaos theory contributed two of the following theoretical

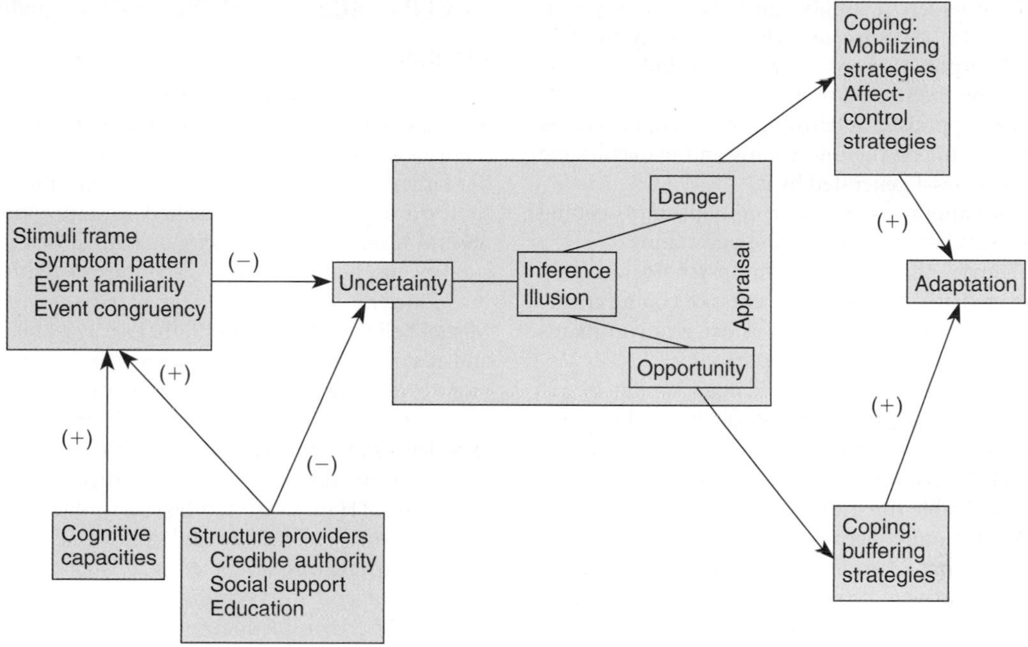

FIG. 28.1 Model of perceived uncertainty in illness. (From Mishel, M. H. [1988]. Uncertainty in illness. *Image: The Journal of Nursing Scholarship, 20*(4), 226.)

assumptions that replace the linear stress to coping to adaptation outcome portion of the model as follows:

- People, as biopsychosocial systems, typically function in far-from-equilibrium states.
- Major fluctuations in a far-from-equilibrium system enhance the system's receptivity to change.
- Fluctuations result in repatterning, which is repeated at each level of the system.

In Mishel's reconceptualized theory, neither the antecedents to uncertainty nor the process of cognitive appraisal of uncertainty as danger or opportunity change. However, uncertainty over time, associated with a serious illness, functions as a catalyst for fluctuation in the system by threatening one's preexisting cognitive model of life as predictable and controllable. Because uncertainty pervades nearly every aspect of a person's life, its effects become concentrated and ultimately challenge the stability of the system. In response to the confusion and disorganization created by continued uncertainty, the system ultimately must change to survive.

Ideally, under conditions of chronic uncertainty, a person gradually moves away from an evaluation of uncertainty as aversive to adopt a new view of life that accepts uncertainty as a part of reality (Fig. 28.2). Thus uncertainty, especially in chronic or life-threatening illness, can result in a new level of organization and a new perspective on life, incorporating the growth and change that result from uncertain experiences.

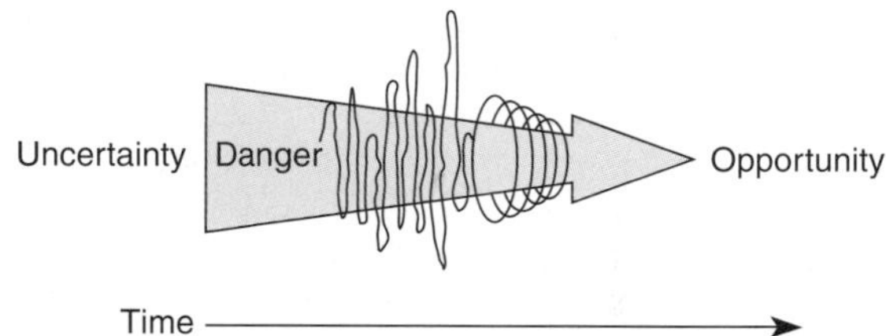

FIG. 28.2 Reconceptualized model of uncertainty in chronic illness. (Copyright Merle Mishel, 1990.)

THEORETICAL ASSERTIONS

Mishel asserted the following (1988, 1990):

- Uncertainty occurs when a person cannot adequately structure or categorize an illness-related event because of the lack of sufficient cues.
- Uncertainty can take the form of ambiguity, complexity, lack of or inconsistent information, or unpredictability.
- As symptom pattern, event familiarity, and event congruence (stimuli frame) increase, uncertainty decreases.

- Structure providers (credible authority, social support, and education) decrease uncertainty directly by promoting interpretation of events, and indirectly by strengthening the stimuli frame.
- Uncertainty appraised as danger prompts coping efforts directed at reducing the uncertainty and managing the emotional arousal generated by it.
- Uncertainty appraised as opportunity prompts coping efforts directed at maintaining the uncertainty.
- The influence of uncertainty on psychological outcomes is mediated by the effectiveness of coping efforts to reduce uncertainty appraised as danger or to maintain uncertainty appraised as opportunity.
- When uncertainty appraised as danger cannot be reduced effectively, coping strategies can be used to manage the emotional response.
- The longer uncertainty continues in the illness context, the more unstable the individual's previously accepted mode of functioning becomes.
- Under conditions of enduring uncertainty, individuals may develop a new, probabilistic perspective on life, which accepts uncertainty as a natural part of life.
- The process of integrating continual uncertainty into a new view of life can be blocked or prolonged by structure providers who do not support probabilistic thinking.
- Prolonged exposure to uncertainty appraised as danger can lead to intrusive thoughts, avoidance, and severe emotional distress.

LOGICAL FORM

As a middle-range theory derived from and applicable to clinical practice, Mishel's uncertainty in illness theory is an exemplar of the multiple steps required to develop theory with both heuristic and practical value. Neither purely inductive nor deductive, Mishel's theoretical work initially arose from questioning the nature of an important clinical problem, followed by systematic qualitative and quantitative inquiry and careful application of theory borrowed from other disciplines. Since publication of the original theory in 1988, Mishel and others have carried out numerous empirical tests of the relationships among the major constructs in the model, applying and largely confirming the theory in illness contexts. Mishel's reconceptualization of the theory in 1990 was deductive in that it was developed from principles of chaos theory and was confirmed by empirical evidence from qualitative studies that suggested that people's responses to uncertainty changed over time within the context of serious chronic illnesses. Thus Mishel's theory represents the bidirectional process in which theory informs and is informed by research.

ACCEPTANCE BY THE NURSING COMMUNITY

Practice

Mishel's theory describes a phenomenon experienced by acute and chronically ill individuals and their families. The theory has its beginning in Mishel's own experience with her father's battle with cancer. During his illness, he began to focus on events that seemed unimportant to those around him. When asked why he had chosen to focus on such events, he replied that when these activities were being done, he understood what was happening to him. Mishel believed this was her father's way of taking control and making sense out of an overwhelming situation. She knew early in the development of her concept and theory that nurses could identify the phenomenon from their experiences in caring for patients.

Several nurses have moved the theory from research to practice. Hansen and colleagues (2012) synthesized findings from qualitative studies to yield a typology of patient experiences of uncertainty that guides nursing engagement and intervention. Similarly, the theory has been used in recommendations for the practice of critical, cardiac, medical-surgical, and enterostomal nursing care (Carroll, McGillion, & Arthur, 2014; Hilton, 1992; Righter, 1995).

Based on a review of the database of Managing Uncertainty in Illness Scale users (Mishel, 1997b), master's-prepared clinicians seek to understand the experience of uncertainty in a variety of clinical settings and patient populations. The scale and theory are used by clinicians from 16 countries.

Education

The theory has been widely used by graduate students as the theoretical framework for theses and dissertations, as the topic of concept analysis, and for the critique of middle-range nursing theory. Mishel uses the theory as an exemplar to illustrate how theory guides the development of nursing interventions in her doctoral-level courses. Mishel frequently presents nursing lectures, seminars, and symposia nationally and internationally, sharing her empirical findings and the process of theory development for faculty and students.

Research

As described previously, a large body of knowledge has been generated by researchers using the uncertainty in illness theory and scales. Mishel's program of research encompassed testing the psychoeducational nursing interventions derived from the theoretical model in samples of adults with breast and prostate cancers. The scales and theory used by nurse researchers and scientists from other disciplines describe and explain psychological responses of people experiencing uncertainty because of illness and test interventions to manage uncertainty in illness contexts. The scales have been translated into 12 languages and applied in research throughout the world. Mishel (1997a, 1999) reviewed research conducted on uncertainty in acute and chronic illness and coauthored a review of the research on uncertainty in childhood illness (Stewart & Mishel, 2000). Current research on uncertainty in illness, though continuing to generate empirical evidence for the theory, is increasingly focused on theory testing of interventions.

FURTHER DEVELOPMENT

Mishel and colleagues have used the original theory as the framework for seven federally funded nursing intervention studies. The intervention has increased cancer knowledge, reduced symptom burden, and improved quality of life in Mexican American, Caucasian, and African American women with breast cancer; in African American and Caucasian men newly diagnosed with prostate cancer; and in those with localized, advanced, or recurrent prostate cancer and their family members (Germino et al., 2013; Gil et al., 2004, 2005, 2006; Mishel et al., 2002, 2003, 2009).

The applicability of the theory to the context of serious childhood illness has been supported in parents of children with HIV infection (Santacroce, Deatrick, & Ledlie, 2002) and in children undergoing treatment for cancer (Lin, Yeh, & Mishel, 2010; Stewart, 2003; Stewart, Lynn, & Mishel, 2010; Stewart et al., 2010). Bailey used the theory to support research in chronic hepatitis C (Bailey et al., 2009, 2010) and has tested an uncertainty self-management intervention in patients awaiting liver transplant and their caregivers.

From qualitative data supporting the reconceptualized theory, Mishel and Fleury (1994) developed the Growth Through Uncertainty Scale (GTUS) to measure the new view of life that can emerge from continual uncertainty. Researchers have also used the reconceptualized theory to understand the uncertainty experience of long-term survivors of breast cancer (Mast, 1998) and individuals with schizophrenia and their family members (Baier, 1995). The reconceptualized theory served as the foundation for Mishel and colleagues' nursing intervention study of women younger than 50 years of age facing the enduring uncertainties inherent in surviving breast cancer. Bailey used the theory and data from qualitative interviews with older men who had elected watchful waiting as treatment for their prostate cancer, to develop a nursing intervention to integrate uncertainty into their lives, view their lives in a positive perspective, and improve their quality of life (Bailey, Wallace, & Mishel, 2007). In the first study of the Uncertainty Management Intervention for Watchful Waiting, men came to see their lives in a new and positive light, reported their quality of life as higher than did the control group, and expected it to be high in the future (Bailey et al., 2004). Wallace (now Kazer) and Bailey conducted a pilot test of a web-based version of the intervention for men with prostate cancer undergoing active surveillance (previously referred to as *watchful waiting*) (Kazer et al., 2011).

The substantial empirical evidence supporting the uncertainty in illness theories provides a strong foundation to extend the theory to intervention development and improve patient and family outcomes. In addition to Mishel's own intervention studies in patients with breast and prostate cancer, several researchers tested interventions to help patients manage uncertainty. Many were directed at reducing sources of uncertainty (Chair et al., 2012; Chiou & Chung, 2012; Faithfull, Cockle-Hearne, & Khoo, 2011; Kazer et al., 2011; Lebel et al., 2014; Muthusamy et al., 2012; Schover et al., 2012). Others focused on the provision of support (Heiney et al., 2012; Maheu et al., 2015) and specific coping strategies (Faithfull, Cockle-Hearne, & Khoo, 2011; Fedele et al., 2013) to help patients manage their uncertainty.

CRITIQUE

Clarity

Uncertainty is the primary concept of this theory and is defined as a cognitive state in which individuals are unable to determine the meaning of illness-related events (Mishel, 1988). The original theory postulates that managing uncertainty is critical to adaptation during illness and explains how individuals cognitively process illness-associated events and construct meaning from them. The original theory's concepts were organized in a linear model around the following three major themes:

1. Antecedents of uncertainty
2. Process of uncertainty appraisal
3. Coping with uncertainty

The framework is clear and easy to follow. The antecedents of uncertainty include the stimuli frame, cognitive capacities, and structure providers. In the linear model, these antecedent variables have both a direct and an indirect inverse relationship with uncertainty.

The second conceptual component of the model is **appraisal**. Uncertainty is seen as a neutral state, neither positive nor negative, until it has been appraised by the individual. Appraisal of uncertainty involves two processes: (1) inference and (2) illusion. Inference is constructed from the individual's personality disposition and includes learned resourcefulness, mastery, and locus of control. These characteristics contribute to an individual's confidence in the ability to handle life events. Illusion is defined as a belief constructed from uncertainty that considers the favorable aspects of a situation. Based on the appraisal process, uncertainty is viewed as either a danger or an opportunity. Uncertainty viewed as a danger results when the individual considers the possibility of a negative outcome. Uncertainty is viewed as an opportunity primarily through the use of illusion, but inference also can lead to the individual appraising the situation as having a positive outcome. In this situation, uncertainty is preferred and the individual remains hopeful.

Coping is the third theme of the original model of uncertainty. Coping occurs in two forms, with the end result of adaptation. If uncertainty is appraised as a danger, then coping includes direct action, vigilance, and seeking information from mobilizing strategies, and it affects management using faith, disengagement, and cognitive support. If uncertainty is appraised as an opportunity, coping offers a buffer to maintain the uncertainty.

The original theory was reconceptualized in 1990 to incorporate the idea that chronic illness unfolds over time, possibly years, and with that, uncertainty is reappraised. The person is viewed as an open system exchanging energy within his or her environment, and, rather than seeking to return to a stable state, chronically ill individuals may move toward a complex world orientation, thus forming new meaning for their lives. If uncertainty is framed as a normal view of life, it becomes a positive force for multiple opportunities with resulting positive mood states. To achieve this, the individual must develop probabilistic thinking, which allows one to examine a variety of possibilities and consider ways of achieving them as the individual envisions a variety of responses and realizes that life changes from day to day.

Mishel described this process as a new view of life in which uncertainty shifts from being seen as a danger to being viewed as an opportunity. To adopt this new view of life, the patient must be able to rely on social resources and health care providers who accept probabilistic thinking. The relationship between the health care provider and the patient must focus on recognizing continual uncertainty and teaching the patient how to use the uncertainty to generate different explanations for events. Hence the importance of structure providers, introduced in the original theory, is maintained in the reconceptualized model.

Despite the complexity and dimensionality of the two models, they are presented clearly and conceptualized comprehensively. Mishel published her measurement model in 1981, her original theoretical model in 1988, and her reconceptualized theory in 1990, and these publications fully explicate the model for application in clinical and research contexts.

Simplicity

The two uncertainty-in-illness models contain concepts comprising relationships that range from simple to complex and direct to indirect. Eleven major concepts are found in the three themes of the original theory, and several new concepts are introduced in the reconceptualized model. The antecedents of uncertainty are concise, and their definitions are clear and simple. The appraisal component is complex because it considers cognitive processes along with beliefs and values held by the individual. The coping phase of the theory is also complex because it is dependent on the appraisal portion of the model and again involves different kinds of strategies targeted toward adaptation. The outcome portion of the model is differentiated into two conceptualizations of the theory, the first relating to patients with acute illness and the second representing an expansion of the model to accommodate patients with chronic illness. Although the models can hardly be called simple, overall the concept definitions and relationships are well operationalized and easily understood.

Generality

The theory explains how individuals construct meaning from illness-related events. It is broad and generalizable and can be used with individuals experiencing illness, as well as with spouses and parents of those experiencing illness-related uncertainty. The concept of credible authority can be applied to physicians, nurses, and other health care workers. The theory can be applied in many areas of nursing practice and has been used by clinicians for acute and chronic illnesses such as cancer, cardiac disease, and multiple sclerosis.

Accessibility

Mishel derived both theoretical models from her program of research. Many of the concepts, assumptions, and relationships among variables draw support from empirical investigation. The concepts are well described, and their relationships are precisely constructed with clear, tested operational definitions. Theory testing occurred in research and clinical settings. The theory led to development and testing of nursing interventions to manage uncertainty.

Importance

Derivable consequences are determined by examining whether a theory guides research, informs practice, generates new ideas, and differentiates the focus of nursing from other professions. Mishel's work represents an exemplar of middle-range theory that informs clinical practice in the encompassing context of acute and chronic illness. The theory has generated considerable empirical research with adults dealing with illness and their family members and continues to stimulate new research directions, such as uncertainty in ill children, in older men electing watchful waiting as the treatment of choice for prostate cancer, and in health care providers informing patients of treatment choices in conditions with uncertain prognoses. Mishel believes that by defining and conceptualizing an important clinical problem, her work supports and enriches nursing practice. The uncertainty in illness theory and its reconceptualization represent frameworks derived from and for practice, a process essential to nursing as a practice discipline.

SUMMARY

The uncertainty in illness theory provides a comprehensive framework within which to view the experience of acute and chronic illness and to organize nursing interventions to promote optimal adjustment. The theory helps explain the stresses associated with the diagnosis and treatment of major illnesses or chronic conditions, the processes by which individuals assess and respond to the uncertainty inherent in an illness experience, and the importance of professional caregivers in providing information and supporting individuals in understanding and managing uncertainty. The reconceptualized theory addresses the unique context of continual uncertainty and thereby expands the original theory to encompass the ongoing uncertain trajectory of many life-threatening and chronic illnesses. The original theory and its reconceptualization are well explicated, deriving support from sound theoretical foundations and extensive empirical confirmation, and it can be applied in illness contexts to support evidence-based nursing practice.

CASE STUDY

Part 1: Original Theory

Rosie, a 45-year-old mother of three, has been diagnosed with stage 3 breast cancer. A mass was detected in her left breast during her annual gynecological appointment, and she has undergone an extensive diagnostic workup, including mammography and sentinel node biopsy. She was referred by her primary physician to a comprehensive breast cancer program at a regional medical center that was 2 hours from her home. The multidisciplinary team has recommended that Rosie undergo preoperative chemotherapy, followed by partial mastectomy and reconstructive surgery. Rosie's husband has accompanied her to most of her medical encounters, but he was unable to attend the final conference, where the treatment recommendations were made.

Lily, the advanced practice nurse coordinating Rosie's care (structure provider–credible authority), directs her interventions toward addressing the many sources of uncertainty for Rosie and her family, including lack of information about treatment options and outcomes (event familiarity), unfamiliarity with the treatment environment (event familiarity), expectations for chemotherapy side effects and postoperative recovery (symptom pattern), effects of treatment on family relationships, and prognosis. In particular, Lily addresses Rosie's many questions about why her treatment plan is different from what her primary physician told her to expect (event congruence) and how she will manage her family life while undergoing treatment. Lily provides an audiotape of the treatment conference so that Rosie's husband (structure provider–social support) can hear what took place and can support Rosie in asking questions and understanding the information provided. Lily's support for Rosie and her family continues throughout Rosie's treatment course, and she periodically reassesses the sources of uncertainty and the strategies that Rosie and her family use to manage them.

Part 2: Reconceptualized Theory

Two years after her breast cancer diagnosis, Rosie returns to the center for a follow-up appointment. Lily asks Rosie to reflect on her cancer experience. Rosie describes the time of diagnosis and treatment as chaotic and dominated by uncertainty, and she wonders how she and her family got through it, but she tells Lily that gradually she came to see the cancer experience as providing new meaning to her life and helping her set priorities. She left a job she was dissatisfied with and now directs her energy toward her relationships with her teenage children. Rosie and her husband recently enjoyed a long-postponed second honeymoon trip to Hawaii. She tells Lily that she now embraces each day as an opportunity to live life and enrich the lives of her children.

CRITICAL THINKING ACTIVITIES

1. You have been assigned to Mrs. Green, a new patient. You want to know about this person's perceptions of the current situation, supportive relationships, and previous experiences with health and illness. What questions would you ask to assess her level of uncertainty?
2. You are working with a young woman who has been living with multiple sclerosis for 6 years. During an exacerbation of her disease, she focuses on her plans for going to law school. One of your colleagues suggests that she may be in denial about the severity of her illness. Use the reconceptualized uncertainty in illness theory to propose an alternative interpretation of her perspective.

POINTS FOR FURTHER STUDY

- Germino, B. B., Mishel, M. H. Crandell, J., et al. (2013). Outcomes of an uncertainty management intervention in younger African American and Caucasian breast cancer survivors. *Oncology Nursing Forum, 40*(1), 82–92.
- Mishel, M. (2008). *The Nurse Theorists: Portraits of Excellence,* vol 2. Athens, OH: Fitne, Inc.
- Research Tested Interventions for Practice (RTIP), NCI. Managing Uncertainty in Older Long-term Breast Cancer Survivors at http://rtips.cancer.gov/rtips/index.do

  Requests for her scales may be sent to the following: Sandy Staley, Department Manager, UNC Philosophy Department, 102 A Caldwell Hall, CB 3125 Chapel Hill, NC 27599-3125; sstaley@email.unc.edu

REFERENCES

Arroll, M., Dancey, C. P., Attree, E. A., Smith, S., & James T. (2012). People with symptoms of Meniere's disease: The relationship between illness intrusiveness, illness uncertainty, dizziness handicap, and depression. *Otology & Neurology, 33*(5), 816–823.

Baier, M. (1995). Uncertainty of illness for persons with schizophrenia. *Issues in Mental Health Nursing, 16*, 201–212.

Bailey, D. E., Barroso, J., Muir, A. J., et al. (2010). Patients with chronic hepatitis C undergoing watchful waiting: Exploring trajectories of illness uncertainty and fatigue. *Research in Nursing and Health, 33*(5), 465–473.

Bailey, D. E., Mishel, M. H., Belyea, M., Stewart, J. L., & Mohler, J. (2004). Uncertainty intervention for watchful waiting in prostate cancer. *Cancer Nursing, 27*(5), 339–346.

Bailey, D. E., Wallace, M., & Mishel, M. H. (2007). Watching, waiting, and uncertainty in prostate cancer. *Journal of Clinical Nursing, 16*, 734–741.

Bailey, D. E., Jr., Landerman, L., Barroso, J., et al. (2009). Uncertainty, symptoms and quality of life in persons with chronic hepatitis C. *Psychosomatics, 50*(2), 138–146.

Baird, D. L., & Eliasziw, M. (2011). Disparity in perceived illness intrusiveness and illness severity between cardiac patients and their spouses. *Journal of Cardiovascular Nursing, 26*(6), 481–486.

Brown, M. A., & Powell-Cope, G. M. (1991). AIDS family caregiving: Transitions through uncertainty. *Nursing Research, 40*, 338–345.

Budner, S. (1962). Intolerance of ambiguity as a personality variable. *Journal of Personality, 30*, 29–50.

Cahill, J., LoBiondo-Wood, G., Bergstrom, N., & Armstrong, T. (2012). Brain tumor symptoms as antecedents to uncertainty: An integrative review. *Journal of Nursing Scholarship, 44*(2), 145–155.

Carroll, S. L., McGillion, M., & Arthur, H. M. (2014). Living with an implantable cardiac defibrillator: A model of chronic uncertainty. *Research and Theory for Nursing Practice, 28*, 71–86.

Carter, B. J. (1993). Long-term survivors of breast cancer. *Cancer Nursing, 16*(5), 354–361.

Chair, S. Y., Chau, M. Y., Sit, J. W. H., Wong, E. M. L., & Chan, A. W. K. (2012). The psychological effects of a videotape educational intervention on cardiac catheterization patients. *Contemporary Nurse, 40*(2), 225–233.

Charmaz, K. (1995). Identity dilemmas of chronically ill men. In D. Sobo & D. F. Gordon (Eds.), *Men's health and illness: Gender, power, and the body* (pp. 266–291). Thousand Oaks, CA: Sage.

Checton, M. G., & Greene, K. (2012). Beyond initial disclosure: The role of prognosis and symptom uncertainty in patterns of disclosure in relationships. *Health Communication, 27*(2), 145–157.

Chiou, C. P., & Chung, Y. C. (2012). Effectiveness of multimedia interactive patient education on knowledge, uncertainty and decision making in patients with end-stage renal disease. *Journal of Clinical Nursing, 21*(9–10), 1223–1231.

Cohen, E. L., Scott, A. M., Record, R., Shaunfield, S., Jones, M. G., & Collins, T. (2016). Using communication to manage uncertainty about cervical cancer screening guideline adherence among Appalachian women. *Journal of Applied Communication Research, 44*(1), 22–39.

Donovan, E. E., LeFebvre, L., Tardif, S., Brown, L. E., & Love, B. (2014). Patterns of social support communicated in response to expressions of uncertainty in an online community of young adults with cancer. *Journal of Applied Communication Research, 42*, 432–455.

Faithfull, S., Cockle-Hearne, J., & Khoo, V. (2011). Self-management after prostate cancer treatment: Evaluating the feasibility of providing a cognitive and behavioural programme for lower urinary tract symptoms. *BJU International, 1107*(5), 783–790.

Fedele, D. A., Hullmann, S. E., Chaffin, M., et al. (2013). Impact of a parent-based interdisciplinary intervention for mothers on adjustment in children newly diagnosed with cancer. *Journal of Pediatric Psychology*, *38*, 531–540.

Fleury, J., Kimbrell, L. C., & Kruszewski, C. (1995). Life after cardiac event: Women's experience in healing. *Heart & Lung*, *24*, 474–482.

Germino, B. B., Mishel, M. H., Crandell, J., et al. (2013). Outcomes of an uncertainty management intervention in younger African American and Caucasian breast cancer survivors. *Oncology Nursing Forum*, *40*(1), 82–92.

Gil, K. M., Mishel, M., Belyea, M., et al. (2004). Triggers of uncertainty about recurrence and long term treatment side effects in older African American and Caucasian breast cancer survivors. *Oncology Nursing Forum*, *31*(3), 633–639.

Gil, K. M., Mishel, M. H., Belyea, M., Germino, B., Porter, L. S., & Clayton M. (2006). Benefits of the uncertainty management intervention for African American and white older breast cancer survivors: 20-month outcomes. *International Journal of Behavioral Medicine*, *13*(4), 286–294.

Gil, K. M., Mishel, M. H., Germino, B., Porter, L. S., Carlton-LaNey, I., & Belyea M. (2005). Uncertainty management intervention for older African American and Caucasian long-term breast cancer survivors. *Journal of Psychosocial Oncology*, *23*(2–3), 3–21.

Hall, D. L., Mishel, M. H., & Germino, B. B. (2014). Living with cancer-related uncertainty: Associations with fatigue, insomnia, and affect in younger breast cancer survivors. *Supportive Care in Cancer*, *22*, 2489–2495.

Hansen, B. S., Rørtveit, K., Leiknes, I., et al. (2012). Patient experiences of uncertainty—a synthesis to guide nursing practice and research. *Journal of Nursing Management*, *20*(2), 266–277.

He, S., You, L.-m., Zheng, J., & Bi, Y.-l. (2016). Uncertainty and personal growth through positive coping strategies among Chinese parents of children with acute leukemia. *Cancer Nursing*, *39*, 205–212.

Heiney, S. P., Adams, S. A., Wells, L. M., Johnson, H., & King, J. M. (2012). Participant evaluation of teleconference support for African American women with breast cancer. *Cancer Nursing*, *34*(2), E24–E30.

Hilton, B. A. (1988). The phenomenon of uncertainty in women with breast cancer. *Issues in Mental Health Nursing*, *9*, 217–238.

Hilton, B. A. (1992). Perceptions of uncertainty: Its relevance to life-threatening and chronic illness. *Critical Care Nurse*, *12*, 70–73.

Hilton, B. A. (1996). Getting back to normal: The family experience during early stage breast cancer. *Oncology Nursing Forum*, *23*, 605–614.

Katz, A. (1996). Gaining a new perspective of life as a consequence of uncertainty in HIV infection. *Journal of the Association of Nurses in AIDS Care*, *7*(4), 51–60.

Kazer, M. W., Bailey, D. E., Jr., Sanda, M., Colberg, J., & Kelly, W. K. (2011). An internet intervention for management of uncertainty during active surveillance for prostate cancer. *Oncology Nursing Forum*, *38*(5), 561–568.

Kim, H. Y., & So, H. S. (2012). A structural model for psychosocial adjustment in patients with early breast cancer. *Journal of Korean Academy of Nursing*, *42*(1), 105–115.

Kim, S. H., Lee, R., & Lee, K. S. (2012). Symptoms and uncertainty in breast cancer survivors in Korea: Differences by treatment trajectory. *Journal of Clinical Nursing*, *21*(7–8), 1014–1023.

Lasker, J. N., Sogolow, E. D., Short, L. M., & Sass, D. A. (2011). The impact of biopsychosocial factors on quality of life: Women with primary biliary cirrhosis on waiting list and post liver transplantation. *British Journal of Health Psychology*, *16*(3), 502–527.

Lazarus, R. S., & Folkman, S. (1984). *Stress, appraisal, and coping*. New York: Springer.

Lebel, S., Maheu, C., Lefebvre, M., et al. (2014). Addressing fear of cancer recurrence among women with cancer: A feasibility and preliminary outcome study. *Journal of Cancer Survivorship*, *8*, 485–496.

Lin, L., Chien, L.-C., Acquaye, A. A., Vera-Bolanos, E., Gilbert, M. R., & Armstrong, T. S. (2015). Significant predictors of patients' uncertainty in primary brain tumors. *Journal of Neuro-Oncology*, *122*, 507–515.

Lin, L., Yeh, C. H., & Mishel, M. H. (2010). Evaluation of a conceptual model based on Mishel's theories of uncertainty in illness in a sample of Taiwanese parents of children with cancer: A cross-sectional questionnaire survey. *International Journal of Nursing Studies*, *47*(12), 1510–1524.

Lin, Y. H. (2012). Comparison of the uncertainty level of radical prostatectomy recipients with or without psychological support. *International Journal of Urological Nursing*, *6*, 76–82.

Maheu, C., Lebel, S., Tomei, C., Singh, M., & Esplen, M. J. (2015). Breast and ovarian cancer survivors' experience of participating in a cognitive-existential group intervention addressing fear of cancer recurrence. *European Journal of Oncology Nursing*, *19*, 433–440.

Mast, M. E. (1998). Survivors of breast cancer: Illness uncertainty, positive reappraisal, and emotional distress. *Oncology Nursing Forum*, *25*, 555–562.

Miles, M. S., Funk, S. G., & Kasper, M. A. (1992). The stress response of mothers and fathers of preterm infants. *Research in Nursing and Health*, *15*, 261–269.

Mishel, M. H. (1981). The measurement of uncertainty in illness. *Nursing Research*, *30*, 258–263.

Mishel, M. H. (1988). Uncertainty in illness. *Image: The Journal of Nursing Scholarship*, *20*, 225–231.

Mishel, M. H. (1990). Reconceptualization of the uncertainty in illness theory. *Image: The Journal of Nursing Scholarship*, *22*, 256–262.

Mishel, M. H. (1997a). Uncertainty in acute illness. *Annual Review of Nursing Research*, *15*, 57–80.

Mishel, M. H. (1997b). *Uncertainty in illness scales manual*. Available upon request from the author at http://nursing.unc.edu/music/instruments.html.

Mishel, M. H. (1999). Uncertainty in chronic illness. *Annual Review of Nursing Research*, *17*, 269–294.

Mishel, M. H., Belyea, M., Germino, B. B., et al. (2002). Helping patients with localized prostate carcinoma manage uncertainty

and treatment side effects—Nurse-delivered psychoeducational intervention over the telephone. *Cancer, 94*, 1854–1866.
Mishel, M. H., & Braden, C. J. (1987). Uncertainty: A mediator between support and adjustment. *Western Journal of Nursing Research, 9*, 43–57.
Mishel, M. H., & Braden, C. J. (1988). Finding meaning: Antecedents of uncertainty in illness. *Nursing Research, 37*, 98–103.
Mishel, M. H., & Fleury, J. (1994). *Psychometric testing of the growth through uncertainty scale*. Unpublished data, University of North Carolina at Chapel Hill.
Mishel, M. H., Germino, B. B., Belyea, M., et al. (2003). Moderators of an uncertainty management intervention for men with localized prostate cancer. *Nursing Research, 52*, 89–97.
Mishel, M. H., Germino, B. B., Lin, L., et al. (2009). Managing uncertainty about treatment decision making in early prostate cancer: A randomized clinical trial. *Patient Education and Counseling, 77*, 349–359.
Mishel, M. H., & Murdaugh, C. L. (1987). Family adjustment to heart transplantation: Redesigning the dream. *Nursing Research, 36*, 332–338.
Mishel, M. H., Padilla, G., Grant, M., & Sorenson, D. S. (1991). Uncertainty in illness theory: A replication of the mediating effects of mastery and coping. *Nursing Research, 40*, 236–240.
Mishel, M. H., & Sorenson, D. S. (1991). Coping with uncertainty in gynecological cancer: A test of the mediating function of mastery and coping. *Nursing Research, 40*, 167–171.
Muthusamy, A. D., Leuthner, S., Gaebler-Uhing, C., Hoffmann, R. G., Li, S. H., & Basir, M. A. (2012). Supplemental written information improves prenatal counseling: A randomized trial. *Pediatrics, 129*(5), e1269–e1274.
Nyhlin, K. T. (1990). Diabetic patients facing long-term complications: Coping with uncertainty. *Journal of Advanced Nursing, 15*, 1021–1029.
O'Brien, R. A., Wineman, N. M., & Nealon, N. R. (1995). Correlates of the caregiving process in multiple sclerosis. *Scholarly Inquiry for Nursing Practice, 9*, 323–342.
Page, M. C., Fedele, D. A., Pai, A. L. H., et al. (2012). The relationship of maternal and child illness uncertainty to child depressive symptomotology: A mediational model. *Journal of Pediatric Psychology, 37*(1), 97–105.
Rains, S. A., & Tukachinsky, R. (2015). Information seeking in uncertainty management theory: Exposure to information about medical uncertainty and information-processing orientation as predictors of uncertainty management success. *Journal of Health Communication, 20*, 1275–1286.
Regan-Kubinski, M. J., & Sharts-Hopko, N. (1995). Illness cognition of HIV-infected mothers. *Issues in Mental Health Nursing, 16*, 327–344.
Righter, B. M. (1995). Ostomy care: Uncertainty and the role of the credible authority during an ostomy experience. *Journal of Wound, Ostomy, and Continence Nursing, 22*(2), 100–104.
Santacroce, S. J., Deatrick, J. A., & Ledlie, S. W. (2002). Redefining treatment: How biological mothers manage their children's treatment for perinatally acquired HIV. *AIDS Care, 14*, 47–60.
Schover, L. R., Canada, A. L., Yuan, Y., et al. (2012). A randomized trial of internet-based versus traditional sexual counseling for couples after localized prostate cancer treatment. *Cancer, 118*(2), 500–509.
Scott, A. M., Martin, S. C., Stone, A. M., & Brashers, D. E. (2011). Managing multiple goals in supportive interactions: Using a normative theoretical approach to explain social support as uncertainty management for organ transplant patients. *Health Communication, 26*(5), 393–403.
Somjaivong, B., Thanasilp, S., Preechawong, S., & Sloan, R. (2011). The influence of symptoms, social support, uncertainty, and coping on health-related quality of life among cholangiocarcinoma patients in northeast Thailand. *Cancer Nursing, 34*(6), 434–442.
Song, L. X., Northouse, L. L., Braun, T. M., et al. (2011). Assessing longitudinal quality of life in prostate cancer patients and their spouses: A multilevel modeling approach. *Quality of Life Research, 20*(3), 371–381.
Step, M. M., & Ray, E. B. (2011). Patient perceptions of oncologist-patient communication about prognosis: Changes from initial diagnosis to cancer recurrence. *Health Communication, 26*(1), 48–58.
Stewart, J. L. (2003). "Getting used to it": Children finding the ordinary and routine in the uncertain context of cancer. *Qualitative Health Research, 13*, 394–407.
Stewart, J. L., Lynn, M. R., & Mishel, M. H. (2010). Psychometric evaluation of a new instrument to measure uncertainty in children and adolescents with cancer. *Nursing Research, 59*(2), 119–126.
Stewart, J. L., & Mishel, M. H. (2000). Uncertainty in childhood illness: A synthesis of the parent and child literature. *Scholarly Inquiry for Nursing Practice, 14*, 299–320.
Stewart, J. L., Mishel, M. H., Lynn, M. R., & Terhorst, L. (2010). Test of a conceptual model of uncertainty in children and adolescents with cancer. *Research in Nursing & Health, 33*(3), 179–191.
Tackett, A. P., Cushing, C. C., Suorsa, K. I., et al. (2016). Illness uncertainty, global psychological distress, and posttraumatic stress in pediatric cancer: A preliminary examination using a path analysis approach. *Journal of Pediatric Psychology, 41*, 309–318.
Tai-Seale, M., Stults, C., Zhang, W. M., & Shumway, M. (2012). Expressing uncertainty in clinical interactions between physicians and older patients: What matters? *Patient Education and Counseling, 86*(3), 322–328.
Van Riper, M., & Selder, F. E. (1989). Parental responses to the birth of a child with Down syndrome. *Loss, Grief, & Care, 3*(3–4), 59–76.
Warburton, D. M. (1979). Physiological aspects of information processing and stress. In V. Hamilton & D. M. Warburton (Eds.), *Human stress and cognition: An information processing approach* (pp. 33–65). New York: Wiley.
Wineman, N. M., O'Brien, R. A., Nealon, N. R., & Kaskel, B. (1993). Congruence in uncertainty between individuals with multiple sclerosis and their spouses. *Journal of Neuroscience Nursing, 25*, 356–361.

BIBLIOGRAPHY

Primary Sources

Book Chapters

Mishel, M. H. (1993). Living with chronic illness: Living with uncertainty. In S. G. Funk, E. M. Tornquist, M. T. Champagne, & R. A. Weise (Eds.), *Key aspects of caring for the chronically ill, hospital and home* (pp. 46–58). New York: Springer.

Mishel, M. H. (1998). Methodological studies: Instrument development. In P. Brink & M. Woods (Eds.), *Advanced design in nursing research* (2nd ed.; pp. 235–282). Beverly Hills, CA: Sage.

Mishel, M. H., & Clayton, M. F. (2008). Uncertainty in illness theories. In M. J. Smith & P. Liehr (Eds.), *Middle range theory in advanced practice nursing* (pp. 55–84). New York: Springer.

Mishel, M. H., Germino, B. G., Belyea, M., et al. (2001). Helping patients with localized prostate cancer: Managing after treatment. In S. G. Funk, E. M. Tornquist, J. Leeman, M. S. Miles, & J. S. Harrell (Eds.), *Key aspects of preventing and managing chronic illness* (pp. 235–246). New York: Springer.

Journal Articles

Amoako, E. P., Skelly, A. H., & Mishel, M. M. (2004). Identifying intervention strategies for older African-American women to manage uncertainty in diabetes. *Diabetes, 53*, A513.

Badger, T. A., Braden, C. J., & Mishel, M. H. (2001). Depression burden, self-help interventions, and side effect experience in women receiving treatment for breast cancer. *Oncology Nursing Forum, 28*, 567–574.

Badger, T. A., Braden, C. J., Mishel, M. H., & Longman, A. (2004). Depression burden, psychological adjustment, and quality of life in women with breast cancer: Patterns over time. *Research in Nursing & Health, 27*, 19–28.

Bailey, D., Stewart, J., & Mishel, M. (2005). Watchful waiting in prostate cancer: Where can older men find support? *Oncology Nursing Forum, 32*, 177.

Bailey, D. E., Barroso, J., Muir, A. J., et al. (2010). Patients with chronic hepatitis C undergoing watchful waiting: Exploring trajectories of illness uncertainty and fatigue. *Research in Nursing and Health, 33*(5), 465–473.

Bailey, D. E., Jr., Wallace, M., Latini, D. M., et al. (2011). Measuring illness uncertainty in men undergoing active surveillance for prostate cancer. *Applied Nursing Research, 24*(4), 193–199.

Braden, C. J., & Mishel, M. H. (2000). Highlights of the self-help intervention project (SHIP): Health-related quality of life during breast cancer treatment. *Innovations in Breast Cancer Care, 5*, 51–54.

Clayton, M. F., Mishel, M. H., & Belyea, M. (2006). Testing a model of symptoms, communication, uncertainty and well-being, in older breast cancer survivors. *Research in Nursing and Health, 29*(1), 18–39.

Farren, A. T. (2010). Power, uncertainty, self-transcendence, and quality of life in breast cancer survivors. *Nursing Science Quarterly, 23*(1), 63–71.

Harris, L., Belyea, M., Mishel, M., & Germino, B. (2003). Issues in revising research instruments for use with Southern populations. *Journal of the National Black Nurses Association, 14*, 44–50.

Hegarty, J. M., Wallace, M., & Comber, H. (2008). Uncertainty and quality of life among men undergoing active surveillance for prostate cancer in the United States and Ireland. *American Journal of Men's Health, 2*(2), 133–142.

Ismail, Z., Kwok-wei So, W., & Wai-Chi Li, P. (2010). Preoperative uncertainty and anxiety among Chinese patients with gynecologic cancer. *Oncology Nursing Forum, 37*(1), E67–E74.

Lai, H. L., Lin, S. Y., & Yeh, S. H. (2007). Exploring uncertainty, quality of life and related factors in patients with liver cancer. *Hu Li Za Zhi, 54*(6), 41–52.

Liao, M. N., Chen, M. F., Chen, S. C., & Chen, P. L. (2008). Uncertainty and anxiety during the diagnostic period for women with suspected breast cancer. *Cancer Nursing, 31*(4), 274–283.

Lien, C., Lin, H., Kuo, I., & Chen, M. (2009). Perceived uncertainty, social support and psychological adjustment in older patients with cancer being treated with surgery. *Journal of Clinical Nursing, 18*(16), 2311–2319.

Liu, L. N., Li, C. Y., Tang, S. T., Huang, C. S., & Chiou, A. F. (2006). Role of continuing supportive cares in increasing social support and reducing perceived uncertainty among women with newly diagnosed breast cancer in Taiwan. *Cancer Nursing, 29*(4), 273–282.

McCorkle, R., Dowd, M., Ercolano, E., et al. (2009). Effects of a nursing intervention on quality of life outcomes in post-surgical women with gynecological cancers. *Psychooncology, 18*(1), 62–70.

McCorkle, R., Jeon, S., Ercolano, E., & Schwartz, P. (2011). Healthcare utilization in women after abdominal surgery for ovarian cancer. *Nursing Research, 60*(1), 47–57.

Mishel, M. H. (1981). The measurement of uncertainty in illness. *Nursing Research, 30*, 258–263.

Mishel, M. H. (1983). Parents' perception of uncertainty concerning their hospitalized child: Reliability and validity of a scale. *Nursing Research, 32*, 324–330.

Mishel, M. H. (1988). Uncertainty in illness. *Image: Journal of Nursing Scholarship, 20*, 225–232.

Mishel, M. H. (1990). Reconceptualization of the uncertainty in illness theory. *Image: Journal of Nursing Scholarship, 22*, 256–262.

Mishel, M. H. (1997). Uncertainty in acute illness. *Annual Review of Nursing Research, 15*, 57–80.

Mishel, M. H. (1999). Uncertainty in chronic illness. *Annual Review of Nursing Research, 17*, 269–294.

Mishel, M. H., Belyea, M., Germino, B. B., et al. (2002). Helping patients with localized prostate carcinoma manage uncertainty and treatment side effects—Nurse-delivered psychoeducational intervention over the telephone. *Cancer, 94*, 1854–1866.

Mishel, M. H., Germino, B. B., Belyea, M., et al. (2003). Moderators of an uncertainty management intervention for men with localized prostate cancer. *Nursing Research, 52*, 89–97.

Mishel, M. H., Germino, B. B., Gilk, K. M., et al. (2005). Benefits from an uncertainty management intervention for African American and Caucasian older long-term breast cancer survivors. *Psychooncology, 14*, 962–978.

Mishel, M. H, Germino, B. B., Lin, L., et al. (2009). Managing uncertainty about treatment decision making in early stage prostate cancer: A randomized clinical trial. *Patient Education and Counseling, 77*(3), 349–359.

Northouse, L. L., Mood, D. W., Montie, J. E., et al. (2007). Living with prostate cancer: Patients' and spouses' psychosocial status and quality of life. *Journal of Clinical Oncology, 25*(27), 4171–4177.

Northouse, L. L., Mood, D. W., Schafenacker, A., et al. (2007). Randomized clinical trial of a family intervention for prostate cancer patients and their spouses. *Cancer, 110*(12), 2809–2818.

Otis-Green, S., Ferrell, B., Sun, V., Spolum, M., Morgan, R., & Macdonald, D. (2008). Feasibility of an ovarian cancer quality-of-life psychoeducational intervention. *Journal of Cancer Education, 23*(4), 214–221.

Porter, L. S., Clayton, M. R., Belyea, M., Mishel, M., Gil, K. M., & Germino B. B. (2006). Predicting negative mood state and personal growth in African American and white long-term breast cancer survivors. *Annals of Behavioral Medicine, 31*(3), 195–204.

Porter, L. S., Mishel, M., Neelon, V., Belyea, M., Pisano, E., & Soo, M. S. (2003). Cortisol levels and responses to mammography screening in breast cancer survivors: A pilot study. *Psychosomatic Medicine, 65*(5), 842–848.

Sammarco, A. (2001). Perceived social support, uncertainty, and quality of life of younger breast cancer survivors. *Cancer Nursing, 24*(3), 212–219.

Sammarco, A. (2003). Quality of life among older survivors of breast cancer. *Cancer Nursing, 26*(6), 431–438.

Sammarco, A. (2009). Quality of life of breast cancer survivors: A comparative study of age cohorts. *Cancer Nursing, 32*(5), 347–356; quiz 357–348.

Sammarco, A., & Konecny, L. M. (2008). Quality of life, social support, and uncertainty among Latina breast cancer survivors. *Oncology Nursing Forum, 35*(5), 844–849.

Sammarco, A., & Konecny, L. M. (2010). Quality of life, social support, and uncertainty among Latina and Caucasian breast cancer survivors: A comparative study. *Oncology Nursing Forum, 37*(1), 93–99.

Schroeder, J. C., Bensen, J. T., Su, L. J., et al. (2006). The North Carolina Louisiana Prostate Cancer Project (PCaP): Methods and design of a multidisciplinary population-based cohort study of racial differences in prostate cancer outcomes. *Prostate, 66*(11), 1162–1176.

Schulman-Green, D., Ercolano, E., Dowd, M., Schwartz, P., & McCorkle R. (2008). Quality of life among women after surgery for ovarian cancer. *Palliative Supportive Care, 6*(3), 239–247.

Stewart, J. L., Lynn, M. R., & Mishel, M. H. (2005). Evaluating content validity for children's self-report instruments using children as content experts. *Nursing Research, 54*, 414–418.

Stewart, J. L., & Mishel, M. H. (2000). Uncertainty in childhood illness: A synthesis of the parent and child literature. *Scholarly Inquiry for Nursing Practice, 14*, 299–320.

Wonghongkul, T., Moore, S. M., Musil, C., Schneider, S., & Deimling, G. (2000). The influence of uncertainty in illness, stress appraisal, and hope on coping in survivors of breast cancer. *Cancer Nursing, 23*(6), 422–429.

Secondary Sources

Selected Publications Citing Mishel's Work

Amoako, E., & Skelly, A. H. (2007). Managing uncertainty in diabetes: An intervention for older African American women. *Ethnicity & Disease, 17*(3), 515–521.

Anderson, G. (2007). Patient decision making for clinical genetics. *Nursing Inquiry, 14*(1), 13–22.

Apostolo, J. L. A., Viveiros, C. S. C., Nunes, H. I. R., & Domingues, H. R. F. (2007). Illness uncertainty and treatment motivation in type 2 diabetes patients. *Revista Latino-Americana De Enfermagem, 15*(4), 575–582.

Artsanthia, J., Mawn, B. E., Chaiphibalsarisdi, P., Nityasuddhi, D., & Triamchaisri, S. K. (2011). Exploring the palliative care needs of people living in Thailand with end-stage renal disease: A pilot study. *Journal of Hospice and Palliative Nursing, 13*(6), 403–410.

Bailey, D. E., Jr., & Wallace, M. (2007). Critical review: Is watchful waiting a viable management option for older men with prostate cancer? *American Journal of Men's Health, 1*(1), 18–28.

Berger, R. J., Corroto, C., Flad, J., & Quinney, R. (2013). Navigating the terrain of medical diagnosis and treatment: Patient decision making and uncertainty. In N. K. Denzin (Ed.), *40th anniversary of studies in symbolic interaction* (vol. 40, pp. 363–394). Bingley, UK: Emerald Group Publishing Limited.

Bishop, M., Stenhoff, D. M., & Shepard, L. (2007). Psychosocial adaptation and quality of life in multiple sclerosis: Assessment of the disability centrality model. *Journal of Rehabilitation, 73*(1), 3–12.

Brashers, D. E., & Hogan, T. P. (2013). The appraisal and management of uncertainty: Implications for information-retrieval systems. *Information Processing & Management, 49*(6), 1241–1249.

Brown, R. T., Fuemmeler, B., Anderson, D., et al. (2007). Adjustment of children and their mothers with breast cancer. *Journal of Pediatric Psychology, 32*(3), 297–308.

Budych, K., Helms, T. M., & Schultz, C. (2012). How do patients with rare diseases experience the medical encounter? Exploring role behavior and its impact on patient-physician interaction. *Health Policy, 105*(2–3), 154–164.

Bunkers, S. S. (2007). The experience of feeling unsure for women at end-of-life. *Nursing Science Quarterly, 20*(1), 56–63.

Carpentier, M. Y., Mullins, L. L., Wagner, J. L., Wolfe-Christensen, C., & Chaney, J. M. (2007). Examination of the cognitive diathesis-stress conceptualization of the hopelessness theory of depression in children with chronic illness: The moderating influence of illness uncertainty. *Childrens Health Care, 36*(2), 181–196.

Christensen, D. (2015). The health change trajectory model: An integrated model of HEA change. *Advances in Nursing Science, 38*, 55–67.

Colagreco, J. P., Bailey, D. E., Fitzpatrick, J. J., Musil, C. M., Afdhal, N. H., & Lai, M. (2014). Watchful waiting: Role of disease progression on uncertainty and depressive symptoms in patients with chronic hepatitis C. *Journal of Viral Hepatitis, 21*(10), 727–733.

Davidson, P. M., Dracup, K., Phillips, J., Padilla, G., & Daly, J. (2007). Maintaining hope in transition: A theoretical framework to guide interventions for people with heart failure. *Journal of Cardiovascular Nursing, 22*(1), 58–64.

Donovan, E. E., Brown, L. E., LeFebvre, L., Tardif, S., & Love, B. (2015). "The uncertainty is what is driving me crazy": The tripartite model of uncertainty in the adolescent and young adult cancer context. *Health Communication, 30*, 702–713.

Donovan-Kicken, E., & Bute, J. J. (2008). Uncertainty of social network members in the case of communication—debilitating illness or injury. *Qualitative Health Research, 18*(1), 5–18.

Drageset, S., Lindstrom, T. C., Giske, T., & Underlid, K. (2011). Being in suspense: Women's experiences awaiting breast cancer surgery. *Journal of Advanced Nursing, 67*(9), 1941–1951.

Elphee, E. E. (2008). Understanding the concept of uncertainty in patients with indolent lymphoma. *Oncology Nursing Forum, 35*(3), 449–454.

Fedele, D. A., Ramsey, R. R., Ryan, J. L., et al. (2011). The association of illness uncertainty to parent and youth adjustment in juvenile rheumatic diseases: Effect of youth age. *Journal of Developmental and Behavioral Pediatrics, 32*(5), 361–367.

Gill, E. A., & Babrow, A. S. (2007). To hope or to know: Coping with uncertainty and ambivalence in women's magazine breast cancer articles. *Journal of Applied Communication Research, 35*(2), 133–155.

Giske, T., & Artinian, B. (2008). Patterns of 'balancing between hope and despair' in the diagnostic phase: A grounded theory study of patients on a gastroenterology ward. *Journal of Advanced Nursing, 62*(1), 22–31.

Giske, T., & Gjengedal, E. (2007). "Preparative waiting" and coping theory with patients going through gastric diagnosis. *Journal of Advanced Nursing, 57*(1), 87–94.

Haugh, K. H., & Salyer, J. (2007). Needs of patients and families during the wait for a donor heart. *Heart & Lung, 36*(5), 319–329.

Hoth, K. F., Wamboldt, F. S., Ford, D. W., et al. (2015). The social environment and illness uncertainty in chronic obstructive pulmonary disease. *International Journal of Behavioral Medicine, 22*, 223–232.

Jordan, A. L., Eccleston, C., & Osborn, M. (2007). Being a parent of the adolescent with complex chronic pain: An interpretative phenomenological analysis. *European Journal of Pain, 11*(1), 49–56.

Ju, H. O., McElmurry, B. J., Park, C. G., McCreary, L., Kim, M., & Kim, E. J. (2011). Anxiety and uncertainty in Korean mothers of children with febrile convulsion: Cross-sectional survey. *Journal of Clinical Nursing, 20*(9–10), 1490–1497.

Kagan, I., & Bar-Tal, Y. (2008). The effect of preoperative uncertainty and anxiety on short-term recovery after elective arthroplasty. *Journal of Clinical Nursing, 17*(5), 576–583.

Kang, Y. (2011). The relationships between uncertainty and its antecedents in Korean patients with atrial fibrillation. *Journal of Clinical Nursing, 20*(13–14), 1880–1886.

Kasper, J., Geiger, F., Freiberger, S., & Schmidt, A. (2008). Decision-related uncertainties perceived by people with cancer: Modeling the subject of shared decision making. *Psycho-Oncology, 17*(1), 42–48.

Kazer, M. W., Bailey, D. E., Jr., Chipman, J., et al. (2013). Uncertainty and perception of danger among patients undergoing treatment for prostate cancer. *Bju International, 111*(3B), E84–E91.

Kosenko, K. A., Hurley, R. J., & Harvey, J. A. (2012). Sources of the uncertainty experienced by women with HPV. *Qualitative Health Research, 22*(4), 534–545.

Lee, Y. L., Santacroce, S. J., & Sadler, L. (2007). Predictors of healthy behaviour in long-term survivors of childhood cancer. *Journal of Clinical Nursing, 16*(11C), 285–295.

Lopez, R. P., & Guarino, A. J. (2011). Uncertainty and decision making for residents with dementia. *Clinical Nursing Research, 20*(3), 228–240.

Maher, K., & de Vries, K. (2011). An exploration of the lived experiences of individuals with relapsed multiple myeloma. *European Journal of Cancer Care, 20*(2), 267–275.

Malbasa, T., Kodish, E., & Santacroce, S. J. (2007). Adolescent adherence to oral therapy for leukemia: A focus group study. *Journal of Pediatric Oncology Nursing, 24*(3), 139–151.

Martens, T. Z., & Emed, J. D. (2007). The experiences and challenges of pregnant women coping with thrombophilia. *Journal of Obstetric Gynecologic and Neonatal Nursing, 36*(1), 55–62.

Mazanec, S. R., Daly, B. J., Douglas, S., & Musil, C. (2011). Predictors of psychosocial adjustment during the postradiation treatment transition. *Western Journal of Nursing Research, 33*(4), 540–559.

Middleton, A. V., LaVoie, N. R., & Brown, L. E. (2012). Sources of uncertainty in type 2 diabetes: Explication and implications for health communication theory and clinical practice. *Health Communication, 27*(6), 591–601.

Mullins, L. L., Wolfe-Christensen, C., Pai, A. L. H., et al. (2007). The relationship of parental overprotection, perceived child vulnerability, and parenting stress to uncertainty in youth with chronic illness. *Journal of Pediatric Psychology, 32*(8), 973–982.

Mutebi, M., & Edge, J. (2014). Stigma, survivorship and solutions: Addressing the challenges of living with breast cancer in low-resource areas. *SAMJ: South African Medical Journal, 104*, 382–382.

Pai, A. L. H., Mullins, L. L., Drotar, D., Burant, C., Wagner, J., & Chaney, J. M. (2007). Exploratory and confirmatory factor analysis of the child uncertainty in illness scale among children with chronic illness. *Journal of Pediatric Psychology, 32*(3), 288–296.

Pelletier, J. (2012). *Appraisal of uncertainty while waiting for a kidney transplant.* Unpublished dissertation, East Carolina University, Greenville, NC.

Penrod, J. (2007). Living with uncertainty: Concept advancement. *Journal of Advanced Nursing, 57*(6), 658–667.

Persson, E., Lindholm, E., Berndtsson, I., Lundstam, U., Hulten, L., & Carlsson, E. (2012). Experiences of living with increased risk of developing colorectal and gynaecological cancer in individuals with no identified gene mutation. *Scandinavian Journal of Caring Sciences, 26*(1), 20–27.

Pickles, T., Ruether, J. D., Weir, L., Carlson, L., & Jakulj, F. (2007). Psychosocial barriers to active surveillance for the management of early prostate cancer and a strategy for increased acceptance. *BJU International, 100*(3), 544–551.

Politi, M. C., Han, P. K. J., & Col, N. F. (2007). Communicating the uncertainty of harms and benefits of medical interventions. *Medical Decision Making, 27*(5), 681–695.

Puterman, J., & Cadell, S. (2008). Timing is everything: The experience of parental cancer for young adult daughters—A pilot study. *Journal of Psychosocial Oncology, 26*(2), 103–121.

Rosen, N. O., Knauper, B., & Sammut, J. (2007). Do individual differences in intolerance of uncertainty affect health monitoring? *Psychology & Health, 22*(4), 413–430.

Ryan, J. L., Ramsey, R. R., Fedele, D. A., Wagner, J. L. Chaney, J. M., & Mullins, L. L. (2011). The relationship of father parenting capacity variables to perceived uncertainty in youth with a chronic illness. *Children's Health Care, 40*(4), 297–310.

Rybarczyk, B., Grady, K. L., Naftel, D. C., et al. (2007). Emotional adjustment 5 years after heart transplant: A multisite study. *Rehabilitation Psychology, 52*(2), 206–214.

Shaha, M., Cox, C. L., Talman, K., & Kelly, D. (2008). Uncertainty in breast, prostate, and colorectal cancer: Implications for supportive care. *Journal of Nursing Scholarship, 40*(1), 60–67.

Shaida, N., Jones, C., Ravindranath, N., et al. (2007). Patient satisfaction with nurse-led telephone consultation for the follow-up of patients with prostate cancer. *Prostate Cancer & Prostatic Diseases, 10*(4), 369–373.

Shih, F. J., Gau, M. L., Kao, C. C., et al. (2007). Dying and caring on the edge: Taiwan's surviving nurses' reflections on taking care of patients with severe acute respiratory syndrome. *Applied Nursing Research, 20*(4), 171–180.

Song, L. X., Northouse, L. L., Zhang, L. L., et al. (2012). Study of dyadic communication in couples managing prostate cancer: A longitudinal perspective. *Psych-Oncology, 21*(1), 72–81.

Sossong, A. (2007). Living with an implantable cardioverter defibrillator: Patient outcomes and the nurse's role. *Journal of Cardiovascular Nursing, 22*(2), 99–104.

Stewart, A. M., Polak, E., Young, R., Schultz, I. Z. (2012). Injured workers' construction of expectations of return to work with sub-acute back pain: The role of perceived uncertainty. *Journal of Occupational Rehabilitation, 22*(1), 1–14.

Taylor, C., Richardson, A., & Cowley, S. (2011). Surviving cancer treatment: An investigation of the experience of fear about, and monitoring for, recurrence in patients following treatment for colorectal cancer. *European Journal of Oncology Nursing, 15*(3), 243–249.

Truitt, M., Biesecker, B., Capone, G., Bailey, T., & Erby, L. (2012). The role of hope in adaptation to uncertainty: The experience of caregivers of children with Down syndrome. *Patient Education and Counseling, 87*(2), 233–238.

Wu, P. X., Guo, W. Y., Xia, H. O., Lu, H. J., & Xi, S. X. (2011). Patients' experience of living with glaucoma: A phenomenological study. *Journal of Advanced Nursing, 67*(4), 800–810.

29

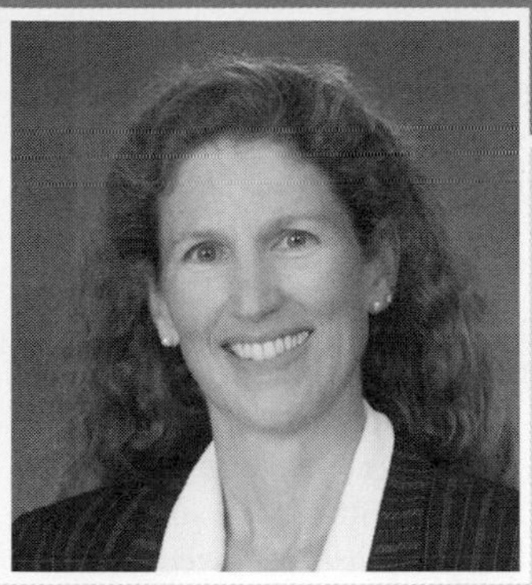

Pamela G. Reed*
(1952–Present)

Self-Transcendence Theory

Pamela G. Reed

"The quest for nursing is to understand the nature of and to facilitate nursing processes."
(Reed, 1997a, p. 77)

CREDENTIALS AND BACKGROUND OF THE THEORIST

Pamela G. Reed was born in Detroit, Michigan, an exciting place to grow up in the 1960s. She married her husband, Gary, in 1973, and they have two daughters. Reed received her bachelor of science degree in nursing from Wayne State University in Detroit, Michigan, in 1974 and earned her master's in nursing in psychiatric–mental health of children and adolescents and in nursing education in 1976. During the interim between earning her master's and doctoral degrees, Reed taught at Oakland University School of Nursing in Rochester, Michigan, and worked part time as a clinical nurse specialist in child-adolescent psychiatric–mental health nursing. Reed received her doctorate in 1982 from Wayne State University with a concentration in nursing theory and lifespan developmental psychology. She pioneered nursing research into spirituality beginning with her doctoral dissertation, directed by Joyce J. Fitzpatrick, focusing on the relationship between well-being and spiritual perspectives on life and death in terminally ill and well individuals. Her self-transcendence theory was a second major scholarly focus from her doctoral studies in nursing and lifespan developmental sciences.

Reed is a professor at the University of Arizona College of Nursing in Tucson, where she also served as Associate Dean for Academic Affairs for 7 years. Her major fields of research include spirituality, mental health in older adults, and ethical dimensions of end-of-life care. Reed developed two widely used research instruments, the *Spiritual Perspectives Scale* and the *Self-Transcendence Scale.* She has published many articles, with recent publications addressing practice knowledge and epistemic justice for nurses and patients. Reed and her coauthor Shearer published *Nursing Knowledge and Theory Innovation: Advancing the Science of Nursing Practice,* promoting a philosophy and methods of practice-based knowledge development. Reed and Shearer are also coeditors of the nursing theory text *Perspectives on Nursing Theory.*

Reed is a fellow in the American Academy of Nursing and a member of a number of professional organizations, including Sigma Theta Tau International, the American Nurses Association, and the Society of Rogerian Scholars. She has been visiting professor at New York University, Duke University, and Florida Atlantic University. She serves on the editorial review boards of several journals and is Contributing Editor for *Nursing Science Quarterly* and *Applied Nursing Research.* Reed recently received a master's of arts degree in philosophy and ethics from the University of Arizona.

THEORETICAL SOURCES

Reed (1991a) developed her self-transcendence theory using the strategy of **deductive reformulation** *to synthesize her theoretical ideas.* This strategy involves a step before synthesizing theoretical ideas, that of modifying or reformulating

*Photo credit: David VanGelder, Tucson, AZ.

existing theories to better align ideas with the theorist's philosophical views and state of the science. To develop self-transcendence theory, lifespan theories on adult social-cognitive and transpersonal development were aligned with the nursing perspective of Martha E. Rogers' (1970, 1980, 1990) conceptual system of unitary human beings. The lifespan perspective of adulthood and aging had mounting scientific evidence that development occurs throughout aging and dying processes and that development occurs by a process of increasing complexity and organization. These ideas were congruent with Rogerian thought and enriched Reed's theory development.

The theoretical work of nursing theorist Martha E. Rogers (1970, 1980, 1990) posits three principles of homeodynamics, which were congruent with the key principles of lifespan developmental theory and science. Rogers' integrality principle identified development as a function of both human and contextual factors; it also identified disequilibrium between person and environment as an important trigger of development. Rogers' helicy principle characterized human development as innovative and unpredictable. This principle is similar to lifespan principles identifying development as nonlinear, continuous throughout the lifespan, and evident in variability within and across individuals and groups. Rogers' resonancy principle described human development as a process of movement that, although unpredictable, had pattern and purpose. Lifespan theorists also proposed that the process of development displayed patterns of complexity and organization. Thus the lifespan developmental perspective was generally congruent with Rogers' ideas, and only minor modifications occurred in the synthesis of theoretical ideas.

Another significant source for self-transcendence theory was evidence from nursing practice and research indicating a relationship between mental health and development; Reed read and observed consistently that those with mental health problems often had fewer developmentally based psychological and cognitive resources to support their well-being. In addition, early research showed that clinically depressed older persons reported fewer developmental resources to sustain their sense of well-being in the face of decreased physical and cognitive abilities than did a matched group of mentally healthy older adults (Reed, 1986b). Also, development in older and oldest-old adults was found to be a nonlinear process of gain and subsequent loss, a process of transforming or trading away old perspectives and behaviors and integrating new views and activities (Reed, 1989, 1991b). Furthermore, Reed's practice knowledge acquired as a clinical nurse specialist in psychiatric–mental health nursing with children and adolescents also supported this idea. Practice knowledge of children and adolescents was modified and applied to adulthood and aging. Similar findings continue to be documented in the literature.

MAJOR CONCEPTS & DEFINITIONS

Vulnerability

Vulnerability refers to awareness that personal or physical well-being is at risk. Life events or crises such as life-threatening illness or loss may increase awareness of personal mortality. This awareness may motivate development or maturation at any developmental stage, including later adulthood and end of life. The concept of vulnerability broadens the awareness of personal mortality situations to include life events such as disability, chronic illness, childbirth and childrearing, and parenting. Self-transcendence is a process of maturing development that occurs within these kinds of contexts (Reed, 1991b).

Self-Transcendence

Self-transcendence is the expansion of self-boundaries multidimensionally such as the following: inwardly (toward greater awareness of one's own beliefs, values, and goals through introspective activities); outwardly (toward others and the environment); temporally (toward integration of past and future in a way that enhances the relative present); and transpersonally (to connect with dimensions beyond the typically discernible world) (Reed, 1991a, 1997b, 2014).

Well-Being

Well-being is "the sense of feeling whole and healthy, in accord with one's own criteria for wholeness and well-being" (Reed, 2014, p. 112). In a *Nursing Science Quarterly* article, "Nursing: The Ontology of the Discipline," Reed described the underlying mechanisms of well-being and proposed nursing to be "the study of nursing processes of well-being" (Reed, 1997a, p. 76). Well-being as a nursing process is described in terms of a synthesis of two kinds of change: changes in complexity in a life (for example, the increasing frailness of advanced aging or the accumulation of losses or significant events in life) tempered by changes in integration (for example, the organization of ideas in constructing meaning from such life events, or the reorganization of aspects in one's life).

MAJOR CONCEPTS & DEFINITIONS—cont'd

Mediating-Moderating Factors

Research findings indicate that self-transcendence is a **mediator** between vulnerability and well-being outcomes. Self-transcendence, then, is a mechanism or process by which individuals can experience well-being in the context of vulnerability. In addition, a variety of personal and contextual variables and their interactions may influence the process of self-transcendence by **moderating** relationships among vulnerability, self-transcendence, and well-being. Examples of these variables include age, gender, cognitive ability, life experiences, health status, spiritual perspectives, social environment, and historical events. These variables may strengthen or weaken relationships between vulnerability and self-transcendence and between self-transcendence and well-being (Reed, 2014). Nursing activities and interventions may be designed to facilitate self-transcendence (as a mediator factor) or to influence moderating factors as they relate to well-being.

USE OF EMPIRICAL EVIDENCE

Self-transcendence theory is grounded in an assumption about the developmental capacity of older adults and the necessity of continued development to maintain mental health and a sense of well-being during the process of aging (Reed, 1983). Therefore Reed's initial research in theory building was conducted with older adults (1986b, 1989, 1991b). An important step in facilitating this research was constructing a measure of this developmental capacity. Reed developed and tested her *Developmental Resources of Later Adulthood* (DRLA) instrument, which was useful in launching empirical study into what would become the self-transcendence theory.

In the first study, Reed (1986b) examined patterns of developmental resources and depression over time in 28 mentally healthy and 28 clinically depressed older adults (mean age, 67.4 years). Levels of developmental resources were measured three times (6 weeks apart) with the 36-item DRLA scale. Healthy adults perceived higher levels of resources across time than did depressed adults. Scores on the Center for Epidemiological Studies Depression (CES-D) scale (Radloff, 1977) were significantly higher in depressed individuals across time than were those of the mentally healthy. Strong relationships between DRLA scores and subsequent CES-D scores indicated that developmental resources influenced mental health outcomes in the healthy group; the reverse relationship found in the depressed group indicated that depression negatively influenced developmental resources in terms of the ability to explore new outlooks on life, to share wisdom and experience with others, and to find spiritual meaning.

In the second study, Reed (1989) explored the degree to which key developmental resources of later adulthood were related to mental health in 30 hospitalized clinically depressed older adults (mean age, 67 years). Participants completed the DRLA and CES-D measures and rated the importance in their current lives of each developmental resource reflected in the DRLA items. An inverse correlation was found between the level of resources and depression. Participants also reported that the resources represented by the DRLA items were highly important in their lives. In addition, key reasons given by participants for their psychiatric hospitalization were congruent with self-transcendence issues significant in later adulthood (e.g., physical health concerns, relationships with adult children, questions about life and death).

During the initial DRLA instrument development and testing, a factor labeled *transcendence* accounted for nearly half of the variance in DRLA scores. In the second study (Reed, 1989), the 15-item transcendence factor was also more highly correlated with the CES-D than was the entire DRLA. Therefore a recommendation for future research was to further examine the psychometric properties of the instrument, with a goal to shorten the DRLA to facilitate ease of administration in clinical settings.

A third study explored patterns of self-transcendence and mental health in 55 independent-living older adults (ranging from 80 to 97 years of age) (Reed, 1991b). In this study, self-transcendence was defined as "the expansion of one's conceptual boundaries inwardly through introspective activities, outwardly through concerns about other's welfare, and temporally by integrating perceptions of one's past and future to enhance the present" (Reed, 1991b, p. 5). Self-transcendence was measured by the newly developed Self-Transcendence Scale (STS), derived from the previously identified transcendence factor in the original DRLA scale. The STS score was inversely correlated with both CES-D and Langner Scale of Mental Health Symptomatology (MHS) scores. The MHS is an index of general mental health on which higher scores indicate impairment in mental health in nonpsychiatric populations (Langner, 1962). In addition, the four patterns of self-transcendence identified by participants (generativity, introjectivity, temporal integration, and body-transcendence) were congruent with Reed's definition of the concept.

In summary, these early studies provided initial evidence for development of the theoretical idea that self-transcendence views and behaviors were, in fact, present in older adults, and that such views and behaviors were strongly positively related to mental health. These findings supported a conceptualization of mental health in later adulthood that went beyond preoccupation with physical and cognitive declines to acknowledge resources that expanded self-boundaries in aging. Since these early studies, many research findings that support this view of self-transcendence theory continue to be published. Several of these studies are cited in the following sections.

MAJOR ASSUMPTIONS

A key assumption underlying self-transcendence theory is based on Rogers' (1970, 1980) conceptualization of human beings as open systems, integral with their environment. However, this openness does not mean that human beings are indistinguishable from their environment. It is known from cognitive science and psychological sciences that individuals perceive or conceive various boundaries between self and environment in distinct ways over development. An assumption underlying Reed's self-transcendence theory is that humans impose conceptual boundaries upon themselves to define their reality and to provide a sense of wholeness and connectedness within themselves and their environment. Self-boundaries fluctuate across the lifespan and are associated with human health and development.

A second major underlying assumption is that self-transcendence is a developmental imperative (Reed, 2014); that is, self-transcendence must be expressed like any other developmental capacity in life for a person to realize a continuing sense of wholeness and connectedness. This assumption is congruent with Frankl's (1969) and Maslow's (1971) conceptualizations of self-transcendence as an innate human characteristic relevant to well-being.

THEORETICAL ASSERTIONS

There are three basic concepts in the self-transcendence theory: vulnerability, self-transcendence, and well-being (Reed, 2014, 2015). Vulnerability is the awareness of personal mortality or some risk to well-being that arises during development and aging and during health events and life crises (Reed, 2014). The concept of vulnerability clarifies that the context within which self-transcendence is realized is not only when confronting end-of-own-life issues but also includes life events such as disability, chronic illness, childbirth, and parenting.

Self-transcendence refers to the fluctuations in perceived boundaries that extend persons beyond their immediate and constricted views of self and the world. The fluctuations are multidimensional: outward (toward awareness of others and the environment), inward (toward greater insight into one's own beliefs, values, and goals), temporal (toward integration of past and future in a way that enhances the relative present), and transpersonal (toward awareness of dimensions beyond the typically discernible world) (Reed, 1997b, 2014).

Well-being is "the sense of feeling whole and healthy, in accord with one's own criteria for wholeness and well-being" (Reed, 2014, p. 112). The theory also allows for additional personal and contextual variables such as age, gender, life experiences, and social environment that can influence the relationships among the three basic concepts. Interventions would focus on nursing activities that facilitate self-transcendence as a process of well-being that occurs in various life contexts.

Four major propositions of the theory were developed based upon several sources. These sources include philosophical assumptions, theoretical and empirical support published in scholarly literature, and practice-based knowledge.

The first proposition is that self-transcendence may be motivated by experiences of vulnerability. *Vulnerability* is defined broadly as it occurs within life events of loss, illness, aging, end-of-life, and other experiences that increase awareness of personal mortality. Individuals may develop or mature in their life perspectives (and increase self-transcendence) as a result of experiencing vulnerabilities. However, without adequate support for development, increased vulnerability may relate to decreased self-transcendence.

The second proposition is that self-transcendence is positively related to well-being (Reed, 1991a). Alternatively, decreased self-transcendence (as in the inability to reach out to others or to accept friendship) is positively related to depression as an indicator of decreased well-being or mental health. An important refinement to self-transcendence theory relates to the mediating effects of self-transcendence.

The third proposition is based on research results accumulated in the past decade. That is, that self-transcendence mediates the relationship between vulnerability and well-being to promote well-being in situations of increased vulnerability. In other words, self-transcendence is an underlying process or mechanism that explains why people may attain well-being when confronted with increased vulnerability.

A fourth set of propositions draws from Rogers' (1980) principle of integrality, which describes an ongoing

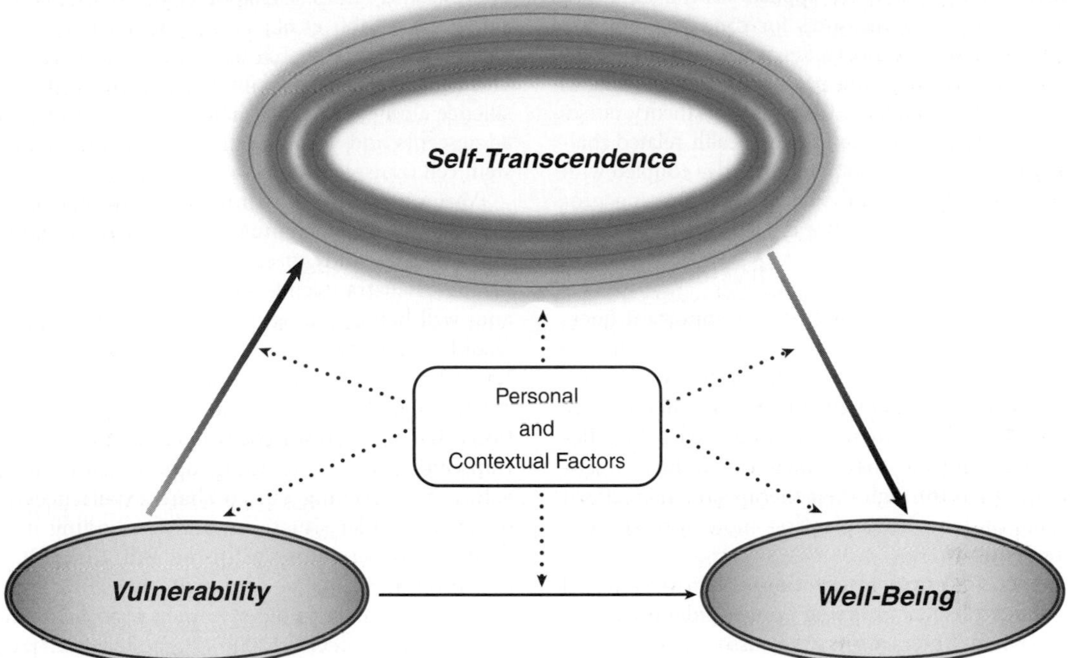

FIG. 29.1 Model of Self-Transcendence Theory. (Used with permission by P. G. Reed. From Reed, P. G. [2014]. The theory of self-transcendence. In M. J. Smith & P. R Liehr [Eds.], *Middle Range Theory for Nursing* [3rd ed.]. New York: Springer.)

person-environment process across the lifespan. Personal and environmental factors function as correlates that may moderate relationships among vulnerability, self-transcendence, and well-being.

In summary, self-transcendence theory proposes the following four sets of relationships (Fig. 29.1):

1. Increased vulnerability is related to self-transcendence. This may be a positive relationship with adequate support.
2. Self-transcendence is positively related to well-being.
3. Self-transcendence also may function as a mediator between vulnerability and well-being.
4. Personal and contextual factors may influence the relationship between vulnerability and self-transcendence and between self-transcendence and well-being.

LOGICAL FORM

Reed's empirical middle-range theory was constructed using the strategy of deductive reformulation in which the logic of inference was primarily deductive—deducing midrange theoretical principles from broader Rogerian and lifespan theories. Analogical reasoning was also used whereby conclusions about self-transcendence are drawn from analyzing comparisons among various theories, including lifespan psychology and nursing on human development and potential for well-being across all phases of life. The key concepts of the theory are related in a clear and logical manner, while allowing for creativity in the way the theory is applied, tested, and further developed. Reed's principal strategy of constructing a nursing theory—from nonnursing theories, a nursing conceptual model, and evidence from practice and research—piqued nurses' interest in developmental perspectives of well-being and provided impetus for further theorizing about the variety of health-related experiences of vulnerability that challenge individuals' well-being.

ACCEPTANCE BY THE NURSING COMMUNITY

The quest for nursing is to facilitate human well-being through what Reed calls "nursing processes," of which self-transcendence is one example (Reed, 1997a). Self-transcendence theory and the STS have been widely used in practice, education, and research. In addition, some researchers have used only the STS to investigate another similar theory. Other investigators have applied self-transcendence theory while using other measures for concepts similar to those in self-transcendence theory. Regardless, research findings overall support a nursing perspective of well-being as promoted by self-transcendence theory. By this theory, nurses facilitate well-being in individuals facing health-related challenges using their nursing practice knowledge coupled with their basic knowledge of individuals' inner nursing processes, of which self-transcendence is a major one.

Practice

From a nursing practice perspective, an important question is whether it is possible for nurses to influence self-transcendence. Although self-transcendence is conceptualized as an inner resource, nurses may still influence this process, because it then influences well-being. Research findings indicate that nurses can influence self-transcendence both through their therapeutic interactions with patients and by implementing more formally designed interventions.

In reference to **nurse interactions**, a cross-sectional study of cognitively intact nursing home residents showed that nurse–patient interactions were associated with increases in the intrapersonal and interpersonal dimensions of self-transcendence (Haugan, 2014; Haugan, Hanssen, & Mokenes, 2013). In addition, there are various healing practices guided by nurse interactions that facilitate self-transcendence by helping individuals to expand personal boundaries in mentally healthy ways (Coward & Reed, 1996; Reed, 1991a). Nurses may facilitate these practices in their interactions with patients. These include journaling, art and music activities; meditation; life review and self-reflection; and religious or other expressions of altruism, faith, and hope.

Specific practices and interventions have been studied for their role in promoting self-transcendence and well-being. Responses of several people with late-stage Alzheimer disease after a "creative bonding" art intervention evidenced increased self-transcendence and well-being (Walsh et al., 2011). A poetry-writing intervention for caregivers of older adults with dementia found themes of self-transcendence in caregivers after the intervention (Kidd, Zauszniewski, & Morris, 2011). A Psychoeducational Approach to Transcendence and Health (PATH) program was found to be a feasible and potentially effective approach to facilitate self-transcendence and promote well-being among community-living older adults (McCarthy et al., 2015). Another creative approach for self-transcendence involves the development of a computer-mediated self-help intervention to facilitate connections among lesbian, gay, bisexual, transsexual, and queer (and/or questioning) (LGBTQ) individuals with shared interests and values (DiNapoli et al., 2014). Haase and her colleagues (Robb et al., 2014) applied her resilience-in-illness model in research to examine a therapeutic music video intervention to facilitate self-transcendence and resilience along with other factors relevant to well-being in adolescents and young adults undergoing hematopoietic stem cell transplantation.

Various **group-based interventions** have been studied for their role in facilitating self-transcendence. In a quasi-experimental study, peer support groups were found to facilitate self-transcendence and promote physical health and well-being among persons with multiple sclerosis (Jadid-Milani et al., 2015). Group psychotherapy (Young & Reed, 1995) and breast cancer support groups (Coward, 1998, 2003; Coward & Kahn, 2004, 2005) are interventions that nurse researchers have used to facilitate self-transcendence by providing opportunities to examine values, for reaching out to share experiences and help others in similar situations, and for finding meaning in their health situations. Stinson and Kirk (2006) used group reminiscence to decrease depression and increase self-transcendence in older women residing in an assisted living facility. McGee (2000) suggested that recovery in alcoholism involves self-transcendence, facilitated by a nurse-designed environment that supports the 12 steps and 12 traditions of Alcoholics Anonymous.

Education

Self-transcendence theory is relevant to nursing education in several ways. First, the theory informs students about a substantive focus of nursing, that of facilitating well-being through resources within the person and creative interactions with nurses. Also, theory-based interventions and nursing interactions can be taught to students for applications in their work with vulnerable individuals.

Second, the concept of self-transcendence has been identified in nursing scholars' writings on the philosophical foundations of nursing as a central concept in nursing (Malinski, 2006; Newman, 1986; Parse, 1981; Rogers, 1970, 1980; Sarter, 1988; Watson, 1979). The concept has historical as well as contemporary relevance in nursing education for promoting understanding of a focus of the discipline.

Third, in addition to the substance of the theory, the theory provides an opportunity to learn about the process of theory development and refinement. Therefore the theory is relevant across the levels of educational content in nursing, from baccalaureate to doctoral level, for practice and research.

Lastly, and importantly, education about self-transcendence theory is relevant in supporting students who, as future nurses, will be confronted with difficult situations that may increase their own vulnerability and affect their well-being. Self-transcendence is a pathway for helping the healer, or healing the healer, so that nurses learn to maintain a healthy lifestyle as they care for others (Conti-O'Hare, 2002). Research findings indicate that nurses can benefit from self-transcendence attitudes and behaviors. For example, a theory-based art activity with older adults at community senior centers helped nursing students expand their own boundaries and acquire more positive attitudes in working with older adults (Chen & Walsh, 2009; Walsh et al., 2008). In other studies, self-transcendence perspectives correlated with lower levels of burnout in hospice and oncology nurses (Hunnibell et al., 2008) with higher levels of work engagement in acute care nurses (Palmer et al., 2010), and with well-being of nurses with alcoholism (McGee, 2000, 2004).

Research

The theory-based practices and interventions addressed in the previous section begin with initial research into potential factors and relationships. This section presents an overview of clusters of research that can provide foundations for subsequent intervention-based research. Studies have focused on certain groups and health experiences, such as individuals with depression and other mental health problems, life-threatening illness, and chronic illness; individuals in long-term care as well as in the community; oldest-old and middle-age adults; and family caregivers.

Initial research focused on depression, with findings supporting significant relationships between self-transcendence and severity or occurrence of depression in older adults (Reed, 1986b, 1989, 1991a). Other research reported similar relationships in depressed older adults (Klaas, 1998; Stinson & Kirk, 2006; Young & Reed, 1995), and middle-age adults (Ellermann & Reed, 2001). In a study among older Taiwanese people living in nursing homes, self-transcendence was strongly and negatively related to depressive symptoms (Hsu et al., 2013). Self-transcendence theory has also been applied to the study of suicidal older adults (Buchanan, Ferran, & Clark,1995). Walton et al. (1991) identified an inverse relationship between self-transcendence and loneliness in healthy older adults.

Several research studies provide evidence to support the association between self-transcendence and increased well-being in populations confronted with life-threatening illness. Results from several studies have demonstrated positive relationships among self-transcendence and well-being or quality of life in persons with human immunodeficiency virus (HIV) or acquired immune deficiency syndrome (AIDS) (Coward, 1994, 1995; Coward & Lewis, 1993; McCormick et al., 2001; Mellors et al., 2001; Mellors, Riley, & Erlen, 1997; Sperry, 2011; Stevens, 1999). Numerous studies have described the significance of self-transcendence in women with breast cancer (Carpenter, Brockopp, & Andrykowski, 1999; Coward, 1990, 1991; Coward & Kahn, 2004, 2005; Farren, 2010; Kinney, 1996; Matthews & Cook, 2009; Pelusi, 1997; Taylor, 2000; Thomas et al., 2010). Other populations in which self-transcendence was found to be significant include elderly men with prostate cancer (Chin-A-Loy & Fernsler, 1998), elders with chronic heart failure (Gusick, 2008), liver transplant recipients (Bean & Wagner, 2006), stem cell transplant recipients (Williams, 2012), and homeless adults (Runquist & Reed, 2007).

Self-transcendence also has been found important for successful aging among those 80 years and older (McCarthy, Ling, & Carini, 2013) and in older adults' perceptions of positive physical and mental health (Bickerstaff, Grasser, & McCabe, 2003; Nygren et al., 2005). It is positively related to engagement in activities of daily living and self-care in noninstitutionalized older adults and healthy middle-aged adults (Coward, 1996; Upchurch,1999; Upchurch & Mueller, 2005).

Among individuals in long-term care or other facilities, self-transcendence is significantly related to well-being. Results from several studies by Haugan and her colleagues consistently support self-transcendence as a significant resource for various dimensions of well-being among cognitively intact older adults in long-term care (Haugan et al., 2013, 2014) and something to be fostered by nurse–patient interaction (Haugan, 2014; Haugan, Hanssen, & Mokenes, 2013). Results from a longitudinal study did not support a direct relationship between self-transcendence and survival of the oldest-old but suggested that self-transcendence facilitated other factors such as social contact, outdoor activities, and other functions that may increase longevity in the presence of life-limiting medical conditions of aging (Norberg et al., 2015).

Several investigators have studied self-transcendence as a component of inner strength (Lundman et al., 2012; Nygren et al., 2005; Viglund et al., 2014) using a theory and measure very similar to that of self-transcendence. They described inner strength as a dynamic and developmental process, measured as an index of sense of coherence, resilience, purpose in life, and self-transcendence (Lundman et al., 2012). Research findings supported the hypothesis that inner strength is at least a partial mediator of the relationship between having a serious disease and self-rated health among older adults.

Moe (2013) and others studied inner strength, with self-transcendence as one of the major components of this concept. Inner strength was measured by the STS and other instruments as related to physical and mental health in a sample of chronically ill oldest-old women and men. A major conclusion was that, although chronically ill oldest-old persons are more vulnerable than younger people, they also have the resource of inner strength to not only cope with life, but to find enjoyment in life. Positive relationships among transcendence and transformation and finding meaning were also described in women living in the community with chronic conditions such as arthritis (Neill, 2002; Shearer, Fleury, & Reed, 2009).

The theory has practice implications for family caregivers. Acton (2003), Acton and Wright (2000), and Kidd, Zauszniewski, and Morris (2011) explored self-transcendence in caregivers of persons with dementia. Acton and Wright (2000) suggested arranging respite care for caregivers so that they have time and energy for transpersonal activities. In describing a case study of a person in the early stages of Alzheimer disease, Vitale, Shaffer, and Fenton (2014) promoted the theory's usefulness in guiding families in ways to enhance well-being in the family member. Self-transcendence was also found to be significant to well-being in caregivers of terminally ill patients who had died within the previous year (Enyert & Burman, 1999; Reed & Rousseau, 2007) and in other groups of bereaved individuals (Joffrion & Douglas, 1994) and those who had lost loved ones from HIV or AIDS (Kausch & Amer, 2007). Kim and colleagues (2011) found significant interdependence within Korean family caregiver–elder dyads on self-transcendence variables and well-being.

FURTHER DEVELOPMENT

Reed's initial conceptualization of self-transcendence focused on later adulthood and identified the importance of personal resources that expand self-boundaries beyond the concerns generated by physical decline resulting from aging or illness. Reed received funding to study self-transcendence as it relates to end-of-life decisions and well-being in patients and their family caregivers. People facing the end of life represent some of the most vulnerable individuals to whom nurses may provide care. Other scholars have broadened the theory to include younger adults with life-limiting conditions that may increase their vulnerability.

Research within the past decade has extended the scope of the theory to include a greater diversity of individuals who experience vulnerability and risks to their well-being—younger and older, patients and nonpatients, and various ethnicities. Examples of research focuses are Japanese hospitalized older adults (Hoshi & Reed, 2011), Korean older adults and their family caregivers (Kim et al., 2011), Amish adults in rural Ohio (Sharpnack et al., 2010, 2011), caregivers of older adults with dementia (Kidd, Zauszniewski, & Morris, 2011), low-income older adults (McCarthy, 2011), older adult residents in Norwegian nursing homes (Haugan, 2014; Haugan et al., 2014), and bullied middle-school boys (Willis & Grace, 2011; Willis & Griffith, 2010). Diverse personal and contextual variables affect the relationship between self-transcendence and well-being across individuals of different ages and life situations.

A recent noteworthy finding is that the accumulation of research results indicates that self-transcendence is a mediator between vulnerability and well-being, suggesting that it may function in interventions to facilitate well-being in individuals' experiences of increased vulnerability. For example, self-transcendence has been found to be a mediator in people with progressive diseases such as multiple sclerosis and systemic lupus erythematosus (Iwamoto, Yamawaki, & Sato, 2011), prostate cancer (Chin-A-Loy & Fernsler, 1998), and oral cancer (Chen, 2012).

Various teams of researchers continue to examine the instrument that measures self-transcendence (the STS) across different groups. Slight modifications have been made in applying it to adolescents, for example. Also, a Swedish group of investigators revised the STS for their sample, reducing the items from 15 to 10 (Lundman et al., 2015). The Scandinavian older adult nursing home population in which Haugan and colleagues (2012) studied self-transcendence generated two key factors in the measure, rather than the single-factor STS developed by Reed. However, Reed recognizes that although there may be many ways to expand boundaries (as it is theorized to be multidimensional, or even pandimensional), the concept of expanded boundaries is basically a single conceptual idea according to self-transcendence theory. Self-transcendence is a rich and somewhat abstract concept and thus may invite diverse interpretations depending on the research context and philosophical views of the investigator. Theory development is a dynamic process of inquiry.

Self-transcendence theory may undergo further refinement as inquiry progresses into other nursing processes of well-being in view of Reed's (1997a) reconceptualization of nursing. By this, Reed suggested broadening the definition of nursing to include not only external sources of nursing activity (the "nurse"), but also to acknowledge the nursing processes *within* human beings. Specifically, Reed defines nursing as a process of well-being that exists within and among human systems, characterized by changing complexity and integration. From this, she proposed self-transcendence as a nursing process. Further explorations into mechanisms of changing complexity and integration should help achieve new theoretical explanations about how self-transcendence emerges and functions in human lives. As the theory of self-transcendence is refined through practice and research, nurses may learn more about human potential for well-being over the lifespan.

CRITIQUE

Clarity

Clarity and consistency are key criteria in the description of and critical reflection on a theory (Chinn & Kramer, 2015). Theory clarity is evaluated by semantic and structural consistency. Semantic consistency evaluates how consistent concepts are used with their definitions and the basic assumptions of the theory. Structural consistency involves assessing congruency among the assumptions, theory purpose, concept definitions, and connections among the concepts. Although the concept of self-transcendence may at first seem too abstract, nurses have been able to appreciate and identify with it, in both their professional and their own lives. Theoretical sources for development of the theory are described clearly across several publications cited in this chapter. The definitions and assumptions about the concepts were straightforwardly derived from lifespan developmental theory and Rogers' science of unitary human beings. In terms of structural consistency, the relationships in schematic models of the theory (see Fig. 29.1) are fully defined, are congruent across theoretical sources, and are described consistently in various chapters published by Reed (2014, 2015). Structural consistency is good in that the identified relationships are logical and consistent.

It is not unusual to find concerns about clarity when a theory incorporates concepts that are somewhat abstract. Overall, however, Reed's theoretical thinking has remained congruent with the original Rogerian and lifespan conceptual views and assumptions underlying the theory. She conceptualized a theory that can be understood by both nurse clinicians and nurse researchers. In addition, many research findings support a strong relationship among the concepts as hypothesized by the theory, supporting the theory's empirical precision.

Simplicity

Reed's middle-range theory is parsimonious, with three major concepts (vulnerability, self-transcendence, and well-being) and their proposed interrelationships. The simplicity of the theory allows for wider application across populations, health experiences, and strategies and goals for well-being. The theory may increase in complexity if needed as specific personal and environmental factors and their relationships to the major concepts are identified in clinical applications. The major concepts and subconcepts (personal and contextual factors) and the number of relationships generated by these concepts are not too numerous yet are sufficient and meaningful in proposing key theoretical propositions.

Generality

The scope and purpose of Reed's theory are such that the theory can be applied to a wide variety of human health situations. The purpose of the theory is to enhance nurses' understanding about processes that promote well-being (Reed, 2014). Initially, Reed's work focused on developmental resources in persons confronted by challenges of later adulthood related to indicators of mental health symptomatology, specifically, clinical depression. In linking self-transcendence to mental health as an indicator of well-being, the scope of the theory expanded to include persons other than older adults who were facing increased vulnerability, such as life-threatening events.

Continued development and testing of the theory led to the specification of self-transcendence as a mediator between vulnerability and well-being, as well as a direct correlate of well-being (Reed, 2014, 2015). The theory is now broader in scope and maintains congruence with a lifespan perspective. The major concepts can be applied to anyone confronted with lifespan and situational events ranging from childbirth and other caregiving experiences, to successful aging, to living with a chronic or serious illness, and end of life. Broadening the scope and purpose of the theory from mental health to well-being increased its generality, resulting in a theory that is applicable in many situations of health and healing.

Accessibility

The criterion of accessibility refers to how well the concepts of the theory are linked to observable, empirical reality and to nursing practice (Chinn & Kramer, 2015). Numerous researchers have identified empirical indicators of the theoretical concepts that are meaningful to their contexts of inquiry. In particular, measurement of self-transcendence has been honed through the development and refinement of Reed's STS. In addition, the STS has been translated into many languages, including Spanish, Swedish, Korean, Mandarin, Iranian, Turkish, French, and Japanese. However, researchers may use other instruments to measure self-transcendence, because the concept lends itself to a variety of approaches and measures that fit the clinical nursing context of interest.

Importance

Self-transcendence theory is a middle-range theory grounded in nursing philosophy and practice and continues to be used in nursing education and tested and extended through research and practice applications. The theory provides insight into human developmental capacities for well-being across health situations relevant to nursing care. Nurses and patients face events that challenge their well-being. Knowledge about self-transcendence can be included in nurses' repertoire for facilitating well-being in times of vulnerability. The abstract yet definable nature of self-transcendence facilitates development of many interventions that may be tested as strategies to promote well-being in a variety of nurse–patient encounters.

SUMMARY

Self-transcendence theory was developed initially using deductive reformulation from lifespan developmental theories, Rogers' conceptual system of unitary human beings, empirical research, and clinical and personal experiences of the theorist. The theoretical concepts are abstract, but concrete subconcepts have been developed and studied extensively in a number of populations. Research findings support the hypothesized relationships among vulnerability, self-transcendence views and behaviors, and well-being. These studies help increase nurses' understanding that regardless of the health situation, people may retain a capacity for personal development and sense of well-being. Self transcendence, as a nursing process both within human beings and as practiced by nurses, is a resource for human well-being and its changing complexity over the lifespan.

CASE STUDY

Mr. Jones is a 65-year-old man whose wife died 6 months ago after a long illness. The couple had been married 45 years, and they were devoted to each other. They had three children who are now in their 30s. Two of the children live several hundred miles away, but one son lives with his wife and two preschool children less than 1 mile from Mr. Jones's home.

Mr. Jones provided much of the care for his wife during her illness. Although her care was time-consuming and fatiguing and kept him at home much of the time, he was grateful that he could care for her. He now is alone in their home, is very lonely and uninterested in preparing meals or eating, and lacks energy to return to his former community and social activities or even to interact with his son and family.

The hospice nurse contacted Mr. Jones for follow-up bereavement counseling. She told him that although he had "passed" a routine physical examination the week before, she was concerned about his continuing sadness and lack of energy. The nurse reassured him that it was not uncommon to grieve for many months after a major loss. She asked him if he thought his wife would have had a similar experience if he had been the first to die. His response was that his wife would have had an even more difficult time adjusting. The nurse and Mr. Jones then spent some time reflecting on his loss and feelings, and talking about his response. The nurse's initial question and Mr. Jones's resulting insight that his grief was not as bad as his wife's would have been helped him transcend his immediate experience of loss and find some meaning in his grief.

This illustration is an example of an inward expansion of self-boundaries indicative of self-transcendence. Other expressions of self-transcendence might help Mr. Jones facilitate his own healing and regain a measure of well-being.

In terms of outward expansion, Mr. Jones, with some encouragement, might reach out to his son's family to begin to reconnect to the world outside himself. Walking to and from his home to theirs could expand his sensory world and provide opportunities to interact with other people and with nature along the way. Spending time with his grandchildren could be enlivening through the joy young children can bring to an older person, as could a sense of satisfaction derived from being helpful to his son and daughter-in-law.

Offering at a future time to use the skills he learned while caring for his wife through volunteering with hospice would be an example of transcending temporally. Integrating his memories of Mrs. Jones into his current life would be another example of temporal self-transcendence.

Transpersonal self-transcendence is another important experience for Mr. Jones. Although he was unable to attend church services for several years, he had in the past found worshiping with others a source of comfort. His spiritual life might even be expanded to consider new spiritual dimensions such as that found in the possibility of "being with" his wife again someday or in some way experiencing her presence in the present. Returning to church or to addressing spiritual dimensions outside of organized worship that relates Mr. Jones's understanding of death to some greater or divine design is another example of transpersonal self-transcendence.

CRITICAL THINKING ACTIVITIES

1. Consider the multidimensional aspect of self-transcendence, and list examples of when you experienced expanded boundaries in your own life. Identify how this expanded awareness influenced your health or sense of well-being in each example.
2. What are some factors in the life of patients you have cared for recently that negatively or positively influenced their self-transcendence? If negative, how might you have facilitated self-transcendence and a more positive outcome?
3. What nursing interventions might facilitate or support self-transcendence in an individual living with a chronic or life-threatening illness? How might you apply the self-transcendence theory to help a frail 95-year-old person living in a nursing home maintain or gain a sense of well-being?

POINTS FOR FURTHER STUDY

- Reed, P. G. (2008). *Reed self-transcendence theory, Nurse Theorists: Portraits of Excellence Vol. II.* Athens, OH: Fitne Productions.
- Reed, P. G. (2010). *Self-transcendence theory and nursing in illness and suffering.* (DVD) For Escola Superior da Saúde Instituto Politécnico de Leiria Research Conference, Lisbon, Portugal.
- Reed, P. G. (2015). The theory of self-transcendence. In M. J. Smith & P. R. Liehr (Eds.), *Middle range theory for nursing* (3rd ed.) (109-139). New York: Springer.
- Reed, P. G., & Shearer, N. B. C. (2011). *Nursing knowledge and theory innovation: Advancing the science of nursing practice.* New York: Springer.

REFERENCES

Acton, G. (2003). Self-transcendent views and behaviors: Exploring growth in caregivers of adults with dementia. *Journal of Gerontological Nursing, 28*(12), 22–30.

Acton, G., & Wright, K. (2000). Self-transcendence and family caregivers of adults with dementia. *Journal of Holistic Nursing, 18*(2), 143–158.

Bean, K., & Wagner, K. (2006). Self-transcendence, illness distress, and quality of life among liver transplant recipients. *Journal of Theory Construction & Testing, 10*(2), 47–53.

Bickerstaff, K. A., Grasser, C. M., & McCabe, B. (2003). How elderly nursing home residents transcend losses of later life. *Holistic Nursing Practice, 17*(3), 159–165.

Buchanan, D., Ferran, C., & Clark, D. (1995). Suicidal thought and self-transcendence in older adults. *Journal of Psychosocial Nursing and Mental Health Services, 33*(10), 31–34, 42–43.

Carpenter, J. S., Brockopp, D., & Andrykowski, M. (1999). Self-transformation as a factor in the self-esteem and well-being of breast cancer survivors. *Journal of Advanced Nursing, 29*(6), 1042–1411.

Chen, S., & Walsh, S. (2009). Effect of a creative-bonding intervention on Taiwanese nursing students' self-transcendence and attitudes toward elders. *Research in Nursing and Health, 32*(2), 204–216.

Chin-A-Loy, S. S., & Fernsler, J. I. (1998). Self-transcendence in older men attending a prostate cancer support group. *Cancer Nursing, 21*(5), 358–363.

Chinn, P. L., & Kramer, M. K. (2015). *Knowledge development in nursing: Theory and process* (9th ed.). St Louis, MO: Mosby-Elsevier.

Conti-O'Hare, M. (2002). *The nurse as wounded healer: From trauma to transcendence.* Sudbury, MA: Jones & Bartlett.

Coward, D. D. (1990). The lived experience of self-transcendence in women with advanced breast cancer. *Nursing Science Quarterly, 3,* 162–169.

Coward, D. D. (1991). Self-transcendence and emotional well-being in women with advanced breast cancer. *Oncology Nursing Forum, 18,* 857–863.

Coward, D. D. (1994). Meaning and purpose in the lives of persons with AIDS. *Public Health Nursing, 11*(5), 331–336.

Coward, D. D. (1995). Lived experience of self-transcendence in women with AIDS. *Journal of Obstetrics, Gynecologic, & Neonatal Nursing, 24,* 314–318.

Coward, D. D. (1996). Correlates of self-transcendence in a healthy population. *Nursing Research, 45*(2), 116–121.

Coward, D. D. (1998). Facilitation of self-transcendence in a breast cancer support group. *Oncology Nursing Forum, 25,* 75–84.

Coward, D. D. (2003). Facilitation of self-transcendence in a breast cancer support group II. *Oncology Nursing Forum, 30*(Part 1 of 2), 291–300.

Coward, D. D., & Kahn, D. L. (2004). Resolution of spiritual disequilibrium in women newly diagnosed with breast cancer. *Oncology Nursing Forum, 31*(2), E24–E31.

Coward, D. D., & Kahn, D. L. (2005). Transcending breast cancer: Making meaning from diagnosis and treatment. *Journal of Holistic Nursing, 23*(3), 264–283.

Coward, D. D., & Lewis, F. M. (1993). The lived experience of self-transcendence in gay men with AIDS. *Oncology Nursing Forum, 20,* 1363–1369.

Coward, D. D., & Reed, P. G. (1996). Self-transcendence: A resource for healing at the end-of-life. *Issues in Mental Health Nursing, 17*(3), 275–288.

DiNapoli, J. M., Garcia-Dia, M. J., Garcia-Ona, L., O'Flaherty, D., & Siller, J. (2014). A theory-based computer mediated communication intervention to promote mental health and reduce high-risk behaviors in the LGBT population. *Applied Nursing Research, 27*(1), 91–93.

Ellermann, C. R., & Reed, P. G. (2001). Self-transcendence and depression in middle-aged adults. *Western Journal of Nursing Research, 23*(7), 698–713.

Enyert, G., & Burman, M. E. (1999). A qualitative study of self-transcendence in caregivers of terminally ill patients. *American Journal of Hospice and Palliative Care, 16*(?), 455–462.

Farren, A. T. (2010). Power, uncertainty, self-transcendence, and quality of life in breast cancer survivors. *Nursing Science Quarterly, 23*(1), 63–71.

Frankl, V. (1969). *The will to meaning*. New York: New American Library.

Gusick, G. M. (2008). The contribution of depression and spirituality to symptom burden in chronic heart failure. *Archives of Psychiatric Nursing, 22*(1), 53–55.

Haugan, G. (2014). Nurse-patient interaction is a resource for hope, meaning in life and self-transcendence in nursing home patients. *Scandinavian Journal of Caring Sciences, 28*(1), 74–88.

Haugan, G., Hanssen, B., & Moksnes, U. K. (2013). Self-transcendence, nurse-patient interaction and the outcome of multidimensional well-being in cognitively intact nursing home patients. *Scandinavian Journal of Caring Sciences, 27*(4), 882–893.

Haugan, G., Rannestad, T., Garåsen, H., Hammervold, R., & Espnes, G. A. (2012). The self-transcendence scale: An investigation of the factor structure among nursing home patients. *Journal of Holistic Nursing, 30*(3), 147–159.

Haugan, G., Rannestad, T., Hammervold, R., Garåsen, H., & Espnes, G. A. (2013). Self-transcendence in cognitively intact nursing-home patients: A resource for well-being. *Journal of Advanced Nursing, 69*(5), 1147–1160.

Haugan, G., Rannestad, T., Hammervold, R., Garåsen, H., & Espnes, G. A. (2014). The relationships between self-transcendence and spiritual well-being in cognitively intact nursing home patients. *International Journal of Older People Nursing, 9*, 65–78.

Hoshi, M., & Reed, P. G. (2011). *Testing the applicability of the self-transcendence scale on Japanese hospitalized elders*. Unpublished paper presented at the Theta Sigma Tau 41st International Biennial Convention, Grapevine, TX. Abstract retrieved from http://hdl.handle.net/10755/201802.

Hsu, Y. C., Badger T., Reed P., & Jones E. (2013). Factors associated with depressive symptoms in older Taiwanese adults in a long-term care community. *International Psychogeriatrics, 25*, 1013–1021.

Hunnibell, L. S., Reed, P. G., Quinn-Griffin, M., & Fitzpatrick, J. J. (2008). Self-transcendence and burnout in hospice and oncology nurses. *Journal of Hospice and Palliative Care, 10*(3), 172–179.

Iwamoto, R., Yamawaki, N., & Sato, T. (2011). Increased self-transcendence in patients with intractable diseases. *Psychiatry and Clinical Neuroscience, 65*, 638–647.

Jadid-Milani, M., Ashktorab, T., Abed Saeedi, Z. & Alavi Majd, H. (2015). The impact of self-transcendence on physical health status promotion in multiple sclerosis patients attending peer support groups. *International Journal of Nursing Practice, 21*(6), 725–732.

Joffrion, L. P., & Douglas, D. (1994). Grief resolution: Facilitating self-transcendence in the bereaved. *Journal of Psychosocial Nursing, 32*(3), 13–19.

Kausch, K. D., & Amer, K. (2007). Self-transcendence and depression among AIDS Memorial Quilt panel makers. *Journal of Psychosocial Nursing & Mental Health Services, 45*(6), 44–53.

Kidd, L. I., Zauszniewski, J. A., & Morris, D. L. (2011). Benefits of a poetry writing intervention for family caregivers of elders with dementia. *Issues in Mental Health Nursing, 32*, 598–604.

Kim, S., Reed, P. G., Hayward, R. D., Kang, Y., & Koenig, H. G. (2011). Spirituality and psychological well-being: Testing a theory of family interdependence among family caregivers and their elders. *Research in Nursing and Health, 34*, 103–115.

Kinney, C. (1996). Transcending breast cancer: Reconstructing one's self. *Issues in Mental Health Nursing, 17*(3), 201–216.

Klaas, D. (1998). Testing two elements of spirituality in depressed and non-depressed elders. *International Journal of Psychiatric Nursing Research, 4*, 452–462.

Langner, T. S. (1962). A twenty-two item screening score of psychiatric symptoms indicating impairment. *Journal of Health and Human Behavior, 3*, 269–276.

Lundman, B., Alex, L., Jonsen, E., et al. (2012). Inner strength in relation to functional status, disease, living arrangements and social relationships among people aged 85 years and older. *Geriatric Nursing, 33*(3), 161–167.

Lundman, B., Årestedt, K., Norberg, A., Fischer, R. S., Norberg, C., & Lövheim, H. (2015). Psychometric properties of the Swedish version of the Self-Transcendence Scale among the oldest old. *Journal of Nursing Measurement, 23*(1), 96–111.

Malinski, V. M. (2006). Rogerian science-based nursing theories. *Nursing Science Quarterly, 19*(1), 7–12.

Maslow, A. H. (1971). *Farther reaches of human nature*. New York: Viking Press.

Matthews, E. E., & Cook, P. F. (2009). Relationships between optimism, well-being, self-transcendence, coping, and social support in women during treatment for breast cancer. *Psycho-Oncology, 18*, 716–726.

McCarthy, V. L. (2011). A new look at successful aging: Exploring a mid-range theory among older adults in a low-income retirement community. *The Journal of Theory Construction and Testing, 15*(1), 17–22.

McCarthy, V. L., Jiying, L., Bowland, S., Hall, L. A., & Connelly, J. (2015). Promoting self-transcendence and well-being in community-dwelling older adults: A pilot study of a psychoeducational intervention. *Geriatric Nursing, 36*(6), 431–437.

McCarthy, V. L., Jiying, L., & Carini, R. M. (2013). The role of self-transcendence. A missing variable in the pursuit of successful aging? *Research in Gerontological Nursing, 6*, 178–186.

McCormick, D. P., Holder, B., Wetsel, M., & Cawthon, T. (2001). Spirituality and HIV disease: An integrated perspective. *Journal of the Association of Nurses in AIDS Care, 12*(3), 58–65.

McGee, E. (2000). Alcoholics Anonymous and nursing: Lessons in holism and spiritual care. *Journal of Holistic Nursing, 18*(1), 11–26.

McGee, E. M. (2004). *I'm better for having known you: An exploration of self-transcendence in nurses.* Unpublished doctoral dissertation, Boston College.

Mellors M. P., Erlen, J. A., Coontz, P. D., & Lucke, K. T. (2001). Transcending the suffering of AIDS. *Journal of Community Health Nursing, 18*(4), 235–246.

Mellors, M. P., Riley, T. A., & Erlen, J. A. (1997). HIV, self-transcendence, and quality of life. *Journal of the Association of Nurses in AIDS Care, 8*(2), 59–69.

Moe, A., Hellzen, O., Ekker, K., & Enmarker, I. (2013). Inner strength in relation to perceived physical and mental health among the oldest old people with chronic illness. *Aging & Mental Health, 17*(2), 189–196.

Neill, J. (2002). Transcendence and transformation in life patterns of women living with rheumatoid arthritis. *Advances in Nursing Science, 24*(2), 27–47.

Newman, M. A. (1986). *Health as expanding consciousness.* St Louis: Mosby.

Norberg, A., Lundman, B., Gustafson, Y., Norberg, C., Fischer, R. S., & Lövheim, H. (2015). Self-transcendence (ST) among very old people—Its associations to social and medical factors and development over five years. *Archives of Gerontology & Geriatrics, 61*(2), 247–253.

Nygren, B., Alex, L., Jonsen, E., Gustafson, Y., Norberg, A., & Lundman, B. (2005). Resilience, sense of coherence, purpose in life and self-transcendence in relation to perceived physical and mental health among the oldest old. *Aging & Mental Health, 9*(4), 354–362.

Palmer, B., Quinn, M. T., Reed, P. G., & Fitzpatrick, J. J. (2010). Self-transcendence and work engagement in acute care staff registered nurses. *Critical Care Nursing, 33*(2), 138–147.

Parse, R. R. (1981). *Man-living-health: A theory of nursing.* New York: Wiley.

Pelusi, J. (1997). The lived experience of surviving breast cancer. *Oncology Nursing Forum, 24*(3), 1343–1353.

Radloff, L. S. (1977). The CES-D scale: A self-report depression scale for research in the general population. *Applied Psychological Measurement, 1*, 385–401.

Reed, P. G. (1983). Implications of the life span developmental framework for well-being in adulthood and aging. *Advances in Nursing Science, 6*(1), 18–25.

Reed, P. G. (1986). Developmental resources and depression in the elderly. *Nursing Research, 35*(6), 368–374.

Reed, P. G. (1989). Mental health of older adults. *Western Journal of Nursing Research, 11*, 143–163.

Reed, P. G. (1991a). Toward a nursing theory of self-transcendence: Deductive reformulation using developmental theories. *Advances in Nursing Science, 13*(4), 64–77.

Reed, P. G. (1991b). Self-transcendence and mental health in the oldest-old adults. *Nursing Research, 40*(1), 5–11.

Reed, P. G. (1997a). Nursing: The ontology of the discipline. *Nursing Science Quarterly, 10*(2), 76–79.

Reed, P. G. (1997b). The place of transcendence in nursing's science of unitary human beings: Theory and research. In M. Madrid (Ed.), *Patterns of Rogerian knowing* (pp. 187–196). New York: National League for Nursing.

Reed, P. G. (2014). The theory of self-transcendence. In M. J. Smith & P. R. Liehr (Eds.), *Middle range theory for nursing* (3rd ed.; pp. 109–139). New York: Springer.

Reed, P. G. (2015). Pamela Reed's theory of self-transcendence. In M. C. Smith & M. E. Parker (Eds.), *Nursing theories and nursing practice* (4th ed.; pp. 411–419). Philadelphia: F. A. Davis.

Reed, P. G., & Rousseau, E. (2007). Spiritual inquiry and well-being in life limiting illness. *Journal of Religion, Spirituality, & Aging, 19*(4), 81–98.

Riegel, K. (1976). The dialectics of human development. *American Psychologist, 31*, 689–699.

Robb, S. L., Burns, D. S., Stegenga, K. A., et al. (2014). Randomized clinical trial of therapeutic music video intervention for resilience outcomes in adolescents/young adults undergoing hematopoietic stem cell transplant: A report from the Children's Oncology Group. *Cancer, 120*(6), 909–917.

Rogers, M. E. (1970). *An introduction to the theoretical basis of nursing.* Philadelphia: F. A. Davis.

Rogers, M. E. (1980). A science of unitary man. In J. Riehl & C. Roy (Eds.), *Conceptual models for nursing practice* (2nd ed., pp. 329–338). New York: Appleton-Century-Crofts.

Rogers, M. E. (1990). Nursing: Science of unitary, irreducible, human beings: Update 1990. In E. A. M. Barrett (Ed.), *Visions of Rogers' science based nursing* (pp. 5–12). New York: National League for Nursing.

Runquist, J. J., & Reed, P. G. (2007). Self-transcendence and well-being in homeless adults. *Journal of Holistic Nursing, 25*(1), 5–13.

Sarter, B. (1988). Philosophical sources of nursing theory. *Nursing Science Quarterly, 1*(2), 52–59.

Sharpnack, P. A., Quinn-Griffin, M. T., Benders, A. M., & Fitzpatrick, J. J. (2010). Spiritual and alternative healthcare practices of the Amish. *Holistic Nursing Practice, 24*(2), 64–72.

Sharpnack, P. A., Quinn-Griffin, M. T., Benders, A. M., & Fitzpatrick, J. J. (2011). Self-transcendence and spiritual well-being in the Amish. *Journal of Holistic Nursing, 29*(2), 91–97.

Shearer, N. B. C., Fleury, J. D., & Reed, P. G. (2009). The rhythm of health in older women with chronic illness. *Research and Theory for Nursing Practice: An International Journal, 23*(2), 148–160.

Sperry, J. J. (2011). *The relationship of self-transcendence, social interest, and spirituality to well-being in HIV/AIDS adults.* Doctoral dissertation. Available from *ProQuest Dissertations and Theses* database. (UMI 3480607.)

Stevens, D. D. (1999). *Spirituality, self-transcendence and depression in young adults with AIDS (Immune deficiency)*. Doctoral dissertation. Available from *ProQuest Dissertations and Theses* database. (UMI 9961253.)

Stinson, C. K., & Kirk, E. (2006). Structured reminiscence: An intervention to decrease depression and increase self-transcendence in older women. *Journal of Clinical Nursing, 15*, 208–218.

Taylor, E. J. (2000). Transformation of tragedy among women surviving breast cancer. *Oncology Nursing Forum, 27*, 781–788.

Thomas, J. C., Burton, M., Quinn-Griffin, M. T., & Fitzpatrick, J. J. (2010). Self-transcendence, spiritual well-being, and spiritual practices of women with breast cancer. *Journal of Holistic Nursing, 28*(2), 115–122.

Upchurch, S. L. (1999). Self-transcendence and activities of daily living: The woman with the pink slippers. *Journal of Holistic Nursing, 17*(3), 251–266.

Upchurch, S. L., & Mueller, W. H. (2005). Spiritual influences on ability to engage in self-care activities among older African Americans. *International Journal of Aging & Human Development, 60*(1), 77–94.

Viglund, K., Jonsén, E., Strandberg, G., Lundman, B., & Nygren, B. (2014). Inner strength as a mediator of the relationship between disease and self-rated health among old people. *Journal of Advanced Nursing, 70*(1), 144–152.

Vitale, S. A., Shaffer, C. M., & Fenton, H. R. A. (2014). Self-transcendence in Alzheimer's disease: The application of theory in practice. *Journal of Holistic Nursing, 23*(4), 347–355.

Walton, C., Shultz, C., Beck, C., & Walls, R. (1991). Psychological correlates of loneliness in the older adult. *Archives of Psychiatric Nursing, 5*(3), 165–170.

Walsh, S. M., Chen, S., Hacker, M., & Broschard, D. (2008). A creative-bonding intervention and a friendly visit approach to promote nursing students' self-transcendence and positive attitudes toward elders: A pilot study. *Nurse Education Today, 28*, 363–370.

Walsh, S. M., Lamet, A. R., Lindgren, C. L., Rillstone, P., Little, D. J., Steffey, C. M., et al. (2011). Art in Alzheimer's care: Promoting well-being in people with late-stage Alzheimer's disease. *Rehabilitation Nursing, 36*(2), 66–72.

Watson, J. (1979). *Nursing: The philosophy and science of caring.* Boston: Little, Brown.

Williams, B. J. (2012). Self-transcendence in stem cell transplantation recipients: A phenomenologic study. *Oncology Nursing Forum, 39*(1), E41–E48.

Willis, D. G., & Grace, P. J. (2011). The applied philosopher-scientist: Intersections among phenomenological research, nursing science, and theory as a basis for practice aimed at facilitating boys' healing from being bullied. *Advances in Nursing Science, 34*(10), 19–28.

Willis, D. G., & Griffith, C. A. (2010). Healing patterns revealed in middle school boys' experiences of being bullied using Roger's Science of Unitary Human Beings (SUHB). *Journal of Child and Adolescent Psychiatric Nursing, 23*(30), 125–132.

Young, C. A., & Reed, P. G. (1995). Elders' perceptions of the role of group psychotherapy in fostering self-transcendence. *Archives of Psychiatric Nursing, 9*(6), 338–347.

30

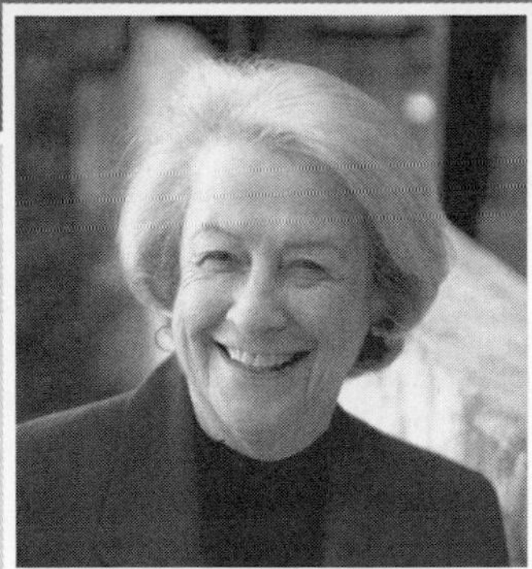

Carolyn L. Wiener*
(1930–Present)

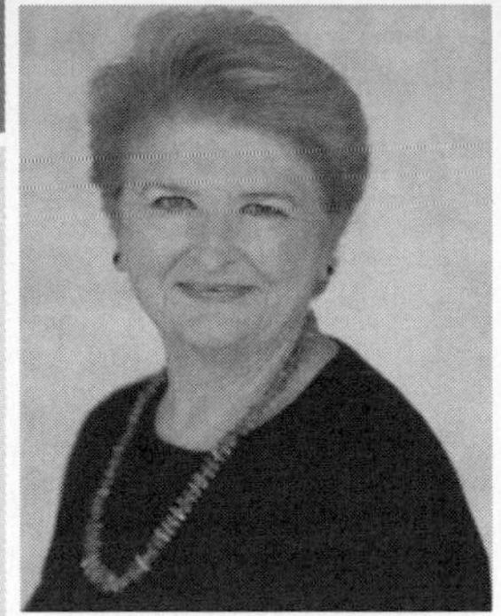

Marylin J. Dodd†
(1946–Present)

Theory of Illness Trajectory

Lisa Kitko, Gwen McGhan, Julie L. Murphy, Cynthia K. Snyder, and Janice Penrod

"The uncertainty surrounding a chronic illness like cancer is the uncertainty of life writ large. By listening to those who are tolerating this exaggerated uncertainty, we can learn much about the trajectory of living."
(Wiener & Dodd, 1993, p. 29)

CREDENTIALS AND BACKGROUND OF THE THEORISTS

Carolyn L. Wiener

Carolyn L. Wiener was born in 1930 in San Francisco. She earned her bachelor's degree in interdisciplinary social science from San Francisco State University in 1972. Wiener received her master's degree in sociology from the University of California, San Francisco (UCSF), in 1975. She remained at UCSF to pursue her doctorate in sociology, which she completed in 1978. After receiving her doctorate degree, Wiener accepted the position of assistant research sociologist at UCSF, where she remained for her entire professional career, attaining the rank of full professor in 1999.

Wiener is Professor Emeritus, Department of Social and Behavioral Sciences at the School of Nursing at UCSF. Her research has focused on organization in health care institutions, chronic illness, and health policy. She taught qualitative research methods, mentored nursing and sociology students and visiting scholars at UCSF, and conducted numerous seminars and workshops, nationally and internationally, on the grounded theory method.

Throughout her career, Wiener's excellence earned her several meritorious awards and honors. In 2001 she gave the opening lecture in an international series titled "Critiquing Health Improvement" at Nottingham University School of Nursing in England. The same year she was an honoree at the UCSF assemblage "Celebrating Women Faculty," an inaugural event honoring women faculty for their accomplishments. Wiener's collaborative relationship with the late Anselm Strauss (cooriginator with Barney Glaser of grounded theory) and her prolific experience in grounded theory methods are evidenced by her invited presentations at the Celebration of the Life and Work of Anselm Strauss at UCSF in 1996, at a conference titled "Anselm Strauss, a Theoretician: The Impact of His Thinking on German and European Social Sciences in Magdeburg, Germany in 1999," and at the First Anselm Strauss Research Colloquium at UCSF in 2005. Wiener was

*Photo credit: Robert Foothorap. From (2001). The UCSF School of Nursing Annual Publication, *The Science of Caring, 13*(1), 7.
†Photo credit: Craig Carlson.

highly sought as a methodological consultant to researchers and students from a variety of specialties.

Dissemination of research findings and methodological papers is a hallmark of Wiener's work. She produced a steady stream of research and theory articles from the mid-1970s. In addition, she authored or coauthored several books (Strauss et al., 1997; Wiener, 1981, 2000; Wiener & Strauss, 1997; Wiener & Wysmans, 1990). Her early works focused on illness trajectories, biographies, and the evolving medical technology scene. From the late 1980s to 1990s, Wiener focused on coping, uncertainty, and accountability in hospitals. Her study examining quality management and redesign efforts in hospitals and the interplay of agencies and hospitals around accountability led to a book, *The Elusive Quest* (Wiener, 2000). In this book, Wiener described the poor fit of quality improvement techniques borrowed from corporate industry in a hospital setting where professionals from diverse disciplines provide highly sophisticated care to patients whose individual biographies defy categorization and whose course of illness is idiosyncratic. Wiener challenged the concept that hospital performance can be, or should be, quantitatively measured. All of Wiener's work is grounded in her methodological expertise and sociological perspective.

Marylin J. Dodd

Marylin J. Dodd was born in 1946 in Vancouver, Canada. She qualified as a registered nurse after studying at Vancouver General Hospital in British Columbia, Canada. She continued her education, earning a bachelor's and a master's degree in nursing from the University of Washington in 1971 and 1973, respectively. Dodd worked as an instructor in nursing at the University of Washington after graduation with her master's degree. By 1977 Dodd returned to academe and completed a doctorate in nursing from Wayne State University. She then accepted the position of Assistant Professor at UCSF. During her tenure there, Dodd advanced to the rank of full professor, serving as Director for the Center for Symptom Management at UCSF. In 2003 she was awarded the Sharon A. Lamb Endowed Chair in Symptom Management at the UCSF School of Nursing. Dr. Dodd is now Professor Emeritus at the UCSF School of Nursing.

Dodd's exemplary program of research focused on oncology nursing, specifically self-care and symptom management. Her outstanding record of funded research provides evidence of the superiority and significance of her work. She skillfully wove modest internal and external funding with 23 years of continuous National Institutes of Health funding to advance her research. Her research trajectory advanced impeccably as she progressively used both descriptive studies and intervention studies through randomized clinical trial methodologies to extend an understanding of complex phenomena in cancer care.

Dodd's research was designed to test self-care interventions (PRO-SELF Program) to manage the side effects of cancer treatment (mucositis) and symptoms of cancer (fatigue, pain). This research, titled "The PRO-SELF: Pain Control Program—An Effective Approach for Cancer Pain Management," was published in *Oncology Nursing Forum* (West et al., 2003). Dodd taught in the oncology nursing specialty. In 2002 she instituted two new courses ("Biomarkers I and II") that were developed by the Center for Symptom Management Faculty Group.

Dodd's illustrious career has merited several prestigious awards. Among these honors, she was recognized as a fellow of the American Academy of Nursing (1986). Her excellence and significant contributions to oncology nursing are evidenced by her having received the Oncology Nursing Society/Schering Excellence in Research Award (1993, 1996), the Best Original Research Paper in Cancer Nursing (1994, 1996), the Oncology Nursing Society Bristol-Myers Distinguished Researcher Career Award (1997), and the Oncology Nursing Society/Chiron Excellence of Scholarship and Consistency of Contribution to the Oncology Nursing Literature Career Award (2000). In 2005 Dodd received the prestigious Episteme Laureate (the Nobel Prize in Nursing) Award from Sigma Theta Tau International. This impressive partial listing of awards demonstrates the magnitude of professional respect and admiration that Dodd garnered throughout her career.

Dodd's record in research dissemination is equally illustrious. Her volume of original publications began in 1975. By the early 1980s, she was publishing multiple, focused articles each year, and this pace only accelerated. She authored or coauthored 130 data-based peer-reviewed journal articles; seven books and many book chapters; and numerous editorials, conference proceedings, and review papers (1978, 1987, 1988, 1991, 1997, 2001, 2004). Her many presentations at scientific gatherings around the world accentuate this work. Dodd has been an invited speaker throughout North America, Australia, Asia, and Europe.

Dodd's service to the university, School of Nursing, Department of Physiological Nursing, and numerous professional and public organizations and journal review boards augments her outstanding record of service to the profession of nursing. In 2015 Dodd was designated as a Living Legend by the American Academy of Nursing. From this brief overview of her amazing career, it is clear that Dodd is an exemplar of excellence in nursing scholarship.

THEORETICAL SOURCES

Although coping with illness has been of interest to social scientists and nursing scholars for decades, Wiener and Dodd clearly explicate that formerly implicit theoretical assumptions have limited the utility of this body of work (Wiener & Dodd, 1993, 2000). Being ill creates a disruption in normal life. Such disruption affects all aspects of life, including physiological functioning, social interactions, and conceptions of self. Coping is the response to such disruption. Because the processes surrounding the disruption of illness are played out in the context of living, coping responses are inherently situated in sociological interactions with others and biographical processes of self. Coping is often described as a compendium of strategies used to manage the disruption, attempts to isolate specific responses to one event that is lived within the complexity of life context, or assigned value labels to the responsive behaviors (e.g., good or bad) that are described collectively as coping. Yet the complex interplay of physiological disruption, interactions with others, and the construction of biographical conceptions of the self warrants a more sophisticated perspective of coping.

The Theory of Illness Trajectory* addresses these theoretical pitfalls by framing this phenomenon within a sociological perspective that emphasizes the experience of disruption related to illness within the changing contexts of interactional and sociological processes that ultimately influence the person's response to such disruption. This theoretical approach defines this theory's contribution to nursing: Coping is not a simple stimulus-response phenomenon that can be isolated from the complex context of life. Life is centered in the living body; therefore physiological disruptions of illness permeate other life contexts to create a new way of being, a new sense of self. Responses to the disruptions caused by illness are interwoven into the various contexts encountered in one's life and the interactions with other players in those life situations.

Within this sociological framework, Wiener and Dodd address serious concerns regarding conceptual overattribution of the role of uncertainty for understanding responses to living with the disruptions of illness (Wiener & Dodd, 1993). An old adage tells us that nothing in life is certain, except death and taxes. Living is fraught with uncertainty, yet illness (especially chronic illness) compounds uncertainty in profound ways. Being chronically ill exaggerates the uncertainties of living for those who are compromised (i.e., by illness) in their capability to respond to these uncertainties. Thus although the concept of uncertainty provides a useful theoretical lens for understanding the illness trajectory, it cannot be theoretically positioned so as to overshadow conceptually the dynamic context of living with chronic illness.

In other words, the illness trajectory is driven by the illness experience lived within contexts that are inherently uncertain and involve both the self and others. The dynamic flow of life contexts (both biographical and sociological) creates a dynamic flow of uncertainties that take on different forms, meanings, and combinations when living with chronic illness. Thus tolerating uncertainty is a critical theoretical strand in the Theory of Illness Trajectory.

*The *Theory of Illness Trajectory* refers to theoretical formulations regarding coping with uncertainty through the cancer illness trajectory. From this perspective, coping is best viewed as change over time that is highly variable in relation to biographical and sociological influences. The trajectory is this course of change, of variability, that cannot be confined to or modeled in linear phases or stages. Rather, the illness trajectory organizes insights to better understand the dynamic interplay of the disruption of illness within the changing contexts of life.

MAJOR CONCEPTS & DEFINITIONS

Life is situated in a biographical context. Conceptions of self are rooted in the physical body and are formulated based on the perceived capability to perform usual or expected activities to accomplish the objectives of varied roles. Interactions with others are a major influence on the establishment of the conception of self. As varied role behaviors are enacted, the person monitors reactions of others and a sense of self in an integrated process of establishing meaning. Identity, temporality, and body are key elements in the biographical context, as follows:

- **Identity**: The conception of self at a given time that unifies multiple aspects of self and is situated in the body
- **Temporality**: Biographical time reflected in the continuous flow of the life course events; perceptions of the past, present, and possible future interwoven into the conception of self
- **Body**: Activities of life and derived perceptions based in the body

Illness, particularly cancer, disrupts the usual or everyday conception of self and is compounded by the perceived actions and reactions of others in the sociological context of life. This disruption permeates the interdependent elements of biography: identity, temporality, and body. This disruption or sense of disequilibrium is marked by a sense of a loss of control, resulting in states of uncertainty.

As life contexts continually unfold, dimensions of uncertainty are manifest, not in a linear sequence of stages or phases, but in an unsettling intermingling of perceptions of the uncertain body, uncertain temporality, and uncertain identity. The experience of illness always is placed within the biographical context—that is, illness is experienced in the continual flow of the life. The domains of

Continued

MAJOR CONCEPTS & DEFINITIONS—cont'd

illness-related uncertainty vary in dominance across the illness trajectory (Table 30.1) through a dynamic flow of perceptions of self and interactions with others.

The activities of life and of living with an illness are forms of work. The sphere of work includes the person and all others with whom he or she interacts, including family and health care providers. This network of players is called the **total organization**. The ill person (or patient) is the central worker; however, all work takes place within and is influenced by the total organization. Types of work are organized around the following four lines of trajectory work performed by patients and families:

1. Illness-related work: Diagnostics, symptom management, care regimen, and crisis prevention
2. Everyday-life work: Activities of daily living, keeping a household, maintaining an occupation, sustaining relationships, and recreation
3. Biographical work: The exchange of information, emotional expressions, and the division of tasks through interactions within the total organization
4. Uncertainty abatement work: Activities enacted to lessen the impact of temporal, body, and identity uncertainty

The balance of these types of work is dynamically responsive, fluctuating across time, situations, perceptions, and varied players in the total organization to gain some sense of equilibrium (i.e., control). This interplay among the types of work creates a tension that is marked by shifts in the dominance of types of work across the trajectory. Recall, however, that the biographical context is rooted in the body. As the body changes through the course of illness and treatment, the capacity to perform certain types of work and, ultimately, one's identity are transformed.

A major contribution of this work was the delineation of types of uncertainty abatement work (Table 30.2). These activities were enacted to lessen the effect of the varied states of uncertainty induced by undergoing cancer chemotherapy. These strategies were highly dynamic and responsive and occurred in varied combinations and configurations across the illness trajectory for different players in the organization. Those enacting these strategies affected the conception of self when they monitored others' responses to the strategy as they attempted to manage living with illness.

TABLE 30.1 Illness Trajectory: States of Uncertainty

Domain	Sources of Uncertainty	Dimensions of Uncertainty
UNCERTAIN TEMPORALITY	Life is perceived to be in a constant state of flux related to illness and treatment.	Loss of temporal predictability prompts concerns surrounding:
Taken-for-granted expectations regarding the flow of life events are disrupted. A temporal disjunction in the biography.	The self of the past is viewed differently (e.g., the way it used to be). Expectations of the present self are distorted by illness and treatment. Anticipation of the future self is altered.	• *Duration:* How long • *Pace:* How fast • *Frequency:* How often the experience of time is distorted (i.e., stretched out, constrained, or limitless)
UNCERTAIN BODY	Faith in the body is shaken (body failure).	Ambiguity in reading body signs. Concerns surrounding:
Changes related to illness and treatment are centered in one's ability to perform usual activities involving appearance, physiological functions, and response to treatment.	The conception of the former body (the way it used to be) comingles with the altered state of the body at present and the changed expectations for how the body may perform in the future.	• What is being done to the body • Jeopardized body resistance • Efficacy and risks of treatment • Disease recurrence
UNCERTAIN IDENTITY Interpretation of self is distorted as the body fails to perform in usual ways, and expectations related to the flow of events (temporality) are altered by disease and treatment.	Body failure and difficulty reading the new body upset the former conception of self. Skewed temporality impairs the expected life course.	Expected life course is shattered. Evidence gleaned from reading the body is not interpretable within the usual frame of understanding. Hope is sustained despite changing circumstances.

TABLE 30.2 Uncertainty Abatement Work

Type of Activity	Behavioral Manifestations
Pacing	Resting or changing usual activities
Becoming "professional" patients	Using terminology related to illness and treatment
	Directing care
	Balancing expertise with supermedicalization
Seeking reinforcing comparisons	Comparing self with persons who are in worse condition to reassure self that it is not as bad as it could be
Engaging in reviews	Looking back to reinterpret emergent symptoms and interactions with others in the organization
Setting goals	Looking toward the future to achieve desired activities
Covering up	Masking signs of illness or related emotions
	Bucking up to avoid stigma or to protect others
Finding a safe place to let down	Establishing a place where, or people with whom, true emotions and feelings could be expressed in a supportive atmosphere
Choosing a supportive network	Selective sharing with individuals deemed to be positive supporters
Taking charge	Asserting the right to determine the course of treatment

USE OF EMPIRICAL EVIDENCE

The Theory of Illness Trajectory was expanded through a secondary analysis of qualitative data collected during a prospective longitudinal study that examined family coping and self-care during 6 months of chemotherapy treatment. The sample for the larger study included 100 patients and their families. Each patient had been diagnosed with cancer (including breast, lung, colorectal, gynecological, or lymphoma) and was in the process of receiving chemotherapy for initial disease treatment or for recurrence. Subjects in the study designated at least one family member who was willing to participate in the study.

Although both quantitative and qualitative measures were used in data collection for the larger study, this theory was derived through analysis of the qualitative data. Interviews were structured around family coping and were conducted at three points during chemotherapeutic treatment. The patients and the family members were asked to recall the previous month and then discuss the most important problem or challenge with which they had to deal, the degree of distress created by that problem within the family, and their satisfaction with the management of that concern.

Meticulous attention was paid to consistency in data collection: Family members were consistent and present for each interview, the interview guide was structured, and the same nurse-interviewer conducted each data collection point for a given family. Audiotaping the interview proceedings, verbatim transcription, and having a nurse-recorder present at each interview to note key phrases as the interview progressed further enhanced methodological rigor. The resultant data set consisted of 300 interviews (three interviews for each of 100 patient-family units) obtained at varied points in the course of chemotherapeutic treatment for cancer.

As the data for the larger study were analyzed, it became apparent to Dodd (principal investigator) that the qualitative interview data held significant insights that could further inform the study. Wiener, a grounded theorist who collaborated with Strauss, one of the method's founders, was subsequently recruited to conduct secondary analysis of interview data. It should be noted that grounded theory methods typically involve a concurrent, reiterative process of data collection and analysis (Glaser, 1978; Glaser & Strauss, 1965). As theoretical insights are identified, sampling and subsequent data collection are theoretically driven to flesh out emergent concepts, dimensions, variations, and negative cases. However, in this project, the data had been collected previously using a structured interview guide; thus this was a secondary analysis of an established data set.

Wiener's expertise in grounded theory methods permitted the adaptation of grounded theory methods for application to secondary data that proved successful. In essence, the principles undergirding analyses (i.e., the coding paradigm) were applied to the preexisting data set. The analytical inquiry proceeded inductively to reveal the core social-psychological process around which the theory is explicated: tolerating the uncertainty of living with cancer. Dimensions of the uncertainty, management processes, and consequences were further explicated, revealing the internal consistency of the theoretical perspective of illness trajectory.

When considering the use of adapted grounded theory methods to analyze preexisting empirical evidence, several insights support the integrity of this work. First, Wiener was well prepared to advance new applications of the method from training and experience as a grounded theorist. The methodological credibility of this researcher supports her extension of a traditional research method into a new application within her disciplinary perspective (sociology). Further support is from the size of the data set: 100 patients and families were interviewed three times each, for a total of 300 interviews, a very large data set for a qualitative inquiry. Oberst (1993) pointed out that given this volume of data, some semblance of theoretical sampling (within the full data set) would likely be permitted by the researchers. But the sheer size of the data set does not tell the whole story.

Sampling patients who had a relatively wide range of types of cancers (ranging from gynecological cancers to lung cancer) and both patients undergoing initial chemotherapeutic treatment and those receiving treatment for recurrence contributed significantly to variation in the data set. These sampling strategies ultimately contributed toward establishing an appropriate sample, especially for revealing a trajectory perspective of change over time. Finally, despite the structured format of the interview, it is important to note that the patients and families dialogued about the previous month's events in a form of "brainstorming" (Wiener & Dodd, 1993, p. 18). This technique allowed the subjects to introduce almost any topic that was of concern to them (regardless of the subsequent structure of the interview). The audiotaping and verbatim transcription of these dialogues contributed to the variation and appropriateness of the resultant data set. Therefore it may be concluded that empirical evidence culled through the interviews conducted in the larger study provides adequate and appropriate data for a secondary analysis using expertly adapted grounded theory methods.

MAJOR ASSUMPTIONS

Person is the focus of this middle-range theory. Middle-range theories address one or more of the paradigm concepts (nursing, person, health, and environment); therefore some are not explicitly addressed. However, the following discussion of theoretical assumptions sheds some light on a theoretical interpretation of these concepts. Wiener and Dodd's Theory of Illness Trajectory explicates major assumptions that reflect its derivation within a sociological perspective (Wiener & Dodd, 1993). Closer examination of each assumption reveals several related basic premises undergirding the theory.

The Theory of Illness Trajectory encompasses not only the physical components of the disease, but also the "total organization of work done over the course of the disease" (Wiener & Dodd, 1993, p. 20). An illness trajectory is theoretically distinct from the course of an illness. In this theory, the illness trajectory is not limited to the person who suffers the illness. Rather, the total organization involves the person with the illness, the family, and health care professionals who render care.

Also, the use of the term *work* is important: "The varied players in the organization have different types of work; however, the patient is the 'central worker' in the illness trajectory" (Wiener & Dodd, 1993, p. 20). This statement reaffirms an earlier assertion in illness trajectory literature (Fagerhaugh et al., 1987; Strauss et al., 1984). The work of living with an illness produces certain consequences that permeate the lives of the people involved. In turn, consequences and reciprocal consequences ripple throughout the organization, enmeshing the total organization with the central worker (i.e., the patient) through the trajectory of living with the illness. The relationship among the workers in the trajectory is an attribute that "affects both the management of that course of illness, as well as the fate of the person who is ill" (Wiener & Dodd, 1993, p. 20).

THEORETICAL ASSERTIONS

The context for the work and the social relationships affecting the work of living with illness in the Theory of Illness Trajectory is based in the seminal work of Corbin and Strauss (1988). As the central worker, actions are undertaken by the person to manage the effects of living with illness within a range of contexts, including the biographical (conception of self) and the sociological (interactions with others). From this perspective, managing disruptions (or coping with uncertainty) involves patient interactions with various players in the organization as well as external sociological conditions. Given the complexity of such interactions across multiple contexts and with the numerous players throughout the illness trajectory, coping is a highly variable and dynamic process.

Originally, it was anticipated that the trajectory of living with cancer had discernible phases or stages that could be identified by major shifts in reported problems, challenges, and activities. This was the rationale for collecting qualitative data at three points during the chemotherapy treatment. In fact, this notion did not hold true: the physical status of the patient with cancer and the social-psychological consequences of illness and treatment were the central themes at all points of measurement across the trajectory.

The authors conceptually equate uncertainty with loss of control, described as "the most problematic facet of living with cancer" (Wiener & Dodd, 1993, p. 18). This theoretical assertion is reflected further in the identification of the core social-psychological process of living with cancer, "tolerating the uncertainty that permeates the disease" (p. 19). Factors that influenced the degree of uncertainty expressed by the patient and family were based in the theoretical framework of the total organization and external sociological conditions, including the nature of family support, financial resources, and quality of assistance from health care providers.

LOGICAL FORM

The primary logical form was grounded theory and inductive reasoning. Analytical reading of the interviews provided insights that led to the identification of the core process that unifies the theoretical assertions: tolerating uncertainty. Systematic coding processes were applied to define the dimensions of uncertainty and management processes used to deal with disease. The findings were then examined for fit within extant theoretical writings to extend understanding of the illness trajectory. The resultant qualitatively derived theory was grounded in the reported experiences of the participants and integrated with illness knowledge trajectories to advance the science.

ACCEPTANCE BY THE NURSING COMMUNITY

Practice

The Theory of Illness Trajectory provides a framework for nurses to understand how cancer patients tolerate uncertainty manifested as a loss of control. Identification of the types of uncertainty is especially useful, because it reveals strategies commonly employed by oncology patients in their attempt to manage their lives as normally as possible in the wake of the uncertainty created by a cancer diagnosis. Awareness of the themes of uncertainty and related management strategies faced by patients undergoing chemotherapy and survivorship and their family members has a significant effect on how nurses subsequently intervene with these compromised patient systems who are managing the work of their illness to "facilitate a less troubled trajectory course for some patients and their families" (Wiener & Dodd, 1993, p. 29). An example is Schlairet and colleagues (2010), who examined the needs of cancer survivors receiving care in a cancer community center using the Theory of Illness Trajectory as a framework. They conclude that nurses need to be aware of the specific needs of cancer survivors so that interventions can be developed to meet their needs (Schlairet, Heddon, & Griffis, 2010).

Education

Wiener and Dodd are highly respected educators who shared their ongoing work through international conferences, seminars, consultations, graduate thesis advising, and course offerings. Incorporation of this work into these presentations not only advances knowledge related to the utility of illness trajectory models but also, perhaps more importantly, demonstrates how data-based theoretical advancement contributes to an evolving program of research in cancer care (Dodd, 1997, 2001). Including the theory in nursing texts on research and theory exposes researchers to the work and those in nursing practice (Wiener & Dodd, 2000).

Research

The theory has been referenced in a limited number of concept analyses or state-of-the-science papers addressing uncertainty (McCormick, 2002; Mishel, 1997; Parry, 2003; Penrod, 2007). Mishel (1997) has praised the broad theoretical focus maintained through the qualitative approach to theory derivation. Much of the work in coping with illness is constrained by the application of Lazarus and Folkman's (1984) framework of problem-based or emotion-based coping; however, in this study, inductive reasoning produced data-based theory that identifies a broad range of strategies related to tolerating and abating uncertainty (Mishel, 1997). The variation and range of abatement strategies identified in this theory are unique and significant contributions to the body of research in coping with the uncertainty of illness. Christensen (2015) attributes the work of Wiener and Dodd to define trajectory and specify management goals across the health change trajectory.

FURTHER DEVELOPMENT

In an earlier response article to the original publication, Oberst (1993) took issue with the delimitation of the concept of uncertainty to loss of control. This criticism was echoed by McCormick (2002), who theoretically positioned loss of control in the uncertainty cycle rather than as a manifestation of a state of uncertainty. In their work on end-of-life caregiving, McGhan and colleagues (2013) and Penrod and colleagues (2012, 2012a, 2011) have posited that minimizing uncertainty by increasing confidence and control is desirable for patients and their family caregivers transitioning through the end-of-life trajectory. Further research on the concept of control is warranted to untangle the conceptual boundaries and linkages with uncertainty throughout the illness trajectory.

Other researchers have criticized the implicit assertion that uncertainty (or loss of control) is always a negative event that requires some form of abatement (Oberst, 1993; Parry, 2003). Oberst (1993) suggested the need for further investigation to differentiate work related to tolerating uncertainty from abatement work to reveal how effective strategies in each type of work affect the sense of uncertainty throughout the trajectory. Parry (2003) studied survivors of childhood cancer and revealed that although uncertain states may be a problematic stressor for some, a more universal theme of embracing uncertainty toward transformational growth was evident in these survivors.

Penrod (2007) clarified the concept of uncertainty with a phenomenological investigation that advanced the concept of uncertainty and identified different types of uncertainty. The experience of living with uncertainty was dynamic in nature with changes in the types and modes of uncertainty, and various types of uncertainty were guided by the primary tenets of confidence and a sense of control.

These insights demonstrate an evolving body of research related to uncertainty, control, and the illness trajectory. Rather than assume that uncertainty is a negative aspect of life, researchers must remain open to all transformational outcomes of living through uncertainty. Wiener and Dodd's original recommendation remains salient, to expand the scope of the illness trajectory framework (Wiener & Dodd, 1993). The illness trajectory theoretical framework is especially useful for understanding the variations in uncertainty and control and for gaining a fuller perspective of the human experience with cancer and other conditions in which the significance of uncertainty and control may vary. The concept of resilience (i.e., thriving in the face of adversity) appears to be a relevant area of inquiry to further expand understanding of positive transformation across trajectories fraught with uncertainty.

CRITIQUE

Clarity

One concern in the clarity in Wiener and Dodd's Theory of Illness Trajectory is the delimitation of the concept of uncertainty to a loss of control. This limited conceptual perspective of uncertainty is clearly set forth in the work; therefore this issue does not create a significant or fatal flaw in the work. The theory is delineated clearly and well supported by previous work in illness trajectories. Propositional clarity is achieved in the logical presentation of relationships and linkages between concepts. The conceptual derivation of managing illness as work is well developed and provides unique insight into the meaning of living through chemotherapy during cancer treatment. The application of the trajectory model is used consistently to demonstrate the dynamic fluctuations in coping, not in clearly demarcated stages or phases, but in situation-specific contexts of the work of managing illness.

Simplicity

This complex theory is interpreted in a highly accessible manner. The Theory of Illness Trajectory adopts a sociological framework that is applied to a phenomenon of concern to nursing: chemotherapeutic treatment of cancer patients and their families. The sense of understanding imparted by the theory is highly relevant to oncology nursing practice. The theory presents an eloquent and parsimonious interpretation of the complexity of cancer work using key concepts with adequate definition; however, review of previous published studies would be very helpful to comprehend the theoretical assertions fully.

Generality

The authors have limited the scope of this theory to patients and families progressing through chemotherapy for initial treatment or recurrence of cancer. The Theory of Illness Trajectory is well defined within this context. The integration of this middle-range theory with other work in illness trajectories and uncertainty theory indicates an emergent fit with other models of illness trajectories and uncertainty. Further theory-building work may produce a broader scope that permits application of the theoretical propositions in other contexts of illness trajectories.

Accessibility

Grounded theory methods rely on the dominance of inductive reasoning—that is, drawing abstractions or generalities from specific situations. Thus the derived theory is rooted in the experiences expressed in the hundreds of interviews with cancer patients and their families. The integration of data-based evidence (e.g., quotes) in the formal description of the theory supports the linkages between the theoretical abstractions and empirical observations. Empirical evidence is presented in a logical, consistent manner that rings true to clinical experiences. Thus the theory is useful to clinicians and holds promise for further research application.

Importance

The importance of the theoretical contributions made by this work, especially types of work and uncertainty abatement strategies during chemotherapy, has been established. The utility of the theory is apparent in cancer treatment, and further theoretical development holds promise of being generalizable to other contexts within cancer care and other illness trajectories. Yet the limited evidence of directly derived consequences related to application of the Theory of Illness Trajectory in practice-based studies in nursing remains problematic. Applicability of this theory to phenomena of concern to nursing has been established by the focus on cancer chemotherapy. Therefore potential utility for guiding nursing practice is demonstrated by the integration of the theory into Dodd's exemplary program of research in cancer care (Dodd, 2001, 2004; Dodd & Miaskowski, 2000; Jansen et al., 2007; Miaskowski, Dodd, & Lee, 2004).

SUMMARY

Wiener and Dodd's Theory of Illness Trajectory is at once complex, yet eloquently simple. The sociological perspective of defining the work of managing illness is especially relevant to the context of cancer care. The theory provides a new understanding of how patients and families tolerate uncertainty and work strategically to abate uncertainty through a dynamic flow of illness events, treatment situations, and varied players involved in the organization of care. The theory is pragmatic and relevant to nursing. The merits of this work warrant attention and use of the theory for practice applications that inform nurses as they interpret and facilitate the management of care during illness.

CASE STUDY

Mr. Miller is a 67-year-old man who has metastatic cancer. His primary caregiver is his wife, Mrs. Miller. Early in the course of treatment in the outpatient cancer care center, the couple focused their questions on the course of the disease, treatment options, and potential side effects of varied treatment options. They were proud of their ability to maintain "normal life" as Mr. Miller continued to work throughout aggressive treatment, taking time off only when the discomforts of treatment were so debilitating that he was physically unable to get to his office. Mr. and Mrs. Miller expressed little emotion throughout the course of treatment; they frequently praised each other's strength and fortitude. During recent visits, Mrs. Miller has become extremely focused on laboratory values and test results, using highly technical language. She has also become adamant that certain staff members must perform certain tasks because "she does it better than anyone."

The Theory of Illness Trajectory helps the clinician to interpret these behaviors and to intervene to help ease transitions across this trajectory. For example, clinicians can identify easily with patients and families who have become "professional patients" as they learn to use complex technical jargon about their treatment, laboratory values, or illness (Wiener & Dodd, 1993, p. 988). Care providers have a tendency to view this behavior as a positive hallmark of assuming self-care and therefore often reinforce such behaviors.

Deeper consideration of the theoretical assertions of the Theory of Illness Trajectory reveals that these behavioral strategies are efforts to tolerate the uncertainty of the illness experience. The confidence built through these socially reinforced behaviors can be converted to guilt very quickly when situations beyond the expertise of the patient or family go awry. Given this perspective, the limitation of this management strategy becomes clear, and intervention is indicated: If patients and families are to manage care effectively, they must be educated proactively to do so (Dodd, 1997, 2001).

In proactively educating the patient-family system, consider the varied domains of uncertainty and the varied forms of uncertainty abatement work. To understand the patient-family trajectory, assessment data are critical. For example, although well-developed protocols for symptom management or palliation are available, such protocols are useless if patients or caregivers fail to describe the extent of symptoms because they perceive these "hassles" or "bothers" as trivial in the face of life-threatening disease. Compounding this issue, nurses may fall into a pattern of focusing on illness-related work, thereby diverting important attention from the other forms of work faced by these patients and their families. Understanding of the varied domains of uncertainty and forms of uncertainty abatement work facilitates a more open dialogue regarding these key areas of concern, allowing the nurse to encourage the patient and caregiver to share more about their experiences to help them through this difficult time.

CRITICAL THINKING ACTIVITIES

1. How does an illness trajectory differ from a course of illness? How do the perspectives align with your views of nursing?
2. Considering your clinical experiences, identify examples of how patients and their families have experienced health-related uncertainty. Did uncertainty seem related to loss of control?
3. As an advanced clinician, you are intimately involved in the work of managing an illness. Based on your understanding of the work of illness management espoused in the Theory of Illness Trajectory, what nursing behaviors exacerbate feelings of loss of control or uncertainty in patients?
4. What factors (personal, environmental, or organizational) contributed to the nursing behaviors observed in question 3? In your practice, what nursing interventions create a less troubling trajectory for patients and families in these situations?

POINTS FOR FURTHER STUDY

- Dodd, M. J. (2001). *Managing the side effects of chemotherapy and radiation therapy: A guide for patients and their families* (4th ed.). San Francisco: UCSF School of Nursing.
- Dodd, M. J., & Miaskowski, C. (2000). The PRO-SELF program: A self-care intervention program for patients receiving cancer treatment. *Seminars in Oncology, 16*(4), 300–308.
- Jansen, C. E., Miaskowski, C. A., Dodd, M. J., & Dowling, G. A. (2007). A meta-analysis of the sensitivity of various neuropsychological tests used to detect chemotherapy-induced cognitive impairment in patients with breast cancer. *Oncology Nursing Forum, 34*(5), 997–1005.
- West, C. M., Dodd, M. J., Paul, S. M., et al. (2003). The PRO-SELF: Pain control program—An effective approach for cancer pain management. *Oncology Nursing Forum, 30*, 65–73.

REFERENCES

Christensen, D. (2015). The health change trajectory model: An integrated model of health change. *Advanced Nursing Science, 38*(1), 55–67.

Corbin, J., & Strauss, A. (1988). *Unending work and care.* San Francisco: Jossey-Bass.

Dodd, M. J. (1978). *Oncology nursing case studies.* New York: Medical Publication Co.

Dodd, M. J. (1987). *Managing the side effects of chemotherapy and radiation therapy: A guide for patients and nurses.* Norwalk, CT: Appleton & Lange.

Dodd, M. J. (1988). *Monograph of the advanced research session at the 13th Annual Oncology Nursing Society's Congress.* Pittsburgh: Oncology Nursing Society.

Dodd, M. J. (1991). *Managing the side effects of chemotherapy and radiation: A guide for patients and their families* (2nd ed.). Englewood, NJ: Prentice-Hall.

Dodd, M. J. (1997). *Managing the side effects of chemotherapy and radiation therapy: A guide for patients and their families* (3rd ed.). San Francisco: UCSF School of Nursing.

Dodd, M. J. (2001). *Managing the side effects of chemotherapy and radiation therapy: A guide for patients and their families* (4th ed.). San Francisco: UCSF School of Nursing.

Dodd, M. (2004). The pathogenesis and characterization of oral mucositis associated with cancer therapy. *Oncology Nursing Forum, 31*(4 Suppl), 5–11.

Dodd, M. J., & Miaskowski, C. (2000). The PRO-SELF program: A self care intervention program for patients receiving cancer treatment. *Seminars in Oncology, 16*(4), 300–308.

Fagerhaugh, S., Strauss, A., Suczek, B., & Wiener, C. (1987). *Hazards in hospital care: Ensuring patient safety*. San Francisco: Jossey-Bass.

Glaser, B. (1978). *Theoretical sensitivity*. Mill Valley, CA: Sociology Press.

Glaser, B., & Strauss, A. (1965). *Awareness of dying*. Chicago: Aldine.

Jansen, C. E., Miaskowski, C. A., Dodd, M. J., & Dowling, G. A. (2007). A meta-analysis of the sensitivity of various neuropsychological tests used to detect chemotherapy-induced cognitive impairment in patients with breast cancer. *Oncology Nursing Forum, 34*(5), 997–1005.

Lazarus, R. S., & Folkman, S. (1984). *Stress, appraisal, and coping.* New York: Springer.

McCormick, K. M. (2002). A concept analysis of uncertainty in illness. *Journal of Nursing Scholarship, 34*(2), 127–131.

McGhan, G., Loeb, S. J., Baney, B., & Penrod, J. (2013). End-of-life caregiving: Challenges, faced by older adult women. *Journal of Gerontological Nursing, 39*(6), 45–54.

Miaskowski, C., Dodd, M., & Lee, K. (2004). Symptom clusters: The new frontier in symptom management research. *Journal of the National Cancer Institute Monographs, 32*, 17–21.

Mishel, M. (1997). Uncertainty in acute illness. *Annual Review of Nursing Research, 15*, 57–80.

Oberst, M. T. (1993). Response to "Coping amid uncertainty: An illness trajectory perspective." *Scholarly Inquiry for Nursing Practice: An International Journal, 7*(1), 33–35.

Parry, C. (2003). Embracing uncertainty: An exploration of the experiences of childhood cancer survivors. *Qualitative Health Research, 13*(1), 227–246.

Penrod, J. (2007). Living with uncertainty: Concept advancement. *Journal of Advanced Nursing, 57*(6), 658–667.

Penrod, J., Baney, B., Loeb, S. J., McGhan, G., & Shipley, P. Z. (2012). The influence of the culture of care on informal caregivers' experiences. *Advances in Nursing Science, 35*(1), 64–76.

Penrod, J., Hupcey, J. E., Baney, B. L., & Loeb, S. J. (2011). End-of-life trajectories. *Clinical Nursing Research, 20*(1), 7–24.

Penrod, J., Hupcey, J. E., Shipley, P. Z., Loeb, S. J., & Baney, B. (2012a). A model of caregiving through the end-of-life: Seeking normal. *Western Journal of Nursing Research, 34*(2), 174–192.

Schlairet, M., Heddon, M. A., & Griffis, M. (2010). Piloting a needs assessment to guide development of a survivorship program for a community cancer center. *Oncology Nursing Forum, 37*(4), 501–508.

Strauss, A., Corbin, J., Fagerhaugh, S., et al. (1984). *Chronic illness and the quality of life.* St Louis, MO: Mosby.

Strauss, A., Fagerhaugh, S., Suczek, B., & Wiener, C. (1997). *Social organization of medical work.* New Brunswick, NJ: Transaction Books.

West, C. M., Dodd, M. J., Paul, S. M., et al. (2003). The PRO-SELF: Pain control program—An effective approach for cancer pain management. *Oncology Nursing Forum, 30*, 65–73.

Wiener, C. (1981). *The politics of alcoholism: Building an arena around a social problem*. New Brunswick, NJ: Transaction Books.

Wiener, C. (2000). *The elusive quest: Accountability in hospitals*. New York: Aldine deGruyter.

Wiener, C., & Strauss, A. (1997). *Where medicine fails* (5th ed.). New Brunswick, NJ: Transaction Books.

Wiener, C., & Wysmans, W. M. (1990). *Grounded theory in medical research: From theory to practice*. Amsterdam: Sivets and Zeitlinger.

Wiener, C. L., & Dodd, M. J. (1993). Coping amid uncertainty: An illness trajectory perspective. *Scholarly Inquiry for Nursing Practice: An International Journal, 7*(1), 17–31.

Wiener, C. L., & Dodd, M. J. (2000). Coping amid uncertainty: An illness trajectory perspective. In R. Hyman & J. Corbin (Eds.), *Chronic illness: Research and theory for nursing practice* (pp. 180–201). New York: Springer.

BIBLIOGRAPHY

Primary Sources

Book Chapters

Dodd, M. J. (1999). Self-care and patient/family teaching. In S. L. Groenwald, M. H. Frogge, M. Goodman, & C. H. Yarbro (Eds.), *Cancer symptom management* (2nd ed., pp. 20–29). Wilsonville, OR: Jones & Bartlett.

Dodd, M. J., & Miaskowski, C. (2003). Symptom management, the PRO-SELF Program: A self-care intervention program. In B. Given, C. Given, & V. Champion (Eds.), *Evidence-based behavioral interventions for cancer patients: State of the knowledge across the cancer care trajectory* (pp. 218–241). New York: Springer.

Journal Articles

Baggott, C., Beale, I. L., Dodd, M. J., & Kato, P. M. (2004). A survey of self-care and dependent-care advice given by pediatric oncology nurses. *Journal of Pediatric Oncology, 21*(4), 214–222.

Chen, L., Miaskowski, C., Dodd, M., & Pantilat, S. (2008). Concepts within the Chinese culture that influence the cancer pain experience. *Cancer Nursing, 31*(2), 103–108.

Cho, M. H., Dodd, M. J., Lee, K. A., Padilla, G., & Slaughter, R. (2006). Self-reported sleep quality in family caregivers of gastric cancer patients who are receiving chemotherapy in Korea. *Journal of Cancer Education, 21*(1 Suppl), S37–S41.

Chou, F., Dodd, M., Abrams, D., & Padilla, G. (2007). Symptoms, self-care, and quality of life of Chinese American patients with cancer. *Oncology Nursing Forum, 34*(6), 1162–1167.

Dodd, M. (2000). Cancer-related fatigue. *Cancer Investigation, 18*(1), 97.

Dodd, M. J. (2002). Defining clinically meaningful outcomes in the evaluation of new treatments for oral mucositis: A commentary. *Cancer Investigation, 20*(5–6), 851–852.

Dodd, M. J., Cho, M. H., Cooper, B., Miaskowski, C., Lee, K. A., & Bank, K. (2005). Advancing our knowledge of symptoms clusters. *Journal of Supportive Oncology, 3*(6 Suppl 4), 30–31.

Dodd, M. J., Dibble, S., Miaskowski, C., et al. (2001). A comparison of the affective state and quality of life of chemotherapy patients who do and do not develop chemotherapy-induced oral mucositis. *Journal of Pain and Symptom Management, 21*(6), 498–505.

Dodd, M. J., Dibble, S. L., Miaskowski, C., et al. (2000). Randomized clinical trial of the effectiveness of 3 commonly used mouthwashes to treat chemotherapy-induced mucositis. *Journal of Oral Surgery, Oral Medicine, Oral Pathology, Oral Radiology, and Endodontics, 90*(1), 39–47.

Dodd, M. J., Janson, S., Facione, N., et al. (2001). Advancing the science of symptom management. *Journal of Advanced Nursing, 33*(5), 668–676.

Dodd, M. J., & Miaskowski, C. (2000). The PRO-SELF program: A self-care intervention program for patients receiving cancer treatment. *Seminars in Oncology, 16*(4), 300–308.

Dodd, M. J., Miaskowski, C., Dibble, S. L., et al. (2000). Factors influencing oral mucositis in patients receiving chemotherapy. *Cancer Practice, 8*(6), 291–297.

Dodd, M. J., Miaskowski, C., Greenspan, D., et al. (2003). Radiation-induced mucositis: A randomized clinical trial of micronized sucralfate versus salt & soda mouthwashes. *Cancer Investigation, 21*(1), 21–33.

Dodd, M. J., Miaskowski, C., & Lee, K. A. (2004). Occurrence of symptom clusters. *Journal of the National Cancer Institute Monographs, 32*, 76–78.

Dodd, M. J., Miaskowski, C., & Paul, S. M. (2001). Symptom clusters and their effect on the functional status of patients with cancer. *Oncology Nursing Forum, 28*(3), 465–470.

Dodd, M. J., Miaskowski, C., Shiba, G. H., et al. (1999). Risk factors for chemotherapy-induced oral mucositis: Dental appliances, oral hygiene, previous oral lesions, and history of smoking. *Cancer Investigation, 17*(4), 278–284.

Edrington, J., Miaskowski, C., Dodd, M., Wong, C., & Padilla, G. (2007). A review of the literature on the pain experience of Chinese patients with cancer. *Cancer Nursing, 30*(5), 335–346.

Edrington, J. M., Paul, S., Dodd, M., et al. (2004). No evidence for sex differences in the severity and treatment of cancer pain. *Journal of Pain and Symptom Management, 28*(3), 225–232.

Facione, N. C., Miaskowski, C., Dodd, M. J., & Paul, S. M. (2002). The self-reported likelihood of patient delay in breast cancer: New thoughts for early detection. *Preventative Medicine, 34*(4), 397–407.

Fletcher, B. S., Dodd, M. J., Schumacher, K. L., & Miaskowski, C. (2008). Symptom experience of family caregivers of patients with cancer. *Oncology Nursing Forum, 35*(2), E23–E44.

Fletcher, B. S., Paul, S. M., Dodd, M. J., et al. (2008). Prevalence, severity, and impact of symptoms on female family caregivers of patients at the initiation of radiation therapy for prostate cancer. *Journal of Clinical Oncology, 26*(4), 599–605.

Hilton, J. F., MacPhil, L. A., Pascasio, L., et al. (2004). Self-care intervention to reduce oral candidiasis recurrence in HIV-seropositive persons: A pilot-study. *Community Dentistry and Oral Epidemiology, 32*(3), 190–200.

Hinds, P. S., Baggott, C., DeSwarte-Wallace, J., et al. (2003). Functional integration of nursing research into a pediatric oncology cooperative group: Finding common ground. *Oncology Nursing Forum, 30*(6), E121–E126.

Jansen, C. E., Miaskowski, C., Dodd, M., & Dowling, G. (2005). Chemotherapy-induced cognitive impairment in women with breast cancer: A critique of the literature. *Oncology Nursing Forum, 32*(2), 329–342.

Jansen, C. E., Miaskowski, C., Dodd, M., Dowling, G., & Kramer, J. (2005). A meta-analysis of studies of the effects of cancer chemotherapy on various domains of cognitive functioning. *Cancer, 104*(10), 2222–2233.

Jansen, C. E., Miaskowski, C., Dodd, M., Dowling, G., & Kramer, J. (2005). Potential mechanisms for chemotherapy-induced impairments in cognitive function. *Oncology Nursing Forum, 32*(6), 1151–1163.

Jansen, C. E., Miaskowski, C. A., Dodd, M. J., & Dowling, G. A. (2007). A meta-analysis of the sensitivity of various neuropsychological tests used to detect chemotherapy-induced cognitive impairment in patients with breast cancer. *Oncology Nursing Forum, 34*(5), 997–1005.

Katapodi, M. C., Facione, N. C., Humphreys, J. C., & Dodd, M. J. (2005). Perceived breast cancer risk: Heuristic reasoning and search for a dominance structure. *Social Science and Medicine, 60*(2), 421–432.

Katapodi, M. C., Facione, N. C., Miaskowski, C., Dodd, M. J., & Waters, C. (2002). The influence of social support on breast cancer screening in a multicultural community sample. *Oncology Nursing Forum, 29*(5), 845–852.

Katapodi, M. C., Lee, K. A., Facione, N. C., & Dodd, M. J. (2004). Predictors of perceived breast cancer risk and the relation between perceived breast cancer screening: A meta-analytic review. *Preventative Medicine, 38*(4), 388–402.

Kim, J. E., Dodd, M., West, C., et al. (2004). The PRO-SELF pain control program improves patients' knowledge of cancer pain management. *Oncology Nursing Forum, 31*(6), 1137–1143.

Krasnoff, J. B., Vintro, A. Q., Ascher, N. L., Bass, N. M., Dodd, M. J., & Painter, P. L. (2005). Objective measures of health-related quality of life over 24 month post-liver transplantation. *Clinical Transplantation, 19*(1), 1–9.

Krasnoff, J. B., Vintro, A. Q., Ascher, N. L., et al. (2006). A randomized trial of exercise and dietary counseling after liver transplantation. *American Journal of Transplantation, 6*, 1896–1905.

Kris, A. E., & Dodd, M. J. (2004). Symptom experience of adult hospitalized medical-surgical patients. *Journal of Symptom Management, 28*(5), 451–459.

Lee, K., Cho, M., Miaskowski, C., & Dodd, M. (2004). Impaired sleep and rhythms in persons with cancer. *Sleep Medicine Reviews, 8*(3), 199–212.

Mandrell, B. N., Ruccione, K., Dodd, M. J., et al. (2000). Consensus statements. Applying the concept of self-care to pediatric oncology patients. *Seminars in Oncology Nursing, 16*(4), 315–316.

McLemore, M. R., Miaskowski, C., Aouizerat, B. E., Chen, L. E., & Dodd, M. (2008). Rules of cell development and their application to biomarkers for ovarian cancer. *Oncology Nursing Forum, 35*(3), 403–409.

Miaskowski, C., Cooper, B. A., Paul, S. M., et al. (2006). Subgroups of patients with cancer with different symptoms experiences and quality-of-life outcomes: A cluster analysis. *Oncology Nursing Forum, 33*(5), E79–E89.

Miaskowski, C., Dodd, M., & Lee, K. (2004). Symptom clusters: The new frontier in symptom management research. *Journal of the National Cancer Institute Monographs, 32*, 17–21.

Miaskowski, C., Dodd, M., West, C., et al. (2001). Lack of adherence with the analgesic regimen: A significant barrier to effective cancer pain management. *Journal of Clinical Oncology, 19*(23), 4275–4279.

Miaskowski, C., Dodd, M., West, C., et al. (2004). Randomized clinical trial of the effectiveness of a self-care intervention to improve cancer pain management. *Journal of Clinical Oncology, 22*(90), 1713–1720.

Miaskowski, C., Dodd, M., West, C., et al. (2007). The use of a responder analysis to identify differences in patient outcomes following a self-care intervention to improve cancer pain management. *Pain, 129*, 55–63.

Miaskowski, C., Mack, K. A., Dodd, M., et al. (2002). Oncology outpatients with pain from bone metastasis require more than around-the-clock dosing of analgesics to achieve adequate pain control. *The Journal of Pain, 3*(1), 12–20.

Molfenter, T., Zetts, C., Dodd., M., Owens, B., Ford, J., & Mccarty, D. (2005). Reducing errors of omission in chronic disease management. *Journal of Interprofessional Care, 19*(5), 521–523.

Schumacher, K. L., Koresawa, S., West, C., Dodd, M., et al. (2002). The usefulness of a daily pain management diary for outpatients with cancer-related pain. *Oncology Nursing Forum, 29*(9), 1304–1313.

Schumacher, K. L., Koresawa, S., West, C., et al. (2005). Qualitative research contribution to a randomized clinical trial. *Research in Nursing & Health, 28*, 268–280.

Schumacher, K. L., Koresawa, S., West, C., Hawkins, C., et al. (2002). Putting cancer pain management regimens into practice at home. *Journal of Pain and Symptom Management, 23*(5), 369–382.

Schumacher, K. L., Stewart, B., Archbold, P., Dodd, M., & Dibble, S. (2000). Family caregiving skill: Development of the concept. *Research in Nursing & Health, 23*, 191–203.

Schumacher, K. L., West, C., Dodd, M., et al. (2002). Pain management autobiographies and reluctance to use opioids for cancer pain management. *Cancer Nursing, 25*(2), 125–133.

Shih, A., Miaskowski, C., Dodd, M. J., Stotts, N. A., & MacPhil, L. (2002). A research review of the current treatments for radiation-induced oral mucositis in patients with head and neck cancer. *Oncology Nursing Forum, 29*(7), 1063–1080.

Shih, A., Miaskowski, C., Dodd, M. J., Stotts, N. A., & MacPhil, L. (2003). Mechanisms for radiation-induced oral mucositis and the consequences. *Cancer Nursing, 26*(3), 222–229.

Tierney, D. K., Facione, N., Padilla, G., Blume, K., & Dodd, M. (2007). Altered sexual health and quality of life in women prior to hematopoietic cell transplantation. *European Journal of Oncology Nursing, 11*(4), 298–308.

Tierney, D. K., Facione, N., Padilla, G., & Dodd, M. (2007). Response shift: A theoretical exploration of quality of life following a hematopoietic cell transplantation. *Cancer Nursing, 30*(2), 125–138.

Villars, P., Dodd, M., West, C., et al. (2007). Differences in the prevalence and severity of side effects based on type of analgesic prescriptions in patients with chronic cancer pain. *Journal of Pain and Symptom Management, 33*(1), 67–77.

Voss, J. G., Dodd, M., Portillo, C., & Holzemar, W. (2006). Theories of fatigue: Application in HIV/AIDS. *Journal of the Association of Nurses in AIDS Care, 17*(1), 37–50.

Voss, J., Portillo, C. J., Holzemer, W. L., & Dodd, M. J. (2007). Symptom cluster of fatigue and depression in HIV/AIDS. *Journal of Prevention and Intervention in the Community, 33*(1–2), 19–34.

Wong, P. C., Dodd, M. J., Miaskowski, C., et al. (2006). Mucositis pain induced by radiation therapy: Prevalence, severity, and use of self care behaviors. *Journal of Pain and Symptom Management, 32*(1), 27–37.

Wood, K. A., Wiener, C. L., & Kayser-Jones, J. (2007). Supraventricular tachycardia and the struggle to be believed. *European Journal of Cardiovascular Nursing, 6*(4), 293–302.

Secondary Sources

Bailey, D. E., Wallace, M., Latini, D. M., Hegarty, J., Carroll, P. R., & Klein, E. A. (2011). Measuring illness uncertainty in men undergoing active surveillance for prostate cancer. *Applied Nursing Research, 24*(4), 193–199.

Chiou, C. P., & Chung, Y. C. (2012). Effectiveness of multimedia interactive patient education on knowledge, uncertainty and decision-making in patients with end-stage-renal-disease. *Journal of Clinical Nursing, 21*(9), 1223–1231.

Flemme, I., Hallberg, U., Johansson, I., & Stromberg, A. (2011). Uncertainty is a major concern for patients with implantable cardioverter defibrillators. *Heart & Lung, 40*(5), 420–428.

Halliday, L. E., Boughton, M. A., & Kerridge, I. (2014). Mothering and self-othering: The impact of uncertain reproductive capability in young women after hematological malignancy. *Health Care for Women International, 35*(3), 249–265.

Halliday, L. E., Boughton, M. A., & Kerridge, I. (2015). Liminal reproductive experiences after therapies for hematological malignancy. *Qual Health Res, 25*(3), 408–416.

Han, P. K., Klein, W. M. P., & Arora, N. K. (2011). Varieties of uncertainty in health care: A conceptual taxonomy. *Medical Decision Making, 31*(6), 828–838.

Hansen, B. S., Rortveit, K., Leiknes, I., et al. (2012). Patient experiences of uncertainty—a synthesis to guide nursing practice and research. *Journal of Nursing Management, 20*(2), 266–277.

Taha, S. A., Matheson, K., & Anisam, H. (2012). Everyday experiences of women posttreatment after breast cancer: The role of uncertainty, hassles, uplifts, and coping on depressive symptoms. *Journal of Psychosocial Oncology, 30*(3), 359–379.

31

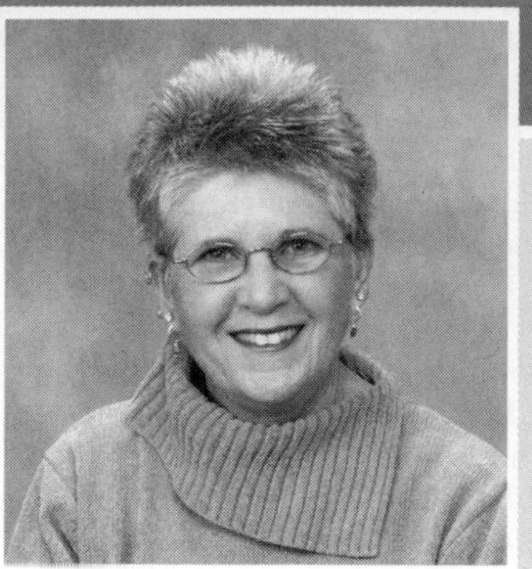

*Georgene Gaskill Eakes**
(1945–Present)

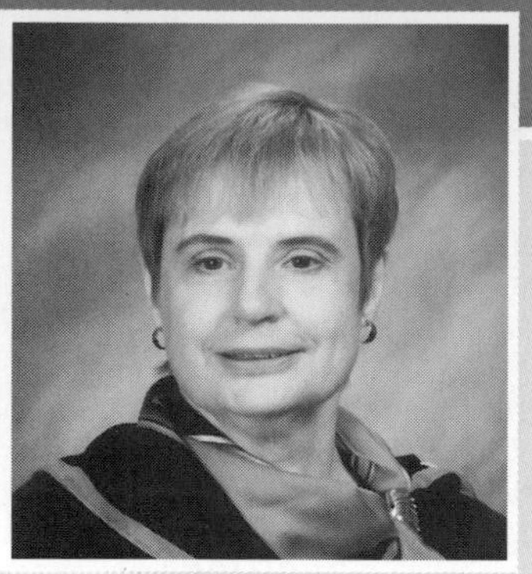

Mary Lermann Burke†
(1941–Present)

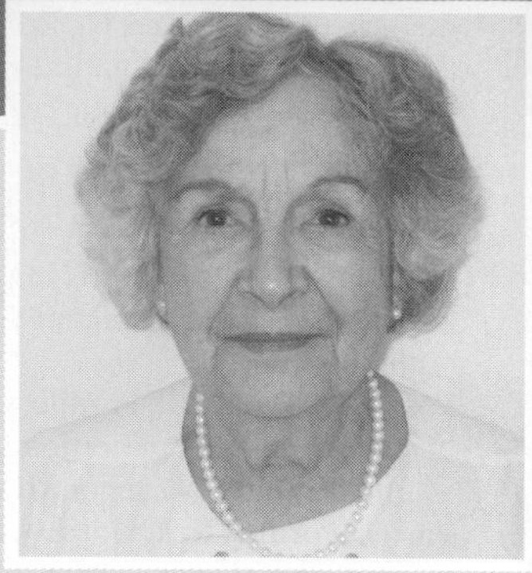

Margaret A. Hainsworth‡
(1931–Present)

Theory of Chronic Sorrow

Ann M. Schreier

"Chronic sorrow is the presence of pervasive grief-related feelings that have been found to occur periodically throughout the lives of individuals with chronic health conditions, their family caregivers and the bereaved."
(Burke, Eakes, & Hainsworth, 1999, p. 374)

CREDENTIALS AND BACKGROUND OF THE THEORISTS

Georgene Gaskill Eakes

Georgene Gaskill Eakes was born in New Bern, North Carolina. She received a Diploma in Nursing from Watts Hospital School of Nursing in Durham, North Carolina, in 1966, and in 1977 she graduated Summa Cum Laude from North Carolina Agricultural and Technical State University with a baccalaureate in nursing. Eakes completed a master's in nursing at the University of North Carolina at Greensboro in 1980, and a doctor of education degree from North Carolina State University in 1988. Eakes was awarded a federal traineeship for her graduate study at the master's level and a graduate fellowship from the North Carolina League for Nursing to support her doctoral studies. She was inducted into Sigma Theta Tau International Honor Society of Nurses in 1979 and Phi Kappa Phi Honor Society in 1988.

Early in her professional career, Eakes worked in both acute and community-based psychiatric and mental health settings. In 1980 she joined the faculty at East Carolina University School of Nursing, Greenville, North Carolina.

Eakes' interest in issues related to death, dying, grief, and loss began in the 1970s, when she sustained life-threatening injuries in an automobile crash. Her near-death experience heightened her awareness of how ill prepared health care professionals and laypeople are to deal with individuals facing their mortality and the general lack of understanding of grief reactions experienced in response to loss situations. Motivated by this insight, she directed her early research efforts to the investigation of death anxiety among nursing personnel in long-term care settings and to the exploration of grief resolution among hospice nurses.

In 1983 Eakes established a twice-monthly community service support group for individuals diagnosed with cancer and their significant others, which she continues to

*Photo credit: Center for Health Sciences Communication, Brody School of Medicine, East Carolina University, Greenville, NC.
†Photo credit: Olan Mills Portrait Studio, Centerdale, RI.
‡Photo credit: Shawn Hainsworth, New York.

cofacilitate. Her involvement with this group alerted her to the ongoing nature of grief reactions associated with diagnosis of potentially life-threatening chronic illnesses. While presenting her dissertation research at a Sigma Theta Tau International research conference in Taipei, Taiwan, in 1989, she attended a presentation on chronic sorrow by Mary Lermann Burke and immediately made the connection between Burke's description of chronic sorrow in mothers of children with a myelomeningocele disability and grief reactions she had observed among cancer support group members.

After the conference, Eakes contacted Burke to explore the possibility of collaborative research endeavors. Subsequent to their discussions, they scheduled a meeting that included Burke and her colleague, Margaret A. Hainsworth, and Carolyn Lindgren, a colleague of Hainsworth. The Nursing Consortium for Research on Chronic Sorrow (NCRCS) was an outcome of this first meeting in the summer of 1989.

Subsequent to NCRCS's establishment, members conducted numerous collaborative qualitative research studies on populations of individuals affected with chronic or life-threatening conditions, on family caregivers, and on bereaved individuals. Eakes focused her individual studies on those diagnosed with cancer, family caregivers of adult mentally ill children, and individuals who have experienced the death of a significant other. From 1992 to 1997, Eakes received three research grant awards from East Carolina University School of Nursing and two research grants from Beta Nu Chapter of Sigma Theta Tau International to support her research endeavors.

In addition to her professional publications, Eakes has conducted numerous presentations on issues related to grief-loss and death and dying to professionals and lay groups at local, state, national, and international levels. She has been heavily involved with the training of sudden infant death syndrome counselors for North Carolina and local and regional hospice volunteers. Eakes is active in efforts to improve the quality of care at the end of life and, toward that end, serves as a member of the Board of Directors of the End of Life Care Coalition of Eastern North Carolina.

In 2002 Eakes received the East Carolina University Scholar Teacher Award in recognition of excellence in the integration of research into teaching practices. In 1999 Eakes received the Best of Image award for theory publication presented by Sigma Theta Tau International Honor Society of Nursing for the publication, "Middle-Range Theory of Chronic Sorrow." She was a finalist for the *Oncology Nursing Forum* Excellence in Writing Award in 1994. Other honors and awards include selection as North Carolina Nurse Educator of the Year by the North Carolina Nurses Association in 1991 and as Outstanding Researcher by Beta Nu Chapter of Sigma Theta Tau International Honor Society for Nurses in 1994 and 1998. Eakes has served as a reviewer for *Qualitative Health Research*, an international, interdisciplinary journal.

Eakes is Professor Emeritus, East Carolina University College of Nursing. Before her retirement she taught undergraduate courses in psychiatric and mental health nursing and nursing research, a master's level course in nursing education, and an interdisciplinary graduate course titled "Perspectives on Death/Dying." Currently, she is the Director of Clinical Education, Vidant Medical Center, in Greenville, North Carolina (G. Eakes, personal communication, 2012).

Mary Lermann Burke

Mary Lermann Burke was born in Sandusky, Ohio, where she grew up. She received a diploma in nursing from Good Samaritan Hospital School of Nursing in Cincinnati in 1962 and a postgraduate certification later that year from Children's Medical Center in District of Columbia. After several years of work experience in pediatric nursing, Burke graduated Summa Cum Laude from Rhode Island College, Providence, with a bachelor's degree in nursing. In 1982 she received her master's degree in parent-child nursing from Boston University. During this program, she received a certificate in Parent-Child Nursing and Interdisciplinary Training in Developmental Disabilities from the Child Development Center of Rhode Island Hospital and the Section on Reproductive and Developmental Medicine, Brown University, in Providence. She received her doctorate of nursing science from Boston University in 1989.

Burke was inducted into Theta Chapter, Sigma Theta Tau, during her master's program at Boston University in 1981 and Delta Upsilon Chapter of Sigma Theta Tau at Rhode Island College in 1988. She received a Doctoral Student Scholarship Award from the Theta Chapter in 1988. She received the 1996 Delta Upsilon Chapter Louisa A. White Award for Research Excellence.

During the period from 1991 through 1996, Burke received four Rhode Island College Faculty Research Grants for studies in the area of chronic sorrow. In 1998 she was awarded a grant from the Delta Upsilon Chapter for initial quantitative instrument development for the study of chronic sorrow. Burke was principal investigator on the Transition to Adult Living Project, funded by a grant from the Department of Health and Human Services, Maternal and Child Health Bureau, Genetics Services Branch, from 1992 through 1995. A New England Regional Genetics Group Special Projects Grant, The Transition to Adult Living Project—System Dissemination of Information, supplemented this in 1995. Burke was co–principal investigator.

In her early career, Burke practiced in the pediatric nursing specialty in both acute and primary settings. She joined the faculty of Rhode Island College Department of Nursing as a clinical instructor in 1980 and became a full-time instructor in 1982, assistant professor in 1987, associate professor in 1991, and professor in 1996. During this period, she taught pediatric nursing in both didactic and clinical courses. She also developed and taught a foundation nursing curriculum course encompassing nutrition, pharmacology, and pathophysiology. She retired from her Rhode Island College faculty position in December 2002.

Burke became interested in the concept of chronic sorrow during her master's degree program while engaged in a clinical practicum at the Child Development Center of Rhode Island Hospital. Working with children with spina bifida and their parents, she developed the clinical hunch that the emotions displayed by the parents were consistent with chronic sorrow as first described by Olshansky (1962). Her master's thesis, *The Concerns of Mothers of Preschool Children With Myelomeningocele,* identified emotions similar to chronic sorrow. She then developed the Burke Chronic Sorrow Questionnaire for her doctoral dissertation research, *Chronic Sorrow in Mothers of School-Age Children With Myelomeningocele.*

In June 1989, Burke presented her dissertation research at the Sigma Theta Tau International Research Congress in Taipei, Taiwan, where she interacted with Dr. Eakes of East Carolina University and Dr. Hainsworth of Rhode Island College. Subsequently, this group became the NCRCS, joined briefly by Dr. Carolyn Lindgren of Wayne State University. Together they developed a modified Burke/NCRCS Chronic Sorrow Questionnaire and conducted individually a series of studies that were analyzed collaboratively. Burke's individual studies in this series focused on chronic sorrow in infertile couples, adult children of parents with chronic conditions, and bereaved parents. The collaboratively analyzed studies resulted in the development of a middle-range theory of chronic sorrow, published in 1998. Members of the Consortium, both individually and collaboratively, presented numerous papers on chronic sorrow at local, state, national, and international conferences and wrote 10 articles published in refereed journals, receiving the Best of Image Award in the Theory Category from Sigma Theta Tau International for their article, "Middle-Range Theory of Chronic Sorrow." More recently, Burke collaborated with Dr. Eakes in the development of the Burke/Eakes Chronic Sorrow Assessment Tool.

Burke is active in numerous professional and community organizations. She is a member of the St. Joseph's Health Services of Rhode Island Board of Trustees. She was awarded the Outstanding Alumna Award for Contributions in Nursing Education by Rhode Island College Department of Nursing and the Rhode Island College Alumni Honor Roll Award (L. Burke, personal communication, 2005).

Margaret A. Hainsworth

Margaret A. Hainsworth was born in Brockville, Ontario, Canada, and grew up in Prescott, Ontario. She entered the diploma school of nursing at the Brockville General Hospital, Brockville, Ontario, graduating in 1953. In 1959 she immigrated to the United States to attend George Peabody College for Teachers in Nashville, Tennessee, receiving a diploma in public health nursing. In 1974 she continued her education at Salve Regina College, Newport, Rhode Island, and received a baccalaureate degree in nursing in 1973 and a master's degree in psychiatric and mental health nursing from Boston College in 1974. She received a doctoral degree in education administration from the University of Connecticut in 1986. In 1988 she was board certified as a clinical specialist in psychiatric and mental health nursing.

She was inducted into Sigma Theta Tau, Alpha Chi Chapter in 1978 and Delta Upsilon Chapter in 1989. In 1976 she was awarded an outstanding faculty award at Rhode Island College. In 1992 she was selected to attend the Technical Assistance Workshop and Mentorship for Nurses in Implementation of the National Plan for Research in Child and Adolescent Mental Disorders that was sponsored by the National Institutes of Health. In 1991 she was selected to review manuscripts for the *Qualitative Health Research* journal. In 1999 Hainsworth was accepted at the Royal Melbourne Institute of Technology in Melbourne, Australia, as a visiting fellow on a faculty exchange program.

Her practice in nursing was in the specialties of public health and psychiatric and mental health nursing. In 1974 she was accepted as a lecturer in the Department of Nursing at Rhode Island College and was promoted to full professor in 1992. Her major area of teaching was psychiatric care that consisted of both classroom lectures and clinical practice. She taught a course titled "Death and Dying" that became an elective in the college's general studies program. Hainsworth always maintained her practice and was employed for 13 years as a consultant at the Visiting Nursing Association. She entered into a private practice at Bay Counseling Association in 1993 and maintained this practice for 5 years.

Her interest in chronic illness and its relationship to sorrow began in her practice as a facilitator for a support group for women with multiple sclerosis. This practice led to her dissertation work, *An Ethnographic Study of Women With Multiple Sclerosis Using a Symbolic Interaction Approach.* This research was accepted for a presentation at the

Sigma Theta Tau Research Congress in Taipei, Taiwan, in 1989. At this conference, she became familiar with the research on chronic sorrow after attending a presentation by Burke.

Building on the work of Burke and Eakes, the NCRCS was established in 1989 to expand the understanding of chronic sorrow. Hainsworth was one of the four cofounders and remained an active member until 1996. The research began with four studies that focused on chronic sorrow in individuals in chronic life situations, and the members of the consortium analyzed data collaboratively. During the 7 years that she was a member, the consortium published 13 manuscripts and presented the findings from their studies at international, state, and regional conferences. In 1999 they were awarded the Best of Image Award in Theory from Sigma Theta Tau International (M. Hainsworth, personal communication, 2005).

THEORETICAL SOURCES

The NCRCS based the middle-range theory of chronic sorrow on two main sources. The work of Olshansky (1962) was cited as the basis of the original concept of chronic sorrow (Eakes, Burke, & Hainsworth, 1998). Lazarus and Folkman's (1984) model of stress and adaptation formed the foundation for the conceptualization of how people cope with chronic sorrow.

The concept of chronic sorrow originated with the work of Olshansky in 1962 (Lindgren et al., 1992). The NCRCS theorists cite Olshansky's observations of parents with mentally retarded children that indicated these parents experienced recurrent sadness and coining of the term *chronic sorrow.* This original concept was described as "a broad, simple description of psychological reaction to a tragic situation" (Lindgren et al., 1992, p. 30)

During the 1980s, other researchers began to examine the experience of parents of children who were either physically or mentally disabled. This work validated a recurrent sadness and a never-ending nature of grief experienced by these parents. Previous to this work, grief had been conceptualized as a process that resolves over time that if unresolved is abnormal according to Bowlby and Lindemann's work (Lindgren et al., 1992). In contrast to that time-bound conceptualization, in the concept of chronic sorrow it is inherent that recurrent sadness is a normal experience (Wikler, Wasow, & Hatfield as cited by Lindgren et al., 1992). Burke, in her study of children with spina bifida, defined chronic sorrow as "pervasive sadness that is permanent, periodic and progressive in nature" (Hainsworth, Eakes, & Burke, 1994, p. 60.)

The NCRCS did not confine their theory to the existence of chronic sorrow but sought to examine the response to grief. This group incorporated Lazarus and Folkman's 1984 work on stress and adaptation as the basis for effective management methods described in their model (Eakes et al., 1998). The disparity encountered and the response to regrief stimulates individual coping mechanisms. There are categories of coping styles or management. Internal coping strategies include action-oriented, cognitive reappraisal, and interpersonal behaviors (Eakes et al., 1998). Thus the middle-range theory of chronic sorrow extended the theoretical base of chronic sorrow to not only the experience of chronic sorrow in certain situations but also the coping responses to the phenomenon.

MAJOR CONCEPTS & DEFINITIONS

Chronic Sorrow

Chronic sorrow is the ongoing disparity resulting from a loss characterized by pervasiveness and permanence. Symptoms of grief recur periodically, and these symptoms are potentially progressive.

Loss

Loss occurs as a result of disparity between the "ideal" and real situations or experiences. For example, there is a "perfect child" and a child with a chronic condition who differs from that ideal.

Trigger Events

Trigger events are situations, circumstances, and conditions that highlight the disparity or the recurrent loss and initiate or exacerbate feelings of grief.

Management Methods

Management methods are means by which individuals deal with chronic sorrow. These may be internal (personal coping strategies) or external (health care practitioner or other persons' interventions).

Ineffective Management

Ineffective management results from strategies that increase the individual's discomfort or heighten the feelings of chronic sorrow.

Effective Management

Effective management results from strategies that lead to increased comfort of the affected individual.

USE OF EMPIRICAL EVIDENCE

Chronic Sorrow

The empirical evidence supporting NCRCS's initial conceptual definition of chronic sorrow was derived from interviews with mothers of children with spina bifida, which Burke (1989) conducted as part of her dissertation research. Through this work, Burke was able to define chronic sorrow as a pervasive sadness and found that the experience was permanent, periodic, and potentially progressive (Eakes et al., 1993). Burke's initial work provided the foundation for subsequent series of studies, including the basis for interview guides used in these studies.

These NCRCS studies involved the following:

- Individuals with:
  - Cancer (Eakes, 1993)
  - Infertility (Hainsworth et al., 1994)
  - Multiple sclerosis (Hainsworth, 1994; Hainsworth et al., 1993) or Parkinson's disease (Lindgren, 1996).
- **Spousal caregivers** of persons with:
  - Chronic mental illness (Hainsworth et al., 1995)
  - Multiple sclerosis (Hainsworth, 1995)
  - Parkinson's disease (Lindgren, 1996)
- **Parental caregivers** of
  - Adult children with chronic mental illness (Eakes, 1995)

Based on these studies, the theorists postulated that chronic sorrow occurs in any situation in which the loss is unresolved. These studies did not demonstrate consistently that the associated emotions worsened over time. However, the theorists concluded that the studies did support the "potential for progressivity and intensification of chronic sorrow over time" (Eakes et al., 1998, p. 180).

The NCRCS theorists extended their studies to individuals experiencing a single loss (bereaved). They found that this population experienced these same feelings of chronic sorrow (Eakes, Burke, & Hainsworth, 1999).

Based on this extensive empirical evidence, the NCRCS theorists refined the definition of chronic sorrow as the "periodic recurrence of permanent, pervasive sadness or other grief-related feelings associated with ongoing disparity resulting from a loss experience" (Eakes et al., 1998, p. 180).

Triggers

Using the empirical data from the series of studies, the NCRCS theorists identified primary events or situations that precipitated the reexperience of initial grief feelings. These events were labeled *chronic sorrow triggers* (Eakes et al., 1993). The NCRCS compared and contrasted the triggers of chronic sorrow in individuals with chronic conditions, family caregivers, and bereaved persons (Burke, Eakes, & Hainsworth, 1999). For all populations, comparisons with norms and anniversaries were found to trigger chronic sorrow. Both family caregivers and persons with chronic conditions experienced triggering with management crises. One trigger unique for family caregivers was the requirement of unending caregiving. The bereaved population reported that memories and role change were unique triggers.

Management Strategies

The NCRCS posited that chronic sorrow is not debilitating when individuals effectively manage feelings. The management strategies were categorized as internal or external. Self-care management strategies were designated as internal coping strategies. The NCRCS further designated internal coping strategies as action, cognitive, interpersonal, and emotional.

Action coping mechanisms were used across all subjects—individuals with chronic conditions and their caregivers (Eakes, 1993, 1995; Eakes et al., 1993, 1999; Hainsworth, 1994, 1995; Hainsworth et al., 1995; Lindgren, 1996). The examples provided are similar to distraction methods commonly used to cope with pain. For instance, "keeping busy" and "doing something fun" are given as examples of action-oriented coping (Eakes, 1995; Lindgren et al., 1992). The NCRCS theorists found that cognitive coping was common, and examples included "thinking positively," "making the most of it," and "not trying to fight it" (Eakes, 1995; Hainsworth, 1994; Lindgren, 1996). Interpersonal coping examples included "going to a psychiatrist," "joined a support group," and "talking to others" (Eakes et al., 1993; Hainsworth, 1994, 1995). Emotional strategy examples included "having a good cry" and expressing emotions (Eakes et al., 1998; Hainsworth et al., 1995). A management strategy was labeled effective when a subject described it as helpful in decreasing feelings of regrief.

External management was described initially by Burke as interventions provided by health professionals (Eakes et al., 1998). Health care professionals assist affected populations to increase their comfort through roles of empathetic presence, teacher-expert, and caring and competent professional (Eakes, 1993, 1995; Eakes et al., 1993, 1999; Hainsworth, 1994, 1995; Hainsworth et al., 1995; Lindgren, 1996).

In summary, an impressive total of 196 interviews resulted in the middle-range theory of chronic sorrow. The theorists summarized a decade of research with individuals with chronic sorrow and found that this phenomenon commonly occurs in persons with chronic conditions, in family caregivers, and in bereaved individuals (Burke et al., 1999; Eakes et al., 1998).

MAJOR ASSUMPTIONS

Nursing

Diagnosing chronic sorrow and providing interventions are within the scope of nursing practice. Nurses can provide anticipatory guidance to individuals at risk. The primary roles of nurses include empathetic presence, teacher-expert, and caring and competent caregiver (Eakes et al., 1998).

Person

Humans have an idealized perception of life processes and health. People compare their experiences both with the ideal and with others around them. Although each person's experience with loss is unique, there are common and predictable features of the loss experience (Eakes et al., 1998).

Health

There is a normality of functioning. A person's health is dependent on adaptation to disparities associated with loss. Effective coping results in a normal response to life losses (Eakes et al., 1998).

Environment

Interactions occur within a social context, which includes family, social, work, and health care environments. Individuals respond to their assessment of themselves in relation to social norms (Eakes et al., 1998).

THEORETICAL ASSERTIONS

1. Chronic sorrow is a normal human response related to ongoing disparity created by a loss situation.
2. Chronic sorrow is cyclical in nature.
3. Predictable internal and external triggers of heightened grief can be categorized and anticipated.
4. Humans have inherent and learned coping strategies that may or may not be effective in regaining normal equilibrium when experiencing chronic sorrow.
5. Health care professionals' interventions may or may not be effective in assisting the individual to regain normal equilibrium.
6. A human who experiences a single or an ongoing loss will perceive a disparity between the ideal and reality.
7. The disparity between the real and the ideal leads to feelings of pervasive sadness and grief (Eakes et al., 1998).

LOGICAL FORM

This theory is based on a series of qualitative studies. Through the analysis of 196 interviews, the middle-range theory of chronic sorrow evolved. With clear empirical evidence, the NCRCS theorists described the phenomenon of chronic sorrow, identified common triggers of regrief, and described internal coping mechanisms and the role of nurses in the external management of chronic sorrow.

ACCEPTANCE BY THE NURSING COMMUNITY

Three perspectives—practice, education, and research—provide a framework for examining the nursing community's acceptance of the NCRCS's work. An examination of each perspective follows.

Practice

Work Original to the Nursing Consortium for Research on Chronic Sorrow

The series of studies by the NCRCS, which form the foundation of the middle-range theory of chronic sorrow (Eakes et al., 1998), are replete with implications for practice. Each article included a section that related the findings to clinical nursing practice (Burke et al., 1999; Eakes, 1993, 1995; Hainsworth, 1994; Hainsworth et al., 1993, 1994, 1995; Lindgren, 1996; Lindgren et al., 1992). The NCRCS work provides suggestions for nurses to assist individuals and family caregivers to manage the milestones or triggering events effectively. More specifically, the work identifies nursing roles as empathetic presence, teacher-expert, and caring and competent professional (Eakes et al., 1993). In addition, the original NCRCS work has provided other authors a basis for publications that are directed to a practice-focused audience.

Literature Derived from the Nursing Consortium for Research on Chronic Sorrow

Several non-NCRCS nurse authors have published articles that cite NCRCS studies directed to practicing clinicians (Gedaly Duff, Stoger, & Shelton, 2000; Gordon, 2009; Joseph, 2012; Kerr, 2010; Marcella-Brienza, 2015; Scornaienchi, 2003, Vitale & Falco, 2014). Other practice-focused literature, although not nurse authored, provided practice guidance that nurses would find useful (Doka, 2004; Harris & Gorman, 2011; Marcella-Brienza, 2015; Rossheim & McAdam, 2010; Weingarten, 2012). Although these works relate to practice, they can also be considered educationally related. The next section presents additional evidence supporting the relevance of the NCRCS's work on chronic sorrow for the educational community.

Education

The use of the NCRCS's work in undergraduate, graduate research, and continuing education lends support for its acceptance by the educational community.

Undergraduate Education: Standardized Nursing Languages

Reviewing the literature on standardized nursing languages reveals that chronic sorrow is a diagnostic category (North American Nursing Diagnosis Association [NANDA], 2014) with related expected outcomes and suggested interventions (Johnson et al., 2011). Comparison of the definitions of chronic sorrow used by NANDA International (NANDA-I) and NCRCS (Eakes et al., 1998) reveals essentially similar dimensions. Several widely used nursing diagnosis textbooks (Ackley & Ladwig, 2013; Carpenito-Moyet, 2014; Doenges, Moorhouse, & Murr, 2016) cite the work of the NCRCS or authors who used the NCRCS's work in the explication of the linkages among chronic sorrow as a diagnostic category, interventions, and outcomes. The linkages among the diagnostic categories of NANDA-I, the Nursing Outcomes Classification (NOC), and Nursing Interventions Classification (NIC) (Johnson et al., 2012) hold educational implications for undergraduate nursing education, because they provide guidance for both nursing students and educators—guidance to nursing students in learning clinical decision processes and to nurse educators teaching clinical decision processes as well as designing curricula. Moreover, the linkages refocus care planning to include attention to outcomes, an essential step in teaching evidence-based practice (Pesut & Herman, 1998).

Graduate Research Education: Nursing

The use of NCRCS's theoretical work in unpublished master's theses and doctoral dissertations and dissertation-related articles provides evidence of its use in graduate nursing education. These studies are categorized here according to graduate level and topic.

- Master's theses:
  - Chronic sorrow in mothers of chronically ill children (Golden, 1994; Shumaker, 1995)
- Doctoral dissertations:
  - Parental caregivers of children with special health care needs (Kelly, 2010)
  - Women treated for cancer who experienced fertility problems and/or premature menopause (Hunter, 2010)
  - Development of *Kendall Chronic Sorrow Instrument* to screen for and measure experience of chronic sorrow (Kendall, 2005)
  - Caregivers of children with sickle cell disease (Neilsen, 2013)

Graduate Research Education: Other Disciplines

Graduate students in other professional disciplines, including education, social work, psychology, education, and family life, have conducted dissertational studies using the NCRCS's work. These unpublished studies, listed here according to topic, hold relevance for nursing practice.

- Individuals with:
  - Chronic back pain (Blair, 2010)
  - Infertility (Casale, 2009)
  - Bipolar disease (Freedberg, 2011)
- Family caregivers of:
  - Young and adolescent children with:
    Multiple disabilities (Parrish, 2010)
    Special health care needs (Kelly, 2010)
    Chronic mental illness (Davis, 2006)
    Autism (Collins, 2008; Monsson, 2010)
  - Adult children with:
    Cerebral palsy (Masterson, 2010; Wee, 2010)

Continuing Education

Several authors used the consortium's work on chronic sorrow in published articles that had, at the time of publishing, continuing education offerings designed for clinicians who work with families with chronically ill members (Doornbos, 1997; Hobdell et al., 2007; Mallow & Bechtel, 1999; Meleski, 2002; Melnyk et al., 2001). Drench's (2003) course for physical therapists and physical therapy assistants presented content on loss and grief that included the NCRCS's work.

Research

A review of published research that has used the NCRCS's work revealed that researchers have extended the work through studies conducted with representatives of populations studied previously and with new populations from international researchers.

- Extension of NCRCS's populations:
  - Multiple sclerosis, individuals and caregivers (Isaksson & Ahlström, 2008; Isaksson, Gunnarsson, & Ahlström, 2007; Liedstrom, Isaksson, & Ahlström, 2008)
  - Neural tube defects, parental caregivers (Hobdell, 2004)
  - Bereavement, parents after stillbirth (Erlandsson et al., 2011).
- Extension of the NCRCS's work to new populations:
  - Individuals:
    Who have human immunodeficiency virus (HIV) (Ingram & Hutchinson, 1999; Lichtenstein, Laska, & Clair, 2002)
    Who are female victims of child abuse (Smith, 2007, 2009)

- Family caregivers of persons with:
  Schizophrenia (Olwit et al., 2015)
- Family caregivers of children with:
  Asthma (Maltby, Kristjanson, & Coleman, 2003)
  Cancer (Nikfarid et al., 2015)
  Diabetes (Bowes et al., 2009; Lowes & Lyne, 2000)
  Disabilities (Mallow & Bechtel, 1999; Patrick-Ott & Ladd, 2010; Whittingham et al., 2013)
  Epilepsy (Hobdell et al., 2007)
  HIV (Mawn, 2012)
  Rare diseases (Glenn, 2015)
  Sickle cell disease (Northington, 2000)

Although most of the authors were from the United States, the literature reflects an international influence, with publications by nurses from Australia (Maltby et al., 2003; Whittingham et al., 2013), New Zealand (Mercer, 2015), Iran (Nikfarid et al., 2015), Sweden (Ahlström, 2007; Isaksson & Ahlström, 2008; Pejlert, 2001), Uganda (Olwit et al., 2015), and the United Kingdom (Bowes et al., 2009; Lowes & Lyne, 2000). Several studies were written by occupational therapists, two by psychologists and one by sociologists, supporting the assertion that the NCRCS work is the basis for international and interdisciplinary research. Application of this middle-range theory to research is seen in current nursing literature (Eakes, 2013).

FURTHER DEVELOPMENT

To date most of the research efforts related to the middle-range theory of chronic sorrow used qualitative methods and focused on identifying the concept's occurrence in other populations. Further development of the theory would be enhanced through instrument development studies, designed to measure the intensity of chronic sorrow at the interval or ratio level. Current instruments, the Burke/Eakes Chronic Sorrow Assessment (Eakes, 2013) and the Kendall Chronic Sorrow Instrument (Kendall, 2005), yield data at the nominal or ordinal level. Ratio or interval chronic sorrow–intensity data would enhance studies designed to measure the effectiveness of nursing roles and interventions in achievement of the outcomes identified in the NOC system, such as "Acceptance: Health Status . . . Depression Level . . . Hope . . . Mood Equilibrium" (Johnson et al., 2012, pp. 220–221). Development of this type of research would provide the empirical support needed for evidence-based nursing practice.

CRITIQUE

Clarity

This theory clearly describes a phenomenon that is observed in the clinical area when loss occurs, and it is certainly evident that it is accepted in nursing practice. As indicated previously, a nursing diagnosis of chronic sorrow is included in the standardized languages of NANDA-I and is defined as cyclical, recurrent, and potentially progressive and, as such, is consistent with the definition of the NCRSC theorists. In each of the published works of these theorists, key concepts are defined, and this middle-range theory describes the proposed relationship between these concepts. The relationship between concepts makes intuitive sense. For example, it is clear that effective management, whether internal or external, will lead to increased comfort, and, conversely, ineffective management will lead to increased discomfort and intensity of chronic sorrow. As a middle-range theory, the scope is limited to explanation of a single phenomenon, that of response to loss, and is congruent with clinical practice experience. As Eakes has stated, the beauty of this middle-range theory is that it rings true with practitioners, students, and educators, as is evident from the continued communication nationally and internationally (G. Eakes, personal communication, May 2012).

One unclear aspect of the theory is an explanation for why not all individuals with unresolved losses experience chronic sorrow. Some, albeit few, of the NCRCS's interviewees did not experience the symptoms labeled as *chronic sorrow.* No further data have been provided about these individuals. Do individuals who do not experience chronic sorrow have different personality characteristics, such as resiliency, or receive different health care interventions at the time of the loss? What would the data from these individuals suggest about coping with ongoing loss?

Another concept that needs clarification is the progression of chronic sorrow. Although chronic sorrow is described as potentially progressive, what is the progression, and is this progression pathological in nature?

Clarification of the categories of internal management strategies is warranted. It is unclear to these reviewers how problem-oriented and cognitive strategies are different. Likewise, the emotive-cognitive, emotional, and interpersonal strategies are not clearly described. There is some obvious overlap between external versus internal management when the word *interpersonal* is used to describe seeking professional help.

Simplicity

The theoretical model of chronic sorrow (Fig. 31.1) enhances the understanding of the relationship between the variables. With this model, it is clear that chronic sorrow is cyclical in nature, pervasive, and potentially progressive. Furthermore, with the subconcepts of internal versus external management and ineffective versus effective management, it is clear what type of assessment and at what

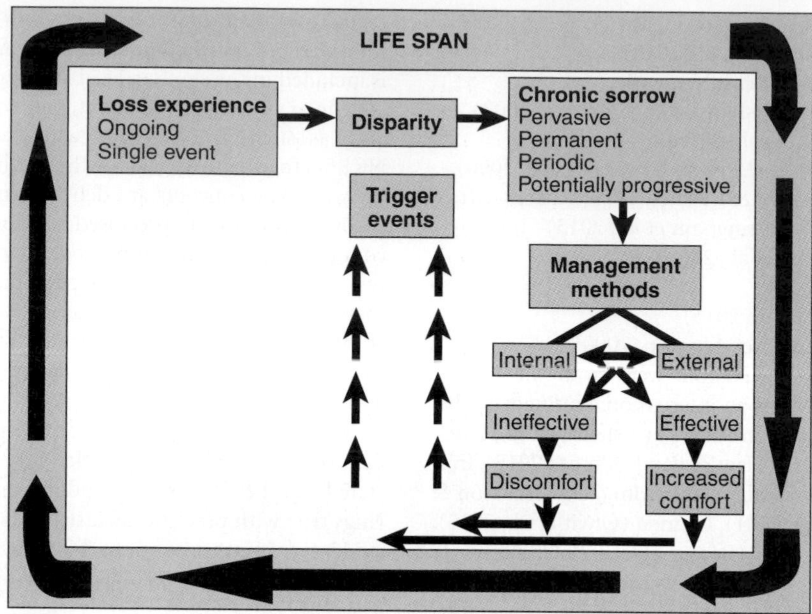

FIG. 31.1 Theoretical model of chronic sorrow. (From Eakes, G.G., Burke, M.L., & Hainsworth, M.A. [1998]. Middle-range theory of chronic sorrow. *Image: The Journal of Nursing Scholarship, 30*[2], 180.)

point appropriate intervention by nurses and other health care providers would be best to prevent chronic sorrow from becoming progressive. With a limited number of defined variables, the theory is succinct and readily understood. As a middle-range theory, it is useful for research design and practice guidance.

Generality

The concept of chronic sorrow began with the study of parents of children with a physical or cognitive defect. The NCRCS theorists, through their generated empirical evidence, expanded the theory to include a variety of loss experiences. The theory clearly applies to a wide range of losses and is applicable to the affected individual as well as to the caregivers and the bereaved. In addition, the theory is useful to a variety of health care practitioners. With these concepts, the unique nature of the experience is captured with the broadness of the concepts such as triggers. The triggers and the management strategies are unique to the individual situation and thus allow the application to a wide variety of situations.

EMPIRICAL PRECISION

As is characteristic of middle-range theory, the limited scope readily allows researchers to study the phenomenon. With a limited number of variables and defined relationships among the variables, researchers are able to generate hypotheses related to the study of nursing interventions that promote effective management strategies for chronic sorrow. These outcome studies provide and add to the foundation of evidence-based practice.

Because the theory was derived from empirical evidence, it has clear utility for further research. The clear definition of chronic sorrow allows the study of individuals with a variety of losses and those loss situations that commonly result in chronic sorrow. In their study of bereaved individuals, Eakes and colleagues (1999) identified symptoms of chronic sorrow in most subjects. Through further study, researchers can devise assessment tools for clinical practice.

DERIVABLE CONSEQUENCES

As a consequence of this rich body of research, chronic sorrow is a widely accepted phenomenon, as is evident by its inclusion in NANDA-I diagnoses. Nurses and other health care professionals have found validity for their experiences with loss in the clinical arena. Subsequently, health care practitioners are able to normalize the experience. As Eakes stated, "chronic sorrow is like the pregnancy experience, it is a normal process in which clients can benefit from guidance and support of health care professionals" (G. Eakes, personal communication, May 2012). Eakes further stated that this experience is unique to each individual and to each situation.

SUMMARY

Loss is an experience common to all individuals. This middle-range theory describes the phenomenon of chronic sorrow as a normal response to the ongoing disparity created by the loss. The major concepts are described and include disparity, triggers, and management strategies (internal and external). The theoretical sources and empirical evidence are described. The chapter presents evidence that the theory is accepted and used in practice, education, and research. It is referenced internationally by nurses and by providers in other disciplines. Suggestions for further development and research are presented. A thorough critique describes the clarity of concepts and the simplicity and the usefulness of the theory for evidence-based research.

CASE STUDY

Susan Jones is a 21-year-old woman who sustained a spinal cord injury at the age of 14 years as a result of a diving accident. She is quadriplegic and attends a local college. Her mother, Mary Jones, is her primary caregiver. Mrs. Jones complains of difficulty sleeping and has frequent headaches. As the nurse, you suspect that Mrs. Jones may be experiencing chronic sorrow.

Using the Burke/NCRCS Chronic Sorrow Questionnaire (caregiver version) as an interview guide, you find evidence of chronic sorrow (Eakes, 1995). Mrs. Jones describes frequent feelings of being overwhelmed. She expresses that she feels both angry at times and heartbroken that her daughter will never have a normal life. She indicates that she has had these feelings off and on since her daughter's accident. Furthermore, she tells you that she sees no end to her caregiving responsibilities. These feelings are strongest when her friends' children get married and get jobs away from home. She copes with these feelings by trying to focus on the positive (her daughter is alive and her sons are doing well) and talking with a few close friends.

You reassure Mrs. Jones that she is not alone in her situation, and that it is normal to have these feelings. In the course of the interview, you find that Mrs. Jones has not sought professional counseling help. Mrs. Jones tells you that she feels better, because this is the first time a health professional has asked her about her feelings. With Mrs. Jones, you begin to strategize on finding respite care and a regular mental health counselor to assist her in coping with chronic sorrow.

CRITICAL THINKING ACTIVITIES

1. Using the middle-range theory of chronic sorrow as a framework, devise one or more hypotheses about parents of children with type 1 diabetes who do or do not attend a support group.
2. Providing a support group is only one possible intervention strategy to assist individuals experiencing chronic sorrow. What outcome measures or objective evaluation would you use to validate the effectiveness of interventions?
3. Compare and contrast the middle range theory of chronic sorrow to Kubler-Ross' stages of grief or to Bowlby's theory of loss.
4. Describe the experience of three individuals with a chronic condition such as multiple sclerosis. Do you think that the theoretical assertions of the middle-range theory of chronic sorrow apply in these situations? State your rationale.

POINTS FOR FURTHER STUDY

- Eakes, G. G. (2013). Chronic sorrow. In S. J. Peterson & T. S. Bredow (Eds.), *Middle range theories: Application to nursing research* (3rd ed., pp. 96–107). Philadelphia: Lippincott Williams & Wilkins.
- Eakes, G. G., & Burke, M. L. (2002). Development and validation of the Burke/Eakes chronic sorrow assessment tool. Unpublished raw data.
- Kendall, L. C. (2005). The experience of living with ongoing loss: Testing the Kendall Chronic Sorrow Instrument. (Doctoral dissertation.) Available from ProQuest Dissertations and Theses database. (UMI No. 3196497.)

REFERENCES

Ackley, B. J., & Ladwig, G. B. (2013). *Nursing diagnosis handbook: An evidence-based guide to planning care* (9th ed.). St Louis, MO: Mosby Elsevier.

Ahlström, G. (2007). Experiences of loss and chronic sorrow in persons with severe chronic illness. *Journal of Nursing and Health Care of Chronic Illness, 16*(3a), 76–83.

Blair, M. B. (2010). *Quality of life despite back pain: A phenomenological study.* (Doctoral dissertation.) Available from *ProQuest Dissertations and Theses* database. (UMI No. 807680746.)

Bowes, S., Lowes, L., Warner, J., & Gregory, J. W. (2009). Chronic sorrow in parents of children with type 1 diabetes. *Journal of Advanced Nursing, 65*(5), 992–1000.

Burke, M. L. (1989). *Chronic sorrow in mothers of school-age children with a myelomeningocele disability.* (Doctoral dissertation.) Available from *ProQuest Dissertations and Theses* database. (UMI No. 303665862.)

Burke, M. L., Eakes, G. G., & Hainsworth, M. A. (1999). Milestones of chronic sorrow: Perspectives of chronically ill and bereaved persons and family caregivers. *Journal of Family Nursing, 5*(4), 374–387.

Carpenito-Moyet, L. J. (2014). *Nursing diagnosis: Application to clinical practice* (13th ed.). Philadelphia: Lippincott Williams & Wilkins.

Casale, A. (2009). *Distinguishing the concept of chronic sorrow from standard grief: An empirical study of infertile couples.* (Doctoral dissertation.) Available from *ProQuest Dissertations and Theses* database. (UMI No. MSTAR_304960139.)

Collins, R. C. (2008). *Raising an autistic child: Subjective experiences of fathers.* (Doctoral dissertation.) Available from *ProQuest Dissertations and Theses* database. (UMI No. MSTAR_89286533.)

Davis, K. L. (2006). *The dynamic factors of chronic sorrow on the life experience of the caregivers of children with chronic mental illness.* (Doctoral dissertation.) Available from *ProQuest Dissertations and Theses* database. (UMI No. 304937755.)

Doenges, M. E., Moorhouse, M. F., & Murr, A. C. (2016). *Nursing diagnosis manual: Planning, individualizing, and documenting client care.* Philadelphia: F. A. Davis.

Doka, K. J. (2004). Grief and dementia. In K. J. Doka (Ed.), *Living with grief: Alzheimer's disease* (pp. 169–175). Washington, DC: Hospice Foundation of America.

Doornbos, M. M. (1997). The problems and coping methods of caregivers of young adults with mental illness. *Journal of Psychosocial Nursing & Mental Health Services, 35*(9), 22–26.

Drench, M. E. (2003). Loss, grief, and adjustment: A primer for physical therapy, part I. *PT: Magazine of Physical Therapy, 11*(6), 50–52, 54–61.

Eakes, G. G. (1993). Chronic sorrow: A response to living with cancer. *Oncology Nursing Forum, 20*(9), 1327–1334.

Eakes, G. G. (1995). Chronic sorrow: The lived experience of parents of chronically mentally ill individuals. *Archives of Psychiatric Nursing, 9*(2), 77–84.

Eakes, G. G. (2013). Chronic sorrow. In S. J. Peterson & T. S. Bredow (Eds.), *Middle range theories: Application to nursing research* (3rd ed., pp. 96–107). Philadelphia: Lippincott Williams & Wilkins.

Eakes, G. G., Burke, M. L., & Hainsworth, M. A. (1998). Middle-range theory of chronic sorrow. *Journal of Nursing Scholarship, 30*(2), 179–184.

Eakes, G. G., Burke, M. L., & Hainsworth, M. A. (1999). Chronic sorrow: The experiences of bereaved individuals. *Illness, Crisis & Loss, 7*(2), 172–182.

Eakes, G. G., Burke, M. L., Hainsworth, M. A., & Lindgren, C. L. (1993). Chronic sorrow: An examination of nursing roles. In S. G. Funk, E. Tornquist, & M. T. Champagne (Eds.), *Key aspects of caring for the chronically ill: Hospital and home* (pp. 231–236). New York: Springer.

Erlandsson, K., Saflund, K., Wredling, R., & Rådestad, I. (2011). Support after stillbirth and its effect on parental grief over time. *Journal of Social Work in End-of-Life & Palliative Care, 7*(2), 139–152.

Freedberg, R. P. (2011). *Living with bipolar disorder: A qualitative investigation.* (Doctoral dissertation.) Available from *ProQuest Dissertation and Theses* database. (UMI No. 900443417.)

Gedaly-Duff, V., Stoger, S., & Shelton, K. (2000). Working with families. In R. E. Nickel & L. W. Desch (Eds.), *The physicians' guide to caring for children with disabilities and chronic conditions* (pp. 31–75). Baltimore: Paul H. Brookes.

Glenn, A. D. (2015). Using online health communication to manage chronic sorrow: Mothers of children with rare diseases speak. *Journal of Pediatric Nursing, 30*(1), 17–24.

Golden, B. A. (1994). *The presence of chronic sorrow in mothers of children with cerebral palsy.* (Unpublished master's thesis.) University of Arizona, Tempe, Arizona.

Gordon, J. (2009). An evidence-based approach for supporting parents experiencing chronic sorrow. *Pediatric Nursing, 35*(2), 115–119.

Hainsworth, M. A. (1994). Living with multiple sclerosis: The experience of chronic sorrow. *Journal of Neuroscience Nursing, 26*(4), 237–240.

Hainsworth, M. A. (1995). Helping spouses with chronic sorrow related to multiple sclerosis. *Journal of Gerontological Nursing, 21*(7), 29–33.

Hainsworth, M. A., Burke, M. L., Lindgren, C. L., & Eakes, G. G. (1993). Chronic sorrow in multiple sclerosis: A case study. *Home Healthcare Nurse, 11*(2), 9–13.

Hainsworth, M. A., Busch, P. V., Eakes, G. G., & Burke, M. L. (1995). Chronic sorrow in women with chronically mentally disabled husbands. *Journal of the American Psychiatric Nurses Association, 1*(4), 120–124.

Hainsworth, M. A., Eakes, G. G., & Burke, M. L. (1994). Coping with chronic sorrow. *Issues in Mental Health Nursing, 15*(1), 59–66.

Harris, D. L., & Gorman, E. (2011). Grief from a broader perspective: Nonfinite loss, ambiguous loss, and chronic sorrow. In D. L. Harris (Ed.), *Counting our losses: Reflecting on change, loss, and transition in everyday life* (pp. 1–13). New York: Routledge/Taylor & Francis Group.

Hobdell, E. (2004). Chronic sorrow and depression in parents of children with neural tube defects. *Journal of Neuroscience Nursing, 36*(2), 82–88, 94.

Hobdell, E. F., Grant, M. L., Valencia, I., et al. (2007). Chronic sorrow and coping in families of children with epilepsy. *Journal of Neuroscience Nursing, 39*(2), 76–82.

Hunter, S. E. (2010). *The emotional and interpersonal aspects of fertility damage and/or premature menopause from cancer treatments.* (Unpublished doctoral dissertation.) University of Auckland, New Zealand. Retrieved from https://researchspace.auckland.ac.nz/handle/2292/6870.

Ingram, D., & Hutchinson, S. A. (1999). Defensive mothering in HIV-positive mothers. *Qualitative Health Research, 9*(2), 243–258.

Isaksson, A. K., & Ahlström, G. (2008). Managing chronic sorrow: Experiences of patients with multiple sclerosis. *Journal of Neuroscience Nursing, 40*(3), 180–191.

Isaksson, A. K., Gunnarsson, L. G., & Ahlström, G. (2007). The presence and meaning of chronic sorrow in patients with multiple sclerosis. *Journal of Clinical Nursing, 16*(11c), 315–324.

Johnson, M., Moorhead, S., Bulechek, G., Butcher, H., Meridean, M., & Swanson, E. (2011). *NOC and NIC linkages to NANDA-I and clinical conditions: Supporting critical reasoning and quality care.* St Louis, MO: Elsevier Mosby.

Joseph, H. A. (2012). Recognizing chronic sorrow in the habitual ED patient. *JEN: Journal of Emergency Nursing, 38*(6), 539–540.

Kelly, M. D. (2010). *Factors that influence the utilization of primary care for children with special health care needs.* (Doctoral dissertation.) Available from ProQuest Dissertations and Theses database. (UMI No. 366434499.)

Kendall, L. C. (2005). *The experience of living with ongoing loss: Testing the Kendall Chronic Sorrow Instrument.* (Doctoral dissertation.) Available from *ProQuest Dissertations and Theses* database. (UMI No. 3196497.)

Kerr, S. L. (2010). A case study on Walker-Warburg syndrome. *Advances in Neonatal Care: Official Journal of the National Association of Neonatal Nurses, 10*(1), 21–24.

Lazarus, R. S., & Folkman, S. (1984). *Stress, appraisal, and coping.* New York: Springer.

Lichtenstein, B., Laska, M. K., & Clair, J. M. (2002). Chronic sorrow in the HIV-positive patient: Issues of race, gender, and social support. *AIDS Patient Care and STDs, 16*(1), 27–38.

Liedstrom, E., Isaksson, A., & Ahlström, G. (2008). Chronic sorrow in next of kin of patients with multiple sclerosis. *Journal of Neuroscience Nursing, 40*(5), 304–311.

Lindgren, C. L. (1996). Chronic sorrow in persons with Parkinson's and their spouses. *Scholarly Inquiry for Nursing Practice, 10*(4), 351–370.

Lindgren, C. L., Burke, M. L., Hainsworth, M. A., & Eakes, G. G. (1992). Chronic sorrow: A lifespan concept. *Scholarly Inquiry for Nursing Practice, 6*(1), 27–42.

Lowes, L., & Lyne, P. (2000). Chronic sorrow in parents of children with newly diagnosed diabetes: A review of the literature and discussion of the implications for nursing practice. *Journal of Advanced Nursing, 32*(1), 41–48.

Mallow, G. E., & Bechtel, G. A. (1999). Chronic sorrow: The experience of parents with children who are developmentally disabled. *Journal of Psychosocial Nursing and Mental Health Services, 37*(7), 31–35, 42–43.

Maltby, H. J., Kristjanson, L., & Coleman, M. E. (2003). The parenting competency framework: Learning to be a parent of a child with asthma. *International Journal of Nursing Practice, 9*(6), 368–373.

Marcella-Brienza, S. (2015). Back to work: Manager support of nurses with chronic sorrow. *Creative Nursing, 21*(4), 206–210.

Masterson, M. K. (2010). *Chronic sorrow in mothers of adult children with cerebral palsy: An exploratory study.* (Doctoral dissertation.) Available from *ProQuest Dissertations and Theses* database. (UMI No. 597186156.)

Mawn, B. E. (2012). The changing horizons of U.S. families living with pediatric HIV. *Western Journal of Nursing Research, 34*(2), 213–229.

Meleski, D. D. (2002). Families with chronically ill children: A literature review examines approaches to helping them cope. *American Journal of Nursing, 102*(5), 47–54.

Melnyk, B. M., Feinstein, N. F., Moldenhouer, Z., & Small, L. (2001). Coping in parents of children who are chronically ill: Strategies for assessment and intervention. *Pediatric Nursing, 27*(6), 548–558.

Mercer, C. J. (2015). The impact of non-motor manifestations of Parkinson's disease on partners: Understanding and application of chronic sorrow. *Journal of Primary Health Care, 7*(3), 221–227.

Monsson, Y. (2010). *The effects of hope on mental health and chronic sorrow in parents of children with autism spectrum disorder.* (Doctoral dissertation.) Available from *ProQuest Dissertations and Theses* database. (UMI No. MSTAR_815245239.)

Nanda, I. (2014). *Nursing diagnoses definitions and classification 2012-2017.* Hoboken, NJ: John Wiley & Sons.

Neilsen, C. M. (2013). *Chronic sorrow and illness ambiguity in caregivers of children with sickle cell disease.* Available from *ProQuest Dissertations & Theses Global.* (No. 1491386440.)

Nikfarid, L., Rassouli, M., Borilmnejad, L., & Alavimajd, H. (2015). Chronic sorrow in mothers of children with cancer. *Journal of Pediatric Oncology, 32*(5), 314–319.

Northington, L. K. (2000). Chronic sorrow in caregivers of school age children with sickle cell disease: A grounded theory approach. *Issues in Comprehensive Pediatric Nursing, 23*(3), 141–154.

Olshansky, S. (1962). Chronic sorrow: A response to a mentally defective child. *Social Casework, 43*, 191–193.

Olwit, C., Musisi, S., Leshabari, S., & Sany, I. (2015). Chronic sorrow: Lived experiences of caregivers of patients diagnosed with schizophrenia in Butabika mental hospital, Kampala, Uganda. *Archives of Psychiatric Nursing, 29*(1), 43–48.

Parrish, R. N. (2010). *Mothers' experiences raising children who have multiple disabilities and their perceptions of the chronic sorrow phenomenon.* (Unpublished doctoral dissertation.) University of North Carolina, Greensburg.

Patrick-Ott, A., & Ladd, L. D. (2010). The blending of boss's concept of ambiguous loss and Olshansky's concept of chronic sorrow: A case study of a family with a child who has significant disabilities. *Journal of Creativity in Mental Health, 5*(1), 74–86.

Pejlert, A. (2001). Being a parent of an adult son or daughter with severe mental illness receiving professional care: Parents' narratives. *Health and Social Care in the Community, 9*(4), 194–204.

Pesut, D. J., & Herman, J. (1998). OPT: Transformation of nursing process for contemporary practice: Outcome-Present State-Test. *Nursing Outlook, 46*(1), 29–36.

Rossheim, B. N., & McAdams, C. R. I. (2010). Addressing the chronic sorrow of long-term spousal caregivers: A primer for counselors. *Journal of Counseling & Development, 88*(4), 477–482.

Scornaienchi, J. M. (2003). Chronic sorrow: One mother's experience with two children with lissencephaly. *Journal of Pediatric Health Care, 17*(6), 290–294.

Shumaker, D. (1995). *Chronic sorrow in mothers of children with cystic fibrosis.* (Unpublished master's thesis.) University of Tennessee, Memphis.

Smith, C. S. (2007). Coping strategies of female victims of child abuse in treatment for substance abuse relapse: Their advice to other women and healthcare professionals. *Journal of Addictions Nursing, 18*(2), 75–80.

Smith, C. S. (2009). Substance abuse, chronic sorrow, and mothering loss: Relapse triggers among female victims of child abuse. *Journal of Pediatric Nursing, 24*(5), 401–412.

Vitale, S. A., & Falco, C. (2014). Children born prematurely: Risk of parental chronic sorrow. *Journal of Pediatric Nursing, 29*(3), 248–251.

Wee, D. (2010). *Acceptability of Stepping Stones Triple P Parenting Program as well as the experience of chronic sorrow and use of coping strategies among parents of children with cerebral palsy: A focus group and survey study.* (Unpublished doctoral dissertation.) University of Queensland, Australia. Retrieved from http://espace.library.uq.edu.au/view/UQ:222537.

Whittingham, K., Wee, D., Sanders, M. R., & Boyd, R. (2013). Predictors of psychological adjustment, experienced parenting burden and chronic sorrow symptoms in parents of children with cerebral palsy. *Child: Care, Health & Development, 39*(3), 366–373.

BIBLIOGRAPHY

Primary Sources

Book Chapters

Eakes, G. G. (2013). Chronic sorrow. In S. J. Peterson & T. S. Bredow (Eds.), *Middle range theories: Application to nursing research* (3rd ed., pp. 96–107). Philadelphia: Lippincott Williams & Wilkins.

Eakes, G. G., Burke, M. L., Hainsworth, M. A., & Lindgren, C. L. (1993). Chronic sorrow: An examination of nursing roles. In S. G. Funk, E. Tornquist, & M. T. Champagne (Eds.), *Key aspects of caring for the chronically ill: Hospital and home* (pp. 231–236). New York: Springer.

Journal Articles

Burke, M. L., Eakes, G. G., & Hainsworth, M. A. (1999). Milestones of chronic sorrow: Perspectives of chronically ill and bereaved persons and family caregivers. *Journal of Family Nursing, 5*(4), 374–387.

Burke, M. L., Hainsworth, M. A., Eakes, G. G., & Lindgren, C. L. (1992). Current knowledge and research on chronic sorrow: A foundation for inquiry. *Death Studies, 16*(3), 231–245.

Eakes, G. G. (1993). Chronic sorrow: A response to living with cancer. *Oncology Nursing Forum, 20*(9), 1327–1334.

Eakes, G. G. (1995). Chronic sorrow: The lived experience of parents of chronically mentally ill individuals. *Archives of Psychiatric Nursing, 9*(2), 77–84.

Eakes, G. G., Burke, M. L., & Hainsworth, M. A. (1998). Middle-range theory of chronic sorrow. *Journal of Nursing Scholarship, 30*(2), 179–184.

Eakes, G. G., Burke, M. L., & Hainsworth, M. A. (1999). Chronic sorrow: The experiences of bereaved individuals. *Illness, Crisis & Loss, 7*(2), 172–182.

Eakes, G. G., Burke, M. L., Hainsworth, M. A., & Lindgren, C. L. (1993). Chronic sorrow: An examination of nursing roles. In S. G. Funk, E. Tornquist, & M. T. Champagne (Eds.), *Key aspects of caring for the chronically ill: Hospital and home* (pp. 231–236). New York: Springer.

Eakes, G. G., Hainsworth, M. E., Lindgren, C. L., & Burke, M. L. (1991). Establishing a long-distance research consortium. *Nursing Connections, 4*(1), 51–57.

Hainsworth, M. A. (1994). Living with multiple sclerosis: The experience of chronic sorrow. *Journal of Neuroscience Nursing, 26*(4), 237–240.

Hainsworth, M. A. (1995). Helping spouses with chronic sorrow related to multiple sclerosis. *Journal of Gerontological Nursing, 21*(7), 29–33.

Hainsworth, M. A., Busch, P. V., Eakes, G. G., & Burke, M. L. (1995). Chronic sorrow in women with chronically mentally disabled husbands. *Journal of the American Psychiatric Nurses Association, 1*(4), 120–124.

Hainsworth, M. A., Burke, M. L., Lindgren, C. L., & Eakes, G. G. (1993). Chronic sorrow in multiple sclerosis: A case study. *Home Healthcare Nurse, 11*(2), 9–13.

Hainsworth, M. A., Eakes, G. G., & Burke, M. L. (1994). Coping with chronic sorrow. *Issues in Mental Health Nursing, 15*(1), 59–66.

Lindgren, C. L. (1996). Chronic sorrow in persons with Parkinson's and their spouses. *Scholarly Inquiry for Nursing Practice, 10*(4), 351–370.

Lindgren, C. L., Burke, M. L., Hainsworth, M. A., & Eakes, G. G. (1992). Chronic sorrow: A lifespan concept. *Scholarly Inquiry for Nursing Practice, 6*(1), 27–42.

Dissertations

Burke, M. L. (1989). *Chronic sorrow in mothers of school-age children with a myelomeningocele disability.* (Doctoral dissertation, Boston University.) *Dissertation Abstracts International, 50*, 233–234B.

Burke, M. L. (1989). *Chronic sorrow in mothers of school-age children with a myelomeningocele disability.* (Doctoral dissertation, Boston University.) *Dissertation Abstracts International, 50*, 233–234B.

Secondary Sources

Books

Roos, S. (2002). *Chronic sorrow: A living loss.* New York: Brunner-Routledge.

Walker, L. O., & Avant, K. C. (2011). *Strategies for theory construction in nursing* (5th ed.). Upper Saddle River, NJ: Pearson/Prentice Hall.

Book Chapters

Roos, S. (2010). The long road to relevance: Disability, chronic sorrow, and shame. In J. Kauffman (Ed.), *The shame of death, grief and trauma* (pp. 171–197). New York: Routledge/Taylor & Francis Group.

Journal Articles

Breen, L. J. (2009). Early childhood service delivery for families living with childhood disability: Disabling families through problematic implicit ideology. *Australasian Journal of Early Childhood, 34*(4), 14–21.

Churchill, S. S., Villareale, N. L., Monaghan, T. A., Sharp, V. L., & Kieckhefer, G. M. (2010). Parents of children with special health care needs who have better coping skills have fewer depressive symptoms. *Maternal and Child Health Journal, 14*(1), 47–57.

Kohlenberg, E., Kennedy-Malone, L., Crane, P., & Letvak, S. (2007). Infusing gerontological nursing content into advanced practice nursing education. *Nursing Outlook, 55*(1), 38–43.

Richardson, M., Cobham, V., Murray, J., & McDermott, B. (2011). Parents' grief in the context of adult child mental illness: A qualitative review. *Clinical Child and Family Psychology Review, 14*(1), 28–43.

Whittingham, K., Wee, D., & Boyd, R. (2011). Systematic review of the efficacy of parenting interventions for children with cerebral palsy. *Child: Care, Health and Development, 37*(4), 475–483.

Zucker, D. M., Dion, K., & McKeever, R. P. (2015). Concept clarification of grief in mothers of children with an addiction. *Journal of Advanced Nursing, 71*(4), 751–767.

Dissertations

Blair, M. B. (2010). *Quality of life despite back pain: A phenomenological study.* (Doctoral dissertation.) Available from *ProQuest Dissertations and Theses* database. (UMI No. 807680746.)

Casale, A. (2009). *Distinguishing the concept of chronic sorrow from standard grief: An empirical study of infertile couples.* (Doctoral dissertation.) Available from *ProQuest Dissertations and Theses* database. (UMI No. MSTAR_304960139.)

Collins, R. C. (2008). *Raising an autistic child: Subjective experiences of fathers.* (Doctoral dissertation.) Available from *ProQuest Dissertations and Theses* database. (UMI No. MSTAR_89286533.)

Davis, K. L. (2006). *The dynamic factors of chronic sorrow on the life experience of the caregivers of children with chronic mental illness.* (Doctoral dissertation.) Available from *ProQuest Dissertations and Theses* database. (UMI No. 304937755.)

Freedberg, R. P. (2011). *Living with bipolar disorder: A qualitative investigation.* (Doctoral dissertation.) Available from *ProQuest Dissertation and Theses* database. (UMI No. 900443417.)

Harris, D. L., & Gorman, E. (2011). Grief from a broader perspective: Nonfinite loss, ambiguous loss, and chronic sorrow. In D. L. Harris (Ed.), *Counting our losses: Reflecting on change, loss, and transition in everyday life* (pp. 1–13). New York: Routledge/Taylor & Francis Group.

Hunter, S. E. (2010). *The emotional and interpersonal aspects of fertility damage and/or premature menopause from cancer treatments.* (Unpublished doctoral dissertation.) University of Auckland, New Zealand. Retrieved from https://researchspace.auckland.ac.nz/handle/2292/6870.

Kelly, M. D. (2010). *Factors that influence the utilization of primary care for children with special health care needs.* (Doctoral dissertation.) Available from *ProQuest Dissertations and Theses* database. (UMI No. 366434499.)

Kendall, L. C. (2005). *The experience of living with ongoing loss: Testing the Kendall Chronic Sorrow Instrument.* (Doctoral dissertation.) Available from *ProQuest Dissertations and Theses* database. (UMI No.3196497.)

Masterson, M. K. (2010). *Chronic sorrow in mothers of adult children with cerebral palsy: An exploratory study.* (Doctoral dissertation.) Available from *ProQuest Dissertations and Theses* database). (UMI No. 597186156.)

Monsson, Y. (2010). *The effects of hope on mental health and chronic sorrow in parents of children with autism spectrum disorder.* (Doctoral dissertation.) Available from *ProQuest Dissertations and Theses* database. (UMI No. MSTAR_815245239.)

Neilsen, C. M. (2013). *Chronic sorrow and illness ambiguity in caregivers of children with sickle cell disease.* Available from *ProQuest Dissertations and Theses Global.* (No. 1491386440).

Northington, L. D. K. (1998). *Chronic sorrow in caregivers of school age children with sickle cell disease: A grounded theory approach.* (Doctoral dissertation.) Available from *ProQuest Dissertations and Theses* database. (UMI No. 304479701.)

Parrish, R. N. (2010). *Mothers' experiences raising children who have multiple disabilities and their perceptions of the chronic sorrow phenomenon.* (Unpublished doctoral dissertation.) University of North Carolina, Greensburg.

Wee, D. (2010). *Acceptability of Stepping Stones Triple P Parenting Program as well as the experience of chronic sorrow and use of coping strategies among parents of children with cerebral palsy: A focus group and survey study.* (Unpublished doctoral dissertation.) University of Queensland, Australia. Retrieved from http://espace.library.uq.edu.au/view/UQ:222537.

32

The Tidal Model of Mental Health Recovery

Nancy Brookes

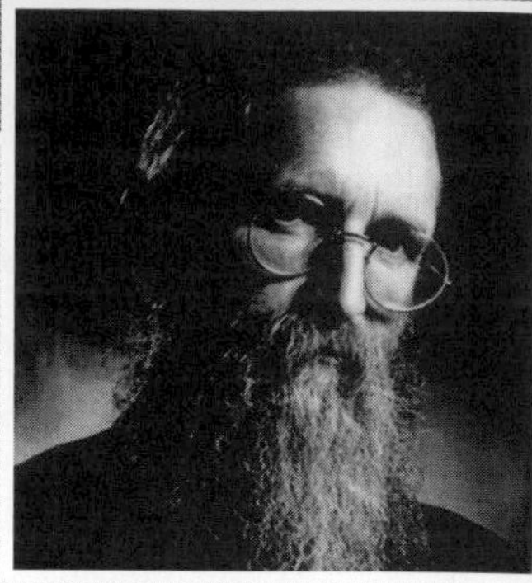

Phil Barker

"Mental illnesses or psychiatric disorders are 'problems of human living'; people find it difficult to live with themselves or to live with others in the social world. A simple idea that becomes complicated when we try to engage with it. Nurses try to help people address these problems of living, in an effort to live through them. Another simple idea, that becomes complicated at the level of practice. All is paradox. If one is to 'care' for another first of all one must encounter the person. One should expect to be surprised even frustrated.

To help someone 'grow and develop'—the essence of the nurturing function of nursing—first we must encounter 'the person.' Such a 'coming together' is necessary if the nurse is to understand the person's needs and the person is to appreciate in what way the nurse might be of help."

(P. Barker, personal communication, April 2016)

BACKGROUND AND CREDENTIALS OF THE THEORIST

Phil Barker was born in Scotland by the sea, and thus began the influence of and interest in water, the ultimate metaphor of life (Barker, 1996a). He credits his father and grandfather with "the warmth of nurture and the discipline of boundaries," who helped him appreciate that "life was an answer waiting for the right question," and he, like them, became a philosopher (Barker, 1999b, p. xii). Life in this context contributed to his evident and enduring curiosity and interest in the philosophy of the everyday. Barker trained as a painter and sculptor in the mid-1960s, and he continues to paint word pictures in metaphor. Barker credits his art school with introducing him to learning from reality, the reality of experience which became the focus of his philosophical inquiries. His fascination with Eastern philosophies, which began at art school, flows through the tidal model with echoes of chaos, uncertainty, change, and the Chinese idea of crisis as opportunity. This early involvement in the arts also helps to explain Barker's view of nursing as the craft of caring (Barker, 2000c, 2000e; Barker & Whitehill, 1997). After a gap of more than 30 years, Barker returned to painting in 2006 and has become a successful, award-wining artist.

Barker's ocean of experience surged in a new direction in 1970, when he took a position as an attendant at the local asylum. His fascination with the human dimension, the lived experience, and the stories of people challenged by mental distress prompted him to relocate his interest in the arts and humanities to *nursing*. Soon after qualifying in 1974, Barker began to study and practice various psychotherapies such as cognitive behavioral therapy and family and group therapy. His doctoral research, begun in 1980, featured cognitive behavioral work with a group of women living with depression (Barker, 1987). However, around this time, Barker became uncomfortable with the application of therapies to people experiencing problems in living, and the "uncertainty principle" resurfaced for him. His curiosity about life and persons provoked questions about the resilience and integrity of the people with whom he was working. Instead of "caring for" or "treating" them, he was learning what it meant to experience distress from the people themselves. He wondered what recovery meant to people. Questions reemerged around the following:

- What it is to be a person?
- What is the proper focus of nursing?
- What are nurses needed for?

During his tenure as Professor of Psychiatric Nursing Practice at the University of Newcastle, began in 1993, these questions framed his research agenda and culminated in the development of the tidal model. As the United Kingdom's first Professor of Psychiatric Nursing Practice, Barker broke the conventional "academic" mold by maintaining his involvement in practice, which led directly to development of the tidal model. Throughout his nursing career, Barker has wondered about the proper focus of psychiatric nursing and the role of care, compassion, understanding, and courage in helping people who are experiencing extreme distress, loss of self, or spiritual crisis (Barker, 1999b). The story knowledge base lies at the heart of the tidal model.

Barker has published in the area of psychiatric and mental health nursing since 1978. A prolific writer, he has published 19 books, more than 50 book chapters, and more than 150 academic papers. In 2006 he received the inaugural "Lifetime Achievement Award" from Blackwell journals, publishers of the *Journal of Psychiatric and Mental Health Nursing,* where he was Assistant Editor for a decade. Barker has held visiting professorships at international universities in Australia (Sydney), Europe (Barcelona), Japan (Tokyo), and Trinity College in Dublin from 2002 to 2007. He is currently an Honorary Professor at the University of Dundee in Scotland and a psychotherapist in private practice.

With his wife and professional partner, Poppy Buchanan-Barker, Barker has conducted recovery-focused workshops and seminars in Australia, Canada, New Zealand, Japan, Finland, Denmark, Turkey, Germany, Ireland, and the United Kingdom. They have further developed the recovery paradigm at Clan Unity, their international mental health recovery and reclamation consultancy in Scotland.

THEORETICAL SOURCES

The tidal model is focused on the fundamental care processes of nursing, is universally applicable, and is a practical guide for psychiatric and mental health nursing (Barker, 2001b). The theory is radical in its reconceptualization of mental health problems as unequivocally *human,* rather than psychological, social, or physical (Barker, 2002b). The tidal model "emphasizes the central importance of developing understanding of the person's needs through collaborative working, developing a therapeutic relationship through discrete methods of active empowerment, establishing nursing as an educative element at the heart of interdisciplinary intervention" (Barker, 2000e, p. 4). It seeks to resolve problems and promote mental health through narrative approaches (Stevenson, Barker, & Fletcher, 2002).

The tidal model is a philosophical approach to recovery of mental health. It is not a model of care or treatment of mental illness, although people described as mentally ill do need and receive care. The tidal model represents a worldview, helping the nurse begin to understand what mental health might mean for the person in care, and how that person might be helped to begin the complex voyage of recovery. The tidal model is not prescriptive. Rather, a set of principles, the Ten Tidal Commitments, serve as a metaphorical compass for the practitioner (Buchanan-Barker & Barker, 2005, 2008). They guide the nurse in developing responses to meet the individual and contextual needs of the person who has become the patient. The experience of mental distress is invariably described in metaphorical terms. The tidal model uses the universal and culturally significant metaphors associated with the power of water and the sea to represent the known aspects of human distress. Water is "the core metaphor for both the lived experience of the person . . . and the care system that attempts to mold itself around a person's need for nursing" (Barker, 2000e, p. 10).

Barker describes an "early interest in the human content of mental distress . . . and an interest in the human (phenomenological) experience of distress," viewed in contexts and wholes rather than isolated parts (Barker, 1999b, p. 13). The "whole" nature of being human is "represented on physical, emotional, intellectual, social and spiritual planes" (Barker, 2002b, p. 233). This phenomenological interest pervades the tidal model with an emphasis on the lived experience of persons, their stories (replete with metaphors), and narrative interventions. Nurses carefully and sensitively meet and interact with people in a "sacred space" (Barker, 2003a, p. 613).

A feature of Barker's nursing practice has been his exploration of the possibilities of genuine collaborative relationships with users of mental health services. In the 1980s, he developed the concept of caring with people, learning that the professional–person relationship could be more mutual than the original nurse–patient relationship defined by Peplau (1969). Barker developed this concept during the 1990s in a working relationship with Dr. Irene Whitehill and others who used mental health services (Barker & Whitehill, 1997). This led to a need for nursing and empowerment studies as well as a commitment to publish the stories of people's experience of madness and their voyage of recovery, complete with personal and spiritual meanings (Barker & Buchanan-Barker, 2004b; Barker, Campbell, & Davidson, 1999; Barker, Jackson, & Stevenson, 1999a). Barker enlisted the support of Dr. Whitehill and other user and consumer consultants to evaluate user-friendly qualities of the original processes of the tidal model. This represents a distinctive feature of continued development of the tidal model.

Barker's long-standing appreciation of Eastern philosophies pervades his work. The work of Shoma Morita is a specific example of how philosophical assumptions of Zen Buddhism integrate with psychotherapy (Morita et al., 1998). Morita's dictum, "do what needs to be done," resonates in many of the practical activities of the tidal model. In contrast to the problem-solving style of much of the west, Morita believed the focus should be on answering the questions:

- What is my purpose in living?
- What needs to be done now?

People have the capacity to live and grow through distress, by doing what needs to be done. For people who are in acute distress, especially when they are at risk to self or others, it is vital that nurses relate directly to the person's ongoing experience. Originally Barker called this process **engagement**, but he has redefined the specific interpersonal process as **bridging**, a supportive human process necessary to reach out to people in distress. This emphasizes the need to creatively build a means of reaching the person, crossing in the process the murky waters of mental distress (Barker & Buchanan-Barker, 2004b).

The tidal model may be viewed through the lens of social constructivism, recognizing that there are multiple ways of understanding the world. Meaning emerges through the complex webs of interaction, relationships, and social processes. Knowledge does not exist independently of the knower, and all knowledge is situated (Stevenson, 1996). Change is the only constant, as meaning and social realities are constantly renegotiated or constructed through language and interaction. Barker believes "all I am is story; all I can ever be is story." As people try to explain to others *who* they are, they tell stories about themselves and their world of experience, revising, editing, and rewriting these stories through dialogue. Barker first discussed this idea in 1994 with his mentor, Hilda (Hildegard) Peplau, who agreed that "people make themselves up as they talk" (Barker, 2003a; Barker & Buchanan-Barker, 2007b).

Barker credits many thinkers with influencing his work, beginning with Annie Altschul and Thomas Szasz. His view of mental health problems as *problems of living* and that it is futile to try to "solve problems in living," popularized by Szasz (1961, 2000) and later Podvoll (1990), is a perspective he prefers to diagnostic labeling and the biomedical construction of people and illness (Barker, 2001c, p. 215). "Life is not a problem to be solved, but something to be lived, as intelligently, as competently, as well as we can, day in and day out" (Miller, 1983, p. 290). The challenge for nursing is to help persons live intelligently and competently.

Travelbee's (1969) concept of the *therapeutic use of self* flows through the tidal model and anchors the proper focus of nursing. The following three main theoretical frameworks underpin the tidal model:

1. Peplau's (1952, 1969) interpersonal relations theory
2. The theory of psychiatric and mental health nursing derived from the Need for Nursing studies
3. Empowerment within interpersonal relationships

The pragmatic emphasis on strengths-based, solution-focused approaches acknowledges the important influence of de Shazer's solution-focused therapy, although there can be no solutions for problems in living, merely pragmatic strategies for living with such problems. The influence of Webster and colleagues, introducing de Shazer's ideas into nursing practice, significantly shaped the development of the tidal model (Webster, Vaughn, & Martinez, 1994). De Shazer's (1994) influence is evident where change and intervention "boils down to stories about the telling of stories, the shaping and reshaping of stories so that troubled people change their story" (p. xvii).

The tidal model draws its core philosophical metaphor from chaos theory, where the "unpredictable yet bounded nature of human behavior and experience can be compared with the flow and power of water" (Barker, 2000b, p. 54). In constant flux, the tides ebb and flow, exhibiting nonrepeating patterns yet staying within bounded parameters (Vicenzi, 1994). Barker (2000b) acknowledges the "complexity [of] both the internal universe of human experience and the external universe, which is, paradoxically, within and beyond the individual, at one and the same time" (p. 52). Within this complex, nonlinear perspective, small changes create later unpredictable changes, a hopeful message that directs nurses and persons to identify small changes and variations. Barker invites nurses to cease the search for certainty, embracing instead the reality of uncertainty. "Know that change is constant," one of the Ten Tidal Commitments, identifies and celebrates change in people, circumstances, relationships, and organizations (Barker, 2003b; Buchanan-Barker & Barker, 2008).

Annie Altschul, "the *Grande Dame* of British psychiatric nursing" (Barker, 2003a, p. 12), and Hilda (Hildegard)

Peplau were Barker's mentors. Altschul's influence, especially her early appreciation of systems theory, is evident in the tidal model, as is her interest in understanding rather than explaining mental distress and her belief that people need more straightforward help than many psychiatric theories suggest. Barker credits Peplau with his becoming "an advocate for nursing as a therapeutic activity in its own right" (Barker, 2000a, p. 617). Peplau introduced her interpersonal paradigm for the study and practice of nursing in the early 1950s and defined nursing as "a significant, therapeutic, interpersonal process" (Peplau, 1952, p. 16). Barker emphasizes that records of the story be recorded in the person's own voice, advancing Peplau's appreciation of the interpersonal process.

The empirically derived interactions framework suggests that improvement in the person's situation and lifestyle is possible and building on strengths is better than focusing on problems. Collaboration is key, participation is the way, and self-determination is the ultimate goal (Barker & Buchanan-Barker, 2004a; Barker, Stevenson, & Leamy, 2000). The strengths base of the tidal model emphasizes searching for and revealing solutions and identifying resources. The theory integrates Barker's Need for Nursing studies, collaboration, empowerment, interpersonal relationships, story, strengths-base, and solution-seeking approaches and is systemic. In the holistic assessment, nurses explore the person's present problems or needs, the scale of these problems or needs, what is currently in a person's life that might help to resolve problems or meet needs, and what needs to happen to bring about change (Barker, 2000e; Barker & Buchanan-Barker, 2007a). Nurses help identify and mobilize a person's strengths and resources, and the person's goals direct the work of the health care team (Barker, 2000e; Stevenson, Jackson, & Barker, 2003). This is a significant reframing of the view of the person-in-care and the proper focus of nursing. The Ten Tidal Commitments support this perspective and direction (Box 32.1).

BOX 32.1 The Ten Tidal Commitments: Essential Values of the Tidal Model

The tidal model draws on values about *relating* to people. These frame our efforts to help others in their moment of distress. These values reflect a philosophy of how we would hope to be treated should we experience distress or difficulty in our lives. As more people around the world have become involved in exploring the tidal model for their work in different settings, the need to reaffirm the core values of the tidal model has become more apparent. We have come to appreciate how *both* the "helper" (whether professional, friend, or fellow traveler) *and* the person need to make a *commitment* to change, which binds them together. The *Ten Tidal Commitments* distil the essence of the value base of the tidal model. These commitments need to be firmly in place for any team or individual practitioner who wishes to develop the practice of the tidal model.

1. **Value the voice:** The person's story is the beginning and endpoint of the whole helping encounter, embracing not only the account of the person's distress, but also the hope for its resolution. The story is spoken by the voice of experience. We seek to encourage the true voice of the person—rather than reinforce the voice of authority.

   Traditionally, the person's story is "translated" into a third-person professional account. This becomes not so much the person's story (*my* story) but the professional team's view of the story *(history)*. The tidal model seeks to help people develop their own unique narrative accounts into a formalized version of *"my story"* by ensuring that all assessments and records of care are written in the person's own "voice." If the person is unable or unwilling to write in his or her own hand, then the nurse records what has been agreed conjointly is important—writing this in the "voice" of the person.
2. **Respect the language:** People develop unique ways of expressing their life stories, representing to others that which the person alone can know. The language of the story—complete with its unusual grammar and personal metaphors—is the ideal medium for illuminating the way to recovery. We encourage people to speak their own words in their distinctive voice.

   Stories written about patients by professionals are traditionally framed by arcane technical language of psychiatric medicine or psychology. Regrettably, people often come to describe themselves in the colonial language of the professionals who have diagnosed them. By valuing—and using—the person's natural language, the tidal practitioner conveys the simplest yet most powerful respect for the person.
3. **Develop genuine curiosity:** The person is writing a life story but is in no sense an "open book." No one can know another person's experience. Consequently, professionals need to express genuine interest in the story

Continued

BOX 32.1 The Ten Tidal Commitments: Essential Values of the Tidal Model—cont'd

so that they can better understand the storyteller and the story.

Often professionals are interested only in "what is wrong" with the person or in pursuing particular lines of professional inquiry—for example, seeking "signs and symptoms." Genuine curiosity reflects an interest in the person and the person's unique experience, as opposed to merely classifying and categorizing features.

4. **Become the apprentice:** The person is the world expert on the life story. Professionals may learn something of the power of that story, but only if they apply themselves diligently and respectfully to the task by becoming apprentice-minded. We need to learn from the person what needs to be done, rather than leading.

   Professionals often talk "as if" they might even know the person better than they know themselves. As Szasz noted: "How can you know more about a person after seeing him for a few hours, a few days, or even a few months, than he knows about himself? He has known himself a lot longer! The idea that the person remains entirely in charge of himself is a fundamental premise" (Szasz, 2000).
5. **Use the available toolkit:** The story contains examples of "what has worked" or beliefs about "what might work" for this person in the future. These represent the main tools to unlock or build the story of recovery. The professional toolkit—commonly expressed through ideas such as "evidence-based practice"—describes what has worked for other people. Although potentially useful, this should be used only if the person's available toolkit is found wanting.
6. **Craft the step beyond:** The professional helper and the person work together to construct an appreciation of what needs to be done "now." Any "first step" is a crucial step, revealing the power of change and potentially pointing toward the ultimate goal of recovery. Lao Tzu said that the journey of a thousand miles begins with a single step. This model would go further: Any journey begins in the *imagination*. It is important to imagine—or envision—moving forward. Crafting the step beyond reminds nurses of the importance of working with the person in the "me now": addressing what needs to be done now, to help advance to the next step.
7. **Give the gift of time:** Although time is largely illusionary, nothing is more valuable. Often, professionals complain about not having enough time to work constructively with the person. Although they may not actually "make" time, through creative attention to their work, professionals often find the time to do "what needs to be done." Here, it is the professional's relationship with the concept of time that is at issue, rather than time itself (Jonsson, 2005). Ultimately, any time spent in constructive interpersonal communication is a gift—for both parties. There is nothing more valuable than the time the helper and the person spend together.
8. **Reveal personal wisdom:** Only the person can know himself or herself. The person develops a powerful storehouse of wisdom through living the writing of the life story. Often, people cannot find the words to express fully the multitude, complexity, or ineffability of their experience, invoking powerful personal metaphors to convey something of their experience (Barker, 2002b). A key task for the professional is to help the person reveal and come to value that wisdom, so that it might be used to sustain the person throughout the voyage of recovery.
9. **Know that change is constant:** Change is inevitable, because change is constant for all people. However, although change is inevitable, growth is optional. Decisions and choices have to be made if growth is to occur. The tasks of the professional helper are to develop awareness of how change is happening and to support the person in making decisions regarding the course of the recovery voyage. In particular, nurses help the person to steer out of danger and distress, keeping on the course of reclamation and recovery.
10. **Be transparent:** If the professional and the person are to become a team, then each must put down their "weapons." In the story-writing process, the professional's pen can all too often become a weapon: writing a story that risks inhibiting, restricting, and delimiting the person's life choices. Professionals are in a privileged position and should model confidence by being transparent at all times, helping the person understand exactly what is being done and why. By retaining the use of the person's own language, and by completing all assessments and care plan records together *(in vivo)*, the collaborative nature of the professional–person relationship becomes even more transparent.

From Buchanan-Barker, P., & Barker, P. (2008). The Tidal Commitments: Extending the value base of mental health recovery. *Journal of Psychiatric and Mental Health Nursing, 15(2)*, 93–100.

MAJOR CONCEPTS & DEFINITIONS

The Theoretical Basis of the Tidal Model*

The tidal model begins from four simple points:

1. The primary therapeutic focus in mental health care lies in the community. A person's natural life is an "ocean of experience." The psychiatric crisis is only one thing, among many, that might threaten to "drown" them. Ultimately, mental health care is aimed to return people to that "ocean of experience," so that they might continue their life voyage.
2. Change is a constant, ongoing process. Although people are constantly changing, this may be beyond their awareness. One of the main aims of the approaches used within the tidal model is to help people develop their awareness of the small changes that, ultimately, will have a big effect on their lives.
3. Empowerment lies at the heart of the caring process. However, people already have their own "power." Nurses need to help people "power up" so they can use their own personal power to take greater charge of their lives, using this in constructive ways.
4. The nurse and the person are united (albeit temporarily) like dancers in a dance. When effective nursing happens, as W. B. Yeats (1928) might have remarked, "How do we tell the dancer from the dance?" This reminds nurses that genuine caring encounters involve "caring with" the person, not just "caring about" the person, or doing things that suggest the nurse is "caring for" them.

The Three Domains: A Model of the Person*

In the tidal model, the person is represented by three personal domains: *self, world,* and *others.* A **domain** is a sphere of control or influence, a place where the person experiences or acts out aspects of private or public life. Simply, a domain is a place where one lives.

The domains are like the person's home address. Their house or flat has several rooms, but the person is not found in each of these rooms all the time; rather the person is sometimes in one room, and sometimes in another. The personal domains are similar. Sometimes the person is mainly in the self domain, and at other times mainly in the world or others domain.

The **self domain** is the private place where the person experiences thoughts, feelings, beliefs, values, and ideas that are known only to the person. In this private world, the distress called "mental illness" is first experienced. All people keep much of their private world secret, only revealing to others what they wish them to know. This is why people are often such a mystery to others, even when they are close friends or relatives.

In the tidal model, the self domain becomes the focus of the nurse's attempts to help the person feel safe and secure, to try to help the person address and begin to deal with the private fears, anxieties, and other threats to emotional stability related to specific problems of living. The main focus is to develop a bridging relationship and to help the person develop a meaningful **personal security plan**. This work is the basis for development of the person's self-help program, which will sustain the person on return to everyday life.

The **world domain** is the place where the person shares some of the experiences from the self domain with other people in the person's social world. When people talk to others about their private thoughts, feelings, beliefs, or other experiences known only to them, they go to the world domain. In the tidal model, the *world domain* is the focus of efforts to understand the person and the person's problems of living. This is done through the use of the Holistic Assessment. At the world domain, we try to help the person begin to identify and address specific problems of living on an everyday basis through **one-to-one sessions**.

The **others domain** is where persons act out everyday life with other people, such as family, friends, neighbors, work colleagues, and professionals. The person engages in different interpersonal and social encounters that may be influenced by others and may, in turn, influence others. The organization and delivery of professional care and other forms of support are in the others domain. However, the key focus of the tidal model is dedicated forms of group work—**discovery**, **information sharing**, and **solution finding**.

By participating in these groups, the person develops awareness of the value of social support, which can be received from and given to others. This becomes the basis of the person's appreciation of the value of mutual support, which can be accessed in everyday life.

Water—A Metaphor*†

The *tidal model* emphasizes the unpredictability of human experience through the core metaphor of water. Life is a journey taken on an ocean of experience. All human development—including the experience of health and illness—involves discoveries made on that journey across the ocean of experience. At critical points in the journey, people may experience storms or piracy. The ship may begin to take in water, and the person may face the prospect of drowning or shipwreck. The person may need to be guided to a safe haven, to undertake repairs, or to recover from the trauma. Once the ship is intact or the

Continued

 **MAJOR CONCEPTS & DEFINITIONS—cont'd**

person has regained his or her sea legs, the journey can begin again as the person sets his or her course on the ocean of experience.

This metaphor illustrates many of the elements of a psychiatric crisis and the necessary responses to this human predicament. "Storms at sea" is a metaphor for problems of living; "piracy" evokes the experience of rape or a "robbery of the self" that severe distress can produce. Many users describe the overwhelming nature of their experience of distress as akin to "drowning," and this often ends in a metaphorical "shipwreck" on the shores of an acute psychiatric unit. A proper "psychiatric rescue" should be akin to "lifesaving" and should lead the person to a genuine "safe haven" where necessary human repair work can take place.

Guiding Principles‡

1. A belief in the virtue of curiosity: The person is the world authority on his or her life and its problems. By expressing genuine curiosity, the professional can learn something of the "mystery" of the person's story.
2. Recognition of the power of resourcefulness: Rather than focusing on problems, deficits, and weaknesses, the tidal model seeks to reveal resources available to the person—both personal and interpersonal—that might help on the voyage of recovery.
3. Respect for the *person's wishes,* rather than being paternalistic or suggesting that one might "know what is best" for the person.
4. Acceptance of the **paradox of crisis** as opportunity: Challenging events in life signal that something needs to be done. This might become an opportunity for a change in life direction.
5. Acknowledging that all goals, obviously, *belong to the person.* These represent the small steps on the road to recovery.
6. The virtue in pursuing elegance: Psychiatric care and treatment are often complex and bewildering. The simplest possible means should be sought that might bring about the changes needed for the person to move forward.

Getting in the Swim—Engagement Beliefs§

When people are in serious distress, they often feel as if they are drowning. In such circumstances, they need a lifesaver. Of course, lifesavers need to engage with the person—they need to get close—to begin the rescue process. To get in the swim and to begin the engagement process, nurses need to believe the following:

- That recovery is possible
- That change is inevitable—nothing lasts
- That ultimately, people know what is best for them
- That people possess all the resources they need to begin the recovery journey
- That the person is the teacher, and nurses, the helpers, are the pupils
- That nurses need to be creatively curious to learn what needs to be done to help the person now

Therapeutic Philosophy

1. *Why this—why now?* The nurse needs to consider, first of all, why the person is experiencing this particular life difficulty now. The focus of care is on what the person is experiencing now and what needs to be done now to address, and hopefully resolve, the problem.
2. *What works?* The nurse needs to ask what works (or might work) for the person under the present circumstances. This represents the person-centered focus of care. Rather than using standardized techniques or therapeutic approaches, which may have general value, the aim is to identify either what has worked for the person in the past or what might work for the person in the immediate future, given their history, personality, and general life circumstances.
3. *What is the person's personal theory?* How does this person understand her or his problems? What sense does the person make of her or his problems? Rather than offering persons professionalized interpretations of their difficulties in the form of theory or diagnosis, the nurse must try to understand how they understand their experience. What is the person's personal theory?
4. *How do we limit restrictions?* What might be the least restrictive means of helping the person address and resolve the difficulties? How little might the nurse do and how much might the person do to bring about meaningful change? Together, these represent the least restrictive intervention.

Continuum of Care

As needs flow with the person across artificial boundaries, care is seamless, with the intention of the person returning to his or her ocean of experience within his or her own community. Across the care continuum, people may need critical or immediate transitional or developmental care. Practical immediate care addresses searching for

MAJOR CONCEPTS & DEFINITIONS—cont'd

solutions to the person's problems, generally in the short term, and focuses upon what needs to be done now. People enter the care continuum for immediate care when experiencing an initial mental health crisis, possibly entering the mental health system for the first time or with people familiar with the system when a crisis occurs. Transitional care addresses the smooth passage from one setting to another, when the person is moving from one form of care to another. Here, nursing responsibilities include liaising with colleagues and ensuring the person's participation in the transfer of care. The other end of the continuum is developmental care, where the focus is on more intensive and longer-term support or therapeutic intervention.

*Barker, P. J., & Buchanan-Barker, P. (2007). *The tidal model: Mental health recovery and reclamation.* Newport-on-Tay, Scotland: Clan Unity International.

†Barker, P. (2000). The tidal model: The lived experience in person-centred mental health care. *Nursing Philosophy, 2*(3), 213–223.

‡Buchanan-Barker, P., & Barker, P. (2008). The Tidal Commitments: Extending the value base of mental health recovery. *Journal of Psychiatric and Mental Health Nursing, 15,* 93–100.

§Barker, P. J., & Buchanan-Barker, P. (2004). Beyond empowerment: Revering the storyteller. *Mental Health Practice, 7*(5), 18–20.

¶Barker, P. J. (2000e). *The tidal model theory and practice.* Newcastle, UK: University of Newcastle.

USE OF EMPIRICAL EVIDENCE

Barker's long-standing curiosity about the nature and focus of psychiatric nursing and the stories of persons-in-care led to the development of a theoretical construction of psychiatric nursing, or a metatheory, that could be further explored through empirical inquiry (Barker, Reynolds, & Stevenson, 1997, p. 663). Over 5 years, beginning in 1995, the Newcastle and North Tyneside research team developed an understanding of what people experiencing problems in living might need from nurses and began using their emergent findings in 1997 as the basis for development of the tidal model. Barker supports learning from using and integrating extant theory and research, as well as the experience of reality—evidence from the most "real" of real worlds (Barker & Jackson, 1997).

The power of the nurse–patient relationship demonstrated through Altschul's pioneering research in the early 1960s and Peplau's paradigm of interpersonal relationships contribute to the empirical base of the tidal model. Altschul's study of nurse–patient interaction in the 1960s provided empirical support for the complex, yet paradoxically ordinary nature of the relationship (Barker, 2002a). Altschul's study of community teams in the 1980s raised questions about the "proper focus of nursing" and the "need for nursing," and both Altschul and Peplau provided evidence related to interprofessional teamwork.

Two of Barker's theory-generating studies provided the empirical base for the tidal model. The Need for Nursing studies (Barker, Jackson, & Stevenson, 1999a, 1999b) examined the perceptions of service users, significant others, members of interprofessional teams, and nurses, and it sought to clarify discrete roles and functions of nursing within an interprofessional care and treatment process and to learn what people value in nurses (Barker, 2001c, p. 215). They demonstrated that professionals and persons-in-care wanted nurses to relate to people in ordinary, everyday ways. There was universal acceptance of special interpersonal relationships between nurses and persons, echoing Peplau's (1952) work. "Knowing you, knowing me" emerged as the core concept in these studies. The nurse is expected to know what the person wants even if it is not verbalized or is not clear, and needs are constantly changing (Jackson & Stevenson, 2004, p. 35). Professional nursing performance is described in three roles identified as (1) ordinary-me, (2) pseudo-ordinary or engineered-me, and (3) professional-me. Relationships are fluid, requiring nurses to toggle, or switch back and forth, from highly professional to distinctly ordinary presentations of self. Relationships differ depending on the required role (Jackson & Stevenson, 1998, 2000). The "pseudo-ordinary or engineered-me is likened to a see-saw" (Jackson & Stevenson, 2004, p. 41). Sometimes people need someone to take care of them, other times someone to take care with them (Barker, Jackson, & Stevenson, 1999a, 1999b). The studies suggested that nurses respond sensitively to persons' and their families' rapidly fluctuating human needs. They need to tune in to what needs to be done now to meet the person's needs (Barker, 2000e). Nurses are translators for the person to the treatment team and the glue that holds the system together (Stevenson & Fletcher, 2002, p. 30).

The second study focused on the nature of empowerment and how this is enacted in relationship between nurses and persons-in-care and resulted in the empowering interactions model (Barker, Stevenson, & Leamy, 2000). This was developed with Flanagan's Critical Incident Technique (Flanagan, 1954) within a cooperative inquiry method (Heron, 1996), using a modified grounded theory approach (Glaser & Strauss, 1967). The study developed Peplau's assumptions about the importance of specific interpersonal transactions, and it provided guidance and strategies for nurses within collaborative nurse–person relationships. Strategies included the following:

- Being respectful of people's knowledge and expertise about their own health and illness
- Putting the person in the driver's seat in relation to the interaction
- Seeking permission to explore the person's experience
- Valuing the person's contribution
- Being curious as a way of validating the person's experience
- Finding a common language to describe the situation
- Taking stock
- Reviewing collaboratively, and inspiring hope through designing a realistic future together

MAJOR ASSUMPTIONS

Two basic assumptions underpin the tidal model. First, change is the only constant. Nothing lasts. All human experience involves flux, and people are constantly changing. This suggests the value of helping people become more aware of how change is happening within and around them (Barker & Buchanan-Barker, 2004a). Second, people are their stories. They are no more and no less than the complex story of their lived experience. The person's story is framed in the first person, and the story of how they came to be here experiencing this problem of living contains the raw material for solutions (Barker & Buchanan-Barker, 2004a).

The tidal model rests on the following assumptions:

- There are such things as psychiatric needs.
- Nursing might in some way meet those needs (Barker & Whitehill, 1997, p. 15).
- Persons and those around them already possess the solutions to their life problems.
- Nursing is about drawing out these solutions (Barker, 1995, p. 12).

The tidal model assumes that when people are caught in the psychic storm of "madness," it is as if they risk drowning in their distress or foundering on the rocks; it is as if they have been boarded by pirates and have been robbed of some of their human identity; it is as if they have been washed ashore on some remote beach, far from home and alienated from all that they know and understand.

Nursing

"Nurses are involved in the process of working with people, their environments, their health *and* their need for nursing" (Barker, 1996a, p. 242). Nursing is continuously changing, internally and in relation to other professions, in response to changing needs and changing social structures. "If any one thing defines nursing, globally, it is the social construction of the nurse's role" (Barker, Reynolds, & Ward, 1995, p. 390). Nursing as nurturing exists only when the conditions necessary for the promotion of growth or development are put in place (Buchanan-Barker & Barker, 2008). Nursing is "an enduring human interpersonal activity and involves a focus on the promotion of growth and development" (Barker & Whitehill, 1997, p. 17) and present and future direction (Barker & Buchanan-Barker, 2007a). Barker extended Peplau's original definition, clarifying the purpose of nursing as *trephotaxis* from the Greek: "the provision of the necessary conditions for the promotion of growth and development" (Barker, 1989, 2009 (p. 5); Buchanan-Barker & Barker, 2003). He emphasizes the distinction between "psychiatric" and "mental health" nursing. When nurses help people *explore* their distress, in an attempt to discover ways of *remedying* or *ameliorating* it, they are practicing *psychiatric nursing.* When nurses help the same people *explore* ways of *growing and developing,* as persons, exploring how they presently *live with* and might move *beyond* their problems of living, they are practicing *mental health nursing* (Barker, 2003a, 2009).

Nursing is a human service offered by one group of human beings to another. There is a power dynamic in the craft of caring; one person has a duty to care for another (Barker, 1996b, p. 4). Nursing is a practical endeavor focused on identifying what people need *now;* collaboratively exploring ways of meeting those needs; and developing appropriate systems of human care (Barker, 1995, 2003a). The proper focus of nursing is the "need" expressed by the person-in-care, which "can only be defined as a function of the relationship between a *person-with-a-need-for-nursing* and a *person-who-has-met-that-need*" (Barker, 1996a, p. 241; Barker, Reynolds, & Ward, 1995, p. 389). "These responses are the phenomenological focus of nursing" (Barker, Reynolds, & Ward, 1995, p. 394)—a focus on human responses to actual or potential health problems (American Nurses Association, 1980). These may range across behavior, emotions, beliefs, identity, capability, spirituality, and the person's relationship with the environment (Barker, 1998a).

Nursing's exploration of the human context of being and caring supports nursing as a form of human inquiry. Being with and caring with people is the process that underpins all psychiatric and mental health nursing, and this process distinguishes nurses from all other health and social care disciplines (Barker, 1997). "Nursing complements other services and is congruent with the roles and functions of other disciplines in relation to the person's needs" (Barker, 2001c, p. 216).

Person

Within the tidal model, interest is directed toward a phenomenological view of the person's lived experience and his or her story (Barker, 1999a, 2000d). "Persons are natural philosophers and meaning makers devoting much of their lives to establishing the meaning and value of their experience and to constructing explanatory models of the world and their place in it" (Barker, 1996b, p. 4). Nurses are able to see and appreciate the world from the person's perspective and share this with the person. People are their stories. "The person's sense of self and the world of experience, including the experience of others is inextricably tied to their life stories and the various meanings they have generated" (Barker, 2001c, p. 219). People are in a constant state of flux, with great capacity for change (Buchanan-Barker & Barker, 2008) and engaged in the process of becoming (Barker, 2000c). They live within their world of experience represented in three dimensions: (1) world, (2) self, and (3) others.

Life is a developmental voyage, and people travel across their "ocean of experience." This voyage of discovery and exploration can be risky, and people have both a fundamental need for security and a capacity to adapt to changing circumstances. The "journey across our ocean of experience depends on our physical body on which we roll out the story of our lives" (Barker & Buchanan-Barker, 2007a, p. 21). The tidal model "holds few assumptions about the proper course of a person's life" (Barker, 2001a, p. 235). Persons are defined in relation, for example, as someone's mother, father, daughter, son, sister, brother, or friend and also in relation with nurses.

Health

Barker provides the provocative definition of health put forth by Illich (1976) as "the result of an autonomous yet culturally shaped reaction to socially-created reality. It designates the ability to adapt to changing environments, to growing up . . . to healing when damaged, to suffering and to the peaceful expectation of death. Health embraces the future . . . includes the inner resources to live with it" (p. 273). Health is a personal task where success is "in large part the result of self-awareness, self-discipline, and inner resources by which each person regulates his/her own daily rhythms and actions, his/her diet, and his/her sexuality" (Illich, 1976, p. 274). Our personhood, connections, and fragility "make the experience of pain, of sickness, and of death an integral part of life" (Illich, 1976, p. 274). Illich's (1976) description illustrates both the *chaotic* and *Zen* sense of "reality." "Health is not 'out-there,' it is not something to be pursued, gained or delivered (health-care). It is a part of the whole task of being and living" (Barker, 1999b, p. 240).

"Health means whole . . . and is likely linked to the way we live our lives, in the broadest sense. This 'living' includes the social, economic, cultural and spiritual context of our lives" (Barker, 1999b, p. 48). The experience of health and illness is fluid. Within a holistic view, people have their own individual meanings of health and illness that we value and accept. Nurses engage with people to learn their stories and their understanding of their current situation, including relationships with health and illness within their worldview (Barker, 2001c). Ill health or illness almost always involves a spiritual crisis or a loss of self (Barker, 1996a). A state of disease is a human problem with social, psychological, and medical relations, a whole life crisis. Nursing with the tidal model is pragmatic and focused upon persons' strengths, resources, and possibilities, maintaining a health orientation; the tidal model is a healthy theory.

Environment

The environment is largely social in nature, the context in which persons travel within their ocean of experience, and nurses create "space" for growth and development. "Therapeutic relationships are used in ways that enhance persons' relationships with their environment" (Montgomery & Webster, 1993, p. 7). Human problems may derive from complex person–environment interactions in the chaos of the everyday world (Barker, 1998b). "Persons live in a social and material world where their interaction with the environment includes other people, groups, and organizations" (Barker, 2003a, p. 67). Family, culture, and relationships are integral to this environment. Vital areas of everyday living, including housing, financing, occupation, leisure, and a sense of place and belonging are facets of environment (Barker, 2001c).

The divide between community and institution is artificial and rejected as needs flow with the person across these boundaries. Much psychiatric and mental health nursing takes place in the most mundane of settings, from day rooms of hospital wards to the living room or kitchen of the person's home (Barker, 1996b). With critical interventions, nurses keep the person and the environment safe and secure. Engagement is critical, and the social environment is critical for engagement. When people are deemed to be at risk, they need to be detained in a safe and supportive environment, a safe harbor until they return to their ocean of experience in the community (Barker, 2003a). "Nurses organize the kind of conditions that help to alleviate distress and begin the longer term process of recuperation, resolution or learning. They help persons to feel the 'whole' of their experience . . . and engender the potential for healing" (Barker, 2003a, p. 9).

THEORETICAL ASSERTIONS

The tidal model is based upon four premises concerning practice, developed in the mid-1990s with the "expert nurse" focus group (Barker, 1997) and validated by a group of former psychiatric patients led by Barker's colleague Dr. Irene Whitehill.

- Psychiatric nursing is an interactive, developmental human activity, more concerned with the future development of persons than the origins or cause of their present mental distress.
- The experience of mental distress associated with a psychiatric disorder is represented through public disturbance or reports of private events that are known only to the person concerned. Nurses help people access, review, and reauthor these experiences.
- Nurses and the people-in-care are engaged in a relationship based upon mutual influence. Change is constant, and within relationships there are changes in the relationship and within the participants in the relationship.
- The experience of mental illness is translated into a variety of disturbances of everyday living and human responses to problems in living (Barker & Whitehill, 1997).

These premises are framed within the wider philosophical and theoretical perspectives, especially the phenomenological assertion that people own their experience; only persons can know their experience and what it means. Mental distress is a symbolic force that is known only, in phenomenological terms, to the person involved. The lived experience is the medium through which we receive important messages about our life and its meaning (Barker, 2001c). Barker views mental distress as part of the whole of the person, not something split off from their "normal" being.

The tidal model assumes and asserts that people know what their needs are, or can be helped to recognize or acknowledge them over time. From that minimally empowered position, people may be helped to meet these needs in the short term. What nurses and everyone else in the person's social world relate to is the expressed behavior. Mental illness is disempowering, and "people who experience any of the myriad threats to their personal or social identities, commonly called *mental illness* or *mental health problems,* experience a human threat that renders them vulnerable." However, "most people are sufficiently healthy to be able to act for themselves and to influence constructively the direction of their lives" (Barker, 2003a, pp. 6–7). Recovery is possible, and people have the personal and interpersonal resources that enable this recovery process (Barker, 2001c).

LOGICAL FORM

The tidal model is logically adequate; the structure of relationships is clear; and the concepts are precise, developed, and developing. It contains broad ideas, addresses many situations of persons with problems in living, follows the logic of experience (Barker, 1996b), and develops practice-based evidence (Barker & Buchanan-Barker, 2005).

Barker and colleagues constructed a metatheory of psychiatric and mental health nursing. Questions about the nature of persons, problems in living, and nursing were followed with systematic inquiry. The theory informs and is shaped by research. The tidal model flows from a particular philosophical perspective and worldview that provides the context for beliefs about persons and nursing.

The theory identifies the core of nursing practice as "knowing you, knowing me." It specifies a nursing focus of inquiry; identifies phenomena of particular interest to nurses; and provides a broad perspective for nursing research, practice, education, and policy. The theory classifies a body of nursing knowledge that is largely story-based. The components are clearly presented and logically derived from clinical observation, practice, theory, research, and philosophy.

The emergent evidence from users of the theory in the United Kingdom, Ireland, Canada, New Zealand, and Scandinavia confirms the importance of the simple affirmation of the personal story, with its emphasis on understanding what is happening for and to the person and what this means for persons, in their own language. Stories generated within the caring context are written in the person's own voice, helping the person to "take back" the personal story, which has been lost from view by becoming a "patient" or "client." Even when the person is severely disabled by problems of living, the nurse keeps the focus on helping the person determine "what needs to be done" and on finding the personal and interpersonal resources necessary to be empowered.

The attempt to understand persons' constructions of their world is expressed through the holistic assessment that helps persons relate their story and explore what needs to be done. Care planning is a collaborative exercise with emphasis on developing an awareness of change and revealing solutions. The celebration of personhood and the holistic narrative approach creates a style of practice of working collaboratively with people. It emphasizes persons' inherent resources and acknowledges change as an enduring characteristic.

ACCEPTANCE BY THE NURSING COMMUNITY

The tidal model appeals to those interested in person-centered care and theory-based practice. The literature illustrates wide acceptance and use of the theory in practice and research around the world. Acceptance of the theory is facilitated by the philosophical, theoretical, research, and practical base, along with clearly stated values and principles.

Practice

The origins of the tidal model lie in work begun in Barker's doctoral research with women with a diagnosis of manic depressive psychosis in the early 1980s and his introduction to the work of Shoma Morita (Reynolds, 1984). The tidal model was developed in practice between 1995 and 1998 in Newcastle, England, and was introduced formally on two acute psychiatric wards. It was subsequently adopted by the Mental Health Program and in 2000 rolled out across nine acute psychiatric wards, their associated community support teams, and one 24-hour facility in the community in the same Mental Health Program (Barker & Buchanan-Barker, 2005). The tidal model became international as interest spread in the United Kingdom first to Ireland, then throughout the world, with nurses from Dublin undertaking short residences in Newcastle with Barker in 1999. In 2001 nurses in New Zealand began to introduce it at a high-security forensic unit (Cook, Phillips, & Sadler, 2005).

Most of the early tidal model developmental work was undertaken in the United Kingdom, with projects ranging across hospital and community services, from acute through rehabilitation, to specialist forensic services and community care. These ranged from metropolitan services in cities like central London and Birmingham, where the clinical populations are socially, culturally, and ethnically diverse, to Cornwall, Glamorgan, and Norfolk, where people from rural English and Welsh communities were served.

The most extensive project was in Scotland, where since 2003 the Glasgow mental health services operated a series of tidal projects, embracing acute, rehabilitation, adolescent, and elder care, in what was the largest mental health service in the United Kingdom (Lafferty & Davidson, 2006). By 2012 the Glasgow projects had extended to include other Scottish centers: Greenock, Inverclyde, Paisley, Fife, and Ayrshire (Henderson, 2013), representing more than a third of the overall population of Scotland.

The Republic of Ireland established a wide range of projects in County Cork, County Mayo, and Dublin, ranging across hospital and community settings. Cork City, Ireland, was the first to introduce and develop the tidal model within community mental health care at Tosnu—Gaelic for "fresh start."

At the Royal Ottawa Mental Health Centre in Canada, three programs implemented the tidal model in September 2002. The Forensic and Mood programs include inpatient wards and outpatient components. The Substance Use and Concurrent Disorders Program included an inpatient ward, outpatient nursing, a day hospital, and a residential program in the community and is the first program of its kind to implement the tidal model. In February 2004 the tidal model was introduced to remaining inpatient wards, including geriatric, crisis and evaluation, general psychiatry in transition, psychosocial rehabilitation, schizophrenia, and youth (adolescents). The Ottawa experience stimulated much interest in the tidal model across Canada and led to developments in many facilities from coast to coast.

In Australia, projects were first established in child and adolescent care in Sydney, with a new development in the area of "justice health." In New Zealand, nurses at *Rangipapa* in Porirua were the first to introduce the tidal model into a forensic setting and the first to investigate the experience with the model from the perspective of staff and clientele (Cook, Phillips, & Sadler, 2005). The tidal model's emphasis on story has proven particularly attractive to the indigenous Maori and Pacific Islands people of New Zealand.

In Japan the tidal model has been the focus of nursing practice since 2002 at the Kanto Medical Center, the largest private psychiatric facility in Tokyo. Dr. Tsuyoshi Akayama, psychiatrist and professor of psychiatry, translated the tidal model training materials into Japanese and taught medical and nursing colleagues how to use the model after his short study tour in Newcastle with Dr. Barker. This was the first formal collaboration between psychiatrists and nurses—nurses had led the implementation in the earlier projects. Dr. Akayama has promoted consideration of the tidal model within the "developing nations" program of the World Psychiatric Association. The Japanese have set a trend for greater interprofessional collaboration, albeit with nursing taking the lead role.

Since 2012 a range of clinical projects have developed across Europe in Germany (Zuaboni, Burr, & Schulz, 2013), Sweden, Denmark, and Switzerland (Zuaboni, 2015), all countries whose philosophical history—especially phenomenology and existentialism—has played a key role in the development of the tidal philosophy. The traditional culture of these countries is, however, changing thanks to immigration and the accommodation of refugees. It will be interesting to see how the "person focus" of the tidal model accommodates these sociocultural changes.

A paper by Kilmer & Lane-Tillerson (2013) describes the use of the tidal model with women experiencing severe emotional problems in relation to fertility treatment. This paper suggests the potential of the tidal model for addressing a range of problems of living beyond the traditional psychiatric and mental health sector. Dos Santos, and colleagues (2015) report on use of the tidal model in Brazil.

The tidal model of mental health recovery is directed toward understanding and further explaining the human condition. Central to this effort is helping people use their voices as the key instrument for charting their recovery from mental distress. The tidal model is a person-centered model of mental health care delivery, which is respectful of culture and creed (Barker & Buchanan-Barker, 2005). This practical theory identifies the concepts necessary to understand the human needs of people with problems in living, and how and what nurses might do to address those needs. The theory systematically explains specific phenomena and suggests the nature of relationships within a particular worldview. Barker, however, has consistently asserted that the theory is "no more than words on paper." It is not a reified work or recipe for practice, but a practical and evolving guide for delivering collaborative, person-centered, strengths-based, and empowering care through relationship.

Education

The holistic, strength-based, narrative tidal model holds great promise for inclusion in educational programs concerned with theory-based practice and person-centered care.

Barker and Buchanan-Barker offer a free training manual for download from their website (www.tidal-model.com). This package is used as the basic preparation for implementation of the model, ensuring fidelity to the values, principles, and processes of the tidal model, while allowing creative, locally relevant implementation. The tidal training manual has now been translated into German, Swedish, Danish, and Spanish by members of nursing teams involved in clinical and educational developments in those countries.

Research

The tidal model developed from a clinical research program, and all teams who introduce it into their practice are encouraged to evaluate its effects within the practice. A research and development consultancy was established as a loose network for tidal model implementation and development projects. The consultancy provides a framework for evaluation of the tidal model in action from the perspective of organizational outcome, professional experience, and user and consumer experience (Barker & Buchanan-Barker, 2005). The important task of evaluating the implementation, processes, and outcomes of the tidal model in practice is ongoing in Canada, Ireland, Japan, Germany, Sweden (Lassenius, 2014), Denmark, Brazil (dos Santos et al., 2015), New Zealand, and across the United Kingdom.

The two earliest evaluation studies (Fletcher & Stevenson, 2001; Stevenson & Fletcher, 2002) explored outcome measures important in evaluating the tidal model and the effects of the tidal model assessment in practice (Stevenson & Fletcher, 2002). Results of both studies indicate an increase in the number of admissions and a decrease in the length of stay. There was a decrease in need for the highest level of observation that correlated with the speed of assessment, and a decrease in incidents of violence, self-harm, and use of restraints. Nurses themselves reported that the tidal model enhanced professional practice and encouraged fuller engagement with persons-in-care. It was useful in helping persons fulfill care plans and enabled nurses to focus their interactions on persons' needs. Support workers were able to help persons identify goals and targets for the day and carry them out; they described the tidal model as "a way of raising their profile and professional esteem" (Stevenson & Fletcher, 2002, p. 35). Similar findings, using the same method, were reported in Birmingham, the second city in England to implement the tidal model (Gordon, Morton, & Brooks, 2005); Glasgow, the largest city in Scotland (Lafferty & Davidson, 2006); and Dublin, Ireland. These studies provide evidence for the implementation of this person-centered theory in practice.

Barker and Walker (2000) studied senior nurses' views of multidisciplinary teamwork in 26 acute psychiatric admission units and the relationship to the care of persons and their families. Although nurses face challenges in implementing "working in partnership," the study provides some direction for further inquiry around the interprofessional nature of the theory.

The transition for nurses to a solution focus in interactions was the subject of study by the Newcastle team (Stevenson, Jackson, & Barker, 2003). Nurses participated in a specially tailored solution educational initiative, and the effects were assessed for both nurses and persons-in-care using multiple data sources. This study provides strong evidence of significant improvement in nurses' solution-focused knowledge, performance, and use in practice. Persons-in-care also found the approach helpful.

The Royal Ottawa Mental Health Centre Tidal Team replicated the Newcastle study and assessed the effect of implementation of the tidal model on selected outcome measures over four periods in the three pioneer programs with similar results, particularly in the Mood Program. They also replicated the Newcastle study over four periods in the Forensic Program at the Brockville site. The Tosnu team completed a user-focused evaluation of the tidal model implementation. In Birmingham, on the Tolkien ward, a 4-month evaluation has been completed and published (Gordon, Morton, & Brooks, 2005). Evaluation work is ongoing at St. Tydfil Hospital in Wales.

In New Zealand, a hermeneutic phenomenological study followed the implementation of the tidal model in a secure treatment unit (Cook, Phillips, & Sadler, 2005). Five themes that reflected meanings attached to providing and receiving care emerged: relationships, hope, human face, leveling, and working together, suggesting positive experiences and outcomes with implementation of the tidal model. The tidal model is set in a research base that provides the possibility of research use or the more contemporary knowledge transfer. Nurses practicing within the tidal model are actively using research in practice and contributing to the development of nursing practice. The tidal model has potential for participatory action research, uncovering knowledge embedded in practice, and developing new knowledge and understandings.

Barker and Buchanan-Barker emphasize that any realistic study of the tidal model in practice must focus on the "workings" of the team, both individually and collectively. It must take into account the organizational context; the support available to the team; the quality of the environment; and the range of other physical, social, and interpersonal factors. As practitioners begin to work in a tidal way, key research questions must focus on "what happens?" in tidal practice.

FURTHER DEVELOPMENT

The tidal model is clear, concepts are defined, and relationships are identified. This enables the identification of areas for further theory development. For example, Barker reframed his original notion of the "logic of experience" as "practice-based evidence." This represents the knowledge of what is possible in this particular situation and what might contribute further to our shared understanding of human helping (Barker & Buchanan-Barker, 2005).

Several other developments characterize the tidal model. It has evolved from the initial acute, inpatient use across the continuum of care, with critical, transitional, and developmental components. The theory has evolved to the tidal model of mental health recovery and reclamation, broadening both its scope and utility. Colleagues in other fields such as palliative care have expressed appreciation of the model and the desire to bring it into their practice settings. Other professions support the values, philosophy, and utility of the tidal model. Mental health user, consumer, and survivor communities around the world are involved in the continuing development of this mental health recovery theory (Barker & Buchanan-Barker, 2005).

Since its inception, the tidal model has gained national and international attention. It continues to be implemented, taught, and studied internationally, with new sites joining from around the world. In November 2003 the tidal model was launched in North America. As new sites implement and study the tidal model, the practical, theoretical, and research base is enriched. In 2003 Barker reaffirmed the values underlying the tidal model in the Ten Tidal Commitments (see Box 32.1). They provide the necessary guidance to pursue and develop the philosophy of the tidal model. Although Barker expects fidelity to the principles and values of the tidal model (Ten Tidal Commitments) in its implementation, he cautions against slavish importation. Rather, implementation needs to be tailored to fit the local context, with the result that each implementation will be unique and contribute to the theory's development. This reflects Barker's appreciation of the concept of practice-based evidence—the art of the possible—that is, developing philosophically and theoretically sound forms of practice that are based on considerations of what is appropriate, meaningful, and potentially effective in any given practice context.

The tidal model is developing across cultures as previously described, with different clinical populations, in a variety of settings. The body of knowledge framed within the tidal model continues to develop, acknowledging the wide range of complex factors that define people and their human experiences—personal history, personal preferences, values and beliefs, social status, cultural background, family affiliations, and community membership (Barker, 2003a).

CRITIQUE

Clarity

The concepts, subconcepts, and relationships are logically developed and clear, and the assumptions are consistent with the theory's goals. The major concepts, subconcepts, and relationships are described carefully, specifically, and metaphorically, though not necessarily concisely. Terms like *problems in living, mental distress,* and *view of people experiencing problems as persons* guide nurses to a proper focus. The identification of human needs rather than psychological, social, or physical needs provides clarity and focus. How nurses see persons and how persons want to be nursed are clearly illustrated through the core category of knowing you, knowing me. Three subcategories, ordinary-me, pseudo-ordinary or engineered-me, and professional-me each have four dimensions: depth of knowing, power, time, and translation (Barker, Jackson, & Stevenson, 1999a; Jackson & Stevenson, 2004).

In practice, using the person's own language, rather than jargon or professional language, contributes to the theory's success and its clarity. Major concepts of collaboration, empowerment, relationships, solution focus, empowering through relationships, narrative, and the use of the term *problems in living* are sufficiently clear and open the theory for use in other areas of nursing and health care.

A number of concepts and relationships are presented elegantly and schematically within the tidal model. The person's unique lived experience is synergistic and reciprocal among the world, self, and others domains that are represented in a triangle (Fig. 32.1). The Holistic Assessment, the person's story, is at the heart of care planning and is represented as a heart. The circle of security assessment and plan surrounds the heart, all of which is surrounded by the interprofessional team circle (Fig. 32.2). The continuum of care (immediate, transitional, and developmental) intersects with the focus of care (Barker, 2000e; Barker & Buchanan-Barker, 2007a) (Fig. 32.3), demonstrating the voyage of the person who enters, progresses through, and exits the service (Fig. 32.4). This easily understood theory is accessible conceptually and linguistically through the use of everyday language.

Simplicity

The tidal model is based upon a few simple ideas about being human and helping one another (Barker, 2000e). It

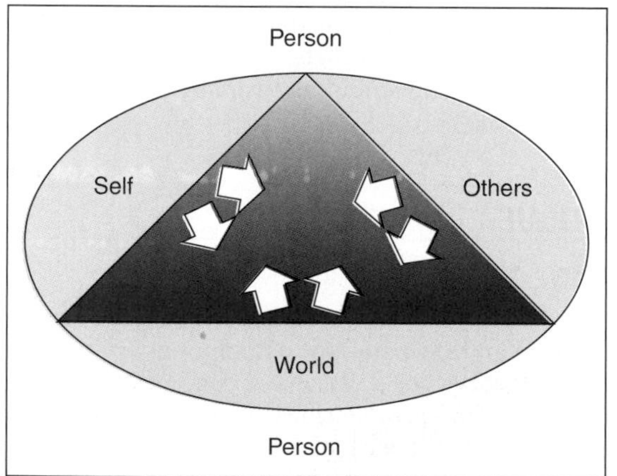

FIG. 32.1 Three dimensions of personhood. (From Barker, P. J., & Buchanan-Barker, P. [2007]. *The tidal model theory and practice* [p. 38]. Clan Unity, Scotland, UK. Copyright Phil Barker & Poppy Buchanan-Barker, 2007.)

is comprehensive, elegant in its simplicity, and at a level of abstraction to guide practice, education, research, and policy. However, the concepts themselves are complex, and the broad relationships among the concepts add to the complexity of the tidal model; people and relationships are inherently complex. Assumptions, concepts, and relationships are described in everyday language and illuminated through metaphor. For example, simply being respectful of the persons' knowledge and expertise about their own health and illness and listening to persons' stories is empowering. Abstract and complex concepts or relationships are expressed metaphorically as in the ebb and flow of the tide. Practical and philosophical, the tidal model provides some direction in operationalizing or using the concepts, but it is careful not to prescribe practice.

Generality

The tidal model is international in scope, suggesting its relevance cross-culturally and cross-nationally. By the beginning of 2004 there were almost 100 tidal model projects in progress in different clinical settings around the world—in Australia, Canada, England, Ireland, Japan, New Zealand, Scotland, and Wales (Barker & Buchanan-Barker, 2005). A wide range of settings and clinical populations are represented in the tidal model projects: rural and urban, acute, crisis and longer-term care wards, private and public facilities, community programs, rehabilitation, forensic, youth, adults, and older adults. The tidal model has been successful across the continuum of psychiatric and mental health care and in a range of practice situations. Universal characteristics of collaboration, empowerment, relationships, stories, and strengths appeal to nurses, service users, and colleagues in other disciplines. The tidal model is consistent with the Ottawa Charter for Health Promotion, in which the process of empowerment and participation is seen as fundamental to good health (World Health Organization, 1986). The Ten Tidal Commitments (Buchanan-Barker & Barker, 2008) provide guidance, direction, and support in using the theory. In Scotland, Lafferty and Davidson (2006) observed that practice with the tidal model helped nurses fulfill the person-centered requirements of the Scottish Mental Health Act. In Canada, the Best Practice Guideline for Person and Family–Centred Care (Registered Nurses' Association of Ontario, 2015) echoes the tidal model, using some of the same language.

Barker acknowledges that to practice within the tidal model, nurses need to believe that recovery is possible and change is inevitable. "The Tidal Model *per se* does not work. The practitioner is the instrument or medium of change" (Buchanan-Barker, 2004, p. 8). Because the tidal

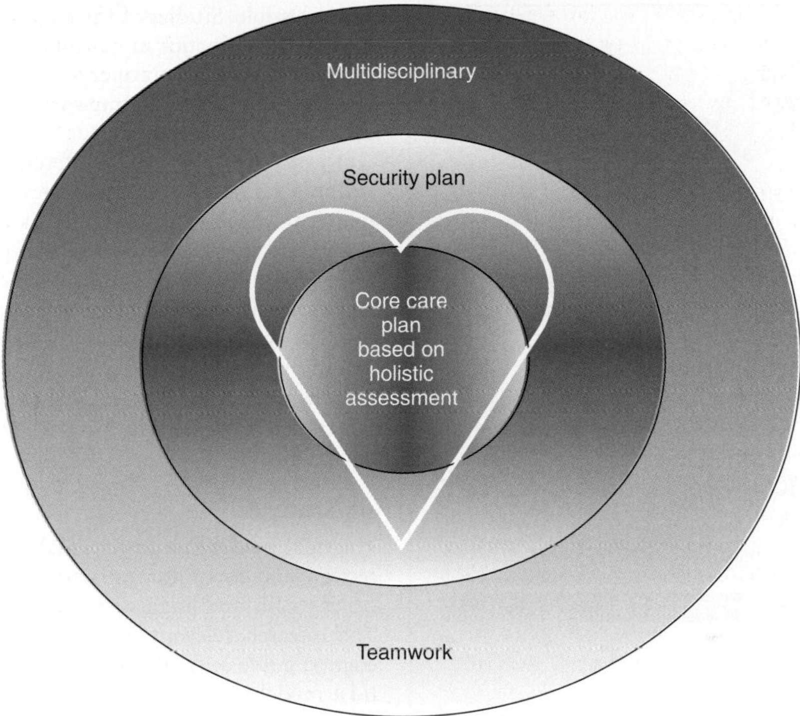

FIG. 32.2 The structure of care. (From Barker, P. J. [2000]. *The tidal model theory and practice* [p. 27]. Newcastle, UK: University of Newcastle. Copyright Phil Barker, 2000.)

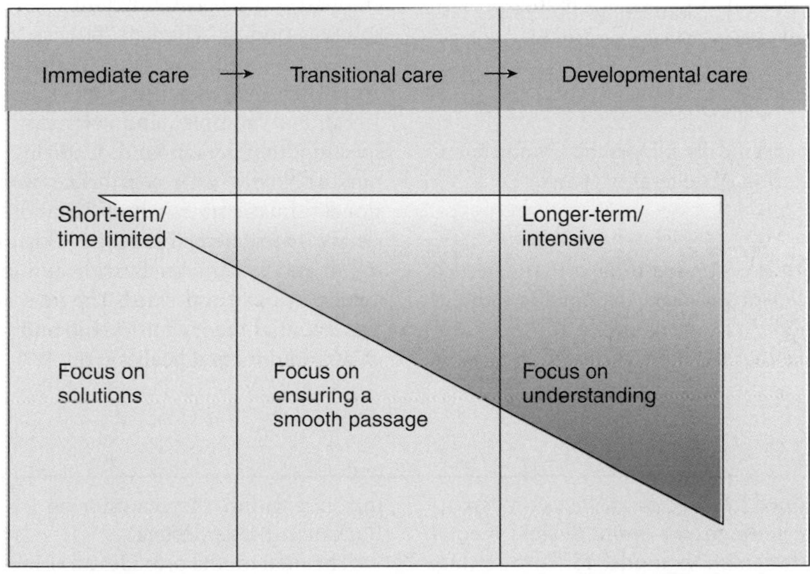

FIG. 32.3 Tidal model care continuum. (From Barker, P. J., & Buchanan-Barker, P. [2007]. *The tidal model theory and practice* (p. 32). Clan Unity, Scotland, UK. Copyright Phil Barker & Poppy Buchanan-Barker, 2007.)

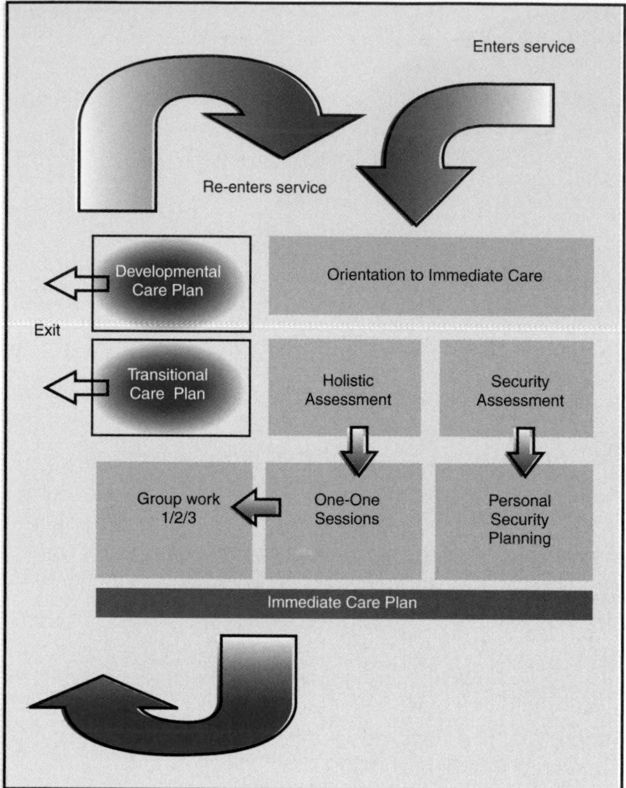

FIG. 32.4 Map of the care continuum. (From Barker, P. J., & Buchanan-Barker, P. [2007]. *The tidal model theory and practice* [p. 37]. Clan Unity, Scotland, UK. Copyright Phil Barker & Poppy Buchanan-Barker, 2007.)

model was developed specifically for psychiatry and mental health care, the criterion of generality is met.

Accessibility

This substantive theory is grounded in data that emerged inductively from studies of the need for nursing. Studies guided by the tidal model suggest its utility and precision and provide confidence that the theory is useful, practical, and accessible. Studies of the effects of implementation of the theory in practice support its utility and precision. The need for nursing, the proper focus of nursing, and the empowering interactions framework provide a strong empirical base for the tidal model.

Nurses working with different clinical populations and in a variety of settings are testing the tidal model in practice. The focus of inquiry is person-centered outcomes and the lived experience of persons collaborating in care. Studies addressing these empowering interactions contribute to empirical adequacy and confidence in this strengths-based, solution-oriented perspective. By making the tidal model manual freely available, centers may have introduced the model to practice entirely without Barker's knowledge. Barker views this as a positive development.

Importance

The tidal model has clearly illustrated that it provides direction and focus for nursing. The theory is accessible conceptually and linguistically and lends itself to research. This research, relevant to nurses' work, contributes knowledge to guide and inform practice. Studies guided by the tidal model also explore its impact and a variety of outcomes. Narrative knowledge derived from the theory advances the practice of nursing, nursing education, nursing research, and policy. The tidal model is represented by a range of "holistic (exploratory) and focused (risk) assessments which generate person-centered interventions that emphasize the person's extant resources and capacity for solution-finding" (Barker, 2001b, p. 82).

Working with the tidal model has enabled nurses to articulate their practice and "invisible skills" (Michael, 1994). For example, empowerment strategies such as respecting the person and inspiring hope give voice to nurses. Nurses gain confidence working as interprofessional team members where their contribution and focus is clearly articulated. Challenges exist at the practical, personal, and system levels with any change, and these are anticipated and addressed. The tidal model is an important and essential theory to develop and guide practice in psychiatry and mental health care.

SUMMARY

The tidal model developed from a discrete focus on psychiatric nursing in acute settings to a more flexible mental health recovery and reclamation model for any setting, relevant to any discipline. It emphasizes empowering forms of engagement or bridging, the importance of the lived experience, and an appreciation of the potential for healing that lies within the reauthoring of the story (Barker & Buchanan-Barker, 2004a).

The tidal model provides an orientation to practice that is research-based, holistic, and person-centered. Keen (in Barker & Buchanan-Barker, 2005, pp. 231–241) describes a "deeply collaborative, person-centered, solution-focused

(McAllister, 2003), narrative-based, pragmatic, and systemic theory." The theory presents assumptions about people, their inherent value, and the value of relating to people in particular ways. It proposes how people might come to appreciate differently, perhaps better, their own value and the unique value of their experience. The tidal model opens possibilities of new ways of being with people in relation. Perhaps some of its appeal is that it harkens back to the values that brought the nurse into nursing in the first place. Although the theory provides direction for practice, education, research, and policy, it challenges nurses to make a shift to commit to change and to grow and develop in enacting the essence of the tidal model, the Ten Tidal Commitments.

CASE STUDY

Scott was a young man described as having a first episode psychosis. He beat his father, who subsequently died. Scott was transferred to a secure unit, where his primary nurse began to explore his story with him through a Holistic Assessment, which represents Scott's world of experience at this moment in time.

How this began: "It all started when my father punched my mother again, he was totally drunk that night. It was so noisy in that room, the TV, the banging, and those voices in my head, they kept yelling at me to do something fast to save my mother. I don't remember exactly what had happened after. I was so confused."

How this affected me: "I don't know. I have been in jail for 4 months before coming here. They told me I killed my father. I don't remember much except that I kept hammering his head; I just remember I was standing in a pool of blood." "They told me my mother is still in the hospital; I haven't seen her since." "I'm scared. I can't sleep."

How I felt in the beginning: It "just devastated me, turned me upside down." "I felt awful even though I hated him so much; he never listened to me; no one ever listened to me or believes me." "I hate him because I watched him beating my mother all my life."

How things have changed over time: "It got worse when my step-brother ran away. My father was a sinner, a drunk, wife beater, even conspired with the Communists. I was not allowed to leave the house except for school, my mother stayed in all day to do farm work, he was the only one that ran errands outside the house." "I've always been a bit scared and angry too."

The effect on my relationships: "I don't have any relationships with anyone; I don't like people because nobody likes me."

How do I feel now? "Well, I feel nervous, very shaky and scared. I don't know what to expect, I don't know what is going to happen." "Confused, I guess, and I'm tired."

What do I think this means? "I don't know, that was my question, maybe I will go back to jail, maybe it means I needed help." "It means I have a lot of challenges to meet."

What does all this say about me as a person? "I just want to be a better person, I want to be well, and I want to take care of my mother."

What needs to happen now? "Well, I suppose I'm here for an assessment."

What do I expect the nurse to do for me? "Continue to talk to me the way you are talking to me. No one ever talks to me like this. You are listening, and it seems like you believe me. This is so different from jail and anywhere else."

The people who are important: "My mother is the only important person in this world. My step-brother came back only for the money."

Things that are important: "Well, able to share with others." "My dog—Pepper, but he is at the Humane Society right now." "I have a really nice picture of me and my mom."

Ideas about life that are important: "Able to fit in."

Evaluating the problems: "My main problems are loneliness and what's going to happen in my future. My whole life is complex!" "I would rate my loneliness as an 8 for distress, an 8 for disturbance, and a 2 for control. My future and what's going to happen would be a 10 for distress, a 10 for disturbance, and I have no control, a 0."

How will I know the problem has been solved? "I'll know the problem has been solved maybe when the voices stop talking to me, when I get out of jail and out of the hospital."

What needs to change for this to happen? "Maybe I need to take medication, maybe I just have to start talking to real people, not the voices."

The nurse recognized that Scott needed some help to feel more emotionally secure. She engaged him in a security assessment and together they developed a Personal Security Plan.

Later in the week, the nurses noted that Scott was spending a lot of time in his room. Instead of encouraging Scott to participate in ward activities, his primary nurse shared her observation and asked Scott how it was helpful to him to spend so much time lying on his bed, alone in the room. Scott's reply was, "The voices don't bother me so much." This opened a conversation, helping the

Continued

CASE STUDY—cont'd

nurse begin to understand what this was like for Scott and what might be helpful for him.

In another conversation, the primary nurse asked "the miracle question." "Suppose that tonight, while you are asleep, the problem you have was miraculously solved. How would you know? What would be the first difference you noticed when you woke up?" Scott's unexpected reply was, "I'd have a friend." By exploring rather than closing down the narrative, the nurse began to involve Scott in "what needed to be done" to help him.

The Holistic Assessment and the Personal Security Plan represent the first steps in helping Scott *reclaim* ownership of the story of his difficulties and distress: beginning to explore what action needs to be taken—by Scott and others—to reduce his distress and address his problems. Within the tidal model, the nurse's focus is pragmatic. By joining with Scott in exploring his difficulties from his perspective, as he describes his experience in his own words, the nurse begins to develop a supportive, empathic relationship. The main aim is to help Scott *make sense* of what has happened to him, rather than telling him, to help him identify what part he has played in the development of his problems, and beginning to work out what needs to be done to address them. When a person like Scott eventually moves out into the everyday world, he will take with him the self-knowledge he has gained through the various relationships established in the individual and group work. Instead of expecting Scott to be passive or compliant, the nurse expects him to participate as fully as possible in constructing the kind of care he needs, establishing ownership not only of his problems but also of the ultimate means of resolving them. This approach clearly makes significant emotional and intellectual demands on both the person and the nurse.

CRITICAL THINKING ACTIVITIES

1. The security plan has two questions: What can I do that will help me to deal with my present problems? What help can others offer that I might find valuable? So what might Scott's security plan look like?
2. Select three or four of the Ten Tidal Commitments, and consider how these might be realized in your practice.
3. Where would you find support for the Ten Tidal Commitments in your workplace?
4. What is the key tidal question?

POINTS FOR FURTHER STUDY

- Barker, P. J. (2003b). *The 10 commitments: Essential values of the tidal model.* http://www.tidal-model.com.
- Barker, P. J., & Buchanan-Barker, P. (2007a). *The tidal model—Mental health recovery and reclamation.* Newport-on-Tay, Scotland: Clan Unity International.
- Buchanan-Barker, P., & Barker, P. (2008). The tidal commitments: Extending the value base of mental health recovery. *Journal of Psychiatric and Mental Health Nursing, 15*(2), 93–100.
- The Tidal Model website at www.tidal-model.com enables accessibility to the international tidal community.

REFERENCES

Allister, M. (2003). Doing practice differently: Solution-focused nursing. *Journal of Advanced Nursing, 41*(6), 528–535.

American Nurses' Association. (1980). *Nursing. A social policy statement.* Kansas City, MO: American Nurses' Association.

Barker, P. J. (1987). *An evaluation of specific nursing interventions in the management of patients suffering from manic-depressive psychosis.* Unpublished PhD thesis, Dundee Institute of Technology, University of Abertay, Scotland.

Barker, P. J. (1989). Reflections on the philosophy of caring in mental health. *International Journal of Nursing Studies, 26*(2), 131–141.

Barker, P. J. (1995). Promoting growth through community mental health nursing. *Mental Health Nursing, 15*(3), 12–15.

Barker, P. J. (1996a). Chaos and the way of Zen: Psychiatric nursing and the "uncertainty principle." *Journal of Psychiatric and Mental Health Nursing, 3*(4), 235–243.

Barker, P. J. (1996b). The logic of experience: Developing appropriate care through effective collaboration. *Australian and New Zealand Journal of Mental Health Nursing, 5*(1), 3–12.

Barker, P. J. (1997). Towards a meta-theory of psychiatric nursing. *Mental Health Practice, 1*(4), 18–21.

Barker, P. J. (1998a). It's time to turn the tide. *Nursing Times, 94*(46), 11–12.

Barker, P. J. (1998b). The future of the theory of interpersonal relations? A personal reflection on Peplau's legacy. *Journal of Psychiatric and Mental Health Nursing, 5*(3), 213–220.

Barker, P. J. (1999a). *Qualitative research in nursing and health care*. London: NT Books.

Barker, P. J. (Ed.). (1999b). *The philosophy and practice of psychiatric nursing*. Edinburgh, Scotland: Churchill Livingstone.

Barker, P. J. (2000a). Commentaries and reflections on mental health nursing in the UK at the dawn of the new millennium: Commentary 1. *Journal of Mental Health, 9*(6), 617–619.

Barker, P. J. (2000b). From chaos to complex order: Personal values and resources in the process of psychotherapy. *Perspectives in Psychiatric Care, 36*(2), 51–57.

Barker, P. J. (2000c). Reflections on caring as a virtue ethic within an evidence-based culture. *International Journal of Nursing Studies, 37*, 329–336.

Barker, P. (2000d). The tidal model: The lived experience in person-centered mental health care. *Nursing Philosophy, 2*(3), 213–223.

Barker, P. J. (2000e). *The tidal model: Theory and practice*. Newcastle, UK: University of Newcastle.

Barker, P. J. (2001a). The tidal model: Developing an empowering, person-centred approach to recovery within psychiatric and mental health nursing. *Journal of Psychiatric and Mental Health Nursing, 8*(3), 233–240.

Barker, P. J. (2001b). The tidal model: Developing a person-centered approach to psychiatric and mental health nursing. *Perspectives in Psychiatric Care, 37*(3), 79–87.

Barker, P. J. (2001c). The tidal model: The lived experience in person-centred mental health nursing. *Nursing Philosophy, 2*(3), 213–223.

Barker, P. J. (2002a). Annie Altschul—An appreciation. *Journal of Psychiatric and Mental Health Nursing, 9*(2), 127–128.

Barker, P. J. (2002b). Doing what needs to be done: A respectful response to Burnard and Grant. *Journal of Psychiatric and Mental Health Nursing, 9*, 232–236.

Barker, P. J. (Ed.). (2003a). *Psychiatric and mental health nursing. The craft of caring*. London: Arnold.

Barker, P. J. (2003b). *The 10 commitments: Essential values of the tidal model*. Retrieved from http://www.tidal-model.com/Ten%20Commitments.htm.

Barker, P. J. (2004, Sept/Oct). Uncommon sense—The tidal model of mental health recovery. *The New Therapist, 33*, 14–19.

Barker, P. J. (Ed). (2009). *Psychiatric and mental health nursing: The craft of caring* (2nd ed.). London: Arnold.

Barker, P., & Buchanan-Barker, P. (2004a). Beyond empowerment: Revering the storyteller. *Mental Health Practice, 7*(5), 18–20.

Barker, P. J., & Buchanan-Barker, P. (2004b). *Spirituality and mental health: Breakthrough*. London: Whurr.

Barker, P. J., & Buchanan-Barker, P. (2005). *The tidal model: A guide for mental health professionals*. London: Brunner-Routledge.

Barker, P. J., & Buchanan-Barker, P. (2007a). *The tidal model—Mental health recovery and reclamation*. Newport-on-Tay, Scotland: Clan Unity International.

Barker, P. J., & Buchanan-Barker, P. (2007b). Words of wisdom. *Nursing Standard, 21*(37), 24–25.

Barker, P., Campbell P., & Davidson B. (1999). *From the ashes of experience: Reflections on madness, recovery and growth*. London: Whurr.

Barker, P. J., & Jackson, S. (1997). No apologies for "imperialist" view [Letter]. *Nursing Standard, 11*(20), 10.

Barker, P., Jackson, S., & Stevenson, C. (1999a). The need for psychiatric nursing: Toward a multidimensional theory of caring. *Nursing Inquiry, 6*(2), 103–111.

Barker, P. J., Jackson, S., & Stevenson, C. (1999b). What are psychiatric nurses needed for? Developing a theory of essential practice. *Journal of Psychiatric and Mental Health Nursing, 6*(4), 273–282.

Barker, P. J., Reynolds, W., & Stevenson, C. (1997). The human science basis of psychiatric nursing: Theory and practice. *Journal of Advanced Nursing, 25*(4), 660–667.

Barker, P. J., Reynolds, W., & Ward, T. (1995). The proper focus of nursing: A critique of the caring ideology. *International Journal of Nursing Studies, 32*(4), 386–397.

Barker, P. J., Stevenson, C., & Leamy, M. (2000). The philosophy of empowerment. *Mental Health Practice, 20*(9), 8–12.

Barker, P. J., & Walker, L. (2000). Nurses' perceptions of multidisciplinary teamwork in acute psychiatric settings. *Journal of Psychiatric and Mental Health Nursing, 7*(6), 539–546.

Barker, P. J., & Whitehill, I. (1997). The craft of care: Towards collaborative caring in psychiatric nursing. In S. Tilley (Ed.), *The mental health nurse. Views of practice and education* (pp. 15–27). Oxford, UK: Blackwell Science.

Buchanan-Barker, P. (2004). The tidal model: Uncommon sense. *Mental Health Nursing, 24*(3), 6–10.

Buchanan-Barker, P., & Barker, P. (2005). The ten commitments: A value base for mental health recovery. *Journal of Psychosocial & Mental Health Nursing, 44*(9), 29–33.

Buchanan-Barker, P., & Barker, P. (2008). The Tidal Commitments: Extending the value base of mental health recovery. *Journal of Psychiatric and Mental Health Nursing, 15*(2), 93–100.

Buchanan-Barker, P., & Barker, P. J. (2003). *Growth and development*. Retrieved from http://www.tidal-model.com/Growth%20and%20Development.pdf.

Cook, N., Phillips, B., & Sadler, D. (2005). The tidal model as experienced by patients and nurses in a regional forensic unit. *Journal of Psychiatric and Mental Health Nursing, 12*, 536–540.

De Shazer, S. (1994). *Words were originally magic*. New York: Norton.

dos Santos, I., Andrade, L., Clos, A., & Nascimento, A. V. (2015). An esthetic and sociopoetic perspective on caring for people with mental disorder: Appropriating the tidal model. *Rev enferm UERJ, 22*(6), 765–770.

Flanagan, J. C. (1954). The critical incident technique. *Psychological Bulletin, 51*, 327–358.

Fletcher, E., & Stevenson, C. (2001). Launching the tidal model in an adult mental health programme. *Nursing Standard, 15*(49), 33–36.

Glaser, B. G., & Strauss, A. L. (1967). *The discovery of grounded theory: Strategies for qualitative research*. Chicago, IL: Aldine/Atherton.

Gordon, W., Morton, T., & Brooks, G. (2005). Launching the tidal model: Evaluating the evidence. *Journal of Psychiatric and Mental Health Nursing, 12*(6), 703–712.

Henderson, J. (2013). How the tidal model was used to overcome a risk-averse ward culture. *Mental Health Practice, 17*, 34–37.

Heron, J. (1996). *Cooperative inquiry: Research into the human condition*. London: Sage.

Illich, I. (1976). *Limits to medicine: Medical nemesis—The expropriation of health*. London: Marion Boyars.

Jackson, S., & Stevenson, C. (1998). The gift of time from the friendly professional. *Nursing Standard, 12*(1), 31–33.

Jackson, S., & Stevenson, C. (2000). What do people need psychiatric and mental health nurses for? *Journal of Advanced Nursing, 31*(2), 378–388.

Jackson, S., & Stevenson, C. (2004). How can nurses meet the needs of mental health clients? In D. Kirby, D. Hart, D. Cross, & G. Mitchell (Eds.), *Mental health nursing—Competencies for practice* (pp. 32–45). Hampshire, UK: Palgrave MacMillan.

Jonsson, B. (2005). *Ten thoughts about time*. London: Constable and Robinson.

Kilmer, D. L., & Lane-Tillerson, C. (2013). When still waters become a soul tsunami: Using the tidal model to recover from shipwreck. *Journal of Christian Nursing, 30*(2), 100–104.

Lafferty, S., & Davidson, R. (2006, March). Putting the person first. *Mental Health Today*, 31–33.

Lassenius, O. (2014). *Being physically active—A bodily anchorage on the journey for recovery in mental ill-health*. Unpublished doctoral thesis, Department of Neurobiology, Karolinska Institute, Stockholm, Sweden.

Michael, S. P. (1994). Invisible skills: How recognition and value need to be given to the "invisible skills" frequently used by mental health nurses, but often unrecognized by those unfamiliar with mental health nursing. *Journal of Psychiatric and Mental Health Nursing, 1*(1), 56–57.

Miller, J. (Ed.). (1983). Objections to psychiatry: Dialogue with Thomas Szasz. In J. Miller (Ed.), *States of mind: Conversations with psychological investigators*. (pp. 270–290). London: British Broadcasting.

Montgomery, C., & Webster, D. (1993). Caring and nursing's metaparadigm: Can they survive the era of managed care. *Perspectives in Psychiatric Care, 29*(4), 5–12.

Morita, M., Kondo, A., Le Vine, P., & Morita, S. (1998). *Morita Therapy and the true nature of anxiety-based disorders (Shinkeishitsu)*. New York: State University of New York Press.

Peplau, H. (1987). Interpersonal constructs for nursing practice. *Nurse Education Today, 7*(5), 201–208.

Peplau, H. E. (1952). *Interpersonal relations in nursing*. New York: Putman.

Peplau, H. E. (1969). Theory: The professional dimension. In C. M. Norris (Ed.), *Proceedings of the first nursing theory conference* (pp. 33–46). Kansas City, KS: University of Kansas Medical Center, Department of Nursing Education.

Podvoll, E. M. (1990). *The seduction of madness: Revolutionary insights into the world of psychosis and a compassionate approach to recovery at home*. New York: HarperCollins.

Registered Nurses' Association of Ontario. (2015). *Best practice guideline: Person and family-centred care*. Toronto, Canada: Author.

Reynolds, D. (1984). *Playing ball on running water: The Japanese way to building a better life*. New York: William Morrow.

Stevenson, C. (1996). The Tao, social constructivism and psychiatric nursing practice and research. *Journal of Psychiatric and Mental Health Nursing, 3*(4), 217–224.

Stevenson, C., Barker, P., & Fletcher, E. (2002). Judgement days: Developing an evaluation for an innovative nursing model. *Journal of Psychiatric and Mental Health Nursing, 9*(3), 271–276.

Stevenson, C., & Fletcher, E. (2002). The tidal model: The questions answered. *Mental Health Practice, 5*(8), 29–38.

Stevenson, C., Jackson, S., & Barker, P. (2003). Finding solutions through empowerment. A preliminary study of a solution-oriented approach to nursing in acute psychiatric settings. *Journal of Psychiatric and Mental Health Nursing, 10*(6), 688–696.

Szasz, T. S. (1961). *The myth of mental illness: Foundations of a theory of personal conduct*. New York: Hoeber-Harper.

Szasz, T. S. (2000). The case against psychiatric power. In P. J. Barker & C. Stevenson (Eds.), *The construction of power and authority in psychiatry*. (pp. 43–56). Oxford, UK: Butterworth-Heinemann.

Travelbee, J. (1969). *Intervention in psychiatric nursing: Process in the one-to-one relationship*. Philadelphia: F. A. Davis.

Vicenzi, A. E. (1994). Chaos theory and some nursing considerations. *Nursing Science Quarterly, 7*(1), 32–44.

Webster D., Vaughn, K., & Martinez, R. (1994). Introducing solution-focused approaches to staff in inpatient settings. *Archives of Psychiatric Nursing, 8*(4), 254–261.

World Health Organization. (1986). *The Ottawa charter for health promotion*. Geneva, Switzerland: Author.

Yeats, W. B. (1928). *The tower*. New York: Macmillan.

Zuaboni, G. (2015). Das Gezeitenmodell: Mit Leadership zu neuen Ufern aufbrechen. *NOVAcura, 2*(1), 15–17.

Zuaboni, G., Burr, C., & Schulz, M. (2013). *Das Gezeiten-Modell: Der Kompass fur eine recovery-orienterte, psychiatrische Pflege*. Bern, Germany: Verlag Hans.

BIBLIOGRAPHY

Primary Sources

Books

Barker, P. (2008). Foreword. In J. Morrissey, B. Keogh, & L. Doyle (Eds.), *Psychiatric/mental health nursing—Concepts, application, challenges and reflections: An Irish perspective*. Dublin, Ireland: Gill & MacMillan.

Barker, P. J. (1997). *Assessment in psychiatric and mental health nursing: In search of the whole person*. Cheltenham, UK: Stanley Thornes.

Barker, P. J. (1999). *The philosophy and practice of psychiatric and mental health nursing*. Edinburgh, Scotland: Churchill Livingstone.

Barker, P. J. (1999). *The talking cures: A guide to the psychotherapies for health care professionals*. London: NT Books.

Barker, P. J. (2009). *Psychiatric and mental health nursing: The craft of caring* (2nd ed.). London: Arnold.

Barker, P. J. (2004). *Assessment in psychiatric and mental health nursing: In search of the whole person* (2nd ed.). London: Nelson-Thornes.

Barker, P. J., & Buchanan-Barker, P. (2004). *Spirituality and mental health: Breakthrough*. London: Whurr.

Book Chapters

Barker, P. J., & Buchanan-Barker, P. (2008). Patiently, telling the story. In T. Warne & S. McAndrew (Eds.), *Creative approaches in health and social care education and practice: Knowing me, understanding you*. (pp. 803–894). Basingstoke, UK: Palgrave Macmillan.

Barker, P. J., & Buchanan-Barker, P. (2008). Spirituality and mental health. In T. Turner & R. Tummey (Eds.), *Critical issues in mental health*. (58–71). Basingstoke, UK: Palgrave Macmillan.

Barker, P. J., & Buchanan-Barker, P. (2008). [tr m. Kayama]. The tidal model of mental health recovery. In Kayama, Noda, Myamoto, & Ohyama (Eds.), *Textbook of psychiatric nursing*. Tokyo: Nankodo (Japanese).

Barker, P. J., Campbell, P., & Davidson, B. (1999). *From the ashes of experience: The experience of recovery from psychosis*. London: Whurr.

Barker, P. J., & Davidson, B. (1998). *Psychiatric nursing: Ethical strife*. London: Arnold.

Barker, P. J., Manos, E., Novak, V., & Reynolds, B. (1998). The wounded healer and the myth of mental well-being: Ethical issues concerning the mental health status of psychiatric nurses. In P. J. Barker & B. Davidson (Eds.), *Psychiatric nursing: Ethical strife*. London: Arnold.

Barker, P. J., & Whitehill, I. (1997). The craft of care: Towards collaborative caring in psychiatric nursing. In S. Tilley (Ed.), *The mental health nurse: Views of practice and education*. Oxford, UK: Blackwell Science.

Buchanan-Barker, P., & Barker, P. (2011). The tidal model. In D. Cooper (Ed.), *Intervention in mental health-substance use*. Oxford, UK: Radcliffe.

Buchanan-Barker, P., & Barker, P. (2012). The tidal model. In D. Cooper & J. Cooper (Eds.), *Palliative care within mental health*. London: Radcliffe.

Journal Articles

Barker, P., & Buchanan-Barker, P. (2004). Bridging: Talking meaningfully about the care of people at risk. *Mental Health Practice, 8*(3), 12–15.

Barker, P., & Buchanan-Barker, P. (2004). Experts without a voice. *Nursing Standard, 18*(50), 22–23.

Barker, P., & Buchanan-Barker, P. (2005). Still invisible after all these years: Mental health nursing on the margins. *Journal of Psychiatric and Mental Health Nursing, 12*, 252–256.

Barker, P. J. (1989). Reflections on the philosophy of caring in mental health. *International Journal of Nursing Studies, 26*(2), 131–141.

Barker, P. J. (1990). The conceptual basis of mental health nursing. *Nurse Education Today, 10*, 339–348.

Barker, P. J. (1990). The philosophy of psychiatric nursing. *Nursing Standard, 3*(12), 28–33.

Barker, P. J. (1993). The Peplau legacy . . . Hildegard Peplau. *Nursing Times, 89*(11), 48–51.

Barker, P. J. (2000). The tidal model of mental health care: Personal caring within the chaos paradigm. *Mental Health Care, 4*(2), 59–63.

Barker, P. J. (2000, Nov/Dec). Turning the tide. *Open Mind, 106*, 10–11.

Barker, P. J. (2000). The virtue of caring. *International Journal of Nursing Studies, 37*, 329–336.

Barker, P. J. (2002). The tidal model: The healing potential of metaphor within the patient's narrative. *Journal of Psychosocial Nursing and Mental Health Services, 40*(7), 42–50, 54–55.

Barker, P. J. (2003). The tidal model: Psychiatric colonization, recovery and the paradigm shift in mental health care. *International Journal of Mental Health Nursing, 12*(2), 96–102.

Barker, P. J., & Buchanan-Barker, P. (2010). The tidal model of mental health recovery and reclamation: Application in acute care settings. *Issues in Mental Health Nursing, 31*, 171–180.

Barker, P. J., & Buchanan-Barker, P. (2011). Mental health nursing and the politics of recovery: A global reflection. *Archives of Psychiatric Nursing, 25*, 350–358.

Barker, P. J., & Cutcliffe, J. (1999). Clinical risk: A need for engagement not observation. *Mental Health Practice, 2*(8), 8–12.

Hungerford, C. (2014). Recovery as a model of care? Insights from an Australian case study. *Issues in Mental Health Nursing, 35*, 156–164.

Simpson, A., & Barker, P. J. (2007). The persistence of memory: Using narrative picturing to co-operatively explore life stories in qualitative inquiry. *Nursing Inquiry, 14*(1), 35–41.

Secondary Sources

Adam, R., Tilley, S., & Pollock, L. (2003). Person first: What people with enduring mental disorders value about community psychiatric nurses and CPN services. *Journal of Psychiatric and Mental Health Nursing, 10*, 203–212.

Biley, F. C. (2010). My life: My encounters with insanity. *Journal of Holistic Nursing, 28*, 150–155.

Bowles, A. (2000). Therapeutic nursing care in acute psychiatric wards: Engagement over control. *Journal of Psychiatric and Mental Health Nursing, 7*, 179–184.

Brookes, N. (2014). The tidal model of mental health recovery. In M. R. Alligood (Ed.), *Nursing theorists and their work* (8th ed., pp. 626–656). St Louis, MO: Mosby.

Brookes, N., Murata, L., & Tansey, M. (2008). Making waves: Implementing the new tidal model of mental health recovery. *Canadian Nurse, 104*(8), 22–27.

Brookes, N., Tansey, M., & Murata, L. (2006). Guiding practice development using the tidal commitments. *Journal of Psychiatric and Mental Health Nursing, 13*, 460–463.

Cameron, D., Kapur, R., & Campbell, P. (2005). Releasing the therapeutic potential of the psychiatric nurse: A human relations perspective of the nurse-patient relationship. *Journal of Psychiatric and Mental Health Nursing, 12*, 64–74.

Clark, G., Ferguson, J., O'Brien, L., Fitzgerald, M., & Vella, N. (2009). Preparing the beach head. An education program in interpersonal skills to prepare for implementation of the tidal model in an adolescent mental health unit. *International Journal of Mental Health Nursing, 18*(Suppl. 1), A4.

Davidson, L. (2005). Recovery, self-management and the expert patient—Changing the culture of mental health from a UK perspective. *Journal of Mental Health, 14*(1), 25–35.

Delaney, K. R. (2012). Moving to a recovery framework of care: Focusing attention on process. *Archives of Psychiatric Nursing, 26*, 165.

Delaney, K. R., & Ferguson, J. (2011). Psychiatric mental health nursing: A dialogue on the nature of our practice. *Archives of Psychiatric Nursing, 25*, 148–150.

Delaney, K. R., & Shattell, M. M. (2011). Special edition: Inpatient psychiatric treatment: Moving the science forward final. *Issues in Mental Health Nursing, 31*, 158–159.

dos Santos, I., & Andrade, L. (2015). Aplicabilidade de teorias de enfermagem na prática cotidiana do trabalho. *Rev enferm UERJ, Rio de Janeiro, 23*(3), 295–296.

Ferguson, J., O'Brien, L., Vella, N., Clark, G., Gillies, D., & Fitzgerald, M. (2009). Implementing the tidal model: Nurses developing a mind to care. *International Journal of Mental Health Nursing, 18*(Suppl. 1), A8.

Fitzgerald, M., O'Brien, L., Ferguson, J., et al. (2009). With partnership in mind . . . bringing the tidal model to life in an adolescent acute inpatient setting: The perspective of the young person and their family or carer. *International Journal of Mental Health Nursing, 18*(Suppl. 1), A8.

Harnett, P. J., & Greaney, A. M. (2008). Operationalizing autonomy: Solutions for mental health nursing practice. *Journal of Psychiatric and Mental Health Nursing, 15*, 2–9.

Hayne, Y. M. (2003). Experiencing psychiatric diagnosis: Client perspectives on being named mentally ill. *Journal of Psychiatric and Mental Health Nursing, 10*, 722–729.

Hosany, Z., Wellman, N., & Lowe, T. (2007). Fostering a culture of engagement: A pilot study of the outcomes of training mental health nurses working in two UK acute admission units in brief solution-focused therapy techniques. *Journal of Psychiatric and Mental Health Nursing, 14*, 688–695.

Jackson, S., & Stevenson, C. (2004). How can nurses meet the needs of mental health clients. In D. Kirby, D. Hart, D. Cross, & G. Mitchell (Eds.), *Mental health nursing—Competencies for practice* (pp. 32–45). Hampshire, UK: Palgrave MacMillan.

Kidd, J. (2010). Cultural boundary surfing in mental health nursing: A creative narration. *Contemporary Nurse, 34*(2), 277–288.

Lipczynska, S. (2011). Recovery from mental illness. *Journal of Mental Health, 20*, 420–422.

McAllister, M., & Moyle, W. (2008). An exploration of mental health nursing models of care in a Queensland psychiatric hospital. *International Journal of Mental Health Nursing, 17*, 18–26.

O'Donovan, A. (2007). Patient-centred care in acute psychiatric admission units: Reality or rhetoric? *Journal of Psychiatric and Mental Health Nursing, 14*, 542–548.

Perraud, S., Delaney, K., Carlson-Sabelli, L., Johnson, M. E., Shepard, R., & Paun, O. (2006). Advanced practice psychiatric mental health nursing, finding our core: The therapeutic relationship in the 21st century. *Perspectives in Psychiatric Care, 42*(4), 215–226.

Thomas, S. P. (2012). New thoughts on talk therapies. *Issues in Mental Health Nursing, 33*, 135–136.

Vella, N., Fitzgerald, M., O'Brien, L., Ferguson, J., Clark, G., & Gillies, D. (2009). Implementing the tidal model: Implications for management and clinical leadership in the delivery of quality care. *International Journal of Mental Health Nursing, 18*(Suppl. 1), A24–A25.

Vella, N., Page, L., Edwards, C., & Wand, T. (2014). Sustaining a culture of practice development in an acute adolescent inpatient mental health unit. *Journal of Child and Adolescent Psychiatric Nursing, 27*, 149–155.

Young, B. B. (2010). Using the tidal model of mental health recovery to plan primary health care for women in residential substance abuse recovery. *Issues in Mental Health Nursing, 31*, 569–575.

33

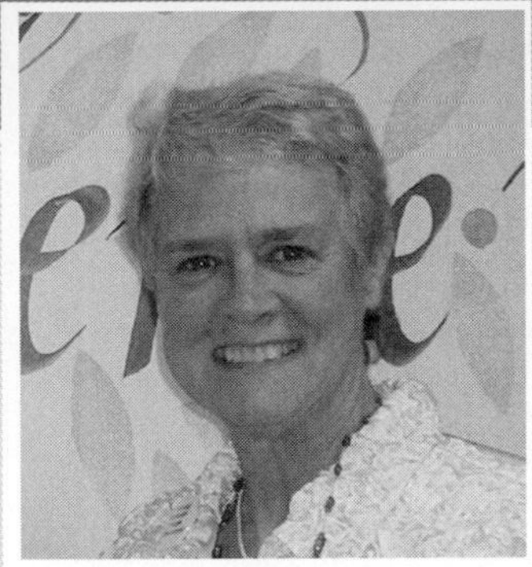

Katharine Kolcaba†
(1944–Present)

Theory of Comfort

*Thérèse Dowd**

"In today's technological world, nursing's historic mission of providing comfort to patients and family members is even more important. Comfort is an antidote to the stressors inherent in health care situations today, and when comfort is enhanced, patients and families are strengthened for the tasks ahead. In addition, nurses feel more satisfied with the care they are giving."
(K. Kolcaba, personal communication, March 7, 2015)

CREDENTIALS AND BACKGROUND OF THE THEORIST

Katharine Kolcaba was born and educated in Cleveland, Ohio. In 1965 she received a diploma in nursing, and she practiced part time for many years in medical-surgical nursing, long-term care, and home care before returning to graduate school. In 1987 she graduated in the first RN to MSN class at Case Western Reserve University (CWRU) Frances Payne Bolton School of Nursing, with a specialty in gerontology. While in school, she job-shared a head nurse position on a dementia unit. It was in this practice context that she began theorizing about the outcome of patient comfort.

Kolcaba joined the faculty at the University of Akron College of Nursing after graduating with her master's degree in nursing. She gained American Nurses Association (ANA) certification in gerontology. She returned to CWRU to pursue her doctorate in nursing on a part-time basis while continuing to teach. Over the next 10 years, she used course work in her doctoral program to develop and explicate her theory in a series of published articles, now summarized in her book (Kolcaba, 2003).

Dr. Kolcaba is retired from the University of Akron as an emeritus associate professor. Her nursing interests include interventions for and documentation of changes in comfort for evidence-based practice. She resides in the Cleveland area with her husband, where she enjoys being near her grandchildren. She represents her company, The Comfort Line, to assist health care agencies implement the theory of comfort on a system-wide basis. She is founder and coordinator of a local parish nurse program and a member of the ANA. Kolcaba continues to work with students and nurses at all levels as they conduct comfort studies.

THEORETICAL SOURCES

Kolcaba began her theoretical work by diagramming her nursing practice, an assignment early in her doctoral studies. When Kolcaba presented her framework for dementia care (Kolcaba, 2003), she was asked, "Have you done a concept analysis of comfort?" Kolcaba replied that she had not but that would be her next step. This question began her long investigation into the concept of comfort.

The first step, the promised concept analysis, began with an extensive review about comfort from the disciplines of nursing, medicine, psychology, psychiatry, ergonomics, and English language (specifically Shakespeare's use of comfort and the *Oxford English Dictionary* [*OED*]). From the *OED*,

*The author wishes to thank Katharine Kolcaba for her assistance with this chapter.

†Photo credit: Barker's Camera Shop, Chagrin Falls, OH.

Kolcaba learned that the original definition of comfort was "to strengthen greatly." This definition provided a wonderful rationale for nurses to comfort patients, because patients would do better and nurses would feel more satisfied.

Historical accounts of comfort in nursing are numerous. Nightingale (1859) declared, "It must never be lost sight of what observation is for. It is not for the sake of piling up miscellaneous information or curious facts, but for the sake of saving life and increasing health and comfort" (p. 70). From 1900 to 1929, comfort was the central goal of nursing and medicine because, through comfort, recovery was achieved (Kolcaba, 2003; McIlveen & Morse, 1995). There were no antibiotics, chemotherapy, or technology to speed up the return to health. Nurses were duty bound to attend to details influencing patient comfort. Aikens (1908) proposed that nothing concerning the comfort of the patient was small enough to ignore. The comfort of patients was nursing's first and last consideration. Good nurses made patients comfortable, and the provision of comfort was a primary determining factor of nurses' ability and character (Aikens, 1908).

Harmer (1926) stated that nursing care was concerned with providing a "general atmosphere of comfort," and that personal care of patients included attention to "happiness, comfort, and ease, physical and mental," in addition to "rest and sleep, nutrition, cleanliness, and elimination" (p. 26). Goodnow (1935) devoted a chapter in her book, *The Technique of Nursing,* to the patient's comfort. She wrote, "A nurse is judged always by her ability to make her patient comfortable. Comfort is both physical and mental, and a nurse's responsibility does not end with physical care" (p. 95). In textbooks dated 1904, 1914, and 1919, emotional comfort was called mental comfort and was achieved mostly by providing physical comfort and modifying the environment for patients (Kolcaba, 2003).

In these examples, comfort is positive, achieved with the help of nurses, and, in many cases, indicates improvement from a previous state or condition. Intuitively, comfort is associated with nurturing activity. From its word origins, Kolcaba explicated its strengthening features, and from ergonomics, its direct link to job performance (progress in therapy). However, often its meaning is implicit, hidden in context, and ambiguous. The concept varies semantically as a verb, noun, adjective, adverb, process, and outcome.

Kolcaba used ideas from three early nursing theorists to synthesize or derive the types of comfort in the concept analysis (Kolcaba, 2003).

- **Relief** was synthesized from the work of Orlando (1961), who posited that nurses relieved the needs expressed by patients.
- **Ease** was synthesized from the work of Henderson (1966), who described 14 basic functions of human beings to be maintained during care.
- **Transcendence** was derived from Paterson and Zderad (1975), who proposed that patients rise above their difficulties with the help of nurses.

Four contexts of comfort, experienced by those receiving care, came from the review of nursing literature about holism (Kolcaba, 2003). The contexts are **physical, psychospiritual**, **sociocultural,** and **environmental** and are defined in Fig. 33.1. The four contexts were juxtaposed with the three types of comfort, creating a taxonomic structure (matrix) from which to consider the complexities of comfort as an outcome.

The taxonomic structure provides a map of the content domain of comfort. It is anticipated that, in the future, researchers will design, modify, or translate comfort questionnaires for their specific population using the taxonomic structure as a guide. The many translations can be found on Kolcaba's website, *The Comfort Line,* where she includes the steps for adaptation of the General Comfort Questionnaire (GCQ).

MAJOR CONCEPTS & DEFINITIONS

In Kolcaba's theory of comfort those receiving comfort measures may be referred to as *recipients, patients, students, prisoners, workers, older adults, communities,* and *institutions.*

Health Care Needs

Health care needs are comfort needs arising from stressful health care situations that cannot be met by recipients' traditional support systems. The needs may be physical, psychospiritual, sociocultural, or environmental. They become apparent through monitoring, verbal or nonverbal reports, pathophysiological parameters, education and support, and financial counseling and intervention (Kolcaba, 2003).

Comfort Interventions

Comfort interventions are nursing actions and referrals designed to address specific comfort needs of recipients, including physiological, social, cultural, financial, psychological, spiritual, environmental, and physical needs (Kolcaba, 2003).

Intervening Variables

Intervening variables are interacting forces that influence recipients' perceptions of total comfort. They consist of past experiences, age, attitude, emotional state, support system, prognosis, finances, education, cultural background, and the totality of elements in the recipients' experience (Kolcaba, 2003). Such intervening variables affect planning and success of patient care interventions. In research, they may be included in the demographic form.

Comfort

Comfort is the immediate state experienced by recipients of comfort interventions. It is the immediate, holistic

MAJOR CONCEPTS & DEFINITIONS—cont'd

experience of being strengthened when one's needs are addressed. The three types of comfort are relief, ease, and transcendence. The four contexts are physical, psychospiritual, sociocultural, and environmental (Kolcaba, 2003) (see these types and contexts in Fig. 33.1).

Health-Seeking Behaviors

Health-seeking behaviors compose a broad category of outcomes related to the pursuit of health as defined by the recipient(s) in consultation with the nurse. The categories were synthesized by Schlotfeldt (1975) and proposed to be internal, external, or a peaceful death. Internal behaviors are those we cannot see, such as surgical healing, T cell formation, or electrolyte balance; external behaviors are those we can see directly such as ambulation or indirectly such as blood pressure. A peaceful death is defined by Kolcaba (2003) as "a death in which conflicts are resolved, symptoms are well managed, and acceptance by the patient and family members allows for the patient to 'let go' quietly and with dignity" (p. 257).

Institutional Integrity

Corporations, communities, schools, hospitals, regions, states, and countries that possess the qualities of being complete, whole, sound, upright, appealing, ethical, and sincere possess **institutional integrity**. As institutions display this integrity, best practices and best policies are in evidence (Kolcaba, 2003).

Best Practices

The use of health care interventions based on evidence to produce the best possible patient and family outcomes is known as **best practices**.

Best Policies

Institutional or regional policies ranging from protocols for procedures and medical conditions to access and delivery of health care are known as **best policies**. Fig. 33.2 illustrates the relationship among institutional integrity, best practices, and best policies.

Type of Comfort

Context in Which Comfort Occurs	Relief	Ease	Transcendence
Physical			
Psychospiritual			
Environmental			
Social			

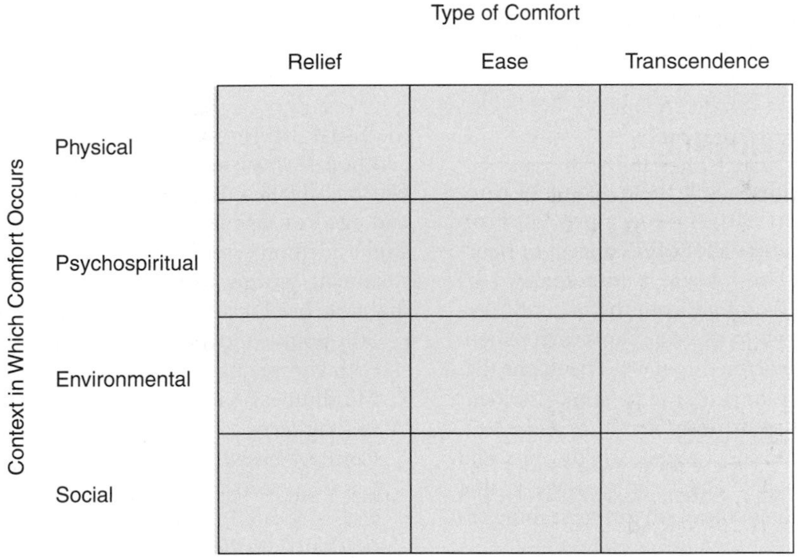

Type of Comfort:
Relief: The state of a patient who has had a specific need met
Ease: The state of calm or contentment
Transcendence: The state in which one rises above one's problems or pain

Context in Which Comfort Occurs:
Physical: Pertaining to bodily sensations
Psychospiritual: Pertaining to internal awareness of self, including esteem, concept, sexuality, and meaning in one's life; one's relationship to a higher order or being
Environmental: Pertaining to the external surroundings, conditions, and influences
Social: Pertaining to interpersonal, family, and societal relationships

FIG. 33.1 Taxonomic structure of comfort. (From Kolcaba, K., & Fisher, E. [1996]. A holistic perspective on comfort care as an advance directive. *Critical Care Nursing Quarterly, 18*[4], 66–76.)

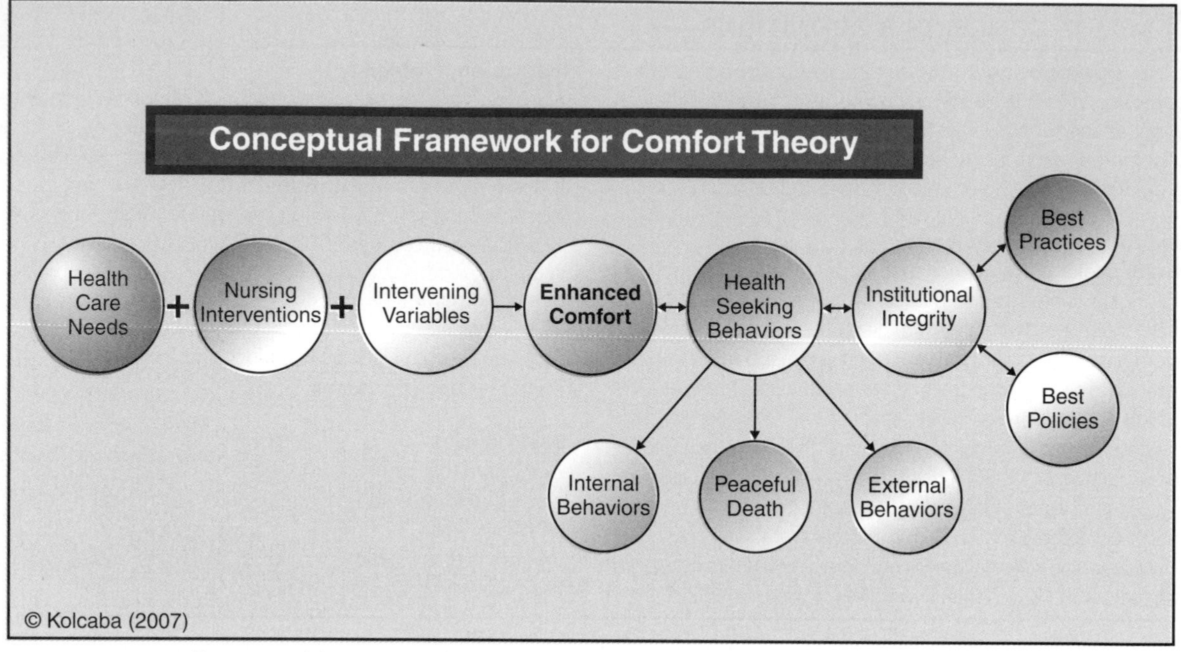

FIG. 33.2 Conceptual framework for the theory of comfort. (Copyright Kolcaba, 2007. Retrieved from www.thecomfortline.com.)

USE OF EMPIRICAL EVIDENCE

The seeds of modern inquiry about the outcome of comfort were sown in the late 1980s, marking a period of collective, but separate, awareness about the concept of holistic comfort. Hamilton (1989) made a leap forward by exploring the meaning of comfort from the patient's perspective. She used interviews to ascertain how each patient in a long-term care facility defined *comfort.* The theme that emerged most was relief from pain, but patients also identified good positioning in well-fitting furniture and a feeling of being independent, encouraged, worthwhile, and useful. Hamilton concluded, "The clear message is that comfort is multi-dimensional, meaning different things to different people" (p. 32).

After Kolcaba developed her theory, she was the first nurse researcher to demonstrate that changes in comfort could be measured using an experimental design (Kolcaba, 2003). In this dissertation study, health care needs were those (comfort needs) associated with a diagnosis of early breast cancer. The holistic intervention was guided imagery, designed specifically for these patients to meet their comfort needs, and the desired outcome was their comfort. The findings revealed significantly higher comfort over time in women receiving guided imagery compared with the usual care group. Kolcaba and associates conducted additional empirical testing of the theory of comfort, which is detailed in her book (Kolcaba, 2003, pp. 113–124) and cited on her website (Kolcaba, 1997). These comfort studies demonstrated significantly higher comfort for the treatment groups over time. Examples of interventions that have been tested recently include the following:

- Still-point induction and massage therapy for patients with chronic pain (Townsend et al., 2014).
- Mindfulness-based stress reduction for elderly residents in long-term care (Kumar, Adiga, & George, 2014).
- Comfort-based nursing care for women with new Cesarean sections (Derya & Pasinliogui, 2015).
- Use of heated blankets to enhance comfort of acute psychiatric patients (Parks et al., 2017).

In each study, interventions were targeted to all attributes of comfort relevant to the research settings, comfort instruments were adapted or translated from the GCQ (Kolcaba, 2003), and there were at least two (usually three) measurement points used to capture changes in comfort over time. Empirical support for the holistic nature of comfort was found in a study of four theoretical propositions (Kolcaba, 2003):

1. Comfort is generally state-specific.
2. The outcome of comfort is sensitive to changes over time.

3. Any consistently applied holistic nursing intervention with an established history for effectiveness enhances comfort over time.
4. Total comfort is greater than the sum of its parts.

Tests on the data set from Kolcaba's earlier study of women with breast cancer supported each proposition. Other areas of study included in the Kolcaba website are burn units, labor and delivery, infertility, nursing homes, home care, chronic pain, pediatrics, oncology, dental hygiene, transport, and those with mental disabilities.

METAPARADIGM DEFINITIONS

Nursing

Nursing is the intentional assessment of comfort needs, the design of comfort interventions to address those needs, and reassessment of comfort levels after implementation compared with a baseline. Assessment and reassessment may be intuitive or subjective or both, such as when a nurse asks if the patient is comfortable. Objective assessments include observations of wound healing, changes in laboratory values, or changes in behavior. Assessment of comfort is achieved through the administration of verbal rating scales (clinical) or comfort questionnaires (research), using instruments developed by Kolcaba (2003).

Patient

Recipients of care may be individuals, families, institutions, or communities in need of health care. Nurses may be recipients of enhanced workplace comfort when initiatives to improve working conditions are undertaken (Boudiab & Kolcaba, 2015).

Environment

The environment is any aspect of patient, family, or institutional settings that can be manipulated by the nurse(s), loved one(s), or the institution to enhance comfort.

Health

Health is optimal functioning of a patient, family, health care provider, or community as defined by the patient or group.

MAJOR ASSUMPTIONS

1. Human beings have holistic responses to complex stimuli (Kolcaba, 2003).
2. Comfort is a value-added holistic outcome that is germane to the discipline of nursing.
3. Comfort is a basic human need that persons strive to meet or have met. It is an active endeavor.
4. Enhanced comfort strengthens patients to engage in health-seeking behaviors of their choice.
5. Patients who are empowered to actively engage in health-seeking behaviors are satisfied with their health care.
6. Institutional integrity is based on a value system oriented to the recipients of care. Of equal importance is an orientation to a health-promoting, holistic setting for families and providers of care.

THEORETICAL ASSERTIONS

The theory of comfort contains three parts or propositional assertions that may be tested separately or as a whole.

Part 1 states that comforting interventions, when effective, result in increased comfort for recipients (patients and families) compared with a preintervention baseline. Care providers may be considered recipients if the institution makes a commitment to the comfort of their work setting. Comfort interventions address basic human needs, such as rest, homeostasis, therapeutic communication, and treatment as holistic beings. Comfort interventions are usually nontechnical and complement the delivery of technical care.

Part 2 states that increased comfort of recipients of care results in increased engagement in health-seeking behaviors (goals) that are negotiated with the recipients.

Part 3 states that increased engagement in health-seeking behavior results in increased quality of care, benefiting the institution and its ability to gather evidence for best practices and best policies.

Kolcaba believes nurses want to practice comforting care and that it can be easily incorporated with every nursing action. She proposes that this type of comfort practice promotes greater nurse creativity and satisfaction, as well as high patient satisfaction. To enhance comfort, the nurse must deliver the appropriate interventions and document the results in the patient record. However, when the appropriate intervention is delivered in an intentional and comforting manner, comfort still may not be enhanced sufficiently. When comfort is not yet enhanced to its fullest, nurses then consider intervening variables to explain why comfort management did not work. Such variables may be abusive homes, lack of financial resources, devastating diagnoses, or cognitive impairments that render the most appropriate interventions and comforting actions ineffective. Comfort management or comforting care includes interventions, comforting actions, the goal of enhanced comfort, and the selection of appropriate health-seeking behaviors by patients, families, and their nurses. Thus comfort management is proposed to be proactive, energized, intentional, and longed for by recipients of care in all settings. It is what nurses do when they practice the art of nursing. To strengthen the role of nurses as comfort agents, documentation of changes in comfort before and after their interventions is essential. For clinical use, Kolcaba suggests asking patients to rate their comfort from 0 to 10, with 10 being the highest possible comfort in a given health care situation. This documentation could be a part of the electronic databases in each institution (Boudiab & Kolcaba, 2015). Note that total comfort may not be possible in most health care situations, but an increase in comfort will nevertheless strengthen patients.

LOGICAL FORM

Kolcaba used three types of logical reasoning in the development of the theory of comfort: (1) induction, (2) deduction, and (3) retroduction (Hardin & Bishop, 2010).

Induction

Induction occurs when generalizations are built from a number of specific observed instances (Hardin & Bishop, 2010). When nurses are earnest about their practice and earnest about nursing as a discipline, they become familiar with implicit or explicit concepts, terms, propositions, and assumptions that underpin their practice. Nurses in graduate school may be asked to diagram their practice as Dr. Rosemary Ellis asked Kolcaba and other students to do, and it is a deceptively easy-sounding assignment.

Such was the scenario during the late 1980s as Kolcaba began. She was head nurse on an Alzheimer unit at the time and knew some of the terms used then to describe the practice of dementia care, such as **facilitative environment, excess disabilities,** and **optimum function**. However, when she drew relationships among them, she recognized that the three terms did not fully describe her practice. An important nursing piece was missing, and she pondered about what nurses were doing to prevent excess disabilities (later naming those actions **interventions**) and how to judge if the interventions were working. Optimum function had been conceptualized as the ability to engage in special activities on the unit, such as setting the table, preparing a salad, or going to a program and sitting through it. These activities made the residents feel good about themselves, as if it were the right activity at the right time. However, those activities did not happen more than twice a day, because the residents couldn't tolerate much more than that. What were they doing in the meantime? What behaviors did the staff hope they would exhibit that would indicate an absence of excess disabilities? Should the term *excess disabilities* be delineated further for clarity? Contemplating these questions led her to reconsider patient care.

Partial solutions to these questions were to (1) introduce the concept of comfort to the original diagram, because this word seemed to convey the desired state for patients when they were not engaging in special activities; (2) divide excess disabilities into physical and mental; and (3) note the feedback loop between comfort and optimum functioning. This thinking marked the first steps toward a theory of comfort and thinking about the complexities of the concept (Kolcaba, 2003).

Deduction

Deduction occurs when specific conclusions are inferred from general premises or principles; it proceeds from the general to the specific (Hardin & Bishop, 2010). The deductive stage of theory development resulted in relating comfort to other concepts to produce a theory. Because the works of three nursing theorists were entailed in the definition of *comfort* (Henderson, 1966; Orlando, 1961; Paterson & Zderad, 1975), Kolcaba looked elsewhere for the common ground needed to unify relief, ease, and transcendence (three major concepts). What was needed was a more abstract and general conceptual framework that was congruent with comfort and contained a manageable number of highly abstract constructs.

The work of psychologist Henry Murray (1938) met the criteria for a framework on which to hang Kolcaba's nursing concepts. His theory was about human needs; therefore it was applicable to patients who experience multiple stimuli in stressful health care situations. Furthermore, Murray's idea about unitary trends gave Kolcaba the idea that, although comfort was state-specific, if comforting interventions were implemented over time, the overall comfort of patients could be enhanced over time. In this deductive stage of theory development, she began with abstract, general theoretical construction and used the sociological process of substruction to identify the more specific (less abstract) levels of concepts for nursing practice.

Retroduction

Retroduction is useful for selecting new phenomena that can be developed further and tested. This type of reasoning is applied in fields that have few available theories (Hardin & Bishop, 2010). Such was the case with outcomes research, which now is centered on collecting databases for measuring selected outcomes and relating those outcomes to types of nursing, medical, institutional, or community protocols. Murray's 20th-century framework could not account for the 21st-century emphasis on institutional and community outcomes. Using retroduction, Kolcaba added the concept of **institutional integrity** to the middle-range theory of comfort. Adding the term extended the theory to consideration of relationships between health-seeking behaviors and institutional integrity. Later, the concepts of **best practices** and **best policies** were linked to institutional integrity (Kolcaba, 2003). Theory-based evidence organizes the knowledge base for best practices and policies (see Fig. 33.2).

ACCEPTANCE BY THE NURSING COMMUNITY

Practice

Many students and nurse researchers have selected this theory as a guiding framework for their studies in areas such as obstetrics (Barbosa et al., 2014), veterans' health (Boudiab & Kolcaba, 2015), postpartum care (Derya & Pasinlioglu, 2015), teaching of nursing students (Goodwin & Candela, 2013), hospice patients (Hansen et al., 2015), cardiac patients (Krinsky, Murillo, & Johnson, 2014), long-term care (Kumar, Adiga, & George, 2014), and prior to anesthesia (Seyedfatemi et al., 2014).

When nurses ask patients or family members to rate their comfort from 0 to 10 before and after an intervention or at regular intervals, they produce documented evidence that significant comfort work is being done. A scale is sensitive to changes in comfort over time (Dowd et al., 2007; Parks et al., 2017). A list of effective comforting interventions for each patient or family member is readily available and communicated.

Perianesthesia nurses have incorporated the theory of comfort into their *Clinical Practice Guidelines* for management of patient comfort. In this setting, comfort management specifies (1) assessing patients' comfort needs related to current surgery, chronic pain issues, and comorbidities; (2) creating a comfort contract with patients before surgery that specifies effective comfort interventions, understandable and efficient comfort measurement, and the type of postsurgical analgesia preferred; (3) facilitating comfortable positioning, body temperature, and other factors related to comfort during surgery; and (4) continuing with comfort management and measurement in the postsurgical period (Wilson & Kolcaba, 2004).

Education

A textbook that is useful for education is the *Nursing Diagnosis Handbook* (Ackley, Ladwig, & Makic, 2017). The nursing diagnoses of Altered Comfort (Kolcaba) and Readiness for Enhanced Comfort (Boudiab) are included in the latest edition. The theory is incorporated in the Nursing Intervention Classification (NIC) and Nursing Outcomes Classification (NOC) handbooks as well. The theory is appropriate for students to use in any clinical setting, and its application can be facilitated by use of the Comfort Care Plans available on Kolcaba's website.

Recently Goodwin and Candela (2013) used the theory of comfort as a transitional philosophy in a group of newly practicing nurses. The new nurses were taught to seek *relief* from stressors, maintain *ease* with their new settings through trusting their staff members, and achieve *transcendence* from their stressors with use of self-comforting techniques. The authors stated that "all participants referred to holistic comfort (HC) as something they still use with both colleagues and patients, implying nurses' application of HC can affect practice outcomes" (p. 618).

Research

An entry in the *Encyclopedia of Nursing Research* speaks to the importance of measuring comfort as a nursing-sensitive outcome (Kolcaba, 2012). Nurses can provide evidence to influence decision making at institutional, community, and legislative levels through studies that demonstrate the effectiveness of comforting care. Kolcaba (2003) called for measurement of comfort in large hospitals and home care to expand the theory and develop the literature on evidence-based comfort.

Using the taxonomic structure of comfort (see Fig. 33.1) as a guide, Kolcaba (2003) developed the GCQ to measure holistic comfort in a sample of hospital and community participants. Positive and negative items were generated for each cell in the taxonomic structure grid. Twenty-four positive items and 24 negative items were compiled with a Likert-type format, ranging from strongly agree to strongly disagree, with higher scores indicating higher comfort. At the end of the instrumentation study with 206 one-time participants from all types of units in two hospitals and 50 participants from the community, the GCQ demonstrated a Cronbach alpha of 0.88.

Researchers are welcome to modify the comfort questionnaires specific to their areas of research. The verbal rating scales and other traditionally formatted questionnaires may be downloaded from Kolcaba's website, where she responds to inquiries about comfort research in support of the use of her theory. Instructions for use of the questionnaires are available on the website. Popularity of the theory seems to be associated with its simplicity and with universal recognition of comfort as a desirable outcome of nursing care for patients and their families.

FURTHER DEVELOPMENT

Kolcaba has persisted in the development of her theory from the original conception as the root of her practice to concept analysis that provided the taxonomic structure of comfort; to development of ways to measure the concept; and currently to its use for practice, education, and research. She uses a full array of approaches to build her theory.

The methodical development and documentation of the concept of comfort resulted in a strong, clearly organized, and logical theory that is readily applied in many settings for education, practice, and research. Kolcaba developed templates for measurement to facilitate application of the comfort theory in additional settings. The comfort management templates she provided for use in practice settings have been helpful to students and faculty members. Outcomes of research have demonstrated the appropriateness of her theory for measuring whole-person changes that were less effectively captured with other types of instruments.

The original theoretical assertion (Part 1) of the theory of comfort has withstood empirical testing. When a comfort intervention is targeted to meet the holistic comfort needs of patients in specific health care situations, comfort is enhanced beyond baseline measurement. Furthermore, enhanced comfort has been correlated with engagement in health-seeking behaviors (Schlotfeldt, 1975). Empirical tests of the theoretical assertions for the second and third parts of the theory should be conducted and published. Outcomes for desirable health-seeking behaviors could include increased functional status, faster progress during rehabilitation, faster healing, or peaceful death when appropriate health-seeking behaviors are negotiated among the patient, family members, and care providers. Institutional outcomes would include decreased length of stay for hospitalized patients, smaller number of readmissions, decreased costs, and achievement of national awards such as the Beacon Award. Kolcaba consults with hospital administrators and staff educators who want to enhance quality of care (Boudiab & Kolcaba, 2015). She views quality care as comforting actions delivered in an intentional manner to create an environment that leads to engagement in health-seeking behaviors.

Kolcaba postulates that intentional emphasis on and support for comfort management by an institution or community increases patient and family satisfaction, because persons are healed, strengthened, and motivated to be healthier. Extending the theory of comfort to the community is also of current interest. It is well known that some communities are more comfortable to live in, go to school in, and grow old in than are others.

An area of interest for further development is the universal nature of comfort. Currently, the GCQ has been translated into Taiwanese, Turkish, Spanish, Iranian, Portuguese, and Italian (see Kolcaba website). Comfort of children has been accurately observed and documented in perioperative settings (Nancy Laurelberry, personal communication, February 2008). Comfort Daisies for children to self-report their comfort (see Kolcaba website) have been tested in a hospital setting (Carrie Majka, personal communication, February 2008).

The theory of comfort has been included in electronic nursing classification systems such as the North America Nursing Diagnosis Association (NANDA) (Ackley, Ladwig, & Makic, 2017), NIC (2008), and NOC (2008). Kolcaba consults with hospitals to include comfort management in their documentation systems (Boudiab & Kolcaba, 2015). Use of the theory has made significant contributions to nursing practice and the discipline. Kolcaba continues to spend time and energy developing and disseminating the theory through presentations, publications, and discussions since retiring from full-time teaching.

The theory of comfort is often used as an organizing framework for Magnet Status certification and other awards for excellence in health care. Nurses often choose this framework because it describes what they want to do for patients and families and what patients want from nurses during their hospitalization. An array of possible uses of the framework components is offered to the hospital, such as Comfort Rounds, performance review criteria, methods of documentation, clinical ladder criteria, and so on. The "value added" benefit when nurses are supported with adequate staffing levels to implement their comforting interventions can be empirically demonstrated through measurement of institutional outcomes such as patient satisfaction, "Best Hospital" designations, and cost savings.

Another way in which comfort theory is appropriate for wide application in a hospital system is to provide a theoretical base to enhance the working environment. Kolcaba collected information about the needs and wants of practicing nurses and arranged them on the taxonomic structure of comfort. From this preliminary work, the Nurses Comfort Questionnaire (NCQ) was developed, which can be used in pilot tests of nurse-inspired changes to the working environment, such as flexible or self-scheduling, mandatory lunch breaks off unit, a pleasant and clean rest area, or debriefing opportunities after difficult patient situations (Boudiab & Kolcaba, 2015; Rondinelli et al., 2015). For an empirical study, nurses would complete the NCQ before the suggested change was implemented and again a few months after implementation to determine whether nurses' comfort had increased over time. Institutional outcomes such as absenteeism, tardiness, or turnover could be added to the study, because comfort theory predicts that these subsequent outcomes would be correlated with enhanced nurse comfort and satisfaction.

CRITIQUE

Clarity

Kolcaba leaves an extensive paper trail of articles that highlight her steps in creating this middle-range theory. They are consistent in terms of definitions, derivations, assumptions, and propositions. Clarity is heightened in her book, which presents the theory and her articles leading to it (Kolcaba, 2003). Kolcaba applies the theory to specific practices using academic, but understandable, language. All research concepts are defined theoretically and operationally.

Simplicity

The theory of comfort is simple, because it is basic to nursing care and the traditional mission of nursing. Its language and application are of low technology, but this does not preclude its use in highly technological settings. There are six variables in the theory, and selected variables may be used for research or educational projects. The main thrust of the theory is for nurses to return to a practice focused on the holistic needs of patients inside or outside institutional walls. Its simplicity allows students and nurses to learn and practice the theory easily (Kolcaba, 2003).

Generality

Kolcaba's theory has been applied in numerous research settings, cultures, and age groups. Her book has been translated into German, Japanese, and Portuguese. The only limiting factor for its application is how well nurses and administrators value addressing the comfort needs of patients. If nurses, institutions, and communities are committed to basic nursing care, the theory of comfort promotes efficient, individualized, holistic practice. The taxonomic structure of comfort facilitates researchers' development of comfort instruments for new settings.

Accessibility

The first part of the theory, asserting that effective nursing interventions offered over time will demonstrate enhanced comfort, has been tested and supported with numerous studies. Furthermore, in the study by Dowd, Kolcaba, and Steiner (2000), enhanced comfort was a strong predictor of increased health-seeking behaviors, meaning when patients are more comfortable, they do better in rehabilitation or recovery. This relationship begins to support the second and third parts of the comfort theory. Comfort instruments have demonstrated strong psychometric properties, supporting the validity of the questionnaires as measures of comfort that reveal changes in comfort over time and support of the taxonomic structure. Verbal rating scales (VRSs) are especially useful for clinical practice; the nurse asks a patient to rate his or her total comfort from 0 (no comfort at all) to 10 (highest comfort possible in this situation). Such ratings are important for documenting effectiveness of nursing interventions by comparing baseline comfort to comfort after nursing care. VRSs are also useful for beginning a conversation with the patient or family members about detractors from total comfort. They have been used in prior research and have strong concurrent validity compared with other comfort questionnaires (Dowd et al., 2007; Parks et al., 2017).

Importance

The theory of comfort describes patient-centered practice and explains how comfort measures matter to patients and family members, their health and satisfaction, and the viability of institutions. The theory predicts the benefit of effective comfort measures (interventions) to enhance comfort and engagement in health-seeking behaviors. The theory of comfort is dedicated to sustaining nursing by bringing the discipline back to its roots. Documentation of comfort strategies and their effects empirically demonstrates the art of nursing. The outcome of comfort describes the effects of memorable helping interactions with patients and family members that go beyond checklists or physician orders. It encompasses the art and science of nursing. Making electronic data systems inclusive of value-added outcomes such as comfort is imperative. Collaboration and the openness of Kolcaba's website facilitates dissemination of the theory for application.

The orientation to patient and family comfort may have been initially present in nursing, but it has become invisible and perhaps less valued by a health care system that values more highly the use of medications and technology. Therefore refocusing on patient and family comfort represents a return to the roots of nursing and also to the need for empirical evidence about the importance of thorough and caring nurses. We can demonstrate through research that comfort is foundational to patient recovery, to other health-seeking behaviors, and to institutional viability. The focus is applicable to other health care professions and ancillary workers. The use of a comfort framework implemented throughout a hospital facilitates everyone being "on the same page." Its concepts are understood and relevant across all health care disciplines.

SUMMARY

From its inception, the theory of comfort focused on what the discipline of nursing does for patients. As the theory evolved, the definition derived from concept analysis expanded to include broader aspects of the patient such as cultural and spiritual aspects. The basic format of the taxonomic structure and conceptual framework did not change. The development of the GCQ was important to validate that the concept can be measured and documented; it is positive; and it is related to desirable patient, family, and institutional outcomes. Comfort theory represents the way most nurses want to practice, and it offers a way to make comfort measures visible through documentation and comfort care plans.

The theory easily guides nurses and other health care professionals in the planning and designing of health care in any setting. It provides a useful framework in education that enables students to organize their assessments and plans of care and learn the art of nursing as well as the science. Comfort theory offers nursing faculty a guide for attending to the comfort needs of students and new graduates as well (Goodwin & Candela, 2013). Expert nurses may demonstrate to other providers in the delivery of care what nurses do beyond the technical aspects of nursing.

In research, testing of the theory has validated improvement in patient comfort after receiving comforting interventions. The concept of comfort accounts for the aspect of quality care that patients describe as "feeling better." Kolcaba has consistently developed and expanded the importance of comfort into all realms of health care. Through her reasoning and interaction with nurses and other health professionals, the concept evolved into patient and health care techniques. Institutions have recognized the value of designing comfort environments for their patients and for their staff. Through Kolcaba's publications and the website activities, the theory of comfort is being used by nurses internationally.

CASE STUDY

A 32-year-old African American mother of three toddlers who is 28 weeks pregnant is admitted to the high-risk pregnancy unit with regular contractions. She is concerned because the plans for her family are not finalized. She has many comfort needs, diagrammed in Table 33.1. When nurses assess for comfort needs in patients, they use the taxonomic structure, or comfort grid, to identify and organize all known needs. Using the comfort grid (see Fig. 33.1) as a mental guide, nurses design interrelated comforting interventions that can be implemented in one or two nurse–patient–family interactions. For this case, some suggestions to individualize the types of comfort interventions that might be considered are presented in Table 33.2.

For clinical use, the nurse might ask the patient to rate her comfort before and after receiving the interventions on a scale from 0 to 10, with 10 being the highest level. To determine whether a specific comforting intervention enhanced the comfort of the patient, a comfort questionnaire is administered, assessing each cell in the comfort grid (see Fig. 33.1). A Likert-type scale with responses ranging from 1 to 6 facilitate a total comfort score. A questionnaire, given to the patient before and after the intervention, demonstrates the level of effectiveness of intervention.

Compare the suggestions for the comfort of this mother of three presented in Table 33.2 with comfort measures you considered as you read the case study of this woman. Are there nursing comfort measures you might add? Explain your addition using Table 33.1.

TABLE 33.1 Taxonomic Structure of Comfort Needs for Case Study

Context of Comfort	Relief	Ease	Transcendence
Physical	Aching back Early strong contractions	Restlessness and anxiety	Patient thinking, "What will happen to my family and to my babies?"
Psychospiritual	Anxiety and tension	Uncertainty about prognosis	Need for emotional and spiritual support
Environmental	Roommate is a primigravida Room is small, clean, and pleasant	Lack of privacy Telephone in room Feeling of confinement with bed rest	Need for calm, familiar environmental elements and accessibility of distraction
Sociocultural	Absence of family and culturally sensitive care	Family not present Language barriers	Need for support from family or significant other Need for information and consultation

TABLE 33.2 Comfort Care Actions and Interventions

Type of Comfort Care Action or Intervention	Example
Standard comfort interventions	Vital signs Laboratory test results Patient assessment Medications and treatments Social worker

TABLE 33.2 Comfort Care Actions and Interventions—cont'd

Type of Comfort Care Action or Intervention	Example
Coaching	Emotional support Reassurance Education Listening Clergy
Comfort food for the soul	Energy therapy such as healing touch if it is culturally acceptable Music therapy or guided imagery (patient's choice of music) Spending time Personal connections Reduction of environmental stimuli

CRITICAL THINKING ACTIVITIES

1. Diagram your practice with concepts. Where is comfort in your diagram? How does it interact with the other concepts?
2. Select a patient and apply the theory of comfort in your nursing practice. How did the theory change your style of practice? Describe your comfort measures in relation to the taxonomic structure? (See Fig. 33.1.)
3. Identify a comfort need you met for someone you cared for recently. How did you know it was successful?
4. Consider how you would apply the theory of comfort in a community setting. What interventions might enhance comfort in an aggregate group? How might you assess effectiveness?
5. Identify an area of nursing practice for comfort research, and explain why it is needed.

POINTS FOR FURTHER STUDY

- Kolcaba, K. (1997). *TheComfortLine.com.* Retrieved from http://www.thecomfortline.com.
- Kolcaba, K. (2003). *Comfort theory and practice: A holistic vision for health care.* New York: Springer.
- Kolcaba, K. (2012). Comfort (including definition, theory of comfort, relevance to nursing, review of comfort studies, and future directions). In J. Fitzpatrick (Ed.), *The encyclopedia of nursing research* (3rd ed., pp. 75-77). New York: Springer.
- Kolcaba, K. video interview. *Nursing theorists: Portraits of excellence, vol. 3,* Fitne, Inc., Athens, OH.

REFERENCES

Aikens, C. (1908). Making the patient comfortable. *The Canadian Nurse, 4*(9), 422–424.

Barbosa, E., deOliveria, F., Guedes, M., et al. (2014). Nursing care for a puerpera based on the theory of comfort. *REME (Revista Mineira De Enfermagem), 18*(4), 850–854. (English translation).

Boudiab, L., & Kolcaba, K. (2015). Comfort theory: Unraveling the complexities of veterans' health care needs. *Advances in Nursing Science, 38*(4), 270–278.

Derya, Y., & Pasinioglu, T. (2015). The effect of nursing care based on comfort theory on women's postpartum comfort levels after Caesarean sections. *International Journal of Nursing Knowledge,* DOI:10.1111/2047–3095, Wiley Online Library.

Dowd, T., Kolcaba, K., & Steiner, R. (2000). Using cognitive strategies to enhance bladder control and comfort. *Holistic Nursing Practice, 14*(2), 91–103.

Dowd, T., Kolcaba, K., Steiner, R., & Fashinpaur, D. (2007). Comparison of healing touch and coaching on stress and comfort in young college students. *Holistic Nursing Practice, 21*(4), 194–202.

Goodnow, M. (1935). *The technique of nursing.* Philadelphia: Saunders.

Goodwin, M., & Candela, L. (2013). Outcomes of newly practicing nurses who applied principles of holistic comfort theory during transition from school to practice: A qualitative study. *Nurse Education Today, 33*(6), 614–619.

Hamilton, J. (1989). Comfort and the hospitalized chronically ill. *Journal of Gerontological Nursing, 15*(4), 28–33.

Hansen, D., Higgins, P., Warner, C., & Mayo, M. (2015). Exploring family relationships through associations of comfort, relatedness states, and life closure in hospice patients: A pilot study. *Palliative and Supportive Care, 13*(2), 305–311.

Hardin, S., & Bishop, S. (2010). Logical reasoning. In M. R. Alligood & A. M. Tomey (Eds.), *Nursing theorists and their work* (7th ed., pp. 26–35). St Louis, MO: Mosby-Elsevier.

Harmer, B. (1926). *Methods and principles of teaching the principles and practice of nursing*. New York: Macmillan.
Henderson, V. (1966). *The nature of nursing*. New York: Macmillan.
Kolcaba, K. (1997). TheComfortLine.com, www.TheComfortLine.com.
Kolcaba, K. (2003). *Comfort theory and practice: A holistic vision for health care*. New York: Springer.
Kolcaba, K. (2012). Comfort (including definition, theory of comfort, relevance to nursing, review of comfort studies, and future directions). In J. Fitzpatrick (Ed.), *The encyclopedia of nursing research* (3rd ed., pp. 75–77). New York: Springer.
Kolcaba, K., & Fisher, E. (1996). A holistic perspective on comfort care as an advance directive. *Critical Care Nursing Quarterly, 18*(4), 66–76.
Krinsky, R., Murillo, I., & Johnson, J. (2014). A practical application of Katharine Kolcaba's comfort theory to cardiac patients. *Applied Nursing Research, 27*(2), 147–150.
Kumar, S., Adiga, K., & George, A. (2014). Effectiveness of mindfulness based stress reduction (MBSR) on stress and anxiety among elderly residing in residential homes. *International Journal of Nursing Care, 2*(2), 81–85.
NANDA; Ackley, B. J., Ladwig, G. B., & Makie, M. B. (2017). *Nursing diagnosis handbook: An evidence-based guide to planning care* (11th ed.). St Louis: Mosby.
NIC; Bulecheck, G. M., Butcher, H. K., & McCloskey-Dochterman, J. (2008). *Nursing interventions classifications* (5th ed., pp. 78–79, 532–533, 578–579). St Louis: Mosby.
NOC; Moorehead, S., Johnson, M., Maas, M. L., & Swanson, E. (2008). *Nursing outcomes classifications* (4th ed., pp. 280–284, 753–756). St Louis: Mosby.
McIlveen, K., & Morse, J. (1995). The role of comfort in nursing care: 1900–1980. *Clinical Nursing Research, 4*(2), 127–148.
Murray, H. (1938). *Explorations in personality*. New York: Oxford Press.
Nightingale, F. (1859). *Notes on nursing*. London: Harrison.
Orlando, I. (1961). *The dynamic nurse-patient relationship: Function, process, and principles*. New York: Putnam.
Parks, M., Morris, D., Kolcaba, K., & McDonald, P. (2017). An evaluation of patient comfort during acute psychiatric hospitalization. *Perspectives in Psychiatric Nursing, 53*(1), 29–37.
Paterson, J., & Zderad, L. (1975). *Humanistic nursing*. New York: National League for Nursing.
Rondinelli, J., Long, K., Seelinger, C., Crawford, C., & Valdez, R. (2015). Factors related to nurse comfort when caring for families experiencing perinatal loss. *Journal for Nurses in Professional Development, 3*(31), 158–163.
Schlotfeldt, R. (1975). The need for a conceptual framework. In P. Verhovic (Ed.), *Nursing research* (pp. 3–25). Boston: Little, Brown.
Seyedfatemi, N., Rafi, F., Rezaei, M., & Kolcaba, K. (2014). Comfort and hope in the preanesthesia stage in patients undergoing surgery. *Journal of Perianesthesia Nursing, 29*(3), 213–220.
Townsend, C., Bonham, E., Chase, L., Dunscomb, J., & McAlister, S. (2014). A comparison of still point induction to massage therapy in reducing pain and increasing comfort in chronic pain. *Holistic Nursing Practice, 2*(28), 78–84.
Wilson, L., & Kolcaba, K. (2004). Practical application of comfort theory in the perianesthesia setting (invited article). *Journal of Perianesthesia Nursing, 19*(3), 164–173.

BIBLIOGRAPHY

Primary Sources

Book Chapters

Kolcaba, K. (2001). Holistic care: Is it feasible in today's health care environment? In H. Feldman (Ed.), *Nursing leaders speak out* (pp. 49–54). New York: Springer.
Kolcaba, K. (2001). Kolcaba's theory of comfort. In D. Robinson & C. Kish (Eds.), *Core concepts in advanced practice nursing* (pp. 418–422). St Louis: Mosby.
Kolcaba, K. (2003). *Comfort theory and practice: A holistic vision for health care*. New York: Springer.
Kolcaba, K. (2010). Katharine Kolcaba's comfort theory. In M. Parker & M. Smith (Eds.), *Nursing theories and nursing practice* (pp. 389–401). Philadelphia: F. A. Davis.
Kolcaba, K. (2017). Comfort. In S. J. Peterson & T. S. Bredow (Eds.), *Middle range theories: Application to nursing research* (4th ed., pp. 196–210). Philadelphia: Lippincott.
Kolcaba, K. (2017). Impaired comfort. In B. Ackley & G. Ladwig (Eds.), *Nursing diagnosis handbook* (pp. 219–222). St Louis: Mosby.
Kolcaba, K., & Kolcaba, R. (2011). Integrative theorizing: Linking middle-range nursing theories with the Neuman systems model. In B. Neuman & J. Fawcett (Eds.), *The Neuman systems model* (5th ed., pp. 299–313). Upper Saddle River, NJ: Pearson.
Kolcaba, K., & Mitzel, A. (2008). Hand massage. In B. J. Ackley, G. B. Ladwig, B. A. Swan, & S. J. Tucker (Eds.), *Evidence-based nursing care guidelines: Medical-surgical interventions* (pp. 402–407). St Louis: Mosby.
Kolcaba, K., & Mitzel, A. (2008). Simple massage. In B. J. Ackley, G. B. Ladwig, B. A. Swan, & S. J. Tucker (Eds.), *Evidence-based nursing care guidelines: Medical-surgical interventions* (pp. 504–508). St Louis: Mosby.
Schuiling, K., Sampselle, C., & Kolcaba, K. (2011). Exploring the presence of comfort within the context of childbirth. In R. Bryar & M. Sinclair (Eds.), *Theory for midwifery practice* (2nd ed., pp. 197–214). Basingstoke, UK: Palgrave Macmillan.

Journal Articles

Dowd, T., Kolcaba, K., & Steiner, R. (2006). Development of an instrument to measure holistic client comfort as an outcome of healing touch. *Holistic Nursing Practice, 20*(3), 122–129.
Kolcaba, K. (1995). The art of comfort care. *Image: The Journal of Nursing Scholarship, 27*(4), 287–289.
Kolcaba, K., & Fox, C. (1999). The effects of guided imagery on comfort of women with early stage breast cancer undergoing radiation therapy. *Oncology Nursing Forum, 26*(1), 67–92.
Kolcaba, K., & Steiner, R. (2000). Empirical evidence for the nature of holistic comfort. *Journal of Holistic Nursing, 18*(1), 46–62.
Kolcaba, K., Tilton, C., & Drouin, C. (2006). Comfort theory: A unifying framework to enhance the practice environment. *Journal of Nursing Administration, 36*(11), 518–544.
Kolcaba, K., & Wilson, L. (2002). The framework of comfort care for perianesthesia nursing. *Journal of Perianesthesia Nursing, 17*(2), 102–114.
Paiva, B., deCarvalho, A., Kolcaba, K., & Paiva, C. (2015). Validation of the holistic comfort questionnaire-caregiver in Portuguese-Brazil in a cohort of informal caregivers of palliative care cancer patients. *Support Care Cancer, 23*(2), 343–351.

Wagner, D., Byrne, M., & Kolcaba, K. (2006). Effect of comfort warming on preoperative patients. *AORN Journal, 84*(3), 1–13.

Cook, C., Clark, T., & Brunton, M. (2014). Optimizing cultural safety and comfort during gynaecological examinations: Accounts of indigenous Maori women. *Nursing Praxis in New Zealand, 30*(3), 19–34.

March, A., & McCormack, D. (2009). Nursing theory-directed health care: Modifying Kolcaba's comfort theory as an institution-wide approach. *Holistic Nursing Practice, 23*(2), 75–80.

Mohammadi, F., Eftekhari, M., Dejman, M., Forouzan, A., & Mirabzadeh, A. (2014). Seeking comfort: Women mental health process in I.R. Iran: A grounded theory study. *International Journal of Preventive Medicine, 5*(2), 217–223.

Norton, E., Holloway, I., & Galvin, K. (2014). Comfort vs risk: A grounded theory about female adolescent behavior in the sun. *Journal of Clinical Nursing, 23*(13-14), 1889–1899.

Slatyer, S., Williams, A., & Michael, R. (2015). Seeking empowerment to comfort patients in severe pain: A grounded theory study of the nurse's perspective. *International Journal of Nursing Studies, 52*(1), 229–239.

34

Postpartum Depression Theory

*M. Katherine Maeve**

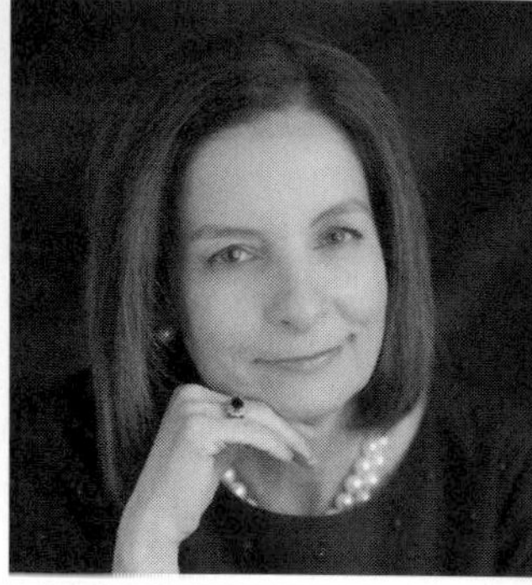

Cheryl Tatano Beck

"The birth of a baby is an occasion for joy—or so the saying goes . . . But for some women, joy is not an option."

(Beck, 2006, p. 40)

CREDENTIALS AND BACKGROUND OF THE THEORIST

Cheryl Tatano Beck graduated from the Western Connecticut State University with a baccalaureate in nursing in 1970. She recognized during her first clinical rotation that obstetrical nursing was to be her lifelong specialty. After graduation, Beck worked as a registered nurse at the Yale New Haven Hospital on the postpartum and normal newborn nursery unit. By 1972, Beck had graduated from Yale University with a master's degree in maternal-newborn nursing and a certificate in nurse midwifery. In 1982 she received a doctorate in nursing science from Boston University.

Beginning at the rank of instructor in 1973, Beck has held academic appointments with increasing rank at several major universities, including the University of Maryland, the University of Michigan, Florida Atlantic University, the University of Rhode Island, and Yale University, and as professor at the University of Connecticut, where she holds a joint appointment in the School of Nursing and School of Medicine. Beck has served as consultant on numerous research projects for universities and state agencies in the northeastern United States. During her career, Beck received more than 30 awards, including Distinguished Researcher of the Year from the Eastern Nursing Research Society in 1999. She was inducted as a fellow in the American Academy of Nursing in 1993.

This body of work resulted in a substantive theory of postpartum depression (Beck, 1993) and the development of the Postpartum Depression Screening Scale (PDSS) (Beck, 2002c; Beck & Gable, 2000) and the Postpartum Depression Predictors Inventory (PDPI) (Beck, 1998, 2002a).

A prolific author and disseminator of her research, Beck has authored more than 100 research-based articles and given research presentations locally, nationally, and internationally. She has served on the editorial boards of nursing journals, including *Advances in Nursing Science, Nursing Research,* and the *Journal of Nursing Education.* Beck serves on the executive board for the Marce Society, an international society for understanding, preventing, and treatment of mental illness associated with childbirth, and on the advisory committee of the Donaghue Medical Research Foundation in Connecticut. Over her career, Beck has received numerous local, national, and international awards for her work. In 2011 Beck received the Best Publication award from Sigma Theta Tau International, Honor Society, *Journal of Nursing Scholarship*-Profession, World Health, and Health Systems, for "International Differences in Nursing Research" coauthored with D. F. Polit. She and her research colleagues received the *Journal of Midwifery & Women's Health* 2012 Article Award for "Postpartum Depressive Symptomatology," a publication of their two-stage national survey results. Also in 2012, she received the Annie Goodrich Distinguished Nurse Lectureship Award.

*The author wishes to thank Dr. Cheryl Tatano Beck for her generosity of spirit in allowing liberties with the interpretation of her life's work. Dr. Beck's work represents an enormous contribution to nursing, made even more remarkable because it did not depend on large amounts of funding from the National Institutes of Health. That alone is an inspiration. Thanks are also extended to Dr. Peggy L. Chinn, who happily has not retired as a mentor or friend.

Many in nursing recognize the classic Polit and Hungler research text, used in many graduate nursing programs. Beck became coauthor of Polit's seventh edition (Polit & Beck, 2003), reflecting Beck's research expertise. In 2011 this text received the *American Journal of Nursing* Book of the Year Award for the ninth edition (Polit & Beck, 2011). Beck has published articles regarding statistical analysis strategies and approaches for qualitative research.

Although Beck conducted seven major studies regarding educational and caring issues with undergraduate nursing students, for more than 3 decades she contributed to knowledge development in obstetrical nursing. Her research career began by studying women in labor, with interest in fetal monitoring. Beck's research focus eventually became the postpartum period and specific studies of postpartum mood disorders.

THEORETICAL AND PHILOSOPHICAL SOURCES

Although Beck does not address caring as a theoretical or philosophical construct specific to her research, she has conducted studies that evidence her belief about the importance of caring in nursing. Beck's use of Jean Watson's caring theory endorses caring as central to nursing, while acknowledging Watson's concern that quantitative methodologies may not adequately reflect the ideal of transpersonal caring. It is obvious throughout Beck's writings, including research reports, that using both quantitative and qualitative methods to advance nursing as a caring profession is desirable and achievable in practice, research, and education.

Because many of the studies used to develop Beck's postpartum depression theory were qualitative in nature, Beck has cited various theoretical sources reflecting the philosophical and theoretical roots of methodologies important for the kind of knowledge developed in each study. Phenomenology was used in the first major study of how women experienced postpartum depression with Colaizzi's (1978) approach. In her next study, Beck used grounded theory as influenced by the theoretical and philosophical ideas of Glaser (1978), Glaser and Strauss (1967), and Hutchinson (1986), all seminal contributors to the evolution of grounded theory in nursing. Throughout all of Beck's work and consistent with feminist theory, there is explicit valuing of the importance of understanding pregnancy, birth, and motherhood through "the eyes of women." Furthermore, Beck acknowledges that childbirth occurs in many simultaneous contexts (medical, social, economic) and that mothers' reactions to childbirth and motherhood are shaped by their contextual responses.

An unusual theoretical source came from the work of Sichel and Driscoll (1999), who developed an earthquake model to conceptualize how interactions between biology and life result in what they term *biochemical loading.* Over time, with constant chemical challenges related to stressors, women's brains may develop a kind of "fault line" that is less likely to remain intact during critical moments in women's lives, such as the challenges women face around childbirth, resulting in a kind of "earthquake." Beck understood Sichel and Driscoll's model to "suggest that a woman's genetic makeup, hormonal and reproductive history, and life experiences all combine to predict her risk of 'an earthquake' which occurs when her brain cannot stabilize and mood problems erupt." Although it is easy to understand the physiological and hormonal challenges of pregnancies for women, Sichel and Driscoll's earthquake model was important in helping Beck to holistically conceptualize the phenomena that might affect the development of postpartum depression for women. Although Beck states that she never experienced postpartum depression after the birth of her own children, those who have may relate to the earthquake metaphor, complete with tremors culminating in postpartum depression or, worse, postpartum psychosis.

Beck has identified Robert Gable as a particularly important source in her work as Professor Emeritus at the University of Connecticut, Neag School of Education. After developing a wealth of knowledge about postpartum depression, the next logical steps for Beck became developing instruments that could predict and screen for postpartum depression. Gable assisted Beck with theoretical operationalization of her theory for practical use. Gable has remained directly involved through the step-by-step development of the PDSS, including the Spanish version (Beck & Gable, 2003).

MAJOR CONCEPTS & DEFINITIONS

Beck's major concepts have undergone refinement and clarification over years of work on postpartum depression. The first two concepts, postpartum mood disorders and loss of control, were developed using phenomenology and grounded theory methods (Beck, 2002b).

Concepts 1 and 2

1. Postpartum Mood Disorders

Postpartum depression and maternity blues have become better delineated over time, as has the understanding of postpartum psychosis. Two other perinatal mood disorders,

Continued

MAJOR CONCEPTS & DEFINITIONS—cont'd

postpartum obsessive-compulsive disorder and postpartum-onset panic disorder, have been identified, as has how these disorders are different and how they are interrelated.

Postpartum Depression

Postpartum depression is a nonpsychotic major depressive disorder with distinguishing diagnostic criteria that often begins as early as 4 weeks after birth. It may also occur anytime within the first year after childbirth. Postpartum depression is not self-limiting and is more difficult to treat than simple depression. Prevalence rates are 13% to 25%, with more women affected who are poor, live in the inner city, or are adolescents. Approximately 50% of all women suffering from postpartum depression have episodes lasting 6 months or longer.

Maternity Blues

Also known as **postpartum blues** and **baby blues**, **maternity blues** is a relatively transient and self-limited period of melancholy and mood swings during the early postpartum period. Maternity blues affects up to 75% of all women in all cultures.

Postpartum Psychosis

Postpartum psychosis is a psychotic disorder characterized by hallucinations, delusions, agitation, and inability to sleep, along with bizarre and irrational behavior. Although postpartum psychosis is relatively rare (1–2 women per 1000 births), it represents a true psychiatric emergency because both mother and baby (and perhaps other children) are in grave danger of harm. Although postpartum psychosis often begins to appear during the first week postpartum, it commonly goes undetected until serious harm has occurred.

Postpartum Obsessive-Compulsive Disorder

Only recently identified, the prevalence rates of **postpartum obsessive-compulsive disorder** have not been reported. Symptoms include repetitive, intrusive thoughts of harming the baby, a fear of being left alone with the infant, and hypervigilance in protecting the infant.

Postpartum-Onset Panic Disorder

Postpartum-onset panic disorder has been identified only recently and is also without reported prevalence rates. It is characterized by acute onset of anxiety, fear, rapid breathing, heart palpitations, and a sense of impending doom.

2. Loss of Control

Loss of control was identified as the basic psychosocial problem in the 1993 substantive theory of Beck's early work. This descriptive theory captured a process women go through with postpartum depression. Loss of control was experienced in all areas of women's lives, although the particulars of the circumstances may be different. The concept of loss of control fit with extant literature and left women with feelings of "teetering on the edge." The process identified consisted of the following four stages:

1. **Encountering terror** consisted of horrifying anxiety attacks, enveloping fogginess, and relentless obsessive thinking.
2. **Dying of self** consists of alarming unrealness, contemplating and attempting self-destruction, and isolating oneself.
3. **Struggling to survive** consisted of battling the system, seeking solace at support groups, and praying for relief.
4. **Regaining control** consisted of unpredictable transitioning, guarded recovery, and mourning lost time.

The conceptual ideas and definitions described previously were used to develop specific foci for testing. Initially, Beck (1998) identified eight risk factors for postpartum depression. Subsequent studies have expanded areas where Beck determined that more conceptual clarity was needed. An important area of change was in reference to marriage. Through research, it was noted that there were two marital factors of concern: marital status and the nature of the marital relationship satisfaction. Two other risk factors identified were socioeconomic status and issues of unplanned and unwanted pregnancies (Beck, 2002b).

Concepts 3–15

Concepts 3–15 are major concepts found to be significant predictors or risk factors for postpartum depression (Beck, 2002b). The most current interpretation of effect size was assigned from a meta-analysis of 138 extant studies and is at the end of each concept definition.

3. Prenatal Depression

Depression during any or all of the trimesters of pregnancy has been found to be the strongest predictor of postpartum depression. (Effect size: Medium)

4. Child Care Stress

Child care stress pertains to stressful events related to child care such as infant health problems and difficulty in infant care pertaining to feeding and sleeping. (Effect size: Medium)

5. Life Stress

Life stress is an index of stressful life events during pregnancy and postpartum. The number of life experiences

MAJOR CONCEPTS & DEFINITIONS—cont'd

and the amount of stress created by each of the life events are combined to determine the amount of life stress a woman is experiencing. Stressful life events can be either negative or positive and can include experiences such as the following:

- Marital changes (e.g., divorce, remarriage)
- Occupational changes (e.g., job change)
- Crises (e.g., accidents, burglaries, financial crises, illness requiring hospitalization)

  (Effect size: Medium)

6. Social Support

Social support pertains to instrumental support (e.g., babysitting, help with household chores) and emotional support. Structural features of a woman's social network (husband or partner, family, and friends) include proximity of its members, frequency of contact, and number of confidants with whom the woman can share personal matters. Lack of social support is when a woman perceives that she is not receiving the amount of instrumental or emotional support she expects. (Effect size: Medium)

7. Prenatal Anxiety

Prenatal anxiety occurs during any trimester or throughout the pregnancy. *Anxiety* refers to feelings of uneasiness or apprehension concerning a vague, nonspecific threat. (Effect size: Medium)

8. Marital Satisfaction

The degree of satisfaction with a marital relationship is assessed and includes how happy or satisfied the woman is with certain aspects of her marriage, such as communication, affection, similarity of values (e.g., finances, child care), mutual activity and decision making, and global well-being. (Effect size: Medium)

9. History of Depression

A woman has a history of depression if there is report of having had a bout of depression before this pregnancy. (Effect size: Medium)

10. Infant Temperament

The **temperament** is the infant's disposition and personality. *Difficult temperament* describes an infant who is irritable, fussy, unpredictable, and difficult to console. (Effect size: Medium)

11. Maternity Blues

Maternity blues was previously defined as a nonpathological condition after giving birth. Prolonged episodes of maternity blues (lasting more than 10 days) may predict postpartum depression. (Effect size: Small to medium)

12. Self-Esteem

Self-esteem is a woman's global feelings of self-worth and self-acceptance. It is her confidence and satisfaction in self. Low self-esteem reflects a negative self-evaluation and feelings about oneself or one's capabilities. (Effect size: Medium)

13. Socioeconomic Status

Socioeconomic status is a person's rank or status in society involving a combination of social and economic factors (e.g., income, education, and occupation). (Effect size: Small)

14. Marital Status

Marital status is a woman's standing in regard to marriage; it denotes whether a woman is single, married or cohabiting, divorced, widowed, separated, or partnered. (Effect size: Small)

15. Unplanned or Unwanted Pregnancy

Unplanned or unwanted pregnancy refers to a pregnancy that was not planned or wanted. Of particular note is the issue of pregnancies that remain unwanted after initial ambivalence. (Effect size: Small)

Concepts 16–22

These final concepts represent the distillation of all predictor and risk factors that are used to screen women for symptoms of postpartum depression in the PDSS (Beck, 2002c).

16. Sleeping and Eating Disturbances

Sleeping and eating disturbances include inability to sleep even when the baby is asleep, tossing and turning before actually falling asleep, waking up in the middle of the night, and difficulty going back to sleep. Even though she is consciously aware of the need to eat, the woman may experience loss of appetite and inability to eat.

17. Anxiety and Insecurity

Anxiety and insecurity includes overattention to relatively minor issues, feelings of jumping out of one's skin, feeling the need to keep moving, or pacing. There is an ever-present feeling of insecurity and a sense of being overwhelmed in the new role of mother.

18. Emotional Lability

A woman experiencing **emotional lability** has a sense that her emotions are unstable and out of her control. It

Continued

 **MAJOR CONCEPTS & DEFINITIONS—cont'd**

is commonly characterized as crying for no particular reason, irritability, explosive anger, and fear of never being happy again.

19. Mental Confusion

Mental confusion is characterized by a marked inability to concentrate, focus on a task, or make a decision. There is a general feeling of being unable to regulate one's own thought processes.

20. Loss of Self

Women sense that the aspects of self that reflected their personal identity have changed since the birth of their infant, so they cannot identify who they really are and are fearful that they might never be able to be their real selves again.

21. Guilt and Shame

A woman experiences **guilt and shame** when she perceives that she is performing poorly as a mother and has negative thoughts regarding her infant. This results in an inability to be open with others about how she feels and contributes to a delay in diagnosis and intervention.

22. Suicidal Thoughts

Women experience **suicidal thoughts** when they have frequent thoughts of harming themselves or ending their lives to escape the living nightmare of postpartum depression.

USE OF EMPIRICAL EVIDENCE

When Beck began to examine postpartum depression in 1993, she noted that only two qualitative studies contributed to the knowledge base of the disorder. Most studies were based upon knowledge developed in disciplines other than nursing. Beck's background as a nurse midwife undoubtedly gave her a view of women throughout the postpartum period that was not commonly available to those in other disciplines involved with women during the perinatal period.

In 1993, after four major studies regarding women in the postpartum period, Beck developed a substantive theory of postpartum depression using grounded theory methodology. The substantive theory was titled "teetering on the edge," with the basic psychosocial problem identified as loss of control.

Since development of the substantive theory, Beck has designed and collaborated with numerous others to refine the theory by examining the experiences of postpartum depression on mother–child interactions, postpartum panic, posttraumatic stress disorder (PTSD), and birth trauma to tease out differences among postpartum mood disorders (postpartum depression, maternity blues, postpartum psychosis, postpartum obsessive-compulsive disorder, postpartum-onset panic disorder). Meta-analyses were conducted on predictors of postpartum depression, the relationship between postpartum depression and infant temperament, and the effects of postpartum depression on mother–infant interaction. In addition, two qualitative metasyntheses were conducted on postpartum depression and mothering multiples.

Beck used 10 qualitative studies of postpartum depression in women from a wide variety of geographical locations and cultures. Women represented in these studies included Black Caribbean, Irish, Indian, Hong Kong Chinese, Hmong, Middle Eastern (living in the United Kingdom), Asian, Portuguese, Australian, Canadian, and African American. These new data were used to compare Beck's original teetering on the edge grounded theory with women in other cultures. Beck found that the theory's modifiability was in keeping with theoretical expectations of a relevant substantive grounded theory. Therefore the theory of "teetering on the edge," with "loss of control" as the basic psychosocial process, was functionally expanded to women in many varied cultures around the world (Beck, 2012).

MAJOR ASSUMPTIONS

Nursing

Beck describes nursing as a caring profession with caring obligations to persons nurses care for, students, and each other. In addition, interpersonal interactions between nurses and those for whom they care are the primary ways nursing accomplishes the goals of health and wholeness.

Person

Persons are described in terms of wholeness with biological, sociological, and psychological components. Furthermore, there is a strong commitment to the idea that persons or personhood is understood within the context of family and community.

Health

Beck does not define *health* explicitly. However, her writings include traditional ideas of physical and mental health. Health is the consequence of women's responses to the contexts of their lives and their environments. Contexts of health are vital to understanding any singular issue of health.

Environment

Beck writes about the environment in broad terms that include individual factors as well as the world outside of each person. The outside environment includes events, situations, culture, physicality ecosystems, and sociopolitical systems. In addition, there is an acknowledgment that women in the childbearing period receive care within a health care environment structured in the medical model and permeated with patriarchal ideology.

THEORETICAL ASSERTIONS

The theoretical assertions within Beck's theory are well represented throughout her writings. She acknowledges the importance of Sichel and Driscoll's (1999) work related to the biological factors involved in postpartum depression in the following assertions:

- The brain can biochemically accommodate various stressors, whether related to internal biology or external events.
- Stressful events (internal or external), particularly over long periods, cause disruption of the biochemical regulation in the brain. The more insults to the brain, the more chronically deregulated the brain becomes. Because an already deregulated brain is challenged again with new stressors (internal or external), it is likely that serious mood and psychiatric disorders will result.
- Women's unique and normal brain and hormonal chemistry result in a vulnerability to mood disorders at critical times in their lives, including after giving birth.
- Postpartum depression is caused by a combination of biological (including genetic), psychological, social, relational, economic, and situational life stressors.
- Postpartum depression is not a homogenous disorder. Women may express postpartum depression with a single symptom but are more likely to have a constellation of varying symptoms. This is related to varying life histories of internal and external stressors.
- Culturally, women are expected to feel happy, look happy, act happy, understand how to be a mother naturally, and experience motherhood with a sense of fulfillment. These expectations make it difficult for women to express genuine feelings of distress.
- The stigma attached to mental illness increases dramatically when a mental illness is related to the birth of a child, leading women to suffer in silence.
- Within a level of prevention framework, postpartum depression can be prevented through identification and mitigation of risk factors during the prepartum period. Postpartum depression can be identified early with careful screening and can be treated effectively. Prevention can alleviate months of suffering and decrease the harmful effects on women, their infants, and their families.
- A number of biological, sociological, and psychological issues and challenges are entirely normal in all pregnancies. These may include fatigue, sleep alterations, questioning one's abilities, and the like. Comprehensive prenatal and postnatal care can eliminate troublesome pathological symptoms and help women normalize expected symptoms, thus reducing the degree of stress they actually experience.

LOGICAL FORM

Beck's postpartum depression theory, as described in previous sections of this chapter, identifies how both inductive and deductive logic significantly contributed to the development of the theory. Chinn and Kramer (2015) identify inductive logic as foundational to qualitative methods, with reasoning from the particular to the general. In contrast, deductive reasoning moves from the general to the particular, drawing conclusions that represent the general.

Because Beck's theory reflects a very complex and focused path in its evolution, it is helpful to be clear about what criteria were used to understand and present the theory. The definition of *theory* currently used is "the creative and rigorous structuring of ideas that project a tentative, purposeful, and systematic view of phenomena" (Chinn & Kramer, 2015, p. 255). Middle-range theories may be derived using grounded theory approaches, and they identify social processes that occur in various social events. For example, Beck's substantive theory of postpartum depression found that loss of control was the basic psychosocial problem facing women, but this problem also occurs in contexts other than the postpartum period.

The evolution of Beck's theory is instructional for several reasons. First, Beck's unceasing, linear, and logical efforts to develop the theory for pragmatic practice concerns led to a theory that addresses a specific practice problem. Because her theory is relatively new, there are fewer contributors to the substance of the theory. Therefore there is opportunity to follow a very clear and focused process of theory development by a scholar who began the work as a young woman. Beck has tested her theory, used it with various populations, developed and tested instruments, and established a work in which other scholars can join her to contribute to the science. Second, Beck's theory of postpartum depression is remarkable as an example of extensive inductive theory development in a specific area of nursing practice addressing a specific patient problem. Although Beck began her work with a global understanding of caring, her focused work on postpartum depression was advanced through the development of a substantive middle-range theory and continues to advance. From the beginning, Beck's goal has been to understand postpartum depression in a way that would allow professionals to develop adequate prevention strategies, develop screening programs for early intervention, and develop adequate treatment strategies to prevent harm to women, their children, and their families. True to her research aims, what began as a descriptive substantive theory of postpartum depression evolved into an extensive research program.

ACCEPTANCE BY THE NURSING COMMUNITY

Practice

As Beck's research findings have been disseminated more widely, the theory and the instruments based on the theory have been used increasingly in nursing practice throughout the United States and globally. The PDSS (2002d) became a standard of care for women in the high-risk obstetrical clinic of the Medical University of South Carolina Hospital (A. Raney, personal communication, April 2004). The clients in this clinic vary in age across the spectrum, come from various ethnic backgrounds, and have a wide range of medical risk factors. She has noted that the tool is a vehicle for opening discussions with women that had not occurred before implementation of the tool. High scores on the PDSS have given physicians evidence to understand how postpartum depression is expressed in their patients, increasing their sensitivity and awareness. Predictably, marshaling of community resources to meet the specific needs of individual clients has been a challenge; however, the landscape for the Charleston community in understanding and responding to the special needs of women during this time has occurred.

Public health initiatives that involve working with new mothers and babies are also using Beck's theory of postpartum depression via the PDSS. For example, the Healthy Start CORPS: Inter-Conceptual Care Case Management Project in North Carolina begins to follow women when they are 6 weeks postpartum. All new clients, many of whom are Native American, are given the PDSS so that intervention and management strategies can be built into plans of care for individual women and their families (L. Baker, personal communication, April 2004). The director of the program emphasizes the ease with which women are able to discuss symptoms of postpartum depression after completing the tool.

Beck's work has also been instrumental in community intervention and education projects such as the Ruth Rhoden Craven Foundation for Postpartum Depression Awareness in South Carolina. Helena Bradford founded this organization because of a tragic postpartum mood disorder within her own family. She advocates for postpartum awareness within her community and conducts support groups (H. Bradford, personal communication, April 2004).

Education

Beck is a frequently invited speaker for professional educational conferences and workshops. Her work is cited in many maternal and newborn nursing texts, such as that of Davidson, London, and Ladewig (2012). At both undergraduate and graduate levels, Beck's work sets the standard for knowledge and understanding about postpartum depression. In addition, Beck's work has been used to educate members of other disciplines, such as physicians, mental health workers, public health professionals, social workers, and those who work in social service agencies that provide protective care for women and children. Beck also brings her work to the general public and policy makers through active community involvement at the local, state, national, and international levels.

Research

As described so far, Beck's postpartum depression theory is a middle-range, practice-level theory. In addition to the continuous studies carried out by Beck, the global literature gives evidence of nurses using her research and research instruments to better understand the experience of pregnancy and improve the care of mothers. For example, Lavoie (2015) reported on a study recently in the *International Journal for Childbirth Education* about caring for breast-feeding women with Five Es—encouragement, empathy, education, engagement, and evaluation—which had a positive effect on postpartum depression.

FURTHER DEVELOPMENT

Beck identified what became another major concept in her theory, as well as a restructuring of postpartum mood disorder definitions. Because of increasing reports of PTSD after childbirth, she has also examined women's experiences of traumatic births (Beck, Driscoll, & Watson, 2014). In this work, birth trauma was defined as "an event occurring during the labor and delivery process that involves actual or threatened serious injury or death to the mother or her infant. The birthing woman experiences intense fear, helplessness, loss of control, and horror" (Beck, 2015, p. 8). She noted that women who actually had been suffering from PTSD were misdiagnosed as having postpartum depression and were treated incorrectly with antidepressant medications. She recommended that the term *postpartum mood disorders* be changed to *postpartum mood and anxiety disorders.* PTSD would then be differentiated as a distinct diagnosis with different treatment approaches. Birth trauma, as a concept, was examined empirically and included predictor and screening instruments as appropriate. Beck and Watson (2010) examined women's experience on the anniversary of their birth trauma, noting that the birthday of a woman's child might represent a time of re-experiencing the trauma all over again (Beck, Driscoll & Watson, 2014).

Researchers have used the PDSS to screen for postpartum depression in a sample acquired on the Internet compared with a community-based sample. Initial results suggested a high degree of internal consistency and construct validity between the two groups. Findings indicated that the Internet group included greater numbers of participation among Hispanic and Asian women, and the Internet group evidenced more risk factors for a postpartum depression diagnosis.

Recent theoretical advancements to Beck's (1993) theory of teetering on the edge are outlined in Beck (2012) where she published what she called "A second grounded theory modification" of her original theory in part to answer the question "Is postpartum depression a Western culture-bound syndrome?" (p. 257). That global work is unique in that it rethinks the concept of postpartum depression through the experiences of women in many countries and continents. Hence Beck began studies of postpartum depression resulting in the second modification of teetering on the edge. Studies were conducted in Australia, Canada, Democratic Republic of the Congo, Ethiopia, Indonesia, Ireland, Taiwan, United Arab Emerites, and the United Kingdom. New dimensions of women in those countries were described, representing a four-stage process of teetering on the edge:

1. **Encountering terror**, evidenced by horrifying anxiety attacks; enveloping fogginess; relentless obsessive thinking; and various somatic expressions
2. **Dying of self**, evidenced by alarming unrealness, contemplating and attempting self-destruction, isolating oneself, and dealing with consequences
3. **Struggling to survive**, evidenced by battling the system, seeking solace at a support group, praying for relief, and developing strategies
4. **Regaining control**, evidenced by unpredictable transitioning, guarded recovery, mourning lost time, and subsequent consequences

Beck (2015) published *A Middle Range Theory of Traumatic Childbirth: The Ever-Widening Ripple Effect.* The second advancement of Beck's original theory was developed using Morse's method of theoretical coalescence on the subject of traumatic childbirth, posttraumatic stress, and secondary traumatic stress. This is an important distinction because many women have seemingly normal births, yet still develop postpartum depression. Given this notion, a traumatic childbirth can be experienced as traumatic psychologically or physically (Beck, 2015).

In this method, formalizing connections with numerous other studies provides what she describes as a "ripple effect" on the original theory. In the course of adding other studies with various groups (such as age differences), studying concepts in different cultures, and perhaps at differing times during their pregnancy, after the birth, and at various points along the first year after birth, the ripples continue.

Women who identified themselves as having had a traumatic birth were assisted in developing their own strategies for making their next delivery different. Three quarters of the women in the study were able to report their subsequent births as healing, bringing them a new sense of empowerment and a spiritual feeling of reverence for their experience (Beck, 2016).

Of particular concern, however, is the ongoing distress women felt for a child who was born from a traumatic experience. Difficulties in the mother–child relationship have been observed, as has a detrimental effect on their cognitive, social, emotional development, and difficulty breast-feeding.

Importantly, the kind of birth that is deemed traumatic has lasting consequences for the fathers or partners, physicians, midwives, nurses, and other personnel who observe the event. Each are vulnerable to and have been found to suffer from ongoing PTSD. Numerous methods to treat PTSD with veterans are recommended for medical personnel as well. Debriefing appears to be a natural and easy way to begin the process for everyone. Debriefing for nurses working in all areas often seems to come naturally.

CRITIQUE

Clarity

Beck's theory evidences a semantic clarity, because concepts are at the practice level and are defined clearly and consistently. Within and between research reports, Beck uses terms, ideas, definitions, and concepts that reflect growth, yet they are defined and easily understood. Her research and writings use both inductive and deductive language, and her verbiage is economical and clear.

Simplicity

Postpartum depression is a complex phenomenon, experientially and theoretically. Yet Beck's theory of postpartum depression follows a logical progression specific to observations made in nursing practice. It is accessible empirically and theoretically. Importantly, concepts and definitions used for predicting a woman's risk for postpartum depression and concepts and definitions used to screen women for symptoms of postpartum depression are explicit, directly meaningful for women, the lay public, and practitioners of nursing and related disciplines.

Generality

Beck has accounted for the complexity of postpartum depression within the expansion of the concepts within the theory. Generality issues relate to how broadly the theory describes human experience, and this is supported by applicability of the theory in different cultural contexts. Chinn and Kramer (2015) note that generality refers to a theory's ability to remain conceptually simple, yet account for a broad range of empirical experiences. Postpartum depression may be thought of as a relatively narrow experience; however, its nature and causation are especially complex. Importantly, Beck studied the experiences of many women and used research from numerous sources that address postpartum depression in various geographical and cultural groups. Embracing findings from these studies to compare and contrast with the extant theory has given new breadth to the theory and significantly affects its generality.

Accessibility

The PDSS has been subjected to a rigorous statistical process for development and standardization. In 2000 Beck and fellow researcher Gable began examining the psychometric properties of the scale with regard to reliability of the measure within developmental and diagnostic samples. Validity analyses were conducted with the two samples, as were procedures used to establish cutoff scores for clinical interpretations. These studies indicated that the PDSS (Beck, 2002c) is a reliable and valid screening instrument for detection of postpartum depression. Beck has two instruments: the PDSS, which is well established, and the PDPI, which has more recently been found valid and reliable in a wide range of studies from 2000 to the present. An important feature of Beck's theory is its immediate accessibility and dynamic potential to affect women's lives.

Importance

The value of Beck's work is of growing importance within nursing and health care disciplines. Perinatal mood disorders are obviously more than transient inconveniences for women and their families. The sequence of events in the life of women points to the extraordinary need for greater awareness and use of Beck's postpartum depression theory and subsequent developments for prevention, identification, early intervention, and treatment.

There is a growing awareness that the responsibility for identification and early intervention of postpartum depression belongs to more than those who are primarily responsible for caring for women during pregnancy and immediately after birth. Because of consistent interactions with mothers, pediatric and neonatal nurses can make valuable contributions to successful interventions for mothers suffering from postpartum depression. Psychiatric nurses might also be able to identify risk in women (or their children) who do not immediately indicate postpartum depression.

However, knowledge about postpartum depression is developing in a way that sheds light on less obvious consequences. Recently postpartum depression has been linked to adverse effects on children's cognitive and emotional development and behavior problems of older children in school. Postpartum depression could have a negative effect on situations such as substance use, traffic accidents, criminal behaviors, domestic violence, progress in school, employment and income, and many others. A growing awareness within nursing, other health care professionals, and the public will allow greater identification of postpartum depression in the many contexts within which people live their lives.

SUMMARY

The development of Beck's postpartum depression theory is the quintessential example of how creative nursing knowledge is developed from nursing observations, using multiple methods and rigorous testing. The theory was influenced by various theoretical and philosophical stances, adding breadth and texture. Maternity nurses are able to read the theory and understand how to apply it in their practice. Beck and others continue to expand the theory by exploring its applicability to different cultures and exploring ways of reaching women who have potential for its benefit.

Increasingly, nurses and the wider society are recognizing that issues of postpartum depression have not been adequately understood or acknowledged. Nursing, like other health care professions, has been shocked by unanticipated events when postpartum depression leads to untoward outcomes that appear in the evening news. Even among nurses and other health professionals, their knowledge does not mitigate the effects of this illness. Tragic news events carried out by troubled mothers point out the importance of this theory. Dr. Cheryl Tatano Beck's work demonstrates how nursing research provides evidence to understand and care for women experiencing postpartum depression. Her research and instruments facilitate detection, early intervention, and treatment.

CASE STUDY

At the tender age of 11 years, Kim was "sold" by her mother to three adult men for an evening of sex and drugs. Kim related that as her mother went out the door, she advised her to "do what they tell you and I'll be back in the morning." Kim was never okay again. Although she did relatively well during the sporadic times she went to school, her life was a series of drug and sex binges. At 17, Kim was in jail and pregnant. She had been arrested several times and released, but the judge insisted that this time she stay incarcerated until after the baby was born to guarantee the baby would be crack-free at birth. Kim's prenatal records, however, did not indicate drug or alcohol use, and neither did her jail records. She adamantly insisted that she never used drugs or alcohol once she found out she was pregnant (late in the first trimester). Through a series of misunderstandings, she was released 2 weeks before the baby's birth. However, Kim did well, continued to stay drug-free, refused medication during labor, and delivered a beautiful healthy baby—a baby whose blood test results were negative for drugs.

Kim recalls that she began motherhood believing this would be the event that would turn her life around. It did for several weeks, but slowly Kim became involved in her old life. She received money to buy clothes and food for her baby. Despite that help, however, Kim had no place to live and no money to support herself. She never held a legal job in her life. She qualified for postpartum medical care for 6 weeks, but after that she was on her own.

When the baby was 7 months old, Kim called a nurse who had once cared for her during her pregnancy and asked for help to give her daughter up for adoption. She believed she would simply never be able to give her baby the life she knew all babies deserved. Kim was using drugs again, and the baby was being kept by whoever was in the mood to do so. Kim absolutely loved this baby, and the choice for adoption came from this love. Kim chose a local Christian adoption agency. Staff there gave her the opportunity to read the profiles of potential families, see pictures of them, and actually choose the family who would raise her baby. Though she did not know the family's name or address, the family and the agency committed to regular photographs and updates about her daughter.

Without resources or support, and without her baby, Kim returned to the only life she had ever known among the only people she really knew. Eighteen months later, Kim gave birth to another baby. This time, she swore things would be different. When this new baby was also about 7 months old, Kim found herself deeply involved in crack use, with her baby being passed around from relative to relative and from friend to friend. Unfortunately, Kim was present during the commission of a violent crime with a predictably tragic outcome. Although Kim did not actually commit this crime, she was present and was ultimately sent to prison.

Kim once remarked that she loved being pregnant, loved giving birth, and loved the idea of being a mother. She said, "It would be great in the beginning, but after a couple of months I'd start feeling bad. It seems like with both my babies that around 6 or 7 months, I just couldn't handle anything."

Although Kim took the baby to a pediatrician for follow-up care, none of those care providers knew her or knew her history—they were primarily concerned with her son's health. Kim's affect was usually very upbeat; she smiled easily. It was not likely that anyone ever asked her any important questions about her life or her experience of being a mother. Kim was, for all intents and purposes, "lost to follow-up."

Kim's story illustrates the kinds of complexities that can make postpartum depression especially challenging for women who live amid drugs and chaos. In the midst of this life, women still want to be good mothers and have the same hopes and same dreams we all have. Drugs, alcohol, crimes, and all the other ways Kim's life was chaotic were the only avenues by which she received services—after-the-fact services.

Interventions by others could have made a difference at many points in Kim's life. One of these points was during her prenatal period. She clearly evidenced most of the risk factors for postpartum depression, despite her cheerful attitude toward the pregnancy. If you had been a nurse caring for Kim during her prenatal care and identified her to be at risk for postpartum depression, what kind of care plan would you have developed before or after her baby's birth? Would you have been willing to intervene on behalf of Kim or her baby, even though their needs occurred within the community and not in the confines of a hospital or office?

CRITICAL THINKING ACTIVITIES

1. Interview a friend or family member about her prenatal and postnatal feelings.
2. Analyze the interview to address the following questions.
   - Did she have feelings that you expected? Did she share any that surprised you?
   - Were her experiences suggestive of risk for postpartum depression?
3. Explore the resources available on the Internet for postpartum women.
4. What resources are available in your community for women with postpartum depression?

POINTS FOR FURTHER STUDY

- Beck, C. T. (1998, 2002a). Postpartum Depression Predictors Inventory (PDPI). Available from *Journal of Obstetric, Gynecologic, & Neonatal Nursing,* published on behalf of the Association of Women's Health, Obstetrics and Neonatal Nurses, by Sage Science Press, an imprint of Sage Publications.
- Beck, C. T., & Gable, R. K. (2000, 2003). *Postpartum Depression Screening Scale (PDSS).* Available through Western Psychological Services, 12031 Wilshire Blvd., Los Angeles, CA 90025–1251.
- Cheryl, T. (2016). Beck interview. *Nursing Theorists: Portraits of Excellence, Vol. III.* Athens, Ohio: Fitne, Inc.

REFERENCES

Beck, C. T. (1993). Teetering on the edge: A substantive theory of postpartum depression. *Nursing Research, 42*(1), 42–48.

Beck, C. T. (1998). Postpartum Depression Predictors Inventory (PDPI). *Journal of Obstetric, Gynecologic, & Neonatal Nursing.*

Beck, C. T. (2002a). Revision of the Postpartum Depression Predictors Inventory (PDPI). *Journal of Obstetric, Gynecologic, and Neonatal Nursing, 31*(4), 394–402.

Beck, C. T. (2002b). Postpartum depression: A meta-synthesis of qualitative research. *Qualitative Health Research, 12*(4), 453–472.

Beck, C. T. (2002c). *Postpartum Depression Screening Scale (PDSS): Manual.* Los Angeles: Western Psychological Services.

Beck, C. T. (2012). Exemplar: Teetering on the edge: A second grounded theory modification. In P. L. Munhall (Ed.), *Nursing research: A qualitative perspective* (5th ed., pp. 257–284). Sudbury, MA: Jones & Bartlett.

Beck, C. T. (2015). A middle-range theory of traumatic childbirth: The ever widening ripple effect. *Global Qualitative Nursing Research.* Vol. 2, open access doi: 1177/2333393615575313.

Beck, C. T. (2016). Posttraumatic stress disorder after birth: A metaphor analysis. *American Journal of Maternal Child Nursing, 41*(2), 76–83.

Beck, C. T., & Gable, R. K. (2000). Postpartum depression screening scale: Development and psychometric testing. *Nursing Research, 49*(5), 272–282.

Beck, C. T., & Gable, R. K. (2003). Postpartum Depression Screening Scale—Spanish version. *Nursing Research, 52*(5), 296–306.

Beck, C. T., Driscoll, J. W., & Watson, S. (2014). *Traumatic childbirth.* New York: Routledge.

Beck, C. T., & Watson, S. (2010). Subsequent childbirth after a previous traumatic birth. *Nursing Research, 59*(4), 241–249.

Chinn, P., & Kramer, M. (2015). *Integrated theory and knowledge development in nursing* (9th ed.). St Louis, MO: Mosby-Elsevier.

Colaizzi, P. (1978). Psychological research as the phenomenologist views it. In R. Valle & M. King (Eds.), *Existential phenomenological alternative for psychology* (pp. 48–71). New York: Oxford University Press.

Davidson, M., London, M., & Ladewig, P. (2012). *Olds' maternal-newborn nursing & women's health across the lifespan* (9th ed.). Upper Saddle River, NJ: Prentice Hall.

Glaser, B. (1978). *Theoretical sensitivity: Advances in the methodology of grounded theory.* Mill Valley, CA: Sociology Press.

Glaser, B., & Strauss, A. (1967). *The discovery of grounded theory.* Chicago: Aldine.

Hutchinson, S. (1986). Grounded theory: The method. In P. Munhall & C. Oiler (Eds.), *Nursing research: A qualitative perspective* (pp. 111–130). Norwalk, CT: Appleton-Century-Crofts.

Lavoie, K. (2015). Five E's to support mothers with postpartum depression for breastfeeding success. *International Journal of Childbirth Education, 30*(2), 55–61.

Polit, D., & Beck, C. T. (2003). *Nursing research: Generating and assessing evidence for nursing practice, North American Edition* (7th ed.). Philadelphia: Lippincott.

Polit, D., & Beck, C. T. (2011). *Nursing research: Generating and assessing evidence for nursing practice, North American Edition* (9th ed.). Philadelphia: Lippincott.

Sichel, D., & Driscoll, J. (1999). *Women's moods.* New York: HarperCollins.

BIBLIOGRAPHY

Beck, C. T. (1992). The lived experience of postpartum depression: A phenomenological study. *Nursing Research, 41,* 166–170.

Beck, C. T. (2003). Recognizing and screening for postpartum depression in mothers of NICU infants. *Advances in Neonatal Care, 3*, 37–46.
Beck, C. T. (2004). Birth trauma: In the eye of the beholder. *Nursing Research, 53*, 28–35.
Beck, C. T. (2004). Posttraumatic stress disorder due to childbirth: The aftermath. *Nursing Research, 53*, 216–224.
Beck, C. T. (2005). Benefits of participating in Internet interviews: Women helping women. *Qualitative Health Research, 15*, 411–422.
Beck, C. T. (2006). Acculturation: Implications for perinatal research. *Maternal Child Nursing, 31*(2), 114–120.
Beck, C. T. (2006). The anniversary of birth trauma: Failure to rescue. *Nursing Research, 55*(6), 381–390.
Beck, C. T. (2006). Pentadic cartography: Mapping birth trauma narratives. *Qualitative Health Research, 16*, 453–466.
Beck, C. T. (2006). Postpartum depression: It isn't just the blues. *American Journal of Nursing, 106*(5), 40–50.
Beck, C. T. (2007). Exemplar: Teetering on the edge: A continually emerging theory of postpartum depression. In P. Munhall (Ed.), *Nursing research: A qualitative perspective* (4th ed., pp. 273–292). Boston: Jones & Bartlett.
Beck, C. T. (2008). The nurses' vantage point. In S. D. Stone & A. E. Menken (Eds.), *Perinatal and postpartum mood disorders: Perspectives and treatment guide for the healthcare practitioner* (pp. 203–217). New York: Springer.
Beck, C. T. (2008). *Postpartum mood and anxiety disorders: Case studies, research, and nursing care*. Washington, DC: Association of Women's Health, Obstetrics, and Neonatal Nursing.
Beck, C. T. (2008). State of the science on postpartum depression: What nurse researchers have contributed. Part 1. *American Journal of Maternal Child Nursing, 33*, 121–126.
Beck, C. T. (2008). State of the science on postpartum depression: What nurse researchers have contributed. Part 2. *American Journal of Maternal Child Nursing, 33*, 151–156, quiz 157–158.
Beck, C. T. (2009). An adult survivor of childhood sexual abuse and her breastfeeding experience: A case study. *American Journal of Maternal Child Nursing, 34*, 91–97.
Beck, C. T. (2009). The arm: There's no escaping the reality for mothers caring for their children with obstetric brachial plexus injuries. *Nursing Research, 58*, 237–245.
Beck, C. T. (2009). Birth trauma and its sequelae. *Journal of Trauma and Dissociation, 10*, 189–203.
Beck, C. T. (2009). Critiquing qualitative research. *AORN Journal, 90*, 543–554.
Beck, C. T. (2009). Viewing the rich, diverse landscape of qualitative research. *Perioperative Nursing Clinics, 4*, 217–229.
Beck, C. T. (2011). Developing a research program using qualitative and quantitative approaches. *Japanese Journal of Nursing Research, 44*, 371–379.
Beck, C. T. (2011). A metaethnography of traumatic childbirth and its aftermath: Amplifying causal looping. *Qualitative Health Research, 21*, 301–311.
Beck, C. T. (2011). Meta synthesis: Helping qualitative research take its rightful place in the hierarchy of evidence. *Japanese Journal of Nursing Research, 44*, 352–370.
Beck, C. T. (2011). Revealing the subtle differences among postpartum mood and anxiety disorders: Phenomenology holds the key. In G. Thomson, F. Dykes, & S. Downe (Eds.), *Qualitative research in midwifery and childbirth: Phenomenological approaches* (pp. 193–214). New York: Routledge.
Beck, C. T. (2011). Secondary traumatic stress in nurses: A systematic review. *Archives of Psychiatric Nursing, 25*, 1–10.
Beck, C. T. (2012). A metaethnography of traumatic childbirth and its aftermath: Amplifying causal looping. *Qualitative Health Research, 21*(3), 301–311.
Beck, C. T., & Barnes, D. L. (2006). Post-traumatic stress disorder in pregnancy. *Annals of the American Psychotherapy Association, summer*, 4–9.
Beck, C. T., & Driscoll, J. W. (2006). *Postpartum mood and anxiety disorders: A clinician's guide*. Sudbury, MA: Jones & Bartlett.
Beck, C. T., Froman, R., & Bernal, H. (2005). Acculturation level and postpartum depression in Hispanic mothers. *American Journal of Maternal Child Nursing, 30*, 299–304.
Beck, C. T., & Gable, R. K. (2001). Comparative analysis of the performance of the Postpartum Depression Screening Scale with two other depression instruments. *Nursing Research, 50*, 242–250.
Beck, C. T., & Gable, R. K. (2001). Ensuring content validity: An illustration of the process. *Journal of Nursing Measurement, 9*(2), 201–215.
Beck, C. T., & Gable, R. K. (2001). Further validation of the Postpartum Depression Screening Scale. *Nursing Research, 50*, 155–164.
Beck, C. T., & Gable, R. K. (2001). Item response theory in affective instrument development: An illustration. *Journal of Nursing Measurement, 9*, 5–22.
Beck, C. T., & Gable, R. K. (2005). The Postpartum Depression Screening Scale (PDSS). In C. Henshaw & S. Elliott (Eds.), *Screening for perinatal depression* (pp. 133–140). London: Jessica Kingley.
Beck, C. T., & Gable, R. K. (2005). Screening performance of the Postpartum Depression Screening Scale—Spanish version. *Journal of Transcultural Nursing, 16*, 331–338.
Beck, C. T., Gable, R. K., Sakala, C., & Declercq, E. R. (2011). Postpartum depressive symptomology: Results from a two-stage U.S. national survey. *Journal of Midwifery & Women's Health, 56*(5), 427–435.
Beck, C. T., Records, K., & Rice, M. (2006). Further validation of the Postpartum Depression Predictors Inventory—Revised. *Journal of Obstetric, Gynecologic, and Neonatal Nursing, 35*, 735–745.
Beck, C. T., & Watson, S. (2008). The impact of birth trauma on breastfeeding: A tale of two pathways. *Nursing Research, 57*, 228–236.
Freda, M. C., Beck, C. T., Campbell, D. E., Dell, D. L., & Ratcliffe, S. (2011). Quality improvement opportunities in postpartum care. In *March of Dimes. Toward improving the outcome of pregnancy III* (pp. 88–100). New York: March of Dimes.
Oppo, A., Mauri, M., Ramacciotti, D., et al. (2009). Risk factors for postpartum depression: The role of the Postpartum Depression Predictors Inventory-Revised (PDPI-R). *Archives of Women's Mental Health, 12*, 239–249.

Segre, L., O'Hara, M., & Beck, C. T. (2010). Nursing care for postpartum depression. Part I: Do nurses think they should offer both screening and counseling? *American Journal of Maternal Child Health Nursing, 35*, 220–225.

Segre, L., O'Hara, M., & Beck, C. T. (2010). Screening and counseling for postpartum depression by nurses Part II: Women's views. *American Journal of Maternal Child Health Nursing, 35*, 280–285.

Bibliography of Research Using the Screening Scale

Baker, L., & Oswalt, K. (2008). Screening for postpartum depression in a rural community. *Community Mental Health Journal, 44*, 171–180.

Boyd, R. C., & Worley, H. (2007). Utility of the Postpartum Depression Screening Scale among low-income ethnic minority women. In A. I. Rosenfield (Ed.), *New research on postpartum depression* (pp. 151–166). Happauge, NY: Nova Science Publishers, Inc.

Callister, L., Beckstrand, R. L., & Corbett, C. (2011). Postpartum depression and help-seeking behaviors in immigrant Hispanic women. *Journal of Obstetric, Gynecologic, & Neonatal Nursing, 40*, 440–449.

Cantilino, A., Carvalho, J. A., Maia, A., Albuquerque, C., Cantilino, G., & Sougey, E. B. (2007). Translation, validation and cultural aspects of Postpartum Depression Screening scale in Brazilian Portuguese. *Transcultural Psychiatry, 44*(4), 672–684.

Clarke, P. (2008). Validation of two postpartum depression scales with a sample of First Nations and Metis women. *Canadian Journal of Nursing Research, 40*, 113–125.

Davis, S., Cross, J., & Link, B. K. (2008). Exploring the Postpartum Adjustment Questionnaire a predictor of postpartum depression. *Journal of Obstetric, Gynecologic & Neonatal Nursing, 37*, 622–630.

De Alencar, A. E., Arraes, L. C., de Albuquerque, E. C., & Alves, J. G. (2008). Effect of kangaroo mother care on postpartum depression. *Journal of Tropical Pediatrics, 55*(1), 36–38.

Karacam, Z., & Kitiis, Y. (2008). The Postpartum Depression Screening Scale: Its reliability and validity for the Turkish population. *Turkish Journal of Psychiatry, 19*(2), 187–196.

Le, H. N., Perry, D. F., & Sheng, X. (2009). Using the Internet to screen for postpartum depression. *Maternal Child Health Journal, 13*, 213–221.

Le, H. N., Perry D. F., & Ortiz G. (2010). The Postpartum Depression Screening Scale-Spanish version: Examining the psychometric properties and prevalence of risk for postpartum depression. *Journal of Immigrant Minority Health, 12*, 249–258.

Li, L., Liu, F., Zhang, H., Wang, L., & Chen X. (2011). Chinese version of the Postpartum Depression Screening Scale: Translation and validation. *Nursing Research, 60*, 231–239.

Pereira, A. T., Bos, S., Marques, M., et al. (2010). The Portuguese version of the postpartum Depression Screening Scale. *Journal of Psychosomatic Obstetrics & Gynecology, 31*, 90–100.

Pereira, A. T., Bos, S. C., Marques, M., et al. (2011). The Postpartum Depression Screening Scale: Is it valid to screen for antenatal depression? *Archives of Women's Mental Health, 14*, 227–238.

Postmontier, B. (2008). Sleep quality with and without postpartum depression. *Journal of Obstetric, Gynecologic, and Neonatal Nursing, 37*, 722–737.

Quelopana, A. M., & Champion, J. D. (2010). Validation of the Postpartum Depression Screening Scale Spanish version in women from Arica, Chili. *Ciencia y Enfermeria, 16*, 37–47.

Zubaran, C., & Foresti, K. (2011). Investigating quality of life and depressive symptoms in the postpartum period. *Women and Birth, 24*, 10–16.

Zubaran, C., Foresti, K., Schumacher, M. V., et al. (2009). Validation of a screening instrument for postpartum depression in Southern Brazil. *Journal of Psychosomatic Obstetrics & Gynecology, 30*, 244–254.

Zubaran, C., Foresti, K., Schumacher, M. V., Amoretti, A. L., Thorell, M. R., & Müller, L. C. (2010). The correlation between postpartum depression and health status. *Maternal Child Health Journal, 14*, 751–757.

Zubaran, C., Schumacher, M. V., Foresti, K., Thorell, M. R., Amoretti, A., & Müller, L. (2010). The Portuguese version of the Postpartum Depression Screening Scale-Short Form. *Journal of Obstetrics and Gynaecology Research, 36*, 950–957.

Zubaran, C., Schumacher, M., Roxo, M. R., & Foresti, K. (2010). Screening tools for postpartum depression: Validity and cultural dimensions. *African Journal of Psychiatry, 13*, 357–366.

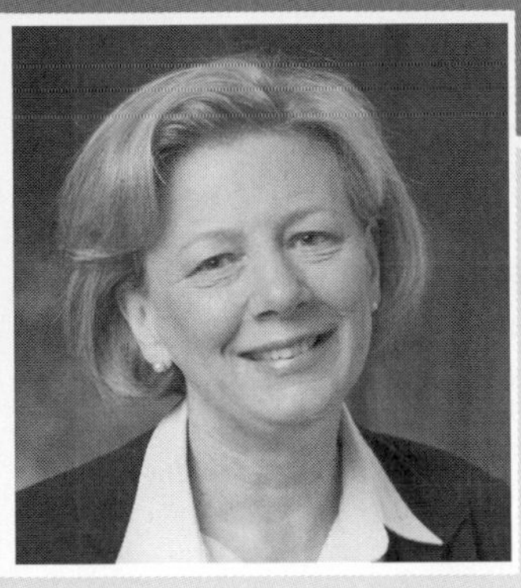
Kristen M. Swanson
(1953–Present)

Theory of Caring

Danuta M. Wojnar

"Caring is a nurturing way of relating to a valued other toward whom one feels a personal sense of commitment and responsibility."
(Swanson, 1991, p. 162)

CREDENTIALS AND BACKGROUND OF THE THEORIST

Kristen M. Swanson, RN, PhD, FAAN, was born in Providence, Rhode Island. She earned her baccalaureate degree (magna cum laude) from the University of Rhode Island, College of Nursing in 1975. She began her career as a registered nurse at the University of Massachusetts Medical Center in Worcester, because the founding nursing administration clearly articulated a vision for professional nursing practice and actively worked with nurses to apply these ideals while working with clients (Swanson, 2001).

As a novice nurse, more than anything Swanson wanted to become a knowledgeable and technically skillful practitioner with a goal of teaching others. Hence she pursued graduate studies in Adult Health and Illness Nursing at the University of Pennsylvania in Philadelphia. After receiving a master's degree in nursing in 1978, she worked briefly as a clinical instructor of medical-surgical nursing at the University of Pennsylvania School of Nursing and subsequently enrolled in the Ph.D. in Nursing program at the University of Colorado in Denver. There she studied psychosocial nursing with an emphasis on the concepts of loss, stress, coping, interpersonal relationships, person and personhood, environments, and caring.

While a doctoral student, as part of a hands-on experience with a self-selected health promotion activity, Swanson participated in a cesarean birth support group focused on miscarriage. The guest speaker, a physician, focused on pathophysiology and health problems prevalent after miscarriage, but women attending the meeting were more interested in talking about their personal experiences with pregnancy loss. That day Swanson decided to learn more about the human experience and responses to miscarrying. Caring and miscarriage became the focus of her doctoral dissertation and subsequently her program of research.

Swanson received an individually awarded National Research Service postdoctoral fellowship from the National Center for Nursing Research, which she completed under the direction of Dr. Kathryn E. Barnard at the University of Washington in Seattle. She joined the faculty at the University of Washington School of Nursing and continued her scholarly work as professor and chairperson of the Department of Family Child Nursing until summer 2009. In addition to teaching and administrative responsibilities at the University of Washington, she conducted research funded by the National Institutes of Nursing Research; published, mentored faculty and students, and served as a consultant at national and international levels. She has been an invited speaker or visiting professor on multiple occasions, including Karolinska Institute in Sweden, IWK (Isaac Walton Killam) Health Centre; a tertiary care hospital for women, children, and families in Halifax, Nova Scotia, Canada; and, most recently, the National Cheng Kung University in Taiwan, Taiwan. While at the University of Washington, from 2004 to 2009 Swanson also held the University of Washington Medical Center Term Professorship in Nursing Leadership. In 2009 she was appointed Dean and Alumni Distinguished Professor at the University of North Carolina (UNC) School of Nursing at Chapel Hill and Associate Chief Nursing

Officer for Academic Affairs at UNC Hospitals. Swanson returned to Seattle in 2014, where she was appointed Dean at Seattle University College of Nursing, a position she holds currently.

Dr. Swanson continues her scholarship, which in recent years shifted to translational research and consulting with various organizations to enact her theory of caring in clinical practice, education, and research. Her service contributions to health care include membership on the Board of Trustees of Swedish Health System in Seattle; Board of Directors for the American Association of Colleges of Nursing (AACN); and editorial board or reviewer for *Journal of Nursing Scholarship, Nursing Outlook, Research in Nursing and Health,* and the *International Journal of Human Caring.* In recognition of many outstanding contributions to the nursing discipline, among other honors, Swanson was inducted as a fellow in the American Academy of Nursing in 1991, received a Distinguished Alumnus Award from the University of Rhode Island in 2002, was selected as a fellow for the Robert Wood Johnson Foundation (RWJF) Nurse Executive Fellows program in 2004, and was selected to serve as a member of the RWJF National Advisory Committee (NAC) to the Faculty Nurse Scholars Program.

THEORETICAL SOURCES

Swanson has drawn on various theoretical sources while developing her theory of caring. She recalls that from the beginning of her nursing career, her education and clinical experience made her acutely aware of the profound difference caring made in the lives of people she served:

> *Watching patients move into a space of total dependency and come out the other side restored was like witnessing miracles unfold. Sitting with spouses in the waiting room while they entrusted the heart (and lives) of their partner to the surgical team was awe inspiring. It was encouraging to observe the inner reserves family members could call upon in order to hand over that which they could not control. It warmed my heart to be so privileged as to be invited into the spaces that patients and families created in order to endure their transitions through illness, recovery, and, in some instances, death.*
>
> ***(Swanson, 2001, p. 412)***

Swanson credits several nursing scholars for insights that shaped her beliefs about the nursing discipline and influenced her program of research. She acknowledges Dr. Jacqueline Fawcett's course on the conceptual basis of nursing practice, which led her to understand the differences between the goals of nursing and other health disciplines, and to realize that caring for others as they go through life transitions of health, illness, healing, and dying was congruent with her personal values (Swanson, 2001). Swanson chose Dr. Jean Watson as her mentor during her doctoral studies. She attributes the emphasis on exploring the concept of caring in her doctoral dissertation to Dr. Watson's influence. However, despite the close working relationship and emphasis on caring in Swanson's dissertation, Swanson's program of research on caring and miscarriage is not an application of Watson's theory of human caring (Watson, 1979, 1988, 1999). Rather, Swanson and Watson each assert that compatibility of findings on caring in their individual programs of research adds credibility to their theoretical assertions (Swanson, 2001). Swanson acknowledges Dr. Kathryn E. Barnard for encouraging her transition from the interpretive to a contemporary empiricist paradigm and for transferring caring knowledge from her phenomenological investigations to intervention research and clinical practice with women who have miscarried.

MAJOR CONCEPTS & DEFINITIONS

Caring

Caring is a nurturing way of relating to a valued other toward whom one feels a personal sense of commitment and responsibility (Swanson, 1991).

Knowing

Knowing is striving to understand the meaning of an event in the life of the other, avoiding assumptions, focusing on the person cared for, seeking cues, assessing meticulously, and engaging both the one caring and the one cared for in the process of knowing (Swanson, 1991).

Being With

Being with means being emotionally present to the other. It includes being there in person, conveying availability, and sharing feelings without burdening the one cared for (Swanson, 1991).

Doing For

Doing for means to do for others what one would do for self if at all possible, including anticipating needs, comforting, performing skillfully and competently, and protecting the one cared for while preserving his or her dignity (Swanson, 1991).

MAJOR CONCEPTS & DEFINITIONS—cont'd

Enabling

Enabling is facilitating the other's passage through life transitions and unfamiliar events by focusing on the event, informing, explaining, supporting, validating feelings, generating alternatives, thinking things through, and giving feedback (Swanson, 1991).

Maintaining Belief

Maintaining belief is sustaining faith in the other's capacity to get through an event or transition and face a future with meaning, believing in other's capacity and holding him or her in high esteem, maintaining a hope-filled attitude, offering realistic optimism, helping to find meaning, and standing by the one cared for no matter what the situation (Swanson, 1991).

USE OF EMPIRICAL EVIDENCE

Swanson formulated her theory of caring inductively, as a result of several investigations. For her doctoral dissertation, using descriptive phenomenology, she analyzed data from in-depth interviews with 20 women who had recently miscarried. As a result of this phenomenological investigation, Swanson proposed two models: (1) the caring model, and (2) the human experience of miscarriage model. The caring model proposed five basic processes *(knowing, being with, doing for, enabling,* and *maintaining belief)* that give meaning to acts labeled as caring (Swanson-Kauffman, 1985, 1986, 1988a, 1988b). This was foundational for Swanson's (1991) middle-range theory of caring.

While a postdoctoral fellow, Swanson conducted a phenomenological study, exploring what it was like to be a provider of care to vulnerable infants in the neonatal intensive care unit (NICU). Swanson (1990) discovered that the caring processes she identified with women who miscarried were also applicable to mothers, fathers, physicians, and nurses who were responsible for care of infants in the NICU. Hence she retained the wording that described the acts of caring and proposed that all-inclusive care in a complex environment embraces balance among caring (for the self and the one cared for), attaching (to others and roles), managing responsibilities (assigned by self, others, and society), and avoiding bad outcomes (Swanson, 1990).

In a subsequent phenomenological investigation conducted with socially at-risk mothers, Swanson (1991) explored what it had been like for these mothers to receive an intense, long-term nursing intervention. Swanson recalls that after this study she was finally able to define caring and refine the understanding of caring processes. Collectively, phenomenological inquiries with women who miscarried, caregivers in the NICU, and socially at-risk mothers formed a basis for expansion of the caring model into the middle-range theory of caring (Swanson, 1991, 1993).

Swanson tested her theory of caring with women who miscarried in investigations funded by the National Institutes of Nursing Research and other funding sources. Swanson's (1999a, 1999b) intervention research (N = 242) examined the effects of caring-based counseling sessions on women coming to terms with loss and emotional well-being during the first year after miscarrying. Additional aims were examination of the effects of passage of time on healing during that first year and development of strategies to monitor caring interventions. This study established that passing of time had positive effects on women's healing after miscarriage; however, caring interventions had a positive effect on decreasing the overall disturbed mood, anger, and level of depression. The second aim was to monitor the caring variable and determine whether caring was delivered as intended. To do so, caring was monitored in the following three ways:

1. Approximately 10% of counseling sessions were transcribed and data were analyzed using inductive and deductive content analysis.
2. Before each caring session, the counselor completed McNair, Lorr, and Droppleman's (1981) Profile of Mood States to monitor whether the counselor's mood was associated with women's ratings of caring after each session, using an investigator-developed Caring Professional Scale.
3. After each session, the counselor completed an investigator-developed Counselor Rating Scale and took narrative notes about her own counseling.

The most noteworthy finding of monitoring caring was that clients were highly satisfied with caring received during counseling sessions, suggesting caring was delivered and received as intended.

Swanson's (1999c) subsequent investigation was a literary meta-analysis on caring. An in-depth review of 130 investigations on caring led Swanson to propose that knowledge about caring may be categorized into five hierarchical domains (levels), and research conducted in any one domain assumes the presence of all previous domains (Swanson, 1999c).

- The first domain refers to the persons' capacities to deliver caring.
- The second domain refers to individuals' concerns and commitments that lead to caring actions.
- The third domain refers to the conditions (nurse, client, organizational) that enhance or diminish the likelihood of delivering caring.
- The fourth domain refers to actions of caring.
- The fifth domain refers to the consequences or the intentional and unintentional outcomes of caring for both the client and the provider (Swanson, 1999c).

Conducting the literary meta-analysis clarified the meaning of the concept of caring as it is used in the nursing discipline and validated the transferability of Swanson's middle-range theory of caring beyond a perinatal context.

Subsequently, Swanson authored or coauthored numerous scholarly articles and book chapters on the application of caring-healing relationships in clinical practice and education or that tested the theory of caring. Swanson coauthored an article on nursing's historical legacy as a caring-healing profession and the meaning, significance, and consequences of optimal healing environments for modern nursing practice, education, and research (Swanson & Wojnar, 2004).

The article presented the core foci of nursing as a discipline: what it means to be a person and experience personhood; the meaning of health at the individual, family, and societal levels; how environments create or diminish the potential for the promotion, maintenance, or restoration of well-being; and the caring-healing therapeutics of nursing. A book chapter followed to enhance nurses' capacity for compassionate caring (Swanson, 2007). In it, Swanson explored how caring matters to the well-being of every person and described conditions that affect the quality of nurse caring ranging from the interpersonal relationships through physical environments to executive or managerial leadership. Swanson's coauthored works have focused on social and economic factors affecting the nurse shortage and quality of care (Grant & Swanson, 2006) and consumer satisfaction with health care (Mowinski-Jennings et al., 2005). Swanson coauthored findings from an investigation that explored soldiers' experiences with caring in military health care settings (Jennings et al., 2005). Findings suggest that quality of care for soldiers is improved by narrowing the gap between what is offered for them as consumers and what they experience when they seek care. Swanson and colleagues explored complementary and alternative medicine (CAM) attitudes and competencies of nursing students and faculty and the results of integrating CAM into the nursing curriculum as a holistic approach to nursing (Booth-Laforce et al., 2010).

In her own program of research, Swanson tested the usability of the theory of caring. In 2003 Swanson and colleagues published results from an investigation on the effects of miscarriage on interpersonal and sexual relationships during the first year after loss from women's perspectives and investigated the context and evolution of women's responses to miscarriage during the first year after loss (Swanson et al., 2007). In 2009 Swanson and her research team published results of a funded intervention study called Couples Miscarriage Healing Project. The purpose was to better understand the effects of miscarriage on men and women as individuals and as couples, to explore the effects of miscarriage on couple relationships, and to identify the best ways of helping men and women heal as individuals and as couples after unexpected pregnancy loss. Study participants (341 heterosexual couples) were randomly assigned to control or one of the following three treatment groups: (1) nurse caring, which entailed attending three counseling sessions with a nurse; (2) self-caring, which involved completing three videos and workbooks; or (3) combined caring, which involved attending one nurse caring session and completion of three videos and workbooks, to determine the most effective way of supporting couples after miscarriage. Interventions, based on Swanson's theory of caring and meaning of miscarriage model, were offered at 1, 5, and 11 weeks after enrollment. Outcomes included depression using the Center for Epidemiologic Studies Scale (CES-D), grief, pure grief (PG), and grief-related emotions (GRE). Differences in rates of recovery were estimated via multilevel modeling conducted in a Bayesian framework. Bayesian odds (*BO*) ranging from 3.0 to 7.9 showed that nurse caring was most effective for accelerating women's resolution of depression. A *BO* of 3.2 to 6.6 favored nurse caring intervention and no treatment over self and combined caring for resolving men's depression. A *BO* of 3.1 to 7.0 favored all three interventions over no treatment for accelerating women's grief resolution, and a *BO* of 18.7 to 22.6 favored nurse caring and combined caring over self-caring or no treatment for resolving men's grief. A *BO* ranging from 2.4 to 6.1 favored nurse-caring and self-caring over combined caring or no treatment for promoting women's resolution of grief-related emotions. A *BO* from 3.5 to 17.9 favored nurse-caring, combined caring, and control over self-caring for resolving men's grief emotions. Nurse-caring had the overall most positive impact on couples' resolution of grief and depression. In addition, grief resolution was accelerated by self-caring for women and combined caring intervention for men. Researchers concluded that applying the theory of caring in clinical practice is an effective strategy to promote healing after unexpected pregnancy loss for women and men as individuals and as couples.

Swanson continues to contribute to research of others, particularly younger scholars whom she mentors. In 2006 Wojnar and Swanson explored why lesbian mothers should deserve special consideration when it comes to healing after miscarriage. As a result, Wojnar, Swanson, and Adolfsson (2011) revised the conceptual model of miscarriage inclusive of the lesbian population for clinical practice and research. Recently Swanson coauthored an article based on the secondary analysis of her data, investigating the influence of gender and reproductive factors on the impact of miscarriage (Huffman, Schwartz, & Swanson, 2015).

Swanson coauthored results from a study that explored the experiences of parents after moderate to severe traumatic brain injury of their child (Roscigno & Swanson, 2011) as well as the quality of life for children after traumatic brain injury (Roscigno et al., 2011), where participants described health and cultural barriers leading to misunderstandings that could be easily prevented. Swanson and colleagues also explored parental grief responses and caring needs in other contexts—for example, grief of parents at risk for giving birth to an extremely premature infant (Kavanaugh et al., 2015).

Likewise, she coauthored an article based on research to investigate experiences of parents whose children were born with a congenital heart defect and required surgery (Wei et al., 2016). Collectively, these works contribute to a growing body of evidence that Swanson's caring theory is being used in a variety of empirical investigations, in addition to education and clinical practice.

MAJOR ASSUMPTIONS

In 1993 Swanson further developed her theory of informed caring by making her major assumptions explicit about the four main phenomena of concern to the nursing discipline: **nursing**, **person-client**, **health**, and **environment**.

Nursing

Swanson (1991, 1993) defines nursing as informed caring for the well-being of others. She asserts that the nursing discipline is informed by empirical knowledge from nursing and related disciplines, as well as "ethical, personal and aesthetic knowledge derived from the humanities, clinical experience, and personal and societal values and expectations" (Swanson, 1993, p. 352).

Person

Swanson (1993) defines persons as "unique beings who are in the midst of becoming and whose wholeness is made manifest in thoughts, feelings, and behaviors" (p. 352). She posits that the life experiences individuals are influenced by are a complex interplay of "genetic heritage, spiritual endowment and the capacity to exercise free will" (Swanson, 1993, p. 352). Hence persons both shape and are shaped by the environment in which they live.

Swanson (1993) views persons as dynamic, growing, self-reflecting, yearning to be connected with others, and spiritual beings. She suggests the following: "spiritual endowment connects each being to an eternal and universal source of goodness, mystery, life, creativity, and serenity. The spiritual endowment may be a soul, higher power/Holy Spirit, positive energy, or, simply grace. Free will equates with choice and the capacity to decide how to act when confronted with a range of possibilities" (p. 352). Swanson (1993) noted, however, that limitations set by race, class, gender, or access to care might prevent individuals from exercising free will. Hence acknowledging free will mandates the nursing discipline to honor individuality and consider a range of possibilities that are acceptable or desirable to those whom the nurses attend.

Moreover, Swanson posits that the other, whose personhood nursing discipline serves, refers to families, groups, and societies. Thus with this understanding of personhood, nurses are mandated to take on leadership roles in fighting for human rights, equal access to health care, and other humanitarian causes. Lastly, when nurses think about the other to whom they direct their caring, they also need to think of self and other nurses and their care as that cared-for other.

Health

According to Swanson, to experience health and well-being is:

> *"to live the subjective, meaning-filled experience of wholeness. Wholeness involves a sense of integration and becoming wherein all facets of being are free to be expressed. The facets of being include the many selves that make us a human: our spirituality, thoughts, feelings, intelligence, creativity, relatedness, femininity, masculinity, and sexuality, to name just a few."*
>
> ***(1993, p. 353)***

Thus Swanson reestablishes well-being as a complex process of curing and healing that includes "releasing inner pain, establishing new meanings, restoring integration, and emerging into a sense of renewed wholeness" (Swanson, 1993, p. 353).

Environment

Swanson (1993) defines environment as situational. She maintains that for nursing it is "any context that influences or is influenced by the designated client" (p. 353). Swanson states there are many influences on environment, such as the cultural, social, biophysical, political, and economic realms, to name only a few. According to Swanson (1993), the terms *environment* and *person-client* in nursing may be viewed interchangeably. For example, Swanson posits, "for heuristic purposes the lens on environment/designated client may be specified to the intraindividual level, wherein the 'client' may be at the cellular level and the environment may be the organs, tissues or body of which the cell is a component" (p. 353). Therefore what is considered an environment in one situation may be considered a client in another.

THEORETICAL ASSERTIONS

Swanson's theory of caring (Swanson, 1991, 1993, 1999a) was empirically derived through phenomenological inquiry. It offers a clear explanation of what it means for nurses to practice in a caring manner and emphasizes that the goal of nursing is promotion of well-being. Swanson (1991) defines caring as "a nurturing way of relating to a valued other toward whom one feels a personal sense of commitment and responsibility" (p. 162).

According to Swanson, a fundamental and universal component of good nursing is caring for the client's biopsychosocial and spiritual well-being. Swanson (1993) asserts that caring is grounded in maintenance of a basic belief in human beings, supported by knowing the client's reality, conveyed by being emotionally and physically present, and enacted by doing for and enabling the client. The caring processes overlap and may not exist in separation. Each is an integral component of the overarching structure of caring (Fig. 35.1). Swanson (1993) noted that the repertoire of caring therapeutics of novice nurses may be limited and restricted by inexperience. Conversely, the techniques and knowledge imbedded in caring of experienced nurses are elaborate and subtle, so caring may go unnoticed by an uninformed observer. Yet Swanson (1993) asserts that, regardless of the years of nursing experience, caring is delivered as a set of sequential processes (subconcepts) created by the nurse's own philosophical attitude (maintaining belief), understanding (knowing), verbal and nonverbal messages conveyed to the client (being with), therapeutic actions (doing for and enabling), and the consequences of caring (intended client outcome).

LOGICAL FORM

Swanson's middle-range theory of caring was developed empirically using an inductive approach. Chinn and Kramer (2015) note, "With induction people induce hypotheses and relationships by observing or experiencing an empiric reality and reaching some conclusion" (p. 184). Swanson's theory was generated from phenomenological investigations with women who experienced unexpected pregnancy loss, caregivers of premature and ill babies in the newborn intensive care unit (NICU), and socially at-risk mothers who received long-term care from master's-prepared nurses. Swanson claims that her in-depth meta-analysis of research on caring has supported the generality of her theory beyond a perinatal context (Swanson, 1999c).

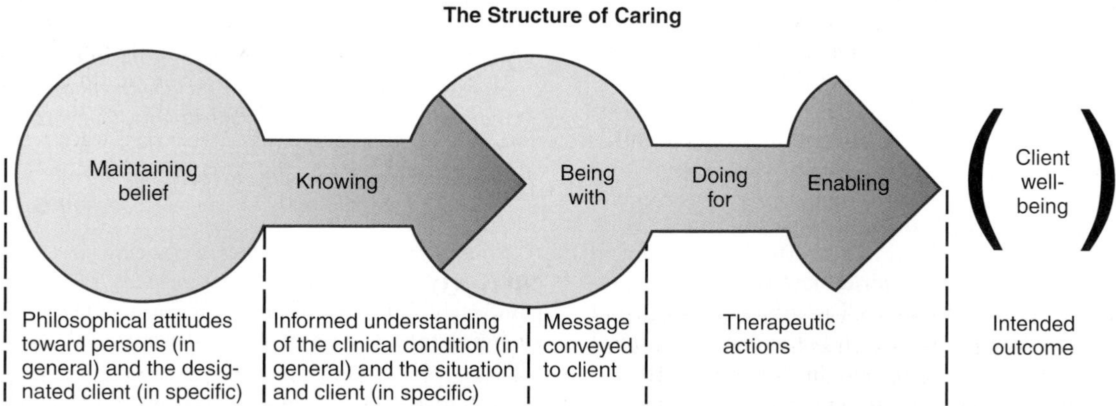

FIG. 35.1 The structure of caring as linked to the nurse's philosophical attitude, informed understandings, message conveyed, therapeutic actions, and intended outcome. (From Swanson, K. M. [1993]. Nursing as informed caring for the well-being of others. *Image: The Journal of Nursing Scholarship, 25*[4], 352–357.)

ACCEPTANCE BY THE NURSING COMMUNITY

Practice

The usefulness of Swanson's theory of caring has been demonstrated in research, education, and clinical practice. The proposition that caring is central to nursing practice had its beginning in the theorist's own insights into the importance of caring in professional nursing practice and in findings from Swanson's phenomenological investigations. Her subsequent investigations demonstrated applicability of the theory of caring in clinical nursing practice, education, and research. Swanson's theory has been embraced as a framework for professional nursing practice in the United States, Canada, and Sweden. An example is the Dalhousie University School of Nursing in Halifax, Nova Scotia, Canada, which selected Swanson's theory of caring to guide the development of future generations of nurses as caring professionals in the early 2000s and continues to this day. Likewise, nurses at the IWK Health Centre in Halifax recognized the traditional legacy of nursing as a caring-healing discipline in 1998 and continue to use Swanson's theory of caring as their framework for professional nursing practice.

Nurse caring is manifested in different ways and practice contexts. For example, in a postpartum context, demonstration of a baby bath to new parents incorporates all five caring processes. The act involves *being with* by demonstrating bathing the newborn to the parents. The unrushed timing of the bath so the infant is awake and parents are present conveys willingness *(doing for or enabling);* and the observing, querying, and involving parents in the task engages them in their own infant's care *(intended outcome)* while acknowledging that they are perfectly capable of caring for their new child and that their preferences matter *(knowing and maintaining belief)*. In carrying out this seemingly simple act, the nurse creates an optimal environment for learning that enables new parents to make decisions about infant care, while leveraging the task as an opportunity to engage in a meaningful social encounter and developing a trusting relationship.

Education

Humane and altruistic caring occurs when the theory is used in various practice areas such as feeding or grooming an incapacitated older adult, monitoring and managing the recovery of a patient who suffered a stroke, or enhancing infant care skills of new parents. Nurse caring, as demonstrated by Swanson in research with women who miscarried, caregivers in the NICU, and socially at-risk mothers, recognizes the importance for nurses to attend to the wholeness of humans in their everyday lives. Thus Swanson's theory offers nurse educators a simple way of initiating students into the profession by immersing them in the language of what it means to be caring and cared for to promote, restore, or maintain the optimal wellness of individuals.

Research

Swanson has persisted in the development of her theory, describing and defining the concept of caring and basic caring processes, instrument development, and testing in intervention research with women and men who have experienced unexpected pregnancy loss. A search of computerized databases (MEDLINE, CINHAL, and Digital Dissertations) indicated that Swanson's work on caring and miscarriage has been cited or otherwise used in more than 190 data-based publications. Examples of applications of Swanson's theory of caring in clinical practice include exploring clinical scholarship in practice (Kish & Holder, 1996); guidelines for nurses working with patients diagnosed with multiple sclerosis (Yorkston, Klasner, & Swanson, 2001); assessing the effects of caring in work with vulnerable populations (Kavanaugh et al., 2006); the importance of creating a caring environment for older adults (Sikma, 2006); Wojnar's (2007) study of lesbian couples who miscarried; Roscigno's research of children who sustained traumatic brain injury (Roscigno et al., 2011; Roscigno & Swanson, 2011), and parents' whose children require surgery for a congenital heart defect (Wei et al., 2016).

FURTHER DEVELOPMENT

Swanson is interested in further development by testing and applying her theory in clinical practice. There is much potential for further development by testing Swanson's theory of caring in various contexts of health and illness. Also, her processes of caring suggest that the theory is applicable in other helping disciplines such as teaching, social work, and medicine as well as additional life situations for nursing.

CRITIQUE

Clarity

The concept of caring and caring processes (knowing, being with, doing for, enabling, and maintaining belief) that are central to the theory are clearly defined and arranged in a logical sequence that describes the processes of caring delivery. Swanson's theory offers clear definitions and contextual linkages with the concepts of the nursing discipline (person, nurse, environment, and health) in nurse–client interactions, thus further explicating the definitions.

Simplicity

A simple theory has a minimal number of concepts. Swanson's theory of caring is simple yet elegant. It brings the importance of caring to the forefront and exemplifies the discipline's values. The main purpose of the theory is the delivery of nursing care focused on the needs of individuals while fostering their dignity, respect, and empowerment. Simplicity and consistent language used to define the concepts and processes allow students and nurses to understand and apply Swanson's theory in their practice.

Generality

Swanson's theory of caring may be applied in research and clinical work with diverse populations. The conditions essential for delivering caring that promotes individuals' wholeness across the lifespan have been described clearly (Swanson, 1999c). Hence the theory is generalizable to nurse–client relationships in many clinical settings.

Accessibility

Swanson's theory of caring concepts and assumptions are grounded in clinical nursing practice and research using an empirical approach. The completeness and simplicity of operational definitions strengthen empirical precision of this theory. Swanson and others have successfully applied her theory in numerous studies. Swanson and her research team tested the theory of caring in a clinical trial with women and men who experienced miscarriage and demonstrated that caring intervention resulted in decreased depressive mood and facilitated healthy grieving for both genders. Swanson has published research guidelines with colleagues for assessing the impact of caring-healing relationships in clinical nursing (Quinn et al., 2003) and developed self-report instruments to measure caring as delivered by health care professionals and by couples to each other (Swanson, 2002). The template for delivering caring-based interventions and the research-based instruments open possibilities for use and further testing with other populations.

Importance

Swanson's theory of caring describes nurse–client relationships that promote wholeness and healing. The theory offers a framework for enhancing contemporary nursing practice, education, and research while bringing the discipline to its traditional values and caring-healing roots. Swanson's theory of caring has been applied to interdisciplinary caring relationships beyond nurse–client encounters. Recent applications in clinical nursing practice show tangible positive results. For example, while at UNC School of Nursing at Chapel Hill as Dean, Swanson focused on intensifying the linkages among nursing education, research, and practice. In partnership with Clinical Professor Dr. Mary Tonges, Chief Nursing Officer and Senior Vice President for Patient Care Services at UNC Hospital, Swanson worked on strengthening the scholarship that supports nursing practice and enhances the relevance of nursing education and research to clinical practice through quality improvement projects. This research partnership resulted in positive outcomes on nursing workplace satisfaction and patient safety. Likewise, more recently, Swanson's theory of caring was applied in clinical practice and evaluated on selected variables at Virginia Mason Medical Center in Seattle, resulting in positive outcomes for patients and nurses. Currently, Swanson is in conversations with the Providence Healthcare System on how to best evolve nursing care within the system to meet populations' health needs in the 21st century.

CASE STUDIES

1. The birth of a child is one of the most memorable experiences in a woman's life. You are a birth unit nurse, and at the change of a shift you are assigned to care for a teen mother who came to the hospital alone and is now in active labor. When you arrive in her room, you notice that she is teary and appears frightened.
   Describe how you would apply Swanson's theory to connect emotionally and deliver caring in your practice with this young mother.
2. A 56-year-old obese man presents in the outpatient clinic. He is experiencing polydipsia and polyuria for over a week. He also reports a weight loss of 5 kg in the past few weeks. He delayed his clinic visit for as long as possible because he feared he may have diabetes like his father and was afraid to face the reality. You check his sugar level and it is 430 mg/dL. The man bursts into tears.
   Describe how you would apply Swanson's theory to help the client face the diagnosis of chronic disease, cope with the disease process, and promote well-being.

CRITICAL THINKING ACTIVITIES

1. Consider Swanson's theory of caring as a framework for your own nursing practice and research in a selected area. How might it be applied?
2. Think about a time when you felt that someone cared about you deeply. Remember what it felt like to experience caring. Now reflect on that experience and review it in the context of the processes of caring in Swanson's theory.
3. Think about an interaction with a client family in your clinical practice that you wish you could change or improve. Use the processes of the theory of caring to critically assess your actions and consider how you might have been more appropriate. What would you change and why?

POINTS FOR FURTHER STUDY

- Swanson, K. M. (1998). Caring made visible. *Creative Nursing, 4*(4), 8–11, 16.
- Swanson, K. M. (1999). Research-based practice with women who have had miscarriages. *Image: The Journal of Nursing Scholarship, 31*(4), 339–345.
- Swanson, K. M. (1999). The effects of caring, measurement, and time on miscarriage impact and women's well-being in the first year subsequent to loss. *Nursing Research, 48*(6), 288–298.
- Swanson, K. M., & Wojnar, D. (2004). Optimal healing environments in nursing. *Journal of Alternative and Complementary Medicine, 10*(1), 43–48.

REFERENCES

Booth-Laforce, C., Scott, C. S., Heitkemper, M. M., Cornman, B. J., Bond, E. F., & Swanson, K. M. (2010). Complementary and alternative medicine (CAM) attitudes and competencies of nursing students and faculty: Results of integrating CAM into nursing curriculum. *Journal of Professional Nursing, 26*(5), 293–300.

Chinn, P. L., & Kramer, M. (2015). *Integrated knowledge development in nursing* (9th ed.). St Louis, MO: Mosby-Elsevier.

Grant, S., & Swanson, K. M. (2006). Steaming the tide of the nursing shortage. *The CERNER Quarterly, 2*(2), 34–35.

Jennings, B. M., Loan, L. A., Heiner, S. L., Hemman, E. A., & Swanson, K. M. (2005). Soldiers' experiences with military health care. *Military Medicine, 170*(12), 999–1004.

Kavanaugh, K., Moro, T. T., Savage, T., & Mehendale, R. (2006). Enacting a theory of caring to recruit and retain vulnerable populations for sensitive research. *Research in Nursing and Health, 29*(3), 244–252.

Kavanaugh, K., Roscigno, C. I., Swanson, K. M., Savage, T. A., Kimura, R. E., & Kilpatrick, S. J. (2015). Perinatal palliative care: Parent perceptions of caring in interactions surrounding counseling for risk of delivering an extremely premature infant. *Palliative Support and Care, 13*(2), 145–155.

Kish, C. P., & Holder, L. M. (1996). Helping to say goodbye: Merging clinical scholarship with community service. *Holistic Nursing Practice, 10*(3), 74–82.

McNair, D. M., Lorr, M., & Droppleman, L. F. (1981). *Profile of mood states: Manual.* San Diego: Educational and Industrial Testing Service.

Mowinski-Jennings, B. M., Heiner, S. L., Loan, L. A., Hemman, E. A., & Swanson, K. M. (2005). What really matters to health care consumers. *Journal of Nursing Administration, 35*(4), 173–180.

Quinn, J., Smith, M., Ritenbaugh, C., & Swanson, K. M. (2003). Research guidelines for assessing the impact of the healing relationship in clinical nursing. *Alternative Therapies, 9*(31), 69–79.

Roscigno, C. I., & Swanson, K. M. (2011). Parent's experiences following children's moderate to severe traumatic brain injury: A clash of cultures. *Qualitative Health Research, 21*(10), 1413–1426.

Roscigno, C. I., Swanson, K. M., Solchany, J., & Vavilala, M. (2011). Children's longing for everydayness: Life following traumatic brain injury in the USA. *Brain Injury, 25*(9), 882–894.

Sikma, S. (2006). Staff perceptions of caring. The importance of a supportive environment. *Journal of Gerontological Nursing, 32*(6), 22–29.

Swanson, K. M. (1990). Providing care in the NICU: Sometimes an act of love. *Advances in Nursing Science, 13*(1), 60–73.

Swanson, K. M. (1991). Empirical development of a middle range theory of caring. *Nursing Research, 40*(3), 161–166.

Swanson, K. M. (1993). Nursing as informed caring for the well-being of others. *Image: The Journal of Nursing Scholarship, 25*(4), 352–357.

Swanson, K. M. (1999a). The effects of caring, measurement, and time on miscarriage impact and women's well-being in the first year subsequent to loss. *Nursing Research, 48*(6), 288–298.

Swanson, K. M. (1999b). Research-based practice with women who have had miscarriages. *Image: The Journal of Nursing Scholarship, 31*(4), 339–345.

Swanson, K. M. (1999c). What's known about caring in nursing: A literary meta-analysis. In A. S. Hinshaw, J. Shaver, &

S. Feetham (Eds.), *Handbook of clinical nursing research* (pp. 31–60). Thousand Oaks, CA: Sage.

Swanson, K. M. (2001). A program of research on caring. In M. E. Parker (Ed.), *Nursing theories and nursing practice* (pp. 411–420). Philadelphia: F. A. Davis.

Swanson, K. M. (2002). Caring Professional Scale. In J. Watson (Ed.), *Assessing and measuring caring in nursing and health science* (pp. 203–206). New York: Springer.

Swanson, K. M. (2007). Enhancing nurses' capacity for compassionate caring. In M. Koloroutis, J. Felgen, C. Person, & S. Wessel (Eds.), *Relationship-based care field guide* (pp. 502–507). Minneapolis: Creative Help Care Management.

Swanson, K. M., Chen, H. T., Graham, J. C., Wojnar, D. M., & Petras, A. (2009). Resolution of depression and grief during the first year after miscarriage: A randomized controlled clinical trial of couples-focused interventions. *Journal of Women's Health and Gender-Based Medicine, 18*(8), 1245–1257.

Swanson, K. M., Connor, S., Jolley, S., Pettinato, M., & Wang, T. J. (2007). Context and evolution of women's responses to miscarriage during the first year after loss. *Research in Nursing and Health, 30*(1), 2–16.

Swanson, K. M., & Wojnar, D. (2004). Optimal healing environments in nursing. *Journal of Alternative and Complementary Medicine, 10*(1), 43–48.

Swanson-Kauffman, K. M. (1985). Miscarriage: A new understanding of the mother's experience. *Proceedings of the 50th Anniversary Celebration of the University of Pennsylvania School of Nursing,* Philadelphia, 63–78.

Swanson-Kauffman, K. M. (1986). Caring in the instance of unexpected early pregnancy loss. *Topics in Clinical Nursing, 8*(2), 37–46.

Swanson-Kauffman, K. M. (1988a). The caring needs of women who miscarry. In M. M. Leininger (Ed.), *Care, discovery and uses in clinical and community nursing* (pp. 55–71). Detroit: Wayne State University Press.

Swanson-Kauffman, K. M. (1988b). There should have been two: Nursing care of parents experiencing the perinatal death of a twin. *Journal of Perinatal and Neonatal Nursing, 2*(2), 78–86.

Watson, J. (1979). *Nursing: The philosophy and science of caring.* Boston: Little, Brown.

Watson, J. (1988). New dimensions of human caring theory. *Nursing Science Quarterly, 1*(4), 175–181.

Watson, J. (1999). *Nursing: Human science and human care: A theory of nursing.* Sudbury, MA: Jones & Bartlett.

Wei, H., Roscigno, C.l., & Swanson, K. M., et al. (2016). Parents' experiences of having a child undergoing congenital heart surgery: An emotional rollercoaster from shocking to blessing. *Heart & Lung, 45*(2), 154–160.

Wojnar, D. M. (2007). Miscarriage experiences of lesbian birth and social mothers: Couples' perspective. *Journal of Midwifery and Women's Health, 52*(5), 479–485.

Wojnar, D., & Swanson, K. M. (2006). Why shouldn't lesbian women who miscarry receive equal consideration? A viewpoint. *Journal of GLBT Family Studies, 2*(1), 1–12.

Wojnar, D., Swanson, K. M., & Aldofsson, A. (2011). Confronting the inevitable: A conceptual model of miscarriage for use in clinical practice and research. *Death Studies, 35*(6), 536–558.

Yorkston, K. M., Klasner, E. R., & Swanson, K. M. (2001). Communication in multiple sclerosis: Understanding the insider's perspective. *American Journal of Speech Language Pathology, 10*(2), 126–137.

BIBLIOGRAPHY

Primary Sources

Book Chapters

Swanson, K. M. (1992). Foreword. In S. Wheeler & M. Pike (Eds.), *Grief ltd. manual.* Covington, IN: Grief Limited.

Swanson-Kauffman, K. M. (1987). Overview of the balancing act: Having it all. In K. Swanson-Kauffman (Ed.), *Women's work, families and health.* New York: Hemisphere. (Reprint of Swanson-Kauffman, K. M. [1987]. Overview of the balancing act: Having it all. *Health Care of Women International, 8*[2–3], 101–108.)

Swanson-Kauffman, K. M., & Roberts, J. (1990). Caring in parent and child nursing. In *Knowledge about care and caring: State of the art and future development.* Washington, DC: American Academy of Nursing.

Swanson-Kauffman, K. M., & Schonwald, E. (1988). Phenomenology. In B. Sarter (Ed.), *Paths to knowledge: Innovative research methods for nursing* (pp. 97–105). New York: National League for Nursing.

Journal Articles

Huffman, C. S., Schwartz, T. A., & Swanson, K. M. (2015). Couples and miscarriage: The influence of gender and reproductive factors on the impact of miscarriage. *Women's Health Issues, 25*(5), 570–578.

Swanson, K. M. (1993). Commentary: The phenomena of doing well in people with AIDS. *Western Journal of Nursing Research, 15*(1), 56.

Swanson, K. M. (1995). Commentary, the power of human caring: Early recognition of patient problems. *Scholarly Inquiry for Nursing Practice, 9*(4), 319–321.

Swanson, K. M. (1998). Caring made visible. *Creative Nursing, 4*(4), 8–11, 16.

Swanson, K. M. (2000). Predicting depressive symptoms after miscarriage: A path analysis based on Lazarus' paradigm. *Journal of Women's Health & Gender-Based Medicine, 9*(2), 191–206.

Swanson, K. M., Karmali, Z., Powell, S., & Pulvermakher, F. (2003). Miscarriage effects on couples' interpersonal and sexual relationships during the first year after loss: Women's perceptions. *Psychosomatic Medicine, 65*(5), 902–910.

Swanson-Kauffman, K. M. (1981). Echocardiography: An access route to the heart. *Critical Care Nurse, 1*(6), 20–26.

Swanson-Kauffman, K. M. (1986). Caring in the instance of unexpected early pregnancy loss. *Topics in Clinical Nursing, 8*(2), 37–46.

Swanson-Kauffman, K. M. (1986). A combined qualitative methodology for nursing research. *Advances in Nursing Science, 8*(3), 58–69.

Swanson-Kauffman, K. M. (1987). Overview of the balancing act: Having it all. *Health Care for Women International, 8*(2–3), 1–8.

Swanson-Kauffman, K. M. (1988). There should have been two: Nursing care of parents experiencing the perinatal death of a twin. *Journal of Perinatal and Neonatal Nursing, 2*(2), 78–86.

Wojnar, D., & Swanson, K. M. (2006). Why shouldn't lesbian women who miscarry receive equal consideration? A viewpoint. *Journal of GLBT Family Studies, 2*(1), 1–12.

Wojnar, D. M., & Swanson, K. M. (2007). Phenomenology: An exploration. *Journal of Holistic Nursing, 25*(3), 172–180; discussion 181–182, quiz 183–185.

Dissertation

Swanson-Kauffman, K. M. (1983). *The unborn one: A profile of the human experience of miscarriage.* Unpublished doctoral dissertation, University of Colorado, Denver.

Newsletters and Reprints

Swanson-Kauffman, K. M. (1984, Spring). A methodology for the study of nursing as a human science. *Alpha Kappa Chapter at Large News, 3.*

Swanson-Kauffman, K. M. (1987). Caring in the instance of unexpected early pregnancy loss. *Counselor Connection, 3*(2), 2–5. (Reprint of Swanson-Kauffman, K. M. [1986]. Caring in the instance of unexpected early pregnancy loss. *Topics in Clinical Nursing, 8*[2], 37–46.)

Swanson-Kauffman, K. M. (1988). Miscarriage: An often-overlooked maternal loss. *Perinatal Newsletter, 2*(3), 1.

Published Abstracts

Swanson, K. M. (1993). Caring as intervention (Abstract). *Communicating Nursing Research, 26*, 299.

Swanson, K. M. (1993). Caring theory: Structure and assumptions (Abstract). *Communicating Nursing Research, 26*, 255.

Swanson, K. M. (1995). Effects of caring on healing post miscarriage (Abstract). *Communicating Nursing Research, 28*, 281.

Swanson, K. M., Kieckhefer, G., Henderson, D., Powers, P., Leppa, C., & Carr, K. (1991). Miscarriage: Patterns of meaning (Abstract). *Communicating Nursing Research, 24*, 110.

Swanson, K. M., Kieckhefer, G., Powers, P., & Carr, K. (1990). Meaning of miscarriage scale: Establishment of psychometric properties (Abstract). *Communicating Nursing Research, 23*, 89.

Swanson, K. M., Klaich, K., & Leppa, C. (1992). A caring intervention to promote well-being in women who miscarry (Abstract). *Communicating Nursing Research, 25*, 365.

Swanson, K. M., Pulvermakher, F., Karmali, Z., & Powell, S. (2001). Effects of miscarriage on couple relationships (Abstract). *Communicating Nursing Research, 34*, 339.

Swanson, K. M., Taylor, G., Shipman, L., Spoor, K., & Zillyet, K. (2002). Miscarriage and healing amongst the Shoalwater (Abstract). *Communicating Nursing Research, 35*, 135.

Swanson, K. M., Wojnar, D. M., Petras, A., Chen, H., & Graham, C. (2008). Effects of caring on couples' grief after miscarriage. *Communicating Nursing Research, 40*, 162.

Swanson-Kauffman, K. M. (1984). A profile of the human experience of miscarriage (Abstract). *Communicating Nursing Research, 6*(3), 46.

Swanson-Kauffman, K. M. (1985). A combined qualitative methodology for nursing research (Abstract). *Communicating Nursing Research, 18*, 57.

Swanson-Kauffman, K. M. (1985). Miscarriage: A new understanding of the mother's experience. *Proceedings of the 50th anniversary celebration of the University of Pennsylvania School of Nursing*, 63–78.

Swanson-Kauffman, K. M. (1986). Work and family: The delicate balance. Symposium (Abstract). *Communicating Nursing Research, 19*, 153–156.

Swanson-Kauffman, K. M. (1988). Empirical development and refinement of a model of caring (Abstract). *Communicating Nursing Research, 21*, 80.

Swanson-Kauffman, K. M. (1989). From phenomenological to experimental design: Qualitative inquiry as a framework for the intervention (Abstract). *Communicating Nursing Research, 22*, 147.

Swanson-Kauffman, K. M., Powers, P., Klaich, K., Lethbridge, D., & Jarrett, M. (1990). Success: As women view it (Abstract). *Communicating Nursing Research, 23*, 59.

Wei, H., Roscigno, C. L., Swanson, K. M., Blacck, B. P., Hudson-Barr, D., & Hanson, C. C. (2016). Parents' experiences of having a child undergoing congenital heart surgery: An emotional rollercoaster from shocking to blessing. *Heart and Lung, 45*(2), 154–160.

36

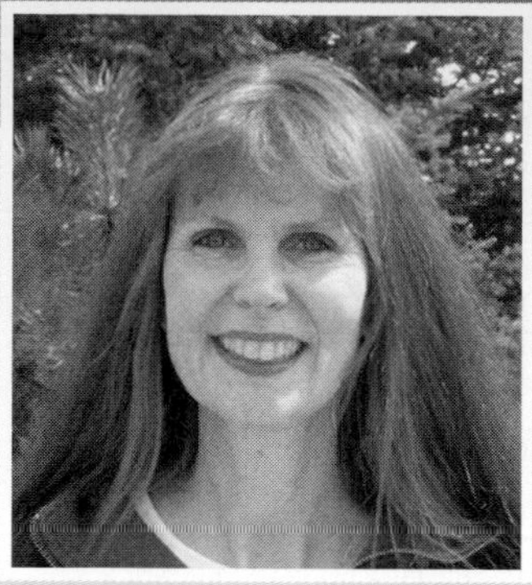

Cornelia M. Ruland
(1954–Present)

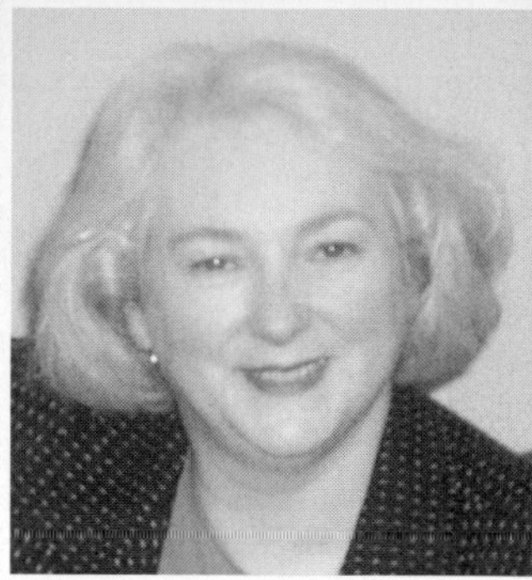

Shirley M. Moore
(1948–Present)

Peaceful End-of-Life Theory

*Dana M. Hansen**

"Standards of care offer a promising approach for the development of middle-range prescriptive theories because of their empirical base in clinical practice and their focus on linkages between interventions and outcomes."

(Ruland & Moore, 1998, p. 169)

CREDENTIALS AND BACKGROUND OF THE THEORISTS

Cornelia M. Ruland

Cornelia M. Ruland received her doctorate in nursing in 1998 from Case Western Reserve University in Cleveland, Ohio. She is Director of the Center for Shared Decision Making and Nursing Research at Rikshospitalet University Hospital in Oslo, Norway, and holds an adjunct faculty appointment in the Department of Biomedical Informatics at Columbia University in New York. Ruland has established a research program on improving shared decision making and patient–provider partnerships in health care and the development, implementation, and evaluation of information systems to support it. She focuses on aspects of and tools for shared decision making in clinically challenging situations: (1) for patients confronted with difficult treatment or screening decisions for which they need help to understand the potential benefits and harms of alternative options and to elicit their values and preferences and (2) preference-adjusted management of chronic or serious long-term illness over time. As primary investigator on a number of research projects, she has received numerous awards for her work.

Shirley M. Moore

Shirley M. Moore is Associate Dean for Research and Professor, School of Nursing, Case Western Reserve University. She received her diploma in nursing from the Youngstown Hospital Association School of Nursing (1969) and her bachelor's degree in nursing from Kent State University (1974). She earned a master's degree in psychiatric and mental health nursing (1990) as well as a doctorate in nursing science (1993) at Case Western Reserve University. She has taught nursing theory and nursing science to all levels of nursing students and conducts a program of research and theory development that addresses recovery after cardiac events. Early in her doctoral

*Previous authors: The author wishes to thank Dr. Patricia Higgins for her important contributions as the previous author of this chapter.

study, Moore was encouraged to not only use theory but to develop it as well. The Rosemary Ellis Theory Conference, held annually for several years at Case Western Reserve University, offered Moore an opportunity to explore theory as a practical tool for practitioners, researchers, and teachers. Influenced by these experiences, Moore assisted in the development and publication of theories such as the one by Ruland and Moore (1998). Moore recognized theory construction as an essential doctoral student skill.

THEORETICAL SOURCES

The peaceful end-of-life theory is informed by a number of theoretical frameworks (Ruland & Moore, 1998). It is based primarily on Donabedian's model of structure, process, and outcomes, which in part was developed from general system theory. General system theory is pervasive in other types of nursing theory, from conceptual models to middle-range and micro-range theories—an indicator of its usefulness in explaining the complexity of health care interactions and organizations. In the peaceful end-of-life theory, the structure-setting is the family system (terminally ill patient and all significant others) that is receiving care from professionals on an acute care hospital unit, and process is defined as those actions (nursing interventions) designed to promote the positive outcomes of the following: (1) being free from pain, (2) experiencing comfort, (3) experiencing dignity and respect, (4) being at peace, and (5) experiencing a closeness to significant others and those who care.

A second theoretical underpinning is preference theory (Brandt, 1979), which has been used by philosophers to explain and define quality of life (Sandoe, 1999), a concept that is significant in end-of-life research and practice. In preference theory, the good life is defined as getting what one wants, an approach that seems particularly appropriate in end-of-life care. It can be applied to both sentient persons and incapacitated persons who have previously provided documentation related to end-of-life decision making. Quality of life, therefore, is defined and evaluated as a manifestation of satisfaction through empirical assessment of such outcomes as symptom relief and satisfaction with interpersonal relationships. Incorporating patient preferences into health care decisions is considered appropriate (Ruland & Bakken, 2001; Ruland, Kresevic, & Lorensen, 1997) and necessary for successful processes and outcomes (Ruland & Moore, 2001).

This theory was derived in a doctoral theory course in which Ruland was a student and Moore was faculty. Middle-range theories were just emerging, and there were few good definitions or examples. The class was challenged to think about the future use and development of middle-range theory for nursing science and practice. The students discussed knowledge sources from which they could derive middle-range theory, such as empirical knowledge, clinical practice knowledge, and synthesized knowledge. Each student was asked to derive a middle-range theory from a knowledge source of choice. Ruland had just completed a major project to develop a clinical practice standard for peaceful end of life with a group of cancer nurses in Norway. The standard was synthesized into the theory of peaceful end of life by Ruland and later was refined with Moore's assistance. This is an example of middle-range theory developed by doctoral nursing students as they study knowledge-development methods. This theory is also an example of middle-range theory development using a standard of practice as a source.

USE OF EMPIRICAL EVIDENCE

The peaceful end-of-life theory is based on empirical evidence from direct experience of expert nurses and review of the literature addressing components of the theory. The group of expert practitioners who developed the standard of care for peaceful end of life had at least 5 years of clinical experience caring for terminally ill patients. The standard of care consisted of best practices based on research-derived evidence in the areas of pain management, comfort, nutrition, and relaxation. This prescriptive theory comprises several proposed relational statements for which more empirical evidence is needed. Explicit hypotheses can be derived from these relational statements to test their usefulness. The authors of the standard of care and authors of the theory attempted to incorporate clearly described, observable concepts and relationships that expressed the notion of caring.

MAJOR CONCEPTS & DEFINITIONS

Not Being in Pain

Being free of the suffering or symptom distress is the central part of many patients' end-of-life experience. Pain is an unpleasant sensory or emotional experience that may be associated with actual or potential tissue damage.

Experience of Comfort

Comfort is defined inclusively, using Kolcaba and Kolcaba's (1991) work as "relief from discomfort, the state of ease and peaceful contentment, and whatever makes life easy or pleasurable" (Ruland & Moore, 1998, p. 172).

Continued

MAJOR CONCEPTS & DEFINITIONS—cont'd

Experience of Dignity and Respect
Each terminally ill patient is "respected and valued as a human being" (Ruland & Moore, 1998, p. 172). This concept incorporates the idea of personal worth, as expressed by the ethical principle of autonomy or respect for persons, which states that individuals should be treated as autonomous agents, and persons with diminished autonomy are entitled to protection (United States, 1978).

Being at Peace
Peace is a "feeling of calmness, harmony, and contentment, [free of] anxiety, restlessness, worries, and fear" (Ruland & Moore, 1998, p. 172). A peaceful state includes physical, psychological, and spiritual dimensions.

Closeness to Significant Others
Closeness is "the feeling of connectedness to other human beings who care" (Ruland & Moore, 1998, p. 172). It involves a physical or emotional nearness that is expressed through warm, intimate relationships.

MAJOR ASSUMPTIONS

Nursing, Person, Health, and Environment

As in other middle-range theories, the focus of the theory of peaceful end of life does not address each metaparadigm concept. The theory was derived from standards of care written by a team of expert nurses who were addressing a practice problem; therefore the metaparadigm concepts explicitly addressed were *nursing* and *person*. The theory addresses the nursing phenomena of complex, holistic care to support persons' peaceful end of life.

Two assumptions of Ruland and Moore's (1998) theory are identified as follows:

1. The occurrences and feelings at the end-of-life experience are personal and individualized.
2. Nursing care is crucial for creating a peaceful end-of-life experience. Nurses assess and interpret cues that reflect the person's end-of-life experience and intervene appropriately to attain or maintain a peaceful experience, even when the dying person cannot communicate verbally.

Two additional assumptions are implicit:

1. Family, a term that includes all significant others, is an important part of end-of-life care.
2. The goal of end-of-life care is not to optimize care, in the sense that it must be the best, most technologically advanced treatment, a type of care that commonly results in overtreatment. Rather, the goal in end-of-life care is to maximize treatment—that is, the best possible care will be provided through the judicious use of technology and comfort measures to enhance quality of life and achieve a peaceful death.

THEORETICAL ASSERTIONS

Six explicit relational statements were identified (Ruland & Moore, 1998) as theoretical assertions for the theory:

1. Monitoring and administering pain relief and applying pharmacological and nonpharmacological interventions contribute to the patient's experience of not being in pain.
2. Preventing, monitoring, and relieving physical discomfort; facilitating rest, relaxation, and contentment; and preventing complications contribute to the patient's experience of comfort.
3. Including the patient and significant others in decision making regarding patient care; treating the patient with dignity, empathy, and respect; and being attentive to the patient's expressed needs, wishes, and preferences contribute to the patient's experience of dignity and respect.
4. Providing emotional support, monitoring and meeting the patient's expressed needs for antianxiety medications, inspiring trust, providing the patient and significant others with guidance in practical issues, and providing the physical presence of another caring person if desired contribute to the patient's experience of being at peace.
5. Facilitating participation of significant others in patient care; attending to significant others' grief, worries, and questions; and facilitating opportunities for family closeness contribute to the patient's experience of closeness to significant others or persons who care.
6. The patient's experiences of not being in pain, comfort, dignity, respect, being at peace, and closeness to significant others or persons who care contribute to the peaceful end of life (p. 174).

LOGICAL FORM

The peaceful end-of-life theory was developed using inductive and deductive logic. A unique feature of the theory is its development from a standard of care. The peaceful end-of-life standard was created by expert nurses in response to a lack of direction for managing the complex care of terminally ill patients. The standard was developed for the surgical gastroenterological care unit in a university hospital in Norway. Thus the standard served as a logical intermediary step linking practice and theory. Standards of care serve as credible, authoritative statements that describe a practitioner's roles and responsibilities and an expected performance level of nursing care by which the quality of practice can be evaluated (American Association of Critical Care Nurses, 1998). In this instance of knowledge development, the standard of care was an interim step that effectively linked clinical practice and theory.

Ruland and Moore (2001) detailed the steps they followed in the development of the standard for peaceful end of life, which included review of relevant literature, clarification of important concepts, and incorporation of clinical practice knowledge. Each step is analogous to those used in theory development. Thus the logic for the development of this theory is straightforward, and the process used is clearly stated.

ACCEPTANCE BY THE NURSING COMMUNITY

Practice

A small but growing number of articles cite the peaceful end-of-life theory. It is included on the Clayton State University School of Nursing Theory Link page, with a link to *American Journal of Critical Care*, End-of-Life Care (Kirchhoff et al., 2000). In addition, Ruland and Moore's innovative development of this theory has been cited in theory construction literature as an important illustration of statement synthesis that occurred before the theory synthesis (Walker & Avant, 2011). Liehr and Smith (1999) refer to the theory's development of a practice standard as a foundation for developing theory, Kehl (2006) cites it in her concept analysis of a "good death," and Baggs and Schmitt (2000) discuss the potential usefulness of the theory as a means to improve end-of-life decision making for critically ill adults. Veillette and colleagues (2010) incorporated the theory into their practice in rural Quebec. Kirchhoff (2002) continued the discussion on creating an environment of care in the intensive care unit that promotes a peaceful death by synthesizing information from three sources:

1. Peaceful end-of-life theory (Ruland & Moore, 1998)
2. Institute of Medicine's definition of peaceful death (Field & Cassell, 1997)
3. Precepts from the American Association of Colleges of Nursing's "Peaceful Death: Recommended Competencies and Curricular Guidelines for End of Life Nursing Care" (1997)

The peaceful end-of-life theory was used to develop a model for holistic palliative care for patients with sickle cell anemia (Wilkie et al., 2010). In Taiwan, Lee and colleagues (2009) cite peaceful end-of-life theory as useful to develop a framework to identify the major barriers of good end-of-life care in an intensive care unit. Lee et al. (2014) tested the validity and reliability of the National Survey of Critical-Care Nurses Regarding End-of-Life Care Questionnaire, which was developed from the peaceful end-of-life theory. The questionnaire incorporates the theory's five concepts: (1) pain management, (2) comfort care, (3) patient respect, (4) peaceful environment, and (5) closeness to significant others.

Education

Peaceful end of life has been integrated into nursing courses for generations with a focus on care of the patient and family. End-of-life content has become more standardized in the form of theory, competencies, and curricular guidelines. Ruland and Moore (1998) provide an example of an early end-of-life theory as attention to hospice and palliative care has developed. Ruland and Moore (1998) were cited by Kirchhoff and colleagues (2000) when end of life was a featured topic of a continuing education (CE) offering for critical care nurses in their online journal.

Research

The peaceful end-of-life theory has gained international recognition as containing key components of a peaceful death. Kongsuwan and colleagues created a conceptual model (Kongsuwan & Touhy, 2009) and conducted qualitative (Kongsuwan & Locsin, 2009) and quantitative research (Kongsuwan et al., 2010) on peaceful death in adult patients in Thailand. Ruland and Moore's (1998) peaceful end-of-life theory served as a comparison model for Kongsuwan and colleagues' work and was cited as possessing qualities essential for a peaceful death that have been identified in many cultures. To continue their work, Kongsuwan and colleagues (2012) compared their findings to concepts identified in the peaceful end-of-life theory and found them to be supported by the theory, indicating that across cultures a peaceful death has significance and similarities.

In Quebec, an ethnographic study was conducted to identify key components of a good death for rural residents, and the authors identified the peaceful end-of-life theory as important to developing an understanding of the concept of a good death (Veillette et al., 2010). Wilkie et al. (2010) studied use of the theory with sickle cell patients. Finally, in 2015, an ethnographic study of hospice patients in Ottawa used the peaceful end-of-life theory to identifying specific attributes at end of life, such as mental awareness, comfort, achieving a sense of closure, and optimizing relationships in facing the end of life (Wright et al., 2015).

FURTHER DEVELOPMENT

Ruland and Moore acknowledge the need for continued refinement and development of the theory. There are a number of potential ideas to advance its development, and testing the theory is in the planning stage; for example, testing the relationships among the five major concepts is a possibility. Another idea is merging some of the process criteria from the three concepts of pain, comfort, and peace to explore outcomes related to physical-psychological symptom management. Concept analysis or mapping could be used to determine whether the process criteria associated with the three concepts are different or sufficiently alike to allow merging. For the concept of pain, two process criteria (monitoring and administering pain relief and applying pharmacological and nonpharmacological interventions) are closely related to the comfort process criterion (preventing, monitoring, and relieving physical discomfort) and the peace process criterion (monitoring and meeting patient's needs for antianxiety medication). Nonpharmacological interventions (e.g., music, humor, relaxation) that serve to distract a dying patient are useful for the relief of pain, anxiety, and general physical discomfort. Future studies are suggested to explore applications of the peaceful end-of-life theory.

CRITIQUE

Clarity

All elements of the theory are stated clearly, including the setting, assumptions, concepts, and relational statements. These concepts vary considerably in their level of abstraction, from more concrete (pain and comfort) to more abstract (dignity).

Simplicity

Despite uncomplicated terms and clear expression of ideas, the theory has been described as one of the higher-level middle-range theories (Higgins & Moore, 2000), primarily because of the level of abstraction of the outcome criteria and the multidimensional complexity expressed in its relational statements.

Generality

The peaceful end-of-life theory has specific boundaries related to time, setting, and patient population. It was developed for use with terminally ill adults and their families who are receiving care in an acute care setting. The concept of peaceful end of life came from a Norwegian context and may not be appropriate for all cultures; however, it has been used for practice and research by nurses in other cultures. Its concepts and relationships resonate with many nurses, and it comprehensively addresses the multidimensional aspects of end-of-life care. For example, the outcome indicators associated with the five concepts address the technical aspect of care:

1. Providing both pharmacological and nonpharmacological interventions for the relief of symptoms
2. Communication for decision making
3. The psychological aspect for emotional support
4. Dignity
5. Respect by treating the patient with dignity, empathy, and respect (Fig. 36.1)

Accessibility

The deductive and inductive logic used to develop this theory provides a solid basis for developing testable hypotheses among the five concepts of the theory. Theoretical congruency is demonstrated through the outcome indicators, all of which are conceptualized from the perspective of the patients and their families.

Importance

As a successful synthesis of clinical practice and scholarly theory development, the peaceful end-of-life theory illustrates a way to bridge the theory–practice–research continuum. Besides addressing an identified need for a comprehensive middle-range theory to guide care of patients in the end-of-life experience, Ruland and Moore's (2001) work clearly illustrates the richness of practice and standards as a source for the development of theory.

All of the outcome indicators are measurable, using qualitative, quantitative, or both methodologies (see Fig. 36.1). Unlike some middle-range theories that have a specific instrument to measure a particular concept, no instrument has been developed by the authors for peaceful end-of-life theory. For future studies among the five concepts, instruments need to be identified to measure hypothesized relationships. Qualitative or mixed methods would be appropriate for investigating the concepts. For example, a phenomenological approach could be used to investigate patient and family perceptions of their opportunities for and satisfaction with family closeness, decision making, or both. Also with attention to linkages, a number of existing instruments have been considered to measure outcome indicators associated with the five concepts (see Fig. 36.1), such as perception of symptoms with the Memorial Symptom Assessment Scale (Portenoy et al., 1994) or the Kolcaba (2003) General Comfort Questionnaire.

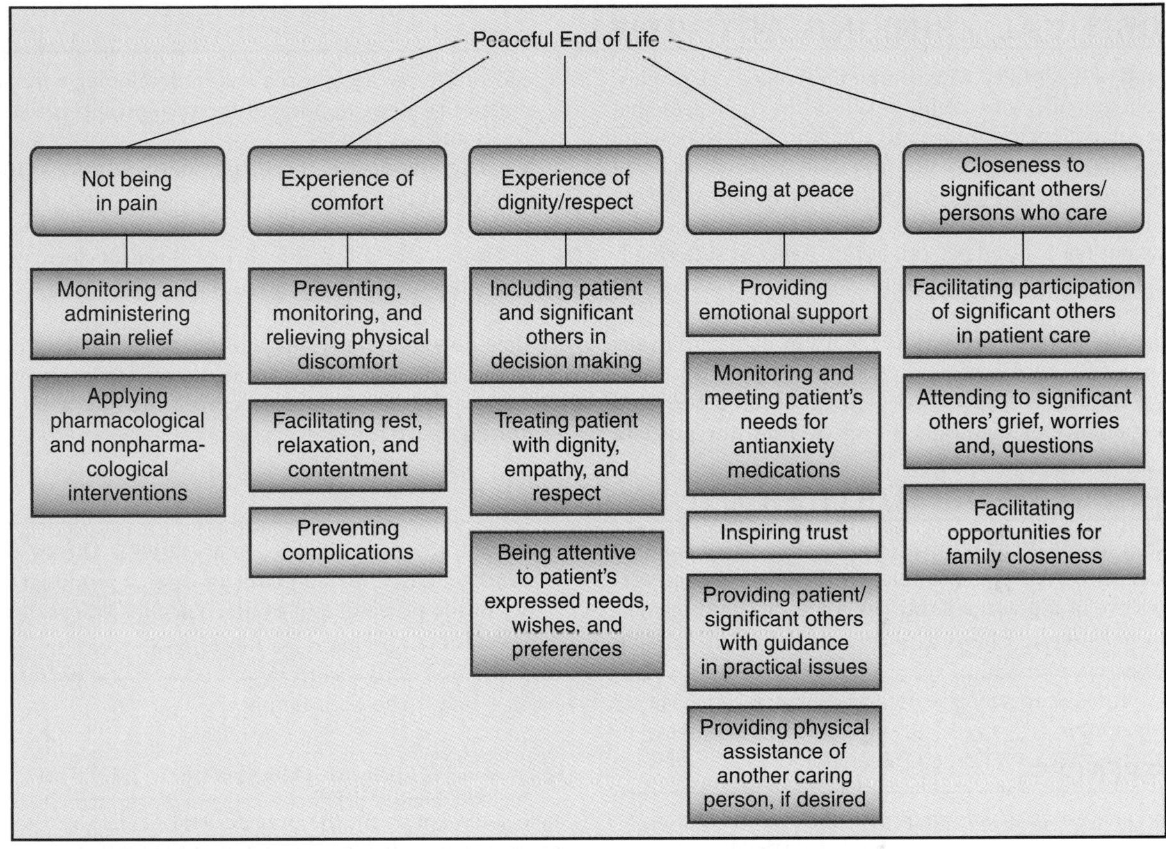

FIG. 36.1 *Relationships among the concepts of the Peaceful End-of-Life Theory.* (From Ruland, C. M., & Moore, S. M. [1998]. Theory construction based on standards of care: A proposed theory of the peaceful end of life. *Nursing Outlook, 46*[4], 174.)

CASE STUDY

Becky is a 66-year-old woman diagnosed with stage 4 congestive heart failure (CHF). She is recently widowed (approximately 6 months ago) and the mother of four devoted young adult children and the grandmother of two. Her youngest daughter (Sue) lives with her and is a student at a local university. Sue has taken leave from the University to care for her mother. Becky has completed her advance directives and is adamant that she not receive extraordinary measures to sustain her life. This has been a difficult issue for her children, because they cannot fathom the loss of another parent. Sue is the durable power of attorney (DPOA) and states she will call 911 in the event her mother stops breathing, even though her mother has a Do Not Resuscitate (DNR) order.

The physician has prescribed home hospice care. The daughter greets the social worker and nurse at the door and insists the word *hospice* is not mentioned to her mother, because it would "kill" her. During the hospice admission, it became clear that Becky understands she is dying and sees how much her children are grieving over the thought of losing another parent. After several weeks on the hospice program, Becky continues to report discomfort, shortness of breath, and difficulty in communicating with her children about her wishes. She is not ready to say good-bye to her children or grandchildren and is afraid to die.

Despite prescribed medication and team-focused care (social worker, nurse, nursing assistant, and clergy), Becky continues to rate her pain level at severe (8–10) and talks about her suffering, fear of death, and concern over what will happen to her family when she is gone. During a team meeting, it was decided to ask Becky to describe three different kinds of pain (physical, emotional, and spiritual). Becky had a physical pain rating of 3–4, and both emotional and spiritual pains were rated as severe (8–10). The adult children continue to ask about treatments that are more aggressive; however, they also state that they do not like to see her suffer.

CRITICAL THINKING ACTIVITIES

The end of life is filled with complex physiological, psychological, spiritual, and family relationship challenges that affect the patient's comfort and ability to achieve peaceful end of life. Unresolved issues in family relationships can lead to complicated grieving for family members before and after the death. Suffering outside of physical discomfort is not readily understood, but the relief of suffering is a fundamental goal of end-of-life care and is necessary to achieve comfort and a peaceful end of life.

1. Use the peaceful end-of-life theory to plan care in the case of Becky above.
2. Use the concepts of "closeness to significant others" and "experience of dignity and respect" from the peaceful end-of-life theory to assist you in developing a nursing practice strategy to address the relationship issues for Becky and her family.
3. What limitations of the theory did you find in these considerations?
4. Identify signs of anticipatory grieving and describe use of the peaceful end-of-life theory to address these issues and achieve a peaceful end of life for Becky and for her family.
5. How do you identify and address issues related to suffering (e.g., emotional, spiritual, and psychological)? Explore the use of peaceful end-of-life theory in your nursing practice.

POINTS FOR FURTHER STUDY

- Kongsuwan, W., Keller, K., Touhy, T., & Schoenhofer, S. (2010). Thai Buddhist intensive care unit nurses' perspective of a peaceful death: An empirical study. *International Journal of Palliative Nursing*, 16(5), 241–247.
- Ruland, C. M., & Moore, S. M. (1998). Theory construction based on standards of care: A proposed theory of the peaceful end of life. *Nursing Outlook, 46*(4), 169–175.

REFERENCES

American Association of Critical Care Nurses. (1998). *Standards for acute and critical care nursing practice*. Aliso Viejo, CA: AACN. Retrieved from http://www.aacn.org.

Baggs, J. G., & Schmitt, M. H. (2000). End-of-life decisions in adult intensive care: Current research base 158 and directions for the future. *Nursing Outlook, 48*(4), 158–164.

Brandt, R. B. (1979). *A theory of the good and the right*. Oxford: Clarendon Press.

Field, M. J., & Cassell, C. K. (1997). *Approaching death: Improving care at the end of life* (IOM report). Washington, DC: National Academy Press.

Higgins, P. A., & Moore, S. M. (2000). Levels of theoretical thinking in nursing. *Nursing Outlook, 48*(4), 179–183.

Kehl, K. A. (2006). Moving toward a peace: An analysis of the concept of the good death. *American Journal of Hospice and Palliative Medicine, 23*(4), 277–286.

Kirchhoff, K. T. (2002). Promoting a peaceful death in the ICU. *Critical Care Nursing Clinics of North America, 14*(2), 201–206.

Kirchhoff, K. T., Spuhler, V., Walker, L., Hutton, A., Cole, B., & Clemmer, T. (2000). End-of-life care: Intensive care nurses' experiences with end-of-life care. *American Journal of Critical Care, 9*(1), 36–42.

Kolcaba, K. (2003). *Comfort theory and practice: A vision for holistic health care and research*. New York: Springer.

Kolcaba, K. Y., & Kolcaba, R. J. (1991). An analysis of the concept of comfort. *Journal of Advanced Nursing, 16*(11), 1301–1310.

Kongsuwan, W., Chaipetch, O., & Matchin, Y. (2012). Thai Buddhist families' perspective of a peaceful death in ICUs. *Nursing in Critical Care, 17*(3), 151–159.

Kongsuwan, W., Keller, K., Touhy, T., & Schoenhofer, S. (2010). Thai Buddhist intensive care unit nurses' perspective of a peaceful death: An empirical study. *International Journal of Palliative Nursing, 16*(5), 241–247.

Kongsuwan, W., & Locsin, R. C. (2009). Promoting peaceful death in the intensive care unit in Thailand. *International Nursing Review, 56*, 116–122.

Kongsuwan, W., & Touhy, T. (2009). Promoting peaceful death for Thai Buddhists; implications for a holistic end of life care. *Holistic Nursing Practice, 23*(5), 289–296.

Lee, J. H., Choi, M., Kim, S., & Beckstrand, R. (2014). Factor structure investigation of perceived facilitators and barriers in end-of-life care among Korean nurses. *Japan Journal of Nursing Science, 11*, 135–143.

Lee, S. Y., Hung, C. L., Lee, J. H., et al. (2009). Attaining good end of life care in intensive care units in Taiwan—The dilemma and the strategy. *International Journal of Gerontology, 3*(1), 26–30.

Liehr, P., & Smith, M. J. (1999). Middle range theory: Spinning research and practice to create knowledge for the new millennium. *Advances in Nursing Science, 21*(4), 81–91.

Portenoy, R. K., Thaler, H. T., Kornblith, A. B., et al. (1994). The Memorial Symptom Assessment Scale: An instrument for the evaluation of symptom prevalence, characteristics and distress. *European Journal of Cancer, 30A*(9), 1326–1336.

Ruland, C. M., & Bakken, S. (2001). Representing patient preference-related concepts for inclusion in electronic health records. *Journal of Biomedical Informatics, 34*(6), 415–422.

Ruland, C. M., Kresevic, D., & Lorensen, M. (1997). Including patient preferences in nurses' assessment of older patients. *Journal of Clinical Nursing, 6*(6), 495–504.

Ruland, C. M., & Moore, S. M. (1998). Theory construction based on standards of care: A proposed theory of the peaceful end of life. *Nursing Outlook, 46*(4), 169–175.

Ruland, C. M., & Moore, S. M. (2001). Eliciting exercise preferences in cardiac rehabilitation: Initial evaluation of a new strategy. *Patient Education and Counseling, 44*(3), 283–291.

Sandoe, P. (1999). Quality of life—Three competing views. *Ethical Theory and Moral Practice, 2*(1), 11–23.

United States, National Commission for the Protection of Human Subjects of Biomedical and Behavioral Research. (1978). *The Belmont report: Ethical principles and guidelines for the protection of human subjects of research*. Bethesda, MD: Superintendent of Documents, U.S. Government Printing Office.

Veillette, A. M., Fillion, L., Wilson, D. M., Thomas, R., & Dumont, S. (2010). La Belle mort en milieu rural: A report of an ethnographic study of the good death for Quebec rural francophones. *Journal of Palliative Care, 26*(3), 159–166.

Walker, L. O., & Avant, K. C. (2011). *Strategies for theory construction in nursing* (5th ed.). Upper Saddle River, NJ: Pearson/Prentice Hall.

Wilkie, D. J., Johnson, B., Mack, A. K., Labotka, R., & Molokie, R. E. (2010). Sickle cell disease: An opportunity for palliative care across the life span. *Nursing Clinics of North America, 45*(3), 375–397.

Wright, D. K., Brajtman, S., Cragg, B., & Macdonald, M. E. (2015). Delirium as letting go: An ethnographic analysis of hospice care and family moral experience. *Palliative Medicine, 29*(10), 959–966.

UNIT VI

The Future of Nursing Theory

- Nursing theoretical systems give direction and create understanding in practice, research, administration, and education.
- Theoretical works of a discipline address pertinent questions, provide frameworks to answer those questions, and develop and test knowledge for evidence-based practice.
- Nursing models and theories exhibit normal science within global communities of scholars whose research and practice contribute scientific achievements and quality practice.
- Expansion of the philosophy of nursing science, qualitative approaches, and quantitative methods has greatly increased the development and use of middle-range theories in nursing research and nursing practice.
- Globalization of nursing and the use of nursing theoretical works by nurse scholars around the world is growing at an exciting rate.

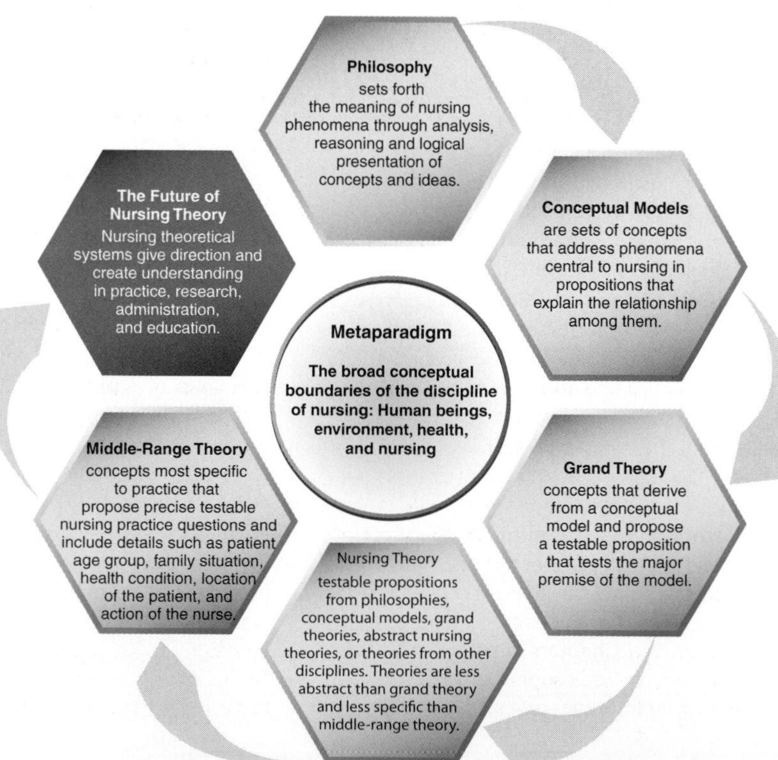
Philosophy
sets forth the meaning of nursing phenomena through analysis, reasoning and logical presentation of concepts and ideas.
Conceptual Models
are sets of concepts that address phenomena central to nursing in propositions that explain the relationship among them.
Grand Theory
concepts that derive from a conceptual model and propose a testable proposition that tests the major premise of the model.
Nursing Theory
testable propositions from philosophies, conceptual models, grand theories, abstract nursing theories, or theories from other disciplines. Theories are less abstract than grand theory and less specific than middle-range theory.
Middle-Range Theory
concepts most specific to practice that propose precise testable nursing practice questions and include details such as patient age group, family situation, health condition, location of the patient, and action of the nurse.
The Future of Nursing Theory
Nursing theoretical systems give direction and create understanding in practice, research, administration, and education.
Metaparadigm
The broad conceptual boundaries of the discipline of nursing: Human beings, environment, health, and nursing

37

State of the Art and Science of Nursing Theory

Martha Raile Alligood

"Nursing theoretical knowledge has demonstrated powerful contributions to education, research, administration and professional practice for guiding nursing thought and action. That knowledge has shifted the primary focus of the nurse from nursing functions to the person. Theoretical views of the person raise new questions, create new approaches and instruments for nursing research, and expand nursing scholarship throughout the world."

(Alligood, 2011, p. 304)

It becomes clear from studying texts such as this one that the understanding and use of nursing theoretical works is increasing globally as never before; pointing the way to new knowledge through research, education, administration, and practice. Reviewers of the eighth edition of this text and published reviews document its contribution to professional nursing. Their suggestions receive careful consideration for each new edition (Dickson & Wright, 2012; Paley, 2006; Smith, 2012). Smith (2012) noted, "The text is significant in that it provides nursing students with an accurate and scholarly reference to identify significant philosophies, models and theories that are pertinent to their own nursing practice" (p. 201). Similarly, Dickson and Wright (2012) concluded, the text "simply and elegantly describes the great progress that nursing as a discipline and profession has accomplished guided by the vision of leading nursing theorists. The scope and depth . . . address the concerns and critics who argue nursing theory is outdated or irrelevant to current practice and research" (p. 204). The chapters in this ninth edition have been updated, maintaining the clarity and integrity of each work while keeping the size of the text workable. Based on reviewer comments, the Unit I content was rearranged to better reflect historical chronological order, and Chapter 5 now introduces the reader to the knowledge structure, chapter content outline, and analysis criteria used in Chapters 6–36 in Units II–V.

The nursing literature for philosophies, nursing models, grand theories, theories, and middle-range theories continues to reflect a philosophy of science that embraces nursing concerns. Theory utilization literature reveals the use of nursing theory to guide practice and highlights Im and Chang's (2012) prediction that "middle range [theory] will play an essential role in nursing research" (p. 162). This global happening portends a very bright nursing theory future.

As in previous editions, the chapters in this ninth edition are written by those who use the theoretical works in their professional practice and research. Nurses around the world are recognizing the vital nature of theoretical works and applying them to their practice, research, education, and administration (Alligood, 2014b; Butts & Rich, 2015; Fitzpatrick & Whall, 2016). This ninth edition continues to clarify the relevance of nursing theoretical works; facilitate their recognition as systematic demonstrations of nursing substance; and inspire their use as frameworks for nursing scholarship in practice, research, education, and administration. Simply put, theoretical framing of patient care guides nursing thought and action for quality practice.

In this final chapter of the text, the future of nursing theory is considered from three related perspectives: the evolving philosophy of science, theory development and use of middle-range theory for practice, and the explosive global recognition and application of nursing theory. First, the philosophy of science continues to open new ways of developing and using nursing theoretical works (Butts & Rich, 2015; Carper, 1978; Chinn & Kramer, 2015; Fawcett & Garity, 2009; Fitzpatrick & Whall, 2016; Wood, 2014) with normal science of the discipline (Kuhn, 1962, 1970). Second, middle-range, practice-level theory reflects the present-day understanding with global expansion and use in all areas of nursing (Butts & Rich, 2015; Fitzpatrick & Whall, 2016; Roy, 2014). Third and finally, the incredible expansion of the use of nursing theoretical works by global nurse scholars highlights the growing awareness of the vital nature of theory for the profession, discipline, and science (Breakey, Corless, & Meedzan, 2015; Fitzpatrick & Whall, 2016; Johnson & Webber, 2015).

PHILOSOPHY OF NORMAL SCIENCE

Many nursing models and theories included in this text exhibit characteristics of Kuhn's (1970) criteria for normal science (Wood, 2014). The characteristics of paradigms that evidence their nature and lead to normal science include the following:

- A community of scholars who base their research and practice on the paradigm
- The formation of specialized journals
- The foundation of specialists' societies
- The claim for a special place in curricula (Kuhn, 1970)

Kuhn (1970) stated, "Paradigms gain their status by being more successful than their competitors in solving a few problems that the group of practitioners have come to recognize as acute" (p. 23). Kuhn (1970) defines normal science as "research firmly based upon one or more past scientific achievements, achievements that some particular scientific community acknowledges for a time as supplying the foundation for its further practice" (p. 10).

Rodgers (2005) describes normal science as "the highly cumulative process of puzzle solving in which the paradigm guides scientific activity and the paradigm is, in turn, articulated and expanded" (p. 100). Rodgers (2005) cites Kuhn's premise that research in normal science "is directed to the articulation of those phenomena and theories that the paradigm supplies" (p. 100).

The conceptual models and grand theories of nursing in this text exhibit these characteristics. Each is unique with ranges of development in these characteristics. Rogers' science of unitary human beings (see Chapter 13) is an excellent example, having generated hundreds of research studies, 13 research instruments, and 12 nursing process clinical tools for practice (Fawcett, 2005; Fawcett & Alligood, 2001). The Society of Rogerian Scholars, founded in 1988, publishes a refereed journal, *Visions: The Journal of Rogerian Nursing Science,* with issues available on the Society of Rogerian Scholars website to foster development of the science and sharing among the community of scholars. Rogerian science is the basis of award-winning texts and curricula for undergraduate and graduate nursing programs (Fawcett & DeSanto-Madeya, 2013). In 2016 the Society of Rogerian Scholars celebrated 35 years of Rogerian conferences, the 30th anniversary of the society, and 25 years of *Visions: The Journal of Rogerian Nursing Science.* Similarly, the International Orem Society for Orem's Self-Care Deficit Theory (see Chapter 14), King International Nursing Group for King's Conceptual System (see Chapter 15), the Neuman Trustee Group and Biennial Symposia for Neuman's Systems Model (see Chapter 16), and the Boston-based Adaptation Research in Nursing Society for Roy's Adaptation Model (see Chapter 17) are productive communities of scholars.

Nursing theories and grand theories that have developed normal science include Boykin and Schoenhofer's theory of nursing as caring (Chapter 19); Meleis' transitions theory (Chapter 20); Pender's health promotion model (Chapter 21); Leininger's theory of culture care (Chapter 22); Newman's theory of health as expanding consciousness (Chapter 23); Parse's theory of humanbecoming (Chapter 24); and Erickson, Tomlin, and Swain's theory of modeling and role-modeling (Chapter 25). Many of these have founded consortia or societies for development of research, presentations, publications, and practice applications.

Increasingly over the past 40 years, the conceptual models of nursing and nursing theory texts have proposed theory-based education, administration, research, and practice. Communities of scholars associated with a model or theory have grown globally as formally organized societies that share knowledge and address questions from research and practice in conferences, on websites, in newsletters, and in journals. The central concepts–person, environment, health, and nursing–have been accepted as such by the discipline of nursing (Fawcett, 1984). Nurses generate theory-based scholarship for research and practice. Work by the communities of scholars in nursing models and theories led to the development of research instruments or clinical measurement tools unique to that paradigm (Fawcett & Alligood, 2001; Fawcett & DeSanto-Madeya, 2013).

EXPANSION OF MIDDLE-RANGE THEORY DEVELOPMENT

Theoretical works provide ways to think about nursing the patient. Johnson and Webber (2015) discuss three significant areas affected by nursing knowledge and dependent on its continued development. They proposed that theory affects recognition of nursing as (1) a profession, (2) a discipline, and (3) a science. Substantive knowledge is the heart for nursing recognition and quality care of patients. Moving nurses beyond functional practice to a professional style of practice requires changing the emphasis from *what nurses do* to a perspective of *the patient.* This requires that practice be systematic and focused on persons. As nurses shift to a professional style of nursing practice, most agree that "nursing knowledge arises from inquiry and guides practice" (Parse, 2008, p. 101).

The increasing use of middle-range theory or situation-specific theory (Alligood, 2010; Meleis, 2012) accentuates the theory-practice connection, opening new insights and vistas for theory development. Classifications are subjective and vary based on the perspective or framework used for the classification. Of greater importance than the classification of a theory is that nurses know the theoretical works of their discipline, recognize them as evidence on which to base practice, teach them to students, and select one for a professional style of practice and improved care.

Nurses eagerly embraced qualitative research approaches to explore questions that quantitative research methods could not answer, and this expanded theory development has led to textbooks devoted to qualitative approach middle-range or situation-specific theories (Meleis, 2012; Peterson & Bredow, 2017; Smith & Liehr, 2014) and middle-range theory texts illustrating quantitative and qualitative methods (Alligood, 2014a; Roy, 2014; Sieloff & Frey, 2007). These new theories expand the volume of practice theory applications. This exciting development continues the work of closing the gap between research and practice coming from quantitative and qualitative methods. Considering nursing knowledge in a generic structure as presented in Fig. 37.1 views knowledge based on the nature of the content within nursing science rather than according to the research methodology. Middle-range theories vary in level of abstraction as the name, middle range, indicates. Actually, this is true for theoretical works in other classifications (philosophies, models, and theories), because they also have similarities and differences in their levels of abstraction (Fawcett & DeSanto-Madeya, 2013). Middle-range theories are recognizable because they include details that are specific to practice, such as the following:

- The situation or health condition involved
- Client population
- Age group
- Location or area of nursing practice
- Action of the nurse
- The nursing intervention (Alligood, 2014c, p. 44)

Application of middle-range theories in nursing practice improves nursing practice quality, whether developed quantitatively or qualitatively. Both approaches are at the practice level, and they produce useful nursing knowledge. Consideration of middle-range theory in a generic structure of knowledge illustrates how theory coming from the quantitative hypothetical-deductive methods or coming from qualitative approaches arrive at knowledge that is at a similar level of abstraction. Despite different philosophical bases, methods, and approaches, the knowledge is at a similar level of abstraction (see Fig. 37.1).

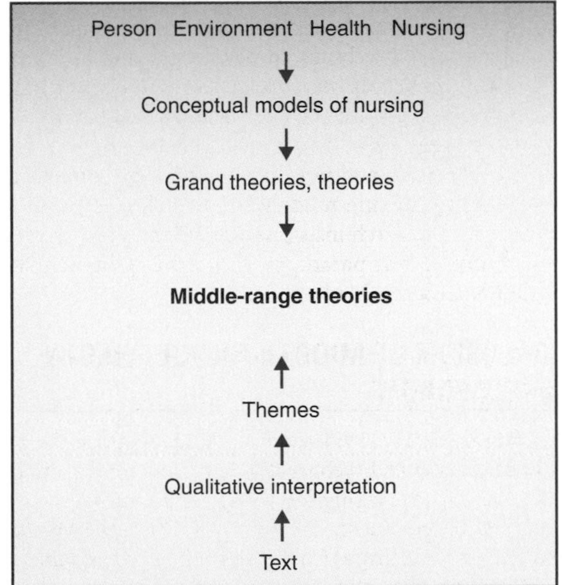

FIG. 37.1 Middle-range theory in a generic structure of nursing knowledge from quantitative research methods and from qualitative research approaches. (Includes data from Fawcett, J. [2005]. *Contemporary nursing knowledge: Nursing models and theories*. Philadelphia: F. A. Davis.)

GLOBAL NURSING SCHOLARS

In addition to the growth stimulated by the expansion of the philosophy of nursing science and the outstanding increase in the development and use of middle-range theories, recently, the major, exciting contribution to the state of the art and science of nursing theory is globalization and communication of knowledge by nursing scholars via the Internet. Although most nursing conceptual model and theory societies or consortia have had international members for years, recent worldwide expansion of theory-guided research and practice reflected in the nursing literature is astounding (Fitzpatrick & Whall, 2016).

Nursing theory societies such as the International Orem Society alternate biennial conferences between the United States and other countries. In 2016 the International Human Caring Conference and the Society of Rogerian Scholars held a joint conference in Boston. Parse's Institute of Humanbecoming and Watson's Consortium on Caring Science draw international applicants each year. The International Biennial Neuman Systems Model Symposium is often held in other countries with global themes such as *Enhancing Global Health with Nursing Theories—NSM* and, in 2015, *Prevention: A Global Perspective.*

These exciting evidences may be attributed to global publications and communication, increased world travel, and translation of nursing theory textbooks into other languages. Nurses around the world are embracing nursing theory as they experience its utility in their research and practice (Bigbee & Illel, 2010). Numerous nursing journals publish articles by international scholars, such as *Journal of Nursing Scholarship, Nursing Science Quarterly, Journal of Advanced Nursing, Advances in Nursing Science, Visions: The Journal of Rogerian Nursing Science,* and *International Journal for Human Caring,* to name a few.

Various editions of this text, *Nursing Theorists and Their Work,* and its companion text, *Nursing Theory: Utilization and Application,* have been published in classical Chinese, Taiwanese, Finnish, German, Indonesian, Italian, Japanese, Korean, Spanish, Swedish, and Portuguese and have international circulation to English-speaking countries. The nursing literature referenced in the updated chapters of this text demonstrate the emergent global use of nursing conceptual models and nursing theories. In addition, this text has for many editions included theoretical works of international theorists: Evelyn Adam, Canada (Chapter 2); Roper, Logan, and Tierney, Scotland (Chapter 2); Katie Eriksson, Finland (Chapter 11); Phil Barker, Ireland (Chapter 32); Kari Martinsen, Norway (Chapter 10); and Nightingale, England (Chapter 6). A PubMed search of nursing theory publications in each language and country possible that was first conducted on October 23, 2008, was updated on August 24, 2012, and was updated once again for this ninth edition of this text on May 16, 2016, continues to confirm persistent growth of nursing theory globally. These many references are evidence that a global consciousness of nursing theory has arrived (Table 37.1).

TABLE 37.1 Global Nursing Theory Publications*

Nursing Theory Publications by Language or Country	Nursing Theory Publications October 23, 2008	Nursing Theory Publications August 24, 2012	Nursing Theory Publications May 16, 2016
English	10,144	12,629	17,932
Japanese	409	413	559
Portuguese	298	376	492
German	295	340	417
French	214	248	338
Korean	79	102	293
Chinese	59	91	320
Dutch	56	56	92
Danish	54	55	85
Spanish	41	59	245
Norwegian	41	41	75
Italian	33	37	60
Sweden	28	28	121
Finnish	24	24	59
Polish	13	14	21
Afrikaans	7	7	15
Russian	3	3	9
Greek	2	2	28
Thai	1	1	142
Turkish	1	1	17
Hebrew	1	1	16
Hungarian	1	2	5
Czeck	1	2	12
Additional languages or countries added in this ninth edition:			
Iran			155
Iraq			13
Jordan			45
Saudi Arabia			10

TABLE 37.1 Global Nursing Theory Publications—cont'd

Nursing Theory Publications by Language or Country	Nursing Theory Publications October 23, 2008	Nursing Theory Publications August 24, 2012	Nursing Theory Publications May 16, 2016
Pakistan			10
Australia			930
Canada			445
New Zealand			145
Zimbabwe			2
Nigeria			9
Kenya			7
Namibia			2
Brazil			233
Mexico			70
Colombia			371
South Africa			88
Israel			84
Ireland			263
Great Britain			898
Wales			241
Scotland			145

*Number of nursing theory publications retrieved by language/country in a PubMed search (updated on May 16, 2016).

Sigma Theta Tau International, with its worldwide membership and international conferences, has contributed to this growth, as has the availability of digitized nursing literature on the Internet. A review of most nursing journals reveals that authorships, location, and research subjects from various world countries have become the norm. Several nursing theory websites provide information, such as the Nursing Theory Link Page maintained by Clayton College and State University Department of Nursing and the Nursing Theory Page maintained by the University of San Diego School of Nursing. Their websites contain links to websites for many theorists and their work.

In conclusion, the state of the art and science of nursing theory is exciting as we witness the phenomenal growth. First, nursing theoretical works are used globally by nurse scholars who collaborate to develop nursing science (Kuhn, 1970). Second, theory development with qualitative research addresses many unanswered nursing questions. New understanding from middle-range theories improves nursing practice. Third, and finally, global nurse scholars are applying nursing theoretical works and contributing new nursing knowledge. Nurses of the world share ideas and knowledge on the Internet (see Fig. 37.1).

This is a crucial time in the history of nursing. As more nurses are prepared with advanced degrees than ever before and many with the nursing practice doctorate (DNP), hospital patient complexity and decreased days in hospital stays challenge nurses to deliver safe, quality care. Similarly, the transformation of nursing education continues to respond to *Educating Nurses* (Benner et al., 2010) and the Institute of Medicine (IOM) report, *The Future of Nursing: Leading Change* (Ellerbe & Regen, 2012).

It is vital that nursing values are maintained and nursing frameworks are taught, learned, and used to continue the growth of nursing knowledge and the discipline (Bigbee & Issel, 2012; McCrae, 2012). As new knowledge is developed and tested in research and applied in practice for quality patient care, disciplinary growth continues (Im & Rendell, 2015). One thing remains true for the nursing profession: "Theory without practice is empty and practice without theory is blind" (Cross, 1981, p. 110).

REFERENCES

Alligood, M. R. (2010). Family healthcare with King's theory of goal attainment. *Nursing Science Quarterly*, *23*(2), 99–104.

Alligood, M. R. (2011). The power of theoretical knowledge. *Nursing Science Quarterly*, *24*(4), 304–305.

Alligood, M. R. (2014a). Areas for further development of theory-based nursing practice. In M. Alligood (Ed.), *Nursing theory: Utilization & application* (5th ed., pp. 414–424). Maryland Heights, MO: Mosby Elsevier.

Alligood, M. R. (2014b). *Nursing theory: Utilization & application* (5th ed.). St Louis, MO: Mosby Elsevier.

Alligood, M. R. (2014c). Philosophies, models, and theories: Critical thinking structures. In M. Alligood (Ed.), *Nursing theory: Utilization & application* (5th ed., pp. 40–62). St Louis, MO: Mosby Elsevier.

Benner, P., Sutphen, M., Leonard, V., & Day, L. (2010). *Educating nurses*. San Francisco: Jossey-Bass.

Bigbee, J. L., & Issel, L. M. (2012). Conceptual models for population-focused public health nursing interventions and outcomes: The state of the art. *Public Health Nursing, 29*(4), 370–379.

Breakey, S., Corless, I., Meedzan, N., & Nicholas, P. (2015). *Global health nursing in the 21st century*. New York: Springer.

Butts, J. B., & Rich, K. L. (2015). *Philosophies and theories for advanced nursing practice* (2nd ed.). Sudbury, MA: Jones & Bartlett.

Carper, B. (1978). Fundamental patterns of knowing. *Advances in Nursing Science, 1*(1), 13–23.

Chinn, P., & Kramer, M. (2015). *Integrated knowledge development in nursing* (9th ed.). St Louis, MO: Mosby Elsevier.

Cross, P. (1981). *Adults as learners*. Washington, DC: Jossey-Bass.

Dickson, V., & Wright, F. (2012). Review of *Nursing theorists and their work* (7th ed.). In M. R. Alligood & A. M. Tomey (Eds.), *Nursing Science Quarterly, 25*(2), 203–204.

Ellerbe, S., & Regen, D. (2012). Responding to health care reform by addressing the institute of medicine report on the future of nursing. *Nursing Administration Quarterly, 36*(3), 210–216.

Fawcett, J. (1984). The metaparadigm of nursing: Present status and future refinements. *Image: The Journal of Nursing Scholarship, 16*(3), 84–89.

Fawcett, J. (2005). *Analysis and evaluation of contemporary nursing knowledge: Nursing models and theories* (2nd ed.). Philadelphia: F. A. Davis.

Fawcett, J., & Alligood, M. (2001). SUHB Instruments: An overview of research instruments and clinical tools derived from the science of unitary human beings. *Theoria: Journal of Nursing Theory, 10*(2), 5–12.

Fawcett, J., & DeSanto-Madeya, S. (2013). *Analysis and evaluation of contemporary nursing knowledge: Nursing models and theories* (3rd ed.). Philadelphia: F. A. Davis.

Fawcett, J., & Garity, J. (2009). *Evaluating research for evidence-based nursing practice*. Philadelphia: F. A. Davis.

Fitzpatrick, J. J., & Whall, A. L. (2016). *Conceptual models of nursing: Global perspectives* (5th ed.). New York: NY, Pearson.

Im, E., & Chang, S. (2012). Current trends in nursing theories. *Image: The Journal of Nursing Scholarship, 44*(2), 156–164.

Im, E., & Rendell, M. O. (2015). The current status of theory evaluation in nursing. *Journal of Advanced Nursing, 71*(10), 2268–2278.

Johnson, B., & Webber, P. (2015). *An introduction to theory and reasoning in nursing* (4th ed.). Philadelphia: Lippincott.

Kuhn, T. S. (1962). *The structure of scientific revolutions*. Chicago: University of Chicago Press.

Kuhn, T. S. (1970). *The structure of scientific revolutions* (2nd ed.). Chicago: University of Chicago Press.

McCrae, N. (2012). Whither nursing models? The value of nursing theory in the context of evidenced-based practice and multidisciplinary healthcare. *Journal of Advanced Nursing, 40*, 346–354.

Meleis, A. I. (2012). *Theoretical nursing: Development and progress* (5th ed.). Philadelphia: Lippincott.

Paley, J. (2006). Book review of *Nursing theorists and their work*. *Nursing Philosophy, 7*(4), 275–280.

Parse, R. R. (2008). Nursing knowledge development: Who's to say how? *Nursing Science Quarterly, 21*(2), 101.

Peterson, S., & Bredow, T. (2017). *Middle range theories* (4th ed.). Philadelphia: Lippincott.

Rodgers, B. L. (2005). *Developing nursing knowledge*. Philadelphia: Lippincott.

Roy, C. (2014). *Generating middle range theory*. New York: Springer.

Sieloff, C. L., & Frey, M. A. (Eds.). (2007). *Middle range theory development using King's conceptual system*. New York: Springer.

Smith, J. M. (2012). Book review of *Nursing theorists and their work* (7th ed.). In M. R. Alligood & A. M. Tomey (Eds.), *Nursing Science Quarterly, 25*(2), 201–202.

Smith, M. J., & Liehr, P. (2014). *Middle range theory for nursing* (3rd ed.). New York: Springer.

Wood, A. (2014). Nursing models: Normal science for nursing practice. In M. R. Alligood (Ed.), *Nursing theory: Utilization & application* (5th ed., pp. 13–39). St Louis, MO: Mosby Elsevier.

INDEX

Q

R

S

U